ACCP Pulmonary Medicine Board Review: 25th Edition

The American Board of Internal Medicine (ABIM) is not affiliated with, nor does it endorse, preparatory examination review programs or other continuing medical education. The content of the ACCP Pulmonary Medicine Board Review: 25th Edition is developed independently by the American College of Chest Physicians (ACCP), which has no knowledge of or access to ABIM examination material.

The views expressed herein are those of the authors and do not necessarily reflect the views of the ACCP. Use of trade names or names of commercial sources is for information only and does not imply endorsement by the ACCP. The authors and the publisher have exercised great care to ensure that drug dosages, formulas, and other information presented in this book are accurate and in accord with the professional standards in effect at the time of publication. However, readers are advised to always check the manufacturer's product information sheet packaged with the respective products to be fully informed of changes in recommended dosages, contraindications, etc., before prescribing or administering any drug.

AMERICAN COLLEGE OF CHEST PHYSICIANS®

Published by the
American College of Chest Physicians
3300 Dundee Road
Northbrook, IL 60062-2348
Telephone: (847) 498-1400; Fax: (847) 498-5460
ACCP Web site: www.chestnet.org

Printed in the United States of America
First Printing
ISBN 978-0-916609-77-1

Contents

Authors

Igor Aksenov, MD, PhD
Pulmonary and Critical Care Medicine Fellow
Division of Pulmonary, Critical Care and Sleep Medicine
University of Florida
Gainesville, FL

W. Michael Alberts, MD, MBA, FCCP
Chief Medical Officer
H. Lee Moffitt Cancer Center
Professor of Oncology and Medicine
Department of Interdisciplinary Oncology
University of South Florida College of Medicine
Tampa, FL

David Ashkin, MD
Medical Executive Director, A. G. Holley State TB Hospital
Florida State TB Health Officer, Florida Department of Health
Adjunct Assistant Professor, Division of Pulmonary and Critical Care Medicine
University of Florida College of Medicine
Gainesville, FL
Visiting Associate Professor, Division of Pulmonary and Critical Care Medicine
University of Miami School of Medicine
Miami, FL

William S. Beckett, MD, FCCP
Associate Professor of Medicine
Harvard Medical School
Primary Care Center
Mount Auburn Hospital
Cambridge, MA

Sidney S. Braman, MD, FCCP
Professor of Medicine
Director, Division of Pulmonary and Critical Care Medicine
The Alpert Medical School of Brown University and Rhode Island Hospital
Providence, RI

David Feller-Kopman, MD, FCCP
Director, Interventional Pulmonology
Associate Professor of Medicine
Johns Hopkins Hospital
Baltimore, MD

Ronald F. Grossman, MD, FCCP
Staff Respirologist
University of Toronto
Chief of Medicine
Credit Valley Hospital
Mississauga, ON, Canada

Richard S. Irwin, MD, FCCP
Professor of Medicine and Nursing
University of Massachusetts
Chair, Critical Care
UMass Memorial Medical Center
Editor in Chief, CHEST
Worcester, MA

David W. Kamp, MD, FCCP
Professor of Medicine
Associate Chief, Division of Pulmonary and Critical Care Medicine
Northwestern University Feinberg School of Medicine
Chicago, IL

Bruce P. Krieger, MD, FCCP
Professor of Medicine
Miller School of Medicine
University of Miami
Associate Medical Director
Critical Care Center
Memorial Hospital
Jacksonville, FL

Teofilo L. Lee-Chiong, Jr., MD, FCCP
Associate Professor of Medicine
Head, Division of Sleep Medicine
Department of Medicine
National Jewish Health
Associate Professor of Medicine
University of Colorado Denver School of Medicine
Denver, CO

Stephanie M. Levine, MD, FCCP
Professor of Medicine
Division of Pulmonary Diseases and Critical Care Medicine
Pulmonary and Critical Care Fellowship Program Director
University of Texas Health Science Center
San Antonio, TX

Joseph P. Lynch III, MD, FCCP
Professor of Clinical Medicine
Associate Chief
Pulmonary, Critical Care Medicine, and Hospitalists
David Geffen School of Medicine at UCLA
Los Angeles, CA

Darcy D. Marciniuk, MD, FCCP
Professor and Vice-Chair, Department of Medicine
University of Saskatchewan, Royal University Hospital,
Saskatoon, SK, Canada

Lisa K. Moores, MD, FCCP
Assistant Dean for Clinical Sciences
Professor of Medicine
The Uniformed Services University of the Health Sciences
Bethesda, MD

Mark J. Rosen, MD, FCCP
Chief, Division of Pulmonary, Critical Care, and Sleep Medicine
North Shore University Hospital and Long Island Jewish Medical Center
Professor of Medicine
Albert Einstein College of Medicine
New Hyde Park, NY

Jay H. Ryu, MD, FCCP
Professor of Medicine
Mayo Clinic College of Medicine
Consultant, Division of Pulmonary and Critical Care Medicine
Director, Interstitial Lung Disease Clinic
Mayo Clinic
Rochester, MN

Steven A. Sahn, MD, FCCP
Professor of Medicine
Director, Division of Pulmonary, Critical Care Medicine,
Allergy and Sleep Medicine
Medical University of South Carolina
Charleston, SC

George A. Sarosi, MD, FCCP
Professor of Medicine
University of Minnesota
Staff Physician
Minneapolis VA Medical Center
Minneapolis, MN

Curtis N. Sessler, MD, FCCP
Orhan Muren Professor of Medicine
Division of Pulmonary and Critical Care Medicine
Virginia Commonwealth University Health System
Medical Director of Critical Care
Medical College of Virginia Hospitals
Richmond, VA

Rakesh D. Shah, MD, FCCP
Chief of Thoracic Radiology
Department of Radiology
North Shore University Hospital
Manhasset, NY

Ulrich Specks, MD
Professor of Medicine
Division of Pulmonary and Critical Care Medicine
Mayo Clinic
Rochester, MN

Michael Strauss, MD
Director
Department of Hyperbaric Medicine
Long Beach Memorial Medical Center
Long Beach, CA

Henry D. Tazelaar, MD, FCCP
Consultant
Mayo Clinic Arizona
Professor of Pathology
Mayo Clinic College of Medicine
Scottsdale, AZ

Janice L. Zimmerman, MD, FCCP
Professor of Clinical Medicine
Weill Cornell Medical College
Head, Critical Care Division
Department of Medicine
Director of MICU
The Methodist Hospital
Houston, TX

DISCLOSURE OF AUTHORS' CONFLICTS OF INTEREST

The American College of Chest Physicians (ACCP) remains strongly committed to providing the best available evidence-based clinical information to participants of this educational activity and requires an open disclosure of any potential conflict of interest identified by our committee members. It is not the intent of the ACCP to eliminate all situations of potential conflict of interest, but rather to enable those who are working with the ACCP to recognize situations that may be subject to question by others. All disclosed conflicts of interest are reviewed by the educational activity course director/chair, the Education Committee, or the Conflict of Interest Review Committee to ensure that such situations are properly evaluated and, if necessary, resolved. The ACCP educational standards pertaining to conflict of interest are intended to maintain the professional autonomy of the clinical experts inherent in promoting a balanced presentation of science. Through our review process, all ACCP CME activities are ensured of independent, objective, scientifically balanced information. Disclosure of any or no relationships is made available for all educational activities.

The following authors of the Pulmonary Medicine Board Review: 25th Edition have disclosed to the ACCP that a relationship does exist with the respective company/organization as it relates to their presentation of material and should be communicated to the participants of this educational activity:

Authors	Relationship
Ronald Grossman, MD, FCCP	Advisory committee: GSK, Bayer, Ortho McNeil, Sanofi Aventis, Wyeth
Teofilo L. Lee-Chiong, Jr., MD, FCCP	Grant Monies (from sources other than industry): NIH Grant Monies (from industry-related sources): Respironics, Restore, Takeda; Consultant fee, speaker bureau, advisory committee, etc: Consultant for Sleep Medicine Clinics (Elsevier)
Darcy D. Marciniuk, MD, FCCP	Grant Monies (from sources other than industry): Canadian Agency for Drugs and Technologies in Health, Canadian Institutes of Health Research, Lung Association of Saskatchewan, Public Health Agency of Canada, Royal University Hospital Foundation, Saskatoon Health Region, Saskatchewan Ministry of Health Grant Monies (from industry-related sources): AstraZeneca, Boehringer-Ingelheim, GlaxoSmithKline, Forest Research, Novartis, Pfizer Fiduciary Position (of any other organization, association, society, etc, other than ACCP): Canadian Thoracic Society Consultant fee, speaker bureau, advisory committee, etc: AstraZeneca, Boehringer-Ingelheim, GlaxoSmithKline, Novartis, Nycomed, Pfizer
Ulrich Specks, MD	Product/procedure/technique that is considered research and is NOT yet approved for any purpose: All medications/interventions used for the treatment of ANCA-associated vasculitis, including cyclophosphamide, methotrexate, azathioprine, mycophenolate mofetil, lefluomide, infliximab, etanercept, abatacept, rituximab, and plasma-exchange represent off-label use for this indication.

The following authors of the Pulmonary Medicine Board Review: 25th Edition have indicated to the ACCP that no potential conflict of interest exists with any respective company/organization, and this should be communicated to the participants of this educational activity:

W. Michael Alberts, MD, FCCP
David Ashkin, MD
William Beckett, MD, FCCP
Sidney Braman, MD, FCCP
Richard Irwin, MD, FCCP
David Kamp, MD, FCCP
Joseph P. Lynch III, MD, FCCP
Lisa Moores, MD, FCCP
Mark Rosen, MD, FCCP
Jay Ryu, MD, FCCP
Steven Sahn, MD, FCCP
George Sarosi, MD, FCCP
Curtis Sessler, MD, FCCP
Ulrich Specks, MD
Henry Tazelaar, MD, FCCP
Janice Zimmerman, MD, FCCP

Needs Assessment

Rely on the ACCP Pulmonary Medicine Board Review: 25th Edition to review the type of information you should know for the Pulmonary Disease Subspecialty Board Examination of the American Board of Internal Medicine (ABIM). Designed as the best preparation for anyone taking the exam, this comprehensive, exam-focused review will cover current critical care literature and management strategies for critically ill patients.

The ABIM Pulmonary Disease Subspecialty Board Examination tests knowledge and clinical judgment in crucial areas of critical care medicine. This premier course will review the information you should know for the exam. Course content mirrors the content of the exam, as outlined by the ABIM, and includes the following topics:

Topic	%
Asthma	7%
Cell/Molecular biology	3.5%
Congenital/neuromuscular/Skeletal	2%
COPD	7%
Critical care. Non-lung	4%
Critical care, lung	9%
ILD-related disorders	6%
Infections	13%
Neoplasms	9%
Obstructive airways disease, other	2%
Occupational and environmental disease	5%
Physiology and metabolism	4%
Pleural disease	5%
Quality, safety and complications	5%
Sleep, Non-respiratory	2%
Sleep, Respiratory	8%
Transplantation	2%
Vascular diseases	2.5%
Total	100%

Target Audience

Physicians in critical care pulmonary medicine
Fellows in critical care and pulmonary medicine
Advanced critical care nurse practitioners
Advanced respiratory therapy practitioners
Physician assistants

General Publications Disclaimer

Participation Opportunities

- ACCP NetWorks—special interest groups within the ACCP that focus on particular areas of chest medicine
- The ACCP Critical Care and Sleep Institutes are centers of excellence merging all programs and resources into central organizational units, providing the ACCP with a strong voice in the future of critical care and sleep medicine.

Critical Care Institute American College of Chest Physicians®   Sleep Institute American College of Chest Physicians®

- Committee and leadership positions
- CHEST Foundation awards in clinical research, leadership in end-of-life care, and humanitarian service
- The CHEST Foundation's Ambassador's Group

Financial Benefits

- Discounts for ACCP courses and products
- Credit card programs
- Discounts for Apple and Dell computers and products.

Point. Click. Access.

Link to the resources you need

www.chestnet.org

Education

- Calendar of upcoming courses, including the annual CHEST meeting and hands-on education opportunities in the ACCP Simulation Center for Advanced Clinical Education
- Online education opportunities and interactive resources, including A Physician's Perspective®
- Self-study products
- Evidence-based clinical practice guidelines

Membership and NetWorks

- Membership information and applications
- ACCP NetWorks and their activities
- Join NetWorks online

Other Resources

- Downloads of consensus statements, ACCP publications, podcasts, and more
- Practice management information
- Access to health-care advocacy updates on socioeconomic and political issues affecting practice and research
- Career Connection employment services
- ACCP product catalog

www.chestfoundation.org

- Award and grant information and applications
- Professional resources
- Patient education products

www.chestjournal.org

- Full articles online
- Numerous tools and features, including Interactive Physiology Grand Rounds
- Article submission information
- Subscription information

THE CHEST FOUNDATION®

Helping You Help Your Patients
Live and Breathe Easier

The CHEST Foundation is the philanthropic arm of the American College of Chest Physicians (ACCP), a 17,500-member international medical specialty society.

The CHEST Foundation mission is to provide resources to advance the prevention and treatment of diseases of the chest. In order to fulfill its mission to advance patient care in cardiopulmonary and critical care medicine, The CHEST Foundation has targeted the following four focus areas:

- Tobacco Prevention
- Humanitarian Service
- Clinical Research
- Critical Care/End-of-Life Care

Tobacco Prevention Education

- The 4th Edition CD-ROM: *Make the Choice: Tobacco or Health?* Speaker's Kit for presentations to health professionals and patients
- *Lung Lessons*[SM] curriculum teaches elementary school children the negative health effects of smoking
- *Lung Lessons*[SM]*: A Presenter's Guide* DVD demonstrates how to teach the *Lung Lessons*[SM] curriculum to children
- *Evils of Tobacco* CD-ROM and video for children and women in India

Critical Care and End-of-Life Care

- The Critical Care Family Assistance Program and replication tool kit to improve coordination of care and communication with ICU staff, patients, and families
- *ICU – Frequently Asked Questions in the ICU* booklet, includes responses to questions that family members have when a family member is admitted to a hospital ICU
- *Stories at the End of Life* booklet series to comfort patients and their family members

Humanitarian Awards

Nearly $1.4 million awarded from 1998 to 2009 to recognize and support volunteer service in over 180 projects/services of ACCP members worldwide

Clinical Research Awards

- Over $5 million conferred from 1998 to 2009 to support promising clinical research
- Distinguished Scholar awards to foster innovation in clinical care to address public health related to chest and critical care medicine

  Eli Lilly and Company Distinguished Scholar in Critical Care Medicine

  GlaxoSmithKline Distinguished Scholar in Respiratory Health

  GlaxoSmithKline Distinguished Scholar in Thrombosis
- Clinical research awards in asthma, COPD, critical care, pulmonary fibrosis, thrombosis, and women's health
- Roger C. Bone Award for Advances in End-of-Life Care
- The CHEST Foundation and ACCP Grant in Venous Thromboembolism
- Alpha-1 Foundation and The CHEST Foundation Clinical Research Award in COPD and Alpha-1 Antitrypsin Deficiency
- The American Lung Association and CHEST Foundation Clinical Investigator Award
- The American Society of Transplantation and The CHEST Foundation Clinical Research Award in Lung Transplantation
- Association of Specialty Professors and The CHEST Foundation of the ACCP Geriatric Development Research Award
- The CHEST Foundation and the LUNGevity Foundation Clinical Research Award in Lung Cancer
- The CHEST Foundation California Chapter Clinical Research/Medical Education Award
- Scientific abstract-related awards

You can support these programs and projects through a tax-deductible donation to The CHEST Foundation. Your gift will help support these programs and resources that help you help your patients live and breathe easier.

Donate online at www.chestfoundation.org.

Unusual Lung Infection, Bronchiectasis, and Cystic Fibrosis

Lisa K. Moores, MD, FCCP

Objectives:

- Compare actinomycosis and nocardiosis infections of the lung
- Discuss the treatment of actinomycosis and nocardiosis infection in the lung
- List the causes of bronchiectasis
- Discuss the therapeutic options for the treatment of bronchiectasis
- Review the genetic aspects of cystic fibrosis
- Discuss the newer therapeutic approaches to the treatment of pulmonary disease in patients with cystic fibrosis

Key words: actinomycosis; bronchiectasis; cystic fibrosis; cystic fibrosis transmembrane regulator; nocardiosis

Unusual Lung Infections

Nocardiosis

Nocardiosis refers to invasive disease caused by members of the genus Nocardia. Respiratory tract disease and extrapulmonary dissemination are the most common manifestations. Pulmonary infection is increasingly seen in immunosuppressed patients, particularly those with defects in cellular immunity. Other presentations include cellulitis, lymphocutaneous syndrome, actinomycetoma, and keratitis. Nocardia species are aerobic, nonmobile, and non-spore-forming organisms that live as soil saprophytes. In tissue specimens, the organisms reveal delicate branching filamentous forms that are Gram-positive and usually acid fast if weak decolorizing agents are used for the stains. Seven species have been associated with human disease. *Nocardia asteroides* is the most common species associated with invasive disease. *Nocardia farcinica* is less common and is associated with dissemination. Other species known to cause human infection are *Nocardia pseudobrasiliensis* and *Nocardia brasiliensis.*

Epidemiology/Pathogenesis: Nocardia species are common natural inhabitants of the soil throughout the world. Epidemics within the hospital environment are rare, and person-to-person transmission has only rarely been suggested. Although Nocardia can occur as a primary pulmonary pathogen in patients with no underlying disease and can complicate surgery or trauma, it is frequently recognized as an opportunistic disease, especially among patients with cell-mediated immune deficiencies, including transplantation (greatest frequency in those who have undergone lung transplantation), lymphoma, and AIDS. High-dose corticosteroids, cytomegalovirus infection in the past 6 months, and high calcineurin inhibitor levels (cyclosporine or tacrolimus) are independent risk factors for Nocardia infection in organ transplant recipients. In HIV-positive persons, nocardiosis most often presents with a $CD4^+$ lymphocyte concentration of <100 cells/μL but can occur in patients with counts <250 cells/μL.

Nocardiosis has also been reported to be associated with pulmonary alveolar proteinosis, mycobacterial diseases, and chronic granulomatous disease. Finally, nocardiosis is not uncommon in patients with COPD receiving long-term corticosteroid treatment, but it is also increasingly being seen in patients with COPD who have received only a recent short course of corticosteroids for an exacerbation. The disease has been reported worldwide and is more common in men than women (approximately 3:1). Most infections result from the inhalation of bacilli. Lesions are characterized by necrotizing abscesses that are not well encapsulated and spread easily. Granuloma formation and fibrosis are infrequent. Because of its propensity for hematogenous dissemination, Nocardia often is associated with metastatic spread, especially to the brain (in up to one third of cases). Chest wall invasion may occur but is uncommon.

Radiographic Manifestations: The chest radiographic patterns are variable. The most frequent manifestation is an airspace consolidation, usually homogeneous, but occasionally patchy. Nodules, either single or multiple, may be confused with metastatic carcinoma. The most common radiographic manifestation is cavitation, which is found in both consolidations and nodules. Pleural involvement with an empyema is present in approximately one third of cases.

Clinical Manifestations: Important features of Nocardia infection include diverse clinical and radiographic presentation, the ability to disseminate to any organ system in the body, and the tendency to relapse or remain unresponsive to therapy. The nonspecific features make diagnosis challenging, and the disease often is not suspected early in the patient's course of symptoms. The median time to diagnosis ranges from 40 to 55 days in reported series. Nocardial pneumonia is the most common respiratory tract presentation. Although the clinical course may be acute in immunosuppressed patients, typically the patients have a subacute presentation consisting of several weeks of symptoms. Cough, purulent sputum, occasional blood-streaked sputum, night sweats, and pleuritic pain are the most common. Superior vena caval syndrome, mediastinitis, and pericarditis have been reported from direct spread from the lungs. Nocardia rarely involves the chest wall. In approximately 50% of pulmonary cases, extrapulmonary dissemination occurs. In a significant number of cases of disseminated disease, the initial respiratory tract involvement does not elicit symptoms. As noted previously, nocardiosis has the propensity for dissemination to the brain, but other extrapulmonary sites include the skin, bone, and muscle. In the CNS, Nocardia brain abscesses may be single or multiple. Nocardia is not usually recovered from the cerebrospinal fluid.

Diagnosis: In most cases of pneumonia, sputum smear findings are negative. Bronchoscopy may be necessary to obtain an adequate specimen for the characteristic Gram-positive filaments that may be acid fast and often take up silver stains. Cultures for Nocardia require special handling because colonies may not appear for 2 to 4 weeks. Blood cultures require incubation aerobically for up to 4 weeks. Advances in DNA extraction and real-time polymerase chain reaction assays may allow for identification of most Nocardia species within hours. The isolation of Nocardia from the sputum in a non-immunosuppressed patient without radiographic abnormalities may represent colonization. However, a sputum culture that is positive for Nocardia in an immunosuppressed patient more often indicates disease. A number of serologic tests have been evaluated, but the diversity of species known to cause disease and the potential lack of sensitivity for detecting an antibody response in immunocompromised patients have limited their practical use.

Treatment: Sulfonamide agents remain the drug of choice for nocardiosis (sulfadiazine or sulfisoxazole, 6 to 8 g/d, then decreasing to 4 g/d as the disease is controlled). The combination of trimethoprim and sulfamethoxazole is thought to be an equally effective alternate choice. Minocycline is an alternative choice for an oral medication in those patients who have sulfa allergies. IV regimens include amikacin, ceftriaxone, cefotaxime, ceftizoxime, and imipenem. Linezolid has now been shown *in vitro* to be highly effective against most strains of Nocardia. However, the high cost and serious potential toxicities currently relegate this agent to refractory cases. Because of the risk of relapse, patients who have intact host defenses are generally treated for 6 to 12 months, whereas immunodeficient hosts and those with CNS involvement are treated for 12 months. When the CNS is involved, treatment with cefotaxime or ceftriaxone in addition to the trimethoprim and sulfamethoxazole is recommended. Surgical drainage should be considered for patients with brain abscesses, empyema, and subcutaneous abscesses. The rate of mortality caused by pulmonary nocardiosis is high (15 to 40%) and increases significantly with CNS involvement. Delay in diagnosis and treatment affects prognosis. It is therefore imperative that practitioners have a high index of suspicion in evaluating patients who are immunosuppressed or who have significant chronic lung disease.

Actinomycosis

Actinomycosis is a slowly progressive infectious disease that is caused by anaerobic or microaerophilic bacteria from the genus Actinomyces.

When they were first described, they were misclassified as fungi. The word actinomycosis is derived from the Greek terms *aktino* (the radiating appearance of the sulphur granule) and *mykos* (mycotic disease). The classic clinical picture is a cervicofacial disease in which the patient presents with a large mass on the jaw. It is now recognized that the organisms colonize in the mouth, colon, and vagina. Infection results from mucosal disruption and can occur at any site in the body. Infection is characterized by a pyogenic response and necrosis, followed by intense fibrosis. Actinomycosis is difficult to diagnose and is often confused with tuberculosis, lung abscess, or malignancy.

Epidemiology/Pathogenesis: The organisms are a normal inhabitant of the human oropharynx and frequently are found in dental caries and at the gingival margins of persons with poor oral hygiene. Actinomycosis is most commonly caused by *Actinomyces israelii.* Actinomycotic infections in the lung are, however, usually polymicrobial. In tissue, actinomycotic infection grows in microcolonies or granules. Because these granules are yellow, they are often called *sulfur granules*, although they contain minimal amounts of sulfa. Actinomycosis of the respiratory tract is acquired most commonly by aspiration, but direct extension of the disease from the head and neck or abdominal cavity can occur. The peak incidence is reported in the fourth and fifth decades of life; nearly all series have reported a male predominance (3:1). The pulmonary form typically constitutes only 15% of reported cases but has been as high as 50% in some series. Most infections occur in individuals who are immunocompetent. However, some cases have been reported in patients with impaired host defenses. Patients with alcoholism and poor dental hygiene are at increased risk. The presentation of pulmonary actinomycosis has changed in recent years to a less aggressive infection, which is likely related to improved oral hygiene and increased use of penicillins, even when the specific diagnosis is not suspected.

Radiographic Manifestations: The usual pattern of acute pulmonary actinomycosis consists of airspace consolidation, commonly in the periphery of the lung and often in the lower lung fields. The typical CT scan feature is a chronic segmental airspace consolidation containing necrotic low-attenuation areas with frequent cavity formation. Other findings include hilar or mediastinal adenopathy, bronchiectasis within the consolidation, and localized pleural thickening and/or effusion. If not treated with appropriate antibiotics, a lung abscess may develop, and the infiltrate may extend into the pleura with an associated empyema. Subsequently, actinomycosis will extend into the chest wall with osteomyelitis of the ribs, abscess formation, and draining sinus formation. CT of the chest may be a more sensitive imaging modality, especially if bone windows are obtained (which might reveal early rib erosion). Actinomycosis often is mistaken for pulmonary carcinoma; the presence of an air bronchogram in the mass lesion should suggest the possibility of a nonneoplastic process. Actinomycosis also can present as an endobronchial infection, which is often associated with a broncholith or other foreign body. Both actinomycosis and nocardiosis often are confused with tuberculosis, cryptococcosis, anaerobic pulmonary infection, bronchogenic carcinoma, and lymphoma.

Clinical Manifestations: Actinomyces most commonly presents as a disease of the cervicofacial region after dental extraction, with osteomyelitis of the mandible or a soft-tissue abscess that drains through the skin. Pulmonary actinomycosis usually presents with an indolent, progressive course. The initial manifestations include a nonproductive cough and low-grade fever, subsequently followed by a productive cough, which can be associated with hemoptysis. With chest wall involvement, pleuritic pain will develop in the patient. Rarely, a sinus tract may appear as a bronchocutaneous fistula. When this occurs, it is highly suggestive of actinomycosis. Late in the disease, the patient may present with weight loss, anemia, and clubbing of the digits.

Diagnosis: A diagnosis of actinomycosis is rarely suspected; in one series, it was suspected on hospital admission in <7% of the patients in whom it was ultimately diagnosed. Because actinomycosis often mimics malignancy, diagnosis may not be made until surgical resection. Because these organisms are normal oropharyngeal flora, isolation in specimens of sputum or bronchial washings is not considered significant, unless sulfa granules are found. Actinomyces are fastidious bacteria that are difficult to culture and, thus, correlation with the clinical and radiographic presentation is essential. Bronchoscopy is usually not diagnostic unless endobronchial disease is present, and samples must be obtained anaerobically with a protected specimen brush and delivered to the laboratory under anaerobic conditions. Histologic examination of lung tissue obtained by either transbronchial lung biopsy or open lung biopsy may be necessary to confirm the diagnosis. There is no reliable serologic test.

Treatment: Untreated, actinomycosis is ultimately fatal, but early treatment can result in cure rates of >90%. Prolonged treatment with high doses of antimicrobial agents is necessary. Penicillin is the drug of choice. Regimens include IV administration of 18 to 24 million units of penicillin for 2 to 6 weeks, followed by oral penicillin for an additional 6 to 12 months. Tetracyclines, erythromycin, clindamycin, imipenem, and chloramphenicol are acceptable alternatives. The organisms generally are not sensitive to the fluoroquinolones, metronidazole, or the aminoglycosides. Whether patients should be treated for the copathogens usually associated with actinomyces is not resolved, but most experts do not recommend the administration of additional antibiotics. Patients with actinomycosis have a tendency to relapse, and prolonged therapy optimizes the likelihood of a cure. However, small trials have shown success with relatively brief courses of therapy (6 weeks). Some cases may require both medical and surgical therapies. Patients with bulky disease should probably not receive short courses of therapy unless surgical debulking is also performed. A comparison of the main features of both actinomycosis and nocardiosis is shown in Table 1.

Bronchiectasis

Bronchiectasis is a syndrome, with many underlying etiologies and associations, that has been defined as an irreversible dilation and destruction of one or more bronchi, and inadequate clearance and pooling of mucus in the airways. Bronchiectasis is also characterized by persistent microbial infection and inflammation with release of microbial toxins and immune mediators. Bronchiectasis often is divided into a form associated with cystic fibrosis (CF) and a non-CF form. Non-CF bronchiectasis will be reviewed first.

Classification

A classification system has been devised by Reed. This system classifies bronchiectasis according to anatomic and morphologic patterns of airway dilatation as follows: (1) cylindrical bronchiectasis, in which there is uniform dilatation of the bronchi which are thick walled and extend to the lung periphery without normal tapering

Table 1. *Distinguishing Features of Nocardiosis and Actinomycosis*

Nocardiosis	Actinomycosis
Gram-positive aerobic*	Gram-positive anaerobic*
Incidence increasing	Incidence decreasing
Male 3:1 predominance	Male 3:1 predominance
Occurs primarily in immunocompromised hosts	Occurs primarily in immunocompetent hosts; alcoholism and poor dental hygiene are risks
Pulmonary manifestations predominate	Pulmonary manifestations in a minority of patients (approximately 15%)
Chest wall involvement is uncommon	Chest wall involvement and bony erosion are common
Metastatic spread (especially to the brain) is common	Metastatic spread is uncommon; spread by direct contiguous invasion
Granuloma formation and fibrosis are rare	Granuloma and intense fibrosis are common; form the characteristic sulfur granule
Diagnosis can usually be made on sputum, BAL fluid, or pleural fluid cultures	Diagnosis often requires cytologic or histologic examination
Treatment with sulfonamides	Treatment with penicillin
Surgical drainage often needed	Often treated successfully with antibiotics alone

*On Gram stain, the two organisms are indistinguishable as branching, Gram-positive filamentous organisms. However, Nocardia species will stain weakly with modified acid-fast stain, whereas actinomycosis will not.

(on a high-resolution CT scan, it has parallel "tram track" lines or "signet ring" appearance); (2) varicose bronchiectasis, which has an irregular and beaded outline of bronchi with alternating areas of constriction and dilatation similar in appearance to saphenous varicosities; (3) cystic bronchiectasis, which is the most severe form and is common in patients with CF, is characterized by bronchial dilation and clusters of round air-filled and fluid-filled cysts, with a honeycomb appearance; and (4) follicular bronchiectasis, which has extensive lymphoid nodules and follicles within thickened bronchial walls. Cystic, cylindrical, and varicose forms may coexist in the same patient. The fourth pattern, follicular bronchiectasis, usually occurs after the occurrence of childhood pneumonia, measles, pertussis, or adenovirus infection. The term *traction bronchiectasis* is a radiologic description of widened airways without thickening, which is in response to surrounding interstitial lung disease. These patients often do not have symptoms related to the bronchiectasis. Although insightful, these definitions are not particularly helpful from a clinical or therapeutic standpoint.

Etiology

The most common causes of non-CF bronchiectasis are listed in Table 2. In general, the etiologies can be categorized as idiopathic, postinfectious, or the result of an underlying anatomic or systemic disease. The number of patients in each category has changed since the introduction of modern antibiotic therapy. Previously, untreated infection was the leading cause of bronchiectasis, but with prompt treatment of infection, it is becoming much less common. In developed countries, the condition is now most often idiopathic in adults. The prevalence of undiagnosed CF is not known, but studies have suggested it is very low. Patients with focal bronchiectasis, which is localized to a segment or lobe, should undergo bronchoscopy to evaluate for and eliminate an obstructing bronchial lesion.

The factor most commonly associated with bronchiectasis in childhood is infection, although it is being seen more commonly in adults now, especially with the increased use of HRCT scanning. Radiographic findings obtained with an HRCT scan of the chest have been described in patients with *Mycobacterium avium* complex (MAC).

Table 2. *Predisposing Factors for Bronchiectasis*

Cause	Disease Example
Localized	Foreign-body aspiration
Mechanical airway obstruction	External compression
	Stenosis
	Lung tumors
Necrotizing pneumonia	
Diffuse	Intraluminal webs
Congenital	Absent cartilage
	Pulmonary sequestrations
CF	
Mucociliary clearance defects	Kartagener syndrome
	Primary cilia dyskinesia
	Young syndrome
Immune disorders	Hypogammaglobulinemia, IgG subclass deficiency, HIV, allergic bronchopulmonary aspergillosis, post-lung transplant
Postinfectious complications	Bacteria
	Mycobacterial infections (tuberculous and NMTb*)
	Whooping cough
	Viral (measles, adenovirus, influenza virus)
Rheumatologic diseases	Rheumatoid arthritis, Sjögren syndrome, inflammatory bowel disease
Sequelae of aspiration or toxic inhalation	
COPD	
Lung fibrosis	Sarcoidosis, after radiation therapy
Miscellaneous	α_1-Antitrypsin deficiency, yellow nail syndrome

*NMTb = non-tuberculosis mycobacteria.

The most notable finding in addition to bronchiectasis is the presence of small nodular opacities or the "tree-in-bud" appearance. Abnormalities most often occur in the lower lung fields. Treatment with multiple antimicrobial agents may lead to the resolution of these abnormalities, but prolonged therapy for up to 18 months may be necessary.

There are an increasing number of immune deficiencies that have been associated with bronchiectasis. Ciliary disorders are considered to be primary disorders of immune defense because airway clearance mechanisms contribute an important component of barrier immunity. Acquired adult-onset hypogammaglobulinemia may involve one or more of the Ig classes. IgG subclass deficiencies may be present even with normal total IgG levels. Patients with HIV infection have been found to have a high incidence of bronchiectasis, which may in part be the result of recurrent bronchopulmonary infections (especially *Pneumocystis jeroveci* pneumonia and *Mycobacterium intracellulare* infection). The bronchiectasis observed in HIV-infected patients is particularly aggressive. Allergic bronchopulmonary aspergillosis (ABPA) predisposes patients to bronchiectasis as a consequence of a persistent complex immune response to airway colonization by Aspergillus. This type of bronchiectasis most commonly involves the central airways, distinguishing it from other types of bronchiectasis. Both ABPA and underlying immunodeficiencies are important diagnoses to consider because the administration of specific therapy may prevent progression of the disease.

Clinical Manifestations

Clinical findings from a retrospective chart review of patients with confirmed bronchiectasis included cough (90%), chronic daily sputum production (76%), dyspnea (72%), hemoptysis (56%), and pleuritic chest pain (46%). Two symptoms that are also very common are rhinosinusitis and fatigue. The most common physical findings were crackles (70%) and wheezing or rhonchi (< 50%). Symptoms is patients with HIV vary somewhat. Daily cough and sputum production have been reported in HIV-positive patients with bronchiectasis confirmed by CT scan in < 39% of cases. The disease is more common in women and most commonly presents in the sixth decade of life.

Pulmonary function study results may be normal if the involvement of bronchiectasis is localized and mild. With diffuse disease, pulmonary function tests may reveal an obstructive ventilatory defect with hyperinflation and impaired diffusing capacity of the lung for carbon monoxide. Airway hyperresponsiveness has been seen in up to 40% of patients with bronchiectasis in some series. However, some patients with diffuse disease may present with a combined obstructive and restrictive ventilatory defect. Pulmonary function tests are not useful in distinguishing bronchiectasis from other obstructive airway diseases. Laboratory studies in patients with bronchiectasis include a mild degree of leukocytosis, usually without a left shift, an increase in the erythrocyte sedimentation rate, mild anemia, and hypergammaglobulinemia.

Radiographic Findings

Routine chest radiograph findings are abnormal in approximately 50% of patients with proven bronchiectasis. The classic finding of tram tracks, representing thickened dilated bronchial walls, is best seen on radiographs obtained from a lateral view. Other findings include hyperinflation and air trapping, increased linear markings, rounded opacities that represent areas of focal pneumonia, and ring shadows that represent dilated airways seen *en face.* HRCT scanning has become the diagnostic standard for the detection of bronchiectasis. It is both highly sensitive and specific for the diagnosis of bronchiectasis.

Today, HRCT scanning is the method used in nearly all cases of bronchiectasis. Given the high sensitivity of HRCT scanning, it has become much easier to diagnose the disorder, which may account for the increased awareness and prevalence of the disease. Standard criteria for the diagnosis of bronchiectasis on HRCT scans have been established. The most specific criteria are an internal bronchus diameter that is wider than its adjacent artery and the failure of the bronchi to taper as they move toward the periphery of the lung parenchyma. Secondary criteria include excessive bronchial wall thickening, impacted mucus, and crowding of the bronchi. Figure 1 shows the characteristic large bronchi in a patient with Kartagener syndrome.

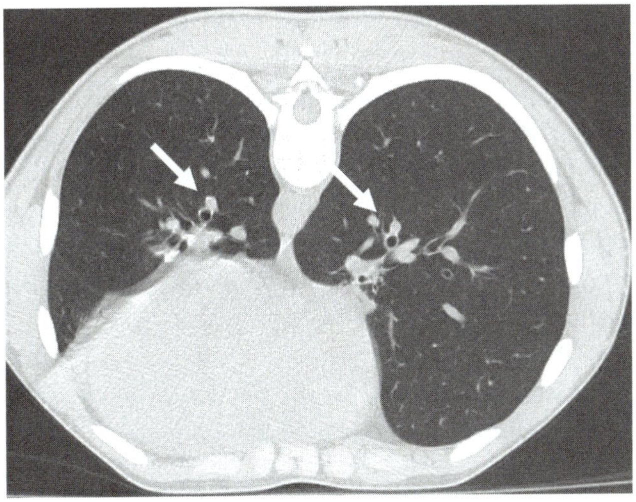

Figure 1. Large internal diameter of the bronchi (greater than the accompanying vessel), which is diagnostic of bronchiectasis (large arrows). From the author's personal files.

Differential Diagnosis

Given the list of possible etiologies, the following information should be obtained in the evaluation of patients with suspected bronchiectasis: age of onset of symptoms; history of frequent upper airway infections; smoking history; history of previous lung surgery; childhood infections (pertussis, pneumonia, measles); pulmonary tuberculosis or atypical mycobacterial infections; atopy or asthma; connective tissue disorders; infertility; reflux symptoms; and risk factors for HIV infection. Bronchiectasis should be distinguished from COPD (particularly chronic bronchitis). Both diseases present with cough, sputum production, wheezing, and dyspnea. Exacerbations are common in both disorders, although the volume of sputum production is greater in patients with bronchiectasis. Recurrent fever and hemoptysis are less likely to be found in patients with chronic bronchitis. The presence of Pseudomonas in the sputum may be helpful to the diagnosis. The incidence of *Pseudomonas aeruginosa* is approximately 31% in patients with bronchiectasis, but only 2 to 4% in patients with COPD. Bronchiectasis also can be confused with interstitial fibrosis, especially in patients with end-state fibrosis who have a honeycomb-like appearance seen on a chest radiograph. This parenchymal honeycomb appearance may mimic the air-filled cysts of bronchiectasis.

Therapy

The objectives of management for bronchiectasis are the relief of symptoms, the prevention of complications, the control of exacerbations, and a reduction in mortality.

Antibiotics: Antibiotics are the cornerstone for the treatment of exacerbations of bronchiectasis. They are used to treat acute exacerbations, to prevent exacerbations, or to reduce the bacterial burden. The bacterial floras include *Streptococcus pneumoniae* and *Haemophilus influenzae*, which can be treated with trimethoprim-sulfamethoxazole, ampicillin-clavulanate acid, or one of the newer macrolide agents. In patients with Pseudomonas colonization, oral therapy requires the use of a fluoroquinolone. In some cases, IV administration of antipseudomonal antibiotics is required. Whether prophylactic antibiotic therapy is necessary remains an unresolved question. Patients who experience frequent exacerbations may benefit from a maintenance regimen, but the evidence for this approach is fairly weak. Strategies for prophylaxis with low-dose antibiotics range from daily to 1 week of each month. Daily, inhaled antibiotic prophylaxis is now recommended in patients with CF who have been colonized with *P aeruginosa* colonization. There is debate as to whether *P aeruginosa* infection has a similar effect on prognosis in patients with non-CF bronchiectasis as in patients with CF. A few small studies suggest that chronic infection with *P aeruginosa* can cause an accelerated decrease in lung function that might be altered by the use of chronic nebulized antibiotic therapy. Large randomized controlled trials, however, are lacking in this population.

Bronchodilators: Most patients with bronchiectasis have significant airway hyperresponsiveness, presumably as a result of transmural airway inflammation. The routine use of bronchodilators has the added potential advantage of the stimulation of mucociliary clearance, which is associated with the use of β-adrenergic agents. Both aerosolized β-agonist therapy and aerosolized anticholinergic therapy should be tried when there is evidence of reversible airway obstruction.

Antiinflammatory Agents: Although intense airway inflammation characterizes bronchiectasis, few studies have looked at the efficacy of corticosteroids in the treatment of this disorder. Inhaled steroids have been suggested as alternative therapy and may be useful in some patients, especially those with significant airway hyperreactivity. It has been shown that inhaled corticosteroids can reduce the levels of inflammatory mediators and improve dyspnea and cough. In addition, inhaled corticosteroids appear to reduce sputum volume and lead to improvements in quality of life. However, a systematic review found no significant improvement in pulmonary function. Short courses of oral corticosteroid therapy often are used during acute exacerbations. Nonsteroidal antiinflammatory agents, such as indomethacin (which is not currently approved in the United States), have been used in Europe, either orally or by inhalation. Leukotriene receptor antagonists may be of benefit in patients with bronchiectasis because they can inhibit neutrophil-mediated inflammation. However, there have been no randomized controlled trials published concerning patients in this population. Macrolides suppress inflammation, independent of their antimicrobial action, and have improved the clinical status and lung function of patients in a few small studies of bronchiectasis. Further study is needed before they can be recommended routinely.

Airway Clearance Techniques: Postural drainage and chest physiotherapy are useful to enhance the gravity-aided clearance of secretions. It is important to consider that patients with non-CF bronchiectasis often have lower-lobe predominate disease, and thus, postural drainage may play a greater role in these patients. Alternative treatment includes the use of a flutter device, a positive expiratory pressure mask, chest oscillation, and humidification of inspired air.

Mucolytic Agents and Hydration: Adequate oral hydration and the use of nebulized solutions may improve airway mucus clearance. Acetylcysteine is beneficial in some patients. To date, there have been no randomized, controlled clinical trials showing mucolytics to be of benefit in the treatment of non-CF bronchiectasis. Recombinant human deoxyribonuclease (rhDNase) breaks down DNA that is released from degenerating bacteria and neutrophils. DNA has a tendency to form thick viscous gels. DNase improves the clearance of secretions and pulmonary function and reduces the number of hospitalizations in patients with CF but has not been found to be useful in non-CF bronchiectasis. One study has suggested that DNase was ineffective and potentially harmful in > 300 adult outpatients with idiopathic bronchiectasis who were in stable condition. Therapy with inhaled mannitol may improve impaired mucociliary clearance by inducing an influx of fluid into the airways and has shown clinical promise inpatients with non-CF bronchiectasis. This is particularly exciting because it is easier to inhale a dry powder than to use a nebulizer.

Exercise Training: The role of pulmonary rehabilitation and inspiratory muscle training has only been investigated in one well-designed trial, but it has been suggested that rehabilitation increases exercise tolerance in patients with bronchiectasis.

Surgery

In patients with localized bronchiectasis, surgical removal of the most affected segment or lobe may be considered. The major indications for surgery include the partial obstruction of a segment or lobe as the result of a tumor or the presence of a highly resistant organism in the affected area, such as MAC or Aspergillus sp. Patients require significant pulmonary function to withstand surgery. Surgery also may be performed for massive hemoptysis in patients with adequate pulmonary reserve, although the increased success of bronchial artery embolization for hemoptysis makes surgery less desirable.

Lung Transplantation

Patients with bronchiectasis and CF initially were considered not to be good transplant candidates because of concerns about overwhelming infection after the use of prolonged immunosuppression. However, double-lung transplantation has been successful in CF patients, and the St. Louis International Transplant Registry lists > 1,000 CF patients and > 200 non-CF bronchiectasis patients who have undergone lung transplantation, with a 1-year survival rate of 72% and a 4-year survival rate of 49% in patients with CF.

Cystic Fibrosis

Genetics

CF is the most common genetic disease in the United States, with an incidence of 1 in 3,000 births in a white population. The incidence is much lower in African-Americans, Asians, Hispanics, and Native Americans. CF is an autosomal-recessive disorder with variable penetrance. Carriers of the CF gene are phenotypically normal. Approximately 5% of persons in the white US population are carriers of the CF gene, and approximately 20,000 individuals are affected by this disorder. The CF gene, which was sequenced in 1989, is located in the long arm of chromosome 7 and encodes for the CF transmembrane regulator (CFTR) protein. The CFTR is located at the cell surface and acts as an ion channel that regulates liquid volume on epithelial surfaces through chloride secretion and the inhibition of sodium absorption.

The CFTR protein may also regulate the function of other epithelial cell proteins. The defective transport of ions across the epithelial membrane leads to thick viscous secretions in many organs and to excessive chloride concentration in the sweat of patients with CF. This abnormality is the basis for the laboratory test that is most frequently performed to diagnose this disorder. The CFTR protein is expressed in all of the epithelial cells affected in patients with CF, including those in the lung, pancreas, sweat glands, and liver. It is also found in the large intestine and testes.

More than 1,600 mutations of the CFTR gene have been described. The ΔF508 mutation is the most common and accounts for approximately 90% of CF chromosomes in patients of northern European descent but only 60% of CF chromosomes worldwide. The mutation is caused by the deletion of a single phenylalanine residue at position 508. CFTR mutations are categorized into six classes:

Class I: absent or defective protein synthesis;

Class II: abnormal processing of transport of the protein to the cell membrane;

Class III: abnormal regulation of CFTR function, inhibiting chloride channel activation;

Class IV: normal amount of CFTR but reduced function (abnormal conductance);

Class V: reduced synthesis of fully active CFTR; and

Class VI: decreased stability of fully processed and functional CFTR.

These multiple mutations lead to varying phenotypic presentations of the disease. Even patients with similar genetic mutations may manifest different clinical manifestations of the disease. The degree of organ involvement and perhaps the disease severity correlate with the individual's sensitivity to the CFTR dysfunction, as well as the amount of functional CFTR, which is influenced by the specific type of mutation. It is now recognized that some patients may present with only one characteristic feature of CF and a borderline abnormal sweat test finding in the presence of either a known CFTR mutation or an abnormal nasal potential difference (PD), which has led to use of the term *atypical* or *nonclassic CF*. Nonclassic CF is often associated with class IV or V mutations. These patients typically present later in life, and will display typical CF symptoms in at least one organ, but often have a normal or borderline sweat chloride test. They are typically pancreatic sufficient and have milder pulmonary disease and a better overall prognosis.

Pathogenesis

CF is initiated by a defect in the gene that is normally responsible for encoding CFTR protein, which is necessary for the flow of electrolytes and fluid across cell membranes. The resultant abnormalities in salt and water transport lead to an alteration in the composition of secretions in the respiratory tract, pancreas, GI tract, sweat glands, and other exocrine tissues. In the lung, these alterations change the properties of the mucus layer lining the epithelia and the composition of the airway surface fluid, ultimately resulting in the clinical features of CF. The net fluid loss on the airway surface leads to the collapse of cilia and impaired mucociliary clearance, persistent bacterial infection, excessive host inflammatory response (characterized by the accumulation of leukocyte-derived DNA and secretions rich in elastase), and airway obstruction, leading to progressive lung destruction. Although bacterial infection clearly leads to an intense inflammatory response, there is mounting evidence that patients with CF have increased basal and inducible airway inflammation independent of infection. Figure 2 summarizes the interaction between airway obstruction, infection, inflammation, and destruction.

Diagnostic Tests

1. Before the mid-1990s, most patients were treated for CF after presenting with typical symptoms. Since that time, newborn screening (NBS) has become much more widespread. Newborns with CF will have increased levels of serum immunoreactive trypsinogen (IRT), which can be detected via a radioimmunoassay or enzyme-linked immunosorbent assay performed on samples of dried blood. After an abnormal IRT, most NBS programs perform DNA testing to identify the known CFTR mutations, although some repeat the IRT after 2 weeks. NBS is not a diagnostic test and thus only identifies newborns at risk for CF. An increased IRT must be followed by direct diagnostic testing (typically with the sweat chloride test). The diagnostic process for screened newborns is shown in Figure 3.
2. Sweat test (pilocarpine iontophoresis): The sweat chloride test remains the "gold standard" diagnostic test because genetic screening only identifies a small number of the most

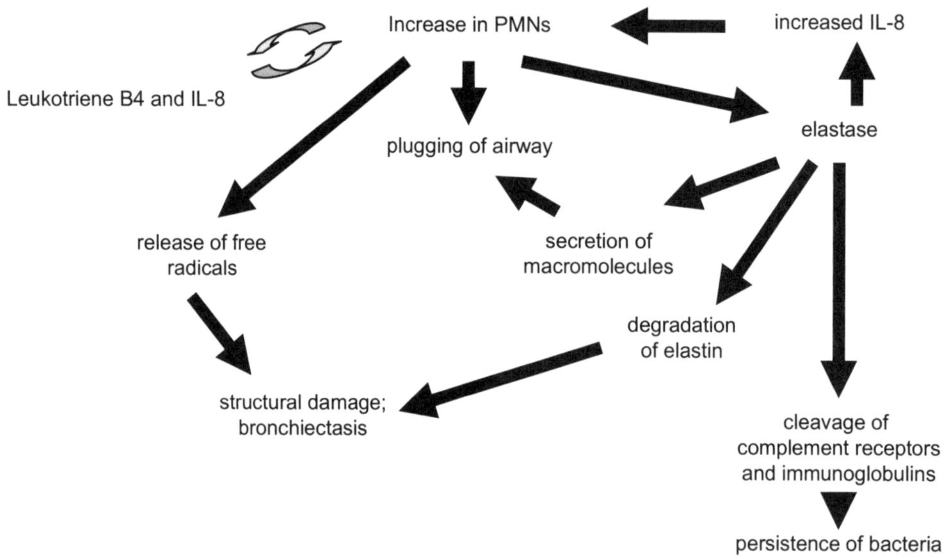

Figure 2. Products of polymorphonuclear neutrophil and their effects on inflammation of the airways in patients with CF. Adapted from Ramsey BW. Management of pulmonary disease in patients with CF. N Engl J Med 1996; 335:179–188.

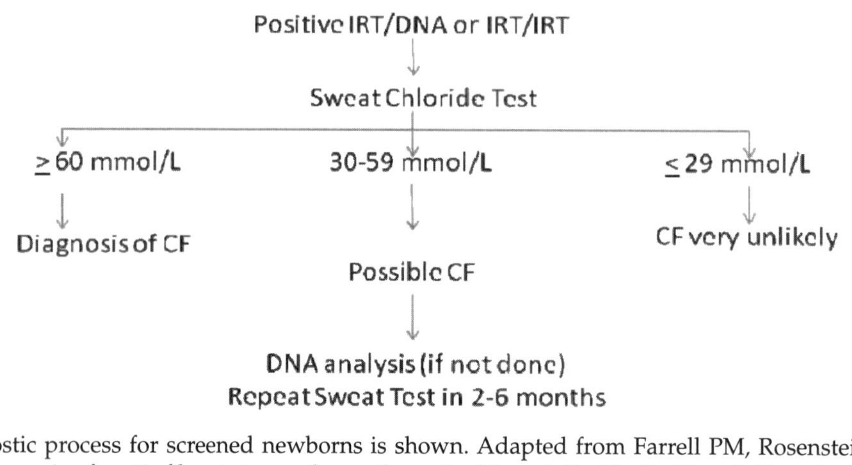

Figure 3. The diagnostic process for screened newborns is shown. Adapted from Farrell PM, Rosenstein BJ, White TB, et al: Guidelines for the diagnosis of cystic fibrosis in newborns through older adults: Cystic Fibrosis Foundation consensus report. J Pediatr 2008; 153:S4–S14.

common mutations. The results of this test are abnormal in the large majority of patients with CF. A chloride level of >60 mEq/dL is usually diagnostic for CF. However, the test must be repeated at least twice, and an adequate sample containing at least 75 mg of sweat must be collected over a 30-min period. Approximately 1% of patients with CF have normal sweat chloride test results. Abnormal sweat test results are seen in patients with other disorders (as listed in Table 3). Therefore, a diagnosis should only be made if the clinical history is suggestive of CF. The current diagnostic criteria for CF are listed in Table 4.

3. Molecular diagnosis: Approximately 1,600 mutations have been identified after sequencing the entire gene in a research laboratory. Genotyping at commercial laboratories usually can identify only 20 to 30 of the most common mutations. This accounts for approximately 90% of CF mutations in the general population.
4. PD across the respiratory epithelium: This is a research tool that may be available at few centers to aid in the diagnosis of CF. The abnormal transport of chloride leads to a very negative PD across the nasal epithelium. The measurement of this PD can establish a CF diagnosis. Nasal perfusion with amiloride hydrochloride and with chloride-free solutions leads to characteristic changes in the PD.

Table 3. *False-Positive Sweat Test Results*

Adrenal insufficiency
Anorexia nervosa
Atopic dermatitis
Autonomic dysfunction
Celiac disease
Familial cholestasis
Fucosidosis
Glucose-6-phosphate dehydrogenase deficiency
Glycogen storage disease, type I
Hypogammaglobulinemia
Hypoparathyroidism
Hypothyroidism (untreated)
Klinefelter syndrome
Mucopolysaccharidosis, type I
Malnutrition
Nephrogenic diabetes insipidus
Nephrosis
Prostaglandin E1 infusion, long-term
Pseudohypoaldosteronism

Table 4. *Criteria for Diagnosis of CF*

Elevated sweat chloride level ≥60 mmol/L on two occasions
or
Identification of mutations known to cause CF in both CFTR genes
or
In vivo demonstration of characteristic abnormalities in ion transport across the nasal epithelium
plus
One or more phenotypical features of CF
Sinopulmonary disease
Characteristic GI or nutritional disorders
Obstructive azoospermia
Salt loss syndrome
or
Sibling with CF
or
Positive NBS result

Nonpulmonary Clinical Manifestations

In the pancreas, dysfunction of the exocrine portion leads to fat malabsorption and malnutrition. Glucose intolerance is present in as many as 50 to 70% of older patients with CF; diabetes mellitus occurs in approximately 15%. Malabsorption of fat-soluble vitamins such as A, D, E, and K can lead to vitamin deficiency and coagulopathy. The liver is affected by biliary cirrhosis as a result of thick secretions in the biliary ducts. This is manifested by abnormal liver function test results. Diffuse liver involvement can lead to portal hypertension.

Meconium ileus is present in approximately 20% of infants with CF and is pathognomonic for this disorder. A similar syndrome occurs in older CF patients caused by inspissated mucus in the GI tract. This results in the distal intestinal obstruction syndrome, often requiring surgical treatment.

Approximately 95% of male patients with CF are infertile. Although sperm maturation is normal, the Wolffian structures often are not developed. The vas deferens is often completely absent. This absence may indicate a role for the CFTR protein in the development of the male genital tract. In fact, in subjects with congenital bilateral absence of the vas deferens but without any other abnormalities of CF, mutations in the CFTR gene have been reported. Women with CF are not infertile, although they may have difficulty conceiving because of thick cervical mucus and/or anovulatory cycles if their nutritional status is poor. Pregnancies can be successful, and pulmonary function has not been found to deteriorate after pregnancy.

Pulmonary Manifestations

The primary cause of morbidity and mortality in CF patients is bronchiectasis and obstructive lung disease. Pulmonary disease is present in 98% of patients with CF by the time they reach adulthood. Despite the great advances in the management of this disorder, the majority of the patients succumb to respiratory complications. A recurrent cough that becomes persistent is often the first manifestation. Airway hyperreactivity and wheezing are common in children. Bronchodilator responsiveness tends to decrease with age, perhaps as a result of the destruction of the cartilage. Pansinusitis with opacification of the paranasal sinuses is a universal finding in patients with CF. Nasal polyps are present in up to 30% of patients with CF.

In patients with CF, the lungs are normal at birth, but infection occurs early in life and is persistent. The abnormal ionic environment and chronic airway obstruction by thick secretions promote colonization with pathogenic bacteria, which leads to the accumulation of inflammatory cells. These cells release inflammatory mediators that cause inflammation and damage to the airway wall, leading to the development of bronchiolitis and subsequently bronchiectasis (Fig 2).

H influenzae, *Staphylococcus aureus* and, later, *P aeruginosa*, are the pathogens that are most commonly found in the airways of patients with CF. The abnormal CFTR may be partly responsible for colonization with Pseudomonas sp because the normal CFTR appears to be involved in the clearance of this organism from the airways. The high sodium content in CF secretions may contribute to chronic infection because low sodium content is required for the effective killing of bacteria in airway epithelia. Colonization with *P aeruginosa* is not benign because it has been found to be an independent risk factor for the accelerated loss of lung function and decreased survival. Colonization with *Burkholderia cepacia* denotes an even worse prognosis.

The mucoid appearance of Pseudomonas is caused by the production of alginate. This bacterium is difficult to eradicate as the result of the poor penetration of antibiotics into purulent airway secretions and to the interference in phagocytic killing by alginate. Bacteria may have native or acquired antibiotic resistance. In addition, the pharmacokinetics differ in patients with CF because the volume of distribution of hydrophilic drugs (*eg*, penicillins, cephalosporins, and aminoglycosides) is increased as the result of decreased amounts of adipose tissue. The renal clearance of aminoglycosides is increased, and therefore, the dosage has to be adjusted, usually at triple the normal dose. Once-daily administration is not recommended.

Management of Pulmonary Disease

Although the focus of this section is on the treatment of pulmonary disease in patients with CF, it should be kept in mind that management in general will be suboptimal unless all aspects of the disease are addressed (*ie*, exocrine pancreatic supplementation, nutritional support, glucose control, psychosocial issues, and treatment compliance). Progress has been made in attempts at addressing the underlying defect of CF with gene therapy, but current clinical treatment is aimed at treating the effects of the CFTR dysfunction—thickened airway mucus, infection, and inflammation.

Clearance of Airway Secretions: The chief nonpharmacologic means of enhancing airway secretion clearance has been chest physiotherapy (either manual or with use of an oscillatory vest) and postural drainage. Other techniques include forced expiratory techniques, positive expiratory pressure, and flutter valves. A Cochrane review in early 2009 noted that there is no high-level evidence that any of these techniques are superior to the others. All patients who produce daily sputum should be instructed in clearance techniques. All of the techniques require a great deal of time, and treatment compliance can be an issue. Therefore, several methods can be introduced to each patient.

Bronchodilator Therapy: As noted previously, many patients with CF will demonstrate a degree of bronchial hyperactivity and reversibility. The obstructive airway disease is typically only partially reversible because the underlying causes include the chronic infection, inflammation, and resulting structural damage. Bronchodilator therapy should be considered in patients who have at least a 10% increase in FEV_1 in response to an inhaled bronchodilator. In addition, bronchodilators often are used in all patients with CF before chest physiotherapy and immediately before the inhalation of hypertonic saline solution, antibiotics, or dornase alfa because these medications have the potential to induce nonspecific bronchial constriction. The role of these medications in improving mucociliary clearance has not been well defined.

Reduction in the Viscosity of Secretions: The increased viscosity of the sputum in patients with CF is caused partly by the presence of many polymorphonuclear neutrophils and their degradation products, including DNA from dying cells. rhDNase I (or dornase alfa) digests extracellular DNA and can help to reduce the viscosity. A metaanalysis of randomized trials of dornase alfa has concluded that treatment improves lung function and is well tolerated. There is some controversy about when to initiate dornase alfa, but most clinicians will consider a trial in patients with documented chronic infection and obstruction in spirometry. A guideline committee for the CF Foundation recommends chronic dornase alfa for all children with CF > 6 years old. The recommended dosage is 2.5 mg/d.

Osmotic Therapy: A decreased amount of airway surface liquid is an important factor in the under lying pathophysiology of CF. Therefore, osmotically drawing water onto the airway surface via inhalation of a hypertonic substance might help to clear secretions and restore mucociliary transport. Inhaled hypertonic saline solution has been used for this purpose in patients with CF, and has been associated with increased mucus clearance and improvement in lung function, and, in one long-term study, with fewer exacerbations requiring antibiotic therapy. Prescribing patterns vary, but twice-daily treatments (4 mL of 7% saline solution) in patients with chronic cough and sputum production should be considered. There have been no randomized controlled trials comparing dornase alfa with hypertonic saline solution. Because the mechanism of action differs somewhat between the two, it is reasonable to assume that they maybe complementary.

Antibiotic Therapy: Patients with CF have frequent exacerbations of infection. Acute exacerbations are manifested by increased cough and sputum volumes, sometimes associated with hemoptysis, and are often accompanied by systemic symptoms such as decreased energy, anorexia, and weight loss. Spirometry demonstrates a decrease in lung function. Parenteral antibiotics are generally administered for 14 to 21 days to reduce the burden of bacteria, to decrease symptoms, and to improve lung function. The most recent respiratory tract cultures should be used to guide therapy. Cephalothin and nafcillin are used for the treatment of infection with *S aureus*, and vancomycin is used for patients with a penicillin allergy. For patients with Pseudomonas sp, an antipseudomonal penicillin is combined with an aminoglycoside. Combination therapy reduces the risk of the development of resistance. Intensified bronchodilator therapy and chest physiotherapy are indicated during the treatment of exacerbations. Therapy with steroids may be used in patients with hyperreactive airways, but it has not been systemically studied.

Chronic infection with Pseudomonas sp is associated with a more rapid decrease in pulmonary function and increased mortality; delaying the onset of chronic infection is critical. When the organism is first isolated, a prolonged course of antibiotics that eradicates the organism has been shown to delay the onset of chronic infection. Repeated attempts to eradicate the organism may also be successful and beneficial. A combination therapy consisting of an oral quinolone and an inhaled aminoglycoside is typically used. Some patients with CF are administered long-term antibiotic therapy in the hopes of suppressing bacterial growth and recurrent infections, although this practice is controversial. The most common current practice involves the use of nebulized antipseudomonal antibiotics in patients with documented chronic infection. The inhaled route is attractive because it allows the delivery of greater concentrations to the airways with low systemic absorption, thus reducing the risk of ototoxicity and nephrotoxicity. A 2009 Cochrane review confirmed that long-term use is associated with improved lung function and a decreased number of hospitalizations.

Antiinflammatory Agents: There is a neutrophil-predominant inflammation in the airways of patients with CF. These neutrophils perpetuate the inflammatory cycle through the release of cytokines, chemotactants, and proteolytic enzymes (Fig 2). As noted earlier, patients with CF have abnormal basal and inducible airway inflammation. This inflammation is not entirely independent from infectious stimulation. When considering potential antiinflammatory strategies, several key concepts must be kept in mind: the inflammatory process is primarily endobronchial; it is characterized by persistent neutrophil influx; intracellular signaling pathways are a key component; the inflammatory response is prolonged and involves heightened oxidative and proteolytic stress.

Several early studies evaluated the effects of systemic glucocorticoids in patients with CF. Although a beneficial effect on lung function was observed in some patients, the adverse effects (glucose intolerance, growth retardation, cataracts) limit widespread use. Therefore, therapy with systemic glucocorticoids is recommended only for patients with asthma or ABPA complicating the disease. There is a lack of good clinical trials of inhaled corticosteroids in patients with CF, and these also are only recommended in patients with asthma or ABPA.

Ibuprofen also has been studied because of its ability to inhibit the migration and activation of neutrophils. In high doses, ibuprofen appears to slow the progressive decrease in lung function, particularly in younger patients with a milder form of disease. The 2009 Cochrane review, which is based on four trials enrolling a total of 287 patients, confirms this finding. The beneficial effects are dependent on achieving adequate serum levels, and thus the drug must be individually dosed based on measured pharmacokinetics (desired peak plasma concentrations between 50 and 100 μg/mL). This therapy has not been used widely (only 6% based on current CF patient registry data) as the result of concerns about the logistics of dosing and fear of GI and renal toxicity. However, several clinical trials have suggested that renal impairment does not occur at an increased rate, and most GI complaints are related to the underlying disease. There is a statistically significant increase in GI bleeding, but the event rates remain very low. The CF Foundation currently recommends high-dose ibuprofen therapy for children 6 to 12 years of age with moderate-to-severe lung disease.

Macrolide therapy was found to be beneficial in patients with panbronchiolitis, which led to empiric use by some physicians in patients with CF. Several well-conducted clinical trials have now shown that the long-term use of azithromycin (which appears to act primarily as an antiinflammatory agent by inhibiting neutrophil migration and elastase production) is associated with improved lung function and a reduction in the number of exacerbations. The CF Foundation currently recommends azithromycin (500 mg po 3 d/wk) for patients with long-term Pseudomonas infection. Before the initiation of therapy, some experts recommend that sputum be examined for nontuberculous mycobacteria because macrolide antibiotics are a vital in the treatment of nontuberculous mycobacteria.

Other antiinflammatory agents are being investigated in patients with CF. Increased oxidative stress and reduced levels of glutathione in the lungs of patients with CF have led to trials of the antioxidant *N*-acetylcysteine, aerosolized glutathione, and oral supplementation with antioxidant vitamins. Evidence suggests that these agents might attenuate lung inflammation, but further study is needed. Pharmacologic therapies that target proinflammatory and regulatory cytokines have been developed for other diseases (rheumatoid arthritis, psoriasis, inflammatory bowel disease). No published data on their use in CF are available. In addition, there is some concern that these agents might overly suppress the inflammatory response, leading to secondary infectious complications. Finding ways to interrupt intracellular signaling pathways that lead to increased inflammation may also be an effective strategy, but more understanding of the complex roles these play in other important cellular mechanisms is needed. The increased levels of neutrophils in the lung lead to massive amounts of proteases that overwhelm native antiproteases. Several trials have examined the use of inhaled α_1-antitrypsin in patients with CF. Although it appears to be well tolerated, no clear benefit on important outcomes have yet been demonstrated. In addition, this therapy is limited by expense, supply, and the risks of using plasma-derived products. Some of this may be overcome in the future with recombinant α_1-antitrypsin.

New Therapies in Development: Because CFTR mutations lead to defective or absent CFTR protein, the most logical way of treating CF would be to replace the CFTR gene to restore normal production. There are multiple steps to achieving this goal: sufficient gene product must be delivered to the primary target cells and it must be incorporated so as to allow normal gene expression. Although progress has been made, gene therapy is still some years away from clinical practice. Other approaches in development include correction of the abnormal protein folding of the CFTR; improvement in the ion channel function; induction of alternative ion channels, and newer antibiotics.

Pulmonary Complications

Hemoptysis: Hemoptysis occurs frequently during bronchitic exacerbations and usually is self-limited. Conservative measures such as bed rest, cough suppression, antibiotics, and correction of coagulopathy, if present, are adequate treatment for most patients. Massive hemoptysis is associated with a high mortality rate but may respond favorably to bronchial artery embolization. It is successful in as many as 90% of cases, but recurrences can occur in approximately 20% of cases. Repeated procedures can be performed if necessary. If this proves unsuccessful, lung resection of the involved lobe may be the only alternative, but it is often difficult to ascertain with certainty which lobe or segment is responsible for the hemorrhage.

Pneumothorax: Spontaneous pneumothorax occurs in approximately 16% of patients with CF. The vast majority of these patients have severe pulmonary involvement antecedent to the pneumothorax, with an FEV_1 of <50% predicted. The average recurrence rate is nearly 50%, and despite treatment, the mortality rate is high at 30 to 60%. This high mortality rate relates more to the severe underlying parenchymal involvement than to the pneumothorax itself. Chemical pleurodesis may be necessary for treating recurrences.

Nontuberculous Mycobacterial Infections: Recently, there has been a marked increase in the isolation of nontuberculous Mycobacterium sp (primarily *Mycobacterium avium* intracellulare complex and *Mycobacterium chelonei*) in adult patients with CF. Several centers have reported positive culture findings from up to 18% of patients studied. Distinguishing airway colonization from infection can be difficult. HRCT scanning may be useful in the evaluation. Nodular opacities or a tree-in-bud appearance suggests the presence of infection rather than colonization. Transbronchial lung biopsies may be required to demonstrate the presence of infection. If pulmonary function declines and atypical Mycobacterium sp are found in cultures from at least three sputum samples, treatment with antimycobacterial agents is recommended.

ABPA: ABPA develops in a small portion of patients in the United States (1.8% in a 1995 report). ABPA should be suspected if there is evidence of bronchospasm, peripheral eosinophilia, sputum cultures positive for *Aspergillus fumigatus*, and an immediate skin test response to *A fumigatus*. Diagnosis is confirmed by total serum IgE levels of >1,000 ng/mL and IgE or IgG specific to *A fumigatus*.

Respiratory Failure and Cor Pulmonale: Respiratory insufficiency develops as lung disease progresses, initially with hypoxemia on exercise, then at rest, and eventually with carbon dioxide retention. Right ventricular failure represents the culmination of the pathologic sequence of lung disease with progressive respiratory failure. In most cases, this process heralds the terminal stage in a patient's course with only limited survival beyond a few months.

Transplantation: Patients with CF are generally good transplant candidates because they are young and otherwise healthy and are used to undergoing complex medical regimens. CF does not develop in the transplanted lung. However, transplantation in CF is not without controversy, especially since some prediction models suggest that transplantation rarely improves survival in CF patients <18 years of age. Others have found that only those patients with a predicted 5-year survival of <50% and without *Burkholderia cepacia* or CF arthropathy are likely to have increased survival. These patients require bilateral lung transplantation using a clamshell incision.

Indications for transplantation include deteriorating respiratory status despite aggressive medical therapy and an FEV_1 of <30% predicted in compliant patients with good nutritional status and no other organ impairments. Patients also can be considered if they manifest major life-threatening pulmonary complications (*eg*, massive hemoptysis), pulmonary hypertension, or increasing antibiotic resistance of bacterial infecting the lungs. The average wait for transplantation is approximately 2 years. In 1997, the actuarial survival rate for CF patients was 72% at 1 year and 49% at 4 years. Female patients and those <18 years of age have a worse prognosis and should be considered for earlier listing.

Contraindications to transplantation include other organ failures, noncompliance with therapy, psychosocial instability, profound malnutrition, or active infection with Aspergillus or atypical Mycobacterium sp. An increased risk for transplantation is associated with colonization with resistant organisms (particularly *B cepacia)*, previous thoracic surgery or pleurodesis, the need for mechanical ventilation, and diabetes mellitus.

Prognosis

Most patients still die of respiratory complications. The degree of pulmonary impairment is predictive of survival. In 1992, Kerem et al published the results of a study that demonstrated that when the FEV_1 decreased to <30% predicted, the 2-year survival rate was <50%. Women appear to experience a greater deterioration of lung function with age.

When the first accurate description of CF was published by Andersen in 1939, >80% of patients died within 1 year of birth. Since then, advances in diagnosis and therapy have been accompanied by a gradual improvement in prognosis and increased survival time. According to data from the CF Patient Registry, the median survival time in the United States was approximately 20 years in 1970 and had increased to 37.4 years by 2007. Recent estimates have projected that children born with CF in the United States today will survive into their sixth decade of life.

Annotated Bibliography

Accurso FJ. Update in CF 2006. Am J Respir Crit Care Med 2007; 175:754–757

CF is a complex inherited disease resulting from abnormalities in the gene that codes for CFTR. The course of CF is surprisingly variable, even when considering CF genotype. This update concisely reviews the latest research on the genetics of airway morphology, infections, effects of the nitric oxide, and assessment of inflammation.

Barker AF, Couch L, Fiel SB, et al. Tobramycin solution for inhalation reduces sputum *Pseudomonas aeruginosa* density in bronchiectasis. Am J Respir Crit Care Med 2000; 162:481–85

More patients treated with tobramycin solution for inhalation than those treated with placebo reported increased cough, dyspnea, wheezing, and noncardiac chest pain, but the symptoms did not limit therapy.

Belkin RA, Henig NR, Singer LG, et al. Risk factors for death of patients with CF awaiting lung transplantation. Am J Respir Crit Care Med 2006; 173:659–666

Precise timing for the listing of CF patients for lung transplantation remains controversial. This retrospective study of patients listed for lung transplantation at four academic medical centers identified risk factors for death while awaiting transplantation. Patients with FEV_1 *>30% predicted had a greater risk of death only when their* $Paco_2$ *was >50 mm Hg, whereas the increased risk of death with* FEV_1 *<30% predicted was not further influenced by the presence of hypercapnia.*

Bilton D. Update on non-cystic fibrosis bronchiectasis. Curr Opin Pulm Med 2008; 14:595–599

This review includes a particularly nice discussion of updates in inherited and noninherited causes of bronchiectasis and insight into the role of nontuberculous mycobacterial and pseudomonal infections in patients with bronchiectasis.

Choi J, Koh WJ, Kim TS, et al. Optimal duration of IV and oral antibiotics in the treatment of thoracic actinomycosis. Chest 2005; 128:2211–2217

IV antibiotic therapy for 2 to 6 weeks followed by 6 to 12 months of oral antibiotic therapy is usually recommended for the treatment of thoracic actinomycosis. However, a retrospective of 28 patients with thoracic actinomycosis showed success with varying treatment regimens. Combined surgical and antibiotic therapy was used in nearly half of the patients. The duration of IV antibiotic therapy ranged from 3 to 17 days, whereas the duration of oral antibiotic therapy ranged from 0 to 534 days. Clinical cures were achieved in 96% of the patients with no clinical evidence of recurrence.

Davis JC, Alton E, Bush A. Clinical review: CF. BMJ 2007; 335:125551–125259

This article includes up-to-date tables with informal evidence grading of management strategies in CF.

Davis PB. Centennial review: CF since 1938. Am J Respir Crit Care Med 2006; 173:475–482

This article summarizes the history of CF since it was distinguished from celiac disease in 1938. The standardization of the sweat test in 1959 allowed the identification of milder cases. In 1983, chloride transport was identified as the basic CF defect. In 1989, the CF gene was discovered. This article is easy to follow and explains concepts in an understandable fashion.

Elkins MR, Robinson M, Rose BR, et al. A controlled trial of long-term inhaled hypertonic saline in patients with CF. N Engl J Med 2006; 354:229–240

Seminal article on the long-term use of hypertonic saline solution in patients with CF.

Farrell PM, Rosenstein BJ, White TB, et al. Guidelines for the diagnosis of cystic fibrosis in newborns through older adults: Cystic Fibrosis Foundation consensus report. J Pediatr 2008; 153:S4–S14

Excellent updated review of the diagnostic tests, including NBS and recommended diagnostic algorithms based upon these tests.

Flotte TR, Laube BL. History and evolution of aerosolized therapeutics. Chest 2001; 120(suppl):124S–131S

Theoretically, CFTR gene replacement during the neonatal period can decrease the rates of morbidity and mortality from CF. In vivo gene transfers have been accomplished in patients with CF. The choice of vector, mode of delivery to the airways, translocation of genetic information, and sufficient expression level of the normalized CFTR gene are issues that are currently being addressed.

Flume PA, Stange C, Ye X, et al. Pneumothorax in CF. Chest 2005; 128:720–728

Pneumothorax is a complication in patients with CF, occurring more commonly in older patients with more advanced lung disease. Approximately 1 in 167 patients will experience this complication each year. The principal risks associated with an increased occurrence of pneumothorax include the presence of P aeruginosa, B cepacia, *or Aspergillus sp in sputum cultures,* FEV_1 *<30% predicted, enteral feeding, Medicaid insurance, pancreatic insufficiency, ABPA, and massive hemoptysis. There is an increased 2-year mortality rate after pneumothorax.*

Flume PA, Yankaskas JR, Ebeling M, et al. Massive hemoptysis in CF. Chest 2005; 128:729–738

Massive hemoptysis is a serious complication in patients with CF, occurring more commonly in older patients with more advanced lung disease. The principal risks associated with an increased occurrence of massive hemoptysis included the presence of S aureus *in sputum cultures and diabetes. There was an increased morbidity (eg, increased hospitalizations and hospital days) and an increased 2-year mortality rate after massive hemoptysis.*

Gilljam M, Ellis L, Corey M, et al. Clinical manifestations of CF among patients with diagnosis in adulthood. Chest 2004; 126:1215–1224

Seven percent of CF patients receive diagnoses in adulthood. Patients with CF presenting in adulthood often have pancreatic sufficiency, inconclusive sweat chloride sweat test results, and a high prevalence of mutations that are not commonly seen in CF diagnosed in childhood. Single-organ manifestations such as congenital bilateral absence of the vas deferens and pancreatitis are seen. The severity of lung disease is variable. Repeated sweat chloride tests and extensive mutation analysis are often required to make a diagnosis.

Husain S, McCurry K, Dauber J, et al. Nocardia infection in lung transplant recipients. J Heart Lung Transplant 2002; 21:354–359

Nocardia infection tended to involve the native lung in single-lung transplant recipients. Trimethoprim-sulfamethoxazole for Pneumocystis carinii *prophylaxis at the doses given was not protective against nocardiosis in these patients.*

Kerem E, Reisman J, Corey M, et al. Prediction of mortality in patients with CF. N Engl J Med 1992; 236:1187–1191

In a cohort of 673 patients with CF, FEV_1 *was predictive of mortality; when it reached <30% of predicted, the 2-year mortality rate exceeded 50%.*

Kim TS, Han J, Koh W, et al. Thoracic actinomycosis: CT features with histopathologic correlation. AJR Am J Roentgenol 2006; 186:225–231

Radiologic, pathologic, and histologic images of patients with pulmonary actinomycosis infection.

Kreider M, Kotloff RM. Selection of candidates for lung transplantation. Proc Am Thorac Soc 2009; 6:20–27

Up-to-date review of general consideration in selecting patients for lung transplantation, as well as specific recommendations for patients with CF.

Mabeza GF, Macfarlane J. Pulmonary actinomycosis. Eur Resp J 2003; 21:545–551

Comprehensive clinical review of the pulmonary manifestations of actinomycosis.

Martinez R, Reyes S, Menendez R. Pulmonary nocardiosis: risk factors, clinical features, diagnosis and prognosis. Curr Opin Pulm Med 2008; 14:219–227

Most current, comprehensive clinical review of pulmonary nocardiosis (including expanded sections on newer diagnostic techniques and new therapeutic options).

McGeinness G, Naidich DP. CT of airways disease and bronchiectasis. Radiol Clin North Am 2002; 40:1–19

This article discusses HRCT findings associated with medium-sized and small airways diseases, focusing on bronchiectasis of both infectious and noninfectious causes.

McMullen AH, Pasta DJ, Frederick PD, et al. Impact of pregnancy on women with CF. Chest 2006; 129:706–711

Concern exists about the impact of pregnancy on the health of women with CF. This study suggests that women with CF who become pregnant experience similar respiratory and health trends compared to nonpregnant women with CF. However, pregnant women used a greater number of therapies and received more intense monitoring of their health.

Moss RB, Rodman D, Spencer LT, et al. Repeated adeno-associated virus serotype 2 aerosol-mediated CF trans-membrane regulator gene transfer to the lungs of patients with CF: a multicenter, double-blind, placebo-controlled trial. Chest 2004; 125:509–521

This eight-center CF gene therapy study determined the safety of repeated doses of aerosolized adeno-associated vector containing CFTR complementary DNA. It showed that the aerosolized viral vector encoding the complete human CFTR DNA was safe and well tolerated. There were trends in improvement in pulmonary function in patients with CF and mild lung disease.

Nichols DP, Konstan MW, Chmiel JF. Anti-inflammatory therapies for cystic fibrosis-related lung disease. Clinc Rev Allerg Immunol 2008; 35:135–153

Comprehensive and up-to-date review of the inflammatory mechanisms in CF. Includes a detailed review of several pharmacologic agents currently use (and those in development) that address these multiple mechanisms.

O'Donnell AE. Bronchiectasis. Chest 2008; 134:815–823

Bronchiectasis is now being recognized with increased frequency around the world. This is a well-written clinical review, including a discussion of pathophysiology and natural history, in addition to reviews of current therapeutic approaches.

O'Donnell AE, Barker AF, Ilowite JS, et al. Treatment of idiopathic bronchiectasis with aerosolized recombinant human DNase I. Chest 1998; 113:1329–1334

rhDNAse was ineffective and potentially harmful in this group of adult outpatients in stable condition with idiopathic bronchiectasis. This contrasts with previously published results that demonstrated the efficacy of rhDNase in patients with CF bronchiectasis.

Ramsey BW. Drug therapy: management of pulmonary disease in patients with CF. N Engl J Med 1996; 335:179–188

Although somewhat out of date, this is an excellent and well-organized approach to the management of pulmonary complications of CF. Includes specific recommendations on antibiotic coverage for acute exacerbations and chronic suppression of pulmonary infections.

Ramsey BW, Pepe MS, Quan JM, et al. Intermittent administration of inhaled tobramycin in patients with CF. N Engl J Med 1999; 340:23–30

This article reports the results of a multicenter trial of intermittent administration of preservative-free preparation of inhaled tobramycin in CF patients with P aeruginosa, *with resultant improvement in pulmonary function and clinical course.*

Ratjen F. New pulmonary therapies for CF. Curr Opin in Pulm Med 2007; 13:541–546

A very current and concise review of new approaches to the management of CF, including gene therapy, CFTR modulation, manipulation of ion channels, and other antiinflammatory and antiinfective medications.

Swensen SJ, Hartman TE, Williams DE. Computed tomographic diagnosis of *Mycobacterium avium*-intracellulare complex in patients with bronchiectasis. Chest 1994; 105:49–52

A clinical study of 100 patients with bronchiectasis with chest CT scan evidence of MAC infection suggests that the presence of multiple small lung nodules on CT scans is predictive of the presence of MAC on culture.

ten Hacken NH, Wijkstra PJ, Kersjens HA. Clinical review: treatment of bronchiectasis in adults. BMJ 2007; 335:1089–1093

Succinct, organized review with evidence tables of differing therapeutic agents.

Vlahakis NE, Aksamit TR. Diagnosis and treatment of allergic bronchopulmonary aspergillosis. Mayo Clin Proc 2001; 76:930–938

ABPA is an underdiagnosed pulmonary disorder in asthmatic patients and patients with CF. If ABPA is diagnosed and treated before the development of bronchiectasis and fibrosis, these complications may be prevented. Total serum IgE and IgE-specific A fumigatus *antibodies establish the diagnosis. Long-term treatment with corticosteroids is often required for management. Itraconazole may be effective as a corticosteroid-sparing agent.*

Yankaskas JR, Marshall BC, Sufian B, et al. CF adult care: consensus conference report. Chest 2004; 125(suppl):1S–39S
This supplement is the most up-to-date summary of the diagnosis and management of CF in the adult but is based on a CF Foundation consensus conference held in 1999.

Yildiz O, Doganay M. Actinomycoses and Nocardia pulmonary infections. Curr Opin Pulm Med 2006; 12:228–234
Well-written, easy-to-understand review and comparison of pulmonary infections related to Actinomyces and Nocardia species.

Notes

Pulmonary Vascular Diseases

Lisa K. Moores, MD, FCCP

Objectives:

- Describe the risk factors and epidemiology of venous thromboembolism (VTE)
- Provide approaches to the diagnosis and treatment of VTE
- Discuss approaches to the prevention of VTE
- Describe the epidemiology and pathophysiology of pulmonary hypertension (PH)
- Describe the steps in the diagnosis of pulmonary arterial hypertension (PAH)
- List the recommended treatment regimens for PH

Key words: anticoagulation; hypercoagulable state; pulmonary arterial hypertension; pulmonary embolism; pulmonary hypertension; thrombolytic therapy; venous thrombosis

VTE

Pulmonary embolism (PE) and deep venous thrombosis (DVT) constitute the spectrum of one disease: venous thromboembolism (VTE). Approximately 79% of patients who present with PE also will have concomitant DVT; conversely, only approximately 50% of patients presenting with DVT will have PE. The estimated annual incidence of VTE in the United States is one episode per 1,000 patients. As many as 3,000,000 people die each year in the United States from acute PE.

Risk Factors

Risk factors associated with VTE often are classified into acquired and genetic factors, and these can overlap in an individual patient. Acquired risks include prolonged immobility or paralysis; cancer; major surgery (particularly, operations involving the abdomen, pelvis, and lower extremities); trauma; obesity; high estrogen states (*ie*, pregnancy, taking birth control pills, and hormone replacement therapy); varicose veins; congestive heart failure; cor pulmonale; myocardial infarction; stroke; fractures of the pelvis, hip, or leg; indwelling femoral vein catheters; inflammatory bowel disease; heparin-induced thrombocytopenia (HIT); and myeloproliferative disorders, such as polycythemia vera and hyperviscosity syndromes. Patients with a history of VTE are at increased risk for recurrence. Congenital or hereditary hypercoagulable states include the following: activated protein C resistance (factor V Leiden mutation); antithrombin III deficiency (can also be acquired with the nephrotic syndrome); protein C deficiency; protein S deficiency; dysfibrinogenemia; disorders of plasminogen and plasminogen activation; the presence of antiphospholipid antibodies and lupus anticoagulant; and hyperhomocysteinemia. Many patients may present with multiple risk factors for VTE that can further increase their likelihood of this complication developing. Examples include the elderly patient with congestive heart failure who sustains a hip fracture and the patient with a myeloproliferative disorder who is undergoing major surgery.

Pathogenesis

The Virchow triad of venous stasis, endothelial vascular injury, and hypercoagulability explains how various processes can interact to overcome antithrombotic defenses resulting in VTE. Vascular stasis predisposes the patient to VTE by allowing activated coagulation factors to remain undiluted and in contact with the vascular endothelium. Vascular trauma or injury, to include the presence of indwelling catheters, presumably initiates thrombosis through the release of tissue factors that activate coagulation proteins. The term *hypercoagulability* refers to abnormal fibrinolytic system pathways or acquired and congenital deficiencies or functional abnormalities that predispose the patient to VTE.

The incidence of cancer is slightly increased in a first episode of DVT (11% vs 9%, respectively) or PE (6% vs 5%, respectively) compared with control subjects. Cancers of the pancreas, liver, ovary, and brain, and metastatic disease account for most of these. This hypercoagulability relates to the effects of tumor cells on thrombin generation and fibrinolysis, as well as to tumor-derived activators of factor X. Because these tumors are most commonly incurable, an exhaustive evaluation for underlying malignancy, apart from routinely obtaining a medical history and conducting a physical examination, is not recommended.

DVT

PE usually arises from the deep venous system of the body as a complication of DVT. Although DVT usually begins in the lower extremities, occasional thrombi form in pelvic veins, renal veins, upper-extremity veins, and the right heart. Most thrombi originate in the soleal veins of the calf, often at sites of decreased blood flow such as the valve cusps or bifurcations. The majority of calf thrombi resolve spontaneously, and PE is uncommon. Approximately 20 to 30% of DVTs propagate to the popliteal, femoral, or iliac veins. An additional 10 to 20% of all DVTs occur in proximal veins without previous calf involvement. Iliofemoral thromboses appear to be the source of most clinically apparent PEs.

The occurrence of DVT can be self-limited, with resolution of the clot in most cases; can embolize resulting in PE; and/or the postthrombotic syndrome of venous insufficiency and the accompanying stasis changes can occur. The postthrombotic syndrome can occur in up to one half of patients with acute DVT. Its frequency is likely reduced by the use of compression stockings for 2 years after the initial event, but the underlying predisposition for the disorder is very poorly understood. Therefore, the prevention of DVT will prevent these complications.

Detection of DVT

The clinical diagnosis of DVT of the lower extremity is insensitive and nonspecific, with DVT rates ranging from 10 to 25% of those suspected of having the disease. Even when the classic signs and symptoms of thrombophlebitis are present, only 45% of patients are found to have DVT by venography. Therefore, patients presenting with suspected DVT should first have the pretest probability of disease determined. The Wells clinical prediction rule (Table 1) has been assessed and validated in multiple studies, and it can accurately categorize patients into low, moderate, or high probability of having the disease. Obtaining a d-dimer level at this point in the evaluation further simplifies the approach and may obviate the need for further testing. Sensitive d-dimer assays (*ie,* enzyme-linked immunosorbent assay [ELISA] or semiquantitative rapid ELISA) have sufficient

Table 1. *Simplified Clinical Model for Assessment of DVT (Wells Rule)**

Clinical Variable	Score
Active cancer (treatment ongoing or within previous 6 mo or palliative)	1
Paralysis, paresis, or recent plaster immobilization of the lower extremities	1
Recently bedridden for ≥3 d or major surgery within the previous 12 wk requiring general or regional anesthesia	1
Localized tenderness along the distribution of the deep venous system	1
Entire leg swelling	1
Calf swelling at least 3 cm larger than that on the symptomatic leg (measured 10 cm below the tibial tuberosity)	1
Pitting edema confined to the symptomatic leg	1
Collateral superficial veins (nonvaricose)	1
Previously documented DVT	1
Alternative diagnosis at least as likely as DVT	−2

*High probability if score is ≥3; moderate if score is 1 to 2; and low if score is ≤0. Adapted from Wells PS, Owen C, Doucette S, et al. Does this patient have deep vein thrombosis? JAMA 2006; 265:199–207.

sensitivity and predictive value to rule out DVT in patients with a low or moderate clinical probability. The false-negative result rate is too high to be useful in patients with a high clinical probability. In those patients and in any patients in the low-risk or moderate-risk groups who have an abnormal d-dimer level, imaging of the extremity is necessary.

The "gold standard" imaging test for DVT is compression ultrasound. The diagnosis of DVT using compression ultrasonography is made by findings such as abnormal compressibility or lack of compressibility of the vein and abnormal Doppler color flow study results. Studies have demonstrated that a lack of compressibility of a vein is highly sensitive ($>95\%$) and specific ($>95\%$) for proximal vein thrombosis. Ultrasound imaging is limited in that it does not detect isolated calf vein thrombi, and serial studies may need to be performed if the initial test result is negative and the clinical probability is high. A repeat study finding that is negative 5 to 7 days later is associated with a $<1\%$ incidence of subsequent VTE during the next 3 months. Other tests used in the evaluation of suspected DVT are shown in Table 2. A recent evaluation of the Prospective Investigation of Pulmonary Embolism Diagnosis (PIOPED) II data as well as metaanalyses of published trials have shown that CT venography is diagnostically equivalent to compression sonography. In patients who also have symptoms suggestive of PE, it may be prudent to perform a single diagnostic test.

PE

Natural History of PE

The resolution of PE with the reestablishment of vascular patency begins almost immediately after PE. The National Institutes of Health trials demonstrated that with heparin therapy alone, the resolution of PEs occurred during the first several weeks after the event, with 36% of the vascular defects resolving by day 5, 52% resolving by day 14, 73% resolving by 3 months, and 76% resolving by 1 year for patients who survive the initial event. Untreated PE has a mortality rate of nearly 30%. If treatment is initiated, the mortality rate is $<8\%$.

Chronic Thromboembolic Pulmonary Hypertension

Chronic thromboembolic pulmonary hypertension (CTEPH) will develop in approximately 3 to 4% of patients with acute PE. It is important to detect this complication because it is the only potentially curable form of severe PH without the need for lung transplantation. A gradual increase in pulmonary vascular resistance occurs in the absence of documented recurrent PE, and it is thought to be related to an increased resistance to flow through the pulmonary arteries that results from the initial obstruction and subsequently from vascular remodeling in small, unobstructed vessels. Risk factors for CTEPH have been identified and include ventriculoatrial shunts, infected

Table 2. *Diagnostic Tests for DVT of the Lower Extremities*

Test	Invasiveness	Complications	Comments
Contrast venography	Most invasive	Phlebitis, allergic reactions, renal failure	Reference or "gold standard"
Radionuclide venography	Less invasive	Minimal	Sensitive for proximal DVT, not commonly used in clinical practice
Impedance plethysmography	Noninvasive	Minimal	Sensitive/specific for proximal DVT, limited in congestive heart failure setting and previous DVT
Fibrinogen scanning	Less invasive	Minimal	Sensitive for calf vein thrombosis, not commonly used in clinical practice
Real-time Doppler ultrasound	Noninvasive	Minimal	Sensitive/specific for proximal DVT, operator dependent; clinical "gold standard"
CT venography	Noninvasive	Allergic reactions	Diagnostically equivalent

pacemakers, splenectomy, previous VTE, recurrent VTE, malignancy, thyroid-replacement therapy, and the antiphospholipid antibody syndrome. Patients who experience a major central thromboembolic event, or have significant hemodynamic compromise on presentation, a documented thrombophilia, or persistent abnormalities seen on lung perfusion studies on follow-up may need to be monitored more closely. Ventilation/perfusion ($\dot{V}/\dot{Q}$) scanning is the screening investigation of choice because many chest radiologists are not familiar with the distinguishing features of CTEPH seen on CT angiography. Patients who are surgical candidates should be referred to a specialty center for the consideration of pulmonary endarterectomy. All patients should receive life-long anticoagulation therapy.

Diagnosis of PE

Clinical Suspicion: The clinical suspicion of PE is often arrived at using an unstructured approach based on a combination of factors, including the presence or absence of identifiable risk factors (*eg*, surgery in the past, obesity, or previous VTE); symptoms (*eg*, dyspnea, pleuritic chest pain, and hemoptysis); physical examination findings (*eg*, tachypnea); the results of basic laboratory studies (*eg*, hypoxemia); and the likely presence of alternative diagnoses (*eg*, asthma, pneumonia, or congestive heart failure). As with DVT, there are now prediction rules that can be applied. The two validated rules are shown in Table 3. It should be emphasized that the tool or approach used is less important than the idea that the clinical pretest probability of disease must be determined in each patient before further testing. As noted in the section on "DVT," moderately to highly sensitive d-dimer assays have a sensitivity of 96 to 98% in patients with suspected PE, which is sufficient to rule out the disease in those patients with an unlikely pretest probability. In patients with a high pretest probability, imaging studies should be performed instead of the d-dimer assay.

Table 3. *Clinical Prediction Rules for Acute PE**

Rule
Canadian (Wells) Clinical Prediction Score
Variable and score
Signs and symptoms of DVT, 3.0
PE as or more likely than an alternative diagnosis, 3.0
Heart rate >100 beats/min, 1.5
Immobilization or surgery in previous 4 wk, 1.5
Previous DVT or PE, 1.5
Hemoptysis, 1.0
Cancer, 1.0
Total score
<2.0, low pretest probability
2.0 to 6.0, moderate pretest probability
>6.0, high pretest probability
Dichotomized Wells score
≤4.0 = PE unlikely
>4.0 = PE likely
Revised Geneva score
Variable and score
Age >65 yr, 1.0
Previous DVT or PE, 3.0
Surgery or lower-limb fracture in previous week, 2.0
Active cancer, 2.0
Unilateral lower limb pain, 3.0
Hemoptysis, 2.0
Heart rate
75 to 94 beats/min, 3.0
≥95 beats/min, 5.0
Pain on leg palpation or unilateral edema, 4.0
Total score
0 to 3, low pretest probability
4 to 10, moderate pretest probability
≥11, high pretest probability

*Adapted from Tapson VF. Acute pulmonary embolism. N Engl J Med 2008; 358:1037–1052.

Diagnostic Imaging Studies for PE

Many studies have been used in diagnosing acute PE. Until the mid-1990s, the first-line imaging study was the $\dot{V}/\dot{Q}$ scan. A normal $\dot{V}/\dot{Q}$ scan finding provides compelling evidence against the diagnosis of PE. In one study of 515 consecutive patients with clinically suspected PE who had anticoagulation therapy withheld on the basis of a normal perfusion scan finding, only 3 patients had symptomatic VTE (PE, 1 patient) during a 3-month follow-up period. When the PIOPED criteria are used, a high-probability $\dot{V}/\dot{Q}$ lung scan finding accompanied with a high prescan clinical suspicion is associated with confirmed PE in >96% of cases. $\dot{V}/\dot{Q}$ scan patterns other than normal or high-probability patterns will require additional diagnostic evaluation.

Spiral CT pulmonary angiography (CTPA) of the pulmonary circulation has emerged as the primary diagnostic method for the evaluation of PE. As a minimally invasive examination, this technique is widely available and has replaced the use of conventional pulmonary angiography in most centers. However, its use in detecting small peripheral PEs is unproven (6% of cases in the PIOPED study). Such small clots may not be important physiologically, but their detection may be important markers for future VTE. Several analyses have suggested that CT scanning may be a more cost-effective initial test for suspected PE compared with the $\dot{V}/\dot{Q}$ lung scan because of its greater sensitivity for PE and its ability to identify alternative diagnoses to PE. In addition, the use of CT scanning for the estimation of clot burden and right ventricular function is emerging as a useful prognostic measure in patients with documented acute PE.

The use of magnetic resonance angiography for the detection of PE is in the initial testing phases. However, the initial results are promising, especially with gadolinium enhancement of the vasculature. A major limitation of the study is the need for an experienced radiologist to interpret the study. In addition, breath holds of 20 to 30 s are required for lung imaging, which limits the efficacy of the test in patients with acute PE. Newer scanners may reduce the need for breath holds beyond 10 to 15 s.

Pulmonary angiography was considered to be the reference "gold standard," especially with the subselective injection of contrast media and the use of magnified views. A negative finding for a pulmonary angiogram with magnification appears to exclude clinically relevant PE, based on data from two follow-up studies. The mortality rate for patients undergoing the procedure is <0.5%, and the morbidity rate is about 5% (usually caused by catheter insertion and contrast reactions). Because of the expense and invasiveness of pulmonary angiography, alternative diagnostic algorithms have been sought. Despite the lack of an independent "gold standard," outcome studies have suggested that spiral CTPA is as accurate as pulmonary angiography. On the basis of the current evidence, the suggested approach for the diagnosis of suspected acute PE is shown in Figure 1.

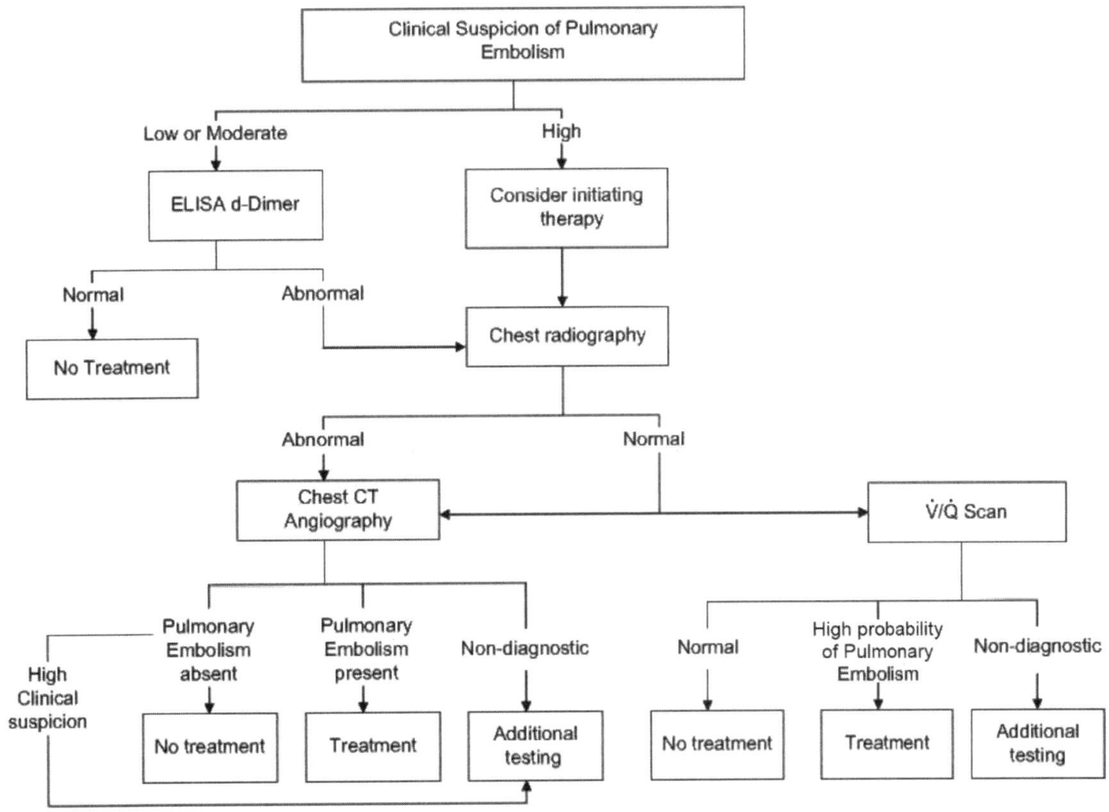

Figure 1. Diagnostic algorithm for acute PE. From: Tapson VF. Acute pulmonary embolism. N Engl J Med 2008; 358:1037–1052.

Treatment of VTE

The goals of short-term treatment of VTE are to reduce the short-term and long-term complications, such as extension of the thrombus, fatal PE, early or late recurrence, postthrombotic syndrome, and CTEPH. When patients present with acute VTE, they should be administered parenteral anticoagulation therapy with IV unfractionated heparin (UFH) or subcutaneous low-molecular-weight heparin (LMWH) or the pentasaccharide fondaparinux. Oral warfarin therapy can be initiated on the first day of treatment. Treatment using both agents should be continued for at least 5 days and until the international normalized ratio stays in the therapeutic range of 2.0 to 3.0 for 2 consecutive days (at which time the heparin or fondaparinux therapy can be discontinued). Compared with treatment of warfarin alone, overlap therapy with heparin reduces the risk of recurrence. A validated weight-based IV nomogram achieves a therapeutic response more effectively than empiric heparin dosing; thus, it is recommended that such a nomogram be used if UFH therapy is used. The most widely used test for monitoring heparin therapy is the activated partial thromboplastin time, which is a global anticoagulation test and does not measure heparin levels. Failure to achieve an adequate anticoagulation response with heparin therapy (*ie*, activated partial thromboplastin time, > 1.5 times control) is associated with the increased recurrence of VTE.

The LMWH preparations and pentasaccharides share advantages over UFH, as follows: greater bioavailability, more predictable dosing, and a lower risk of HIT. These advantages negate the need for monitoring in most instances, although measuring the anti-factor Xa level in morbidly obese patients or in those with significantly impaired renal function can be considered. In patients with suspected or documented HIT, treatment with a direct thrombin inhibitor, such as argatroban or lepirudin, should be considered. Treatment with warfarin should not be initiated until the platelet count has returned to normal, especially in those with active thrombosis, as there is the potential for worsening thrombotic complications.

Bed rest is not recommended for the treatment of acute DVT unless there is significant pain and swelling. Many patients with DVT can be treated entirely as outpatients. Although some patients with PE likely can also be treated as outpatients, the data for this population are less robust. Recently, prognostic scores in patients with acute PE have been developed and validated and may help to accurately identify low-risk patients.

Patients with acute VTE require prolonged anticoagulation to prevent extension and recurrence. The current guidelines recommend 3 months of therapy for patients in whom thrombosis develops in the setting of documented transient risk factors. In patients who experience idiopathic (unprovoked) events, treatment should be given for at least 3 months. At that point, patients should be evaluated for the risk-benefit ratio of continuing therapy indefinitely. Studies suggest that d-dimer levels, persistent thrombus on ultrasound imaging, thrombin levels, and perhaps other markers of chronic inflammation may help to identify those patients who are at the greatest risk of recurrence after stopping anticoagulation therapy, but we are not yet able to use these in a systematic fashion that allows us to individualize the duration of therapy. Therefore, in the absence of a high bleeding risk, most patients with an unprovoked event should receive indefinite therapy. There is no evidence that longer (but finite) initial courses of therapy (such as 6, 12, or 18 months) are more effective than 3 months because the recurrence rates upon discontinuation of therapy are identical. In patients with continuing risk factors (such as active malignancy) and patients who have had a documented recurrent event, long-term (perhaps lifelong) therapy is recommended.

Thrombolytic Therapy

Thrombolytic therapy is approved for the treatment of proximal DVT and massive PE. These agents dissolve thrombi by activating plasminogen into plasmin. Plasmin degrades fibrin to soluble peptides in the presence of a thrombus or hemostatic plug. Streptokinase, urokinase, and tissue plasminogen activator are approved for use in the United States. Thrombolytic treatment of DVT has been associated with decreased pain, swelling, loss of venous values, and a reduced incidence of postphlebitic syndrome. For the treatment of PE, thrombolytic agents produce more rapid resolution of intravascular abnormalities than have been demonstrated by either $\dot{V}/\dot{Q}$ lung scans or pulmonary angiography. However, no proven effect on mortality has yet been demonstrated. Thrombolytic therapy is currently recommended for patients with acute PE who show signs of hemodynamic instability, unless there are major contraindications related to the bleeding risk.

Inferior Vena Cava Interruption

Inferior vena cava interruption is most commonly achieved with the use of an intravascular filter. A randomized trial found that the use of an inferior vena cava filter reduced the rate of PE, had no effect on mortality, and was associated with a greater risk of recurrent DVT. These devices are being used more frequently, especially now that many can be safely retrieved after several months. However, the approved indications remain few, as follows: absolute contraindication to anticoagulation; life-threatening bleeding while receiving anticoagulation; and documented recurrent VTE while receiving therapeutic anticoagulation.

Surgical Embolectomy

This procedure should be reserved for patients with confirmed massive PEs who are hemodynamically unstable and who are not candidates for thrombolysis. The high mortality rates associated with this procedure, especially if cardiopulmonary arrest has occurred, has resulted in a limited enthusiasm for its use. Interventional catheter extraction or fragmentation may become viable options for these patients in the near future.

Prevention of DVT/PE

The rationale for DVT and PE prophylaxis is based on the clinically silent nature of the disease and the high prevalence of DVT among hospitalized patients. There is added importance for prophylaxis when one considers that most patients who die of PE do so within 30 min of the acute event. The strategy used for the prevention of DVT and PE should be based on the patient's level of risk, as suggested by the American College of Chest Physicians Consensus Conference on Antithrombotic Therapy. The current approach involves assessing patient risk by assigning them to a risk group based upon their primary reason for hospitalization.

Low-Risk Patients

These patients can be defined as individuals who are undergoing uncomplicated minor surgery and fully mobile medical patients with no clinical risk factors for VTE. Their risk of DVT without prophylaxis is < 10%, and thus, no specific thromboprophylaxis is recommended.

Moderate-Risk Patients

These patients are most general, open gynecologic or urologic surgery patients or medical patients who are at bed rest (including all critical care patients). Their approximate risk of DVT without prophylaxis is 10 to 40%. These patients should receive prophylaxis with LMWH, low-dose UFH, or fondaparinux. Those with a very high risk of bleeding should receive mechanical thromboprophylaxis.

High-Risk Patients

These are patients undergoing hip or knee arthroplasty, hip fracture surgery, or patients who have had major trauma or spinal cord injury. The recommended prophylaxis is LMWH, fondaparinux, or an oral vitamin K antagonist (international normalized ratio 2 to 3). As in moderate-risk patients, if the bleeding risk is extremely high, mechanical methods of prophylaxis should be used. Pharmacologic prophylaxis should be started as soon as the bleeding risk decreases.

Although VTE is considered to be more common in surgery or trauma patients, 50 to 70% of symptomatic thromboembolic events and 70 to 80% of fatal PEs occur in nonsurgical patients. Hospitalization for an acute medical illness is independently associated with a relative risk for VTE of about 8. Thus, the appropriate prophylaxis of medical inpatients is clearly as important as that in surgical patients.

Several risk factors for VTE have been identified in hospitalized medical patients. Major risk factors include New York Heart Association (NYHA) functional class III and IV heart failure, COPD exacerbations, and sepsis. Additional risk factors include advanced age, history of VTE, cancer, stroke with lower-extremity weakness, end-stage renal disease, and bed rest. Many medical patients have multiple risk factors. Unfortunately, no systematic way of combining these to identify risk categories in medical patients has been accepted and validated. Therefore, medical patients are generally classified as low risk if they are fully mobile and have no additional risk factors for VTE. All other medical patients are considered to be at moderate risk and should receive thromboprophylaxis as noted previously.

Pulmonary Hypertension (PH)

PH is a hemodynamic state that is defined by a mean pulmonary artery pressure (PAP) of $>$25 mm Hg at rest or $>$30 mm Hg during exercise, which is shared by many conditions. PH was previously categorized into primary or secondary PH, based on the absence or presence of identifiable causes or associated conditions. A revised classification system that acknowledged the separation of disorders directly affecting the arterial tree from disorders affecting the venous circulation or those affecting the circulation by altering respiratory function was proposed in 1998. A revision of this classification was proposed at the Third-World Conference on Pulmonary Hypertension, held in Venice, Italy, in 2003 (Table 4). The major changes noted in these revisions were as follows: (1) abandonment of the term *secondary PH* and (2) the replacement of the term *primary PH* with *idiopathic pulmonary arterial hypertension* (IPAH) or, when supported by genetic testing, *familial pulmonary arterial hypertension* (FPAH).

PAH is a subset of PH that is defined as a mean PAP of $>$25 mm Hg at rest or $>$30 mm Hg during exercise with a normal pulmonary capillary wedge pressure ($<$15 mm Hg) and a lesion localized to the pulmonary arteriole. IPAH is an uncommon disorder affecting women more commonly than men during the ages 20 to 40 years. In approximately 6% of patients, there is a family history of PAH (*ie,* FPAH), which has been found to be related to 1 of $>$70 identified mutations in the gene-encoding bone morphogenetic protein receptor type II (BMPR2), which is localized to chromosome 2q33. Sporadic mutations in this gene are seen in up to 25% of patients with IPAH. Asymptomatic carriers

Table 4. *Revised Nomenclature and Classification of PH (2003) from the Third-World Conference on Pulmonary Hypertension**

- WHO group I
  - PAH
    - IPAH
    - FPAH
- Associated with
  - Collagen vascular disease
  - Congenital systemic to pulmonary shunts (large, small, repaired, or nonrepaired)
  - Portal hypertension
  - HIV infection drugs and toxins
  - Other (glycogen storage disease, Gaucher disease, hereditary hemorrhagic telangiectasia, hemoglobinopathies, myeloproliferative disorders, splenectomy)
- Associated with significant venous or capillary involvement
  - Pulmonary venoocclusive disease
  - Pulmonary capillary hemangiomatosis
- WHO group II
  - Pulmonary venous hypertension
  - Left-sided atrial or ventricular heart disease
  - Left-sided valvular heart disease
- WHO group III
- Pulmonary hypertension associated with hypoxemia
  - COPD
  - Interstitial lung disease
  - Sleep-disordered breathing
  - Alveolar hypoventilation disorders
  - Chronic exposure to high altitude
- WHO group IV
- PH caused by chronic thrombotic and/or embolic disease
  - Thromboembolic obstruction of proximal pulmonary arteries
  - Thromboembolic obstruction of distal pulmonary arteries
  - Pulmonary embolism (tumor, parasites, foreign material)
- WHO group V
  - Miscellaneous
  - Sarcoidosis, histiocytosis X, lymphangiomatosis, compression of pulmonary vessels (adenopathy, tumor, fibrosing mediastinitis)

*Adapted from Rubin LJ. Diagnosis and management of pulmonary arterial hypertension: ACCP evidence-based clinical practice guidelines. Chest 2004; 126(suppl):7S–10S.

of the BMPR2 gene often have an abnormal increase in pulmonary artery (PA) pressures in response to exercise and, given additional environmental or genetic stimuli, may develop overt disease. Thus, genetic testing and counseling should be offered to patients with either IPAH or FPAH and their families. The lack of a single genetic mutation, the low penetrance of overt PAH in BMPR2 mutation carriers, and the lack of a single environmental stimulus have led to the development of the multiple-hit hypothesis in the etiology of PAH (Fig 2).

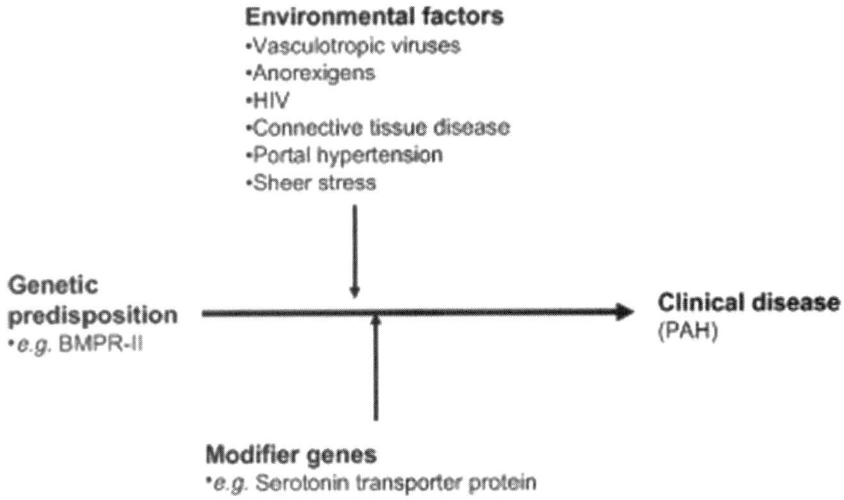

Figure 2. Multiple-hit hypothesis of pathogenesis of PAH: BMPR-II, bone morphogenic protein receptor type 2. From Gabbay E, Reed A, Williams TJ. Assessment and treatment of pulmonary arterial hypertension: an Australian perspective in 2006. Intern Med J 2006; 37:38–48.

PAH related to risk factors or associated conditions is a heterogeneous group of disorders, including connective tissue disease, congenital systemic pulmonary shunt, portal hypertension, HIV infection, drugs and toxin, and those conditions such as hemoglobinopathies and myeloproliferative disorders. The use of appetite-suppressant drugs for >3 months has been associated with a 30-fold increase in the risk of development of PH. Hepatosplenic schistosomiasis may account for one of the most prevalent forms of PAH worldwide. The World Health Organization (WHO) also suggests that other appetite stimulants such as amphetamines may have a very likely causative role in PH.

Pathogenesis

The current understanding of PAH is as a vasoproliferative disease invoked by mitogenic stimuli. The pathogenesis of PAH is complex and poorly understood and, as mentioned previously, includes both genetic and environmental factors that alter vascular structure and function. The vascular changes involve the pulmonary arteriole, and they are characterized by vasoconstriction, vascular remodeling with intimal and medial proliferation, the formation of plexiform lesions, and thrombosis (Fig 3). These changes lead to progressive obstruction of flow, increased pulmonary vascular resistance, and eventual right heart failure and death. Because the number of patients who respond significantly to acute vasodilator challenge is very low, the contribution of vasoconstriction relative to vascular remodeling is minimal.

The main cellular changes involve smooth muscle cells, fibroblasts, endothelial cells, and platelets. The following three pathways are important: prostacyclin (prostaglandin 12), nitric oxide (NO)–cyclic guanosine monophosphate-phosphodiesterase 5, and endothelin. An imbalance between the up-regulated vasoconstrictive/proproliferative endothelin system and the down-regulated vasodilatory/antiproliferative/antithrombotic NO and prostaglandin 12 systems

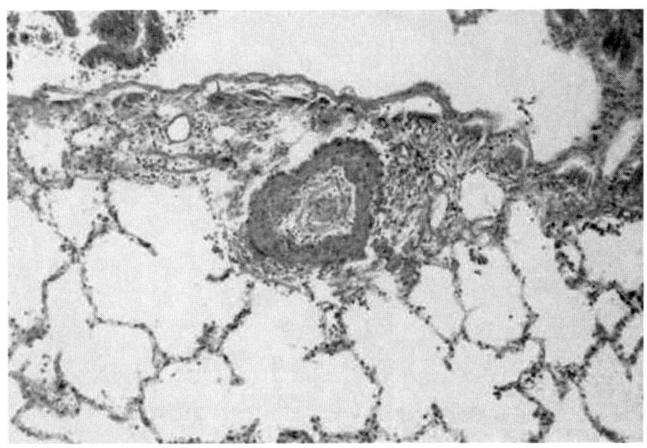

Figure 3. Typical micrograph of a lung from a patient with PAH. The patient has normal alveolar structures but a small PA, in which the lumen is occluded by concentric fibrosis. The artery also has increased medial smooth muscle and a reactive adventitia. Dilated small vessels border the airway above the artery. From Newman JH, Phillips JA, Loyd JE. Pulmonary hypertension. Ann Intern Med 2008; 148:278–283.

is a key contributor. Platelets likely play an important role as procoagulants by increasing the platelet release of serotonin, vascular endothelial growth factor, and platelet-derived growth factor.

Clinical Features

PH frequently presents with nonspecific symptoms (Table 5). The most common symptoms are dyspnea on exertion, fatigue, and syncope, resulting from reduced cardiac output during activity. Patients may also occasionally present with angina-like chest pain with normal coronary arteries. This chest pain may reflect right ventricular ischemia. Hemoptysis as a consequence of pulmonary vascular rupture is rare but may be a catastrophic event. The Raynaud phenomenon is seen in approximately 2% of patients with IPAH but is a frequent finding in cases of PH associated with connective tissue diseases such as scleroderma. The physical examination findings are nonspecific but may give clues to a secondary cause of PH. With more advanced disease, the physical examination reveals signs of right ventricular dysfunction. The ECG most often reveals right atrial or right ventricular hypertrophy and right-axis deviation. The chest radiograph shows an enlarged cardiac silhouette that is consistent with right ventricular hypertrophy, with enlarged pulmonary arteries.

Diagnostic Approach

The most important step in the diagnosis of PAH is to suspect its presence. As noted, the symptoms are vague and nonspecific, and PAH should be considered in any patient with unexplained dyspnea on exertion (and perhaps in all those patients with an unexplained isolated reduction in diffusing capacity). There are no early symptoms of PAH, and thus, annual screening in high-risk populations should be considered. Risk groups thought to benefit from screening include patients with known genetic mutations, first-degree relatives of patients with PAH, patients with scleroderma, patients with portal hypertension before liver transplantation, and patients with congenital systemic to pulmonary shunts. The best screening test for the detection of PAH is a transthoracic echocardiogram (TTE). TTE is also a valuable tool to detect features of left-sided heart disease or intracardiac shunts. Increased PA systolic pressure raises the possibility of PH but is clearly not specific for PAH. If the TTE confirms increased PAP, further testing to identify the underlying cause is warranted.

Table 5. *Signs and Symptoms of PH*

Signs	Symptoms
Jugular vein distention	Dyspnea or exertion
Prominent right ventricular heave	Fatigue
Accentuated pulmonic valve component (P_2)	Syncope
Right-sided third heart sound (S_3)	Anginal chest pain
Tricuspid insufficiency murmur	Hemoptysis
Hepatomegaly	Raynaud phenomenon
Peripheral edema	

Spirometry, diffusing capacity, arterial blood gas measurement, and CT scan of the lung can be performed to exclude underlying respiratory disease and/or hypoxemia. When suggested by history, an overnight polysomnography can be performed to assess for severe sleep apnea. The tests for underlying liver disease, HIV, and autoimmune diseases are noninvasive and should be performed in most patients with unexplained PH. A $\dot{V}/\dot{Q}$ scan should be performed to evaluate for potential CTEPH because patients who qualify for thromboendarterectomy can have a dramatic improvement with this procedure.

Right-heart catheterization is the "gold standard" for diagnosis and should be performed in all patients with suspected PH, especially if specific treatment is planned. Cardiac catheterization is indicated to establish severity and prognosis, measure wedge pressure, exclude congenital heart disease, and test the response to selective pulmonary vasodilators (*eg*, inhaled NO or IV adenosine or epoprostenol). Most authors recommend heart catheterization of both the right and left sides. Left-sided heart catheterization can evaluate for coronary artery disease, as well as measure left ventricular end-diastolic pressure. Right-heart catheterization measurements should include sequential oxygen saturation for the presence of an intracardiac shunt, pulmonary angiography for thromboembolic PH, hemodynamic measurements including PAPs, PA occlusion pressure, and cardiac index. A positive response to therapy with vasodilators is defined as a decrease in mean PA pressure of >10 mm Hg to reach a mean PA pressure of <40 mm Hg, with an increased or unchanged cardiac output. Very few patients show a short-term response, but a negative challenge result will obviate a trial of calcium-channel blockers.

Measurement of Exercise Capacity

Formal assessment of exercise capacity is an integral part of the evaluation. A 6-min walk test usually is performed to determine the degree of exercise limitation because it has proven to be reproducible and to correlate well with other measures of functional status. This test has been very useful in monitoring the response to therapy and has often been used as a primary end point in clinical trials. Importantly, it has been found to be an independent predictor of survival in patients with PAH.

Treatment of PAH

No treatment for PAH has been found to achieve a cure for this devastating disease. There are six main types of treatment for PAH. The first is prevention. Because some forms of PAH have clear causal mechanisms, these factors should be eliminated where possible. The second line of treatment is screening of high-risk patients (as previously discussed) because it is generally believed that earlier diagnosis and treatment may improve outcomes. The third is to optimize the therapy for any related diseases, such as heart failure, hypoxemia, sleep disorders, or collagen vascular diseases. The fourth line of therapy is supportive—directed at the consequences of PAH. General measures include pneumococcal and influenza vaccinations in addition to the avoidance of pregnancy, high-altitude exposure, tobacco, and medications such as appetite suppressants, decongestants, and nonsteroidal antiinflammatory agents. In addition, the following supportive treatments are available:

1. Anticoagulation: Patients with PAH should receive long-term anticoagulation therapy. Patients with this condition are prone to thromboembolism, in part caused by reduced PA blood flow, right ventricular dilation, venous insufficiency, and inactivity. The range of anticoagulation that is recommended is an international normalized ratio of 1.5 to 2.5.
2. Oxygen: All patients with PAH and documented hypoxemia should receive supplemental oxygen to maintain an oxygen saturation of >90%.
3. Diuretics: Careful diuresis is indicated in patients with evidence of right ventricular failure.
4. Inotropic agents: There are no data on the long-term use of inotropic therapy for PAH. Some authors have suggested the use of digitalis because it may improve right ventricular function. The use of cardiac glycosides is controversial because of the lack of well-designed randomized controlled trials in this population.

The fifth line of treatment is vascular-targeted therapy aimed at reversing or reducing vasoconstriction, endothelial cell proliferation, and smooth-muscle cell proliferation. In patients who exhibit evidence of an acute hemodynamic response to vasodilator challenge testing, long-term treatment with orally administered calcium-channel blockers in relatively high doses can occasionally produce a sustained hemodynamic response with a reduction in PAP and an increased cardiac output. This group of responders not only shows improvement in symptoms in exercise tolerance, but they also have increased survival. Unfortunately, calcium-channel blockers have no antiproliferative effect, and thus, only a small subset of patients will benefit from long-term use. In patients who do not show a reduction in PAP (with the administration of vasodilators) during right-heart catheterization, it is not beneficial and is potentially dangerous to initiate therapy with calcium-channel blockers. Significant adverse effects include systemic hypotension, pulmonary edema, and right ventricular failure.

Current US Food and Drug Administration-approved and investigational therapies aimed at reducing endothelial and smooth-muscle cell proliferation target the following three major pathways involved in the pathogenesis of PAH: prostacyclin, NO, and endothelin. Continuous IV epoprostenol, subcutaneous and IV treprostinil, and inhaled iloprost are prostanoids that have been shown to improve exercise capacity, functional capacity, hemodynamics and, in the case of epoprostenol, survival. In the NO pathway, sildenafil (which inhibits phosphodiesterase 5) has demonstrated improvement in exercise capacity, functional status, and hemodynamics. Bosentan is an oral nonselective endothelin receptor antagonist; sitaxsentan and ambrisentan are selective endothelin A receptor antagonists. These therapies have been shown to improve exercise capacity, functional status, and time to clinical worsening. Bosentan has also been shown to improve hemodynamics. Two studies have shown improved survival with bosentan therapy compared with historical control subjects. Although many of the trials that use these classes of medications were not powered to detect an improvement in survival, a recent metaanalysis suggests that the rate of mortality is lower in patients treated with targeted therapies.

The approach to the use of these agents in PAH is typically based on their functional class, as defined by the WHO classification system, which is a modification of the NYHA functional class system for heart failure (Table 6). In general, patients who are in functional class I receive general care only, although trials with early use of specific therapy are currently underway. Oral therapies are considered to be first-line agents for patients who are in functional class II and class III, whereas parental therapies generally are reserved for patients who are in class IV. There is no clear consensus as to which agent to start first, nor is there any current consensus as to the role of combination therapy.

Few studies have been published that directly compare individual medications or classes of medications. Multidrug treatment is appealing because the three classes of medications approved by the Food and Drug Administration exert their effects by different mechanisms. The use of two or more drugs may allow for dosing below the levels that cause important side effects. A few small studies have confirmed this theory, but more data are needed before firm recommendations can be made. Authors of the American College of Chest Physicians evidence-based guideline published updated guidance for medical therapy for PH in June 2007. Their overall recommended approach is shown in Figure 4. If pharmacologic treatment fails, surgical (the sixth line) treatment (lung transplantation or atrial septostomy) should be considered.

Prognosis

Median duration of survival of patients diagnosed with PAH between 1980 and 1985 was 2.8 years. Since that time, survival has improved. Patients without evidence of right ventricular failure may survive >10 years. Responders to calcium-channel blockers have a 95% 5-year survival rate. Patients in NYHA classes II and IV who have been treated with epoprostenol have a 5-year survival rate that is twice that of matched control patients.

Patients with evidence of right heart failure have a much lower survival rate. Posttreatment markers of poor prognosis included persistent increases in right atrial pressure, low cardiac index, low mixed venous oxygen saturation, continued functional class III or IV symptoms, poor exercise capacity (6-min walk test distance <380 m), and

Table 6. *WHO Classification of Functional Status of Patients with PH**

Class 1	Patients with PH but without resulting limitation of physical activity. Ordinary physical activity does not cause undue dyspnea or fatigue, chest pain, or near syncope.
Class 2	Patients with PH resulting in slight limitation of physical activity. These patients are comfortable at rest, but ordinary physical activity causes undue dyspnea or fatigue, chest pain, or near syncope.
Class 3	Patients with PH resulting in marked limitation of physical activity. These patients are comfortable at rest, but less than ordinary physical activity causes undue dyspnea or fatigue, chest pain, or near syncope.
Class 4	Patients with PH resulting in inability to perform any physical activity without symptoms. These patients manifest signs of right-heart failure. Dyspnea and/or fatigue may be present at rest, and discomfort is increased by any physical activity.

*Modified from the NYHA classification of patients with cardiac disease. From McGoon, Gutterman D, Steen V, et al. Screening, early detection, and diagnosis of pulmonary arterial hypertension: ACCP evidence-based clinical practice guidelines. Chest 2004; 126:18S.

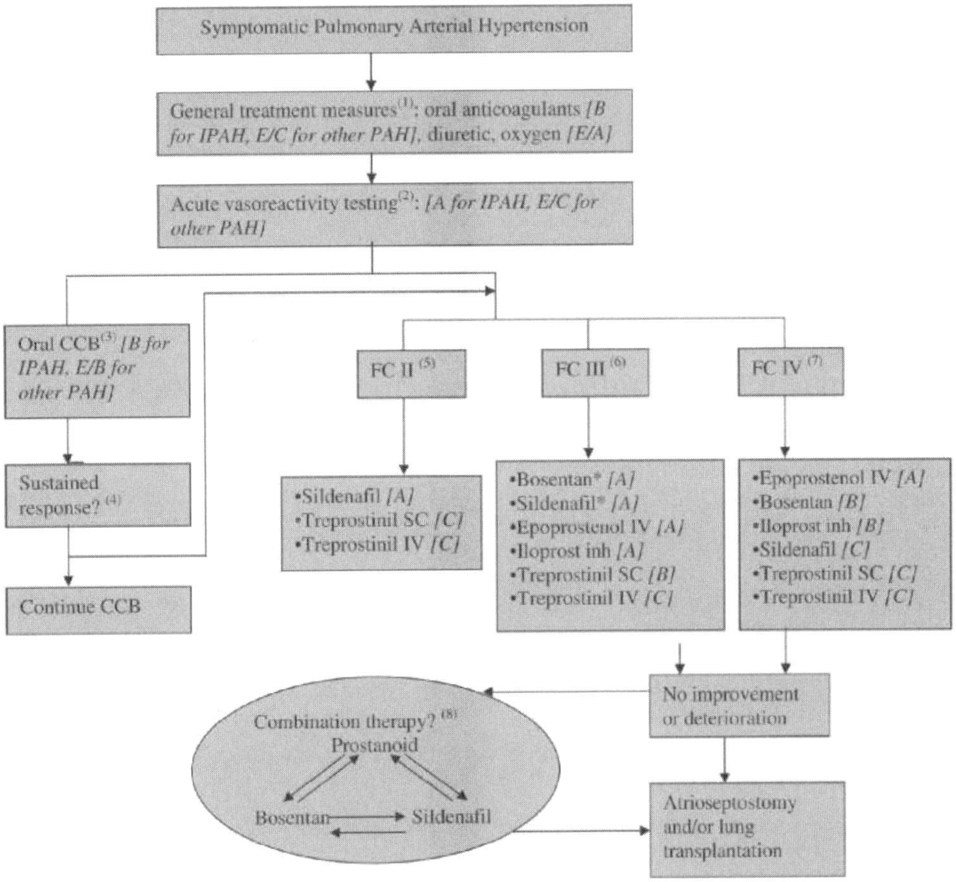

* Not in order of preference.

Figure 4. Treatment algorithm for PAH. The recommended therapies presented in this algorithm have been evaluated mainly in those patients with IPAH or PAH associated with connective tissue disease or anorexigen use. Extrapolation to other forms of PAH should be made with caution. Country-specific regulatory agency approval status and functional class indications for PAH medications vary. From: Badesch DB, Abman SH, Simonneau G, et al. Medical therapy for pulmonary arterial hypertension: updated ACCP evidence-based clinical practice guidelines. Chest 2007; 131:1917–1928.

increased serum B-type natriuretic peptide levels. Patients with persistent poor functional class or exercise capacity, severely reduced right heart function, a right atrial pressure > 15 mm Hg, or cardiac index < 2l/min/m² should be considered for lung transplantation. Either single- or double-lung transplantation are options, but surgeons in most centers prefer double transplantation because of concerns about postoperative reperfusion injury after a single-lung transplant. Experience has shown that lung transplant recipients with primary PH have survival rates of 73% at 1 year, 55% at 3 years, and 45% at 5 years. Obliterative bronchiolitis is a common complication in transplant patients with PAH. The recurrence of PAH after lung transplantation has not been reported in the transplanted lung.

Annotated Bibliography

Badesch DB, Abman SH, Ahearn GS, et al. Medical therapy for pulmonary arterial hypertension: ACCP evidence-based clinical practice guidelines. Chest 2004; 126(suppl):35S–62S

This article was included in the July 2004 supplement to CHEST, which was devoted to the diagnosis and management of PAH. Patients with IPAH should undergo acute vasoreactivity testing with use of a short-acting agent such as IV epoprostenol or adenosine or inhaled NO. Patients with IPAH should receive anticoagulation with warfarin.

Badesch DB, Abman SH, Simonneau G, et al. Medical therapy for pulmonary arterial hypertension: updated ACCP evidence-based clinical practice guidelines. Chest 2007; 131:1917–1928

This article is an update to the one before it, taking into account the rapidly evolving field of therapeutic trials in PAH. The authors give a nice review of the current evidence for each potential agent and a suggested algorithm for their use in patients with PAH.

Budhiraja R, Hassoun PM. Portopulmonary hypertension: a tale of two circulations. Chest 2003; 123:562–576

Pulmonary involvement is common in patients with portal hypertension and can manifest in diverse ways. Changes in pulmonary arterial resistance, manifesting either as the hepatopulmonary syndrome or portopulmonary hypertension, have been increasingly recognized. Portopulmonary hypertension is defined as an elevated PAP in the setting of increased pulmonary vascular resistance and normal wedge pressure in a patient with portal hypertension.

Decousus H, Leizorovicz A, Parent F, et al. A clinical trial of vena caval filters in the prevention of pulmonary embolism in patients with proximal deep-vein thrombosis. N Engl J Med 1998; 338:409–415

In high-risk patients with proximal DVT, the initial beneficial effect of vena caval filters for the prevention of PE was counterbalanced by an excess of recurrent DVT without any difference in mortality.

DeMonye W, Sanson BJ, MacGillavry MR, et al. Embolus location affects the sensitivity of a rapid quantitative d-dimer assay in the diagnosis of pulmonary embolism. Am J Respir Crit Care Med 2002; 165:345–348

d-dimer concentration and the accuracy of d-dimer assays are dependent on embolus location; smaller, subsegmental emboli may be missed when d-dimer assays are used as the sole test to exclude PE.

Douketis JD, Kearon C, Bates S, et al. Risk of fatal pulmonary embolism in patients with treated venous thromboembolism. JAMA 1998; 279:458–462

Among patients with symptomatic PE or DVT who are treated with anticoagulation therapy for 3 months, the occurrence of fatal PE is rare during and after anticoagulant therapy. However, patients presenting with PE are more likely to die of recurrent PE than are patients presenting with DVT.

Gabbay E, Reed A, Williams TJ. Assessment and treatment of pulmonary arterial hypertension: an Australian perspective in 2006. Intern Med J 2007; 37:38–48

This article, although focusing on the Australian experience in managing patients with PH, is a very nice overview of the current classification, pathogenesis, diagnosis, and treatment of PH.

Galie N, Rubin LJ, eds. Pulmonary arterial hypertension: epidemiology, pathobiology, assessment, and therapy. J Am Coll Cardiol 2004; 43(suppl):1S–90S

This entire supplement is devoted to PH, with articles by noted authorities.

Geerts WH, Bergqvist D, Pineo GF, et al. Prevention of venous thromboembolism. American College of Chest Physicians evidence-based clinical practice guidelines. 8th ed. Chest 2008; 133:381S–453S

Evidence-based recommendations on prevention of VTE in all surgical and medical populations. Excellent review of the literature on risk, risk stratification, and preventive strategies.

Goldhaber SZ, Grodstein F, Stampfer MJ, et al. A prospective study of risk factors for pulmonary embolism in women. JAMA 1997; 277:642–645

Obesity, cigarette smoking, and hypertension were associated with an increased risk of PE in women. Control of these risk factors could decrease the risk of PE among women.

Hayashino Y, Goto M, Noguchi Y, et al. Ventilation-perfusion scanning and helical CT in suspected pulmonary embolism: meta-analysis of diagnostic performance. Radiology 2005; 234:740–748

Helical CT scanning has better discriminatory power than $\dot{V}/\dot{Q}$ scanning for excluding PE, but the two tests have a similar discriminatory power in the diagnosis of PE when the $\dot{V}/\dot{Q}$ scan results disclose a "high probability."

Heit JA, Kobbervig CE, James AH, et al. Trends in the incidence of venous thromboembolism during pregnancy or postpartum: a 30-year population-based study. Ann Intern Med 2005; 143:697–706

Among pregnant women, the greatest risk for PE and VTE is during the postpartum period. Prophylaxis should be especially targeted to postpartum women.

Highland KB. Pulmonary arterial hypertension. Am J Med Sci 2008; 335:40–45

This is an excellent succinct, current review of PH by a clinical expert in the field.

Humbert M. Update in Pulmonary Hypertension 2008. Am J Respir Crit Care Med 2009; 179:650–656.

This article summarizes the advances in pulmonary hypertension as reported in the medical literature over the past 24 months.

Kearon C, Kahn SR, Agnelli G, et al. Antithrombotic therapy for venous thromboembolic disease. American College of Chest Physicians evidence-based clinical practice guidelines. 8th ed. Chest 2008; 133:454S–545S.

Comprehensive evidence-based literature review and graded recommendations on treatment of DVT and PE.

Kearon C, Ginsberg JS, Hirsh J. The role of venous ultrasonography in the diagnosis of suspected deep venous thrombosis and pulmonary embolism. Ann Intern Med 1998; 129:1044–1049

Venous ultrasonography is a valuable test for the diagnosis and management of patients with suspected DVT or PE. However, the following factors reduce the positive predictive value of venous ultrasonography for detecting acute thromboembolism: asymptomatic for DVT, low clinical suspicion for DVT, abnormality confined to a short segment of a proximal vein, abnormality confined to the calf veins; history of VTE, negative result of another test that is sensitive for DVT (such as d-dimer), and low prevalence of DVT in a referral population. (With one or more of the aforementioned factors, venography or other testing should be considered to exclude the possibility of a false-positive test result.)

Mandel J, Mark EJ, Hales C A. Pulmonary venoocclusive disease. Am J Respir Crit Care Med 2000; 162:1964–1973

This review summarizes the current state of knowledge regarding pulmonary venoocclusive disease.

McGoon M, Gutterman D, Steen V, et al. Screening, early detection, and diagnosis of pulmonary arterial hypertension: ACCP evidence-based clinical practice guidelines. Chest 2004; 126(suppl):14S–34S

A comprehensive evidence-based review and recommendations on the diagnostic approach to patients with suspected PH.

McGoon MD, Kane GC. Pulmonary hypertension: diagnosis and management. Mayo Clin Proc 2009; 84:191–207

This is a recent, well-organized clinical review that includes discussion of several controversial issues, such as the importance of mild or exercise-induced PAH, disproportionate PAH, assessment of therapeutic efficacy, combination therapy, and the management of the symptoms other than dyspnea (angina, syncope, and arrhythmias).

McNeil K, Dunning J. Chronic thromboembolic pulmonary hypertension (CTEPH). Heart 2007; 93:1152–1158

A description of the natural history, pathophysiology, diagnosis, and treatment of CTEPH are included. The authors underscore the fact that this disease is more common than previously thought, and they stress the importance of identifying it in patients with newly diagnosed PH.

Moores LK, Holley AB. Computed tomography pulmonary angiography and venography: diagnostic and prognostic properties. Semin Respir Crit Care Med 2008; 29:3–14

An up-to-date review of the diagnostic accuracy and utility, as well as the prognostic features, of spiral CT angiography and venography.

Moores LK, Jackson WL Jr, Shorr AF, et al. Meta-analysis: outcomes in patients with suspected pulmonary embolism managed with computed tomographic pulmonary angiography. Ann Intern Med 2004; 141:866–874

The rate of subsequent VTE after negative results of spiral CTPA is similar to that seen after negative results on conventional pulmonary angiography. It appears safe to withhold anticoagulation therapy after negative CTPA results.

Newman JH. Pulmonary hypertension. Am J Respir Crit Care Med 2005; 172:1072–1077

This "Centennial Review" discusses the birth of modern cardiopulmonary medicine, including pulmonary circulation, primary PH, and hypoxemia associated with PH.

Newman JH, Phillips JA, Loyd JE. Narrative review: the enigma of pulmonary arterial hypertension; new insights from genetic studies. Ann Intern Med 2008; 148:278–283

A short, easily understandable description of the discovery and meaning of genetic predispositions to the development of PAH.

Quinlan DJ, McGuillan A, Eikelboom JW. Low-molecular-weight heparin compared with intravenous unfractionated heparin for treatment of pulmonary embolism: a meta-analysis of randomized, controlled trials. Ann Intern Med 2004; 140:175–183

LMWH appears to be similar to UFH in safety and efficacy for the treatment of either symptomatic or asymptomatic PE.

Quiroz R, Kucher N, Zou KH, et al. Clinical validity of a negative computed tomography scan in patients with suspected pulmonary embolism: a systematic review. JAMA 2005; 293:2012–2017

A negative CT scan finding is as accurate as pulmonary angiography in ruling out suspected PE. A negative CT scan finding in a low-risk patient rules out PE, whereas a negative CT scan finding in a high-risk patient may require further confirmation.

Rubin LJ. American College of Chest Physicians. Diagnosis and management of pulmonary arterial hypertension: ACCP evidence-based clinical practice guidelines. Chest 2004; 126(suppl):75S–105S

In this brief introduction to the guidelines, Dr. Rubin gives an excellent review of the evolution and current classification of PH.

Schulman S, Granqvist S, Holmstrom M, et al. The duration of oral anticoagulant therapy after a second episode of venous thromboembolism. N Engl J Med 1997; 336:393–398

Prophylactic anticoagulation that was continued for an indefinite period after a second episode of VTE was associated with a much lower rate of recurrence during 4 years

of follow-up than treatment for 6 months. However, there was a trend toward a greater risk of major hemorrhage when anticoagulation was continued indefinitely.

Sorensen HT, Mellemkjaer L, Steffensen FH, et al. The risk of a diagnosis of cancer after primary deep venous thrombosis or pulmonary embolism. N Engl J Med 1998; 338:1169–1173

Among 15,348 patients with DVT and 11,305 patients with PE, there were 1,727 cases of cancer. The expected number of cancer cases was 1,372 based on national statistics from Denmark (ratio of observed/expected number of cancer cases, 1.3; 95% confidence interval, 1.21 to 1.33). Forty percent of patients with a diagnosis of cancer within 1 year of hospitalization for VTE had distant metastases at the time of the diagnosis of cancer. The authors conclude that an aggressive search for hidden cancer in patients presenting with VTE is not warranted.

Stein PD, Fowler SE, Goodman LR, et al. Multidetector computed tomography for acute pulmonary embolism. N Engl J Med 2006; 354:2317–2327

In patients with suspected acute PE, multidetector CT angiography (CTA) in combination with venous phase multidetector CT venography (CTV) was more sensitive than CTA alone for diagnosing PE. However, it only increased the negative predicted value from 95 to 97% overall. Therefore, the added dose of radiation from CTV may not be justified when added to the dose from CTA. The multidetector CTA may be accurate enough to eliminate PE, at least in patients with low-to-intermediate clinical probability of PE.

Stein PD, Hull RD, Patel KC, et al. D-dimer for the exclusion of acute venous thrombosis and pulmonary embolism: a systematic review. Ann Intern Med 2004; 140:589–602

For the diagnosis of DVT, the ELISA and quantitative rapid ELISA are more sensitive than latex and whole-blood agglutination assays. For the diagnosis of PE, the ELISA and quantitative rapid ELISA are more sensitive than semiquantitative latex and whole-blood agglutination assays.

Stein PD, Woodard PK, Weg JG, et al. Diagnostic pathways in acute pulmonary embolism: recommendations of the PIOPEDII investigators. Am J Med 2006; 119:1048–1055

The PIOPED II investigators recommend a stratification of patients with suspected PE according to a clinical probability assessment. The investigators conclude that the sequence of diagnostic test for patients with suspected PE will depend on the clinical circumstances.

Swensen SJ, Sheedy PF, Ryu JH, et al. Outcomes after withholding anticoagulation from patients with suspected acute pulmonary embolism and negative computed tomographic findings: a cohort study. Mayo Clin Proc 2002; 77:130–138

Results showed that the incidence of overall DVT, PE, or fatal PE among patients with suspected acute PE, negative CT scan results, and no other evidence of VTE is low. Withholding anticoagulation therapy in these patients appears to be safe.

Tapson VF. Acute pulmonary embolism. N Engl J Med 2008; 358:1037–1052

An updated review of the epidemiology, diagnosis, treatment, and prevention of acute PE from an international expert in the field.

Tillie-Leblong I, Marquette C-H, Perez T, et al. Pulmonary embolism in patients with unexplained exacerbation of chronic obstructive pulmonary disease: prevalence and risk factors. Ann Intern Med 2006; 144:390–396

This study showed a 25% prevalence of PE in patients with COPD hospitalized for severe exacerbation of unknown origin.

Van Belle A, Buller HR, Huisman MV, et al. Effectiveness of managing suspected pulmonary embolism using an algorithm combining clinical probability, d-dimer testing, and computed tomography. JAMA 2006; 295:172–179

This study assessed the clinical effectiveness of a simplified algorithm using a clinical decision rule, d-dimer testing, and CT scanning in patients with suspected PE. The use of this algorithm was associated with a low risk for subsequent fatal and nonfatal VTE.

Wells PS, Ginsberg JS, Anderson DR, et al. Use of a clinical model for safe management of patients with suspected pulmonary embolism. Ann Intern Med 1998; 129:997–1005

Among inpatients and outpatients with suspected PE, only 3 of 665 patients (0.5%; 95% confidence interval, 0.1 to 1.3%) with low or moderate pretest probability and a non—high-probability $\dot{V}/\dot{Q}$ lung scan finding who were considered to be negative for PE had PE or DVT during a 90-day follow-up. These data suggest that the management of patients with suspected PE on the basis of pretest probability and the results of $\dot{V}/\dot{Q}$ lung scanning is safe.

Wells PS, Owen C, Doucette S, et al. Does this patient have deep vein thrombosis? JAMA 206; 295:199–207

This article is part of the rational clinical examination series in JAMA and uses a case scenario to walk the reader through the approach to the evaluation of a patient with suspected DVT. In so doing, the authors have also performed a systematic review of the literature regarding clinical prediction rules and d-dimer levels and applied these data in the context of clinical decision making.

Wood KE. Major pulmonary embolism: review of a pathophysiologic approach to the golden hour of hemodynamically significant pulmonary embolism. Chest 2002; 121:877–905

This is an extensive review of a pathophysiologic approach to hemodynamically significant PE. The article also discusses risk gratification in part based on right ventricular dysfunction. Thrombolytic therapy is acknowledged as a treatment of choice with embolectomy for those patients in whom thrombolysis is contraindicated.

Notes

Lung Cancer

W. Michael Alberts, MD, MBA, FCCP

Objectives:

- Outline the various causes of lung cancer and the types of clinical and radiographic presentations peculiar to each cell type
- Review the paraneoplastic syndromes associated with lung cancer
- Place in perspective the appropriate use of laboratory studies, imaging techniques, and diagnostic approaches to patients with lung cancer
- Review the results of various treatment modalities for both small cell and non-small cell lung cancers

Key words: non-small cell lung cancer; paraneoplastic syndromes; screening; small-cell lung cancer; solitary pulmonary nodule; staging; treatment

---

The statistics are no doubt familiar but, nonetheless, staggering: An estimated 215,020 individuals in the United States will receive a diagnosis of lung cancer in 2009. More disconcerting is that 161,830 individuals will succumb to the disease within 1 year. The numbers from abroad are no more comforting (and, in many cases, more ominous). It has been estimated that 1 to 2 million people worldwide die of this disease each year.

Lung cancer is currently the leading cause of cancer deaths in both men and women in the United States. Deaths from lung cancer in women surpassed those from breast cancer in 1987 and are expected to account for approximately 26% of all cancer deaths in women in 2009. Thirty-one percent of cancer deaths in men are attributable to lung cancer. Lung cancer causes more deaths than the next four most common cancers combined (colon, 49,962; breast, 40,930; pancreas, 34,290; and prostate, 28,660). Fortunately, the death rate from lung cancer in men in the United States began to decrease in 1991, which is reflective of a decrease in smoking that began in the 1950s. The mortality rate in women has reached a plateau. The anticipated decrease has lagged behind the decrease in men, likely to the result of smoking prevalence among women. Currently, approximately 20% of adults in the United States smoke (23.9% of men and 18.1% of women). Lung cancer is now more prevalent in ex-smokers than active smokers.

The status of the treatment of lung cancer is no more encouraging. The expected 5-year survival for the diagnosis of lung cancer is 16% as compared with 65% for colon cancer, 89% for breast cancer, and nearly 100% for prostate cancer. Furthermore, progress in treatment has been slow. The current overall 5-year survival rate of 16% is only slightly better than the 8% survival rate of the early 1960s. Even when a small primary tumor (<3 cm in diameter) is diagnosed "early" and no apparent metastatic spread is found (*ie*, stage IA), the expected 5-year survival is significantly <100%, with the authors of most studies reporting only 65%. The 5-year survival for other potentially resectable lesions is even worse (IB = 57%, IIA = 55%, IIB = 39%, and IIIA = 23%). When diagnosed "late" with documented extrathoracic spread, the disease is incurable, with an expected 5-year survival of <1%. The median survival of patients with untreated metastatic non-small cell lung cancer is 4 to 5 months, with a survival rate at 1 year of 10%.

Before reviewing the subject at hand, it must be said that much of the effort evidenced in this review might not be necessary but for the real culprit, namely tobacco and tobacco products. Tobacco use is the leading cause of preventable death in this country and accounts for one of every five deaths. Half of regular smokers die prematurely of a tobacco-related disease. Not to minimize the efforts of clinicians and clinical researchers, but the "biggest bang for the buck" comes in the form of lung cancer prevention. Whether primary, secondary, or tertiary, the prevention of cigarette smoking has the biggest potential to improve the dismal statistics associated with this cancer.

Etiology of Lung Cancer

Tobacco causes 80 to 90% of all lung cancers. There is a clear dose–response relationship between the number of cigarettes smoked per day and the incidence of lung cancer. Cigarette smoking causes damage to the DNA in the cells of the bronchial epithelium. There are >20 known carcinogens in tobaccos smoke. Nicotine, itself, does not appear to be carcinogenic but leads to smoking addiction. The risk of dying in white men is decreasing as the result of lower rates of smoking. The increasing rate in women parallels their increasing use of cigarettes. The risk of lung cancer increases, in cigar and pipe smokers, depending on inhalation practices. The effect of pipe and cigar use on the risk of lung cancer is generally similar to that of light cigarette smoking. Smokeless tobacco products (*eg*, chewing tobacco and snuff) are carcinogenic for the upper aerodigestive tract but not for the lungs.

Passive Smoking

It is estimated that up to 25% of lung cancer in nonsmokers comes from passive exposure to cigarette smoke, which translates into an estimate that passive smoking causes approximately 1.6 to 5% of all lung cancers. Passive smoke differs significantly from mainstream smoke inhaled by the active smoker and may be even more carcinogenic. Several studies show that spouses of smokers have a twofold to threefold increased risk of lung cancer.

Other Carcinogens for Lung Cancer

Other carcinogens include asbestos, radon daughters, a variety of polycyclic hydrocarbons, cadmium, chloromethyl ethers (especially for small cell lung cancer), chromium, nickel, and inorganic arsenic. It has been conjectured that air pollution may promote the action of other carcinogens but may not be carcinogenic alone. As risk factors for lung cancer, most, if not all, of these environmental factors either require or are markedly augmented by concomitant exposure to cigarette smoke.

Dietary Factors

Dietary factors are thought possibly to decrease the risk of lung cancer. Vitamin A intake is inversely associated with lung cancer risk, especially among cigarette smokers. The constituents of green and yellow vegetables, such as beta-carotene and selenium, appear to have potential as protective agents against lung cancer. More than 30 case–control and cohort studies have suggested that people who eat more vegetables and fruit have a lower risk of lung cancer than those who eat fewer such foods or who have lower beta-carotene concentrations in their blood.

These observations stimulated several large, controlled trials of beta-carotene supplementation. Most trials do not support the observed beneficial association or a role for supplemental beta-carotene in the prevention of lung cancer. Instead, the same studies provide striking evidence of an excessive lung cancer incidence in smokers (an adverse effect). This finding stresses the importance of establishing the efficacy of chemoprevention agents in carefully conducted clinical trials.

Genetic Lesions and the Molecular Pathogenesis of Lung Cancer

It is becoming apparent through candidate gene and genome-wide approaches that clinically evident lung cancers have accumulated numerous (perhaps ≥20) clonal genetic and epigenetic alterations in a multistep process. These alterations include the classical genetic abnormalities of tumor suppressor gene inactivation and overactivity of growth-promoting oncogenes. These changes lead to the so-called "hallmarks of lung cancer": (1) abnormalities in self-sufficiency of growth signals, (2) evading apoptosis, (3) insensitivity to antigrowth signals, (4) limitless replicative potential, (5) sustained angiogenesis, and (6) tissue invasion and metastases. These findings may have important clinical ramifications.

Advances in cell and molecular biology have increased our understanding of the multiple events that lead to the development of lung cancer. The field cancerization theory suggests that multiple genetic abnormalities occur throughout the respiratory epithelium as a result of long-term carcinogen exposure. Mutations may occur during adult life as a result of cigarette smoking, but it is also possible that some of them may be acquired during embryonic development of the bronchial epithelium.

Inherited Predisposition to Lung Cancer

A predisposition to early age of onset of lung cancer may be inherited in a Mendelian codominant fashion. COPD is associated with the development of lung cancer, and there appears to be a familial correlation with the development of such respiratory disease. Inheritance of an abnormality in carcinogen metabolism is another possibility. Inheriting genes predisposing to malignancy usually results in a high rate of secondary tumors (lung, head and neck, esophagus, and other organs). For example, patients cured of laryngeal tumors have an increased risk of lung cancer.

Lung Cancer in Never Smokers

A small proportion of patients with lung cancer do not have a significant history of cigarette use (defined as <100 cigarettes in a lifetime). In the United States, 10 to 15% of lung cancer occurs in never smokers (5 to 10% in men and 15 to 25% in women). This rate is greater than that of ovarian cancer or Hodgkin disease. Worldwide, 15% of men and 53% of women with lung cancer are never-smokers.

The cause of lung cancer in never-smokers is uncertain. Speculation surrounds environmental tobacco smoke, cooking fumes, indoor air quality, genetic factors, occupational exposures, hormonal factors, and oncogenic viruses. The study of the molecular basis for oncogenesis has led to speculation that lung cancer in never smokers and lung cancer in smokers may be different disease entities.

Smoking Cessation

Smokers should be offered counseling and nicotine-replacement therapy (NRT) at every visit. "Treating Tobacco Use and Dependence—2008 Update" was released and posted by the US Public Health Service Commissioned Corps in May of 2008. This document provides the latest information and techniques.

Psychological and behavioral techniques, such as delivering a strong personalized message, arranging intensive counseling (both individual and group), providing self-help material, referring to a tailored self-help programs, encouraging the use of telephone "Quit-lines" (telephone therapy is now accessible in every state at 1-800-Quit now), using aversive smoking techniques, and exercise, have proven to be of benefit. Conversely, the use of hypnosis or acupuncture has not proven to be beneficial.

Pharmacotherapy in the form of NRT is beneficial. NRT may be delivered in the form of a gum, a patch, a nasal spray, an inhaler, or as lozenges. Both bupropion, an antidepressant that inhibits the reuptake of dopamine and norepinephrine, and varenicline, a partial nicotine agonist at a subtype of the nicotinic acetylcholine receptor, have been shown to be effective. A recent study demonstrated smoking abstinence from weeks 9 to 12 of a 3-month study of 44% for users of varenicline, 30% for bupropion, and 18% for placebo. Nausea occurs in 30 to 50% of patients on varenicline. In addition, there have been recent alerts from the US Food and Drug Administration on the use of varenicline. There may be an increased risk of neuropsychiatric symptoms, including agitation, depressed mood, suicidal ideation, and worsening of preexisting psychiatric disease.

Combination therapy may be more effective. For example, the use of a baseline patch plus NRT boost (gum, lozenge, spray) is common. A baseline patch and oral bupropion plus NRT boost may be helpful for heavy smokers. Pharmacotherapy doubles the cessation success rate at 6 months when compared with placebo. On occasion, long-term therapy may be necessary.

Classification of Lung Cancer

World Health Organization Histologic Class

An important distinction is to separate small cell lung cancer (SCLC; 15 to 18% of all lung cancers) from non-small cell bronchogenic carcinomas (82 to 85%). Approximately 10% of SCLCs are combined with non-small cell lung cancer (NSCLC) components. The management approach to SCLC is significantly different from that for all subtypes of non-small cell bronchogenic carcinomas. Small-cell carcinoma is generally regarded as a disorder for which surgery is not indicated.

Microscopically, SCLC in made up of small, round cells with large nuclei that stain blue when hematoxylin and eosin is used. Histologically, they are characterized by scant cytoplasm, fine chromatin, and nuclear molding. "Crush artifact' is commonly noted. SCLC arises from neuroendocrine cells and stains positive for synaptophysin, chromogranin A, and neuron-specific enolase. SCLC is so strongly associated with cigarette smoking that such a diagnosis in a nonsmoker should be questioned.

All other cell types of bronchogenic carcinoma, depending on their stage, can potentially be managed surgically with the potential for cure. Non-small cell carcinomas are split into squamous cell (29% of the total); adenocarcinoma, including bronchioloalveolar cell carcinoma (32% of the total), large-cell carcinoma (9% of the total), and undifferentiated (11% of total). Non-small cell lung carcinomas are believed to arise from lung epithelial cells. They express cytokeratin in a distinct pattern (negative for CK20 and positive for CK7) and are commonly positive for thyroid transcription factor 1.

Adenocarcinomas are the least closely associated with cigarette smoking and most commonly arise in the lung periphery from epithelial cells involved in gland formation. They may grow in acinar, papillary, bronchioloalveolar, or solid growth patterns, often in association with the production of mucus. Up to 50% of patients have never smoked, and 80% present with metastatic disease.

Bronchioloalveolar cell carcinoma (BAC) often is characterized as a subtype of adenocarcinoma. BAC is the most common type of lung cancer in never-smokers. BAC tumors grow in lepidic fashion, spreading along the lining of alveolar air spaces, and there is no invasion of the stroma, pleura, or lymphatics. Where such invasion occurs, the disease process is termed *adenocarcinoma mixed type with a predominant BAC pattern*. BAC often is very slow growing and commonly spreads within the lung through the airways. BAC is divided into three subtypes: mucinous, nonmucinous, and a mixed type.

Squamous cell carcinoma is characterized by keratin formation, intercellular bridging, and a nonglandular appearance. Squamous cell lung cancer typically arises within the major bronchi near the center of the chest. A total of 95% of patients with squamous cell are smokers, and 60% present with metastatic disease.

Large cell carcinoma lacks the features of either a squamous cell or an adenocarcinoma. This tumor is a more poorly differentiated form of NSCLC. Large cell tumors that express neuroendocrine tumor markers are less responsive to chemotherapy than SCLC and carry a poor prognosis compared with other types of NSCLC.

Other cell types constitute a small minority of all lung neoplasms. For example, carcinoid tumors may arise in the lung. These tumors have a neuroendocrine phenotype, like SCLC, but grow slowly, rarely metastasize, and the treatment is often surgery alone. These tumors are composed of small, round blue cells but can be differentiated from SCLC by their low-grade appearance and lack of mitotic figures. Carcinoid tumors tend to be highly resistant to radiation therapy and chemotherapy and are therefore best treated by surgery. More aggressive carcinoid tumors with an intermediate number of mitotic figures are termed atypical carcinoids. These tumors are faster growing and have the potential for metastatic spread. Fortunately, atypical carcinoid tumors of the lung are more responsive to chemotherapy and radiation therapy.

Preinvasive lesions have been identified. These include squamous dysplasia/carcinoma in situ (leading to squamous cell carcinoma), atypical adenomatous hyperplasia (leading to adenocarcinoma), and diffuse idiopathic pulmonary neuroendocrine cell hyperplasia (leading to carcinoid).

International Staging System for Lung Cancer

Lung cancers are staged by the TNM system (T = 5 primary tumor, N = 5 regional lymph nodes, M = presence or absence of distant metastases). The TNM system, developed in the late 1940s, is used as a guide to estimate prognosis, to select treatment options, and to report outcomes. Several changes were made to the staging system in 1997. These changes were made to more closely align patient clinical presentation to appropriate treatment options and expected outcomes. The seventh edition of the TNM Classification of Malignant Tumors is expected to be published in 2009.

Stage I Patients Redefined: Only T1N0M0 (stage IA) and T2N0M0 (stage IB) patients are now included in stage I. T1N1M0 is now placed in stage II. The prognosis for survival with N1 involvement is significantly worse, especially in the case of adenocarcinoma, than when there is no lymph node involvement. The prognosis for 5-year survival, with surgical resection, is 70 to 80% for T1N0M0 patients and 50 to 60% for T2N0M0 patients.

Stage II Patients: The survival pattern for T1N1M0 (stage IIA) patients more closely resembles the survival patterns for patients with stage II lung cancer than stage I subsets. Stage IIB includes T2N1M0 and T3N0M0. T3N0M0 was moved from stage IIIA to IIB reflecting a prognosis more similar to other stage II tumors.

Stage III Patients: Tumors staged in this grouping are very heterogeneous. The 10% of patients with NSCLC who present with stage IIIA cancer are described by the American College of Chest Physicians (ACCP) guidelines as "perhaps the most therapeutically challenging and controversial subset" of lung cancer patients, because they fit between the generally resectable stage I and stage II tumors and the generally unresectable stage IIIB and stage IV cases.

Although not recognized by the American Joint Committee on Cancer's Cancer Staging Manual, for treatment purposes, patients with N2 disease may be artificially classified into four subgroups:

- $IIIA_1$: incidental nodal metastases found on final pathologic examination of the resection specimen;
- $IIIA_2$: nodal metastases (single station) recognized intraoperatively;
- $IIIA_3$: nodal metastases (single or multiple station) recognized by prethoracotomy staging; and
- $IIIA_4$: bulky or fixed multistation N2 disease.

Stage IIIA Patients: Patients with involvement of the ipsilateral mediastinal lymph nodes (N2 disease) are categorized as IIIA patients. A better outcome is anticipated for these patients than when mediastinal node metastasis is more extensive (N3 disease). Patients with IIIA tumors (IIIA1, IIIA2, and IIIA3 after neoadjuvant) may potentially undergo complete resection. If nonoperative therapy is appropriate, randomized controlled trials have shown that chemotherapy and radiation therapy improve survival over the use of radiation therapy alone. The role of surgical resection as an adjunct to this combined method of treatment is still not clear.

Stage IIIB Patients: Stage IIIB patients include those with T4 tumors (T4 is for tumors of any size that invade the mediastinum or involve the heart, great vessels, trachea, esophagus, vertebral body, or carina; or for the presence of a malignant pleural effusion) and with any N3 metastases (contralateral mediastinal lymph nodes, contralateral hilar lymph nodes, ipsilateral or contralateral scalene, or supraclavicular nodes), but with M0 disease. Selected stage IIIB patients (good performance status) typically are treated with chemoradiation.

Stage IV Patients: Stage IV patients include those with any T designation and any N involvement accompanied by spread to different lobes of the lung than the site of the primary tumor or, by way of the bloodstream, to distant sites within the body.

Exceptions for SCLC: The TNM and staging systems (I-IV) are appropriate for SCLC. Many physicians, however, use the old Veteran's Administration staging system, the reason being that there is less variation in survival for the stages described by the TNM system when applied to SCLC. Therefore, the more detailed TNM system offers no advantage. Both treatment options and prognosis can be adequately communicated by the use of a two-stage system. In the two-stage system developed by the Veteran's Administration Lung Cancer study group, small cell lung cancer is staged as "limited disease" or "extensive disease." Limited disease for SCLC (30% of patients) typically is defined as no detectable disease outside of the hemithorax, with or without ipsilateral, mediastinal, hilar, or supraclavicular lymph nodes. Patients with unilateral pleural effusion also have been classified as having limited disease. Extensive disease (70% of patients) is any disease occurring beyond the sites listed for limited disease.

Proposals for the Seventh Edition of the TNM Classification and Stage Groupings: The International Association for the Study of Lung Cancer (IASLC) recently has issued recommendations for the seventh Edition of the TNM Classification and Stage Groupings of Lung Cancer based on an intensive and validated analysis of a database that included >100,000 patients. The recommended changes in the T classification are to subclassify T1 into T1a (≤2 cm) and T1b (>2–≤3 cm) and T2 into T2a (>3–≤5 cm) and T2b (>5–≤7 cm) and to reclassify T2 tumors >7 cm into T3. Furthermore, with additional nodules in the same lobe as the primary tumor, T4 would be reclassified as T3. With additional nodules in another ipsilateral lobe, M1 would be reclassified as T4. With pleural dissemination, T4 would be reclassified as M1.

The IASLC recommends that the current N descriptors should be maintained and that revisions to should include grouping cases with malignant pleural effusions and cases with nodules in the contralateral lung in the M1a category, and cases with distant metastases should be designated M1b. In addition, cases with nodule(s) in the ipsilateral (nonprimary lobe) currently staged M1 should be reclassified as T4M0.

Recommendations for revisions to the stage groupings include additional cutoffs for tumor size, with tumors >7 cm moving from T2 to T3; reassigning the category given to additional pulmonary nodules in some locations; and reclassifying pleural effusions as an M descriptor. In addition, IASLC suggested that T2bN0M0 cases be moved from stage IB to stage IIA, T2aN1M0 cases from stage IIB to stage IIA, and T4N0-1M0 cases from stage IIIB to stage IIIA.

Clinical Features of Lung Cancer

Lung cancer symptoms may range from none to such problems as cough, hemoptysis, dyspnea, fever, and hoarseness. Only 5 to 10% of cases are asymptomatic at discovery, and 15% have extrapulmonary symptoms as the first clue to the diagnosis. The most common symptoms are listed to follow: cough (75%), dyspnea (60%), chest pain (45%), hemoptysis (35%), other pain (25%), clubbing (22%), hoarseness (18%), dysphagia (2%), and wheezing (2%). Items that should be included in the history include weight loss, focal skeletal pain, chest pain, headache, syncope, seizure, extremity weakness, and change in mental status.

Resectable lung cancer will seldom be diagnosed based on the history. Approximately 50% will have demonstrable metastatic lesions or evidence of unresectability at the time of first diagnosis. Further testing will reveal that another 15% are unresectable. Finally, another 5 to 10% will be found to be unresectable at surgery. Thus, only 25 to 30% of cases are potentially curable by surgery.

Physical examination findings usually parallel the symptoms. The physical examination will become positive only late in the course. If the first clue to the diagnosis comes from the physical examination, it is probably too late to expect any chance for cure. Items that should be included in the physical include lymphadenopathy, hoarseness, superior vena cava syndrome, bone tenderness, hepatomegaly, focal neurologic signs, papilledema, and soft-tissue mass.

Regional Spread of Tumor

Typical symptoms, when the lung cancer has spread to the mediastinum, include dysphagia (from esophageal compression or involvement) and the development of effusions (from lymphatic obstruction). Cardiovascular involvement can be associated with arrhythmias and heart failure (from pericardial involvement). The pericardium or the myocardium is involved in 15 to 35% of patients (autopsy data), but the frequency of clinical symptoms is unknown. Malignant pericardial effusion with tamponade may develop.

The superior vena cava syndrome is more common if the primary tumor is on the right side. In NSCLC (usually squamous) the obstruction develops slowly, allowing development of a collateral venous system evident at the time of physical examination. Edema and suffusion may also be present.

Regional nervous system involvement includes Horner syndrome (unilateral dilated pupil, enophthalmos, facial dryness, and ptosis) seen with superior sulcus (Pancoast) tumors. Symptoms include shoulder pain, with radiation to the ulnar nerve distribution of the arm and often with radiographic destruction of the first and second ribs.

Hoarseness is caused by involvement of the recurrent laryngeal nerve. This is more common on the left side because of the longer course of the nerve. Phrenic nerve paralysis produces elevation of the hemidiaphragm and the potential for dyspnea.

Malignant Pleural Effusions

These effusions can compromise lung function by compressing the lung. Malignant pleural effusions may be highly symptomatic, with shortness of breath and pain. Among NSCLCs, the frequency is highest with large-cell carcinoma (67%), followed by adenocarcinoma (60%) and squamous cell carcinoma (34%). However, because of the greater frequency of adenocarcinoma, this is the cell type most likely to be associated with a malignant pleural effusion.

Metastatic Disease Outside the Thorax

At autopsy, the frequency of extrathoracic metastases is 54% for squamous cell carcinoma, 82% for adenocarcinoma, and 86% for large-cell carcinoma. At the time of presentation, most small-cell carcinoma has already spread outside the thorax, although it may not be clinically evident, even after all applicable staging maneuvers have been completed.

Bone marrow involvement is encountered in 15 to 25% of patients with SCLC at the time of diagnosis. Cortical bone involvement occurs in approximately 22% of patients with SCLC and is the isolated site of metastatic disease in 10%. The CNS is commonly involved by metastatic lung cancer. The brain is involved in approximately 10% of cases of SCLC at presentation, but 30% of patients will have parenchymal brain metastases sometime during the course of disease.

For NSCLC, the most common cell types to involve the brain are adenocarcinoma and large-cell carcinoma. Spinal cord involvement usually is preceded by back pain, followed by symptoms and signs of compression (bladder/bowel dysfunction, or paraplegia). Carcinomatous meningitis is less common and usually causes death within 4 to 6 weeks.

Constitutional symptoms and signs include anorexia and weight loss (31% at time of presentation); weakness; fever (21% of cases, caused by tumor); and clubbing (29%). Cutaneous manifestations of lung cancer are uncommon but include skin metastases, acanthosis nigricans, bullous lesions (erythema multiforme), dermatomyositis, scleroderma, and tylosis (hyperkeratosis of the palms and soles). Vascular and hematologic manifestations of lung cancer include anemia, thrombophlebitis (especially migratory), disseminated intravascular coagulopathy, nonbacterial thrombotic endocarditis with arterial emboli, granulocytosis, and leukoerythroblastosis.

Paraneoplastic Syndromes

Paraneoplastic syndromes can be found in both SCLC and NSCLC but are more common in the former. They may be attributable to secretion of biologically active peptides and hormones, or as a result of tumor-related immune events. Parathyroid hormone secretion with hypercalcemia is a phenomenon associated with squamous cell lung cancer, whereas most of the other paraneoplastic syndromes are far more commonly seen with SCLC. It is estimated that approximately 20% of patients with SCLC will present with some type of paraneoplastic syndrome sometime during the course of the disease. The reason SCLC is more frequently accompanied by paraneoplastic syndromes is unclear; it may be related to its putative cell of origin, the APUD cell, which is of neuroendocrine origin, thus enabling it to elaborate a number of hormones and other biologically active proteins.

Specific Syndromes

Parathyroidlike Hormone: Hypercalcemia is more common from this cause than from skeletal metastases. Parathyroidlike syndrome is unusual in patients with SCLC; if hypercalcemia is observed in this setting, consider a coexistent non-small-cell histology, coexisting hyperparathyroidism, or transformation from SCLC to NSCLC. Hypertrophic pulmonary osteoarthropathy is seen more often in adenocarcinoma (1 to 10% of cases).

Antidiuretic Hormone: Syndrome of inappropriate antidiuretic hormone (SIADH) is the most common paraneoplastic syndrome in SCLC. Approximately 5 to 10% of patients present with this syndrome. An additional 40 to 50% of patients can be shown to have subclinical abnormalities compatible with SIADH on appropriate clinical testing. The source of the ADH can be the primary tumor and/or the metastases. Laboratory abnormalities include hyponatremia, increased excretion of sodium in the urine, normal volume status and adrenal/renal function, and failure to excrete maximally diluted urine with water challenge.

Adrenocorticotropic Hormone: SCLC is the most common tumor associated with ectopic corticotropin production. Approximately 3 to 7% of patients with SCLC will have Cushing syndrome, but a much greater percentage have a subclinical form (11 to 72% by radioimmunoassay). The clinical features of Cushing syndrome tend to be masked by anorexia and significant weight loss. Severe weakness and the profound mineralocorticoid effects of edema, hypertension, and hypokalemia are more common. The potassium level is <3.0 mEq/L in 70 to 90% of patients. Hyperpigmentation occurs in approximately 25 to 30% of patients. The calcitonin level is elevated in 38 to 67% of all patients with lung cancer, but SCLC is associated with the greatest frequency. Calcitonin causes an immediate calciuresis, but it does not produce symptoms.

Paraneoplastic Neurologic Syndromes: Neuromyopathies are most commonly associated with SCLC. The incidence of neuromyopathies for all lung cancers is 10%. Multiple small brain metastases, carcinomatous meningitis, and spinal cord or peripheral nerve compression by tumor can all mimic neuromyopathies, as can diabetes and use of steroids. Other considerations before diagnosing a neuromyopathy as caused by the lung cancer itself are syndrome of inappropriate ADH and infectious agents (progressive multifocal leukoencephalopathy).

The carcinomatous neuromyopathy can occasionally present up to 1 year before the clinical diagnosis of SCLC, but it usually is apparent at the initial presentation. Side effects of chemotherapy (*eg*, Vinca alkaloids and *cis*-platinum) may be confused with paraneoplastic neurologic syndromes.

Peripheral neuropathy is the most common neurologic syndrome in SCLC, occurring in nearly 100% of patients sometime during its course. It is probably related to the high-frequency use of Vinca alkaloids. Perhaps an underlying subclinical neuropathy exists in most patients with SCLC and the Vinca alkaloids precipitate this to the point where it can be clinically detected. The most common symptoms are decreased sensation and paresthesias in the extremities.

Dementia is the most common encephalopathy in SCLC. It is characterized by forgetfulness, loss of memory, or confusion. A response to treatment of SCLC is not necessarily associated with improvement in dementia. There is also a greater incidence if prophylactic whole-brain irradiation is used.

Subacute Cerebellar Degeneration: Bilateral symmetrical truncal and extremity ataxia are characteristic features. Dysarthria and tremors also are seen frequently. The clinical course is usually rapid, with the patient requiring a wheelchair within weeks or months.

Eaton-Lambert Syndrome: The clinical picture is very similar to myasthenia gravis, with proximal muscle weakness and easy fatigability. Symptoms are more pronounced in the lower extremities, with difficulty in walking, climbing stairs, and getting up from a chair. An electromyogram clearly distinguishes this syndrome from myasthenia gravis in that there is facilitation of muscular action potentials with repeated stimulation. Unlike the other neuromyopathies, the Eaton-Lambert syndrome frequently responds to treatment of the tumor.

Early Detection and Screening for Lung Cancer

In the 1970s, the National Cancer Institute supported three mass-screening programs at three major institutions (Johns Hopkins, the Mayo Foundation, and Memorial Sloan-Kettering Cancer Center). No mortality difference was observed between the screened and the control groups even with extended follow-up through 1996. As a result of these and other studies, no organizations currently recommend screening.

The NCI studies screened men who were at high risk (smokers >45 years of age who smoked one or more packs per day for at least 20 years). In the John Hopkins and Memorial Sloan Kettering projects, annual chest radiographs in a control group were compared with chest radiographs and cytology in an experimental group. Cytology was not associated with a different outcome over chest radiographs alone, but long-term survival in both studies was about three times greater than predicted from other data.

Two randomized trials (the aforementioned Mayo study and a Czechoslovakian study) compared regular and frequent rescreening chest radiographs in an experimental group with sporadic and/or infrequent rescreening in a control group. Both studies demonstrated a striking advantage for screening with regard to stage distribution, resectability, survival, and fatality, but mortality was somewhat greater in the screened groups. Thus, it can be stated that intensive screening (every 4 months, compared with annual) with chest radiographs and sputum cytology does detect lung cancer earlier. The mortality rate from lung cancer, despite its earlier detection and diagnosis, was not significantly different in the screened group compared with the control group. The better survival rate may be a function of earlier lead time.

A survival benefit, as opposed to a mortality benefit, with screening compared with no screening may be anticipated because of several potential inherent biases. Lead-time bias is defined as apparent improved survival by earlier diagnosis with screening even when the outcome, death caused by lung cancer, remains unchanged. Length-time bias has the effect of improving apparent survival by selecting cancers that, by their slow growth, have a good prognosis compared with cancers found by symptoms. Overdiagnosis bias improves the apparent overall survival by the identification of cancer that, in the absence of screening, would have gone undetected because the cancer would neither cause symptoms nor death because of its indolent nature.

The failure to improve mortality by screening patients for lung cancer with plain chest radiographs and sputum cytology led to an indifference to screening for >2 decades. There is now a renewed interest in screening, particularly for high-risk populations (smokers, especially those with airflow obstruction demonstrated by spirometry) because of two new methods to screen for lung cancer: low-dose spiral CT and autofluorescence bronchoscopy.

Low-dose CT scanning allows imaging of the entire chest with a single breath hold with low radiation exposure. An observational study published in 2006 reported on 31,567 asymptomatic persons at risk for lung cancer screened by low-dose CT. Screening resulted in a diagnosis of lung cancer in 484 participants, and 412 (85%) had clinical stage I disease. The results confirmed that annual spiral CT screening can detect lung cancer at a stage when surgical resection is possible. This detection and subsequent treatment results in an improvement in apparent survival but does not confirm or refute a mortality ("true survival" as opposed to "apparent survival") benefit.

A study published in 2005 reported on low-dose CT screening coupled with sputum cytology screening on 1,520 smokers older than the age of 50 years and found noncalcified lung nodules in 66% over the course of 1 year. There were 25 prevalence cases and incidence cases of lung cancer; CT alone detected 23 of the cases. Twenty-two patients underwent surgical resection that is thought to be curative; 7 of the patients underwent resection of benign nodules. The authors conclude that the use of spiral CT can detect early-stage lung cancers but caution that this does not necessarily translate into decreased mortality. They were particularly concerned about the high false-positive rate.

Although these studies and others suggest that lung cancer can be identified and at an earlier stage by low-dose CT screening, many caution that this screening method is not yet ready for widespread application. The high rate of abnormal screens, most of which are false- positive, creates a necessity for follow-up CT scanning, subspecialty consultations, and other testing that creates a high total cost for such screening. The National Cancer Institute has commissioned a randomized prospective controlled trial, aiming to enlist 50,000 current or former smokers who will be followed up for 8 years after three annual screening low-dose CTs. Half the subjects will be randomized to be screened with CT imaging, and the other half by standard chest radiographs. Until the results of this and other longer-term studies are available, there should be caution and reservations about spiral CT screening. Screening with low-dose spiral CT should be conducted in the context of well-designed clinical trials.

A second screening method that holds promise for the detection of early-stage lung cancers is autofluorescence bronchoscopy, which is also undergoing extensive early multicenter trials for smokers with obstructive lung disease and identified carcinoma cells or severe dysplasia in sputum samples. Dual screening with both autofluorescence bronchoscopy and low-dose spiral CT may someday become the norm for patients at high risk for lung cancer. However, now is not the time to begin such dual screening outside the context of well-designed clinical trials, pending the outcome of additional studies to prove efficacy, cost-efficiency, and a mortality benefit for patients who undergo such screening.

Solitary Pulmonary Nodule

Solitary pulmonary nodules (SPNs) are seen on a plain chest radiograph, are <3 cm in diameter, and are rounded or slightly ovoid. They are located in the lung parenchyma, and there are no other associated abnormalities on the plain chest radiograph. Granulomas and hamartomas constitute 40 to 60% of all SPNs and are the leading cause of SPNs in persons < 35 years of age. In older patients, especially those with a history of cigarette smoking, the key concern is whether the SPN represents a malignancy. Availability of an old chest radiograph/CT that shows the same lesion, stable or nearly stable in size for at least 2 years, will often be a key arbiter of the proper treatment in such a situation. Malignant lesions have a doubling time of between 30 and 500 days, whereas benign lesions may double in < 30 days or show no growth over the course of 2 years.

Although SPNs, especially those ≥2 cm in diameter, can be definitively diagnosed as malignant with bronchoscopy (> 65% yield) or transthoracic fine-needle biopsy (> 85% yield), it is the rare patient who will truly benefit from such an approach. Generally speaking, when the SPN is strongly suspected to be malignant, it should be resected both for definitive diagnosis and for cure (assuming it turns out to be malignant). Exceptions, in which a lesser invasive procedure is justifiable, include patients who are poor surgical candidates or situations in which the surgeon or patient refuses surgery. In these cases, an invasive diagnostic procedure less than a thoracotomy is appropriate to define the nature of the lesion and to facilitate alternative treatment planning (external beam radiation therapy).

The probability of malignancy varies from 10 to 70%, depending on the patient population. The probability can be estimated from the smoking history, age, size of the lesion, and a history or previous malignancy. Clinicians should estimate the pretest probability of malignancy either qualitatively by using their clinical judgment or quantitatively by using a validated model. SPNs that have a lower pretest probability (*ie*, < 5%) for malignancy may be monitored by follow-up serial CT scans to assess stability. A reasonable schedule is at 3 months for the first follow-up scan, at 6 months for the second, a third at 1 year, and a fourth at 24 months. For SPNs that have an intermediate probability of cancer (*ie*, 5 to 60%), additional testing (*eg*, positron emission tomography [PET] imaging, transthoracic fine-needle aspiration biopsy, bronchoscopy) is advised. For SPNs that have a high probability of cancer (*ie*, > 60%), excisional biopsy with an intraoperative frozen section examination is advised.

The Role of Diagnostic Tests

A complete history and physical examination remain the key elements in the choice of all laboratory studies for staging the cancer; particularly performance status, a history of weight loss, symptoms and signs suggestive of metastatic disease, and the function of the vocal cords and diaphragm.

Past and Current Chest Radiographs: Consider whether the abnormality has been stable during a 2-year span; if it is stable, then it is almost always associated with a benign lesion (less certain if the lesion is a GGO). Certain types of calcifications within a lesion indicate that it is benign, *eg*, concentric lamellated rings. Remember, however, that not all calcified lesions are benign.

Screening Blood Work and Other "Routine" Studies: Simple blood work is indicated as part of the pretreatment assessment of all patients known or strongly suspected of having lung cancer on the basis of their clinical and radiographic presentation. Appropriate studies and the rationale for doing them include a CBC count (anemia is a poor prognostic indicator); urinalysis (may identify a renal paraneoplastic syndrome); serum liver function tests (alkaline phosphatase, alanine aminotransferase, total bilirubin, aspartate aminotransferase to screen for the presence of liver metastases—if liver function tests are abnormal, additional investigation is warranted, but liver enzymes are rarely abnormal unless there are extensive metastases); serum calcium test (to screen for parathyroid-like hormone syndrome and bone metastases); serum creatinine (many chemotherapeutic agents are nephrotoxic); and serum albumin (a low value is a poor prognostic factor). No other laboratory tests are routinely recommended, although a creatinine clearance may be needed if chemotherapy is contemplated because many chemotherapeutic agents used in the treatment of lung cancer are nephrotoxic.

Sputum Cytology: Sputum cytology may be diagnostic in up to 20% of cases (74% of in central lesions and 5% of peripheral lesions) and is therefore a reasonable first step in selected cases.

Flexible Bronchoscopy: For central (endoscopically visible) cancer, flexible bronchoscopy is 90 to 95% sensitive (or greater). The main goal is to establish a diagnosis and distinguish SCLC from NSCLC. For peripheral tumors, flexible bronchoscopy has a reasonable sensitivity (60 to 75%) if the tumor is ≥2 cm in diameter and fluoroscopy is used. Flexible bronchoscopy is especially important before thoracotomy for NSCLC with curative intent to judge the proximal extent of the tumor for transection of the bronchus and to look for an occult central or contralateral second primary (1 to 3% frequency). Flexible bronchoscopy can often be done by the surgeon at the same anesthetic sitting, just prior to thoracotomy (especially when the tumor is peripheral in its location).

Transbronchial Needle Aspiration: A transbronchial needle aspiration (TBNA) biopsy of the mediastinal/hilar lymph nodes can stage the extent of the disease at the same time the diagnosis is made. This biopsy is more important when stage IIIA disease is suspected than in any other situation. Some centers have a consistently greater yield than others (depending on technique). A greater yield can be expected if the TBNA is guided by findings from CT than if done "blindly" or as a routine part of every procedure. The TBNA specimen should be obtained first, so as to avoid contamination with possible false-positive results. The need to perform TBNA is predicated, at least in part, on the institutional philosophy of whether stage IIIA NSCLC is a surgically resectable disease.

Endobronchial Ultrasound-Guided Needle Aspiration: Ultrasound-guided transbronchial aspiration (EBUS) of lymph nodes is proving to be a valuable minimally invasive method of sampling suspicious nodes. In experienced hands, EBUS guidance may allow sampling of level 2, 4R, 7, 10, and 11 lymph nodes.

Transesophageal ultrasound-guided needle aspiration *(EUS)*: Ultrasound-guided transesophageal aspiration of mediastinal lymph nodes that are not accessible by flexible bronchoscopy (or cervical mediastinoscopy) is proving to be a valuable minimally invasive method of sampling suspicious nodes. A false-negative rate of up to 23% is a potential drawback. In experienced hands, EUS guidance is especially useful for sampling level 4L, 7, 8, and 9 lymph nodes. Some have opined that EBUS plus EUS may allow near-complete minimally invasive mediastinal staging in patients with lung cancer.

Fine-Needle Aspiration: Percutaneous fine-needle aspiration biopsy has a greater sensitivity (90 to 95%) than bronchoscopy for malignant peripheral solitary nodules, especially if the diameter is <2 cm. A pneumothorax can be expected in 20 to 25% of patients; a chest tube will be required in 5% of all patients treated this way. Nondiagnostic results may not obviate the need for thoracotomy if the lesion is likely malignant. Bronchoscopy is still needed before thoracotomy (at the same anesthetic sitting, however) to exclude a second primary.

Specific indications for fine-needle aspiration include pulmonary masses in a patient unable to undergo a curative thoracotomy (because of compromised pulmonary function, medical contraindications to thoracotomy, or refusal of thoracotomy) who needs a definitive tissue diagnosis; an undiagnosed localized or worsening pneumonic infiltrate in an immunocompromised patient despite standard antibiotic therapy; a history of another malignancy and an abnormality on chest radiograph; and the evaluation of other masses on a chest radiograph or CT scan (*eg*, mediastinal masses) that need to be histologically evaluated to develop a therapeutic plan.

Thoracentesis/Pleural Biopsy: In the setting of lung cancer, a pleural effusion usually indicates that the cancer has seeded the pleura and the patient is not a candidate for curative treatment. There are occasional exceptions, however. Some pleural effusions will be parapneumonic in nature (benign), when a tumor obstructs a more centrally located bronchus with a postobstructive pneumonitis. Likewise, there are rare situations in which a patient's lymphatics will be obstructed by a tumor that involves the more central lymph nodes, impeding fluid transfer through the pleural space with a benign effusion as a result. Therefore, it is important to sample the pleural fluid and to study it cytologically to determine if the tumor has seeded the pleural space, rendering the patient incurable. Cytologic analysis of a pleural effusion ultimately proven to be malignant is associated with a 50 to 60% true-positive yield. A second cytologic analysis of the fluid should be done for those whose first pleural fluid specimen is negative for malignant cells. Closed needle biopsy of the pleura adds only approximately 8% to the overall yield for malignancy, so it is generally not recommended as part of the approach to a patient with a suspected malignant pleural effusion. Instead, for patients with two negative cytologic studies of their pleural fluid, a thoracoscopy should be done, because the true-positive yield when malignancy is present is approximately 98 to 99%.

Bone Scan: There is general agreement that radionuclide scans of the bones are not warranted during a preoperative evaluation unless symptoms, signs, or abnormal blood test results raise a suspicion of metastatic involvement of the bones. There are many other bone disorders that can give rise to one or more focal areas of increased uptake; thus, the false-positive rate is unacceptably high when bone scans are performed routinely. Bone scans should be done when the clinical evaluation reveals bone pain, pathologic fractures, and/or an elevated alkaline phosphatase or serum calcium level. Additionally, a bone scan can be obtained when nonspecific findings indicate the presence of metastatic disease.

The increasing availability of whole-body PET scans in the evaluation of the patient with lung cancer may soon affect the frequency with which bone scans are ordered. A recent study has found PET scans to be 90% sensitive and 98% specific in the search for bony metastases whereas comparable figures for radionuclide bone scanning are 90% sensitive and 61% specific.

Bone Marrow Aspiration and Biopsy: This test is not performed as part of NSCLC staging. For SCLC, the incidence of bone marrow involvement is 15 to 25% at the time of diagnosis. Therefore, bilateral bone marrow aspiration and biopsy will show a greater incidence of involvement. The procedure is not recommended for routine use. Bone marrow involvement usually occurs in the setting of other metastatic disease. The bone marrow is the sole site of metastatic disease in 4 to 10% of patients at the time of initial presentation.

Staging the Mediastinum

CT assessment is much more sensitive than radiographs to detect direct extension of the primary tumor and regional lymph node enlargement. In the absence of distant metastases or inadequate cardiopulmonary reserve, chest CT is generally though to be an integral part of the pretreatment planning. Situations in which a chest radiograph alone is adequate include obvious metastatic bone lesions or the presence of large, bulky contralateral mediastinal lymph nodes. The sensitivity and specificity of determining mediastinal lymph node involvement is a function of the cut point chosen. With a short axis diameter >1.0 cm defined as abnormal, the sensitivity and specificity are at best approximately 80%. (Some studies list 40 to 70%.) Because of their imperfect specificity, however, abnormal mediastinal CT findings in an otherwise operable patient should never preclude thoracotomy unless pathologically confirmed.

MRI: MRI is not better than CT for the evaluation of mediastinal metastases. It is more expensive than CT, but it can be of particular value in selected cases, such as determining whether the chest wall is invaded when the tumor is shown to be contiguous by plain chest radiograph or by CT assessment. MRI may also display invasion of vascular structures in the mediastinum with greater specificity than is possible with CT.

Position Emission Tomography Scanning: There are a number of published studies that indicate that PET scanning is more sensitive and more specific than CT for staging the mediastinum in lung cancer. PET is a metabolic imaging technique based on the function of a tissue rather than its anatomy. It is useful to differentiate neoplastic from normal tissue, but it is not infallible because some non-neoplastic diseases and infections may be positive on PET imaging. Size limitations are also an issue, with the lower limit of resolution of PET scanning at approximately 1 cm. The sensitivity of PET scanning for mediastinal nodes is approximately 85 to 91%, and specificity is approximately 86 to 88% from combined studies. Thus, PET has both greater sensitivity and specificity for evaluation of mediastinal lymph node staging than CT scanning (sensitivity of 75% and specificity of 66% in a recent study). For metastatic disease to the bone, the PET is up to 90% sensitive and 98% specific, whereas bone scanning is 90% sensitive but only 68% specific. Decision analyses demonstrate that the use of fluorodeoxyglucose–PET may reduce overall costs of medical care by identifying patients with false-negative CT scans in the mediastinum or otherwise-undetected sites of metastases. The advent of fused CT-PET images may prove to be a significant advance.

Although a negative mediastinal PET (NPV of 87 to 100%) may obviate the need for mediastinoscopy before thoracotomy, a positive mediastinal PET (positive predictive value of 74 to 80%) should not be taken as a sign of unresectability because there is a possibility of false-positive results on PET. Cost and availability of PET scanning still limit the use of this promising modality.

Cervical Mediastinoscopy: The diagnostic yield ranges from 10 to 75%, depending on (1) the histologic type of tumor, (2) the size and location of the primary tumor, and (3) the extent of the disease. The value of mediastinoscopy in the preoperative evaluation is related directly to the therapeutic philosophy of the surgeon. If involvement of the mediastinum indicates that the tumor is not resectable, the surgeon will perform mediastinoscopy (or insist on some other sampling procedure of the mediastinum) routinely. Those who resect mediastinal involvement with curative intent will use mediastinoscopy less frequently. At the time of mediastinoscopy, the pretracheal/paratracheal lymph nodes can be sampled, as well as some of the subcarinal nodes (right at the bifurcation) and the azygous nodes (primarily levels 2, 4, and 7). Mediastinoscopy helps to exclude thoracotomy for patients with marginal chances for survival after thoracotomy: those with poor performance status, advanced age, or poor pulmonary function.

Anterior Mediastinotomy: Anterior mediastinotomy is performed by resecting the second costal cartilage on either side. There is usually better exposure and less likelihood of surgical misadventure (uncontrollable bleeding) than with mediastinoscopy. At the time of mediastinotomy, the surgeon can sample the paratracheal, azygous, superior hilar nodes on the right side, and the nodes in the aortopulmonary window and the anterior mediastinum on the left side. The pretracheal, left paratracheal, and subcarinal lymph nodes cannot be sampled with this approach, however. The morbidity and mortality are essentially nil with transbronchial/transcranial needle aspiration. The morbidity is 2% with mediastinoscopy or mediastinotomy. The false-negative rate is much greater with needle aspiration, generally approximately 8% with mediastinoscopy or mediastinotomy, but it may be as much as 20% in some series.

Supraclavicular/Scalene Node Biopsy: This is not routine in the absence of palpable adenopathy. It is not of value in patients with peripheral tumors. Its value in patients with central tumors, especially adenocarcinoma or those of unknown histologic type, is still debated. An alternative is needle aspiration/cytology in palpably enlarged lymph nodes.

Other Radionuclide Scans: Brain and liver scans have been replaced by CT assessment of these organs in patients with suspicious clinical findings, abnormal laboratory test results, or intermediate or advanced stages of tumor.

Imaging to Detect Occult Extrathoracic Metastases

Patients undergoing surgical therapy for NSCLC have occult metastatic disease 20% of the time in the adrenal glands, liver, kidney, and/or brain.

Brain CT Imaging and MRI: Some studies suggest an increased utility of brain imaging, even in the absence of symptoms or signs of CNS metastases, for patients with stage IB or greater tumors, adenocarcinoma, and/or undifferentiated carcinoma/large-cell carcinoma. If a comprehensive clinical evaluation is negative, however, patients with NSCLC will be found to have brain metastases by CT assessment only 3% of the time. MRI, particularly when enhanced with gadolinium, is more sensitive than CT.

Brain imaging in patients with NSCLC should be performed for patients with headaches or for those with nonspecific findings that suggest widespread disease if metastatic disease has not been found elsewhere. A brain CT scan (or preferably an MRI) usually os warranted for patients with SCLC.

Hepatic and Adrenal (Abdominal) CT Imaging: The liver is one of the most frequent sites of metastatic involvement in SCLC, seen in 15 to 28% of patients at the time of presentation and 6 to 10% of patients as the sole site of metastatic disease. The use of screening liver function tests help to determine which patients have metastatic liver disease, both for SCLC and NSCLC. In NSCLC the absence of hepatomegaly or discrete intrahepatic masses on physical examination plus normal liver function test results indicate that hepatic CT imaging should not be done routinely. Conversely, routine hepatic imaging is more reasonable for patients with SCLC, as involvement is so common and hepatic CT imaging provides useful information for staging and monitoring response to therapy. CT imaging is much superior to radionuclide imaging, particularly when contrast material is injected intravenously. Chest CT, done properly, will extend into the upper abdomen and provide imaging of the adrenal glands and the upper part of the liver.

There are major pitfalls of CT in both organs, however. Cysts and hemangiomas within the liver are quite common. They usually are indistinguishable from metastases on CT imaging. When this happens, an ultrasound study will help to differentiate. Needle biopsy of the liver, or occasional open liver biopsy, may be needed before denying an otherwise resectable patient with NSCLC the chance for a curative thoracotomy.

Adrenal adenomas occur in up to 2 to 10% of the population and look just like metastases in the adrenal by CT imaging. Thus, CT-guided needle aspiration biopsy to prove they are metastases is essential in NSCLC, provided this is the only site of extrathoracic disease, before denying an otherwise resectable patient with NSCLC the opportunity for curative resection.

Tumor Markers: No tumor marker is useful to screen for lung cancer in the general smoking population. Markers that have been studied include carcinoembryonic antigen (CEA), total sialic acid, lipid bound sialic acid, subunits of human chorionic gonadotropin, β_2-microglobulin, lipotropin, calcitonin, and parathyroid hormone. The routine monitoring of any of these substances is not recommended in the screening, staging, or evaluation of disease progression.

The CEA level may have prognostic value in the follow-up of patients with NSCLC after surgery, because a level > 15 ng/mL before surgery is associated with a reduced possibility of a successful resection. During follow-up, patients with an elevated CEA level relapse more often than patients with CEA levels that remain normal.

Determination of Resectability and Operability

In contemplating potential surgery, one must ask two questions: is the tumor resectable and is the patient operable. The answer to the first question should be apparent after the workup and basically depends on whether all tumor tissue can be removed at the time of surgery. It is a search for metastatic disease, for there is no benefit from debulking lung cancer. The answer to the second question depends most heavily on the overall health of the patient. In other words, can the patient withstand the stress of surgery and do the potential benefits of the surgery outweigh the risks?

Operability usually relates to the functional capacity of the cardiorespiratory system. Cardiorespiratory problems account for at least three-fourths of postoperative morbidity and mortality. Cardiac complications cause approximately 20% of postoperative deaths. A history of cardiac disease doubles the risk of major morbidity (18% vs 9%). Pulmonary complications, however, are more common than cardiac problems.

The preoperative physiologic assessment of a patient being considered for surgical resection of lung cancer must consider the immediate perioperative risks from comorbid cardiopulmonary disease, the long-term risks of pulmonary disability, and the threat to survival due to inadequately treated lung cancer. As with any planned major operation, especially in a population predisposed to atherosclerotic cardiovascular disease by cigarette smoking, a cardiovascular evaluation is an important component in assessing perioperative risks. Measuring the FEV_1 and the diffusing capacity of the lung for carbon monoxide DLCO measurements should be viewed as complementary physiologic tests for assessing risk related to pulmonary function. If there is evidence of interstitial lung disease on radiographic studies or undue dyspnea on exertion, even though the FEV_1 may be adequate, a DLCO should be obtained.

In patients with abnormalities in FEV_1 or DLCO identified preoperatively, it is essential to estimate the likely postresection pulmonary reserve. The amount of lung function lost in lung cancer resection can be estimated by using either a perfusion scan or the number of segments removed. A predicted postoperative FEV_1 or DLCO $< 40\%$ indicates an increased risk for perioperative complications, including death, from lung cancer resection. Exercise testing should be performed in these patients to further define the perioperative risks before surgery.

Formal cardiopulmonary exercise testing is a sophisticated physiologic testing technique that includes recording the exercise ECG, heart rate response to exercise, minute ventilation, and oxygen uptake per minute, and allows calculation of maximal oxygen consumption ($\dot{V}o_2max$). Risk for perioperative complications can generally be stratified by $\dot{V}o_2max$. Patients with preoperative $\dot{V}o_2max > 20$ mL/kg/min are not at increased risk of complications or death; $\dot{V}o_2max < 15$ mL/kg/min indicates an increased risk of perioperative complications; and patients with $\dot{V}o_2max < 10$ mL/kg/min have a very high risk for postoperative complications. Alternative types of exercise testing include stair climbing, the shuttle walk, and the 6-min walk. Although often not performed in a standardized manner, stair climbing can predict $\dot{V}o_2max$. In general terms, patients who can climb five flights of stairs have $\dot{V}o_2max > 20$ mL/kg/min. Conversely, patients who cannot climb one flight of stairs have $\dot{V}o_2max < 10$ mL/kg/min. Data on the shuttle walk and 6-min walk are limited, but patients who cannot complete 25 shuttles on two occasions will have $\dot{V}o_2max$ $O_2max < 10$ mL/kg/min. Desaturation during an exercise test has been associated with an increased risk for perioperative complications

Morbidity and Mortality After Surgery: The overall 30-day operative mortality rate is 3.7%. Age is an important variable: for patients <60 years old, the mortality rate is 1.3%; between 60 and 69 years, 4.1%; and >70 years, 7.1%. Some studies indicate a lower mortality, even among octogenarians, when resection does not require more than a lobectomy. The extent of resection also influences mortality: pneumonectomy, 6.2%; lobectomy, 2.0%; and lesser resections, 1.4%. Microscopic tumor at the bronchial margin does not appear to preclude prolonged survival. Microscopic extramucosal spread to peribronchial tissues is associated with much poorer outcome.

NSCLC with solitary cerebral metastases is a special situation because of the potential for cure in a few patients with resection of both the metastasis (which should be addressed first) and the primary tumor. A recent randomized trial suggests that surgical resection of the brain metastasis followed by cranial irradiation is associated with better survival and much better control of neurologic symptoms than cranial irradiation alone. It is important to recognize that not all pulmonary cancers in previously treated patients with NSCLC represent recurrence of the original tumor. Surgical resection with curative intent is sometimes possible for these patients.

Treatment

SCLC

SCLC, more than other solid tumors, acts as a systemic disease, and therefore, the cornerstone of therapy is chemotherapy. Combinations of active drugs are more effective than any single agent. Drugs active as single agents typically are chosen for combination therapy, such as cisplatin, carboplatin, etoposide, docetaxel, and irinotecan. The response rate to first-line chemotherapy is excellent (>80%), so much so that the superior vena cava syndrome attributable to SCLC may be treated with chemotherapy.

First-Line Chemotherapy: Platinum-based chemotherapy is the mainstay of treatment for SCLC. This class of drugs is most commonly combined with etoposide. Carboplatin plus etoposide appears to be as effective as cisplatin plus etoposide but is less toxic (except for increased myelosuppression). Treatment is given for four to six cycles, which takes about 4 to 5 months to complete. Newer agents are under investigation and may replace current programs because of greater efficacy and lesser toxicity. Recent studies have suggested that irinotecan plus cisplatin is an effective treatment. Initial response rates for extensive disease may be 60 to 85%, with a complete remission in 20 to 30%. Median survival among those treated is 6 to 12 months. Two-year survival is 20%, and 5-year survival is <5%.

Chemotherapy doses have been escalated up to those requiring bone marrow transplant rescue without any benefit. This strategy has failed. Maintenance chemotherapy beyond four to six cycles only adds toxicity and expense without benefit. The hypothesis that emergence of drug-resistant tumor cells can be minimized by rapid alteration of equally effective non--cross-resistant combinations of drugs has been tested. As yet, there has been no evidence of benefit from the use of this strategy.

Second-Line Regimens: Despite high initial response rates to chemotherapy (complete response in 45 to 75% of patients with limited disease and 20 to 30% in extensive disease), the response duration is usually short. In general, the progression-free period is 4 months for extensive disease and 12 months for limited disease. It goes without saying, however, that when the relapse appears, the prognosis is grim, with a median survival time of 3 to 4 months. Palliation is usually the goal.

Those who relapse ≥3 months after first-line therapy may be retreated with the same induction regimen used initially. The chance of a second response is approximately 50%. Those who relapse <3 months after first-line therapy and are in satisfactory clinical condition should be offered a second-line regimen. No single second-line treatment is standard. A number of single agents and combinations may be used but a response is found in <10%.

A number of recent studies have looked at topotecan as a second-line therapy. This drug has now been approved as second-line therapy. Response to topotecan in patients with a relapse ≥3 months after therapy is 25 to 35%. Enrollment in clinical trials is encouraged.

Limited-Stage Disease: Combined Modality Treatment: Disease confined to one hemithorax (without distant metastasis) and the mediastinum, which can be encompassed within a radiation therapy treatment field, is treated with concurrent chest radiation and chemotherapy. This produces superior survival compared with sequential therapy or chemotherapy alone. Concurrent radiation with the induction phase of chemotherapy is judged "best" at the present time, as there seem to be greater response rates for local control of intrathoracic disease. Patients so-treated have a median survival of 16 to 24 months, a response rate of 65 to 90%, a complete response rate of 45 to 70%, and 20% may be alive at 5 years. Hyperfractionated concurrent radiation (smaller fractions delivered twice daily) results in a slightly superior survival as compared with standard daily fractionation.

Extensive-Stage Disease: chemotherapy: Chemotherapy alone is used. Radiotherapy is not usually administered because patients with metastatic disease usually relapse in the site of previous metastases, even if they achieve a complete remission. The cause of death in these patients is usually widespread metastatic involvement, and not disease in the chest. Treatment is primarily aimed at the systemic disease, and the patient usually receives chemotherapy alone. Radiation may palliate symptoms, but it does not prolong survival.

Surgery: The role of surgery in patients known to have small cell lung cancer is controversial. Many would say that surgery is never indicated. No randomized trial has shown a survival advantage in patients with SCLC who receive surgical treatment. A few highly selected nonrandomized trials, however, have reported 5-year survivals in the 25 to 40% range. A recent report that pooled the available studies found a 5-year survival of 40 to 53%, which is clearly impressive. Taking this into account, the ACCP Guidelines suggest that in patients documented to have clinical T1 or T2, NO tumors, surgery is an option in selected cases and should be followed by platinum-based chemotherapy.

Prophylactic Cranial Irradiation: The ACCP guidelines suggest that prophylactic cranial irradiation (PCI) should be offered to patients with either limited or extensive stage disease who achieve a complete response to first-line therapy. The argument for PCI suggests that in those who achieve complete remission, there is a 60% chance that CNS metastases will develop within 2 to 3 years of starting treatment. The high rate of CNS failures can be attributed to the fact that most chemotherapy agents do not adequately penetrate the blood–brain barrier. The brain is a sanctuary site. Once overtly present, although often responding to chemotherapy or radiation therapy (XRT), the patient is rarely if ever cured. The chance of developing a risk for CNS metastasis can be cut in half by delivering whole brain radiation to about 2,500 to 3,000 cGy. In addition, one study found a modest improvement in 3-year survival from 15 to 21%.

The argument against PCI suggests that whole-brain XRT may result in a decrease in neuropsychological functioning. Several prospective studies, however, have now shown that patients treated with PCI do not have detectably different neuropsychological functioning than patients not treated, at least in a 2-year follow-up. Any decrease in functioning appears not to be caused by PCI but by other treatment components or may be a part of the disease.

NSCLC

- To oversimplify, for stage Ia And Ib, the treatment is surgery.
- For stage IIa and IIb, the treatment is surgery.
- For stage IIIA, the treatment is surgery for some, neoadjuvant therapy followed by surgery for some, and chemotherapy/radiation therapy for some.
- For stage IIIb, except for some T4N0M0, the treatment is chemotherapy and XRT, preferably concurrently, if possible.
- For stage IV, the treatment is "best supportive care" or chemotherapy.

Surgery: Surgery is the most effective method for curing NSCLC. Surgical treatment for cure is predicated on achieving a complete resection (R0 resection). Lobectomy is the most widely used operation. Pneumonectomy must be performed to remove all known tumor in 10 to 55% of patients. There is increasing interest in the use of conservative resections. The minimal operation encompassing all the known areas of disease is used, conserving pulmonary tissue and pulmonary function. Wedge resections, segmental resections, and sleeve lobectomies are increasingly more common. Resection via thoracoscopy has been used, but complete dissection of lymph nodes is not possible (and is clearly an important part of optimal lung cancer surgery). No matter what the extent of lung tissue resection, careful intraoperative staging is needed, including frozen sections of biopsies of surgical margins and lymph nodes. More aggressive resections may include the chest wall, diaphragm, and lower roots of the brachial plexus, and occasionally portions of the atria. Resection of ipsilateral mediastinal lymph nodes (N2 disease) is possible.

There are a few unique situations such as T3/ NI/MO, which is a IIIA tumor. The guidelines suggest that those with T3N1 tumors be treated the same way as patients with stage II disease. These tumors are grouped as IIIA by virtue of a 5-year survival more in keeping with other IIIA tumors (29% when staged pathologically and opposed to 39 to 55% for stage IIB and IIA, respectively). Additionally, a T4/N0,1,2,3/MO is stage IIIB tumor, but surgery is an appropriate approach in those very few patients who are T4N0 because of either satellite tumor nodules within the primary tumor lobe or carinal involvement.

NSCLC of the superior sulcus (Pancoast tumor) is uncommon. For such tumors demonstrated to be without mediastinal node involvement, preoperative concurrent chemotherapy plus radiation therapy, followed by surgical resection, provides the best long-term survival.

Radiation Therapy: Radiotherapy has a role in early, medically inoperable, and locally advanced unresectable NSCLC, in the palliation of advanced lung cancer of all types, and in the adjuvant treatment of limited stage SCLC. Radiation therapy is clearly inferior to surgery in the curative treatment of NSCLC (15 to 35% cure rate). The limitations of radiation therapy relate to the tolerance of pulmonary tissues because nearly any tumor can be eradicated by irradiation given sufficiently high doses. Selected reports indicate a high cure rate for early-stage lung cancers, but these studies are uncontrolled. Radiation therapy leads to a loss of lung function and is a poor choice for patients who are inoperable because of insufficient pulmonary reserve. Standard therapy consists of approximately 60 Gy, with the dose divided among 30 sessions during a period of 6 weeks, although greater doses have been used. Technological improvements in XRT delivery, such as three-dimensional conformal radiation therapy, intensity modulated radiation therapy, and stereotactic radiosurgery may allow the delivery of higher doses of radiation to the tumor.

There is no established role for preoperative radiation therapy in patients with operable lung cancer, although uncontrolled studies suggest a benefit from preoperative radiation therapy for patients with Pancoast tumors. There is no role for postoperative radiation therapy for patients without nodal involvement.

The effect of prophylactic cranial radiation is pronounced in preventing clinical brain metastases in patients with adenocarcinoma (0% vs 29%) but still not considered standard therapy. There is no apparent survival benefit, however, and significant neuropsychological deficits may develop. Palliative radiation is clearly beneficial in the management of specific symptoms, such as pain control, hemoptysis, superior vena cava syndrome, and atelectasis.

Chemotherapy: Chemotherapy agents available in the 1980s were relatively ineffective, producing response rates of ≤15%. The combination of two active agents produced only marginally better response rates of 20%. Moreover, these slight gains were accompanied by significant toxicity and risk. As a result, many physicians adopted an attitude of "therapeutic nihilism" (not without merit) and routinely recommended no therapy beyond "best supportive care" for most patients. A 1992 state-of-the-art review of chemotherapy for patients with lung cancer concluded that the impact of chemotherapy on survival had not been demonstrated and that "it is difficult to recommend incorporating chemotherapy into the standard care of patients with disseminated NSCLC."

Several years later, in 1995, a metaanalysis of clinical trials that compared best supportive care with cisplatin-based combination chemotherapy demonstrated a slight benefit for the latter, with an increased median survival of 1.5 months and a 10% improvement in 1-year survival. Later in the 1990s, a number of new agents (taxanes, gemcitabine, vinorelbine, and irinotecan) became available. When combined with platinum compounds, these agents produced response rates of up to 60%, median survival of >12 months, and 1-year survival rates of 50% or better in Phase II trials.

Unfortunately, as is usually the case, recently published Phase III trials have yielded less optimistic results. A recent study compared four commonly used treatment regimens (cisplatin plus paclitaxel, cisplatin plus gemcitabine, cisplatin plus docetaxel, carboplatin plus paclitaxel). The response rate (>50% reduction in measurable disease) for all 1,155 eligible patients was 19%, with a median survival of 7.9 months, a 1-year survival of 33%, and a 2-year survival rate of 11%. None of the combinations offered a significant advantage over the others.

Despite the modest benefit, more recent metaanalyses and randomized trials have suggested that chemotherapy should be considered in patients with stage IV NSCLC who have a good performance status (ECG/Zubrod 0, 1, 2, or ≥70% on the Karnofsky scale). This therapy may modestly prolong survival, reduce symptoms, and improve quality of life with an acceptable level of risk. The cost of chemotherapy compares with that of other accepted medical interventions and may be less than best supportive care. It can be fairly concluded, however, that in 2009, state-of-the-art standard chemotherapy treatment for this population provides a median survival of approximately 8 to 12 months (a mere 3- to 4-month extension over nontreated) and a 1-year survival rate of 33% (as compared with 10% in untreated). This modest benefit must be weighed against a 3 to 5% risk of chemotherapy-related death, most often the result of infections during periods of neutropenia.

Preoperative ("Neoadjuvant") Therapy: This term refers to the use of nonsurgical therapy as initial treatment for cases in which surgery is a suboptimal initial approach. Neoadjuvant therapy might result in both tumor shrinkage and early eradication of systemic micrometastases. Several studies, although not all, have suggested that patients with stage IIIA NSCLC who are given several cycles of chemotherapy followed by surgical resection (postoperative treatment such as radiation therapy or more chemotherapy has been variable in these studies), have a survival advantage over those treated without the addition of preoperative chemotherapy. Preoperative chemotherapy ("neoadjuvant chemotherapy") is best considered an investigational approach requiring further validation in controlled trials before it is incorporated as the new standard of practice for such patients.

Postoperative ("Adjuvant") Therapy: This refers to the use of radiation or chemotherapy to improve survival after a tumor has been completely resected. Genuine promise exists that systematic adjuvant chemotherapy will increase the cure rate in "operable" NSCLC. Because modern combination chemotherapy produces remission in 40 to 50% of good performance status patients with metastatic NSCLC and because adjuvant chemotherapy increases survival in other common malignancies (colorectal and breast cancer), it is logical to suspect that adjuvant chemotherapy may prolong survival in NSCLC. In theory, chemotherapy with a cytotoxic agent may eliminate micrometastases, improving survival.

The International Adjuvant Lung Cancer Trial evaluated the impact on survival of three to four cycles of adjuvant cisplatin-based chemotherapy after complete resection compared with resection and no chemotherapy. Chemotherapy significantly improved survival rates by 3% at 2 years and 5% at 5 years (70% vs 67% at 2 years; 45% vs 40% at 5 years; $p < 0.03$) and disease-free survival by 6% at 2 years and 5% at 5 years (61% vs 55% at 2 years; 39% vs 34% at 5 years; $p < 0.003$). The authors of a metaanalysis published in 2006 found an overall 5.5% survival advantage. The stage II subset demonstrated a 27% reduction in risk. The stage IB subset trended positive but the benefit was not statistically significant. Unfortunately, there was a negative impact in the stage IA subset. The ACCP Guidelines recommend that adjuvant chemotherapy be considered in completely resected stage II and stage IIIA patients who can tolerate chemotherapy.

On the basis of these and other trials, most consider the controversy surrounding adjuvant chemotherapy to be over and state that that adjuvant platinum-based chemotherapy should be recommended after complete resection of selected NSCLC in patients with a good performance status. It is important to remember that the potential improvement in overall survival comes at the cost of possible increased morbidity and even mortality.

The results of adjuvant radiotherapy have been variable, with some trials showing a benefit, whereas most showing none. The authors of a large metaanalysis published in 1998 suggested that postoperative radiotherapy was actually detrimental with an increase in relative risk of death. The risk was most marked in stage I patients but not statistically significant in N2 patients. One must say, however, that the data used in the analysis was variable and often dated. A recent update of this metaanalysis in 2005 continues to show decreased survival for N0 and N1 patients. Another significant study concluded that adjuvant radiotherapy improves local control in patients with N2 disease but did not improve overall survival. The ACCP Guidelines recommend against adjuvant radiation in completely resected stage I and II lung cancer but recommend that adjuvant XRT be considered in completely resected stage IIIA disease to reduce local recurrence. Postoperative radiotherapy is, however, indicated for incompletely resected disease and when surgical margins are positive but re-resection is not feasible.

Stage IIIA Disease

The 10% of patients with NSCLC who present with stage IIIA cancer are described by the ACCP guidelines as "perhaps the most therapeutically challenging and controversial subset" of lung cancer patients because they fit between the generally resectable stage I and stage II tumors and the unresectable stage IIIB and stage IV cases. An approach is the combination of induction chemotherapy or chemoradiotherapy followed by surgery, but this has not been widely used for long enough to provide reliable data involving large groups of patients.

Patients with N2 disease may be divided into four subgroups for the purpose of treatment:

- $IIIa_1$: incidental nodal metastases found on final pathologic examination of the resection specimen;
- $IIIa_2$: nodal metastases (single station) recognized intraoperatively;
- $IIIa_3$: nodal metastases (single or multiple station) recognized by prethoracotomy staging;
- $IIIa_4$: bulky or fixed multistation N2 disease.

Patients with incidental N2 disease (stages $IIIA_1$ and $IIIA_2$) can undergo resection as planned if only one nodal station is involved and the nodes and primary tumor are all technically resectable. The guidelines also recommend performing a mediastinal lymphadenectomy. Those patients who are completely resected may benefit from adjuvant cisplatin-based chemotherapy.

In those patients in whom complete resection is not possible, the ACCP Guidelines recommend aborting the planned surgery but conducting systematic mediastinal lymph node sampling or complete mediastinal lymph node dissection. Adjuvant radiation therapy may reduce the risk of local recurrence in selected patients.

Potentially resectable N2 disease (stage $IIIA_3$) should be treated with two or more modalities, according to the guidelines because surgery alone has a poor prognosis. Multidisciplinary evaluation of each patient will assist in determining the best treatment plan.

Bulky N2 disease (stage IIIA$_4$) traditionally was treated with radiation alone until the advent of more effective platinum-based chemotherapy regimens made the combination of both therapies feasible. The guidelines recommend using both modalities in patients with good performance status.

Stage IIIB Disease

Significant advances in the management of "unresectable" locally advanced NSCLC (stage IIIB and many IIIA patients) have been made. The older traditional standard treatment of radiation alone has been replaced by chemoradiotherapy. Although consensus exists that chemoradiotherapy is superior, major issues that remain unresolved are: sequential vs concurrent modality treatment; induction chemotherapy vs concurrent treatment; and the specific choice of dose and schedule of chemotherapeutic agents to be used with radiation. One common regimen is cisplatin plus etoposide plus radiation concurrently. Results of the RTOG 9410 trial showed that concurrent chemoradiotherapy was associated with better survival rates than sequential therapy. The improved outcome comes at a cost. Patients treated concurrently have a greater rate of acute side effects, and severe esophagitis is common.

Stage IV Disease

Single-agent chemotherapy is of little value. The most active traditional drugs include cisplatin and vinblastine. In recent years, several new drugs have demonstrated activity, such as vinorelbine, paclitaxel, docetaxel, carboplatin, topotecan, and gemcitabine. Combination chemotherapy offers a small survival advantage compared with best supportive care. Two of the best regimens are carboplatin plus paclitaxel and cisplatin plus gemcitabine. These therapies are cost effective compared with best supportive care. They should be offered to ambulatory patients. However, nonambulatory (poor performance status; Eastern Cooperative Oncology Group status >2 or greater) patients have greater toxicity and lower response rates. Consequently, they may be managed with single-agent therapy or best supportive care.

Patients with stage IV disease should be limited to three or four (perhaps up to six) cycles of two-agent chemotherapy. Because virtually all treatment for stage IV disease fails, second-line therapy often will be necessary. Studies have suggested that single-agent docetaxel or pemetrexed (and perhaps other agents) may offer some survival benefit. Erlotinib is approved for the treatment of patients with locally advanced or metastatic NSCLC after failure of first-line or second-line chemotherapy. The use of this drug conveys a small survival benefit (6.7 vs 4.7 months with placebo).

A recent study has shown that the addition of bevacizumab to carboplatin and paclitaxel conveys a 2-month survival benefit (10.2 vs 12.5 months) over carboplatin and paclitaxel alone. Bevacizumab is a humanized monoclonal antibody that targets the vascular endothelial growth factor (VEGF). By preventing the growth factor from interacting with endothelial cell, tumor-induced angiogenesis is theoretically hampered. Hemoptysis has been noted and is more commonly seen in patients with squamous cell histology. As a result, patients with squamous cell histology have been excluded from recent trials

Virtually all patients with stage IV disease will experience recurrence. In appropriate patients, a second- or third-line chemotherapy regimen may be used. In this setting, docetaxel has an 8.8% response rate, and the median survival is improved by 2.2 months. Similar results have been shown for pemetrexed and erlotinib in this setting.

Targeted Therapy: A promising area of research emanates from the study of tumor cell biology and the molecular mechanisms of oncogenesis. The recognition that alterations in proteins and genes involved in cell signaling, the cell cycle, and the control of programmed cell death has suggested that therapies targeted directly at the molecular alterations inherent in neoplastic cells may lead to reversal of the malignant phenotype. Such "targeted therapy" is distinguished by inhibition of specific pathways and processes in the cancer cell rather than a generalized attack on cell proliferation characterized by standard cytotoxic chemotherapy. A number of such "targeted therapies" are under active investigation. As an example, gefitinib and erlotinib affect signal transduction initiated by the binding of epidermal growth factor to cell surface receptors.

The initial trials of epidermal growth factor receptor (EGFR)-blocking agents revealed that these agents were not uniformly effective. A closer look at the data indicated that patients with certain clinical characteristics (never smokers, women, Asian ethnicity, and adenocarcinoma) may exhibit dramatic results. This important clinical observation led to a search for predictors of responsiveness to these agents. Research focused on the detection of EGFR mutations. Mutations have been demonstrated in the first four exons (18 to 21) of the EGFR-TK domain. The highest frequency of EGFR mutations has been demonstrated in those patients with clinical characteristics that predict TKI response.

Multiple prospective trials have demonstrated that patients whose tumors harbor these genetic changes have a collective response rate of nearly 75% to EGFR-TK inhibitors. In addition, it has been shown that increased EGFR gene copy number (as determined by fluorescent *in situ* hybridization) is a positive predictor of EGFR-TKI response. Interestingly, a mutated K-*ras* gene (*KRAS*) is a strong predictor of nonresponse to EGFR inhibitors. Tumors rarely have mutations in both EGFR and *KRAS*. K-*ras* is a critical downstream effector of the EGFR pathway that has been found to be mutated in 15 to 30% of adenocarcinomas and in associated with tobacco smoking.

Another target is neoangiogenesis. An increased blood supply is necessary for tumor growth beyond a certain volume. Tumor-derived and stromal-derived VEGF binds to receptors on endothelial cells triggering intracellular pathways that lead to endothelial cell proliferation and increased permeability. Countering this process, as an example, bevacizumab (a humanized anti-VEGF monoclonal antibody) binds to and neutralizes VEGF, thus preventing the initiation of the signaling pathway that leads to angiogenesis. Many other drugs targeting many other molecular level processes are under study.

Tailoring therapy based on genetic or protein expression profiles of individual tumors and utilizing targeted therapy based on this information has significant theoretical promise and may prove to be a significant advance.

Personalized Therapy: Recent studies have suggested that tailoring chemotherapy based on the individual's tumor profile may be efficacious. One such study based therapy on whether the tumor overexpressed ribonucleotide reductase subunit 1 (RRM1) and excision repair cross-complementing group 1 (ERCC1). RRM catalyzes the biosynthesis of deoxyribonucleotides from corresponding ribonucleotides. RRM1, the regulatory subunit of RRM, plays a role in suppressing tumor cell migration and metastasis formation. It is the molecular target of gemcitabine. High expression of RRM1 correlates negatively with gemcitabine efficacy (ie, tumors with low RRM1 expression responded better to treatment compared with tumors with high levels of expression). ERCC1 is a DNA damage repair gene that encodes the 5 endonuclease of the nucleotide excision repair complex. Increased ERCC1 predicts resistance to cis-platin. In this study, selection of double-agent chemotherapy based on RRM1 and ERCC1 expression proved feasible and also effective when compared with historical controls in a Phase II study (eg, survival at 1 year was 59% vs a historical survival of 33%). Phase III studies are underway.

Prognosis

SCLC

With changes in the treatment during the past 15 to 20 years, the median survival time has increased from <3 months to approximately 1 year. For patients with limited disease, the median survival ranges from 1 to 2 years, and approximately 10 to 20% remain alive at 2 years. There is a potential for long-term cure. Thirty percent of patients with small-cell carcinoma die of local tumor complications, and 70% die of carcinomatosis. Fifty percent of patients with small-cell carcinoma have brain metastases at autopsy.

NSCLC

The most important determinant of survival duration is stage of the disease. Seventy-five percent of patients with squamous cell carcinoma die of complications of the thoracic tumor, as only 25% have extrathoracic dissemination at autopsy. Forty percent of patients with adenocarcinoma and large-cell carcinoma die of intrathoracic complications, whereas 55% have distant metastases. Fifty percent of patients with large-cell carcinoma and adenocarcinoma have brain metastases at autopsy. CNS deaths are seen in 8 to 9% of patients with large-cell carcinoma and adenocarcinoma. Two percent of CNS deaths are found in patients with squamous cell carcinoma. Thus, there is a clear distinction between squamous cell carcinoma and other forms of lung cancer in terms of the mode of death. Local/regional disease dominates squamous cell carcinoma. Carcinomatosis dominates the latter groups of patients. The median survival with metastatic NSCLC varies from 6 weeks to more than 1 year, depending on the initial Karnofsky performance status (the most important variable), the extent of disease, and the presence or absence of weight loss in the 6 months before diagnosis. Biological prognostic factors, including mutation of the tumor suppressor gene (p53), activation of K-*ras* oncogenes, and other biological markers, may have significant value in predicting a poor prognosis

Lung Cancer as a Second Primary

This disease may occur after a previous diagnosis of nonpulmonary primary cancer (which is the case in up to 9.7% of all lung cancer patients). Lung cancer may occur as a second or even a third primary tumor after successful treatment of a previous primary lung cancer. Subsequent lung cancers may be any cell type, but the second tumor is usually NSCLC. This is a particular problem in long-term survivors of combined modality treatment for small-cell carcinoma (up to 4.4 per person per year). This underscores the need for patients with a lung cancer to stop smoking cigarettes. The ACCP Guidelines recommend that, after successful surgery, patients be examined and undergo an imaging study every 6 months for 2 years then yearly thereafter.

Conclusion

Although a 5-year survival of 16% is meager and still dismal, the near doubling of the 5-year survival rate (when compared with the 1950s) has provided some room for optimism and has begun to shift the nihilism associated with lung cancer treatment into a guarded optimism. In addition, a number of promising new drugs have been incorporated into clinical trials, and many more are in the pipeline. Specifically targeted biological therapies are particularly promising. New diagnostic modalities, such as PET, are finding widespread use and may alter our diagnostic and therapeutic algorithms. New surgical procedures and techniques have been developed and perfected. Safer and more effective methods of delivering radiation are coming into clinical use and the medical community is hopeful that lung cancer screening will prove to convey a mortality benefit and be cost effective. Even with all this, it must be said once more that all the research, all the clinical care, and even this review would not be necessary, if we could find a way to eliminate the problem of tobacco.

Annotated Bibliography

Reviews

Herbst RS, Heymach JV, Lippman SM. Molecular origins of cancer: lung cancer. N Engl J Med 2008; 359:1367–1380

This review focuses on the major advances in the molecular study of the origins and biology of lung cancer.

Molina JR, Yang P, Cassivi SD, et al. Non-small cell lung cancer: epidemiology, risk factor, treatment and survivorship. Mayo Clin Proc 2008; 83:584–594

Excellent short review.

Spira A, Ettinger DS. Multidisciplinary management of lung cancer. N Engl J Med 2004; 350:379–392

Concise review of radiotherapy, chemotherapy, and the combination in the treatment of lung cancer.

Subramanian J, Govidan R. Lung cancer in never smokers: a review. J Clin Oncol 2007; 25:561–570

Although up to 90 % of lung cancer is "smoking assisted," lung cancer in never smokers is being recognized more frequently.

Screening

Bach PB. Lung cancer screening. J Natl Compr Canc Netw 2008; 6:271–275

Bach PB, Jett JR, Pastorino U, et al. Impact of computed tomography screening on lung cancer outcomes. JAMA 2007; 297:1–9

Henschke CI, Yankelevitz DF, Libby DM, et al. Survival of patients with stage I lung cancer detected on CT screening. N Engl J Med 2006; 355:1763–1771

CT screening can identify lung cancers when they are small and predominantly stage I. It is hoped that the randomized controlled trials currently underway will provide evidence relating to the important issue of mortality benefit.

Midthun DE, Swensen SJ, Hartman TE, et al. Lung cancer screening results: easily misunderstood. Mayo Clin Proc 2007; 82:14–15

Excellent short reviews of the arguments for and against screening for lung cancer with a discussion of future methods.

Staging

Mountain CF. Revisions in the international system for staging lung cancer. Chest 1997; 111:1710–1717

Mountain CF. Regional lymph node classification for lung cancer staging. Chest 1997; 111:1718–1723

Classic articles that describe important modifications in the TNM system for staging patients with lung cancer.

Rami-Porta R, Ball D, Crowley J, et al. The IASLC lung cancer staging project: proposals for the revision of the T descriptors in the forthcoming (seventh) edition of the TNM classification for lung cancer. J Thorac Onc 2007; 2:593–602

Rami-Porta R, Crowley JJ, Goldstraw P. The revised TNM staging system for lung cancer. Ann Thorac Cardiovasc Surg 2009; 15:4–9

Proposals for changes in the descriptors and staging of lung cancer.

Clinical Practice Guidelines

Alberts WM, American College of Chest Physicians. Diagnosis and management of lung cancer: ACCP evidence-based guidelines. Chest 2007; 132:1S–422S

Clearly and simply, the "gold standard." The second edition of the Guidelines was published in 2007 as a supplement to CHEST.

British Thoracic Society guidelines: guidelines on the selection of patients with lung cancer for surgery. Thorax 2001; 56:89–108

This guideline addresses the work-up necessary to answer the questions of resectability and operability

Ettinger DS, Akerley W, Bepler G, et al. Non-small cell lung cancer. Clinical practice guidelines in oncology. J Natl Compr Canc Netw 2008; 6:228–269

Clinical Practice Guidelines from a well-respected organization presented in an algorithm type format.

Pfister DG, Johnson DH, Azzoli CG, et al. American Society of Clinical Oncology Treatment of unresectable non-small-cell lung cancer guideline: update 2003 J Clin Onc 2004; 22:330–353

Update of the consensus based ASCO Guidelines first published in 1997. Excellent discussion of the recent literature on the diagnosis and management of unresectable disease.

Smoking

Ebbert JO, Sood A, Hays JT, et al. Treating tobacco dependence: review of the best and latest treatment options. J Thorac Oncol 2007; 2:249–256

Wilson JF. In the clinic. Smoking cessation. Ann Intern Med 2007; 146:ITC2-1–ICT2-16

Quick reviews of the latest treatment options.

Treatment

Alberts WM. Follow-up and surveillance of the patient with lung cancer: what do you do after surgery? Respirology 2007;12:16–21

Discussion of the appropriate follow-up for patients after definitive surgical treatment monitoring for recurrence of the original tumor and for the potential development of a second primary

Molina JR, Adjei AA, Jett JR. Advances in chemotherapy of non-small cell lung cancer. Chest 2006; 130:1211–1219

Concise discussion of the history and current state-of-the-art of chemotherapy in the management of lung cancer.

Price A. State of the art radiotherapy for lung cancer. Thorax 2003; 58:447–452

Concise discussion of current indications for radiation therapy and the methods of delivery.

Schiller JH, Harrington D, Belani C, et al. Comparison of four chemotherapy regimens for advanced non-small-cell lung cancer. N Engl J Med 2002; 346:92–98

This study compared four commonly used chemotherapy doublets and found that no combination provided superior results.

Silvestri GA, Rivera MP. Targeted therapy for the treatment of advanced non-small cell lung cancer. Chest 2005; 128:3975–3984

Cytotoxic chemotherapy has likely reached a plateau in efficacy. Fortunately, the study of molecular oncogenesis has suggested targets for future drug development.

Visbal AL, Leight NB, Feld R, et al. Adjuvant chemotherapy for early-stage non-small cell lung cancer. Chest 2005; 128:2933–2943

New addition to treatment guidelines.

Targeted and Personalized Therapy

Bepler G, Begum M, Simon GR. Molecular analysis-based treatment strategies for non-small cell lung cancer. Cancer Control 2008; 15:130–139

Hodkinson PS, MacKinnon A, Sethi T. Targeting growth factors in lung cancer. Chest 2008; 133:1209–1216

Personalized treatment regimens and the use of targeted agents may prove to be a major advance in the treatment of lung cancer.

Small Cell Lung Cancer

Kalemkerian GP, Akerley W, Downey RJ, et al. Small cell lung cancer. Clinical practice guidelines in oncology. J Natl Compr Canc Netw 2008; 6:294–314

Clinical Practice Guideline from a well-respected organization presented in an algorithm type format.

Sher T, Dy GK, Adjei AA. Small cell lung cancer. Mayo Clin Proc 2008; 83:355–367

Discussion of the currently recommended treatment for limited and extensive small cell lung cancer.

Hypersensitivity Pneumonitis

W. Michael Alberts, MD, MBA, FCCP

Objectives:

- Discuss the features of dusts and particulate matter that dictate possible clinical manifestations
- Identify the most common causes and the usual clinical presentation of hypersensitivity pneumonitis
- Describe those clinical syndromes that are similar to hypersensitivity pneumonitis but are clinically distinct entities
- Review the most likely pathogenetic mechanisms and the continuing gaps in our understanding
- Outline an approach to the diagnosis of the disease

Key words: allergic alveolitis; farmer's lung; inhalation fever; organic dust toxic syndrome; pigeon breeder's disease

---

Inspired air may contain a wide variety of potentially harmful substances. These substances may be in the form of aerosols, gases, vapors, fumes, or particulate matter. Inhaled particles may cause respiratory system dysfunction as the result of an irritant, toxic, or hypersensitivity effect. Hypersensitivity pneumonitis (HP) is one type of hypersensitivity reaction caused by the inhalation of particulate matter. The type of hypersensitivity reaction that develops in response to inhaled particles is dependent on a number of factors, such as the size of the particle, the concentration of the particles, the duration of exposure, the frequency of exposure, the nature of the substance, and individual susceptibility.

A major factor is the size of the particle. Inhaled particles of >10 μm in diameter are intercepted by the nose and never reach the tracheobronchial tree. In the nose, they are cleared by the usual mechanisms or cause such problems as allergic rhinitis. Particles between 5 and 10 μm impact on the tracheobronchial mucosa. Here, they may be cleared by the ciliary transport mechanism or cause extrinsic asthma. Particles between 0.3 and 5 μm may escape deposition and reach the alveolar spaces. Here, they may be cleared by pulmonary macrophages or cause a hypersensitivity reaction. The hypersensitivity reaction that develops in the alveoli and terminal bronchioles is HP. Particles <0.3 μm will normally act as vapors or fumes and are exhaled in the expired gas.

Definition

HP is an immunologic-induced, non-IgE-mediated inflammatory lung disease resulting from the sensitization and subsequent recurrent exposure to any of a wide variety of inhaled organic dusts. The disease is a diffuse, predominantly mononuclear inflammation of the lung parenchyma, particularly the terminal bronchioles, interstitium, and alveoli. There is little, if any, involvement of the larger airways. The lymphocytic inflammation and monocyte accumulation often organize into granulomas and may progress to fibrosis. The disease is caused by the inhalation of an organic dust in a sensitized individual. Recently, the definition has been broadened to include some diseases caused by inorganic chemicals that are capable of serving as haptens. These reactive chemicals join native airway proteins to form the complete antigen. HP is also known as extrinsic allergic alveolitis. Previously considered a rare disease, HP may be more common than previously estimated.

Etiology

Since the original description of farmer's lung by Campbell in 1932, >300 different occupational and environmental sources of antigen exposure have been identified. HP was once thought to be primarily an occupational hazard. The disorder is now known to be a recreational, avocational, and general environmental hazard as well. The list of offending agents seems to be ever-expanding. The associated diseases often have been given colorful and descriptive names. For example, bagassosis is caused by exposure to moldy sugar cane, maple bark stripper's disease is caused by exposure to a fungus found under the bark (*Cryptostroma corticale*), paprika slicer's lung is caused by exposure to *Mucor stolinfer*, and duck fever is caused by exposure to duck feathers. The main etiologic agents are microbial spores, animal products (*eg*, avian-related antigens), and saprophytic fungi.

Farmer's lung is the best known of the HP syndromes. Farmer's lung is caused by the inhalation of one of the thermophilic actinomycetes, such as *Faenia rectivirgula* (also known as *Micropolyspora faeni* or *Saccharopolyspora rectivirgula*) and *Thermoactinomyces vulgaris*. These ubiquitous unicellular organisms usually are thought of as fungi but, in reality, are bacteria. These organisms grow exuberantly in hay that has not been properly dried or stored. Farm workers are exposed when the stored hay is subsequently raked or turned over. Thermophilic actinomycetes also have been isolated from the soil, manure, and grain compost.

The thermophilic actinomycetes also grow in air conditioners, home humidifiers, hot air furnaces, swimming pools, hot tubs, and fireplace flues. When HP is acquired by these routes, the disease may be termed forced air disease or more commonly humidifier lung. Common to all is the presence of warm stagnant water.

Another common mode of acquiring HP is the inhalation of animal products (*eg*, serum proteins, urine proteins, dried excrement, feathers, egg whites, and bloom). The best-known example is pigeon breeder's disease (or bird fancier's lung), but also gerbil keeper's lung, turkey handler's lung, and pituitary snuff taker's lung.

HP may be caused by exposure to true fungi. Examples include malt worker's lung caused by *Aspergillus clavatus*; cheese worker's lung caused by *Penicillium caseii;* and suberosis caused by *Penicillium frequetans* growing on moldy cork. A unique form of disease recently has been described in Japan, occurring in summer. Summer-type HP is associated with contamination of homes with *Trichosporon asahii* or *Trichosporon mucoides*.

Highly reactive chemicals that are capable of forming hapten-protein complexes with airway proteins have been shown to cause HP. HP associated with exposure to toluene diisocyanate, diphenyl methane diisocyanate, hexamethylene diisocyanate, and trimellitic anhydride have been described.

A number of ingested drugs have also been shown to cause an "HP-like illness." The best characterized is probably amiodarone, but also gold, minocycline, procarbazine, hydrochlorothiazide, among others. In general, these reactions are not considered HP as the inciting agent is administered systemically and the pathogenesis is likely different.

During the past several years, >100 cases of HP have been reported in workers using water-based metalworking fluids in the automotive industry. An HP-like syndrome may develop after exposure to aerosolized *Mycobacterium avium*-intracellulare. Many exposures come from the use of recreational hot tubs, thus the common term *hot tub lung*. Separating actual infection from an immunologic response to the organism often is difficult.

Epidemiology

The incidence of HP in exposed populations varies widely. A survey of >1,000 farmers in Wisconsin revealed precipitins in 8.5%. Clinical manifestations of the disease occurred in nearly one half of the precipitin-positive group. In another study, the prevalence of farmer's lung in three agricultural areas of Scotland ranged from 2.3 to 8.6%. Studies of pigeon breeder clubs have found precipitins in 40 to 50% of members and disease manifestations in from 6 to 21%. Reports of outbreaks of HP resulting from microbially contaminated office buildings and industrial sites have reported attack rates of 15% and up to 70% of those exposed.

Because the disease is present in only a small minority of identically exposed individuals, host factors must be important. The reason for individual sensitivity is unknown. A number of studies have confirmed that HP occurs more frequently in nonsmokers than in smokers. The mechanism for this effect is not known. Atopic patients are not at increased risk. Concomitant viral infections with exposure may play a role

A related unanswered question is the frequency with which undiagnosed HP presents as end-stage idiopathic pulmonary fibrosis (IPF). It has been estimated that 10% of patients referred to National Jewish in Denver with IPF had histologic features suggestive of HP.

Related Disorders

Several disorders often are confused with HP. Silo filler's disease (not to be confused with farmer's lung) is an acute toxic lung injury caused by the inhalation of nitrogen dioxide. Nitrogen dioxide develops as a result of an interaction of nitric oxide and freshly stored silage. This chemical, when inhaled, will affect the terminal airways of all who are sufficiently exposed, regardless of previous exposure or sensitization. This is, in essence, a chemical burn manifesting as bronchitis, bronchiolitis, or acute respiratory distress syndrome.

Organic dust toxic syndrome (ODTS) is an inflammatory pneumonitis that develops when a massive dose of organic dust is inhaled. This disorder was originally termed *pulmonary mycotoxicosis* by Emanuel in 1975 to describe fever and cough in Wisconsin dairy farmers. The term *ODTS* has been described as "clumsy and ugly." As a result, some prefer to use the term *inhalation fever* to describe this and related illnesses. Clinically, ODTS resembles HP with symptoms that are flu-like and dominated by fever and chills. ODTS, however, does not require previous sensitization, and most of the time this disorder will develop in subjects who are sufficiently exposed. The attack rate can be 70% or greater, given sufficient exposure. No long-term effects have been documented, and complete recovery may be expected. In fact, the afflicted worker should be able to work with the dust again, if the levels are kept low. This may be very important in rendering employment advice.

Bacterial endotoxins, mycotoxins, or spores that reach the terminal airspaces may provoke an intense inflammatory reaction. This reaction may be caused by the direct activation of the alternate complement pathway and/or stimulation of the production of proinflammatory cytokines. ODTS is most commonly recognized in an agricultural setting. Exposure to dusts in swine-confinement and poultry-raising buildings and exposure to grain dust, resulting in grain fever, are common forms of the disorder. The National Institute of Occupational Safety and Health has estimated that up to 30 to 40% of all heavily exposed workers, predominantly in the agricultural sector, might experience ODTS after organic dust inhalation. ODTS is distinct from HP and far more common.

ODTS, or inhalation fever, also has been reported with exposure to contaminated humidifier water as found in industrial humidifiers, air conditioning units, central heating and humidification systems, and cool mist home vaporizers. Although HP (termed *humidifier lung*) has been acquired by this route, sufficient evidence has shown that inhalation fever (termed *humidifier fever*) is a separate and distinct entity. Humidifier fever is an ill-defined feeling of malaise, fever, cough, and myalgia. These flu-like symptoms resolve within 24 h. Symptoms tend to be worse at the beginning of the work week (much like byssinosis). There are no radiographic changes or long-term effects. One theory of pathogenesis is that recirculated water becomes contaminated by Gram-negative organisms that produce endotoxin. Subsequent inhalation of the endotoxin triggers the clinical syndrome.

Metal fume fever is a nonspecific, self-limited acute illness that resembles an attack of influenza. The syndrome is chiefly caused by exposure to zinc oxide. The most common modern industrial activity associated with zinc oxide fume inhalation is electric arc welding on galvanized steel. Although the data are sparse, metal fume fever also has been reported to occur after exposure to copper, magnesium, antimony, and iron. The pathogenesis is believed to be a direct toxic effect rather than a hypersensitivity reaction. Polymer fume fever is a similar syndrome resulting from exposure to combustion products of polymers and reactive chemicals used in polymer production.

Ornithosis (not to be confused with pigeon breeder's disease) is an infectious disease acquired by inhaling contaminated droppings. The illness is usually caused by *Chlamydia psittaci*. The disease usually resembles a flu-like illness but may be a fulminant toxic syndrome.

Clinical Presentation

The clinical picture of HP is very similar regardless of the inciting agent. Although there is considerable overlap and an individual patient may be difficult to categorize, it is conceptually expedient to describe three forms of the disease, namely acute, subacute, and chronic. Some authors list two forms by combining the acute with the subacute form. The chronic form, in turn, appears to be the final common pathway for either multiple episodes of acute HP or prolonged subacute disease.

Acute HP is commonly caused by a brief-but-intermittent intense exposure. Abrupt onset of symptoms occurs 4 to 8 h after exposure. The illness resembles the "24-h flu" with cough, dyspnea, tachypnea, diffuse end inspiratory rales, chills, fever, malaise, diaphoresis, headache, and myalgias. The clinical picture is often mistaken for a viral or *Mycoplasma pneumonia*. Symptoms last for 12 to 24 h, with a peak at 8 to 12 h after exposure. Between attacks, the patient is usually asymptomatic. In most instances, the acute febrile episode occurs after each contact with the responsible antigen.

Subacute HP is likely attributable to a less intense but more prolonged exposure. The disease is insidious, and symptoms resemble progressive chronic bronchitis with chronic cough, exertional dyspnea, malaise, anorexia, fatigue, and weight loss. Symptoms are much less specific and do not readily associate themselves with exposure to inhaled substances. This form of the disease presents a diagnostic challenge to even the most astute clinician. Nevertheless, subacute disease must be recognized because it may progress to the chronic form if avoidance of the responsible agent is not practiced.

Chronic HP may be the final result of inadequately treated or unrecognized acute or subacute disease. Signs and symptoms of chronic HP are those of any chronic interstitial pulmonary fibrosis in which irreversible lung damage has occurred. At this stage, the entire picture is indistinguishable from end-stage IPF of any cause.

Pathogenesis

The pathogenesis of HP is complex and incompletely understood. This is an area of intense controversy and ongoing research. The final story is not in at this time, but there is much speculation. In fact, several mechanisms may be involved. We do know that HP occurs in the setting of exposure to dust and particles of the correct size and composition. Particles must be approximately between 0.5 and 5 μm. Particles must be capable of providing an antigenic stimulus for not all particles of this size will cause the syndrome. Particles must be relatively resistant to degradation so that the antigen can persist long enough in lung tissue to allow sensitization. The patient must have been sensitized during a previous exposure. The period of sensitization is variable and may be as short as several months or may require a number of years of exposure. Not all of those exposed will become sensitized, and the disease may not occur, upon being re-exposed, in all who do. Individual susceptibility is important but not well characterized.

Current speculation suggests that the pathogenesis may involve both immune complex-mediated disease and cell-mediated immunity, perhaps in a sequential fashion. Immune complex mechanisms may initiate and mediate the acute syndrome. There is little to suggest that type I or type II immune mechanisms are involved.

BAL studies in humans have provided some insights into possible pathogenetic mechanisms. Fluid analysis <48 h after the last exposure is characterized by neutrophilia. Fluid analysis, >2 to 5 days after last exposure, may reveal T-cell differential counts of as high as 70 to 80%. There appears to be a preferential expansion of CD8+ cells (suppressor/cytotoxic T cells). HP has therefore been termed a *T-suppressor cell alveolitis*.

Recent studies have suggested that proinflammatory cytokines and chemokines are involved in pathogenesis. These substances activate alveolar macrophages, cause an influx of CD8+ lymphocytes, facilitate granuloma formation, and promote the development of fibrosis. Interferon gamma, interleukin-10, tumor necrosis factor-α, and transforming growth factor-β have been implicated.

In summary, it is clear that a type III or a type IV reaction alone cannot explain all the observed phenomena, and there is little evidence for a type I or type II reaction. As a result, a possible scenario is that an immune complex-mediated hypersensitivity reaction initiates acute lung injury and induces the syndrome. This is followed by T-cell-mediated hypersensitivity mechanisms that perpetuate the acute injury and induce the inflammation, granuloma formation, and interstitial fibrosis seen in subacute and chronic disease. Once again, this is an active area of ongoing research. The pathogenetic mechanisms discussed may or may not prove to be correct.

Diagnosis

No single clinical feature or laboratory test result is diagnostic of the disease. The diagnosis should therefore be made from a combination of characteristic symptoms, physical findings, radiographic changes, pulmonary function test results, and immunologic test results. Of prime importance is a high index of suspicion. In patients with recurrent bouts of an influenza-like illness or in patients with active interstitial lung disease, a complete occupational, avocational, and environmental history is vital.

Laboratory studies are neither sensitive nor specific. In the setting of acute disease, a mild leukocytosis (25,000 mL) with a left shift is usually seen. Eosinophilia is variable. Increased erythrocyte sedimentation rate, rheumatoid factor, and antinuclear antibody levels are common. A nonspecific polyclonal increase in gamma globulins often is noted. IgE levels are normal.

The chest radiograph is variable, and normal radiographs do not rule out the disease. In one study, 4% of acute cases of farmer's lung had normal radiographs and another 40 to 45% had minimal changes that might have otherwise been overlooked. In acute or subacute disease, a fine soft poorly defined reticulonodular pattern (often described as "alveolar mottling") is noted. The mottling is less distinct than miliary tuberculosis and is widespread or predominantly located in the lower lung fields. Another common picture is scattered patchy interstitial infiltrates that may coalesce. Segmental or lobar consolidation is unusual. Pleural effusions, thickening, and hilar adenopathy are rare. The degree of radiographic abnormalities correlates poorly with symptoms. The symptoms often are worse than the chest radiograph as opposed to *Mycoplasma pneumonia* in which the chest radiograph may look "worse" than the patient. The chest radiograph usually returns to normal in several days to weeks after an acute episode.

High-resolution CT (HRCT) may be helpful, although no single pathognomonic feature identifies the syndrome. Some believe that HRCT can be used to distinguish IPF from HP in most, but not all cases. Authors of one studied noted that desquamative interstitial pneumonitis looked like acute or subacute HP. Chronic HP looked like IPF. These investigators concluded that a lung biopsy specimen was still the "gold standard" for diagnosis.

Characteristic findings in subacute HP on HRCT included the following: poorly defined centrilobular micronodules, widespread ground-glass opacities, a mosaic attenuation on inspiratory images, and air trapping on expiratory CT images. A predominance of disease in upper and middle lung zones often is mentioned. A pattern of centrilobular ground-glass nodules is fairly specific for the diagnosis of HP with the appropriate clinical history.

In chronic stages, the chest radiograph is indistinguishable from diffuse interstitial fibrosis of any cause. A reticular pattern throughout the lung fields and/or honeycombing is common. Diffuse volume loss is evident, and features of right ventricular enlargement and pulmonary hypertension may dominate the film. In some cases, upper lung zones contract with upward retraction of the pulmonary arteries. The final appearance may be indistinguishable from tuberculosis, sarcoidosis, ankylosing spondylitis, and eosinophilic granuloma, all of which are in the differential for upper lung zone fibrosis. The HRCT picture of chronic HP is that of reticulation superimposed on the findings of subacute HP.

Pulmonary function testing most commonly suggests a restrictive ventilatory impairment, although obstructive and mixed patterns occasionally are noted. In acute disease, the forced vital capacity is commonly approximately 80% of predicted. Decreased flow rates in concert with volumes (*ie*, a normal ratio) are usually noted. The diffusing capacity is reduced (commonly about 60% of predicted). Decreased lung compliance and a decreased Po_2 with an increased alveolar-arterial oxygen pressure difference gradient are noted. Pulmonary function usually returns to normal between episodes of acute disease but may require several weeks to completely recover. Progressive and irreversible restrictive changes are found in the chronic form of the disease.

Skin testing is neither appropriate nor practical in most patients. Few antigens are available and, where available, they often are nonspecifically irritating, not well standardized, and/or impure. Where good antigens are available, an immediate wheal-and-flare reaction is observed in 80%. This reaction is not IgE mediated and is either nonspecific or IgG4 mediated. A classic Arthus skin reaction may be noted 6 to 8 h after placement but delayed skin reactions are rarely, if ever, seen

Precipitating antibodies were once believed to be the *sine qua non* of the disease. They are now more useful in establishing evidence of exposure to specific antigens. Serum precipitins are antigen-specific complement-fixing antibodies of the IgG class, although IgM and IgA have also been detected. Precipitating antibody to the offending agent is found in 90 to 100% of patients with clinical disease. False-negative results are likely to be caused by methodologic problems or an inability to define the relevant antigen. Serum precipitins may disappear over time. Antibodies persist for at least a year, and many are present at 3 years after cessation of exposure. There are a number of commercially available farmer's lung and bird fancier batteries. These batteries are not for screening purposes nor are they useful in the absence of a clinical suspicion of HP. Reference laboratories may be able to prepare antigens for testing from dust extracts or fungal cultures.

Although the composition of BAL fluid varies with the stage of the disease, certain findings have been suggested as being of clinical use. There is an increase in lymphocytes in HP vs non-HP patients (65% vs 6%). Moreover, HP appears to be mainly characterized by a low $CD4^+/CD8^+$ ratio. In contrast, a high $CD4^+/CD8^+$ ratio frequently is found in sarcoidosis. The presence of plasma cells in BAL fluid samples is highly suggestive of HP. BAL has also been touted as useful in separating IPF from HP. BAL fluid analysis in patients with IPF commonly reveals a neutrophil predominance as opposed to the lymphocyte predominance in HP. Unfortunately, BAL findings do not distinguish disease from exposure, $CD4^+/CD8^+$ ratios vary widely (and are not stable over time), do not correlate with disease activity, and do not serve as prognostic indicators. These latter findings would suggest that BAL analysis may not fulfill its early diagnostic promise.

A biopsy may not be necessary but often is useful in establishing a diagnosis. Unfortunately, histopathology varies depending on the stage of the illness and is distinctive but not diagnostic. Lung tissue usually is obtained by open biopsy rather than transbronchial lung biopsy. Very few biopsies have been performed during the acute form of the disease. Where available, they have shown alveolar and interstitial accumulation of polymorphonuclear leukocytes, fluid, and macrophages. One of the most characteristic features is a centrilobular distribution of changes.

More often, biopsies are conducted in the subacute or chronic phases. At this stage of the disease, biopsy specimens show a predominant lymphocyte, plasma cell, and macrophage infiltration in the alveolar wall and interstitium. Seventy percent show noncaseating granulomas described as less compact and less well defined than those seen in sarcoidosis. Sixty-five percent show varying degrees of fibrosis. Foam cells are seen in 65%. Foam cells are large foamy histiocytes representing activated macrophages. Fifty percent of specimens show bronchiolitis obliterans. Vasculitis and eosinophils are distinctly unusual. The typical biopsy specimen is best described by the finding of cellular bronchiolitis, a bronchiolocentric lymphocytic interstitial pneumonitis, and poorly formed noncaseating granulomas.

Inhalation challenge tests are rarely performed but may be available in specialized centers. These challenge tests are not as well standardized, as is the case for asthma. Each test must be individualized. The test is not to be taken lightly, as the reaction may be quite severe. Once a reaction is established, bronchodilators are of little benefit. Corticosteroids must be used. Outside of research settings, it would be difficult to recommend testing. In general, after a simulated exposure, the patient is observed for 12 to 24 h. Reproduction of the clinical syndrome is a positive test. Some or all of the following parameters are monitored: temperature, WBC count, lung volumes, physical examination, carbon monoxide diffusing capacity, arterial blood gases, and spirometry.

In summary, the diagnosis of HP may be challenging. A high degree of suspicion bolstered by a compatible history may permit a presumptive diagnosis. Removal of the suspected antigen source or avoidance by the patient followed by resolution of symptoms is very strong circumstantial evidence. The authors of several recent articles have emphasized the difficulties encountered in making the diagnosis.

In 1997, Schuyler and Cormier suggested six major and three minor criteria for the diagnosis. A diagnosis of HP may be confirmed if four of the major and two of the minor criteria are present. Major criteria are as follows: (1) symptoms compatible with HP, (2) evidence of exposure to appropriate antigen by history or detection of antibody in serum and/or BAL fluid, (3) findings compatible with HP on chest radiograph or HRCT, (4) BAL fluid lymphocytosis, (5) histologic changes compatible with HP, and (6) positive "natural challenge" (*ie*, reproduction of symptoms and laboratory abnormalities after exposure to the suspected environment). Minor criteria are (1) bibasilar rales, (2) decreased diffusing capacity, and (3) arterial hypoxemia.

In 2003, the Hypersensitivity Pneumonitis Study Group attempted to develop a clinical prediction rule for this diagnosis. Six significant predictors were identified: (1) exposure to a known offending antigen, (2) positive precipitating antibodies to the offending antigen, (3) recurrent episodes of symptoms, (4) inspiratory crackles on physical examination, (5) symptoms occurring 4 to 8 h after exposure, and (6) weight loss.

Treatment

The key is prevention and avoidance of reexposure is the top priority. This may require a job change, discarding a hobby, or moving to a new home. These changes may not be well received by the patient. In one study, 75% of pigeon breeders with disease were still breeding (pigeons, that is) at a 10-year follow-up. Changes in industrial procedures have proven beneficial. For example, maple bark stripper's disease has all but vanished because of the adoption of alternate work procedures. The act of spraying bagasse with dilute propionic acid has decreased the incidence of bagassosis. Improvements in ventilation, air filtering systems, or masks may help in some circumstances.

For symptomatic relief of the inflammatory pneumonitis, antipyretics and supplemental oxygen may be needed. Bronchodilators generally are not beneficial. Corticosteroids, such as prednisone at 0.5 to 1 mg/kg/d for 1 to 4 weeks, may decrease toxicity of the acute form but probably offer no long-term advantage. Recurrence of acute farmer's lung, however, may be more common in patients treated with corticosteroids suggesting that this treatment may also suppress the counterregulatory aspects of the immune response in these patients. Longer periods of treatment may be necessary for the subacute form (up to 3 to 6 months), but once again, these are of variable and questionable benefit. Once the chronic phase has developed, any treatment is of marginal benefit.

Prognosis

Prognosis is incompletely understood. In the acute form, recovery is usually complete. Symptoms have usually disappeared in 12 to 48 h, but fatigue, lassitude, and exertional dyspnea may last for several weeks. The patient usually is asymptomatic between attacks. In the subacute form, recognition is crucial. With avoidance, signs and symptoms may completely disappear. In one study, 30 to 60% of patients with farmer's lung who continued to be exposed were disabled in 5 years and 10 to 15% were dead. However, this also means that 40 to 70% did not suffer clinical deterioration despite continued exposure. A study in pigeon breeders in Mexico demonstrated a 5-year mortality of 30%. Some patients with HP, for example, pigeon breeders, may experience progression of the disease despite avoidance of repeated exposure. In the chronic form, progressive functional deterioration to respiratory insufficiency is likely, but progression to end-stage disease is not a uniform finding.

Building-Related Lung Disorders

Americans generally spend > 90% of their time indoors, and more than half of the workforce now works primarily in offices or commercial buildings. Therefore, it is not surprising that the quality of indoor air has become an important public concern. A number of well-publicized outbreaks of work-related illness acquired from the indoor work environment have heightened the public awareness of this issue.

Unfortunately, the popular media has begun to lump all signs and symptoms related to the indoor working environment under the catchy but somewhat inflammatory term, *sick building syndrome*. There are, however, a number of clinical syndromes associated with indoor working environment that are distinctly different in terms of diagnosis, prognosis, and management. The sick building syndrome is but one of these syndromes. A more inclusive term, *building-related illness*, better describes the entire spectrum of disorders acquired in the indoor working environment.

The building-related illnesses may be further classified or into the following: (1) specific disorders and (2) nonspecific disorders (*ie*, sick building syndrome). Specific disorders are characterized by well-defined signs, symptoms, and laboratory findings. A specific cause can be established and a long recovery time is the norm. Examples would include HP, humidifier fever, asthma, and various respiratory tract infections. Conversely, nonspecific building-related disorders are characterized by nonspecific symptoms and variable signs. There are no characteristic laboratory findings, and no single cause can be identified. Symptoms appear soon after arriving at work, worsen during the day, and dramatically disappear on leaving the building.

Worldwide, it has been estimated that in 25% of the investigations of apparent outbreaks of building-related illness, a specific cause can be identified, such as microbial contamination of humidification systems or the accumulation of motor vehicle exhausts. The remaining 75% of outbreaks are unexplained and are considered to be due to the sick building syndrome. In a review of 356 cases of building-related illness in the United States, the National Institute for Occupational Safety and Health found that 39% involved identifiable contaminants and 50% were associated with inadequate provision of fresh air with no identifiable contaminants. In 11%, no cause was found.

Building-Related Illness: Specific Disorders

These disorders are conditions with a uniform clinical picture attributable to a specific identifiable cause. The symptoms of specific building-related disorders are due to identifiable allergens, toxins, or infectious agents that may be identified by appropriate laboratory tests or identification of the source in the building. In turn, the treatment of these disorders hinges on removing the source rather than merely altering building ventilation. The etiology of the specific disorders may be categorized into those caused by the following: (1) antigens and organic dusts, (2) infectious agents, and (3) toxins and irritants.

Building-Related Illness: Sick Building Syndrome

In the 1970s, a remarkably consistent pattern of complaints from office workers began to surface: dry eyes, dry skin, stuffy nose, fatigue, and headache. This was the time of the energy crisis, and newly constructed or remodeled buildings were being designed with energy efficiency in mind. Most of these buildings had no windows that opened, and outside air was provided only through a recirculating air-conditioning system. Moreover, ventilation standards had been lowered from 20 cubic feet of outdoor air per minute per occupant to 5 cubic feet per minute per occupant. This lower standard is below the circulation rate of 15 cubic feet per minute per occupant, which is necessary to ensure a CO_2 level of $<1{,}000$ parts per million. A CO_2 level of $<1{,}000$ parts per million ppm generally is believed to indicate an adequate fresh air supply. As a result, the building-related symptoms were assumed to be attributable to lower rates of ventilation that resulted in inadequate dilution of irritants. The eye, nose, and throat irritation, headache, and difficulty concentrating that occurred in workers in these buildings came to be called the sick building syndrome.

In the 1990s, similar complaints were heard from occupants of many buildings, regardless of design, age, or geography. The World Health Organization estimated that 30% of newly constructed or remodeled buildings are associated with health and discomfort problems and that between 10 and 30% of the occupants of these buildings may develop symptoms of sick building syndrome.

The World Health Organization has defined the sick building syndrome as follows: an excess of work-related irritations of the skin and mucous membranes and other symptoms, including headache, fatigue, and difficulty concentrating, reported by workers in modern office buildings. Because most of these symptoms are commonly experienced by the general population, an outbreak of sick building syndrome is defined by an excessive reporting of one or more symptoms by the occupants of a building. Excessive is defined as in excess of what would ordinarily be expected as the "background" level of such complaints. It has been estimated that the *background rate* of similar vague symptoms in any population of people is 10 to 20%. In addition, symptoms must be work-related. Symptoms must develop after coming to work, worsen during work, and disappear on leaving work. Finally, there should be no evidence of apparent nonoccupational cause (such as a preexisting medical condition) nor an obvious exposure to occupational toxic materials.

Core symptoms of sick building syndrome are remarkably consistent and consist of lethargy; mucous membrane irritation (dry throat, stuffy nose); headache; eye symptoms (itchy, irritated, watery); and dry skin. These symptoms are not the result of tissue damage detectable by physical examination or laboratory tests. The most commonly reported symptoms are mucous membrane irritation (46%), headache (43%), and lethargy (57%). These symptoms, although not threatening, can be very unpleasant, disruptive to work and home life, cause lost work time and decreased productivity, and create concern about more serious health problems.

Annotated Bibliography

Reviews

Ismail T, McSherry C, Boyd G. Extrinsic allergic alveolitis. Respirology 2006; 11:262–268

Kurup VP, Zacharisen, Fink JN. Hypersensitiviy pneumonitis. Ind J Chest Dis Allied Sci 2006; 48:115–128

Madison JM. Hypersensitivity pneumonitis. Clinical perspectives. Arch Pathol Lab Med 2008; 312:195–198
Short but comprehensive review.

Salvaggio JE. Hypersensitivity pneumonitis. J Allergy Clin Immunol 1987; 79:558–571
"Classic" review of the subject.

Diagnosis

Glazer CS, Rose CS, Lynch DA. Clinical and radiologic manifestations of hypersensitivity pneumonitis., J Thorac Imaging 2002; 17:261–272

Krasnick J, Meuwissen HJ, Nakao MA, et al. Hypersensitivity pneumonitis: problems in diagnosis. J Allergy Clin Immunol 1996; 97:1027–1030
Through a discussion of a challenging case, the authors describe the difficulties encountered in the diagnosis of HP.

Lacasse Y, Selman M, Costabel U, et al. Clinical diagnosis of hypersensitivity pneumonitis. Am J Respir Crit Care Med 2003; 168:952–958
Members of the Hypersensitivity Pneumonitis Study Group attempt to develop a clinical prediction rule for diagnosis.

Schuyler M, Cormier Y. The diagnosis of hypersensitivity pneumonitis. Chest 1997; 111:534–536
Since the clinical and laboratory findings of HP overlap with those of many other pulmonary disease, the diagnosis can be difficult. The authors of the editorial suggest major and minor criteria that should be present in a patient with this disorder.

Silva CI, Churg A, Muller NL. Hypersensitivity pneumonitis: spectrum of high-resolution CT and pathologic findings. Am J Roentgenol 2007; 188:334–344
There are several high-resolution CT findings that are typical of HP.

Pathology

Barrios RJ. Hypersensitivity pneumonitis. Histopathology. Arch Pathol Lab Med 2008; 132:199–203

Churg A, Muller NL, Flint J, et al. Chronic hypersensitivity pneumonitis. Am J Surg Pathol 2006; 30:201–208

Takemura T, Akashi T, Ohtani, et al. Pathology of hypersensitivity pneumonitis. Curr Opin Pulm Med 2008; 14:440–454.
Discussion of the pathologic features of this disease.

Mechanism

McSharry C, Anderson K, Bourke SJ. Takes your breath away—the immunology of allergic alveolitis. Clin Exp Immunol 2002; 128:3–9
Useful discussion of the current thinking on pathogenesis.

Woda BA. Hypersensitivity pneumonitis. An immunopathology review. Arch Pathol Lab Med 2008; 132:204–205
Recent thoughts on the still incompletely understood pathogenesis.

Inhalation Fever (ODTS)

Linaker C, Smedley J. Respiratory illness in agricultural worker. Occup Med 2002; 52:451–459
Inhalation fever (ODTS) may be more common than HP. These reviews highlight the distinct nature of these disorders.

Seifert SA, Von Essen AS, Jacobitz K, et al. Organic dust toxic syndrome: a review. J Toxicol Clin Toxicol 2003; 41:185–193

Building-Related Illness

Alberts WM. Building-related illness. J Respir Dis 1994; 15:899–910

Brooks SM, Spaul W, McCluskey JD. The spectrum of building-related airways disorders. Chest 2005; 128:1720–1727

Burge PS. Sick building syndrome. Occup Environ Med 2004; 61:185–190

Jones TF, Craig AS, Hoy D, et al. Mass psychogenic illness attributed to toxic exposure at a high school. N Engl J Med 2000;342:96–100 (editorial: Wessely S. Responding to mass psychogenic illness. N Engl J Med 2000; 342:129–130)

Report and discussion of a nonspecific building-related disorder. Excellent discussion of physiologic symptoms in a psychogenic disorder.

Menzies D, Bourbeau J. Building-related illnesses. N Engl J Med 1997; 337:1524–1530

All four are short reviews of the entire spectrum of building-related illnesses, including the sick building syndrome. The first is a classic.

Eosinophilic Lung Diseases

W. Michael Alberts, MD, MBA, FCCP

Objectives:

- Highlight the heterogeneous nature of these disorders and suggest a usable classification system
- Discuss important aspects of the eosinophil
- Review diseases that involve the eosinophil and the airways
- Discuss known parenchymal lung disorders that are associated with peripheral and/or tissue eosinophilia
- Highlight the idiopathic eosinophilic lung diseases

Key words: acute eosinophilic pneumonia; allergic bronchopulmonary aspergillosis; chronic eosinophilic pneumonia; eosinophil; Loeffler pneumonia

The eosinophilic lung diseases are a heterogeneous group of clinical entities in which there is an increased number of eosinophils in the airways and/or lung parenchyma. These disorders may or may not be accompanied by peripheral eosinophilia. The presence of eosinophils does not establish a cause-and-effect relationship. In some cases, the eosinophil is merely a part of the inflammatory process and may even be present to protect host tissues. In other cases, the eosinophil appears to be directly responsible for the tissue damage.

Classification of the Eosinophilic Lung Syndromes

There have been many attempts to create a clinically useful classification system. In the 1950s, the first classification system was based on Crofton's five syndromes, marked by peripheral blood eosinophilia and pulmonary infiltrates. The five categories were as follows: (1) simple pulmonary eosinophilia, (2) prolonged pulmonary eosinophilia, (3) pulmonary eosinophilia associated with asthma, (4) tropical eosinophilia, and (5) pulmonary eosinophilia with polyarteritis nodosa. These are the so-called *PIE syndromes* (pulmonary infiltrates with eosinophilia) as coined by Reeder and Goodrich.

In the 1960s, a new group of diseases was included. These disorders had increased parenchymal eosinophils but did not necessarily have peripheral blood eosinophilia. A lung biopsy specimen was needed to identify these disorders. Chronic eosinophilic pneumonia, as reported by Carrington, is an example. In the 1980s, additional diseases were added to this heterogeneous collection of syndromes by virtue of their association with an increased percentage of eosinophils in BAL specimens; "acute eosinophilic pneumonia" is an example.

Currently, there is no universally accepted or optimal way to classify these disorders. In their state-of-the-art review, Allen and Davis state that an improved understanding of the role of cytokines and the other factors that control eosinophil traffic in the lung may ultimately permit a scientifically plausible classification of these disorders. One suggested classification scheme is listed in Table 1 and will be used in this review.

Table 1. *Classification Scheme*

- Airway disorders
  - Asthma
  - Eosinophilic bronchitis
  - Allergic bronchopulmonary aspergillosis
  - Bronchocentric granulomatosis
- Interstitial disorders
  - Secondary (associated with known underlying disease processes)
    - Bacterial infections (*eg*, brucellosis, mycobacterial)
    - Fungal infections (*eg*, Coccidiomycosis and Aspergillus)
    - Interstitial lung diseases
      - Idiopathic pulmonary fibrosis
      - Sarcoidosis
      - Systemic lupus erythematosus
      - Eosinophilic granuloma
    - Hypereosinophilic syndrome
    - AIDS-associated *Pneumocystis carinii* pneumonia
    - Parasitic infections
    - Pulmonary vasculitis
    - Hodgkin disease
    - Drug reactions
    - Lung cancer
    - Others
  - Primary (idiopathic eosinophilic pneumonia)
    - Simple pulmonary eosinophilia
    - Chronic eosinophilic pneumonia
    - Acute pulmonary pneumonia

The Eosinophil

The eosinophil is a polymorphonuclear leukocyte that is produced in the bone marrow. The individual cell is 12 to 15 μm in diameter. The nucleus has two lobes. There is abundant endoplasmic reticulum and an active Golgi apparatus. Eosinophils contain three different types of granules: two smaller granule populations and one larger eosin-specific granule population. There are approximately 200 of these larger granules per cell. The larger granules are responsible for the characteristic red staining. The eosin-specific granule has a very characteristic electron microscopic appearance. The internal core of the eosin-specific granule is comprised primarily of major basic protein. Major basic protein is an arginine-rich, highly cationic polypeptide that is highly toxic to parasites, tumor cells, and respiratory epithelial cells. The cell contains other cationic proteins, such as eosinophil cationic protein, eosinophil peroxidase, eosinophil-derived neurotoxin, and several collagenases. Another unique constituent of this cell is the membrane associated Charcot-Leyden crystal protein.

Differentiation of the eosinophil in the bone marrow is under the control of interleukin (IL)-3, IL-5, and granulocyte macrophage colony-stimulating factor. There are two populations of circulating eosinophils that differ in their biochemical makeup and their functional activities. They are termed *normodense cells* and *hypodense cells*. An increased proportion of hypodense cells can be found both in the tissues and blood in eosinophilic disorders. These cells are more metabolically active and may represent "activated" cells.

The eosinophil is primarily a tissue cell. After a brief time in the peripheral circulation (usually 13 to 18 h), the cell moves into tissues and organs throughout the body. There are 100 to 400 times as many eosinophils in the tissues as compared with the circulation at any one time. The eosinophil tends to settle in submucosal areas of organs exposed to the environment such as the lungs, the GI tract, and the genitourinary tract. The movement of eosinophils into the tissues is controlled by many factors. Known chemotactic factors include complement components, histamine, eosinophil chemotactic factor of anaphylaxis, platelet-activating factor, leukotrienes, lymphokines, tumor-associated factors, and IL-5.

There are several teleological theories of eosinophil function: host defense against parasites, modulator of inflammation, and tissue-destructive cell. The host defense theory builds on the well-established clinical observation that the tissue invasive stages of parasitic infection are associated with a striking peripheral eosinophilia. *In vitro* studies have shown that eosinophils can degranulate into and kill parasites. The modulator of inflammation theory holds that the eosinophil protects host tissues by dampening the damaging effects of inflammation. Eosinophils contain a variety of substances that have been shown to dampen or modulate the effect of various inflammatory mediators. Eosinophils tend to encircle areas of acute and chronic inflammation, perhaps representing an attempt to contain inflammation. The tissue-destructive cell theory holds that the eosinophil is activated at sites of inflammation and is directly responsible for the damage of host tissues.

Eosinophilic Lung Diseases

Airway Disorders

Asthma: Peripheral eosinophilia is present in many asthmatics and is independent of the type of asthma (intrinsic vs extrinsic). Eosinophil counts may in fact be used to follow the course of the disease in a given patient. In many cases, there is a quantitative linear relationship between the eosinophil count and the degree of expiratory airflow limitation.

Eosinophilic Bronchitis (Without Asthma): Eosinophilic bronchitis with a high percentage of eosinophils (approximately 40%) in sputum is a well-recognized cause of chronic cough. This entity is responsive to corticosteroid treatment. In contrast to patients with asthma, those with nonasthmatic eosinophilic bronchitis do not have variable airflow limitation or bronchial hyperresponsiveness.

Fungus-Induced Asthmatic Reactions: Inhalation of fungal spores by the asthmatic may result in several types of reactions: (1) IgE-mediated allergic rhinitis and asthma and (2) allergic bronchopulmonary mycosis. Fungal IgE-mediated asthma is a noninfectious disease resulting from the immune response of the atopic host. The response to inhaled fungal spores or mycelial antigens resembles the response to other inhalant allergens, such as house dust mite. Allergic bronchopulmonary mycosis is an "infectious disease" characterized by periods of persistent fungal growth or colonization of the respiratory tract. Both types of disorders can cause longstanding asthmatic manifestations in susceptible individuals.

Allergic Bronchopulmonary Aspergillosis: Allergic bronchopulmonary aspergillosis (ABPA) is the most common type of allergic bronchopulmonary mycosis. ABPA is a complication of allergic asthma in which the ubiquitous fungus, *Aspergillus fumigatus*, colonizes the lower respiratory tract. Patients with cystic fibrosis are particularly vulnerable. ABPA may be found in up to 15% of patients with cystic fibrosis and 2 to 28% of asthmatics. An ABPA-like disorder may be caused by other fungi such as *Candida albicans*, Helminthosporium species, and *Curvularia lunata*. Each of these organisms is capable of hyphal growth at body temperature. The hyphae persist in the airways and continually release antigens. The antigen combines with specific IgG and IgE to cause actual tissue damage. This tissue damage may result in permanent damage, as evidenced by proximal bronchiectasis and irreversible airways obstruction.

Bronchocentric Granulomatosis: Bronchocentric granulomatosis (BG) is a rare granulomatous disorder characterized by granuloma formation and necrosis centered on and limited to bronchi and bronchioles. Vasculitis is not a major component. BG may be a nonspecific response to a number of substances. A surgical biopsy specimen is required for diagnosis. The disease is defined by morphologic criteria and is not a clearly defined clinical syndrome. It has been debated whether BG is a separate disease entity or purely a pathologic description of one of the limited ways in which bronchi and bronchioles respond to injury.

Parenchymal Disorders (Associated With Other Known Disease Entities)

Interstitial Lung Diseases: Increased BAL eosinophils (>5%) may be present in approximately 10 to 20% of interstitial lung diseases. Common interstitial diseases associated with increased BAL eosinophils include idiopathic pulmonary fibrosis, sarcoidosis, systemic lupus erythematosus, and eosinophilic granuloma. The pathogenetic importance of eosinophils in these disorders is unknown. The presence of BAL eosinophilia in idiopathic pulmonary fibrosis may correlate with clinical deterioration and may predict a poor response to therapy.

Drug Reactions: A number of drugs have been associated with the PIE syndrome. Most have been reported as isolated cases, such as nitrofurantoin, sulfasalazine, phenytoin, bleomycin, and tetracycline. The reactions are generally mild and, therefore, little is known about the pathologic condition of the pulmonary infiltrates or even whether the reaction involves eosinophilic lung inflammation. Most patients with drug-induced eosinophilic lung disease will improve by simply discontinuing the medication. In severe or persistent cases, corticosteroids have been used with some success.

Pulmonary Vasculitis: Eosinophils may be associated with lung lesions that accompany pulmonary vasculitis syndromes. Pulmonary vascular inflammation is found most frequently as a manifestation of primary systemic vasculitis but also occurs in association with a number of conditions, including rheumatologic disorders (*eg*, systemic lupus erythematosus and polymyositis); chronic infection; lymphoma; sarcoidosis; and extrinsic allergic alveolitis. Primary vasculitic processes affecting the lung include giant cell arteritis, pulmonary capillaritis, Takayasu arteritis, and those associated with circulating antibodies to neutrophil cytoplasmic enzymes (*eg*, Churg-Strauss syndrome, Wegener granulomatosis, and microscopic polyangiitis).

The Churg-Strauss syndrome, also known as *allergic granulomatosis* and *angiitis*, is a rare but distinctive disorder. Patients with the Churg-Strauss syndrome generally have long-standing established asthma and a dramatic peripheral eosinophilia. Manifestations of the disease appear to be attributable to a granulomatous inflammatory response that results in vascular necrosis, primarily involving the lungs. An open lung biopsy specimen usually is necessary for diagnosis. In the past, the pathophysiology of this disorder was presumed to be caused by immune complex deposition in the walls of small- and medium-sized arteries and veins. More recent speculation involves the role of *anti-neutrophilic cytoplasmic antibody* (ANCA) and the characteristic vasculitis. The association with asthma and eosinophilia is unexplained.

Clinical features include asthma, a history of atopic disease, fever, malaise, and weight loss. Systemic manifestations of the illness may include upper airway involvement (sinusitis, rhinitis, nasal polyps); skin changes (nodules, purpura, urticaria); arthralgias; myalgias, mononeuritis multiplex; abdominal symptoms (pain, diarrhea, bleeding); cardiac findings (heart failure, pericarditis, hypertension); and microscopic hematuria. Chest radiographs commonly reveal patchy and transient infiltrates, but large and small nodules also have been reported. Thin-section CT findings include bilateral subpleural consolidation with lobular distribution, centrilobular nodules (especially within the ground-glass opacity), or multiple nodules, especially in association with bronchial wall thickening. Pleural effusions may be noted in one-third of cases. The effusions are exudative and may contain a significant number of eosinophils. Common laboratory abnormalities include leukocytosis with marked eosinophilia, a high percentage of BAL eosinophils, prolonged erythrocyte sedimentation rate, and anemia. The IgE level is often markedly increased and appears to correlate with disease activity. In Churg-Strauss syndrome, the prevalence of a positive serum ANCA result ranges from 44 to 66%. The p-ANCA pattern is often present as opposed to the c-ANCA observed in Wegener granulomatosis.

Clinically, there are three distinct phases: (1) a prodromal phase that may persist for many years, consisting of asthma, often preceded by allergic rhinitis; (2) a second phase of marked peripheral blood eosinophilia and eosinophilic tissue infiltrates resembling Loeffler syndrome, or chronic eosinophilic pneumonia, which may recur during a period of years; and (3) a third, life-threatening vasculitic phase.

Survival is dramatically enhanced with treatment. In the past, without treatment, 50% of patients died within 3 months of onset. Myocardial involvement was the most frequent cause of death. In patients treated with corticosteroids, a mean survival of 9 years has been reported. Corticosteroids alone usually are effective in the treatment of Churg-Strauss syndrome. The addition of oral cyclophosphamide may reduce the rate of relapse but has not been shown to improve survival. In patients who fail to respond to corticosteroid therapy, however, "pulse" methylprednisolone, azathioprine, or cyclophosphamide may be effective. It is important to separate the Churg-Strauss syndrome from other necrotizing vasculitides, such as Wegener granulomatosis and polyarteritis nodosa, which may require treatment with cytotoxic agents.

The association of leukotriene antagonists with the Churg-Strauss syndrome originally described in patients taking zafirlukast has now been recognized to occur with montelukast as well and is therefore most likely an uncommon but documented class association with an incidence of approximately 1 in 20,000 patients. The pathophysiology is unknown, but these patients may have had a primary eosinophilic infiltrative disorder that had been clinically recognized as asthma, was quelled by steroid treatment, and was unmasked after corticosteroid withdrawal facilitated by the initiation of the leukotriene inhibitor.

Parasitic Disease: PIE syndrome may develop in conjunction with a number of parasitic infections. In the United States, the most common infections are caused by Strongyloides, Ascaris, Toxocara, and Ancylostoma. The syndrome may arise because of the presence of the parasite in the lung at certain stages of its life cycle. At this point, eosinophils may be recruited to the lung to kill the parasite. Eosinophils have been shown to be present in the lung, however, when parasites are not demonstrable, which suggests that immunologic mechanisms may be involved. GI symptoms usually dominate the clinical picture of parasitic infestation. Respiratory symptoms of cough and wheezing are usually mild. The lung disease commonly resolves with therapy directed at the specific parasite. Corticosteroids usually are not needed.

The most serious and best-characterized parasitic eosinophilic lung disease is tropical pulmonary eosinophilia. This disorder is caused by the filarial worms *Wuchereria bancrofti* and *Brugia malayi*. These organisms are found primarily in India, Africa, South America, and Southeast Asia. Microfilariae released from adult worms cause an intense inflammatory reaction in the lung. This reaction commonly causes nocturnal cough, dyspnea, wheezing, fever, weight loss, and malaise. A history of residence in a filarial endemic region and a finding of peripheral eosinophilia >3,000/mm^3 should initiate a consideration of this disease. Cases of tropical pulmonary eosinophilia typically have been reported to masquerade as acute or refractory asthma. The recommended treatment is diethylcarbamazine. If left untreated or treated late, the disease may lead to long-term sequelae of pulmonary fibrosis or chronic bronchitis with chronic respiratory failure.

Idiopathic Hypereosinophilic Syndrome: Idiopathic hypereosinophilic syndrome is a rare illness of unknown etiology. This disorder affects multiple organ systems, primarily as the result of the infiltration of mature eosinophils. This disorder is likely related to unchecked T-cell secretion of IL-3, IL-5, or granulocyte macrophage colony-stimulating factor. Specific diagnostic criteria for the hypereosinophilic syndrome have been established: (1) peripheral eosinophilia (>1,500 cells per microliter) for 6 months; (2) involvement of various organ systems with evidence of end organ damage; and (3) no evidence of parasitic, allergic, vasculitic, or other known causes of eosinophilia.

The illness may be mild or fatal. The major cause of morbidity and mortality is cardiac disease where endocardial fibrosis; restrictive cardiomyopathy; valvular damage (supportive structures around the valves, especially the mitral valve, are prone to fibrosis); and mural thrombus formation occur. Lung involvement occurs in 40% of cases. Symptoms are nonproductive cough and dyspnea. The chest radiograph may show pulmonary edema and pleural effusions associated with cardiac dysfunction but may also reveal interstitial infiltrates presumably due to perivascular eosinophilic infiltration or fibrosis. Patients usually are treated with oral corticosteroids, but only about 50% will have a good clinical response. Other drugs, such as busulfan, interferon alfa, and hydroxyurea, may be used in steroid-unresponsive patients. Advances in molecular diagnostics have enabled the identification of subtypes of the hypereosinophilic syndrome that may respond to imatinib, a small molecule tyrosine kinase inhibitor. Additionally, studies have reported success in treatment with the use of mepolizumab, which is a monoclonal antibody against IL-5.

Miscellaneous: Bronchogenic carcinoma occasionally is associated with lung and peripheral eosinophilia. Eosinophils have been shown to invade the tumor, which suggests that eosinophils may be involved in host defense against tumors. Hodgkin disease may be associated with peripheral, BAL, and lung eosinophilia. Fungal disease may be associated with peripheral eosinophilia. Peripheral blood eosinophilia is noted in the majority of cases of primary coccidiomycosis. Pulmonary eosinophilic infiltrates may be noted on biopsy specimen or BAL. Administration of corticosteroids to patients early in their infection can result in an acceleration of the infection with possible fatal dissemination. In AIDS-associated *Pneumocystis carinii* pneumonia, 15% of patients had BAL eosinophils >5%. A number of other diseases have been reported to be associated with pulmonary infiltrates and blood or alveolar eosinophilia. They include bronchiolitis obliterans organizing pneumonia, ulcerative colitis, mycobacterial infection, Sjögren syndrome, and postradiation fibrosis.

Parenchymal Disorders (Idiopathic)

Simple Pulmonary Eosinophilia (Loeffler pneumonia): Simple pulmonary eosinophilia was originally described by Loeffler in 1932. This disorder is characterized by migratory pulmonary infiltrates accompanied by peripheral eosinophilia. Respiratory symptoms are minimal or absent. Malaise, fever, and cough may be noted. At times, the chest radiographic pattern may be almost diagnostic, with transitory and migratory ill-defined peripheral, nonsegmental, and relatively homogeneous densities. By definition, the disease resolves within 4 weeks. Afflicted patients have an excellent prognosis. Complete resolution with or without treatment is the rule. In the original description of this disorder, most of the patients likely had a parasitic infection or a drug reaction. Currently, it is estimated that up to one-third of cases do not have a clinically identifiable cause. This latter group is included in the idiopathic eosinophilic pneumonias. Apparent simple pulmonary eosinophilia, however, should be viewed as a sign of possible underlying disease. A careful search for parasitic infection or drug reaction should be pursued.

Chronic Eosinophilic Pneumonia: Although uncommon, this entity is the best characterized of the idiopathic eosinophilic pneumonia syndromes. Both histologic and BAL studies strongly implicate the eosinophil in the pathogenesis of the disorder. A recent study found strikingly increased levels of IL-5, IL-6, and IL-10 in BAL fluid recovered from involved lung segments. No such increase was noted in serum or uninvolved lung segments. Furthermore, the presence of circulating immune complexes, increased levels of IgE, and a frequently positive rheumatoid factor suggest an immunopathogenic mechanism.

Chronic eosinophilic pneumonia (CEP) is a serious disease that requires specific treatment. The disease usually affects middle-aged atopic women, but it has been reported in both sexes and all ages. Onset of the disorder is insidious with progressive respiratory and constitutional symptoms. In one study, symptoms have been present for an average of 7.7 months before the correct diagnosis is made. The most common symptoms are cough, dyspnea, fever, night sweats, malaise, and weight loss. Asthma is present in 50 to 60% of patients and is usually of recent onset. Laboratory evaluation may reveal increased IgE levels, and the levels may correspond to the clinical activity. Peripheral eosinophilia occurs in up to 88%.

Diffuse peripherally based infiltrates in the outer two thirds of the lung fields are found in 63% of patients. On occasion, the chest radiograph may be so characteristic as to be diagnostic. Bilateral peripheral or pleural-based dense infiltrates without segmental or lobar distribution may be noted. These infiltrates may form a pattern described as "the photographic negative of pulmonary edema." Unfortunately, <50% of patients demonstrate this classic plain radiographic picture. A CT scan will reveal peripheral infiltrates in all afflicted. Biopsy specimens show interstitial and alveolar eosinophils that are degranulated. Common findings include eosinophilic microabscesses (which are aggregates of necrotic eosinophils surrounded by a rim of palisading histiocytes), low-grade vasculitis, and interstitial fibrosis. BAL specimens usually show eosinophilia that average 44%.

Fewer than 10% of patients will have spontaneous resolution, and deaths from CEP have been reported. The disease responds quickly and dramatically to corticosteroid therapy. The patient may become asymptomatic in hours or a few days. The prognosis is excellent, but treatment for prolonged periods is usually necessary, at least 6 months. Steroid therapy must be tapered slowly as the disease tends to relapse. If a relapse occurs, treatment must be continued for a prolonged period before trying to taper again.

Acute Eosinophilic Pneumonia: In 1989, several well-documented cases of acute respiratory failure associated with increased BAL or tissue eosinophils were reported. The cause is unknown but may be a unique hypersensitivity reaction to an inhaled antigen. Various drug toxicities have been reported to produce this syndrome. The following diagnostic criteria have been suggested: (1) acute febrile illness of <5 days in duration, (2) hypoxemic respiratory failure, (3) diffuse mixed alveolar and interstitial chest radiographic infiltrates, (4) BAL eosinophilia (>25%), (5) no apparent infectious etiology, (6) rapid and complete response to corticosteroid therapy, and (7) no relapse after discontinuing corticosteroid therapy. Recent studies have suggested that new cigarette smokers may be at increased risk.

Patients typically present with an acute febrile illness accompanied by myalgias, pleuritic chest pain, and hypoxemic respiratory failure, often requiring mechanical ventilation. Clinically, there is little to distinguish acute eosinophilic pneumonia from an acute infectious process or ARDS. It is the BAL that provides the clue to the diagnosis. Peripheral blood eosinophil percentage is usually normal, but a very high percentage of BAL eosinophils is characteristic, with an average of 42% in one series. Small-to-moderate pleural effusions are frequent. Fluid analysis may reveal a high percentage of eosinophils.

Patients usually respond rapidly to high doses of corticosteroids, usually within 24 to 48 h. The dose is then tapered, but treatment is usually continued for 2 to 4 weeks. Most patients survive and recover normal lung function. Acute eosinophilic pneumonia is a diagnosis of exclusion. An infectious etiology should be pursued even after corticosteroid therapy is begun. It is especially important to look closely for disseminated fungal disease in all patients and *P carinii* in the HIV-positive patient.

Conclusion

In these disorders, teleologically, the eosinophil may be: (1) a "good guy," (2) a "bad guy," or (3) an "innocent bystander." The eosinophil may be a good guy. The "host defense" theory builds on the clinical observation that the tissue invasive stages of parasitic infections are associated with a striking eosinophilia. *In vitro* studies have shown that eosinophils can kill parasites. Conversely, the eosinophil may be a bad guy. The eosinophil is activated at sites of inflammation and thus may be responsible for the actual tissue damage. Alternatively, the eosinophil may be an innocent bystander. The appearance of the cell may be part of the body's attempt to dampen or contain the effects of inflammation—the so-called *modulator of inflammation theory*.

Whatever the function of the eosinophil, it is important to remember that the disease processes lumped together as the eosinophilic lung diseases are a heterogeneous group of diseases. In an attempt to categorize these disorders, we may have either appropriately or artificially connected them by their association with the eosinophil.

Annotated Bibliography

"State-of-the-Art" Review

Allen JN, Davis WB. Eosinophilic lung diseases. Am J Respir Crit Care Med 1994; 150:1423–1438
Most authoritative and complete, yet readable, review of the eosinophilic lung diseases. This article should be in your reprint collection as a ready reference.

Jeong YJ, Kim KI, Seo IJ, et al. Eosinophilic lung diseases: a clinical, radiologic, and pathologic overview. Radiographic 2007; 27:617–637
More recent comprehensive review highlighting the radiologic manifestations.

The Eosinophil

Afshar K, Vucinic V, Sharma. Eosinophil cell: pray tell us what you do! Curr Opin Pulm Med 2007; 13:414–421
This review concentrates on the cell rather than the clinical syndromes.

Short Reviews

Alberts WM. Eosinophilic interstitial lung disease. Curr Opin Pulm Med 2004; 10:419–424

Katz U, Shoenfeld Y. Pulmonary eosinophilia. Clin Rev Allerg Immunol 2008; 34:367–371

Wechsler ME. Pulmonary eosinophilic syndromes. Immunol Allergy Clin North Am 2007; 27: 477–492
Shorter reviews with emphasis on the recent literature.

Acute Eosinophilic Pneumonia

Allen J. Acute eosinophilic pneumonia. Semin Respir Crit Care Med 2006; 27:142–147
Short recent review of this entity.

Allen JN, Pacht ER, Gadek JE, et al. Acute eosinophilic pneumonia as a reversible cause of noninfectious respiratory failure. N Engl J Med 1989; 321:569–574

Badesch DB, King TE, Schwarz MI. Acute eosinophilic pneumonia: a hypersensitivity phenomenon? Am Rev Respir Dis 1989; 139:249–252
Original descriptions of the "newest" idiopathic eosinophilic pneumonia.

Chronic Eosinophilic Pneumonia

Alam M, Burki NK. Chronic eosinophilic pneumonia. N Engl J Med 1969; 280:787–798
Original description of the most common idiopathic eosinophilic pneumonia syndrome.

Carrington CB, Addington WW, Goff AM, et al. Chronic eosinophilic pneumonia: a review. South Med J 2007; 100:49–53
Short recent review.

Bronchocentric Granulomatosis

Ortiz-Saracho J, Vidal R, Delgado E, et al. Bronchocentric granulomatosis in a non-asthmatic patient without etiologic agent. Respiration 1996; 63:129–132
In a report of a nonasthmatic patient with bronchogenic granulomatosis, the authors discuss different proposed pathogenetic mechanisms.

Ward S, Heyneman LE, Flint JDA, et al. Bronchocentric granulomatosis: computed tomographic findings in five patients. Clin Radiol 2000; 55:296–300
Discussion of the radiographic findings in this rarely diagnosed disorder.

Allergic Bronchopulmonary Aspergillosis

Lazarus AA, Thilagar B, McKay SA. Diagnosis and treatment of allergic bronchopulmonary aspergillosis. Mayo Clin Proc 2001; 76:930–938

More comprehensive review of the topic.

Vlahakis NE, Aksamit T. Allergic bronchopulmonary aspergillosis. Dis Mon 2008; 54:547–564

Short, but complete, update of this entity. Suitable for a quick review.

Classics in Eosinophilic Pneumonia

Crofton JW, Livingstone JL, Oswald NC, et al. Pulmonary eosinophilia. Thorax 1952; 7:1–35

First attempt to categorize a group of disorders that shared the features of pulmonary infiltrates and peripheral eosinophilia.

Reeder WH, Goodrich BE. Pulmonary infiltration with eosinophilia (PIE syndrome). Ann Intern Med 1952; 36:1217–1240

Reeder and Goodrich coined the term PIE syndrome *in this article.*

Churg-Strauss Syndrome

Alberts WM. Pulmonary manifestations of the Chrug-Strauss syndrome and related idiopathic small vessel vasculitis syndromes. Curr Opin Pulm Med 207; 12:445–450

Excellent short reviews of the pertinent literature with an emphasis on the thoracic manifestations.

Choi YH, Im JG, Han BK, et al. Thoracic manifestations of Churg-Strauss syndrome: radiologic and clinical findings. Chest 2000; 117:117–124

Noth I, Strek ME, Leff AR. Churg-Strauss syndrome. Lancet 2003; 361:587–594

Brief, readable review of this rare disorder.

Parasitic and Tropical Pulmonary Eosinophilia

Chitkara RK, Krishna G. Tropical pulmonary eosinophilia: pathogenesis, diagnosis, and management. Curr Opin Pulm Med 2007; 13:428–432

Review of eosinophilia and pulmonary eosinophilia associated with parasites.

Vijayan VK. Parasitic pulmonary eosinophilia. Semin Respir Crit Care Med 2006; 27:171–184

Excellent discussion of a rare, but becoming more common, cause of eosinophilia.

Nonasthmatic Eosinophilic Bronchitis

Gonlugur U, Gonluger TE. Chronic cough due to nonasthamatic eosinophilic bronchitis. Chest 2006; 129:116S–121S

An underrecognized cause of chronic cough.

Brightling CE. Eosinophilic bronchitis without asthma. Int Arch Allergy Immunol 2008; 147:1–5

Asthma

Sidney S. Braman, MD, FCCP

Objectives:

- Understand the epidemiology of asthma and the contributions of genetic predisposition and environmental factors
- Learn the pathology and pathophysiology of asthma and the importance of inflammatory mechanisms of this disease
- Appreciate the risk factors for asthma and the causes of exacerbation of symptoms
- Be able to objectively and accurately diagnose this disease
- Learn the strategies of treating asthma based on the National Institutes of Health NAEPP (*National Asthma Education and Prevention Program)* guidelines

Key words: asthma; atopy; diagnosis; epidemiology; pathophysiology; treatment

Definition of Asthma

A universally accepted definition of asthma was elusive for most of the 20th century. Many of the clinical and physiologic features appeared to overlap with other diseases of the airways. Although the inflammatory nature of asthma was known in the latter part of the 19th century and was even reported in Sir William Osler's *Textbook of Medicine* during that time period, this important distinctive aspect of asthma was put aside for most of the 20th century.

The definition instead emphasized the clinical and physiologic consequences of reversible bronchospasm and bronchial hyperresponsiveness (BHR). This emphasis resulted in controversy because these two major features of asthma are found in other common pulmonary conditions such as COPD and acute viral tracheobronchitis. During the past decade or so, the emphasis in asthma research and patient care has again shifted to inflammation and the recognition that this distinct feature allows for a more precise definition of this disease.

An expert panel of the National Institutes of Health has provided us with the most widely accepted definition of asthma. The first report of this group was published in 1991. It is often referred to as the *NAEPP Asthma Guidelines.* It was updated as the "Expert Panel Report 3" in 2007. The guidelines define asthma as

> a chronic inflammatory disease of the airways in which many cells play a role, in particular, mast cells, eosinophils, and T lymphocytes. In susceptible individuals this inflammation causes recurrent episodes of wheezing, breathlessness, chest tightness, and cough, particularly at night and/or in the early morning. These symptoms are usually associated with widespread but variable airflow limitation that is at least partially reversible either spontaneously or with treatment. This inflammation also causes an associated increase in airway hyperresponsiveness to a variety of stimuli.

Pathophysiology

Asthma is caused by a complex interaction of cells, mediators, and cytokines that results in inflammation. This interaction causes the following important pathophysiologic changes in asthma patients: airway smooth-muscle contraction, hypertrophy and hyperplasia, microvascular leakage, activation of airway neurons, stimulation of mucus-secreting cells, disruption of the ciliated epithelium, and the laying down of collagen in the lamina reticularis of the basement membrane layer. The characteristic cellular changes involve the following: (1) constitutive cells such as epithelial cells, mucous glands, endothelial cells, and myofibroblasts; (2) resident cells such as bone marrow-derived mast cells and macrophages; and (3) infiltrating cells such as eosinophils, CD4 (helper-cell) T lymphocytes, neutrophils, basophils, and platelets. These inflammatory cells, including histamine, platelet-activating factor, and a number of derivatives of the arachidonic cascade such as prostaglandin (PG) D_2 and the cysteinyl leukotriene (LT) C_4, LTD_4, and LTE_4, are capable of generating a wide variety of mediators that can induce bronchoconstriction. A number of typical histopathologic findings can be found in the airways of patients with asthma.

Histopathologic Findings

Infiltration of the airways by inflammatory cells such as mast cells, eosinophils, activated T lymphocytes, and neutrophils can be demonstrated by bronchial biopsies and inferred by demonstrating increased numbers of these cells in BAL fluid. The extensive bronchial wall infiltration by eosinophils may be accompanied in severe cases by eosinophilic infiltration of the alveolar septae and adjacent arteries. The number of activated lymphocytes found in bronchial biopsy specimens has been correlated with the number of local activated eosinophils and the severity of asthma.

Specific cytokines, most of which are products of lymphocytes and macrophages, appear to direct the movement of cells to the site of airway inflammation. They also activate the cells, causing them to release their mediators. For example, interleukin (IL)-3, IL-5, and granulocyte-macrophage colony-stimulating factor direct eosinophils to release a number of mediators from their preformed granules. These mediators are major basic protein, eosinophil cationic protein, eosinophil-derived neurotoxin, and eosinophil peroxidase. All have inflammatory effects that contribute to the pathogenesis of asthma.

Mast cells, usually as a result of IgE-mediated stimulation, also release preformed mediators, such as histamine and proteases (*eg*, tryptase, chymotryptase, carboxypeptidase, and kininogenase) and further act as a regulator of inflammation by producing cytokines that promote eosinophil infiltration and activation. Several mast-cell products (histamine, LTC_4, and PGD_2) are smooth-muscle constrictors and, hence, induce bronchoconstriction. LTs also cause increased mucus secretion. Increased vascular permeability is caused by histamine, LTC_4, platelet-activating factor, and bradykinin.

Denudation of the airway epithelium can lead to airway edema and the loss of substances in the mucosa that protect the airway. Epithelial damage promotes BHR because access by irritating substances to sensory nerve endings is increased. Similarly, aeroallergens can more readily penetrate the airways. It is believed that eosinophil-derived basic proteins, together with partial reductive products of oxygen and proteases, contribute to epithelial fragility. Regeneration first appears as simple or stratified squamous epithelium before differentiation and maturation to new ciliated and mucus (goblet) cells.

One of the characteristic findings in patients with severe asthma is the presence of tenacious mucus plugs in the airways. There are approximately 20 mammalian mucin genes. There are identified with the letters MUC followed by a number. MUC5AC is the principal mucin up-regulated by asthma inflammation. Strategies to suppress mucin secretion may be possible in the future. Death from asthma usually occurs from blockage of the airways by diffuse mucus plugging. In fatal asthma, evidence shows >98% of the airways are occluded to some extent with mucus. The presence of mucus is associated with hyperplasia and metaplasia of goblet cells; it may cause lung hyperinflation caused by the trapping of air or, when more severe and located in central airways, can cause atelectasis.

Edema of the airway mucosa is caused by increased capillary permeability with leakage of serum proteins into the interstitium. A number of cell-derived mediators are capable of inducing edema formation, including histamine, PGE, LTC_4, LTD_4, LTE_4, platelet-activating factor, and bradykinin. The intense mucosal thickening in asthma contributes to the airway wall thickness and, therefore, airway wall narrowing.

Growing evidence points to asthma as a disease of airway wall restructuring that involves the activation of the epithelial mesenchymal trophic unit (EMTU). Inflammatory cells and mediators interact with the EMTU to cause the changes we refer to as *airway remodeling*. The airway epithelium becomes an important source of mediators, growth factors, and chemokines that perpetuate the inflammatory and repair response. Biopsy studies in patients with chronic asthma have shown a number of pathologic changes that support the hypothesis of increased release of fibroproliferative and fibrogenic growth factors in *in vivo* models of asthma. Growth factors that are thought to be important in asthma include fibroblast growth factor-2, insulin-like growth factor-1, platelet-derived growth factor, endothelin-1, and transforming growth factor-β.

Thickening of the reticular basement membrane, the laminar reticularis, is observed with light microscopy, is a constant feature of asthma, and is diagnostic of the disease. In other chronic respiratory diseases such as COPD, bronchiectasis, and tuberculosis, basement membrane thickening appears to be more focal and variable.

There is evidence of increased bronchial smooth-muscle mass that contributes considerably to the thickness of the airway wall. The smooth muscle of asthmatic patients does not behave abnormally after isolation; there is no correlation between airway hyperresponsiveness *in vivo* and increased airway muscle sensitivity measures *in vitro*. New evidence suggests that the smooth-muscle cell may secrete cytokines and chemokines and express cellular adhesion molecules. Therefore, the smooth muscle that traditionally has been thought of only as a passive effector cell of asthma, responsible for bronchomotor tone, may also contribute to the inflammation of asthma. This immunomodulatory function of the smooth muscle is similar to that found in epithelial cells. There is also evidence that smooth-muscle cells in the airways are capable of producing growth factors that can themselves promote proliferation in an autocrine manner. The airway architecture is changed by the deposition of type III and V collagen and fibronectin beneath the basement membrane. This deposition has been referred to as subepithelial fibrosis. Increased numbers of myofibroblasts are also seen in the reticular layer in biopsy material obtained from asthmatic patients. There is a microvascular component to airway remodeling in asthma, with evidence of angiogenesis in biopsy material and increased levels of vascular endothelial growth factor in BAL fluid and sputum.

The structural changes that occur in the airways of asthmatic patients are likely to be detrimental and contribute to fixed airway narrowing. This is particularly true in patients with severe asthma. Biopsy studies have shown the changes of airway remodeling in such patients despite treatment with high doses of inhaled and oral corticosteroids. Thickening the inner airway wall may also amplify the degree of luminal narrowing for a given degree of smooth-muscle shortening, which might result in an exaggerated narrowing of the airway after a bronchoconstricting stimulus. It has been argued that some aspects of remodeling have beneficial effects, as follows: stiffening the airway may result in decreased compressibility allowing the airways to better resist dynamic compression; and extra connective tissue surrounding the smooth-muscle cells may provide a radial constraint to maximal shortening.

Physiologic Mechanisms

Neurogenic Influences: There is growing evidence that the neural control of the airways is abnormal in patients with asthma and that neurogenic mechanisms may augment or modulate the inflammatory response. The autonomic nervous system regulates many aspects of airway function, such as airway tone, airway secretions, blood flow, microvascular permeability, and the release of inflammatory cells. A primary defect in autonomic control, the β-adrenergic receptor theory, has been postulated for asthma. It is more likely, however, that autonomic dysfunction is a secondary defect caused by inflammation or by the effects of treatment. For instance, inflammatory mediators can modulate the release of neurotransmitters from airway nerves such as irritant receptors and C-fiber endings. They can also directly act on autonomic receptors such as those that cause reflex bronchoconstriction from gastroesophageal reflux.

There is also evidence that the nonadrenergic, noncholinergic nervous system is important in the pathogenesis of asthma. As the airway epithelium becomes denuded, sensory nerve endings may become exposed, causing a release of potent neuropeptides such as substance P, neurokinin A, and calcitonin gene-related protein. These neuromediators can lead to bronchoconstriction, microvascular leakage, and mucus hypersecretion.

This neurogenic inflammation of the airways, triggered by sensitized sensory nerve endings, has been postulated to cause airway "hyperalgesia" and result in symptoms such as cough and chest tightness. Nitric oxide (NO) also appears to be one of the neurotransmitters of the nonadrenergic, noncholinergic system and is an important braking mechanism that can initiate bronchodilation.

BHR: Airway inflammation is thought to be a key factor in producing BHR, which is a cardinal feature of asthma. This inflammation can be described as an exaggerated bronchoconstrictive response by the airways to a variety of stimuli such as aeroallergens, histamine, methacholine, cold air, and environmental irritants. It is not clear whether bronchial hyperreactivity is acquired or is present at birth and genetically determined to appear with the appropriate stimulus. It is thought that airway inflammation is the stimulus for BHR because it may be induced by a number of inciting events. These events include viral respiratory infections, an IgE-mediated allergic reaction, and the inhalation of noxious agents such as ozone or sulfur dioxide. Antiinflammatory agents such as inhaled corticosteroids (ICS) are effective in reducing BHR.

The degree of BHR can be determined in the pulmonary function laboratory by standard inhalation challenge testing. The methacholine and histamine inhalation challenges are the most frequently used clinical tools to determine the presence and degree of BHR. Cold air and hypotonic saline solution challenges also are performed. Although the end result of this testing, airway narrowing, is the same for these provocative agents, the mechanisms that cause the airways to constrict vary. Methacholine and histamine act directly on airway smooth muscle. Exercise and hyperosmolar or hypoosmolar solutions act indirectly by releasing pharmacologically active substances from mediator-secreting cells such as mast cells. Sulfur dioxide and bradykinin act by directly stimulating airway sensory nerve endings.

The inhalation of hypertonic saline solution or mannitol and adenosine 5′-monophosphate have been advocated as producing more diagnostic provocation for asthma than histamine or methacholine but have not attained widespread use clinically. The degree of BHR usually correlates with the clinical severity of asthma and the medication needs of the patient. In addition, fluctuations of diurnal peak flow measurements correlate with the degree of BHR.

Airway Obstruction: Airway obstruction is another cardinal feature of asthma. The causes of airflow limitation in patients with asthma are listed in Table 1. During an acute asthma attack, lung hyperinflation occurs. This results in an increase in lung elastic recoil forces, which act on the airways to prevent further narrowing. This occurs because of the interdependence of lung volume and airway caliber because parenchymal attachments cause greater tethering of the airways at greater lung volumes.

Table 1. *Causes of Airflow Limitation in Asthma*

Acute bronchoconstriction
Mucus plugging of airways
Bronchial wall edema
Inflammatory cell infiltration
Airway wall remodeling (fibrosis)
Smooth-muscle hypertrophy
Uncoupling of elastic recoil forces

Inflammation of the bronchial wall, however, may uncouple the mechanical linkage between the parenchyma and the airway, which may contribute to airway narrowing and also to BHR. During an acute attack of asthma, airway resistance increases, and all measures of airflow (*eg*, peak expiratory flow rate [PEFR], FEV_1, FEV_1/FVC ratio, and specific conductance) are abnormal. During remission, the results of these tests may be normal, and yet considerable dysfunction may be present in peripheral airways. Studies in which the authors used a wedged bronchoscope technique have shown that peripheral resistance can be 10-fold greater than that in healthy subjects. There is evidence that this resistance is linked to BHR. In many asthmatic patients, particularly children and younger adults with milder disease, airflow obstruction is completely reversible. In most elderly asthmatic patients and those of any age group with more severe and persistent symptoms, airflow obstruction is only partially reversible despite continuous intense antiinflammatory and bronchodilator therapy, including large doses of oral corticosteroids. The reasons for these permanent physiologic changes remain obscure, and it is suspected that airway remodeling is, at least in part, responsible.

Atopic Asthma

Atopy may be defined as the largely genetic susceptibility for developing IgE directed to epitopes expressed on common environmental allergens such as dust mites, animal proteins, pollens, and fungi. Atopic (allergic) reactions in the upper airways (*eg*, nose and sinuses) and lower airways are both important in the pathogenesis of asthma. The term *extrinsic asthma* has been used to describe asthma that is triggered by exposure to inhaled aeroallergens. Cellular responses may occur with the first exposure to a specific antigen in such genetically predisposed individuals. The antigen is trapped in airway mucus and is exposed to underlying epithelial cells and resident dendritic (Langerhans) cells. As the antigen penetrates beneath the mucosa, it is likely exposed to granulocytes and tissue macrophages and eventually enters the lymphatic system after enzymatic degradation.

In performing these functions, antigen-presenting cells (APCs) are setting the stage for subsequent lymphocyte activation to occur. It is not definitely known which cells are the APCs. There is a key role for naive $CD4^+$ T thymocytes (called *TH0 cells*). As they come in contact with the antigen on the APCs, these lymphocytes become differentiated and activated ($CD4^+/CD25^+$ state). The specific subclass of TH0 cells that become differentiated during this allergic reaction are called *TH2 cells* and are to be distinguished from the TH1 subclass that is associated with the delayed hypersensitivity reaction. The TH2 subclass is associated with the release of specific ILs and other cytokines that are responsible for episodic and chronic allergic reactions. For example, in the sensitization stage, the release of IL-4 enhances the synthesis of IgEs by antigen stimulated B lymphocytes (plasma cells). IgE infiltrates the airways and becomes fixed to mast cells, basophils, and dendritic cells through high-affinity cell surface receptors. This step sets the stage for the acute allergic response with the inhalation of more antigens.

This reaction can be divided into an early (minutes after exposure) bronchospastic response and a late (hours after exposure) inflammatory response. First, the antigen bridges to at least two IgE antibodies. Then, mast-cell degranulation and synthesis of proinflammatory molecules occurs. The synthesized mediators are IL-3, IL-4, IL-5, tumor necrosis factor (TNF)-α, granulocyte-macrophage colony-stimulating factor, and arachidonic acid derivatives LTs, PGD_2, and thromboxane A_2. The late-phase response is initiated by mast-cell mediators as follows: IL-5 is a chemoattractant for eosinophils, IL-3 and IL-5 are chemoattractants for basophils, LTB_4 appears to attract neutrophils, and TNF-α increases the number of adhesion molecules on endothelial cells that enhance the adhesion of leukocytes.

The formation of antigen-specific IgE antibody usually does not occur until the second or third year of life. The prevalence of allergic asthma is, therefore, less common during infancy. Allergen exposure during infancy to cat antigen has been shown to be a predictor of skin test sensitivity and asthma at age 6 years. The prevalence of atopy increases throughout childhood and adolescence and peaks in the second decade of life. Sensitization to indoor aeroallergens (*eg*, dust mites, cockroaches, molds, and animals) and outdoor aeroallergens (*eg*, pollens and molds) may be an important cause of acute and chronic recurrent symptoms in patients in these age groups. Often allergic asthma has a well-defined seasonal variation; avoidance of the offending antigen may result in a dramatic improvement of symptoms and in pulmonary function and BHR.

Nonatopic Asthma

The term *intrinsic asthma* is used to describe patients who have none of the typical features of atopy, including a positive family history of allergy and asthma, positive immediate hypersensitivity reactions to skin-prick tests after exposure to a variety of aeroallergens, and an increased serum IgE level. Usually, such patients are older than atopic asthmatic patients and have a later onset of asthma. Bronchial biopsy studies in patients with intrinsic asthma have been compared with a group of patients with extrinsic asthma with a comparable severity of symptoms. There is a more intense inflammatory cell infiltrate in the bronchial mucosa of the intrinsic asthmatic patients with leukocytes, macrophages, and CD3 and CD4 cells. Patients with intrinsic asthma have an exaggerated T-cell response to maintain the same degree of symptoms and BHR. This may mean that intrinsic asthma may involve activation by an as-yet unidentified antigen. Putative nonallergic antigens that may cause such reactions include viral antigens or inappropriately recognized "self-antigens."

Risk Factors for Asthma

Genetics of Asthma

Although it is generally agreed that there is a major hereditary contribution to the etiology of asthma, the inheritance patterns are complex, and asthma cannot be simply classified as having an autosomal-dominant, autosomal-recessive, or sex-linked mode of inheritance. This may be in large part caused by the marked heterogeneity of the asthma phenotype. For example, the role of contributing factors such as atopy, viruses, aspirin sensitivity, exercise, and occupational exposure differs greatly among patients with asthma. Variability in clinical symptoms, severity of disease, degree of BHR, and response to therapy are other examples of disease heterogeneity. However, genetic studies have discovered multiple chromosomal regions that may contain genes that contribute to asthma. High serum IgE levels have been linked to chromosomes 5q, 11q, and 12q. Clinically, there is a strong correlation between BHR and increased IgE levels, and evidence shows there is coinheritance of genes for atopy and BHR found on these same chromosomes.

Population studies that have conducted genome-wide screens have contributed to our understanding of the inheritance of asthma. They have shown the linkage of asthma, BHR, total IgE levels, and elevated eosinophil counts to multiple chromosomal regions. Chromosomes 2q, 3p, 5q, 6p, 12q, 13q, 19q, and 21q are likely to contain genes for allergy and asthma. These genome screens also have found numerous loci that contain potential candidate genes that can regulate the immune response of asthma. For example, genes that regulate IgE production, β_2-adrenergic and glucocorticoid receptor function, and the inflammatory mediator response have been found. They may be important in determining genetic susceptibility, responses to environmental stimuli, and responses to treatment.

After the identification and characterization of the β-receptor gene, variants of the gene were evaluated to see whether they could be responsible for the expression of asthma. One mutation (the substitution of glycine for arginine at position 16) was associated with more severe asthma and especially with more severe nocturnal symptoms. This mutation causes an increase in the degree of agonist-promoted down-regulation of receptor expression. Studies by researchers in China have shown that the increased risk for the development of asthma in homozygotes for this allele is profoundly affected by cigarette smoking. Another mutant at position 27 renders the receptor more resistant to β-agonist down-regulation and has been associated with less intense BHR in patients with asthma. Genes determining the specificity of the immune response also may be important to the pathogenesis of asthma. Genes located on the human leukocyte antigen complex may govern the response to aeroallergens in some individuals. Genes on chromosomes 11, 12, and 13 may direct the control of proinflammatory cytokines. Chromosome 12, for example, contains genes that encode for interferon-7, mast-cell growth factor, insulin-like growth factor, and NO synthase. Polymorphisms of the *IL4RA* gene have been associated with severe exacerbations and poor lung function, and the *ADAM33* gene, which is expressed on smooth-muscle cells, fibroblasts, and myofibroblasts and plays a role in cell signaling, appears to be a susceptibility gene for asthma and is associated with an accelerated decrease in lung function. It should be noted that despite many encouraging reports, most studies on the genetics of asthma that show an association between asthma-related phenotypes and alleles within a specific gene have generally lacked statistical power.

Sex and Race

Childhood asthma is more prevalent in boys, but this prevalence is reversed in puberty and adulthood. The overall prevalence, therefore, is greater in female individuals. Black race/ethnicity is associated with a greater risk of asthma death, independent of socioeconomic status and education. The greater incidence of asthma that has been observed with urbanization suggests that environmental factors maybe as important as genetic and racial factors. In fact, subjects of different races acquire the risk of the population to which they move.

Environmental Factors

Allergens and occupational factors are considered to be the most important causes of asthma. Several epidemiologic studies have shown a correlation between allergen exposure and the prevalence of asthma and the improvement of asthma when allergen exposure ceases. Important indoor allergens include domestic (house dust) mites; animal allergens (*eg*, cats, dogs, and rodents); cockroach allergen; and fungi (Alternaria, Aspergillus, Cladosporium, and Candida sp). House dust is composed of several organic and inorganic compounds, including insects and insect feces, mold spores, mammalian dander, pollen grains, fibers, mites, and mite feces. Outdoor allergens include pollens (mainly from trees, weeds, and grasses); fungi; molds; and yeasts. Occupational asthma is discussed in a later section.

Air Pollution

Both outdoor and indoor pollutants contribute to worsening asthma symptoms by triggering bronchoconstriction, increasing BHR, and enhancing responses to inhaled aeroallergens. The two main outdoor pollutants are industrial smog (sulfur dioxide particulate complex) and photochemical smog (ozone and nitrogen oxides). Whether long-term exposure is further injurious is not clear. Modern construction techniques have been suspected of causing greater indoor air pollution. In energy-efficient buildings, there is 50% less turnover of fresh air. Indoor pollutants include cooking and heating fuel exhausts as well as insulating products, paints, and varnishes that contain formaldehyde and isocyanates. Long-term passive cigarette smoke exposure has been linked to new-onset asthma in children and adults as well as worsening asthma symptoms in those with preexisting asthma. The effect of cleaning solutions and sprays in the home a number of times a week has been linked to an increased risk of asthma developing. Health-care professionals also have increased odds of asthma developing when exposed to aerosolized irritants, cleaning solutions, nebulized medications, and powdered latex gloves. Nurses show the greatest risk; there is a correlation with the length of time on the job.

Respiratory Infections

The role of respiratory infections in the pathogenesis of asthma has been under intense investigation. It has been established that viral respiratory infections are common precipitators of asthma. Whether they can initiate the disease *de novo* is suspected but has not been strongly suggested. There are strong data to suggest that some of the atypical bacteria, such as *Chlamydia pneumoniae* and *Mycoplasma pneumoniae*, also may be involved. These organisms are temporally related to exacerbations of asthma and can be found by the use of polymerase chain reaction techniques to be present in bronchial biopsy specimens obtained from patients with chronic stable asthma. There have also been reports of asthma appearing for the first time after an active infection with both of these organisms, as well as significant improvement in lung function and symptoms with antimicrobial therapy directed to these organisms. In one prospective study, *M pneumoniae* or *C pneumoniae* was found in the airways of >60% of a group of stable patients with chronic asthma. Therapy with the macrolide antibiotic clarithromycin improved lung function and decreased tissue expression of IL-5 in those patients who were polymerase chain reaction positive to these organisms. This finding suggests that antibiotic use in some patients with persistent asthma may help to control the disease.

Allergic Rhinitis

Nasal and sinus diseases are common comorbidities in patients with asthma. Allergic rhinitis (AR) and asthma commonly occur together; >40% of children with AR have asthma. Furthermore, the presence of AR in a child <7 years of age predicts future asthma; smokers with AR have a threefold increased risk for developing asthma. Whether this risk is because AR and asthma are the same disease process or are two different diseases that affect the same susceptible population is not known. The fact that the eosinophilic and lymphocytic inflammation in the upper and lower airways are the same, and also that the severity of both diseases occurs in parallel, support the former theory. It has been discovered that patients with AR, despite the paucity of pulmonary symptoms, have abnormal lung function and, when tested with methacholine or histamine, demonstrate BHR. Exhaled NO also has shown to be increased in such patients, and bronchial biopsies have demonstrated eosinophils and mast cells. There has been considerable interest in whether treatment of the upper airway improves asthma control. Retrospective studies suggest it, but prospective studies have been disappointing.

Other Factors

A number of interesting epidemiologic associations have come to light concerning the risk of the development of asthma and atopy. For instance, being underweight and being overweight are both associated with an increased risk of the development of asthma. There is some evidence that weight loss in obese asthmatic patients is associated with improved symptoms and lung function, especially PEFR variability. Growing up on a farm decreases the risk of atopy and allergic rhinitis in adulthood, suggesting that environmental factors may have a lifelong protective effect against the development of allergy. In developing countries, the move to cities is associated with a switch from biomass fuels such as wood, charcoal, and animal wastes to gas and electricity. The use of modern fuels has been associated with an increased rate of allergic sensitization and symptoms. Studies indicate a reverse relationship between family size and asthma. This finding and others suggest that the exposure of young children to older children at home or to children at day-care centers protects against the development of asthma. There has been some suggestion that the use of dietary antioxidants may protect against the development of asthma. In one study, for example, the severity of asthma was negatively associated with the consumption of red wine. This is another bit of evidence to suggest that flavonoids and other dietary antioxidants may protect against asthma.

The Natural History of Asthma

The most reliable information on the natural history of asthma comes from large community surveys. Comparisons from country to country and even within the same country are difficult to make because of the varying criteria used to make the diagnosis and the inclusion of cigarette smokers who might also have underlying COPD. The peak prevalence of asthma in all studies is in childhood and is approximately 10% of the population. This rate decreases to approximately 5 to 6% in adolescence and early adulthood, when remission rates are quite high. The prevalence increases again during later adulthood to 7 to 9%.

The relationship of atopy and asthma has been carefully studied. In children and adults, the presence of bronchial hyperreactivity correlates with the presence and number of positive immediate hypersensitivity skin test results to inhalant allergens. The presence of positive skin test results in infants of allergic parents correlates with the onset of asthma in later childhood, and the number of positive skin test results shows a correlation with the severity of asthma in childhood and early adulthood. Studies correlating skin test reactivity to house dust mite exposure and asthma also strongly implicate atopy in the pathogenesis of asthma. One alternative theory is that there is one common mechanism involved in the development of both IgE-mediated hypersensitivity and bronchial hyperreactivity or that the two may be related by genetic linkage. This would suggest that there is not a causal relation between atopy and asthma and would explain why certain patients (intrinsic asthmatic patients) have no allergic basis for their asthma.

It has been stated that most patients with asthma during childhood will outgrow it by early adulthood. Statistics show that this is true in only 30 to 50% of children with asthma and is more likely in male patients than in female patients. Lung growth appears to be relatively normal in children with asthma but can be reduced in some with more severe and persistent symptoms. Even in those who become asymptomatic at puberty, lung function frequently remains abnormal, and cough and BHR persist. The following three features of childhood asthma may predict those who are more likely to have persistent symptoms into adulthood: severe atopy determined by skin testing; a marked degree of bronchial reactivity; and difficult-to-control asthma. This is particularly evident in young girls. Elevations in serum IgE levels, eosinophilia, and skin test reactivity to aeroallergens are seen in children with persistent wheezing from early childhood to later childhood but not in those who wheeze in the first 6 years of life but outgrow their wheezing by age 6 years (*ie*, transient wheezers).

In adulthood, there is a steady incidence of new-onset asthma through patients of all ages, even in elderly patients. Many patients begin with recurrent wheezing after respiratory viral infections. This pattern may gradually or abruptly develop into persistent wheezing and often severe, poorly responsive disease. At other times, asthma develops explosively, with no previous respiratory symptoms, immediately after the onset of a typical viral respiratory infection. Longitudinal studies of asthmatic patient populations have shown that although remission from asthma is common in the second decade, it is much less common in older age groups, although it still may be as high as 20 to 30%. Asthmatic subjects who have severe symptoms, reduced ventilatory function, and a concomitant diagnosis of COPD are much less likely to experience remission. Not infrequently, heavy cigarette smokers in whom COPD has developed may also manifest acute bronchospasm that is responsive to therapy with inhaled bronchodilators. This pattern is similar to that seen with asthma. Because of the underlying emphysema and chronic bronchitis, these patients have an element of irreversible airflow obstruction, and they often are labeled as having asthmatic bronchitis to distinguish them from those with pure asthma and to identify the irreversible component of their disease. Unlike some adult asthmatic patients, those patients with asthmatic bronchitis will not ever have a complete remission of their disease. Asthma may also result from exposure to occupational hazards. Remission usually occurs when the patient is removed from the offending environment, but unfortunately, this is not always the case.

Clinical Features of Asthma

Symptoms of Asthma

The typical triad of symptoms of asthma is wheezing, shortness of breath, and cough with or without sputum production. These symptoms are not specific for asthma and can be seen in other acute and chronic airway diseases. For example, an acute viral tracheobronchitis associated with or after typical upper respiratory infection symptoms can cause the asthma triad of symptoms and can be associated with BHR for up to 6 weeks. Unlike asthma, these symptoms usually resolve completely over time. COPD caused by emphysema and chronic bronchitis can also cause typical asthma symptoms, and the distinction between these conditions can become quite difficult, especially when COPD is complicated by acute viral or irritant-induced bronchospasm.

In general, the symptoms of asthma are considerably more episodic and of more sudden onset than those of COPD, and periods of prolonged remission are typical. Attacks of asthma are likely to be provoked by known aeroallergens, especially in the younger atopic population. It is not unusual for asthmatic patients to have a history of wheezing and shortness of breath after exposure to household pets such as cats and dogs. Sensitivity to rats, guinea pigs, and other small animals may similarly develop in animal handlers and laboratory workers. Asthma may occur seasonally, such as during ragweed season in the fall or during flower and tree blooming in the spring. It is believed that exposure to household mites that live in bedding, in floor rugs, and on other fabrics found in the house also is a major cause of asthma symptoms, especially in warmer climates that favor their growth. Similarly, in areas of the inner city, especially where poverty is found, cockroach exposure is an important inciting agent of atopic asthma.

The immediate hypersensitivity reaction (atopic reaction) has two phases, an immediate reaction that causes symptoms within minutes after exposure and a delayed reaction that occurs up to 6 h after exposure. Sometimes exposure to an aeroallergen results in a predominantly delayed allergic reaction. The patient may not recognize the offending agent since the exposure has occurred many hours previously.

Typically, the triad of symptoms of asthma presents simultaneously, but this is not always the case. There is evidence that some patients with asthma perceive their symptoms poorly. In studies of acutely ill asthmatic patients, up to 10% of them have no shortness of breath and complain only of wheezing and cough. The reasons for the lack of dyspnea remain obscure, but the following several observations are relevant:

- Asthmatic subjects have a greater threshold for tolerating resistive loads than normal subjects.
- Asthmatic subjects with greater resting baseline airflow obstruction are less likely to perceive worsening lung function after a cholinergic inhalation challenge.
- Symptoms caused by a precipitous decrease in lung function caused by the immediate hypersensitivity reaction are better perceived than those that may occur as a result of a slower equal decline in lung function caused by the late-onset reaction.
- Abnormalities in the perception of asthma symptoms have important therapeutic implications, *eg*, an asthmatic patient who is not able to

detect increased airway resistance will not reach for appropriate medication when necessary.

- Finally, it has been postulated that poor perception of asthma in some patients may be responsible for fatal and near-fatal attacks, especially in the elderly because impaired perception of bronchospasm is also a feature of aging. Objective monitoring of airway function by means of spirometry and peak flowmeters is essential for asthma prevention.

Other variant manifestations of asthma also occur. Patients with asthma may present with only cough or dyspnea as isolated symptoms. A nonproductive cough may be present for years as a sign of asthma before the full triad of symptoms begins. Cough is probably caused by the stimulation of airway sensory nerves by inflammatory mediators. The asthmatic cough is often provoked by respiratory irritants such as cigarette smoke and by cold air, laughter, and cough itself. Many times, a single cough will begin a series of violent coughing paroxysms that may last for many minutes and lead to exhaustion. Cough may be provoked also by deep inhalation and by forced exhalation. This mechanism may be useful as a bedside test because a coughing paroxysm induced by a deep-breathing maneuver suggests hyperreactive asthmatic airways.

Because patients with isolated cough or dyspnea may have normal findings on pulmonary function studies, reversible airflow obstruction may not be possible to document. In such cases, bronchoprovocation testing with histamine or methacholine may be useful in making the proper diagnosis. Other symptoms of asthma are chest tightness, substernal pressure, chest pain, and nocturnal awakenings. These symptoms are more likely to be confused with cardiac disease, especially ischemic heart disease, in the older individual. Gastroesophageal reflux also causes a feeling of chest tightness in addition to heartburn. Reflux can exacerbate asthma, especially in children, and sometimes the treatment of reflux can result in improvement of asthma. In patients with symptomatic reflux, upper respiratory symptoms are very common, and they can be confused with the symptoms of asthma. For example, cough may be the sole presenting manifestation of gastroesophageal reflux. Symptoms of nasal and laryngeal irritation are common to both gastroesophageal reflux and asthma, and objective measures of airway disease can be helpful in distinguishing the two.

Physical Signs of Asthma

The physical findings associated with acute bronchospasm of asthma are (1) the direct result of diffuse airway narrowing and hypersecretion of mucus, and (2) the indirect result of reflex influences from an increase in the work of breathing, increased metabolic demands on the body, and diffuse sympathetic nervous discharge. Tachypnea and tachycardia are universal features of acute asthma. The average respiratory rate is between 25 and 28 breaths/min, and the average pulse rate is 100 beats/min. Respiratory rates of >30 breaths/min and heart rates of >120 beats/min are not uncommon and may be seen in as many as 25 to 30% of patients.

Sinus tachycardia is also a known complication of asthma therapy that occurs with the use of drugs such as sympathomimetics and theophylline. Usually, however, because airway function improves with sympathomimetic treatment, sinus tachycardia actually improves rather than worsens. In patients with acute asthma, premature ventricular contractions occur occasionally, whereas atrial arrhythmias are extremely uncommon. Other ECG abnormalities seen in acute severe asthma include P-pulmonale, right axis shift, right bundle-branch block, and right ventricular strain.

Diffuse musical wheezes are characteristic of asthma, but their presence or intensity does not reliably predict the severity of asthma. By the time wheezing can be detected by stethoscope, peak flow rates may be decreased by as much as $\geq 25\%$. In general, wheezing during inspiration and expiration, loud wheezing, and high-pitched wheezing are associated with greater airway obstruction. In very severe cases, wheezing may be absent. This suggests very poor air movement and impending respiratory failure.

A prolonged phase of exhalation is typically seen, as is chest hyperinflation. These are the result of airflow obstruction and trapped air, respectively. Accessory muscle use, pulsus paradoxus, and diaphoresis are associated with severe airflow obstruction, although their absence does not rule out a severe attack. Cyanosis and signs of acute hypercarbic acidosis, such as mental obtundation, are absent in all but extreme cases. Accessory muscle use and pulsus paradoxus are caused by large negative changes in intrapleural pressure, and they may not be manifest in the patient with rapid, shallow breathing. They are reported to be present in 30 to 40% of patients with acute asthma.

Objective Measures of Asthma and Asthma Severity

The use of objective measurements of pulmonary function is important in patients with asthma because the perception of asthma symptoms often is poor and the physician's findings on physical examination may either overestimate or underestimate the severity of the airflow obstruction. The following four tests of pulmonary function are extremely useful for establishing the diagnosis of asthma and/or for following the clinical course of the patient once the diagnosis has been made: (1) spirometry, (2) PEFR measurements with a peak flowmeter, (3) arterial blood gas analysis, and (4) bronchoprovocation testing.

During an acute attack of asthma, on average the FEV_1 is reduced to approximately 30 to 35% of predicted, and the FVC to approximately 50% of predicted. The FEV_1 in absolute terms is reduced to approximately 1 L. The PEFR is reduced to approximately 150 L/min. Reversible airflow obstruction is characteristic of asthma and can be demonstrated by spirometry: a >15% improvement in the FEV_1 (and an absolute value >200 mL) 5 to 10 min after treatment with a short-acting inhaled β-agonist generally is accepted as a significant change. Alternatively, after outpatient treatment, a >15% improvement in the FEV_1 between office visits proves the presence of reversible airway disease and supports a diagnosis of asthma.

Short-term home monitoring with the PEFR meter can be useful in the diagnosis of asthma and identification of environmental triggers of asthma and also can be used to detect early signs of deterioration when symptoms change. Long-term monitoring is useful for those with severe brittle asthma and for those who have a poor perception of asthma symptoms. Peak flow measurements ideally should be performed early in the morning (when measurements tend to be lowest) and in the evening (when they should be highest), 5 to 10 min after the patient inhales a β-agonist. Each patient should establish a personal best PEFR after a period of maximal therapy. The severity of asthma is reflected not only by the level of baseline obstruction but also its variability during a 24-h period. A zone system has been provided by the NAEPP guidelines for patient ease, as follows: green is 80 to 100% of the personal best and shows good control; yellow is 50 to 80% of the personal best and signals caution that asthma is not under sufficient control, and red is <50% of personal best and signifies danger and the need for immediate physician intervention.

A diurnal variation in PEFR of 20% is diagnostic of asthma. The magnitude of peak flow variability is in general proportional to the severity of the disease. A high degree of variability signals unstable asthma that demands increased medication. Virtually all asthmatic patients have hypoxemia during an acute exacerbation; the more severe the attack, the lower the arterial oxygen tension. Arterial blood gas analysis is helpful during a severe attack. During an acute attack, an assessment of oxygen saturation by transcutaneous oximetry is helpful to ensure adequate oxygenation. The mechanism of arterial hypoxemia is ventilation/perfusion mismatch. Areas with low ventilation/perfusion ratios cause hypoxemia and are caused by bronchospasm, mucus plugging, and mucosal swelling from inflammation.

Hypocarbia and respiratory alkalosis are present in approximately 75% of patients with acute asthma. When the obstruction worsens and the FEV_1 approaches about 15 to 20% of predicted, the Pco_2 normalizes. Carbon dioxide retention occurs when the FEV_1 reaches <15% of predicted and the absolute FEV_1 is very severely reduced to ≤0.5 L. Acute respiratory acidosis results. This occurs in approximately 10% of asthmatic patients who seek emergency care. The mechanism of carbon dioxide retention in patients with severe asthma is severe ventilation-perfusion mismatch. High ventilation/perfusion ratios result in dead space or wasted ventilation. As the work of breathing increases and carbon dioxide production rises, the lungs become incapable of removing the carbon dioxide that is produced, and respiratory acidosis occurs.

It is believed that respiratory muscle fatigue also contributes to respiratory failure and, in extreme cases, sudden respiratory muscle failure can result in acute cardiopulmonary arrest. Superimposed metabolic acidosis is observed on blood gas analysis in severe cases. This may be the result of lactic acidosis caused by vigorous muscle contraction or to inadequate cardiac output and may possibly be seen as a complication of excessive symptomatic use. Inhalation challenge testing is useful in some patients when the diagnosis of asthma is not secure. This occurs when the patient has normal peak flow rates and spirometry findings yet typical asthma symptoms are present. In such cases, an FEV_1 response to an inhaled bronchodilator cannot be used as a criterion for asthma. If the fluctuation in diurnal PEFR is also not useful, methacholine or histamine bronchoprovocation testing can be helpful. Low concentrations of the agonist are inhaled after baseline spirometry ensures normal or nearly normal airway function.

Gradually increasing doses are administered, either by tidal volume breathing or by single deep breaths from a dosimeter, and the forced spirogram is repeated after each dose. A calculation of the FEV_1 at the administration of each dose produces a dose-response curve. If the FEV_1 decreases 20% below baseline at any standard dose, the test result is positive. An inhaled β-agonist is administered, which promptly returns lung function to baseline. A positive methacholine challenge result is typical of asthma, but it is not specific because it can be seen in a number of other inflammatory airway diseases and in patients who have allergic rhinitis without asthma. A normal response to methacholine or histamine is incompatible with asthma, and an alternative diagnosis should be considered.

Exercise testing is a form of bronchoprovocation testing that is especially useful in children. Using a standard 6-min protocol, a 15% decrease in FEV_1 or a 20% decrease in PEFR from baseline 5 to 15 min after exercise is considered to be diagnostic. Although the presence and quantification of various inflammatory cells and mediators in sputum and body fluids have been used to reflect the activity of inflammation in asthma, there is unfortunately there are no biomarkers of disease activity that can be used clinically. NO is a reactive gas that is formed from arginine through the action of NO synthase. In asthma, there is some evidence that this enzyme is up-regulated, and elevated levels of NO have been detected in the exhaled air of asthmatic subjects. Exhaled NO is well established as a marker of eosinophilic inflammation and has been shown to correlate with sputum eosinophil counts, BHR, serum IgE levels asthma symptoms and lung function tests. It has been shown to be a fairly effective screening tool with a sensitivity of 88% when there are levels of ≥20 parts per billion in patients with asthma symptoms. Unfortunately, exhaled NO levels do not correlate with disease severity, but serial measurements may aid in monitoring disease activity. They have shown promise, for example, in identifying pending exacerbations of asthma. A standardized method of measurement must be carefully followed to prevent spurious results. The availability of a low-cost, hand-held analyzer may lead to more use, especially when adequate reimbursement by insurance companies is available.

The Treatment of Asthma

There are both short-term and long-term therapeutic objectives for every asthmatic patient. The short-term objectives are the control of immediate symptoms and the response to decreasing peak flow rate measurements. Long-term objectives are those directed at disease prevention because there are now well-proven strategies to avoid serious exacerbations of acute bronchospasm that often lead to ED visits or hospitalization. To meet these therapeutic objectives, four components of asthma care should be addressed. First, the optimal treatment of asthma depends on a careful assessment of the patient's symptoms as well as objective monitoring by office spirometry and home PEFR measurements. Second, the treatment of asthma with bronchodilator and antiinflammatory medications is tailored to the patient's needs and relies on a staging system that is based on the symptoms and objective measures of lung function. Third, measures should be taken to avoid exposure to respiratory allergens and irritants that can cause the worsening of symptoms, including the avoidance of outdoor allergens such as ragweed, grass, pollens, and molds and indoor allergens such as animal dander, house-dust mites, and cockroach antigen. When exposure cannot be avoided, allergen immunotherapy should be considered, although this modality is somewhat controversial. Indoor irritants such as smoke from cigarettes and wood-burning stoves, strong odors, and cleaning solutions are particularly troublesome. Fourth, patient education can be a powerful tool in asthma control. Family members also can be helpful, especially with children and elderly adults. Active participation by a patient in monitoring lung function, the avoidance of provocative agents, and decisions regarding medications provide asthma management skills that give that patient the confidence to control his or her own disease.

Medications for Asthma

Antiinflammatory Agents: Antiinflammatory agents are capable of reducing airway inflammation and thus improving lung function, decreasing bronchial hyperreactivity, reducing symptoms, and improving the overall quality of life. Corticosteroids are the most useful antiinflammatory agents. They act by preventing the migration and activation of inflammatory cells, interfering with the production of PGs and LTs, reducing microvascular leakage, and enhancing the action of β_2-adrenergic receptors on airway smooth muscle.

Corticosteroids are available for oral, parenteral, and inhaled use. Oral preparations such as prednisone are useful for the treatment of acute exacerbations of asthma that are unresponsive to bronchodilator therapy. Doses of 40 to 60 mg/d are administered until the patient responds, and then the dosage can be slowly tapered down. Often, poorly controlled asthma requires daily or every-other-day maintenance therapy with prednisone in dosages of 10 to 15 mg. IV corticosteroids, usually administered as methylprednisolone, 60 to 80 mg every 6 to 8 h for 1 or 2 days, are effective within 4 to 6 h of administration in preventing further progression of the severe asthma exacerbation that requires hospitalization.

ICS are safe and effective treatment for moderate-to-severe asthma and have been in use for > 20 years. Formulations of beclomethasone, triamcinolone, flunisolide, fluticasone, budesonide, and ciclesonide can reduce airway inflammation with one to several months of treatment. Several studies have shown that the therapeutic effects of ICS are imparted in active cigarette smokers. The long-term use of ICS has been associated with a good safety profile. High doses of inhaled steroids (*eg*, > 1,000 μg/d) are capable of causing hypophysea l–pituitary–adrenal axis suppression. Local adverse effects such as hoarseness, dysphonia, cough, and oral candidiasis do occur but can usually be avoided by the use of a spacer or holding chamber and by rinsing the mouth after each use. Oral and parenteral corticosteroids are associated with many side effects such as the risk of osteoporosis, cataracts, diabetes mellitus and, rarely, depression of immunity to infection. Attempts to reduce dependence on oral corticosteroids should be made, especially by the use of inhaled agents.

Cromolyn sodium and nedocromil sodium are two antiinflammatory agents that are available in inhaled form and have an extremely good safety profile. A 4- to 6-week trial may be useful to determine their effectiveness in the prevention of asthma symptoms. These agents are capable of preventing allergen-induced bronchospasm. LT pathway modifiers (LPMs) are also medications that are considered to be asthma controllers. There are two subclasses, as follows: the 5-lipoxygenase inhibitors, which inhibit the cysteinyl LTs and also LTB_4, and the LTD_4 receptor antagonists (LTRAs) of the cysteinyl LTs LTC_4, LTD_4, and LTE_4. These agents have been shown to be effective in preventing allergen-induced asthma, exercise-induced asthma (EIA), and aspirin-induced bronchospasm and allergic rhinitis. The use of antihistamines with the LPMs provides a more complete protection to allergen challenge. Studies comparing the LPMs with low-dose ICS have favored the latter with respect to FEV_1; however, symptom scores, daily β_2-agonist use, and patient preferences are similar. The use of LPMs also may reduce asthma exacerbation rates and the need for steroid bursts.

The authors of several studies examined the role of LTRAs as steroid-sparing agents. In patients whose symptoms were well controlled on an ICS/LABA combination, switching to a regimen of LTRA/LABA resulted in greater numbers of treatment failure (26% vs 9%), showing clear inferiority of the LTRA/LABA combination. In a large randomized trial of asthmatic patients with poorly controlled symptoms, an LTRA (or theophylline) did not add any benefit when added to existing treatment regimens. There is some evidence that the use of LTRAs in active smokers may improve outcomes compared with the use of an ICS.

The LPMs are generally very safe, which has led to more use in younger asthmatics, especially <4 years of age. The rare cases of Churg-Strauss vasculitis have occurred in patients with severe steroid-dependent asthma who have had a recent steroid taper. Because this form of vasculitis has been seen in patients in whom inhaled steroids have been substituted when oral steroids have been tapered, the reaction may not be specific to the LT-modifying agents.

Omalizumab, a humanized murine monoclonal antibody that inhibits the binding of IgE to mast cells by forming complexes with circulating free IgE, has been shown to be effective in the treatment of patients with atopic asthma. The reduction of free IgE in the circulation leads to a down-regulation of basophil and mast-cell receptors. This further reduces the potential for mast cell/basophil activation and the subsequent release of inflammatory mediators. Randomized, controlled trials have been conducted in patients with moderate-to-severe asthma. The agent has been shown to reduce the asthma exacerbation rate and the use of ICS. Many patients are able to completely eliminate the need for corticosteroid therapy. Symptom scores and quality-of-life indexes also improve. The medication must be administered by injection twice a month, and many patients can be taught self-administration. The drug is well tolerated, with serious adverse events rarely reported. The US Food and Drug Administration (FDA) issued a warning regarding omalizumab in 2007 after it was notified of case reports of anaphylaxis after injection of this agent. The reaction may occur at random time points and not just after the first injection. Physicians are advised to have epinephrine available for such an adverse reaction after treatment, and patients should carry an epinephrine kit after leaving the office.

Bronchodilators: Inhaled short-acting β-adrenergic agonists (SABAs) are the treatment of choice for the acute exacerbation of asthma symptoms. Inhaled agents can be delivered by metered-dose inhaler, dry-powder capsules, and compressor-driven nebulizers. Long-acting β-agonists (LABAs) may be helpful for long-term maintenance therapy and also used to control nocturnal symptoms. Studies of inadequately controlled asthmatic patients have shown a benefit to adding a LABA to a moderate-dose ICS regimen rather than doubling the dose of the ICS, adding theophylline, or adding an LPM. However, because of potential safety concerns with LABA therapy, the most recent NAEPP guidelines (Expert Panel Report 3) retracted previous recommendations to give a low-dose ICS/LABA combination in preference over doubling the dose of an ICS. The Global Initiative for Asthma (GINA) guidelines have not made this change because of the robust literature supporting combination therapy superiority.

The safety of LABA therapy was questioned mainly as a result of a study called the *SMART trial*, a 28-week randomized observational study in which the authors found a small but statistically significant increase in respiratory-related and asthma deaths in patients receiving salmeterol. A subgroup analysis suggested that the risk was greater in African Americans. A *post hoc* analysis suggested that deaths were mainly found in patients who were not receiving effective controller medication. It has been argued that the bronchodilator effect of the LABA offered symptomatic relief, thereby masking inflammation and worsening the disease.

The need for regularly scheduled doses of SABAs should alert the physician to the need for more intense antiinflammatory medication. Regularly scheduled doses of SABA agents have been associated with diminished control of asthma and heightened bronchial reactivity. In addition, epidemiologic evidence has linked excessive β-agonist use to increased mortality. Ideally, SABA therapy should be prescribed for acute symptom relief on an as-needed basis.

With the discovery and sequencing of the β-agonist receptor gene (*ADRB2*), interest has turned to the role of β-adrenergic polymorphisms in the control of asthma. The variant at amino acid position 16 (Gly16Arg) has received the most clinical attention. Most studies have shown no influence on bronchodilator responses. Prospective studies such as the β-Adrenergic Response by Genotype Study study have shown that patients homozygous for Arg16 have worse asthma control when treated with regularly scheduled short acting β-antagonist, albuterol, than those asthmatics homozygous for Gly 16. The effect of continuous long acting β-adrenergic therapy on asthma control is less clear. Numerous large retrospective pharmacogenetic analyses have failed to show an effect in all racial groups and in children and adults.

Theophylline is an effective bronchodilator and has antiinflammatory properties. It is available as a sustained-release preparation and can be taken once or twice daily. The monitoring of theophylline blood levels is important to avoid toxicity, especially in the elderly, who are more prone to adverse effects. GI side effects are seen with mild toxicity and blood levels in the range of 20 to 30 μg/mL. Serious cardiac arrhythmias and seizures may occur with blood levels in excess of this range. A blood level of 8 to 15 μg/mL is generally considered to be therapeutic.

Inhaled anticholinergic agents such as ipratropium produce bronchodilatation by reducing vagal tone and are widely used in patients with COPD. They may be useful in combination with β-agonists for a severe acute exacerbation of asthma. Their role in long-term maintenance therapy for asthma has not been established. They may be tried as a substitute bronchodilator when side effects preclude the use of β-agonists, although it must be remembered that they have a slower onset of action of 30 to 60 min until the maximal effect is produced.

Treatment Protocols for Asthma

A global strategy for asthma management and prevention has been offered in the NAEPP guidelines. The most recent 2007 NAEPP guidelines (Expert Panel Report 3) have offered two new treatment plans. Treatment protocols use step-care pharmacologic therapy based on the intensity of asthma symptoms and future risk as measures of control and the clinical response to these interventions. As symptoms and lung function worsen, step-up or add-on therapy is administered. As symptoms improve, therapy can be stepped down.

Asthma Severity: The severity classification and recommended treatment protocols are listed in Table 2.

Asthma Control: The classification of asthma by severity has proven useful when decisions are being made about management at the time of the initial assessment of a patient. Asthma severity, however, involves both the severity of the underlying disease and its responsiveness to treatment. This classification of severity is no longer recommended as the basis for ongoing treatment decisions in the new NAEPP guidelines. Instead, the concept of asthma control has been suggested as a basis for treatment decisions. The term *control* refers to control of the manifestations of disease, including symptoms, effects on the quality of daily living, and use of rescue medication. A periodic assessment of asthma control is useful and strongly recommended. The new classification of asthma control is listed in Table 3.

Table 2. *Asthma Treatment by Severity of Disease*

Mild intermittent asthma
- Severity: symptoms <2 times/wk nocturnal symptoms <2 times/mo FEV_1 and PEFR $>80\%$ of predicted; PEFR variability $<20\%$
- Treatment: NEAPP guidelines call this step 1 therapy: inhaled SABA as needed

Mild persistent asthma
- Severity: symptoms <2 times/wk and <1 time/d; nighttime symptoms >2 times/mo; FEV_1 and PEFR $>80\%$ of predicted; PEFR variability of 20 to 30%.
- Treatment: step 2 therapy: Begin antiinflammatory therapy; low-dose ICS are preferred, or consider a LPM or cromolyn. Use short-acting β-agonist as needed for quick relief; however, increased use means need for additional controller therapy.

Moderate persistent asthma
- Severity: daily symptoms and daily use of rescue β-agonist; >2 exacerbations/wk and 1 nighttime exacerbation/mo; FEV_1 and PEFR of 60 to 80% of predicted; PEFR variability $>30\%$.
- Treatment: Step therapy is advised in the 2007 NAEPP guidelines. Adding an LABA is given equal weight to increasing to medium-dose ICS; if symptoms still persist, may increase dose of ICS or add LABA, whichever applies, or medium-dose ICS with LPM or consider theophylline; continue a SABA for short-term relief. Step 5 is high-dose ICS plus LABA and consider omalizumab.

Severe persistent asthma
- Severity: continuous symptoms; limited physical activity; frequent exacerbations; frequent nighttime symptoms; FEV_1 and PEFR $<60\%$ of predicted; PEFR variability $>30\%$.
- Treatment: high-dose ICS, LABA, possibly theophylline, oral corticosteroids, and consider omalizumab.

Table 3. *Classification of Asthma Control in Youths >12 Years of Age and Adults*

Characteristics	Controlled (All of the Following)	Not Well Controlled (Any Measure Present in Any Week)	Very Poorly Controlled
Daytime symptoms	None (≤2/wk)	>2 times/wk	Throughout day
Interference with normal activities	None	Any	Extremely limited
Nocturnal symptoms/awakening	<2 times/ mo	1 to 3 times/wk	>4 times/wk
Need for SABA (rescue treatment)	None (≤2/wk)	>2 times/wk	Several times a day
Lung function (PEFR or FEV_1)	>80% of predicted or personal best	60 to 80% of predicted or personal best	<60% of predicted or personal best
Validated questionnaire (*eg*, Asthma Control Test score)	>20	16 to 19	≤15

Step-down Care. There are no hard and fast rules on stepping down asthma care when asthma control is improved. Studies conducted by the Asthma Clinical Research Centers have shown that patients with mild persistent asthma controlled with a low dose of ICS do better with continuation of the corticosteroid than switching to a LTRA but do as well when switched to a once-a-day regimen of ICS/LABA. In another study with similar patients, as-needed use of a ICS/SABA combination did as well as daily ICS twice daily with less total inhaled corticosteroid use, but patients randomized to as-needed SABA did worse. The use of an ICS/LABA combination concurrently as a scheduled maintenance controller and as an as needed controller reliever is another new approach (not approved by the FDA in the United States). The use of a budesonide/formoterol combination product in this manner has led to fewer exacerbations and better lung function.

Asthma Syndromes

EIA

Nearly all asthmatic patients experience increased bronchospasm after vigorous exercise at some point in their history (*ie*, EIA). If they are tested in the pulmonary function laboratory while not receiving medication, 70 to 80% of patients will show a characteristic decrease in peak flow or FEV_1 immediately after a 6- to 8-min exercise challenge. During exercise, patients seem to be protected as the airways actually dilate, possibly attributable to the presence of circulating catecholamines. Symptoms of cough and shortness of breath parallel the decrease in lung function that usually reaches its peak response 5 to 10 min after exercise. Often patients hear no wheezing during the attack, and in some patients, atypical presentations of chest tightness or chest pain alone will occur. A cardiac workup may often precede pulmonary testing in such patients. The symptoms usually abate without treatment, although the administration of a short-acting β-agonist immediately returns lung function to normal. Occasionally, the attack after exercise can be very severe and may require emergency treatment.

The mechanisms that cause exercise-induced bronchospasm in susceptible patients (*eg*, asthmatic patients, some patients with allergic rhinitis, and patients with cystic fibrosis) have been intensely studied. As ventilation increases with exercise, cooler, dryer air is drawn into the airways in greater quantities. This action causes heat and water loss from the airways into the airstream. Airway cooling and mucosal drying are thought to trigger mast cells to release their mediators. The greater the heat and water loss, the greater the degree of bronchospasm. A number of factors may enhance or reduce the risk of exercise-induced bronchospasm, including the following:

- Patients with poorly controlled asthma are more likely to have EIA.
- Exercise in cold, dry air is more likely to cause EIA.
- Running, especially outdoors, is more likely to cause EIA than other activities such as swimming.
- The greater the intensity of the exercise, the more likely the bronchospasm.
- Bronchoconstriction becomes less intense during a second challenge if performed an hour or

so after the first. An intense warm-up period 30 to 60 min before competitive sports can be helpful.

- Pretreatment can effectively block exercise-induced bronchospasm in >90% of patients. β-agonists are the first choice for treatment, and cromolyn is a good alternative. They can be used together if needed.

Nocturnal Asthma

Exacerbations of wheezing and shortness of breath are a common cause of sleep deprivation in asthma patients and tend to be underreported by patients and overlooked by physicians. Even patients who have mild disease that is apparently controlled by medication may awake at least one time during the night because of their asthma. Deaths from asthma have been increasing in many countries during the past few decades, and most of these deaths from asthma occur at night between midnight and 8:00 AM. The mechanisms of nocturnal asthma are not completely understood. Bronchial biopsy specimens have not shown increases in T cells, eosinophils, or mast cells at 4:00 AM in asthmatic patients with nocturnal asthma. Transbronchial biopsy specimens have shown accumulations of eosinophils and macrophages in alveolar and peribronchial tissue in these patients, leading to the concept that adventitial inflammation in the peripheral airways leads to excessive airway narrowing. This leads to an altered airway-parenchymal interdependence and the loss of the normal elastic recoil forces that normally keeps the airways open.

It has been observed that lung function has a definite circadian rhythm and that PEFRs are highest at 4:00 PM and lowest at 4:00 AM. Healthy individuals show a fluctuation of only about 8%, whereas many asthmatic patients can, during periods of unstable symptoms, show as much as a 50% variation in peak expiratory rates in a 24-h period. This variation can result in frequent nocturnal awakenings and the need for frequent rescue therapy. Sustained-release theophylline has proven to be a valuable tool in the control of nocturnal asthma, and LABAs such as oral extended-release albuterol and inhaled salmeterol are also helpful. Because research with transbronchial biopsy specimens has shown that the levels of inflammatory cells are greatest at 4:00 AM, the key to controlling nocturnal asthma is the control of the inflammatory response with ICS or, if necessary, oral corticosteroids.

Aspirin-Induced Asthma

Acute idiosyncratic reactions to aspirin may result in either acute bronchospasm or urticaria/angioedema, rarely both together. Aspirin-induced asthma is a syndrome that predominantly affects adults rather than children and nonatopic individuals. One third of patients, however, may manifest positive immediate skin-test hypersensitivity to inhaled aeroallergens. The disease usually evolves during the course decades and first begins as chronic nonallergic perennial rhinitis, often complicated by nasal polyposis and recurrent bacterial sinusitis. Asthma then appears, is often severe and unremitting, and requires treatment with systemic steroids.

The symptoms of rhinosinusitis, however, may continue to be more troubling to the patient than the asthma. Although aspirin may have previously been tolerated, suddenly acute bronchospasm develops in the patient 30 min to several hours after ingesting a standard dose of oral aspirin. The use of aspirin also may be associated with flushing of the face and ocular and nasal congestion. Cross-sensitivity occurs with the use of other nonsteroidal antiinflammatory drugs such as indomethacin, naproxen, ibuprofen, sulindac, and piroxicam, all of which are inhibitors of PG synthesis from the cyclooxygenase pathway of arachidonic acid metabolism. Noninhibitors such as sodium salicylate, salicylamide, propoxyphene, and acetaminophen do not cause the reaction.

It is believed that, by blocking the cyclooxygenase pathway, arachidonic acid metabolism is preferentially shifted to the 5-lipoxygenase pathway to produce LTs, including the cysteinyl LTs LTC_4, LTD_4, and LTE_4. They are potent inflammatory mediators that can induce bronchoconstriction, mucous secretion, bronchial wall edema, and swelling of the nasal mucosa. They are also potent chemokines for eosinophils. There is a fourfold increase in urinary LTE_4 levels after aspirin provocation in the aspirin-sensitive patient. It has also been shown that aspirin-sensitive patients have increased expression of the cysteinyl LT receptor CysLT1 on leukocytes from nasal mucosalbiopsy specimens compared with those who do not have this syndrome. The precise mechanism for this syndrome is not known. The overexpression of the enzyme LTC_4 synthase has been reported, and some studies have described polymorphisms of the LTC_4 synthase promoter region.

The prevalence of aspirin-induced bronchospasm in the population of asthmatic patients depends on the population studied. Approximately 3 to 5% of hospitalized asthmatic patients report a history of a reaction to aspirin. This number is greater at highly specialized referral centers at which patients with the most severe asthma are cared for. The treatment is, of course, the avoidance of aspirin and nonsteroidal antiinflammatory drugs with known cross-reactivity. For the occasional patient who needs these drugs, oral desensitization protocols using gradually increasing doses of aspirin are effective. With the use of aspirin desensitization, approximately two thirds of the patients report a significant improvement in their rhinosinusitis, and approximately one half have improvement in their asthma. The addition of LT inhibitors (*eg*, zileuton) and receptor antagonists (*eg*, montelukast) as therapeutic options for asthma is important because the agents have been shown to block aspirin-induced bronchospasm in sensitive patients.

Occupational Asthma

Asthma that is precipitated by a particular occupational environment and not to stimuli outside of the workplace is called *occupational asthma.* The following two types have been described: (1) asthma that follows a latent period of exposure to either a high-molecular-weight or a low-molecular-weight "sensitizing" antigen and (2) asthma that follows exposure to workplace irritants. One form of irritant-induced asthma is called *reactive airways dysfunction syndrome*, a condition that usually results from the sudden inhalation of a large dose of a highly irritating substance. Occupational asthma associated with a latency period causes asthma by immunologic events that affect only a small proportion of exposed subjects.

Although some compounds induce asthma through the production of specific IgE antibodies, the immunologic mechanisms responsible for other agents have not been identified. The reaction between specific IgE antibodies and antigens may cause an isolated early asthmatic reaction that occurs within a few minutes after the occupational exposure. It typically reaches a maximum within 30 min and subsides within 1 to 1.5 h. Also, a biphasic reaction may occur, and the spontaneous recovery may be followed by a late bronchospastic reaction 4 to 6 h after exposure. This reaches maximal intensity within 8 to 10 h and subsides after 24 to 48 h. When an isolated late reaction occurs, the affected individual may be away from the workplace, making the diagnosis less obvious. The presence of sensitization to occupational agents can be detected by skin tests, radioallergosorbent tests, or enzyme-linked immunosorbent assay, which can strongly support the diagnosis. Unfortunately, there are very few standardized commercially available materials for skin tests or for radioallergosorbent tests in patients with this disorder.

The following six major categories of agents have been described in the pathogenesis of occupational asthma:

1. Exposure to animals, shellfish, fish, and arthropods can cause asthma in farmers, laboratory workers, grain handlers, and poultry workers.
2. Exposure to wood, plants, and vegetables can cause asthma in woodworkers, carpenters, grain handlers, bakers, and tobacco workers.
3. Enzymes and pharmaceuticals are known to cause asthma in pharmaceutical workers, pharmacists, and detergent industry workers.
4. Low-molecular-weight chemicals cause asthma in solderers, spray painters, chemical manufacturers, polyurethane manufacturers, and electronics workers.
5. Metals and metal salts such as aluminum, chromium, cobalt, nickel, and platinum fumes can cause asthma in electroplaters, hard metal workers, polishers, and solderers.
6. Dusts, fumes, and gases may cause asthma via a sudden, high-concentration exposure, usually as the result of an accident in the workplace or via less severe repetitive exposures.

Estimates of the prevalence of occupational asthma vary, but it is estimated that 2 to 15% of all cases of adult-onset asthma occur from workplace exposure. Seeking the occupational causes of asthma in the patient's history can be very rewarding and can lead to primary prevention by the avoidance of the offending environment.

Cough-Variant Asthma

At times, cough may be the sole presenting manifestation of asthma, and the characteristic findings of variable airflow obstruction may not be present. Such patients represent a subgroup of patients with asthma, rather than being asthmatic patients who cough. As a result, cough-variant asthma (CVA) is significantly underdiagnosed. Prospective studies have shown that asthma is among the most common causes of chronic cough (24 to 29%) in adult nonsmokers.

There is evidence that cough receptors in the airways are separate from bronchoconstrictive receptors, and this may explain why such patients do not wheeze. Cough receptors are more abundant in the central airways. Patients with CVA have demonstrated heightened sensitivity of their cough reflexes, whereas those with the typical form of asthma do not differ from healthy volunteers when cough reflex sensitivity is experimentally measured. Methacholine sensitivity, on the other hand, occurs less often in patients with CVA when compared with those with typical asthma. The cough receptors are presumably stimulated by inflammatory cell mediators that are released by airway inflammation. Subepithelial layer thickening, which is a pathologic feature of airway remodeling that is thought to be caused by chronic inflammation, is present in CVA.

The diagnosis of CVA should be suspected in a patient who has a chronic cough, usually present for months and even years, and no obvious cause seen on the chest radiograph. The history is often suggestive in that the patient coughs vigorously after exposure to fumes, cigarette smoke, and other irritants and often after laughter and exercise. The diagnosis is supported by a positive response to bronchial inhalation challenge with methacholine, histamine or exercise, and is confirmed by a clinical response to bronchodilators and/or antiinflammatory agents. Most patients will respond to treatment with the use of inhaled bronchodilators and ICS. A subgroup of patients will require the addition of LT receptor antagonists and/or a short course of oral corticosteroids. A negative methacholine inhalation challenge test result essentially excludes asthma from the differential diagnosis of chronic cough.

Allergic Bronchopulmonary Aspergillosis

Allergic bronchopulmonary aspergillosis (ABPA) is a syndrome most commonly found in patients with asthma and cystic fibrosis. Patients present with wheezing, fleeting, pulmonary infiltrates, and expectoration of brown mucus plugs. ABPA is suspected on clinical grounds, and the diagnosis is confirmed by radiologic and serologic testing. In the United States, the accepted criteria for diagnosis are as follows: (1) asthma, (2) immediate cutaneous reactivity to *Aspergillus fumigatus*, (3) precipitating (IgG) antibodies to *A fumigatus*, (4) elevated total serum IgE levels (>1,000 ng/mL), (5) elevated serum IgE antibodies to *A fumigatus*, (6) proximal bronchiectasis, (7) infiltrates seen on the chest radiograph, and (8) peripheral eosinophilia with radiographic infiltrates.

A radiologic classification of ABPA has been proposed: ABPA-S (seropositive) and ABPA-CB (central bronchiectasis). Patients with ABPA-S represent the earliest form of disease, and the clinical outcome is more favorable. The presence of central bronchiectasis, often accompanied by central mucoid impaction of the bronchus, is an independent predictor of failure to achieve long-term remission.

It is wise to diagnose ABPA early and begin the treatment of patients to prevent the development of bronchiectasis. The mainstay of treatment for ABPA is oral corticosteroids to control the asthma symptoms as well as the immunologic response to the Aspergillus antigens. Usually, prednisone, 40 to 60 mg, is required for complete clearing. The use of low-dose corticosteroids has been associated with relapse and corticosteroid dependence, and ICS are ineffective. On effective therapy the IgE concentration should decrease in 1 to 2 months, and a subsequent increase suggests recurrence of the disease. The goal is to decrease the IgE level by 30 to 50%. Azoles such as itraconazole have also shown effectiveness in the treatment of this condition and usually are reserved for relapses or corticosteroid dependency.

Gastroesophageal Reflux and Asthma

The prevalence of gastroesophageal reflux in asthma is quite high and has been discovered in as many as 30 to 90% of patients. In patients with reflux symptoms, 24-h pH monitoring has proven reflux to be present in >80% of patients. Even when reflux symptoms are not present, reflux can be demonstrated with this study nearly 30% of the time. Asthmatic patients have been shown to have decreased lower esophageal sphincter pressures when compared with healthy individuals. Medications such as theophylline and β-agonists can lower the lower esophageal sphincter as can certain foods, such as those with a high fat content, chocolate, caffeinated beverages, alcohol, and peppermint. In addition, the administration of prednisone orally has been shown to increase esophageal acid contact time.

A large study of veterans showed that patients with significant esophageal disease, such as erosive esophagitis and/or esophageal stricture, had a 1.5 odds ratio of having asthma compared with healthy subjects. In patients with difficult-to-control asthma, reflux should be considered as a possible triggering agent. A favorable asthma response to antireflux medical therapy has been shown to occur, especially in patients with reflux symptoms, but also in as many as 24% of patients with no reflux symptoms. Unfortunately, such studies have not shown consistent results. A trial of therapy with a proton-pump inhibitor used in high doses (*eg*, omeprazole, 20 mg bid) may be necessary and has been shown to be more effective than the use of histamine type 2 blocker therapy. Consensus has not been reached on the role of surgery when medical therapy fails. The following two possible mechanisms of gastroesophageal reflux-induced asthma exacerbation have been proposed: (1) a vagally mediated reflex caused by acid in the esophagus, which stimulates sensory mucosal receptors, and (2) microaspiration into the upper airway, which stimulates other vagally mediated reflexes. With either mechanism, heightened cholinergic tone could result in significant bronchoconstriction.

Corticosteroid-Resistant Asthma

Patients with severe unremitting asthma symptoms despite the use of high doses of corticosteroids have been termed *corticosteroid-resistant asthmatic patients* when no confounding factors have been discovered. These factors include poor adherence to recommended therapy, uncontrolled gastroesophageal reflux, unrecognized food or environmental antigen exposure, aspirin-sensitive asthma, ABPA, systemic vasculitis, and fixed airway disease secondary to COPD. By definition, such patients have an FEV_1 <75% of predicted, with a failure to improve by 15% after an adequate dose and duration of glucocorticoid therapy (*eg*, 40 mg/d of prednisone for 1 to 2 weeks); are clinically resistant to corticosteroid therapy; and have a longer duration of asthma, lower morning lung function, and a greater degree of bronchial reactivity than corticosteroid-sensitive asthmatic patients.

Although some abnormalities have been demonstrated in other tissues, such as the cutaneous vasoconstrictor responses to beclomethasone dipropionate, metabolic effects suggesting glucocorticoid resistance in other tissues such as bone have not been seen, and the hypothalamic pituitary adrenal axis response in such patients has been shown to be normal. Glucocorticoid resistance probably is produced by a number of heterogeneous mechanisms. It is thought that the major mechanisms for resistance occur distal to the nuclear translocation step. The management of patients with glucocorticoid-resistant asthma presents a difficult challenge as there are no effective and well-tolerated alternatives to therapy with steroids. Methotrexate and cyclosporine have been used.

Fatal and Near-Fatal Asthma

Despite our better understanding of the pathogenesis of asthma and more effective treatment programs, the rates of morbidity and mortality associated with this condition still remain a problem in most countries in the industrialized world. Many factors have been proposed to explain this dilemma. These factors include poor compliance with medication and asthma monitoring; an underestimation by the patient and physician alike of the severity of the asthma; poor long-term access to medical care, especially for the poor; and overreliance on inhaled β-agonist therapy. Near-fatal and fatal attacks of asthma are the result of acute hypercarbic respiratory acidosis; fatalities rarely are caused by serious cardiac arrhythmias.

Despite severe degrees of acidosis, even to pH levels of <7.0, recovery can be rapid and complete.

In fact, there is evidence that when the asthma attack is sudden and respiratory failure occurs within a few hours, recovery too is rapid. Improvement occurs more rapidly than when the asthma attack has been slowly progressive over days. The term *sudden asphyxic asthma* has been given to such explosive attacks. There is evidence that such patients are immunohistologically different in that their airways have a relative paucity of eosinophils and a larger number of neutrophils compared with the classic asthma picture. Typically, in patients who die of asthma, the lungs are overinflated, and both large and small airways are filled with plugs consisting of a mixture of mucus, serum proteins, inflammatory cells, and cell debris. Microscopically, there is infiltration of the airway lumen and wall with eosinophils and mononuclear cells. This is accompanied by vasodilation, evidence of microvascular leakage, and epithelial cell sloughing.

The most commonly identified causes of near-fatal asthma are listed in Table 4. Risk factors for fatal or near-fatal asthma are as follows: (1) high medication use (three or more medications), (2) overuse of inhaled β-agonist agents, (3) a history of recurrent hospitalizations, (4) previous occurrences of life-threatening attacks, and (5) marked fluctuations in morning and evening peak flow rate measurements. In addition, investigations have shown that patients with near-fatal attacks have abnormal respiratory control mechanisms such as a blunted perception of dyspnea and a reduced hypoxic ventilatory response to hypoxia. They are also more likely to have a drinking problem, to smoke cigarettes, and to have family problems.

Asthma management plans are becoming popular, especially with high-risk patients. Studies have shown that death from asthma can be reduced by the use of a peak flowmeter, a written action plan, and oral glucocorticoids prior to a severe attack. The risk of death is enhanced by the use of a nebulizer for symptomatic relief in the month before death. Because blood levels of albuterol are 2.5 times greater in patients dying of asthma compared with control subjects, closer supervision of β-agonist use should reduce asthma mortality. Structured educational plans to teach management may also offer improved mortality statistics in asthma patients.

Table 4. *Identified Causes of a Near-Fatal Asthma Attack*

Environmental allergen exposure
Upper respiratory viral infection
Aspirin and nonsteroidal antiinflammatory drug ingestion
Profound emotional upsets
β-Blocker drugs
Exposure to indoor air pollutants
Air pollution after a thermal inversion

Annotated Bibliography

Abramson MJ, Bailey MJ, Couper FJ, et al. Are asthma medications and management related to deaths from asthma? Am J Respir Crit Care Med 2001; 163:12–18

A questionnaire was administered to the next-of-kin of patients who had died of asthma. Smoking, drinking, and family problems were more likely among patients dying of asthma than in a group of control subjects. The risk of death was reduced by the use of a peak flowmeter in the previous year. The use of oral glucocorticoids also appeared to reduce the risk of death. The risk of death was increased by the use of a nebulizer for symptomatic relief in the previous month. Blood albuterol levels were considerably greater in patients dying of asthma, suggesting that albuterol overuse is a marker for asthma mortality.

Adams RJ, Fuhlbrigge A, Guilbert T, et al. Inadequate use of asthma medication in the United States: results of the asthma in America National Population survey. J Allergy Clin Immunol 2002; 110:58–64

This study is based on a cross-sectional national telephone survey. It reveals that appropriate therapy for asthma remains inadequate. Antiinflammatory therapy is still greatly underused, especially in socioeconomically disadvantaged groups.

Agarwal R, Gupta D, Aggarwal AN, et al. Allergic bronchopulmonary aspergillosis: lessons from 126 patients attending a chest clinic in north India. Chest 2006; 130: 442–448

This article describes the clinical findings in 126 cases of ABPA. A total of 27% of the patients had ABPA-S (serologic positivity alone) and the remainder had ABPA-CB (with central bronchiectasis); many of the latter had other radiologic findings such as patchy infiltrates and atelectasis. This study showed no significant difference between the stages of ABPA and the duration of illness, the severity of asthma, and the serologic findings (ie, absolute eosinophil count, total IgE levels, and IgE levels for A fumigatus*). All patients went into "remission" at 6 weeks on corticosteroids. Twenty-five patients had a "relapse" during the course of their treatment. One hundred nine patients had "complete remission," 17 patients were classified as having "glucocorticoid-dependent*

ABPA," and 7 patients were classified as having "end-stage ABPA."

Barnes PJ. The cytokine network in asthma and chronic obstructive pulmonary disease. J Clin Invest 2008; 118:3546–3556

This article discusses how cytokines orchestrate the chronic inflammation and structural changes of the respiratory tract in both asthma and COPD and have become important targets for the development of new therapeutic strategies in these diseases.

Barnes PJ, Adcock IM. How do corticosteroids work in asthma? Ann Intern Med 2003; 139:359–370

Corticosteroids suppress a number of pathways of chronic inflammation in asthma. Inflammatory genes are regulated by proinflammatory transcription factors such as nuclear factor-κB and activator protein-1. These factors can switch on gene transcription. Corticosteroids act to suppress the action of these factors. This review discusses the mechanisms involved.

Bateman ED, Boushey HA, Bousquet J, et al. Can guideline-defined asthma control be achieved? Am J Respir Crit Care Med 2004; 170:836–844

*This is the Gaining Optimal Asthma Control study, which examined the use of inhaled ICS/LABAs such as fluticasone and salmeterol for the treatment of asthma. This study specifically looked at the guideline-defined approach, using dose escalation as necessary to achieve improved asthma care. The study looked at increasing the dose of ICS alone or increasing the dose of ICS and coupling it with a LABA for asthma control. Total control was achieved across all levels of treatment in 41% vs 28% of patients, respectively, at 1 year for ICS-LABA therapy vs ICS therapy alone. Asthma was well controlled (*ie, *nearly totally controlled) in 71% vs 59% of patients, respectively. This study confirmed that guideline-derived asthma control can be achieved in a majority of patients; however, the asthma of a significant percentage of patients cannot even be well controlled with this combination therapy.*

Berry MA, Hargadon B, Shelley M, et al. Evidence of a role of tumor necrosis factor alpha in refractory asthma. N Engl J Med 2006; 354:697–708

*A double-blind, placebo-controlled study was conducted in patients with severe asthma to determine the effect of blocking TNF-α with etanercept. When etanercept was added to usual care, significant improvements in FEV_1 and BHR were found. Further studies are needed because the study group was quite small (*ie, *10 patients). Blocking TNF-α may prove to be an effective disease-modifying strategy for asthma.*

Blaiss MS. Management of rhinitis and asthma in pregnancy. Ann Allergy Asthma Immunol 2003; 90(suppl): 16–22

This report from the FDA, the American College of Allergy, Asthma, and Immunology, and the American College of Obstetricians and Gynecologists underscores the important differences in pregnant and nonpregnant patients. For pregnant women with asthma, inhaled cromolyn should be the first-line therapy, followed by inhaled budesonide if symptoms worsen. Other agents, such as salmeterol, LT modifiers, and the newer ICS, may be considered if the patient had a good response to these drugs before pregnancy.

Blitz M, Blitz S, Beasely R, et al. Inhaled magnesium sulfate in the treatment of acute asthma. Cochrane Database Syst Rev. Issue 4, 2005

This Cochrane Database review concludes that nebulized inhaled magnesium sulfate in addition to a β-agonist for the treatment of an acute asthma exacerbation appears to have benefits with respect to improved pulmonary function. In patients with severe asthma, there is a trend toward benefit in terms of hospital admissions.

Borish L. Allergic rhinitis: systemic inflammation and implications for management. J Allergy Clin Immunol 2003; 112:1021–1031

This review of the inflammatory mechanisms of allergic rhinitis reminds us that some inflammatory cells and mediators may pass into the bloodstream and create a systemic reaction. It offers justification for the use of LT modifiers to treat the systemic antiinflammatory effects of rhinitis.

Boulet LP, Lemière C, Archambault F, et al. Smoking and asthma: clinical and radiologic features, lung function, and airway inflammation. Chest 2006; 129:661–668

This study shows that compared with nonsmoking asthma patients, smoking asthma patients have features similar to what could be found in patients with early stages of COPD.

Braman SS, Hanania NA. Asthma in older adults. Clin Chest Med 2007; 28:685–702

This review underscores the differences between asthma in the young and elderly. Airflow obstruction in the elderly is often difficult to reverse, and many elderly patients have fixed airway disease, even with maximum therapy. Pitfalls in asthma therapy in treating the elderly are discussed as well as differences in pathogenesis.

Chalmers GW, Macleod KJ, Little SA, et al. Influence of cigarette smoking on inhaled corticosteroid treatment in mild asthma. Thorax 2002; 57:226–230

This study showed that active cigarette smoking impairs the efficacy of short-term ICS treatment in patients with mild asthma. This study obviously has important implications for patients with mild asthma who smoke.

Chung KF. Individual cytokines contributing to asthma pathophysiology: valid targets for asthma therapy? Curr Opin Invest Drugs 2003; 4:1320–1326

This article reviews the evidence for cytokine-targeted therapy. IL-4, IL-5, and IL-13 contribute to the inflammation of asthma; the inhibition of these cytokines might be useful in the future.

Cochrane MG, Bala MV, Downs KE, et al. Inhaled corticosteroids for asthma therapy: patient compliance, devices, and inhalation technique. Chest 2000; 117: 542–550

This article presents a systematic literature review concerning compliance, inhalation techniques, and ICS devices for the treatment asthma.

Compalati E, Penagos M, Tarantini F, et al. Specific immunotherapy for respiratory allergy: state of the art according to current meta-analyses. Ann Allergy Asthma Immunol 2009; 102:22–28

A meta analyses of studies that met the inclusion criteria, five evaluating sublingual immunotherapy and two evaluating subcutaneous immunotherapy, reported a reduction in symptom and medication scores. The authors conclude that according to evidence-based criteria, specific immunotherapy can be recommended for the treatment of respiratory allergy because of its efficacy in reducing asthma and rhinitis symptoms and that future methodologic approaches that consider safety and costs should corroborate this positive evaluation.

Cote J, Bowie DM, Robichaud P, et al. Evaluation of two different educational interventions for adult patients consulting with an acute asthma exacerbation. Am J Respir Crit Care Med 2001; 163:1415–1419

These authors show that a structured educational plan emphasizing self-capacity to manage asthma exacerbation and the use of peak flow rate reduce the morbidity of patients with asthma.

Creticos PS, Reed CE, Norman PS, et al. Ragweed immunotherapy in adult asthma. N Engl J Med 1996; 334:501–506

This article examined the efficacy of immunotherapy for asthma in ragweed-sensitive patients. Patients were followed up for 2 years of treatment. Although immunotherapy for adults in this study had positive effects and produced objective measures of improvement of asthma and allergy during the first year of therapy, the improvement was not sustained during the second year.

Currie GP, Devereux GS, Lee DK, et al. Recent developments in asthma management. BMJ 2005; 330:585–589

This is an evidence-based review of developments from the past few years in asthma management. It is a comprehensive literature search up to 2005 on a number of approaches to asthma therapy including allergen avoidance, dietary manipulation, asthma action plans, and pharmacologic management. It is an up-to-date review with excellent references.

Dicpinigaitis PV. Cough: 4: cough in asthma and eosinophilic bronchitis. Thorax 2004; 59:71–72

This author discusses the difference between CVA and eosinophilic bronchitis. The main distinction is that the former is associated with BHR. Eosinophilic bronchitis patients have a negative methacholine challenge result. Evidence suggests that LT receptor antagonists might be useful in treating CVA. Eosinophilic bronchitis responds to therapy with ICS.

Dicpinigaitis PV. Chronic cough due to asthma: ACCP evidence-based clinical practice guidelines. Chest 2006; 129(suppl):75S–79S

Asthma should be considered a potential etiology in any patient with chronic cough. A subgroup of asthmatic patients presents with CVA. This group of patients has only cough with no other asthma symptoms. The cough should respond to standard antiasthma therapy. This article is taken from the American College of Chest Physicians Evidence-Based Practice Guidelines on Cough, which was published in 2006.

Donohue JF. The expanding role of long-acting β-agonists. Chest 2000; 118:283–285

The author summarizes the use of salmeterol, an LABA, for hospital inpatients. He first provides evidence that salmeterol users are at no greater risk for asthma-related hospitalizations, emergency department visits, or ICU stays. The treatment of an acute asthma attack is not compromised by maintenance therapy with this long-acting agent. In addition, salmeterol can be safely used for the treatment of acute exacerbation of COPD along with albuterol. Minimal cardiac effects are seen in most patients; however, there are very few data on this subject in patients with preexisting heart disease. Careful monitoring is urged if both agents are used.

Drazen J. Asthma and the human genome project: summary of the 45th annual Thomas L. Petty Aspen Lung Conference. Chest 2003; 123(suppl):447S–449S

This article discusses more recent thinking on the genetics of asthma.

Forbes L. Do exogenous estrogens and progesterone influence asthma? Thorax 1999; 54:265–267

This interesting article discusses the influence of estrogens and progesterone on asthma. The author believes that there was no convincing evidence to suggest that hormonal contraceptives either exacerbate or improve asthmatic symptoms. Their use in patients with severe asthma or those with premenstrual exacerbations of asthma will require future clinical trials. The author concludes that, "[a]t the present [time,] there is not enough evidence to suggest any change to current prescribing practice."

Gern JE. Viral respiratory infection and the link to asthma. Pediatr Infect Dis J 2004; 23(suppl):S78–S86

Acute asthma symptoms have been correlated with a variety of viral pathogens. Most commonly, it is respiratory syncytial virus in infancy and rhinovirus in older children. This article enhances our knowledge of how viruses can adversely affect lung or immune development in asthma patients.

Grau RG. Churg-Strauss syndrome: 2005–2008 update. Curr Rheumatol Rep. 2008; 10:453–458

This article provides a recent update on this disease.

Greenstone IR, Ni Chroinin MN, Masse V, et al. Combination of inhaled long-acting β_2-agonists and inhaled steroids versus higher dose of inhaled steroids in children and adults with persistent asthma. Cochrane Database Issue 4, 2005

This Cochrane Database review presents data on the use of high-dose ICS vs ICS plus LABA. It concludes that the combination of LAB A and ICS leads to greater improvement in lung function, symptoms, and the use β_2-agonists for rescue. There are also fewer withdrawals from poor asthma control when the combination therapy is used. However, in head-to-head comparison, the combination of LABA and ICS vs greater-dose ICS showed no significant differences for the prevention of exacerbations requiring systemic corticosteroids.

Harding SM. Recent clinical investigations examining the association of asthma and gastroesophageal reflux. Am J Med 2003; 115(suppl):39S–44S

This article reviews the association between gastroesophageal reflux disease and asthma. Esophageal acid may alter BHR. Medical and surgical therapy for gastroesophageal reflux disease may improve asthma outcomes in selected patients.

Holgate ST, Chuchalin AG, Herbert J, et al. Efficacy and safety of a recombinant anti-immunoglobulin E antibody (omalizumab) in severe allergic asthma. Clin Exp Allergy 2004; 34:632–638

This study investigated the role of omalizumab, the IgG monoclonal antibody, in patients with severe allergic asthma that is refractory to corticosteroid therapy. In this 16-week study, the primary end point was corticosteroid withdrawal. Anti-IgE therapy led to greater reductions in ICS dosage compared with placebo. It also led to significantly improved symptoms, lung function, quality of life, and reduced control or medication use.

Holgate ST, Davies DE, Puddicombe S, et al. Mechanisms of airway epithelial damage: epithelial-mesenchymal interactions in the pathogenesis of asthma. Eur Respir J 2003; 44(suppl):24S–29S

The authors provide evidence that asthma is a disease of airway wall restructuring that engages activation of the EMTU. Activation of this unit provides a stimulus for altered airway wall structure and function and may explain the decline in lung function observed over time with asthma. In asthma patients, the epithelium shows considerable evidence of injury and activation as well as goblet-cell metaplasia. The altered epithelium becomes an important source of mediators, chemokines, and growth factors that sustain ongoing inflammation. Injury to the epithelial cells is thought to result in increased release of fibroproliferative and fibrogenic growth factors. This results in the deposition of interstitial collagens in the lamina reticularis, the deposition of collagen in the submucosa, smooth-muscle hyperplasia, and microvascular neuronal proliferation.

Israel E, Deykin A, Mitra N, et al. Use of regularly scheduled albuterol treatment in asthma: genotype-stratified, randomised, placebo-controlled cross-over trial. Lancet 2004; 364:1505–1512

Genetic polymorphisms of the β-adrenergic receptor have been described. Homozygosity for arginine (Arg/Arg) rather than glycine (Gly/Gly) predicts adverse events with asthma. This is a prospective clinical trial in patients with mild asthma that show that when albuterol was kept to a minimum, patients with Arg/Arg genotype had an increase in morning peak flow rate, whereas the change in patients with Gly/Gly genotype was not significant. Patients with Gly/Gly genotype using regularly scheduled albuterol had an improvement in PEFR. By contract, the Arg/Arg genotype group had lower morning peak flow rates during the treatment with albuterol. This suggests that bronchodilator treatments avoiding albuterol may be appropriate for patients with Arg/Arg genotype.

Jones SL, Kittelson J, Cowan JO, et al. The predictive value of exhaled nitric oxide measurements in assessing changes in asthma control. Am J Respir Crit Care Med 2001; 164:738–743

ENO has been confirmed as a marker of airway inflammation. It is present in greater concentrations in steroid-naive asthmatic patients compared with healthy control individuals. This group of investigators measured exhaled NO in 75 asthmatic subjects with mild-to-moderate asthma. ICS therapy was withdrawn and loss of asthma control ensued. There were highly significant correlations between exhaled NO and symptoms, sputum eosinophils, and BHR. Exhaled NO had an 80 to 90% predictive value for the loss of asthma control. It has also been previously confirmed that exhaled NO is closely related to several other markers of asthma control such as asthma symptoms, dyspnea score, and daily use of rescue medication. This technique is noninvasive and can be performed repeatedly. It appears that a change in the exhaled NO levels measured over time could be useful in monitoring asthma control.

Källén B. The safety of asthma medications during pregnancy. Exp Opin Drug Saf 2007; 6:15–26

This article reviews the literature on asthma or use of antiasthmatic drugs during pregnancy.

Lee-Wong M, Dayrit FM, Kohli AR, et al. Comparison of high-dose inhaled flunisolide to systemic corticosteroids in severe adult asthma. Chest 2002; 122: 1208–1213

High-dose ICS are as effective as systemic corticosteroids in the 7 days after hospital admission for severe asthma.

Le Gall C, Pham S, Vignes S, et al. Inhaled corticosteroids and Churg-Strauss syndrome: a report of five cases. Eur Respir J 2000; 15:978–981

The association of Churg-Strauss syndrome with LPMs has been well documented. This group presents five cases of Churg-Strauss syndrome in severe steroid-dependent asthmatic subjects in which the use of ICS allowed systemic corticosteroid withdrawal. It gives further evidence for systemic steroid withdrawal as a cause of Churg-Strauss syndrome since these patients were not receiving LPMs.

Leone FT, Fish JE, Szefler SJ, et al. Systematic review of the evidence regarding potential complications of inhaled corticosteroid use in asthma: collaboration of American College of Chest Physicians, American Academy of Allergy, Asthma, and Immunology, and American College of Allergy, Asthma, and Immunology. Chest 2003; 124:2329–2340

This multisociety report discusses the complications of ICS use in asthma patients. ICS use is not associated with a reduction in bone density in children with asthma. This can be said in adults but less conclusively. The risk of cataracts may be negligible in young asthmatic patients but it may be increased in older patients. The risk of glaucoma may be small, and further study is warranted. Therapy with ICS in children is associated with a decrease in short-term growth rates in children, but the overall effect is small and may not be sustained with long-term therapy. The risk of skin thinning and easy bruising is elevated in patients receiving ICS.

Lima JJ, Blake KV, Tantisira KG, et al. Pharmacogenetics of asthma. Curr Opin Pulm Med 2009; 15:57–62

This article discusses genetic variations in patient responses to drugs, including topics of β-agonist polymorphisms and responses to corticosteroids and LT antagonists.

Malo JL, Lemiere C, Gautrin D, et al. Occupational asthma. Curr Opin Pulm Med 2004; 10:57–61

This article reviews some of the more recent information regarding the pathophysiology, diagnosis, and prevention of occupational asthma. High-molecular-weight inhaled antigens work through an IgE mechanism. The second category of agents that induce occupational asthma are low-molecular-weight agents. They are generally chemicals, and the pathophysiology is not as well understood. There is little evidence for an IgE-mediated mechanism. The effects of exposure to isocyanates, the chemical most frequently responsible for occupational asthma, may work through the overproduction of matrix metal-loproteinase-9, which may cause symptoms and BHR. There is a predominant sputum neutrophilia after exposure to isocyanates. Specific inhalation challenges represent the "gold standard" for the diagnosis of occupational asthma. When not available, the serial recording of PEFRs has been advocated. The risk for men is greatest among bakers, laundry workers, shoemakers, animal skin and hide workers, and metal plating and coating workers. For women, the greatest risks are for shoemakers, railway station personnel, jewelry engravers, engine room crews, foundry molders, round-timber workers, and bakers. Results indicate that respiratory symptoms and airway responsiveness to methacholine persist in subjects who are removed from exposure to the isocyanates for >10 years.

Matricardi PM, Rosmini F, Panetta V, et al. Hay fever and asthma in relation to markers of infection in the United States. J Allergy Clin Immunol 2002; 110:381–387

This study shows that hay fever and asthma were less common in participants who were seropositive for hepatitis A, Toxoplasma gondii, *and herpes simplex virus 1 compared with seronegative participants. This finding suggests that the acquisition of certain infections, primarily food-borne and orofecal infections, is linked with a lower probability of having hay fever and asthma. These data are from the National Health and Nutrition Examination Study III.*

McFadden ER Jr. Acute severe asthma. Am J Respir Crit Care Med 2003; 168:740–759

This review discusses the current therapeutic options for the acute exacerbation of asthma. Seventy to 80% of patients in emergency departments clear within 2 h with standard care. The relapse rate is between 7% and 15%. The 20 to 30% of patients who are resistant to β-agonist therapy in the emergency department slowly reverse their condition over 36 to 48 h but require intensive treatment with corticosteroids.

McFadden ER Jr., Zawadski DK. Vocal cord dysfunction masquerading as exercise-induced asthma. Am J Respir Crit Care Med 1996; 153:942–947

This article discusses an interesting group of patients and extends the syndrome of vocal cord dysfunction to those who have only exercise-induced symptoms. Although the combination of exertion and wheezing suggests EIA, when patients presented in this article underwent clinical and physiologic evaluations, including bronchoprovocation testing, asthma was ruled out. Laryngoscopy was helpful in diagnosing vocal cord dysfunction.

McParland BE, Macklem PT, Pare PD. Airway remodeling: friend or foe? J Appl Physiol 2003; 95:426–434

In asthmatic patients, chronic inflammation of the airway wall results in an abnormal repair process. Changes that occur include subepithelial fibrosis, smooth-muscle hyperplasia and hypertrophy myofibroblast hyperplasia, epithelial hypertrophy, and mucus gland and goblet-cell hyperplasia. Collectively, these changes are called airway remodeling. *These structural changes are thought to be detrimental as they contribute to fixed airway narrowing. Thickening of the inner airway wall may also amplify the degree of luminal narrowing for a given degree of smooth-muscle shortening. This might result in an exaggerated narrowing of the airway after a bronchoconstricting stimulus. It has been argued that some aspects of remodeling have beneficial effects: stiffening the airway may result in decreased compressibility allowing the airways to better resist dynamic compression; and extra connective tissue, surrounding the smooth-muscle cells may provide a radial constraint to maximal shortening.*

Mitsunobu F, Tanizaki Y. The use of computed tomography to assess asthma severity. Curr Opin Allergy Clin Immunol 2005; 5:85–90

Chronic inflammation in asthma can lead to airway remodeling and airway narrowing. This can be quantified by the use of CT scanning. High-resolution CT scanning is a useful tool for imaging the airways of asthmatic patients. Asthmatic patients have thicker airways compared with control subjects. The thickness is related to disease severity, airflow obstruction, and airway reactivity. This is a new tool for assessing asthma severity.

Moore WC. Update in asthma 2007. Am J Respir Crit Care Med 2008; 177:1068–1073

This review discussed the articles published in 2007 in this respiratory journal.

Morgan WJ, Crain EF, Gruchalla RS, et al. Results of a home-based environmental intervention among urban children with asthma. N Engl J Med 2004; 351: 1068–1080

This group looked at a cohort of children with atopic asthma. A controlled trial of environmental intervention to reduce allergies and environmental smoke that included the reduction of exposure to indoor allergens, including cockroach and dust mite allergens, resulted in reduced asthma-associated morbidity.

Morgan WJ, Stern DA, Sherrill DL, et al. Outcome of asthma and wheezing in the first 6 years of life: follow-up through adolescence. Am J Respir Crit Care Med 2005; 172:1253–1258

The authors found that in children who start having asthma-like symptoms before the preschool years, the prevalence of wheezing and the levels of lung function are established by age 6 years and do not appear to change significantly by age 16 years. Transient early wheezers (ie, children who wheeze during early life but who were not wheezing at age 6 years) were no more likely to wheeze after age 6 years than healthy children. These children have lower lung function before the transient wheezing and continue to have lower levels of lung function through adolescence. It is known from other studies that COPD is more likely to develop during later adult years in individuals who enter adult life with lung function deficits. Whether early wheezing predicts COPD is not known. The study also showed that deficits in lung function that are observed in children with asthma are not the consequence of ongoing disease, but rather are due to changes before the age of 6 years. Although the transient wheezers have lower lung function that is present as early as the first 3 months of life, they do not have the elevations in serum IgE levels, eosinophilia, and skin test reactivity to aeroallergens that are seen in those with persistent wheezing from early childhood to later childhood.

Murphy VE, Clifton VL, Gibson PG. Asthma exacerbations during pregnancy: incidence and association with adverse pregnancy outcomes. Thorax 2006; 61:169–176

This article reminds us that exacerbations during pregnancy occur primarily in the late second trimester. The major triggers are viral infection and nonadherence to ICS therapy. Women who have an exacerbation during pregnancy are at a significantly increased risk of having a low-birth-weight baby compared to women without asthma.

Murugan A, Prys-Picard C, Calhoun WJ. Biomarkers in asthma. Curr Opin Pulm Med. 2009; 15:12–18

This article reviews the current literature about the use of biomarkers for the diagnosis and monitoring of asthma. To date, evidence suggests that exhaled NO may become a clinical test for asthma control. The article discusses the limitation of this measurement and recent clinical trials showing some promise.

Nathan RA, Sorkness CA, Kosinski M, et al. Development of the asthma control test: a survey for assessing asthma control. J Allergy Clin Immunol 2004; 113: 59–65

The NAEPP guidelines have concentrated on a classification of asthma that is static and does not really discuss asthma control and response to therapy. This asthma control test presents a scoring system for asthma control that includes five items for gauging the status of current asthma. These include asthma symptoms, the use of rescue medications, and questions regarding the impact of asthma on everyday functioning. This is a brief, easy-to-administer, patient-based index of asthma control.

National Asthma Education and Prevention Program. Expert panel report 3: guidelines for the diagnosis and management of asthma. Bethesda, MD: National Institutes of Health, August 2007

This guideline should be on the bookshelf of every pulmonologist. This particular report is the most recent update of the first report published in 1991. This updated report is posted on the Internet (http://www.nhlbi.NAEPP.gov/guidelines/asthma/index.htm). Key differences in the report include the following comments: (1) The critical role of inflammation has been further substantiated, but evidence is emerging for considerable variability in the pattern of inflammation, thus indicating phenotypic differences that may influence treatment responses. (2) Gene-by-environmental interactions are important to the development and expression of asthma. Of the environmental factors, allergic reactions remain important. Evidence also suggests a key and expanding role for viral respiratory infections in these processes. (3) The onset of asthma for most patients begins early in life, with the pattern of disease persistence determined by early, recognizable risk factors, including atopic disease, recurrent wheezing, and a parental history of asthma. (4) Current asthma treatment with antiinflammatory therapy does not appear to prevent progression of the underlying disease severity. (5) The key elements of assessment and monitoring are refined to include the separate, but related, concepts of severity, control, and responsiveness to treatment. Classifying severity is emphasized for initiating therapy; assessing control is emphasized for monitoring and adjusting therapy. Asthma severity and control are defined in terms of two domains: impairment and risk. (6) The distinction between the domains of impairment and risk for assessing asthma severity and control emphasizes the need to consider separately asthma's effects on quality of life and functional capacity on an ongoing basis (ie, in the present) and the risks it presents for adverse events in the future, such as exacerbations and progressive loss of pulmonary. (7) Emphasis on the many potential points of care and sites available in which to provide asthma education, including review of new evidence regarding the efficacy of asthma self-management and education outside the usual office setting. (8) Greater emphasis on the two aspects of the written asthma action plan—(a) daily management and (b) how to recognize and handle worsening asthma. Use of the terminology "written asthma action plan" encompasses both aspects. This change addresses confusion over the previous guidelines' use of different terms. One term is now used for the written asthma action plan, although in some studies cited, investigators may have used a variation of this term. (9) New sections on the impact of cultural and ethnic factors and health literacy that affect delivery of asthma self-management education. (10) Information about asthma medications has been updated based on review of evidence published since 1997. This updated report (Expert Panel Report 3) continues to emphasize that the most effective medications for long-term therapy are those shown to have antiinflammatory effects. (11) New medications—immunomodulators—are available for long-term control of asthma. (12) New data on the safety of LABAs are discussed, and the position of LABA in therapy has been revised). The most significant difference is that for youths ≥ 12 years of age and adults who have moderate persistent asthma or asthma inadequately controlled on low-dose ICS, the option of increasing the dose of medium-dose ICS should be given equal weight to the option of adding LABA to low-dose ICS. (13) The estimated clinical comparability of different ICS preparations has been updated. The significant role of ICS in asthma therapy continues to be supported.

Nelson HS, Weiss SC, Bleecker ER, et al. The Salmeterol Multicenter Asthma Research Trial: a comparison of usual pharmacotherapy for asthma or usual pharmacotherapy plus salmeterol. Chest 2006; 129:15–26

The safety of salmeterol vs placebo was studied in a 28-week randomized observational study. In a telephone follow-up, it was found that there were small but statistically significant iincreases in respiratory-related and asthma deaths in the population of patients receiving placebo. Subgroup analysis suggested that the risk was greater in African Americans. A post hoc analysis was conducted to explore the effect of ICS use on the results of this trial, often called the SMART trial. *The number of deaths that occurred in patients who were not receiving ICS at baseline was greater in the salmeterol group, suggesting a relationship. The study was not designed to evaluate the effects of ICS therapy; therefore, adequate conclusions could not be drawn. The study raised the alert that therapy with LABAs may have adverse effects in some populations. Further studies need to clarify the veracity of these findings. In the meantime, the US Food and Drug Administration has placed a warning on the package insert because of this study.*

Newman KB, Mason UG III, Schmaling KB. Clinical features of vocal cord dysfunction. Am J Respir Crit Care Med 1995; 152:1382–1386

This article reviews vocal cord dysfunction in asthmatic and nonasthmatic patients. All patients had laryngoscopic evidence of paradoxical vocal cord motion with inspiratory and/or early expiratory vocal cord adduction. The patients were predominantly women and had a misdiagnosis of asthma for an average of almost 5 years. Many were steroid dependent, and medical utilization was enormous. Twenty-eight percent of the patients had been intubated. This study helps to define the historical and clinical features of vocal cord dysfunction.

Ngoc LP, Gold DR, Tzianabos AO, et al. Cytokines, allergy, and asthma. Curr Opin Allergy Clin Immunol 2005; 5:161–166

This article is a review of more recent articles on the relation ship of cytokines to allergy and asthma. It discusses the immune mechanisms involved in the phenotypic expression of allergic diseases, including the allergen-specific T-helper type 2 responses that release IL-4, IL-13, and IL-5.

O'Bryne PM, Bisgaard H, Godard PP, et al. Budesonide/formoterol combination therapy as both maintenance and reliever medication in asthma. Am J Respir Crit Care Med 2005; 171:129–136

This group hypothesized that the conditions of patients receiving low-dose ICS/LABA therapy whose asthma was not under good control would be improved with as-needed ICS/LABA (ie, budesonide/formoterol) therapy rather than short-acting β_2*-agonist reliever medication. In a double-blind randomized study of 2,760 patients with asthma, the budesonide/formoterol maintenance therapy plus relief medication prolonged the time to first exacerbations and resulted in a 45% lower exacerbation risk vs therapy with budesonide/formoterol plus a short-acting* β_2*-agonist. The therapy also improved symptoms, nighttime awakenings, and lung function.*

O'Byrne PM, Inman MD. Airway hyperresponsiveness. Chest 2003; 123(suppl):411S–416S

This is a review of the features of airway hyperresponsiveness, a feature that is constant in asthma. Measurements of airway responsiveness are useful in making a diagnosis of asthma, especially when symptoms are present and there is no airflow obstruction.

O'Byrne PM, Pedersen S. Measuring efficacy and safety of different inhaled corticosteroid preparations. J Allergy Clin Immunol 1998; 102:879–886

This is a review of ICS therapy in patients with asthma. An excellent section on potential systemic effects is also included. Differences in pharmacologic properties among the ICS are discussed.

Panettieri RA Jr. Airway smooth muscle: an immunomodulatory cell. J Allergy Clin Immunol 2002; 110: S269–S274

The airway smooth muscle is a major effector cell of asthma that is responsible for bronchomotor tone. Some evidence suggests that it also may be active in secreting cytokines and chemokines and also may express cellular adhesion molecules. Growth factors may be formed from airway smooth-muscle cells, and hence, an autocrine-like proliferative response may occur.

Pearlman DS. Pathophysiology of the inflammatory response. J Allergy Clin Immunol 1999; 104:S132–S137

This article provides a review of the pathophysiology of the atopic inflammatory response. An in-depth discussion of antigen sensitization and the subsequent cytokine response is provided.

Phipps P, Garrard CS. The pulmonary physician in critical care: acute severe asthma in the intensive care unit. Thorax 2003; 58:81–88

This review discusses the approach to status asthmaticus in the ICU, including a good discussion on modes of ventilation, ventilator setting, and the use of extrinsic positive end-expiratory pressure. Other modalities, including the use of helium, magnesium sulfate, and inhalation anesthetic agents, also are discussed.

Restrepo RD, Peters J. Near-fatal asthma: recognition and management. Curr Opin Pulm Med 2008; 14: 13–23

This review discusses recent advances in our understanding of the pathophysiology, diagnosis, and treatment of near-fatal asthma

Ringdal N, Chuchalin A, Chovan L, et al. Evaluation of different inhaled combination therapies (EDICT): a randomised, double-blind comparison of Seretide (50/250 microg bd Diskus vs formoterol (12 microg bd) and budesonide (800 microg bd) given concurrently (both via Turbuhaler) in patients with moderate-to-severe asthma. Respir Med 2002; 96:851–861

This study was the first comparison of LABA/ICS combination therapies. Salmeterol plus fluticasone was at least as effective as formoterol plus budesonide in improving pulmonary function despite a lower corticosteroid dose. The former combination also significantly reduced exacerbation rates and nocturnal symptoms. More studies are needed to confirm these results.

Rodrigo GJ, Rodrigo C, Pollack CV, et al. Use of helium-oxygen mixtures in the treatment of acute asthma: a systematic review. Chest 2003; 123:891–896

This study discusses the use of helium in the treatment of acute asthma and concludes that evidence does not provide support for heliox mixtures in patients with acute severe asthma. Conclusions, however, are based on small studies.

Salvi SS, Krishna MT, Sampson, et al. The anti-inflammatory effects of leukotriene-modifying drugs and their use in asthma. Chest 2001; 119:1533–1546

This article reviews the beneficial effects of LT-modifying drugs in the management of all grades of asthma severity. It concludes that certain patient groups, such as those with EIA or aspirin-induced asthma, may be particularly suitable for such therapy.

Schaub B, von Mutius E. Obesity and asthma, what are the links? Curr Opin Allergy Clin Immunol 2005; 5:185–193

This article reviews the relationship between obesity and asthma. A number of prospective studies have shown that weight gain can antedate the development of asthma. Several hypotheses have been proposed to explain the epidemiologic associations and are discussed in this article, including airway mechanics, influences on immune responses, and hormonal influences. Particularly, the diminished tidal lung expansion in overweight individuals may partially account for the findings. Studies in animal models have indicated that elevations of IL-6 levels may contribute to and up-regulate inflammation in the airways. The levels of the hormone leptin, a member of the IL-6 family, are increased in obese persons. Leptin may have an effect on inflammation by promoting the release of IL-6 from macrophages in lymphocytes. Other potential factors also are discussed.

Sciurba FC. Physiologic similarities and differences between COPD and asthma. Chest 2004; 126(suppl): 117S–124S

There are significant differences in the physiologic consequences of COPD in asthma, as described in this article. However, it also takes a closer inspection of the literature and reveals significant overlaps between the two conditions. It reminds us that there is a subgroup of COPD patients that has features indistinguishable from asthma.

Sears MR, Greene JM, Willan AR, et al. A longitudinal, population-based, cohort study of childhood asthma followed to adulthood. N Engl J Med 2003; 349:1414–1422

The outcome of childhood asthma is reported in this population-based study. The risk factors for the persistence and relapse of asthma into adulthood are described. In this study, more than one in four children had wheezing that persisted from childhood to adulthood or that relapsed after remission. The factors predicting persistence or relapse were sensitization to house dust mites, airway hyperresponsiveness, female sex, smoking, and early age at onset. These findings, together with persistently low lung function, suggest that outcomes in adult patients with asthma may be determined primarily in early childhood.

Shore SA, Drazen JM. β-Agonists and asthma: too much of a good thing? J Clin Invest 2003; 112:495–497

This interesting article discusses a theory of why a paradoxical response sometimes develops in asthmatic patients who receive long-term treatment with short-acting β-agonists.

Sin DD, Sutherland ER. Obesity and the lung: 4. Obesity and asthma. Thorax 2008; 63:1018–1023

This review examines the clinical and epidemiological relationship between obesity and asthma and the purported mechanisms that may link these two processes together.

Smith AD, Cowan J, Brassett K, et al. Exhaled nitric oxide: a predictor of steroid response. Am J Respir Crit Care Med 2005; 172:453–459

Patients with asthma symptoms who had not previously received a diagnosis of asthma were studied to determine whether exhaled NO measurements would predict steroid-responsive phenotypes. Levels of exhaled NO proved to be more sensitive and specific for identifying steroid responders than was FEV_1 percentage of predicted, peak flow variability, or tests of BHR.

Smith AD, Cowan J, Brassett K, et al. Use of inhaled nitric oxide measurements to guide treatment of chronic asthma. N Engl J Med 2005; 352:2163–2173

These authors determined whether measurements of the fraction of exhaled NO constitute a noninvasive marker of inflammation that may be a useful alternative for the adjustment of ICS treatment. A threshold of ≥ 15 parts per billion of exhaled NO was used to increase the dose of ICS. They found that with fraction of exhaled NO measurements maintenance doses of ICS could be significantly reduced without compromising asthma control.

Smith AD, Taylor DR. Is exhaled nitric oxide measurement a useful clinical test in asthma? Curr Opin Allergy Clin Immunol 2005; 5:49–56

This is a good review on the use of exhaled NO measurements in the management of asthma. Epidemiologic data confirm that exhaled NO measurements reflect the presence and severity of airway inflammation in asthma patients. Reference values and thresholds for an abnormal test need to be agreed on internationally.

Sont JK, Willems LNA, Bel EH, et al. Clinical control and histopathologic outcome of asthma when using airway hyperresponsiveness as an additional guide to long-term treatment. Am J Respir Crit Care Med 1999; 159:1043–1051

This group of investigators explored whether a treatment strategy aimed at reducing airway hyperresponsiveness added to the strategies used in the asthma guidelines would provide more effective control of asthma and greater improvement in chronic airway inflammation. They did show that reducing airway hyperresponsiveness led to more effective control of asthma. This implies that the monitoring of airway hyperresponsiveness (by repeated bronchial inhalation challenge) may improve the long-term management of asthma.

Suissa S, Ernst P, Benayoun S, et al. Low-dose inhaled corticosteroids and the prevention of death from asthma. N Engl J Med 2000; 343:332–336

This important article gives evidence that the regular use of low-dose ICS is associated with a decreased risk of death from asthma.

Sur S, Crotty TB, Kephart GM, et al. Sudden-onset fatal asthma: a distinct entity with few eosinophils and relatively more neutrophils in the airway submucosa? Am Rev Respir Dis 1993; 148:713–719

This study determined the histologic differences in the airways of patients who died of sudden-onset asthma (<1 h) compared with those who had the more commonly seen slow-onset asthma. Patients with slow-onset asthma had more eosinophils and fewer neutrophils than patients with sudden-onset asthma. The authors concluded that sudden-onset asthma is immunohistologically distinct from the slow-onset type because of these differences in eosinophilic and neutrophilic airway infiltration. They raise the possibility that the mechanisms involved in these two distinct forms of asthma are different.

Sutherland ER, Martin RJ. Asthma and atypical bacterial infection Chest. 2007; 132:1962–1966

This article reviews the basic and clinical science that implicates the atypical bacterial pathogens M pneumoniae *and* Chlamydophila *(formerly* Chlamydia*)* pneumoniae *as potentially important factors in asthma. Although their exact contribution to asthma development and/or persistence remains to be determined, evidence links them to new-onset asthma and asthma exacerbations.*

Szczeklik A, Stevenson DD. Aspirin-induced asthma: advances in pathogenesis, diagnosis, and management. J Allergy Clin Immunol 2003; 111:913–921

This article discusses aspirin-induced asthma, including the clinical presentation and the molecular biology. It concludes that aspirin-induced asthma runs a protracted course even if therapy with cyclooxygenase-1 inhibitors is avoided. Aspirin desensitization followed by daily aspirin treatment is a valuable therapeutic option.

Tan WC. Viruses in asthma exacerbations. Curr Opin Pulm Med 2005; 11:21–26

This review discusses the role of viruses as triggers for acute exacerbations of asthma. The application of molecular diagnostic methods has shown that rhinovirus is the most common cause but coinfection is frequent. Viruses provoke asthma attacks by additive or synergistic interactions with allergen exposure or air pollution. Respiratory viruses cause asthma exacerbations by triggering the recruitment of T-helper type 2 cells into the lung.

Tarlo SM, Balmes J, Balkissoon R, et al. Diagnosis and management of work-related asthma: American College of Chest Physicians Consensus Statement. Chest 2008; 134(3 suppl):1S–41S

This review replaces a previous American College of Chest Physicians Consensus Statement on asthma in the workplace was published in 1995. This current Consensus Statement was written by a panel of experts, including allergists, pulmonologists, and occupational medicine physicians, The Consensus Document defined work-related asthma to include occupational asthma (ie, asthma induced by sensitizer or irritant work exposures) and work-exacerbated asthma (ie, preexisting or concurrent asthma worsened by work factors). The Consensus Document focuses on the diagnosis and management (including diagnostic tests, and work and compensation issues), as well as preventive measures.

Turner WS, Palmer LJ, Rye PJ, et al. The relationship between infant airway function, childhood airway responsiveness and asthma. Am J Respir Crit Care Med 2004; 169:921–927

This study sought to determine whether there are early life factors that can predict the development of asthma later in childhood. A total of 243 Australian children were prospectively studied during the course of 11 years. The presence of wheezing at age 11 years was associated with lower lung function during infancy and was independent of increased airway responsiveness and atopy at a younger age. This suggests that intrinsic disturbances in lung function, possibly related to lung development, maternal factors, and/or environmental factors close to the time of birth, have a role in the later development of asthma. Ongoing atopy and BHR predicted wheezing that persisted from ages 4 to 6 years to age 11.

Van Hove CL, Maes T, Joos GF, Chronic inflammation in asthma: a contest of persistence vs resolution. Allergy 2008; 63:1095–109

Recent investigations have highlighted that endogenous antiinflammatory mediators and immune-regulating mechanisms are important for the resolution of inflammatory processes. A disruption of these mechanisms can be causally related not only to the initiation of unnecessary inflammation, but also to the persistence of several chronic inflammatory diseases. This article discusses these potential mechanisms with asthma.

Vonk JM, Jongepier H, Panhusen CIM, et al. Risk factors associated with the presence of irreversible airflow limitation and reduced transfer coefficient in patients with asthma after 26 years of follow up. Thorax 2003; 58:322–327

Fixed airflow obstruction develops in some asthmatic patients. In this study, after 20 to 30 years of follow-up, adults with a history of asthma were reexamined to assess the risk factors for the development of irreversible airway obstruction and low diffusing capacity. In this study, irreversible airflow obstruction developed in 16% of patients. This was associated with a lower FEV_1 *(percentage of predicted), a lower level of BHR, less reversibility at initial testing, and with less use of corticosteroids at follow-up.*

Walker S, Monteil M, Phelan K, et al. Anti-IgE for chronic asthma. Cochrane Database Syst Rev (database online). Issue 3, 2004

This Cochrane Database report discusses the use of recombinant humanized monoclonal antibody directed against IgE. This therapy (called omalizumab) is significantly more effective than placebo at increasing the number of patients who are able to reduce or withdraw from therapy with ICS. It also reduces the number of asthma exacerbations.

Wark PA, Gibson PG, Wilson AJ. Azoles for allergic bronchopulmonary aspergillosis associated with asthma. Cochrane Database Syst Rev (database online). Issue 34, 2004

This review concludes that itraconazole modifies the immunologic action associated with ABPA and improves clinical outcomes.

Wenzel S. Severe/fatal asthma. Chest 2003; 123(suppl): 405S–410S

This is a discussion of severe fatal asthma, including the genetic and environmental factors that are responsible. It discusses the pathologic findings, including eosinophilic inflammation, structural changes, and distal disease.

Wenzel S. Severe asthma in adults. Am J Respir Crit Care Med 2005; 172:149–160

This is a pulmonary perspective on severe asthma, which disproportionately consumes health-care resources related to this disease. Early-onset severe asthma is a more allergic associated disease. Severe asthma with persistent eosinophilia (either early onset or late onset) is more symptomatic and has more near-fatal events. At least 50% of patients with severe asthma have little identifiable inflammation. Steroid resistance in severe asthma is also discussed in this article.

Wenzel SE, Szefler SJ, Leung DY, et al. Bronchoscopic evaluation of severe asthma. Am J Respir Crit Care Med 1997; 156:737–743

This study was designed to evaluate the type of airway inflammation in patients with severe asthma who are receiving high-dose oral glucocorticoids. Eosinophils were not found in healthy control individuals or patients with severe asthma but were seen in patients with moderate asthma. In contrast, patients with severe asthma demonstrated a greater concentration of neutrophils in BAL fluid. Findings suggest that inflammation remains in symptomatic patients with severe asthma despite glucocorticoid treatment.

West PM, Fernandez C. Safety of COX-2 inhibitors in asthma patients with aspirin hypersensitivity. Ann Pharmacother 2003; 37:1497–1501

This study concludes that cyclooxygenase-2 inhibitors provide a potentially safe alternative for the treatment of inflammatory conditions in patients with aspirin-induced asthma.

Notes

Cardiopulmonary Exercise Testing

Darcy D. Marciniuk, MD, FCCP

Objectives:

- Provide a brief overview of normal exercise physiology and responses
- Outline the indications, conduct, and interpretation of cardiopulmonary exercise testing
- Highlight characteristic responses commonly demonstrated by patients with various disorders frequently assessed by the pulmonologist

Key words: cardiopulmonary exercise testing; exercise; interpretation; pulmonary function laboratory; pulmonary function testing

---

Exercise in the normal human involves the effective integration of respiratory, cardiovascular, neuromuscular, and metabolic functions. The organs involved in these varied and important roles have a sizeable reserve, with the consequence that clinical manifestations of a disease state or abnormality may not become readily apparent until the functional capacity of the organ(s) is markedly impaired. When this manifestation occurs, patients often experience the distressing and disabling symptoms of shortness of breath with activity and exercise limitation. Cardiopulmonary exercise testing (CPET) has secured an essential role in our practice of clinical medicine by allowing the clinician to objectively evaluate these important functions and symptoms.

Objective assessment and measurement of various parameters during exercise, which places an increased physiologic demand on the functional reserve capacity of these organs, can also provide a sensitive method for the early detection of abnormal function and response(s). The results from exercise testing parallel functional capacity and quality of life more closely than measurements obtained only at rest, and they have been shown to accurately predict important outcomes, such as the rate of mortality, in a variety of patients and clinical circumstances. Although the use of CPET has been previously viewed as being merely interesting in the hands of a few individuals, CPET is now cemented into mainstream clinical practice. In view of these meaningful benefits, the conduct and interpretation of CPET is now an essential competency for practicing pulmonologists.

Normal Exercise Physiology

Knowledge and a thorough understanding of normal exercise physiology are essential for the appropriate interpretation of exercise responses in disease. Although relevant principles of normal exercise physiology will be briefly summarized, a comprehensive review of this subject topic is beyond the intent of this course and syllabus. The reader is encouraged to consult more detailed appropriate source literature and documents on this topic (see the references section).

To meet the increased metabolic demands of exercise, the respiratory and cardiovascular systems must be able to augment oxygen delivery to the working skeletal muscles. Oxygen transport in the body depends on a series of linked mechanisms that can be schematically expressed as follows (adapted from Jones; 1). Potential factors that may affect these mechanisms are shown in parentheses, but these are not inclusive:

Inspired O_2
(altitude)
↓
Respiratory ventilation
(alveolar ventilation, distribution)
↓
Respiratory gas exchange
(diffusion, ventilation/perfusion)
↓
Arterial O_2
(oxygen capacity, saturation)
↓
Cardiac output
(SV, cardiac frequency)
↓

Circulation and muscle blood flow
(peripheral vascular resistance)
↓
O_2 extraction
(capillary-tissue diffusion)
↓
Muscle O_2 utilization → O_2 stores
(respiratory enzymes)
↓
Venous O_2

Similarly, the removal of carbon dioxide (CO_2), which is a byproduct of metabolism, can be expressed with the following scheme (adapted from Jones; 1):

CO_2 production (aerobic, anaerobic)
↓→ CO_2 stores
Muscle blood flow and circulation
↓
Venous CO_2
↓
Venous return
(cardiac output)
↓
Respiratory gas exchange
(ventilation/perfusion)
↓
Respiratory ventilation
(alveolar ventilation, distribution)
↓
Expired CO_2

Understanding the cardiorespiratory and metabolic responses to exercise is further facilitated by closer examination of the direct physiologic determinants of oxygen uptake ($\dot{V}o_2$) and carbon dioxide output ($\dot{V}co_2$) as depicted in the following equations. The cardiovascular responses are represented by rearrangement of the Fick equation:

$$(1)\ \dot{V}o_2 = Q_T\,(Cao_2 - Cvo_2)$$

or

$$(2)\ \dot{V}o_2 = (HR \cdot SV)\,(Cao_2 - Cvo_2)$$

where Qt is cardiac output, the product of stroke volume (SV) and heart rate (HR), and $Cao_2 - Cvo_2$ is the oxygen content difference between systemic arterial and mixed venous blood.

Meanwhile, when the inspired CO_2 concentration is negligible, the respiratory response to exercise can be represented by the following equation:

$$(3)\ \frac{V_A = k \cdot \dot{V}co_2}{Paco_2}$$

or

$$(4)\ \frac{\dot{V}_E = k \cdot \dot{V}co_2}{Paco_2\,(1 - V_D/V_T)}$$

where $\dot{V}_E$ is minute ventilation, the sum of alveolar ventilation (V_A) and dead space ventilation (V_D). V_D/V_T is the ratio of physiologic dead space to tidal volume. These relationships are used to understand the ventilatory response during exercise because $\dot{V}_E$ and V_A are associated more closely to $\dot{V}co_2$ than to $\dot{V}o_2$. Graphical representations of how the respiratory and cardiovascular systems respond to meet the demands of exercise in the normal human are shown in Figures 1 and 2.

These relationships and equations also serve to illustrate and emphasize the integrative aspects of exercise, which result in the total response being greater than could be supported by any individual contribution alone. For instance, oxygen supply in a fit athlete may increase to >20 times the resting oxygen consumption (*ie*, from 0.25 L/min at rest to >5.0 L/min at peak exercise). This net increase

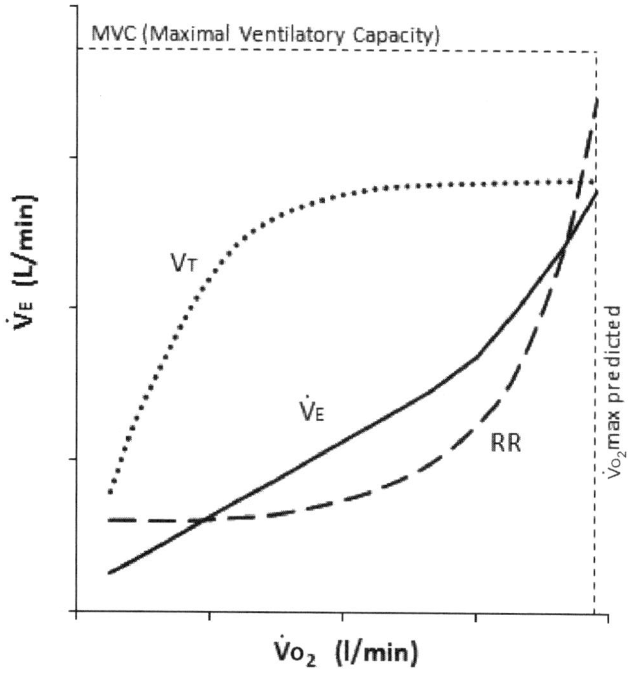

Figure 1. Respiratory system responses during exercise.

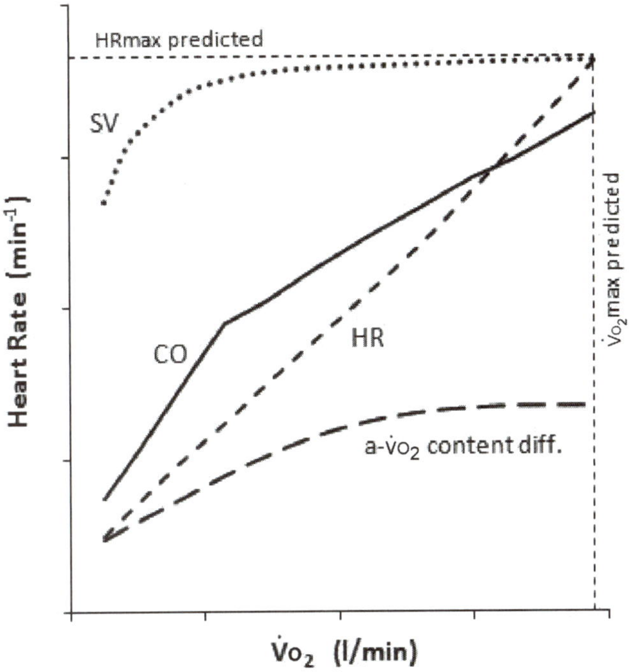

Figure 2. Cardiovascular system responses during exercise.

is not brought about by a 20-fold increase in any one mechanism but rather is shared between mechanisms. For example, the increase in $\dot{V}$E during exercise occurs not only because of the typical hyperventilation (attributable to metabolic acidosis) at the end of exercise but also because of a significant decrease in VD/VT during exercise.

The fractional changes in various components of the cardiovascular and respiratory systems during exercise are summarized in Figure 3, which shows representative data from a population of normal middle-aged men. These data illustrate the major demands placed on cardiorespiratory function during exercise, and they exemplify the significant reserve that exists to meet the increased demands of exercise. These demands are met by increases in ventilation (breathing frequency and VT) and cardiac output (HR and SV) as well as by redistribution of blood to the exercising muscles. In addition, VD decreases as VA becomes more efficient. The $\dot{V}o_2$ increases with increasing exercise and, in some fit and motivated individuals, reaches a plateau near the end of exercise. Meanwhile, as CO_2 production continues, further fueled by anaerobic respiration and progressive increases in lactate production later in exercise, the respiratory exchange ratio (RER) increases in the normal human. The peak $\dot{V}o_2$ is usually determined by the capacity of the cardiovascular system to deliver oxygen to the working muscles. Except in well-trained athletes and perhaps the fit elderly, gas exchange remains well preserved during exercise, although the hyperventilation induced by lactic acid production typically results in a slight decrease in $Paco_2$ and an increase in Pao_2.

Clinical Indications for CPET

The indications for CPET are varied and depend on the clinical setting and question(s) to be addressed. Shortness of breath with exercise and limitation of activity are cardinal and common symptoms of dysfunction and are therefore some

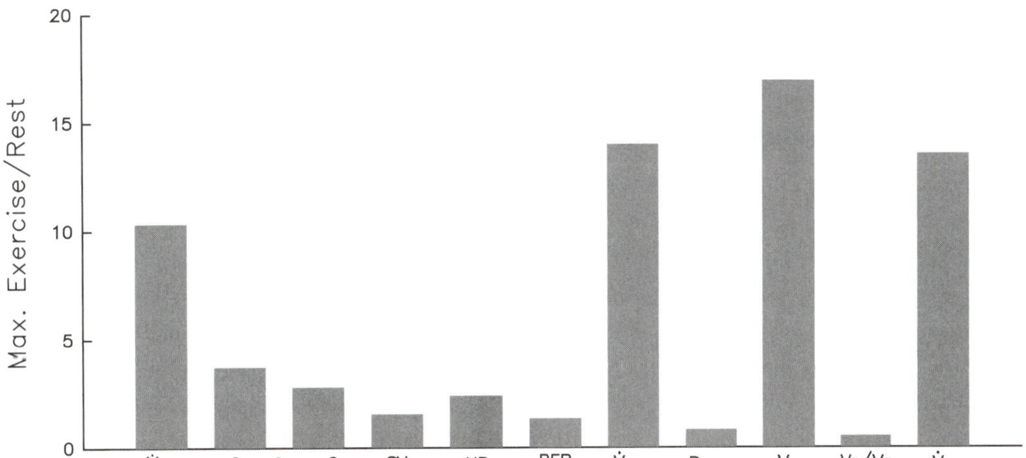

	$\dot{V}o_2$ (L/min)	QT (L/min)	Cao_2-Cvo_2 (ml/L)	SV (ml)	HR (min^{-1})	RER	$\dot{V}co_2$ (L/min)	$Paco_2$ (mmHg)	VA (L/min)	VD/VT	$\dot{V}$E (L/min)
Rest	0.29	5.8	50	77	75	0.83	0.24	40	5.2	0.34	7.9
Maximal	3.00	21.6	140	120	180	1.12	3.36	33	88	0.18	107

Figure 3. Relationship between resting and maximal exercise values in normal humans. Adapted from Gallagher.[2]

of the most frequent reasons for testing in the clinical laboratory. CPET also has significant utility in distinguishing normal from abnormal responses and in establishing cardiovascular from respiratory causes for activity limitation.

Our understanding of the clinical utility of CPET is also increasing as further work is published demonstrating the prognostic value of exercise testing in various clinical settings.[1,3,4,5] Results from exercise testing have been shown to correlate with important clinical outcomes, including rate of mortality, in COPD, interstitial lung disease (ILD), cystic fibrosis, primary pulmonary hypertension, and chronic heart failure. Generally accepted clinical indications for CPET are listed in Table 1.

Equipment, Conduct, and Measurements

Exercise testing is most commonly performed with either a stationary cycle ergometer or a motorized treadmill. Both cycle ergometer and treadmill testing are appropriate, although the cycle ergometer is used more frequently. The cycle ergometer allows for a direct measurement of work rate, has less potential for the creation of artifacts, and seems to be better tolerated by patients, particularly those with significant lower-limb joint problems. Alternatively, the treadmill yields greater values for the peak $\dot{V}O_2$ (approximately 8 to 12%) and is better accepted by fit normal subjects.[5]

Specialized equipment is required for CPET, necessitating both increased cost and expertise. Although reliable and user-friendly equipment is now available as the result of advances in technology, these advances also have ushered in a multitude of confusing numbers and graphs that this new equipment now produces. Similar to pulmonary function testing equipment, exercise testing equipment systems, whether mixing chamber or breath-by-breath ones, require meticulous calibration procedures to ensure that measurements are and remain accurate and precise. In addition to daily calibration, routine physiologic calibration should be performed. This calibration is best undertaken by having a healthy staff member exercise at several constant work rates for a specified duration while $\dot{V}E$, $\dot{V}O_2$, and $\dot{V}CO_2$ are measured. This procedure might entail measurements after 4 to 6 min each of rest, 50 W and 100 W. Values should remain consistent (< 5% variation) with measurements collected previously under identical circumstances. If not, the cause of any discrepancy must be investigated and corrected. The ventilatory measurements unique to CPET are listed in Figure 4, in which measured variables are denoted by solid lines, whereas derived variables are denoted by dashed lines.

In addition to the aforementioned measurements, the PaO_2 (arterial sampling) or arterial oxygen saturation (SpO_2; *ie*, oxygen saturation by pulse oximetry) work rate (cycle ergometer), BP (cuff sphygmomanometer), heart rate/rhythm (ECG), and symptoms of shortness of breath and leg fatigue (modified Borg scale or visual analog scale) are measured. The reason(s) for stopping exercise should always be noted.

Together, these measurements allow for a comprehensive evaluation of behaviors during exercise and for the determination of various derived variables that provide additional information in the interpretation process. However, as noted, it is important to be focused on the overriding principles, values, and relationships of both normal and abnormal responses rather than become confused and misled by the often-unnecessary plethora of confusing numbers and graphs.

Cycle ergometers and treadmills should undergo periodic calibration, although this calibration is typically necessary only every few years or if the equipment has been moved. The manufacturer should be contacted to facilitate these procedures, which are more detailed and require more specialized expertise and techniques.

The patient should wear comfortable clothes and shoes, and he or she should refrain from heavy activity or meals for 2 h before testing. All testing

Table 1. *Clinical Indications for CPET**

Objective assessment of symptoms
Evaluation of severity of impairment
Appraisal of contributors to exercise limitation
Early detection of disease or impairment
Assessment of response to therapy
Disability assessment
Assessment/titration of supplemental oxygen therapy
Identification of exercise-associated bronchoconstriction
Preoperative risk and transplantation assessment

*Adapted from Palange et al[4] and Weisman et al.[5]

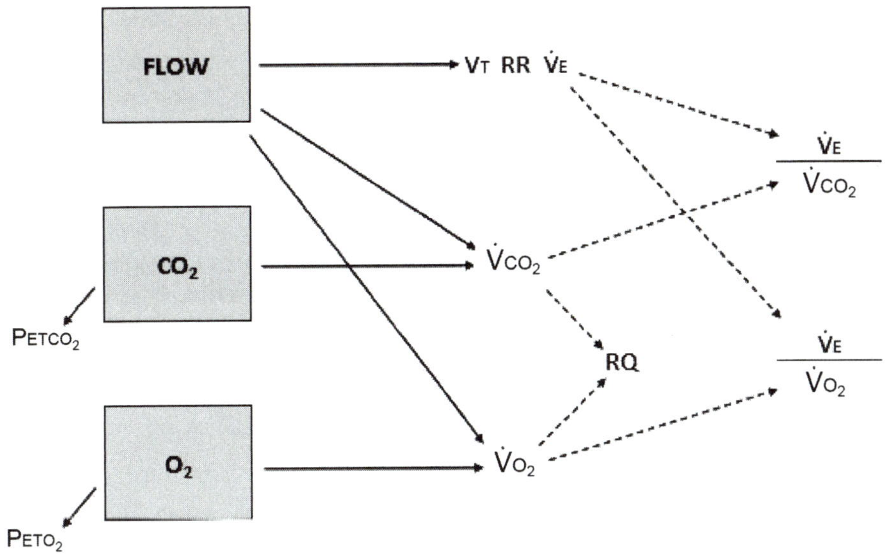

Figure 4. Measured and derived ventilatory measurements.

procedures should be explained, and informed consent should be obtained. A brief review of the clinical history and a physical examination should be performed. Baseline spirometry is measured, and the patient should be familiarized with use of the equipment before the test. If a cycle will be used, the seat and handlebars should be adjusted for comfort. In the case of a treadmill, the patient should be shown how to get on and off the moving belt comfortably and safely.

The choice of which test to perform depends in large part on the clinical question being addressed. Maximal symptom-limited incremental protocols are most commonly performed. Endurance exercise protocols often are conducted in clinical trials to determine a treatment effect, and they may have clinical utility in the individual patient when the clinician is assessing a response to an intervention. They are often completed at a constant work rate (approximately 75% of the maximal work rate is typical) and continued until the patient is no longer able to exercise. Exercise challenge testing frequently is performed to objectively assess for the presence of exercise-induced bronchoconstriction (EIB). The test is performed to illicit approximately 6 min of very intense exercise associated with high levels of $\dot{V}_E$. Spirometry is then performed after exercise at frequent intervals (1, 5, 10, 15, 20, and 30 min are recommended), with a decrease in the FEV_1 of 10% indicating possible and 15% probable EIB.[6] Readers are asked to consult referenced guideline statements for further information and detail regarding the conduct of this specialized testing.[5,6]

The performance and conduct of the 6-min walk distance test will not be addressed in this chapter, but it is discussed in more detail elsewhere.[7] However, timed walk tests (typically 6 min or 12 min) are the standard "simple" test for the assessment of activity limitation. They are safe and practical, and they tend to mimic activities of daily living. Their utility has been confirmed to improve with standardization, although they are susceptible to a training effect (similar to other tests). Their major limitation is they provide restricted information regarding physiologic contributors and mechanisms of exercise limitation. Nonetheless, they have become embedded in our field because of the meaningful information they yield.[8,9]

Shuttle walk tests are emerging as another option in this setting, and reports[10,11] have validated their usefulness in detecting a treatment effect. The obstacle to more widespread use at this time relates to a lack of familiarity. However, as further reports validating their utility are published, our understanding of the role of both incremental and endurance shuttle walk test protocols will mature.

In short, CPET is the current "gold standard" for assessing exercise performance. It allows determination of mechanistic insights, recognition of coexistent and multiple exercise-limiting factors, and provides a thorough evaluation of respiratory responses and constraint. Both incremental and endurance protocols may be used, and the results from endurance exercise testing have been found to be more responsive to a treatment effect than either incremental exercise or 6-min walk testing. If a thorough evaluation of exercise performance is required, particularly in patients with multiple comorbidities, CEPT remains the testing method of choice.

CPET is safe, with the risk of death for patients approximating 2 to 5 per 100,000 exercise tests performed.[5] These risks can be minimized by a number of practical and common sense precautions, including the following:

- direct physician supervision (the importance of this cannot be overemphasized) and a thorough understanding of the contraindications to undergoing testing, as well as the indications for terminating exercise testing;
- appropriate cardiac and BP monitoring;
- resuscitation equipment and expertise; and
- accurate Sao_2 monitoring and availability of supplemental oxygen.

Specific contraindications for testing are listed in Table 2. Indications for prematurely terminating CPET are listed in Table 3.

Specific Variables Assessed During Exercise

Although a discussion of individual measurements is presented, it is important to recognize that CPET involves their collective integration for interpretation. In many instances, specific individual measurements are of lesser importance and are dictated by the clinical question being addressed and, in part, by responses demonstrated by the patient during testing.

Table 2. *Contraindications to CPET*

Unstable angina or recent acute coronary syndrome
Uncontrolled arrhythmias causing symptoms or hemodynamic compromise
Active endocarditis, myocarditis, or pericarditis
Symptomatic, severe aortic stenosis
Poorly or uncontrolled heart failure
Acute pulmonary embolism or infarction
Thrombosis of the lower limbs
Suspected dissecting aortic aneurysm
Uncontrolled asthma
Pulmonary edema
Significant hypoxemia

Table 3. *Indications for Terminating CPET in the Clinical Laboratory**

Unstable angina or chest pain suggestive of myocardial ischemia
ECG changes suggestive of ischemia, complex ectopy, or second- or third-degree heart block
Systolic BP decrease $>$20 mm Hg from highest value
Systolic BP $>$250 mm Hg, diastolic BP $>$120 mm Hg
Desaturation to $<$80%
Sudden pallor or dizziness
Mental confusion
Signs of respiratory failure

*Adapted from Weisman et al.[5]

$\dot{V}o_2$

$\dot{V}o_2$ is determined by cellular oxygen demand and maximal oxygen transport (see the section "Normal Exercise Physiology"). It is typically presented together with work rate, and it increases nearly linearly as external work increases. The slope of this relationship reflects the efficiency of metabolic conversion of energy to work and the mechanical efficiency of the musculoskeletal system. Values of 8.5 to 11.0 mL/min/W are normal for the $\Delta\dot{V}o_2/\Delta$ work rate relationship and are unaffected by age, height, or sex. Although obese individuals may have an increased ratio, the slope of that relationship remains normal.

As exercise progresses, $\dot{V}o_2$ increases until one of more of its determinants approach limitation (HR, SV, or tissue extraction), at which time the $\dot{V}o_2$/work rate may begin to plateau. This plateau has been used as the best evidence of maximum $\dot{V}o_2$, which is the "gold standard" used for assessing cardiorespiratory fitness. However, in the clinical setting, a plateau may not be reached, and the peak $\dot{V}o_2$ is often used for this purpose. The peak $\dot{V}o_2$ is often normalized for body size by dividing it by weight in kilograms. Unfortunately, normalization by body weight in obese individuals may provide a falsely low value. Although use of the lean body mass or height may be more desirable, there is no consensus on how best to account for body size.

A reduced peak $\dot{V}O_2$ is the starting point for interpretation, and underlying causes responsible for reduced exercise capacity are determined by inspecting the pattern of responses in other variables. The peak $\dot{V}O_2$ should be expressed as both an absolute value and also as a percentage of the predicted value.

$\dot{V}CO_2$

$\dot{V}CO_2$ is determined by factors similar to $\dot{V}O_2$, but because CO_2 is more soluble, $\dot{V}CO_2$ is more closely related to $\dot{V}E$ than to $\dot{V}O_2$. Importantly, the body uses CO_2 to compensate for acute metabolic acidosis, which contributes to the $\dot{V}CO_2$ vs work intensity relationship above the point of anaerobic metabolism. An accurate measurement of $\dot{V}CO_2$ is important because it serves in the calculation of several meaningful derived variables. Moreover, because $\dot{V}E$ is so closely related to $\dot{V}CO_2$, it is helpful to analyze $\dot{V}E$ in relation to $\dot{V}CO_2$.

RER

The RER is the ratio of $\dot{V}CO_2/\dot{V}O_2$, which under steady-state conditions approximates the respiratory quotient. An RER of 1.0 indicates metabolism by primarily carbohydrates, 0.7 by primarily fat, and 0.8 by primarily protein. Values >1.0 may indicate carbohydrate metabolism but also CO_2 derived from lactic acidosis or, importantly, hyperventilation. The RER should be reported as a function of the $\dot{V}O_2$.

Anaerobic Threshold

Anaerobic threshold (AT), also often referred to as the *lactate threshold* or *gas exchange threshold*, is considered an indicator of the onset of metabolic acidosis caused predominantly by increased arterial lactate during exercise. The AT should be expressed as a percentage of the peak $\dot{V}O_2$. In normal individuals, the AT occurs at 50 to 60% of peak $\dot{V}O_2$, with the range of normal being 40 to 80%. The AT is affected by the type of exercise (lower for arm vs leg exercise) and method of testing (lower for cycle vs treadmill testing). From a practical point of view, the AT denotes the upper limit of exercise intensity that can be accomplished aerobically, and exercise above the AT is associated with a progressive decrease in exercise tolerance.

Invasive methods for measuring the AT include arterial blood sampling of lactate or bicarbonate. There are various proposed methods for estimating the AT noninvasively (Fig 5), including the ventilatory equivalents method ($\dot{V}E/\dot{V}O_2$, $\dot{V}E/\dot{V}CO_2$, end-tidal PO_2 [$PETO_2$], and end-tidal PCO_2 [$PETCO_2$]) and the V-slope method ($\dot{V}CO_2$ vs $\dot{V}O_2$). Confirmatory evidence is provided by noting the change in slope of the $\dot{V}E$ vs $\dot{V}O_2$ relationship, and when the RER approximates 1.

Like the peak $\dot{V}O_2$, a reduced AT is nonspecific and requires inspection of other variables to determine the underlying etiology of the reduction. Values $>40\%$ may be witnessed with a wide variety of cardiovascular, respiratory, and musculoskeletal conditions. In some patients with severe respiratory limitation (for example, severe COPD), the AT cannot be determined noninvasively.

HR and HR/$\dot{V}O_2$

In normal healthy individuals, HR increases linearly with increasing exercise and $\dot{V}O_2$. Predicted maximal HR is often estimated by 220 – age, but this equation may underestimate maximal HR in the elderly. The difference between predicted maximal HR and the observed maximal HR is called the *HR reserve*. In normal individuals, there is little or no HR reserve at the end of exercise, which suggests a maximal or near-maximal patient effort. Peak HR may be reduced in a variety of cardiovascular conditions (including with pharmacologic agents) or in a submaximal study, but if a patient achieves predicted maximal HR, it suggests that cardiovascular function contributed to exercise limitation. In this instance, examination of other variables (*ie*, $\dot{V}O_2$, AT) will assist in the determination of whether this occurrence was normal or abnormal.

The slope of the HR-$\dot{V}O_2$ relationship is a function of SV; the greater the SV, the lower the HR (Figs 2 and 6). In patients with significant lung disease, the opposite may be seen, often reflecting deconditioning, mechanical ventilatory limitation, or potentially the hemodynamic consequences of dynamic hyperinflation.

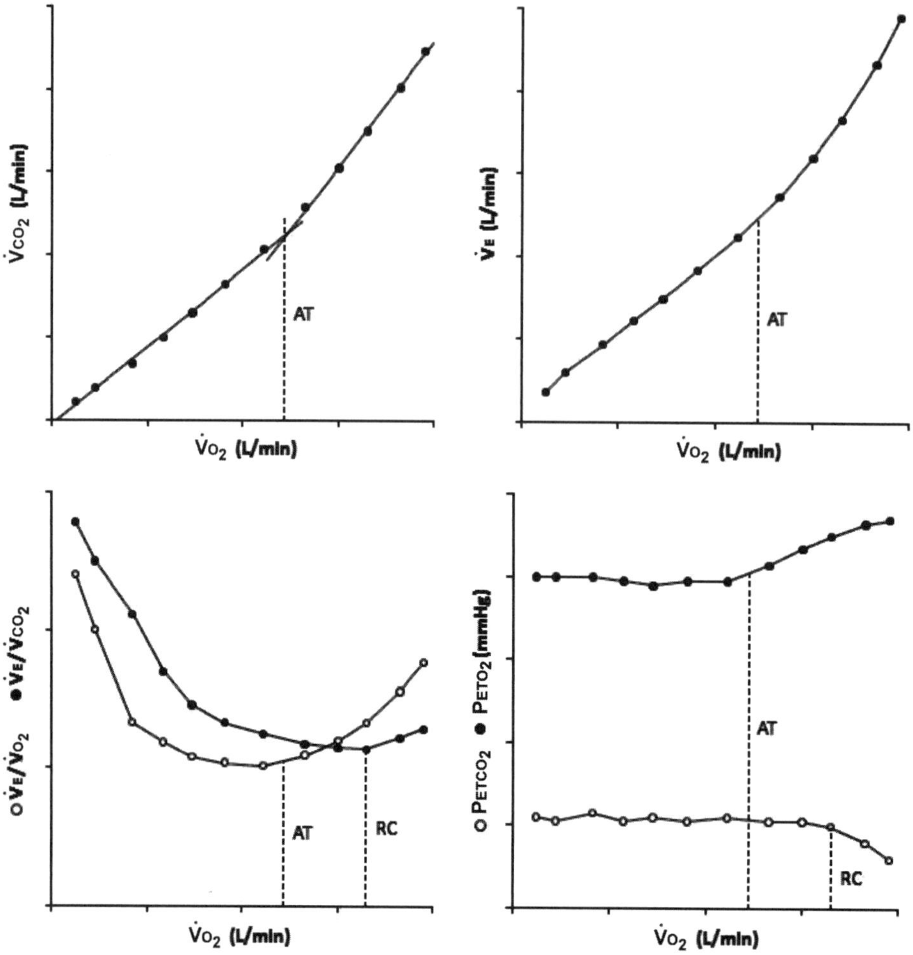

Figure 5. Noninvasive estimations of the AT.

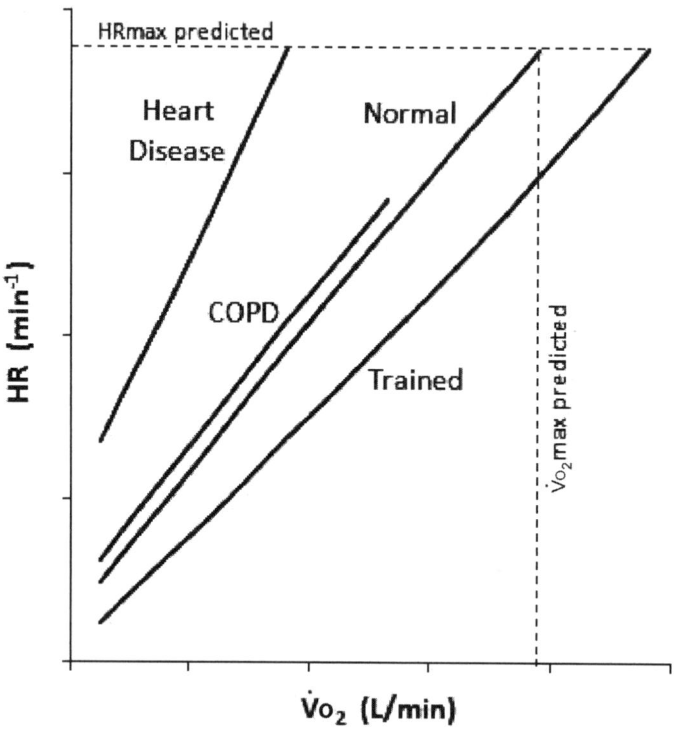

Figure 6. Cardiovascular responses during exercise in different clinical situations.

Oxygen Pulse

The ratio of $\dot{V}O_2$ to HR is referred to as the *oxygen pulse* and is often used as a correlate of SV during exercise. Although under ideal conditions this relationship generally holds true (see equations 1 and 2), in many settings the variable must be used with caution. The assumptions in the equations are not valid in the presence of significant desaturation or with impaired skeletal muscle oxygen extraction. A low oxygen pulse may therefore not only reflect cardiovascular disease but also deconditioning, early exercise termination caused by respiratory factors, symptoms or submaximal effort, and/or the presence of arterial oxygen desaturation.

BP

Systolic BP typically increases progressively during exercise as $\dot{V}O_2$ increases, whereas diastolic BP typically increases only slightly or remains relatively unchanged. Abnormal patterns of response during exercise include an exaggerated increase, a reduced increase, or a decrease. Exaggerated increases are found with resting hypertension, but in those without a known diagnosis, they may also predict the future onset of resting hypertension. A reduced increase may suggest underlying cardiovascular or sympathetic control abnormalities. A decreasing BP during exercise is very serious, and it is an indication for immediate termination of the test. If a decrease occurs, serious efforts to exclude heart failure, ischemia, or outflow tract obstruction should be undertaken.

Breathing Pattern and Ventilation

The increase in $\dot{V}E$ with exercise is accompanied by increases in both the depth and frequency of breathing (Fig 1). Increases in VT are primarily responsible for the increase in $\dot{V}E$ at low levels of exercise, but as exercise progresses, both VT and respiratory rate increase. At 70 to 80% of peak exercise, increases in $\dot{V}E$ are achieved primarily by increases in respiratory rate.

There are various methods used to estimate peak $\dot{V}e$, including actual measurement of the maximal voluntary ventilation. Predicted maximal $\dot{V}e$ may also be estimated with various equations, most commonly the $FEV_1 \times 37$ to 40. Unfortunately, none of these methods are perfect, and a pressing need exists for enhancements in this area. The use of the maximal voluntary ventilation is limited by concerns regarding patient effort and repeatability and with the unique breathing strategy adopted during the maneuver that does not parallel the strategy used during exercise. Equations are therefore most commonly used, but they may be less suited for patients with neuromuscular disorders or respiratory muscle weakness. Despite these limitations and regardless of the method used, estimating the peak $\dot{V}e$ has significant clinical utility and has withstood the test of time.

The terms *breathing reserve* or *ventilatory reserve* are used to denote the relationship between predicted peak $\dot{V}e$ and the actual measured peak $\dot{V}e$, displayed both as an absolute value (in liters) and as a percentage of the predicted peak $\dot{V}e$. Patients with respiratory disease characteristically have reduced ventilatory capacity and increased ventilatory demand, resulting in reduced ventilatory reserve. Ventilatory demand is usually increased both at rest and during exercise in patients with COPD, ILD, and pulmonary vascular disease, for example, as the result of ventilation/perfusion inequality and increased VD/VT, hypoxemia, and/or increased stimulation of lung receptors (which serves to increase ventilation). It is also dependent on other factors such as metabolic requirements, lactic acidosis, behavioral factors, deconditioning, body weight, and mode of testing. In most healthy adults, peak $\dot{V}e$ at the end of exercise approaches 70% of the maximal $\dot{V}e$, although this percentage may be greater with increased fitness and with aging (Fig 7). In patients with significant respiratory disease and mechanical abnormalities, the patient's end-of-exercise $\dot{V}e$ may reach or even exceed the predicted maximal peak $\dot{V}e$. A plot of $\dot{V}e$ vs either $\dot{V}CO_2$ or $\dot{V}O_2$ is acceptable for the graphical representation of ventilatory data.

Ventilatory Equivalents for $\dot{V}O_2$ and $\dot{V}CO_2$

The ratio of $\dot{V}E$ to $\dot{V}O_2$ is called the *ventilatory equivalent for oxygen* and the ratio of $\dot{V}E$ to $\dot{V}CO_2$ is called the *ventilatory equivalent for CO_2*. They are both related to VD/VT and are greater as VD/VT increases. They also both increase with hyperventilation. Normal responses for these variables are

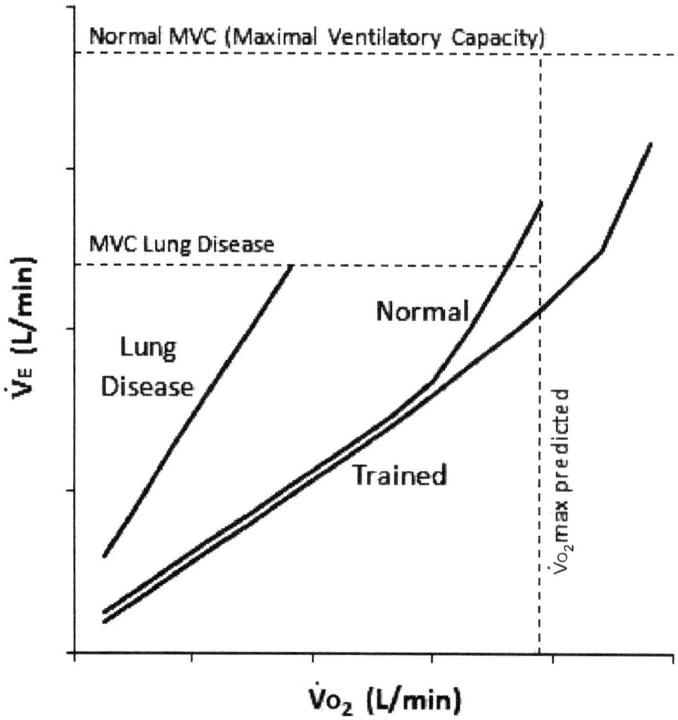

Figure 7. Respiratory responses during exercise in different clinical situations.

shown in Figure 5 (bottom left). The initial increase in the $\dot{V}E/\dot{V}O_2$ (while the $\dot{V}E/\dot{V}CO_2$ has still not increased) that typically occurs in concert with metabolic acidosis is different than the pattern demonstrated with hyperventilation (attributable to anxiety, pain, or hypoxemia), whereby both the $\dot{V}E/\dot{V}O_2$ and the $\dot{V}E/\dot{V}CO_2$ increase together. The subsequent increase in the $\dot{V}E/\dot{V}CO_2$ represents the respiratory compensation associated with a decrease in the $PaCO_2$ and the $PETCO_2$.

The $\dot{V}E/\dot{V}CO_2$ is usually <34 at the AT and usually <37 to 40 at the end of exercise. Increased values reflect either an increased VD/VT or a low $PaCO_2$. A lack of an increase with exercise reflects either insensitivity to the stimulus of metabolic acidosis, or an inability of the respiratory system to respond to that stimulus (*ie*, significant COPD).

$PETO_2$ and $PETCO_2$

The characteristic response of these variables during exercise is shown in Figure 5 (bottom right). The period of increasing $PETO_2$ with relatively stable $PETCO_2$ has been termed *isocapnic buffering*. A high $\dot{V}E/\dot{V}CO_2$ without a corresponding decrease in $PETCO_2$ suggests increased VD/VT, whereas a decrease in $PETCO_2$ when the $\dot{V}E/\dot{V}CO_2$ is high suggests hyperventilation.

Flow-Volume Curves

Although first reported in 1961, flow-volume curves during exercise were not adopted nor well studied until the 1990s. Since that time, our insight of their usefulness to better understand respiratory responses and symptoms during exercise has grown (12). This greater understanding, coupled with advances in technology, has led to the routine analysis of flow-volume curves during exercise. The added value garnered from their use relates to their ability to provide information about the overall breathing strategy adopted by patients during exercise. They also enable an appreciation of the behavior of operational lung volumes, including the end-expiratory lung volume (derived from the total lung capacity and the inspiratory capacity) and the end-inspiratory lung volume. Additionally, analysis of flow-volume curves provides an objective assessment of the presence and degree of flow limitation during exercise.

In patients with significant disease, there are a number of characteristic patterns of response in lung volumes that differ from normal patients

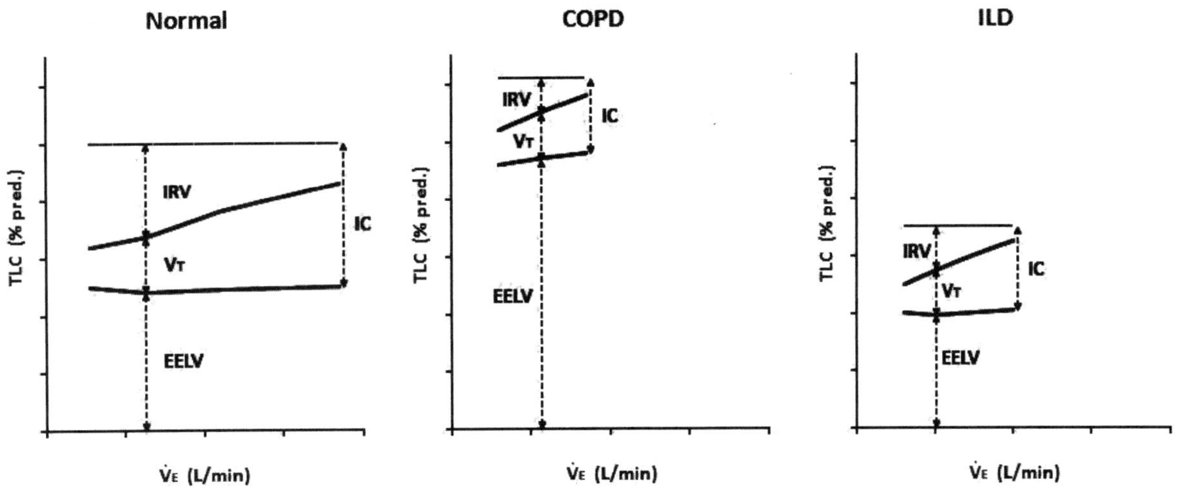

Figure 8. Behavior of operational lung volumes during exercise.

(Fig 8: volume vs V̇E; Fig 9: flow vs volume). In addition to COPD and ILD, patients with significant obesity and central airway obstruction also demonstrate distinguishing responses.[13] Analysis of flow-volume curves during exercise is also especially useful in helping to assess a therapeutic response.[14,15]

In these examples, the end-expiratory lung volume, the inspiratory reserve volume, and the presence/absence of flow limitation serve to distinguish the various disease states from normal, these changes being unique and characteristic. The value of flow-volume curves during exercise is being further studied, and it is likely that additional indications and applications such as using them to better estimate maximal ventilatory capacity may be adopted.

Pao_2, Sao_2, and Alveolar-Arterial Po_2

Normal exercise responses are enabled by efficient gas exchange. Arterial hypoxemia is uncommon during exercise in normal humans, but it may occur in some elite or aging athletes during high-intensity exercise. Inefficient gas exchange is demonstrated by the alveolar-arterial oxygen pressure difference, or $P(A\text{-}a)o_2$, gradient and by the Pao_2. A significant widening of the gradient and decrease in the Pao_2 are abnormal, and they are most characteristic of ILD and significant right-to-left shunts as well as some patients with COPD and pulmonary vascular disease (PVD). A reduced Pao_2 with a normal $P(A\text{-}a)o_2$ may be seen in processes associated with abnormal respiratory control and in a hypoxic environment (*ie*, altitude), although the

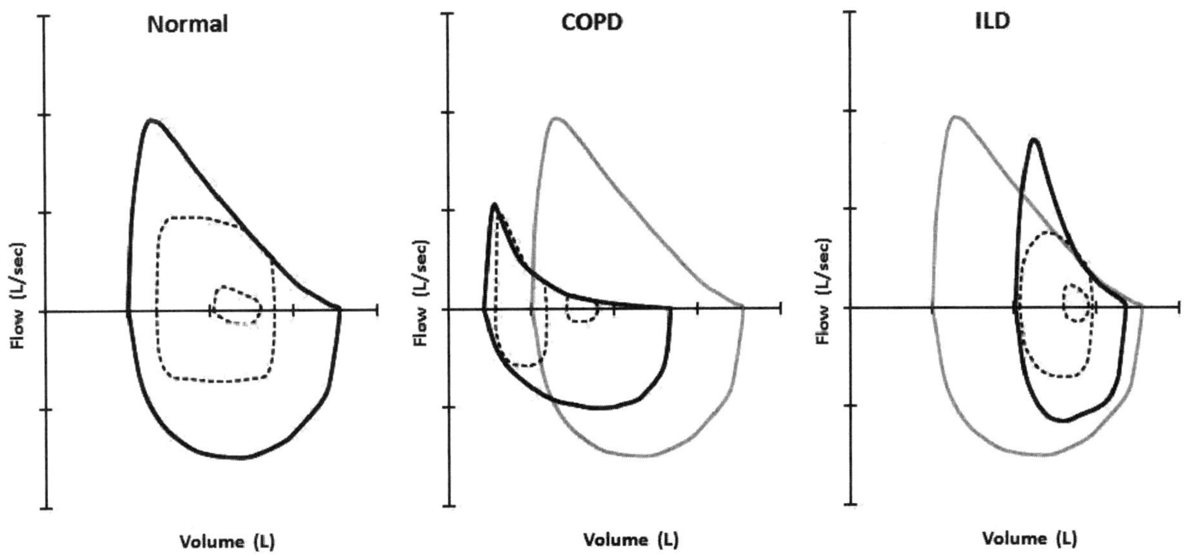

Figure 9. Maximal and tidal flow-volume curves at rest and during exercise.

latter is rarely reproduced in the clinical laboratory. A reduced Pao_2 with an abnormally widened $P(A\text{-}a)o_2$ would suggest worsening ventilation/perfusion inequalities, right-to-left shunt, and/or diffusion limitation, potentially accompanied by a decrease in the mixed venous Po_2.

The $P(A\text{-}a)o_2$ is normally <10 mm Hg at rest but may normally increase to >20 mm Hg during exercise. Values >35 mm Hg are abnormal and indicate possible gas exchange abnormalities. Occasionally, a less-than-optimal substitute, Spo_2, is used as an alternative to arterial blood gas sampling. In the normal individual, both the Pao_2 and the Spo_2 are not appreciably different during exercise when compared with rest.

VD/VT

VD/VT is another index of gas exchange efficiency. An increase in VD/VT represents an increased inefficiency of ventilation, which requires an increase in $\dot{V}E$ to maintain $Paco_2$. VD/VT is highly dependent on the breathing pattern because a rapid shallow breathing pattern increases VD/VT without any other abnormalities. The VD/VT is calculated from the $Paco_2$ and the $PECO_2$ using the following equation:

$$(5)\ V_D/V_T = \frac{(Paco_2 - P_{ECO_2})}{Paco_2}$$

where the $PECO_2$ is the mixed expired CO_2 value of alveolar and dead space gas. VD/VT is obtained directly by collecting expired gas and measuring its CO_2 concentration. This test can easily be performed with a mixing chamber or, for breath-by-breath systems, after determination of the $\dot{V}E/\dot{V}co_2$ ratio. Approaches that substitute end-tidal Pco_2 for $Paco_2$ yield unreliable results, particularly in disease, because pulmonary gas exchange abnormalities in themselves affect the difference between $Paco_2$ and $PETco_2$.

At rest, the VD/VT may normally be approximately 0.30 and decrease to approximately 0.10 to 0.15 at the end of exercise. Patients with respiratory disease may have at rest either normal or increased values that fail to decrease normally during exercise. In some instances, the VD/VT will increase during exercise in patients with significant disease. However, the VD/VT is neither sensitive nor specific for lung disease and, thus, an isolated abnormality should be interpreted with caution. This finding also emphasizes the importance of evaluating the patterns of response from a collection of variables rather than reacting to just a single measurement.

Symptoms During Exercise

Patients often report that breathlessness and/or leg fatigue limits their exercise, although other reasons such as musculoskeletal complaints and exhaustion are also reported. Objective evaluation of these end points is valuable, and the use of either a visual analog scale[16] or a modified Borg scale[17] is recommended. These scales have shown to be repeatable and responsive and are commonly used in clinical laboratories. The reproducibility of results obtained from these scales can be enhanced by providing a consistent set of written instructions to the patient prior to testing. As noted, the reason(s) for discontinuing exercise should be recorded. The value of these ratings is further enhanced when relationships such as $\dot{V}E$ or work rate vs dyspnea or leg fatigue are examined, particularly in serial studies or after interventions.

Reference Values

The selection of appropriate reference values for use in interpreting CPET is essential. The reader is advised to consult source references[1, 5, 18] for guidance in selecting which reference values may be most appropriate for their specific clinical laboratory.

Reproducibility of CPET Results

Whenever serial testing is undertaken, for example, to assess the response to therapy, the variability of the measurements during CEPT must be considered before a beneficial, detrimental, or no effect can be concluded. The coefficient of variation (ratio of the SD to the mean, expressed as a percentage) reported for serial measurements during maximal testing in the same subject are as follows (range of reported values listed):

$\dot{V}o_2$	3.0–8.4%	$\dot{V}co_2$	5.0–9.6%
HR	1.4–8.6%	$\dot{V}E$	5.0–12.3%
AT	9.2–13.0%	Systolic B/P	2.2–6.7%
Sao_2	2.5%	Duration (work rate)	3.6–13.8

It should be understood that the variability depends on a number of factors, such as the population studied, the type of testing performed, and the specific variable examined. However, it appears reasonable to assume that differences in most measurements obtained during CEPT should exceed approximately 12 to 20% to be considered clinically significant (*ie*, twice the coefficient of variation) and not caused by inherent variability alone.

Interpretation and Reporting of CPET

Interpretation of CPET begins with the requisition form. Requisition forms should be designed to encourage the requesting physician to provide as much clinical information as is reasonable to enable the interpretation to be valuable. This information will enhance the ability of the reporting physician to provide the most meaningful interpretation possible from the available measured data. There are a number of important fundamental questions that the reporting physician must address when interpreting CPET (19), including the following:

1. Are the results normal or abnormal?
2. How limited is the patient?
3. What factors are responsible for the limitation?
4. What abnormal patterns of response are demonstrated?
5. What clinical disorders may result in these patterns of response?

Determining whether a test is physiologically maximal is necessary in excluding potential underlying diseases or abnormalities. Useful indicators may include the following:

1. A plateau of peak $\dot{V}O_2$, or peak $\dot{V}O_2$ is achieved.
2. Maximum work rate is achieved.
3. HR or $\dot{V}E$ reach predicted maximum.
4. RER $>$1.15.
5. Blood lactate level $>$4 (mmol/L).
6. Patient exhaustion.

The clinician must also decide on contributors to exercise limitation and whether they are normal (*ie*, appropriate) or abnormal. Potential factors that may contribute to limit exercise include the following:

1. Cardiovascular function.
2. Respiratory mechanics (and/or respiratory muscle function).
3. Arterial hypoxemia.
4. Dyspnea.
5. Unfitness/deconditioning.
6. Musculoskeletal disorders, peripheral vascular disease.
7. Other factors, *ie*, motivation, secondary gain, and technical factors.

Although responses during exercise may vary in normal individuals, and the range of normal is quite broad, an understanding of "normalcy" and normal exercise physiology is essential for the recognition of disease. This understanding is essential for the appropriate interpretation of CPET. Suggested normal values for various measurements obtained during CPET are listed in Table 4.

In interpreting CPET, it is important to focus on what is most important; patterns of responses during exercise and the reason(s) for testing. This focus will ensure that a correct and meaningful interpretation will result. The multitude of both graphical and numerical results and an overreliance and overdependence on complicated algorithms has contributed to confusion. They distract and deter us from cardinal measurements and relationships, the fundamental importance of patient's symptoms during exercise, and the basic physiologic principles that would help us to better understand and appreciate the role and benefit (as well as the limitations) of exercise testing in clinical practice. They also detract from the practical reality that, unlike in textbooks, guideline statements, and/or the lecture hall, CPET is never ordered nor interpreted in isolation. It should be requested and its results translated within the context of all available clinical information from the patient, with the specific goal of addressing the question(s) being asked. CPET does not replace common sense, starting with the clinical assessment of the patient. For example, there are more appropriate methods than CPET to differentiate COPD from ILD. To aid in achieving this goal, the characteristic patterns of response during exercise demonstrated in various disease states are noted in Table 5. These values highlight the importance of understanding that no single measurement is diagnostic of any specific disease entity.

Summary

CPET typically involves the measurement of respiratory gas exchange ($\dot{V}O_2$, $\dot{V}CO_2$, $\dot{V}E$, and other

Table 4. *Suggested Normal Values for Selected CPET Variables**

Variable	Normal Value
Peak $\dot{V}O_2$	>85% predicted
AT	>40% predicted peak $\dot{V}O_2$
Peak HR	>90% predicted peak HR
HR reserve	>15 beats/min
BP	<200/90 mm Hg
Oxygen pulse ($\dot{V}O_2$/HR)	>80% predicted
Peak $\dot{V}E$	<85% (peak $\dot{V}E$/predicted peak $\dot{V}E$)
Ventilatory reserve	>11 L (predicted peak $\dot{V}E$ [minus] peak $\dot{V}E$)
RR	<60 breaths/min
$\dot{V}E/VCO_2$	<34 at AT; <37–40 at end of exercise
VD/VT	<0.30
PaO_2	>80 mm Hg
SaO_2 desaturation	<5%
$P(A\text{-}a)O_2$	<35 mm Hg
HR	1.4 to 8.6%
AT	9.2 to 13.0%
$\dot{V}CO_2$	5.0 to 9.6%
$\dot{V}E$	5.0 to 12.3%
Systolic BP	2.2 to 6.7%
Duration (work rate)	3.6 to 13.8%

*Adapted from Weisman et al.[5]

variables) while the ECG, BP, SpO_2, and perceived exertion (Borg scale) is monitored during a maximal symptom-limited incremental exercise test on a cycle ergometer or on a treadmill. In some circumstances, a constant workload exercise test (based on maximal test results) may be performed. Measurement of arterial blood gases provides more detailed information on pulmonary gas exchange. Resting and exercise tidal flow-volume loops should also be monitored to accurately assess/understand the degree of ventilatory constraint.

CPET provides a global assessment of the integrative exercise responses that are not adequately reflected by measurement of individual organ system function at rest: Resting values cannot reliably predict exercise performance and functional capacity. CPET is safe, comorbidities can be identified, and enhanced understanding and insight into

Table 5. *Characteristic Patterns of Response During Exercise Demonstrated in Various Disease States**

Variable	Congestive Heart Failure	COPD	ILD	Pulmonary Vascular Disease	Deconditioned
Peak $\dot{V}O_2$	↓	↓	↓	↓	↓
AT	↓	v or indeterminate	↓	↓	↔ or ↓
Peak HR	v	↔ or ↓	↓	↔ or ↓	↔ or ↓
Oxygen pulse	↓	↔ or ↓	↔ or ↓	↓	↓
Peak $\dot{V}E$/maximal voluntary ventilation	↔ or ↓	↑	↔ or ↑	↔	↔
$\dot{V}E/\dot{V}CO_2$	↑	↑	↑	↑	↔
VD/VT	↑	↑	↑	↑	↔
PaO_2	↔	v	↓	↓	↔
$P(A\text{-}a)O_2$	↔	v	↑	↑	↔

*Adapted from several sources.[4,5,18,20,21] ↓ = decreased; ↔ = unchanged from normal; ↑ = increased; v = variable.

various responses, including exercise limiting factors, is possible. Importantly, CPET promotes an integrative approach to assessing metabolic, ventilatory, and cardiac function and reserve. Although technically more demanding than simpler tests, the use of CPET provides the clinician with a measurement of the peak $\dot{V}o_2$ (and relationships involving the peak $\dot{V}o_2$), which remains the "gold standard" for assessing aerobic exercise capacity.

Acknowledgment

The author is indebted to Mr. R. Clemens for his expert assistance in the preparation and review of the figures and the manuscript.

References

1. Jones NL. Clinical exercise testing. 4th ed. Philadelphia, PA: Saunders, 1997
2. Gallagher CG. Exercise and chronic obstructive pulmonary disease. Med Clin N Am 1990; 74:619–641
3. Palange P. The prognostic value of exercise testing. Breathe 2009; 5:229–234
4. Palange P, Ward SA, Carlsen K-H, et al. Recommendations on the use of exercise testing in clinical practice—ERS Task Force. Eur Respir J 2007; 29:185–209
5. Weisman IM, Beck K, Casaburi R, et al. American Thoracic Society/American College of Chest Physicians joint statement on cardiopulmonary exercise testing. Am J Respir Crit Care Med 2003; 167:211–277
6. American Thoracic Society. ATS statement: guidelines for methacholine and exercise challenge testing—1999. Am J Respir Crit Care Med 2000; 161:309–329
7. American Thoracic Society. ATS statement: guidelines for the six-minute walk test. Am J Respir Crit Care Med 2002; 166:111–117
8. Marciniuk DD, Butcher SJ, Reid JK, et al. The effects of helium-hyperoxia on 6-min walking distance in COPD: a randomized, controlled trial. Chest 2007; 131:1659–1665
9. Celli BR, Cote CG, Marin JM, et al. The body-mass index, airflow obstruction, dyspnea and exercise capacity index in chronic obstructive pulmonary disease. N Engl J Med 2004; 350:1005–1012
10. Pepin V, Brodeur J, Lacasse Y, et al. 6-minute walking versus shuttle walking: responsiveness to bronchodilation in chronic obstructive pulmonary disease. Thorax 2007; 62:291–298
11. Brouillard D, Pepin V, Milot J, et al. Endurance shuttle waling test: responsiveness to salmeterol in COPD. Eur Respir J 2008; 31:579–584
12. Johnson BD, Weisman IM, Zeballos RJ, et al. Emerging concepts in the evaluation of ventilatory limitation during exercise: the exercise tidal flow-volume loop. Chest 1999; 116:488–503
13. Babb TG. Mechanical ventilatory constraints in again, lung disease, and obesity: perspectives and brief review. Med Sci Sports Exerc 1999; 31: S12–S22
14. Maltais F, Marciniuk DD, Hernandez P, et al. Improvements in symptom-limited exercise performance over 8 h with once-daily tiotropium in patients with COPD. Chest 2005; 128:1168–1178
15. O'Donnell DE, Sciurba F, Celli B, et al. Effect of fluticasone propionate/salmeterol on lung hyperinflation and exercise endurance in COPD. Chest 2006; 130:647–656,
16. Gift AG. Visual analogue scales: measurement of subjective phenomena. Nurs Res 1989; 38:286–288
17. Borg GA. Psychophysical bases of perceived exertion. Med Sci Sports Exerc 1982; 14:377–381
18. Wasserman K, Hansen JE, Sue DY, et al. Principles of exercise testing and interpretation. 4th ed. Philadelphia, PA: Lippincott Williams and Wilkins, 2005
19. Younes M. Interpretation of clinical exercise testing in respiratory disease. Clin Chest Med 1984; 5:189–206
20. Marciniuk DD, Gallagher CG. Clinical exercise testing in interstitial lung disease. Clin Chest Med 1994; 15:287–303
21. Marciniuk DD, Gallagher CG. Clinical exercise testing in chronic airflow limitation. Med Clin N Am 1996; 80:565–587

Notes

Hypercapnic Respiratory Failure

Mark J. Rosen, MD, FCCP

Objectives:

- Understand the determinants of $Paco_2$ and the types of physiologic derangements that lead to hypercapnia
- Review specific neurologic and muscular disorders that cause respiratory failure
- Discuss respiratory muscle function and the assessment of respiratory muscle strength
- Outline the types of situations in which an imbalance between the work of breathing and energy supply to respiratory muscles leads to fatigue
- Discuss how hypercapnia may occur when excessive concentrations of inspired oxygen are administered to susceptible persons

Key words: hypercapnia; neuromuscular diseases; respiratory failure; respiratory muscles

Components of the Respiratory System

The respiratory system can be considered as two distinct parts: the lungs and a ventilatory pump. Disorders of the lungs interfere with gas exchange, manifested mainly by hypoxemia. Disorders of the pump impair ventilation, manifested by hypercapnia. Arterial carbon dioxide is related to carbon dioxide output ($\dot{V}co_2$) by metabolism and is removed by alveolar ventilation ($\dot{V}A$). $\dot{V}A$ is the total minute ventilation ($\dot{V}E$) minus dead space ventilation ($\dot{V}D$). $Paco_2$ is determined by the following: $Paco_2 = K(\dot{V}co_2/\dot{V}A)$, where K = 0.863 mm Hg; ($\dot{V}A = \dot{V}E - \dot{V}D$) or, rearranged, $Paco_2 = K(\dot{V}co_2/\dot{V}E\,(1 - \dot{V}D/\text{tidal volume [VT]})$.

Increased $\dot{V}co_2$

Hypercapnia may occur when $\dot{V}co_2$ increases without a corresponding increase in $\dot{V}A$. $\dot{V}co_2$ increases in proportion to the metabolic rate, as with fever and exercise. Carbohydrate utilization also increases the respiratory quotient (or $\dot{V}co_2$ /oxygen consumption) compared with fat and protein metabolism, producing more carbon dioxide for each calorie expended. In patients with limited ventilatory reserve, an increase in $\dot{V}co_2$ may culminate in an increase in $Paco_2$.

Reduced $\dot{V}A$

Any disorder causing a reduction in $\dot{V}A$ will increase $Paco_2$. This occurs with three types of pathophysiologic derangements:

- $\dot{V}E$ (the product of respiratory rate and VT) is reduced.
- VT is reduced. Even if the overall $\dot{V}E$ is normal or high, the portion of each breath that is distributed to anatomic or physiologic dead space (dead space fraction, or $\dot{V}D/VT$) increases, and $\dot{V}A$ is reduced. If $\dot{V}E$ does not increase proportionally, $Paco_2$ increases. This occurs commonly in patients with rapid, shallow breathing patterns.
- $\dot{V}D/VT$ increases, with normal or high $\dot{V}E$ and VT. An extreme example would be a patient with fixed $\dot{V}E$ who has a massive pulmonary embolism. Here, although $\dot{V}E$ and VT remain the same, the increase in $\dot{V}D/VT$ that results from the newly underperfused lung units reduces $\dot{V}A$ and increases $Paco_2$.

Disorders of Ventilation

Central Control

The medullary central controller sends signals that set the respiratory rate and VT. This center receives inputs from higher CNS centers, peripheral chemoreceptors, and receptors in the lungs, chest wall, and airways. The carbon dioxide sensor (chemoreceptor) is located in the medulla and responds to changes in pH of extracellular fluid. Oxygen sensors in the carotid body and aortic body sense changes in Po_2. Disorders of central respiratory control include the following: (1) congenital central hypoventilation syndrome (CCHS, or

Ondine's curse) and inborn failure of autonomic control of breathing, linked to mutations in the PHOX2B gene; (2) central sleep apnea; (3) overdoses with narcotics or sedatives; (4) diseases of the medulla (infarct, tumor); (5) hypothyroidism; (6) metabolic alkalosis, in which the $Paco_2$ usually increases 0.7 to 0.8 mm Hg for every 1.0 mEq/L increase in plasma bicarbonate; and (7) rabies.

Rabies is a viral infection transmitted in the saliva of infected mammals that causes an encephalomyelitis that is almost always fatal. In North America, bats are implicated in transmission in >90% of cases. The virus may involve the entire nervous system in infected persons, and respiratory failure may occur from either central respiratory depression or ascending spastic paralysis, which occurs in 20% of cases. Postexposure prophylaxis with rabies immune globulin and rabies vaccine is recommended for the unvaccinated person who is exposed to bat saliva. Because the consequences of rabies are so devastating, postexposure prophylaxis should be considered even if a bite cannot be reasonably excluded.

Motor Neurons

Interruption of transmission impulses from the respiratory centers to the respiratory muscles also leads to hypoventilation. Motor neuron diseases include the following: (1) spinal cord injury, especially at the C3 level; (2) tetanus; and (3) diseases involving the anterior horn cells, including amyotrophic lateral sclerosis (ALS) and poliomyelitis. In tetanus, the anaerobe *Clostridium tetani* may inoculate a disruption of the skin barrier and elaborate the exotoxin tetanospasmin, which reaches the spinal cord by retrograde axonal transport and blocks the release of inhibitory transmitters. Trismus is often the first symptom, which progresses to spastic paralysis, especially of the laryngeal and respiratory muscles, causing respiratory failure that may persist for several months. Subcutaneous injection of heroin, or "skin popping," accounted for the increasing incidence of tetanus and would botulism in California since 1997. In surgical wound infection, contraction of the muscles surrounding the wound could be the first sign. The disease is preventable through vaccination; patients with tetanus should be treated with wound care, tetanus immune globulin to neutralize remaining exotoxin, support of ventilation and hemodynamics, and medications to suppress muscle rigidity.

ALS is characterized by the presence of dysarthria, tongue atrophy and fasciculations, amyotrophy (muscle atrophy), extremity fasciculations, weakness, and hyperreflexia. The diagnosis of ALS is confirmed with electrophysiologic studies. Although new cases of poliomyelitis are almost unheard of in developed nations, late manifestations may occur many years after the primary infection. The "postpolio syndrome" may occur in up to half of the survivors of paralytic poliomyelitis, with the onset of new weakness or abnormal muscle fatigue, muscle atrophy, or generalized fatigue. Muscle weakness may even lead to respiratory failure in a few patients.

Peripheral Neuropathy

Disorders of the peripheral nerves commonly cause hypercapnic respiratory failure. Guillain-Barré syndrome (GBS) is the most common cause of acute generalized paralysis after the virtual elimination of poliomyelitis around the world. There are at least four subtypes of GBS; the most common is an acute, inflammatory demyelinating polyradiculopathy; others are acute motor and sensory neuropathies (alone or together), acute pandysautonomic forms, and overlap syndromes. GBS is believed to be the result of an aberrant T-cell response to a previous infection, leading to a macrophage-mediated destruction of myelin. The majority of cases involve either a flu-like illness or gastroenteritis within the previous 6 weeks, and approximately one fourth of patients with GBS, especially those with axonal forms of the disease, have had a recent infection with *Campylobacter jejuni*.

The lipopolysaccharide of *C jejuni* cell walls shares similar antigens with peripheral nerve gangliosides. Patients usually present with ascending paralysis, paresthesias, and hypoflexia or areflexia. The disorder usually is diagnosed by finding electromyography (EMG) evidence of conduction block in motor nerves. Cerebrospinal fluid studies typically show few or no cells, increased protein after 1 to 2 weeks, and circulating or cerebrospinal fluid antiganglioside antibodies in some patients. Plasmapheresis and infusion of γ-globulin appear to be equally effective, and the combination of both treatments confers no additional benefit. There is no established role for therapy with corticosteroids in this disorder.

Critical illness polyneuropathy (CIP) is an acute sensory-motor disorder that mainly affects the lower limbs of critically ill patients. It may be the consequence of microcirculatory damage caused by decreased perfusion or endothelial injury from a systemic inflammatory cytokine response. Critical illness myopathy (CIM) is an acute myopathy that causes weakness and paralysis in critically ill patients and that usually occurs with CIP. Because CIP and CIM usually overlap, the term *critical illness polyneuromyopathy* is often used. Sepsis, multiorgan failure, and hyperglycemia often are cited as risk factors but cannot be confirmed because of methodologic limitations of investigations into these disorders.

These patients often present with "weaning problems" after sepsis resolves, typically with flaccid paresis that spares the cranial muscles, muscle atrophy, and reduced or absent deep tendon reflexes. EMG shows axonal neuropathic and/or myopathic patterns, and muscle biopsies (when performed) show denervation atrophy. If the patient survives the critical illness, the syndrome may resolves over weeks to months, but many patients remain permanently disabled. There is no specific treatment, but efforts to prevent this disorder include minimizing the use of corticosteroids, and some studies have suggested that rigorous glycemic control is associated with a reduced incidence.

Unusual causes of neuropathy include diphtheria, porphyria, and tick paralysis. Exposure to toxins also may cause severe neuropathy and paralysis. For example, fugu, a puffer fish, elaborates a potent neurotoxin, and ingestion of improperly prepared fugu sushi accounts for approximately 50 deaths in Japan each year.

Neuromuscular Junction

Disorders/particulars interfering with transmission of impulses at the neuromuscular junction include the following:

Myasthenia Gravis: In this disease, binding of IgG antibodies to the postsynaptic acetylcholine receptor induces complement-mediated receptor destruction and skeletal muscle weakness. Most cases are idiopathic, but the disease may be induced by penicillamine and transiently exacerbated by corticosteroids. The diagnosis is supported by the following: (1) impaired neuromuscular transmission on EMG, with decremental response to repetitive stimulation; (2) clinical response to cholinergic agents (edrophonium); and (3) the presence of acetylcholine receptor antibodies in the serum (85 to 90% of patients with generalized weakness). Myasthenia gravis is associated with both benign and malignant thymoma. Treatments include cholinergic drugs, corticosteroids for mild-to-moderate disease (and sometimes with other immunosuppressive agents), and plasma exchange or IV Ig for patients with severe weakness. Plasma exchange and IV Ig are equally effective in exacerbations of myasthenia gravis, and the role of these treatments in chronic disease is unproven. Even in the absence of thymoma, thymectomy is generally recommended for patients with generalized myasthenia gravis between puberty and 60 years of age because it is associated with a greater likelihood of remission or improvement.

Eaton-Lambert Syndrome: This paraneoplastic disorder often is associated with small cell carcinoma of the lung. Weakness is mainly proximal and spares the ocular and bulbar muscles. Unlike myasthenia, EMG in Eaton-Lambert syndrome shows an incremental pattern with repetitive stimulation.

Organophosphates: Organophosphates, a component of some insecticides, inhibit choline-esterase.

Botulism: The spores of *Clostridium botulinum* generate a potent neurotoxin that causes a potentially lethal, descending flaccid paralysis. Patients typically present with oculomotor palsies, progressing to facial muscle paralysis and difficulty swallowing, and then limb and respiratory muscle weakness and paralysis. Although botulism is best known to be acquired by ingestion of preserved food containing preformed toxin, a similar syndrome may occur when the organism is inoculated into a wound or other devitalized tissue; it may also be acquired by inhalation, making it a potential bioterrorist weapon. Similar to tetanus, a dramatic increase in reported cases of wound botulism was linked to subcutaneous or IM injection of "black tar" heroin in California. Like Eaton-Lambert syndrome, there is augmentation of muscle action potential with repetitive nerve stimulation, although to a lesser degree. The diagnosis is established by identifying the toxin in the serum, stool, or wound, or the organism in stool or wound. Treatment includes debridement, botulinum antitoxin, and supportive care.

Prolonged Muscle Weakness: Prolonged muscle weakness after nondepolarizing neuromuscular blocking agents is common. Discontinuing mechanical ventilation may be delayed, and weakness may persist for months. Two types of neuromuscular dysfunction occur. Persistent blockade of the neuromuscular junction may occur as the result of accumulation of the drug or active metabolites, especially in patients with renal failure. This occurs more commonly with aminosteroid agents (pancuronium and vecuronium), in which renal excretion of active metabolites is important, than with the benzylisoquinolone agents (atracurium, doxacurium, and cisatracurium), which are inactivated spontaneously in the blood. The second is an acute, generalized, necrotizing myopathy that clinically resembles and may be indistinguishable from CIM in the absence of these agents, except that these patients generally have intact sensation, usually have greater creatine kinase levels, and nerve conduction is normal. This complication is most common in patients who are receiving high doses of corticosteroids along with neuromuscular blocking agents, including the benzylisoquinolones. Treatment is supportive, but patients maybe incapacitated for months after recovery from the acute illness. Minimizing the dose and duration of paralytic agents and corticosteroids is the best way to prevent this complication.

Respiratory Muscles

The respiratory muscles perform the work of breathing. The diaphragm is the most important inspiratory muscle, responsible for 60 to 90% of work of breathing at rest. Contraction of the costal component displaces abdominal viscera downward and lifts the lower rib cage; the crural component displaces abdominal viscera downward. The external intercostals, scaleni, and sternocleidomastoids comprise the accessory muscles of inspiration and are used when $\dot{V}_E$ is increased or when the diaphragm is weak or fatigued. Contraction of these muscles elevates the rib cage.

The expiratory muscles (internal intercostal and abdominal) are not used during resting breathing because exhalation is passive. However, they contract actively when $\dot{V}_E$ is increased and are essential to the cough reflex. The internal intercostals depress the ribs, and the abdominal muscles depress the lower ribs and pull the abdominal wall inward.

Muscle Weakness

Weakness is defined as a reduced capacity of a rested muscle to generate an expected force. Weakened inspiratory muscles may be incapable of performing the work of breathing, leading to hypercapnia. Expiratory muscle weakness impairs the cough reflex, promoting retention of secretions and pneumonia. Causes of muscle weakness are listed in Table 1.

As part of normal aging, respiratory muscle strength generally declines in parallel with overall muscle performance. Malnutrition causes all muscles, including those of respiration, to become atrophic and weak, causing predisposition to respiratory failure. Respiratory muscles may become weak as the result of denervation, myopathy, and endocrinopathies. Metabolic disorders, including severe abnormalities in serum potassium, magnesium, and phosphate, may interfere with contractile function, causing inadequate $\dot{V}_E$ and

Table 1. *Causes of Respiratory Muscle Weakness*

Aging
Malnutrition
Denervation
Myopathy
Muscular dystrophy
Polymyositis
Drug-induced (neuromuscular blocking agents, corticosteroids)
Endocrinopathy (hyperthyroidism, Cushing syndrome)
Metabolic
Hypokalemia
Hyperkalemia
Hypophosphatemia
Hypomagnesemia
Hypermagnesemia
Acidosis
Hyperinflation

hypercapnia. When acidosis impairs the contractile force of respiratory muscles, a positive feedback loop of respiratory muscle weakness and respiratory acidosis may be established.

Hyperinflation places the inspiratory muscles at mechanical disadvantage, largely because of a reduction in muscle length. Inspiratory muscle weakness with hyperinflation is more pronounced in acute disorders like severe asthma than in COPD. With time, remodeling of sarcomeres restores them to normal length, and the proportion of slow-twitch muscle fibers increases. These adaptive responses improve contractile function and increase resistance to fatigue. Also, many patients with COPD lose weight; these patients have increased circulating levels of tumor necrosis factor-α, which promotes muscle wasting and weakness. The benefits of lung volume reduction surgery (LVRS) in patients with severe COPD are probably attributable to enhanced ventilatory pump function; LVRS reduces hyperinflation and air trapping, improving diaphragm mechanics and increasing $\dot{V}_A$.

Assessment of Respiratory Muscle Strength

In clinical practice, the strength of respiratory muscles usually is measured with maximal pressures at the mouth against a closed airway (maximum inspiratory pressure, maximum expiratory pressure). The "gold standard" measurement, used more in scientific investigations than in clinical practice, is transdiaphragmatic pressure (Pdi) during a maximal inspiratory effort. Pdi is calculated as the difference between abdominal pressure measured with a gastric balloon catheter, and pleural pressure measured in the esophagus.

Respiratory Muscle Fatigue

Fatigue is defined as a reduced capacity to generate an expected force, which is corrected with rest. Fatigue can be classified as central, transmissional, and contractile. Central fatigue describes a reversible decrease in central neural respiratory drive caused by overuse of muscles. It may be motivational when strength can be restored by voluntary effort and *nonmotivational* when strength is not restored by increased effort but the muscle responds normally to electrical stimulation. Central fatigue is probably a consequence of reflex inhibition, influenced by afferent and cortical signals, perhaps endogenous opioids. Transmission fatigue is a reversible, exertion-induced impairment of neural transmission; its pathophysiology and significance are unknown.

Contractile fatigue is a reversible impairment in contractile response to neural impulses not caused by drugs or alteration in length/tension or force/velocity relationships. It occurs when energy demands on contracting muscles exceed the energy supply. Energy demand is a function of the work of breathing ($\dot{V}_E$, compliance, and resistance) and the efficiency of the respiratory system. Fatigue typically occurs when the tension time index is >0.15. The tension-time index is defined as follows: Pdi/maximal Pdi × T_I/T_T, where T_I = duration of inspiration, and T_T = duration of one respiratory cycle.

Put more simply, fatigue occurs when Pbreath/MIP × T_I/T_T is excessive, where Pbreath = inspiratory pressure for a given breath, and MIP = maximal inspiratory pressure. Therefore, a weak muscle (where maximal Pdi and MIP are reduced) is more likely to fatigue and fail than a normal muscle.

The efficiency of inspiratory muscle contraction is impaired by lung volume, the presence of neuromuscular disease, and malnutrition. Body position also influences contractile efficiency; inspiration requires less effort in the upright position because the abdominal contents are displaced downward by gravity, unloading the diaphragm. Patients with lung disease and an increased work of breathing usually are more comfortable in an upright compared with supine position. This is especially true for patients with massive obesity, when assuming the supine position may precipitate respiratory arrest because the diaphragm cannot overcome the intolerable load imposed by the weight of the abdominal contents.

The energy supply to muscles varies directly with blood flow. Shock often culminates in respiratory failure because blood flow and oxygen supply to contracting respiratory muscles are reduced. In cardiogenic shock, hypercapnic respiratory failure occurs because pulmonary edema increases the work of breathing, and impaired hemodynamic function reduces blood flow to the respiratory muscles. Hypoxemia may compromise oxygen supply to respiratory muscles, but hypoxemia alone does not usually cause muscle fatigue; oxygen consumption can be maintained by increased cardiac output and augmented oxygen extraction from capillary blood.

When respiratory muscles are fatigued, the EMG power spectrum is shifted, with increased low-frequency and decreased high-frequency components. Dyspnea and tachypnea are common. Respiratory alternans, the alternating recruitment and derecruitment of the diaphragm and other inspiratory muscles, often precedes the onset of paradoxical abdominal motion with respiration.

Treatment of fatigue depends on correcting the underlying disorders and rest. If the underlying condition that provoked muscle fatigue is not readily reversible, the patient will require mechanical ventilation until adequate rest is achieved. Pharmacologic approaches to improve respiratory muscle function have been investigated. Although aminophylline, digoxin, and dobutamine have all been demonstrated to increase the contractility of the diaphragm, their clinical utility in patients with respiratory muscle fatigue is unproven. Similarly, the role of strength and endurance training of the respiratory muscles has been under investigation for decades, but there is still no good evidence to support its use.

Hypercapnia With Oxygen Administration

Excessive oxygen administration may worsen preexisting hypercapnia, especially in patients with COPD. Mechanisms include the following: (1) increased physiologic dead space. This factor is an important one, but the precise explanation for this phenomenon is not completely understood; (2) attenuation of hypoxic ventilatory drive; patients with chronic hypercapnia become insensitive to increments in $Paco_2$; and (3) the Haldane effect, in which oxygen releases co_2 bound to hemoglobin, increasing $Paco_2$.

Primary Disorders of the Chest Wall

Severe kyphoscoliosis, obesity, thoracoplasty, and pleural thickening all may cause hypoventilation by one of two general mechanisms, which can be categorized as "can't breathe" and "won't breathe." Significant increase in the work of breathing caused by severe mechanical derangements of the chest wall may lead to reduced V_Ts and increased $\dot{V}_D/V_T$ (can't breathe). Many patients with chest wall restriction have central carbon dioxide nonresponsiveness, either as a primary disorder or to compensate for increased work of breathing (won't breathe). In acute illness, respiratory muscle fatigue imposed by increased work of breathing may precipitate frank hypercapnic respiratory failure.

The interplay of increased work of breathing and diminished respiratory drive is a prominent feature of the obesity-hypoventilation syndrome (OHS), defined as a combination of obesity (body mass index > 30 kg/m^2) and hypercapnia ($Paco_2$ > 45 mm Hg) during wakefulness in the absence of other known causes of alveolar hypoventilation. In many patients, severe obesity is associated with chronic daytime hypercapnia and hypoxemia, erythrocytosis, and right ventricular failure. Most (but not all) patients with OHS also have obstructive sleep apnea, but only a minority of obese patients with obstructive sleep apnea have OHS. Patients with OHS have a blunted central drive in response to hypercapnia and hypoxemia, possibly related to decreased circulating levels or receptor hyporesponsiveness to leptin, a hormone that acts on the hypothalamus to suppress appetite and probably also on central respiratory centers to maintain hypercapnic ventilatory responses. Obesity-related upper airway narrowing, dependent atelectasis, and excessive loading of respiratory muscles may all be contributing factors.

Annotated Bibliography

Caruana-Montaldo B, Gleeson K, Zwillich CW. The control of breathing in clinical practice. Chest 2000; 117:205–225

Review of the physiology of each component of the integrated systems that control breathing, with cases illustrating disorders of these systems.

Laghi F, Tobin MJ. Disorders of the respiratory muscles. Am J Respir Crit Care Med 2003; 168:10–48

Very thorough review of the role of respiratory muscles in acute respiratory failure; specific neuromuscular diseases; and the influence of chest wall, systemic diseases, and surgery on respiratory muscle function.

Weinberger SE, Schwartzstein RM, Weiss JW. Hypercapnia. N Engl J Med 1989; 321:1223–1231

Concise summary of mechanisms, specific disorders, and therapeutic strategies.

Neuromuscular Disorders

Bunch TJ, Thalzi MK, Pillikka PA, et al. Respiratory failure in tetanus: case report and review of a 25-year experience. Chest 2002; 122:1488–1492

Centers for Disease Control and Prevention. Human rabies: Alberta, Canada, 2007. MMWR Morb Mortal Wkly Rep 2008; 57:197–200

Describes clinical picture, management, and prevention strategies.

Cherington M. Clinical spectrum of botulism. Muscle Nerve 1998; 21:701–710

Deem S, Lee CM, Curtis JR. Acquired neuromuscular disorders in the intensive care unit. Am J Respir Crit Care Med 2003; 168:735–739

Hermans G, Wilmer A, Meersseman W, et al. Impact of intensive insulin therapy on neuromuscular complications and ventilator dependency in the intensive care unit. Am I Respir Crit Care Med 2007; 175:480–489

Horowitz BZ. Botulinum toxin. Crit Care Clin 2005; 21:825–839

Hughes RAC, Cornblath DR. Guillain-Barré syndrome. Lancet 2005; 366:1653–1666

Jubelt B, Agre JC. Characteristics and management of postpolio syndrome. JAMA 2000; 26:412–414

Latronico N, Peli E, Botteri M. Critical illness myopathy and neuropathy. Curr Opin Crit Care 2005; 11:126–132

Leatherman JW, Fluegel WL, David WS, et al. Muscle weakness in mechanically ventilated patients with severe asthma. Am J Respir Crit Care Med 1996; 153:1686–1690

Muscle weakness occurred in 20 of 69 patients who received both a neuromuscular blocking agent and corticosteroids compared with none of the 38 patients who received corticosteroids alone. Weakness correlated with the duration of paralysis, and the incidence of weakness was not reduced in patients who received atracurium compared with those who received pancuronium or vecuronium.

Pujar T, Spinello IM. A 38-year-old woman with heroin addiction, ptosis, respiratory failure and proximal myopathy. Chest 2008; 134:867–870

Concise review with table summarizing the differential diagnosis of neuromuscular diseases that cause respiratory failure.

Schweickert WD, Hall J. ICU-acquired weakness. Chest 2007; 131:1541–1549

Schwendimann RN, Burton E, Minagar A. Management of myasthenia gravis. Am J Ther 2005; 12:262–268

These articles are cited because they are relatively current and offer detailed discussions regarding neuromuscular disorders that may cause respiratory failure.

Werner SB, Passaro D, McGee J, et al. Wound botulism in California, 1951–1998: recent epidemic in heroin injectors. Clin Infect Dis 2000; 31:1018–1024

The upsurge in diagnoses have been attributed to subcutaneous drug injection (skin popping). Abscess formation and devitalized tissue provide a favorable milieu for growth of the organism. This article also provides a concise review of other paralytic diseases discussed in this chapter.

Respiratory Muscles

American Thoracic Society/European Respiratory Society. Skeletal muscle dysfunction in chronic obstructive pulmonary disease: a statement of the American Thoracic Society and European Respiratory Society. Am J Respir Crit Care Med 1999; 159(Suppl):S1–S40

Comprehensive review of mechanisms.

Cohen CA, Zagelbaum G, Gross D, et al. Clinical manifestations of inspiratory muscle fatigue. Am J Med 1982; 73:308–316

Progression of clinical findings leading to respiratory failure.

Criner G, Cordova FC, Leyenson V. Effect of lung volume reduction surgery on diaphragm strength. Am J Respir Crit Care Med 1998; 157:1578–1585

Lando Y, Boiselle PM, Shade D, et al. Effect of lung volume reduction surgery on diaphragm length in severe chronic obstructive pulmonary disease. Am J Respir Crit Care Med 1999; 159:796–805

Polkey MI, Moxham J. Clinical aspects of respiratory muscle dysfunction in the critically ill. Chest 2001; 119:926–939

Reviews respiratory muscle physiology, evaluation of muscle dysfunction, and disorders that lead to prolonged ventilator dependency.

Roussos C, Macklem PT. The respiratory muscles. N Engl J Med 1982; 307:786–797

Develops the concept of "pump failure," reviewing the physiology and clinical features of muscle mechanics, energetics, and fatigue.

Shade D, Cordova F, Lando Y, et al. Relationship between resting hypercapnia and physiologic parameters before and after lung volume reduction surgery in severe chronic obstructive pulmonary disease. Am J Respir Crit Care Med 1999; 159:1405–1411

These three studies from the same center show that LVRS increases the length of the diaphragm and improves its strength, the changes correlate with postoperative *improvements in exercise capacity and maximum voluntary ventilation, and patients with hypercapnia have reductions in $Paco_2$ as ventilatory pump function and $\dot{V}E$ improve.*

Hypercapnia After Oxygen Administration

Aubier M, Murciano D, Milic-Emili J, et al. Effects of the administration of O_2 on ventilation and blood gases in patients with chronic obstructive pulmonary disease during acute respiratory failure. Am Rev Respir Dis 1980; 122:747–754

Hanson CW, Marshall BE, Frasch HF, et al. Causes of hypercarbia with oxygen therapy in patients with chronic obstructive pulmonary disease. Crit Care Med 1996; 24:23–28

This study uses a computer model of the pulmonary circulation with data from the study of Aubier et al to evaluate the factors contributing to hypercarbia after oxygen administration in patients with COPD. The discussion offers a lucid explanation of the pathophysiology of this phenomenon.

Robinson TD, Freiberg DB, Regnis JA, et al. The role of hypoventilation and ventilation-perfusion redistribution in oxygen-induced hypercapnia during acute exacerbations of chronic obstructive pulmonary disease. Am J Respir Crit Care Med 2000; 161:1524–1529

These studies exploring the mechanisms of hypercapnia after oxygen administration in patients with COPD. The former shows that increased wasted ventilation is the major factor whereas the latter holds that both increased dead space and reduced total ventilation are responsible.

OHS

Kessler R, Chaouat A, Schinkewitch P, et al. The obesity-hypoventilation syndrome revisited: a prospective study of 24 consecutive cases. Chest 2001; 120: 369–376

Most patients with OHS also have obstructive sleep apnea. In addition to daytime hypercapnia, OHS is likely associated with pulmonary hypertension and severe hypoxemia.

Malhotra A, Hillman D. Obesity and the lung: 3—obesity, respiration and intensive care. Thorax 2008; 63:925–931

Thorough review of physiology and complications of obesity with a broad discussion of critical illness in these patients.

Mokhlesi B, Tulaimat A. Recent advances in obesity hypoventilation syndrome. Chest 2007; 132:1322–1336

Reviews pathophysiology and treatment options.

Thoracic Imaging

Rakesh D. Shah, MD, FCCP

Objectives:

- Review the basic plain radiograph and cross-sectional anatomy and pathology of the tracheobronchial tree, lobar atelectasis, and the mediastinum
- Evaluate the role of CT pulmonary angiography in the diagnosis of both acute and chronic pulmonary thromboembolic disease
- Review the current methods for evaluation of solitary pulmonary nodule
- Learn to interpret high-resolution CT scan images in patients with diffuse lung disease

Key words: chest imaging; CT pulmonary angiography; high-resolution CT scan; positron emission tomography

This chapter is divided into six broad sections: (1) evaluation of the nonneoplastic diseases of the tracheobronchial tree, (2) lobar atelectasis, (3) evaluation of mediastinal structures and pathology, (4) CT pulmonary angiography in the diagnosis of acute and chronic thromboembolic disease, (5) current concepts in the evaluation of solitary pulmonary nodule, and (6) high-resolution CT (HRCT) scan findings in patients with diffuse lung disease.

Tracheobronchial Tree

Focal or diffuse lesions of the tracheobronchial tree are produced by a variety of diseases. The etiologies include infection, malignancy, trauma, collagen vascular disease, and idiopathic entities such as amyloidosis and tracheobronchopathia osteochondroplastica. These conditions may produce symptoms of cough, dyspnea, wheezing, or stridor. Despite significant symptomatology, airway abnormalities frequently are not apparent or often are overlooked on chest radiographs, which results in a delay of the diagnosis. CT scan of the chest is the imaging modality of choice if there is a clinical suspicion of tracheobronchial abnormality. The following is a brief description of the important nonneoplastic diseases that are associated with tracheal narrowing.

Tracheal Stenosis

Most tracheal stenoses are complications of tracheal intubations. Narrowing occurs at the thoracic inlet where the cuff has been inflated for tracheostomy or intubation. As the cuff pressure exceeds the capillary pressure, blood supply to the tracheal mucosa is compromised. This compromise leads to inflammation, followed by ulceration and necrosis. Eventually, scarring occurs and leads to stenosis. On CT, 1- to 2-cm long circumferential narrowing of the trachea is noted at the thoracic inlet.

Tracheobronchomalacia

Tracheobronchomalacia is a condition defined by excessive expiratory collapse of the trachea and bronchi. It is a result of weakness of the airway walls or supporting cartilage. Some cases are congenital in nature; however, most cases are acquired and are caused by previous intubation, trauma, infection, or chronic inflammation. On CT, diagnosis is suggested when greater than a 50% decrease in the cross-sectional area of the airway lumen is noted on dynamic expiratory images.

Saber-Sheath Trachea

Saber-sheath trachea is characterized by marked decrease in the transverse diameter of the intrathoracic trachea associated with an increase in its sagittal diameter. Changes in tracheal configuration are a result of abnormal intrathoracic transmural pressures. It is found in men who smoke and have COPD.

Tracheobronchopathia Osteochondroplastica

It is a rare, benign disease characterized by development of osseous or cartilaginous nodules within the anterolateral walls of the trachea. The posterior membrane of the trachea is spared because of the absence of cartilage in this area. It occurs in men older than 50 years and usually is detected incidentally. On CT, calcified nodules protruding into the tracheal lumen are noted. Resultant tracheal narrowing may be present.

Relapsing Polychondritis

Relapsing polychondritis is a rare inflammatory disease that affects the cartilages of the ear, nose, respiratory tract, and joints. It is characterized by repeated episodes of cartilaginous inflammation, leading to loss of structure and fibrosis. The respiratory tract is affected in approximately one half of all the patients. On CT, thickening of the anterolateral tracheal wall with sparing of the posterior membrane is noted. Resultant luminal narrowing and airway collapse are best demonstrated on dynamic expiratory CT scans.

Amyloidosis

Amyloidosis is a rare condition characterized by deposition of insoluble protein in the extracellular tissues. It may involve any portion of the respiratory tract. Within the lung parenchyma, abnormal amyloid deposition can appear as single or multiple nodules or diffuse interstitial opacities. Deposits within the tracheobronchial tree lead to concentric or nodular thickening of the tracheal submucosa with resultant narrowing of the lumen. Calcification and/or ossification of the lesions may occur.

Wegener Granulomatosis

It is a necrotizing granulomatous vasculitis that involves the upper and lower respiratory tract. Involvement of the lung parenchyma shows multiple nodules with or without cavitation. Involvement of the tracheobronchial tree is rare and usually presents late in the disease. On CT, circumferential thickening, ulceration, and luminal narrowing of the trachea are noted.

Mounier-Kuhn syndrome (Tracheobronchomegaly)

Tracheobronchomegaly, also referred to as *Mounier-Kuhn syndrome*, is a rare condition characterized by diffuse dilatation of the trachea and the main bronchi. It is thought to result from atrophy of muscular and elastic tissue found in both trachea and main bronchi. On CT, thin wall trachea with scalloped or corrugated appearance, increased tracheal diameter of >3 cm, and diverticulosis are present.

In summary, diagnosis of the nonneoplastic diseases of the tracheobronchial tree requires knowledge of the anatomy, and observation of the following on CT scans:

1. Is the trachea dilated or narrowed?
2. If there is thickening of the airway wall? If so, is it focal or diffuse? Is the thickening at the thoracic inlet or not?
3. Is there stenosis? If so is it focal or diffuse?
4. Is calcification present or not?
5. Is ulceration present or not?
6. Is the posterior membrane involved or spared?
7. Is there collapse of the tracheal wall on dynamic expiratory images?

The differential diagnosis can be significantly narrowed once the above questions have been answered.

Atelectasis

Atelectasis is defined as decrease in volume of lung or a portion of the lung. Resorption, passive, cicatrization, and adhesive are the four types of atelectasis that can be explained by the mechanism in which the loss of lung volume occurs. Resorptive atelectasis is the most common type and results from absorption of gas from the alveoli when the communication between the alveoli and the trachea is obstructed by an endobronchial lesion or a mucus plug. Passive atelectasis is caused by extrinsic pressure on the lung from a large pleural effusion, pneumothorax, or mass resulting in collapse. *Cicatrisation* atelectasis occurs in patients with scarring or pulmonary fibrosis. The exact mechanism of adhesive atelectasis is poorly understood but is thought to be caused by widespread collapse of alveoli. It is usually seen in patients with respiratory distress syndrome and in those who are recovering from surgery.

Lobar atelectasis may be complete or partial. The most common cause of lobar atelectasis is obstruction by a central endobronchial lesion. However, in hospitalized patients and particularly in those who are intubated, a mucus plug is the most common cause of partial or lobar atelectasis. Primary and secondary signs on chest radiograph help identify the atelectasis and site of endobronchial obstruction. The major sign of lobar atelectasis is opacification of the affected lobe due to airlessness and displacement of the interlobar fissure. Secondary signs of atelectasis include displacement of the mediastinal structures, elevation of the hemidiaphragm, decrease in the distance of the intercostals spaces, displacement of the hila, and compensatory overinflation of the remaining lung. Discussion of the major and minor radiographic features of the main lobar atelectasis follow.

Right Upper Lobe Atelectasis

On the frontal chest radiograph, the right upper lobe collapses superiorly and medially, creating a wedge-shaped opacity in the upper right hemithorax. The major fissure is displaced anteriorly and the minor fissure is displaced upward. Right upper lobe collapse secondary to a central carcinoma may produce a characteristic appearance on the frontal chest radiograph, termed the "reverse S-sign" of Golden. On the lateral projection, the collapsed lobe may appear as a triangular opacity with its apex at the hilum and its base at the apex of the hemithorax.

Left Upper Lobe Atelectasis

When the left upper lobe collapses, the frontal chest radiograph demonstrates a hazy opacification in the left perihilar area with partial obscuration of the left heart border. Sometimes, the resultant overinflation of the superior segment of the left lower lobe inserts between the apex of the atelectatic upper lobe and the aortic knob, creating a sharp lucent interface called the *Luftsichel sign*. On the lateral radiograph, there is forward displacement of the major fissure that is almost parallel to the anterior chest wall.

Lower Lobe Atelectasis

The pattern of lower lobe collapse is similar in both lungs because of the equivalent anatomy bilaterally. Both lower lobes collapse posteromedially and inferiorly. On the frontal radiograph, a triangular opacity is visualized in the paraspinal location of the lower hemithorax, while on the lateral projection, increased opacity overlying the lower thoracic vertebral bodies and loss of visualization of the posterior left hemidiaphragm are noted.

Right Middle Lobe Atelectasis

On the frontal chest radiograph, the right middle lobe collapse shows a vague opacity in the lower right hemithorax with obliteration of the right heart border. On the lateral projection, the collapse is seen as a linear band or triangular opacity overlying the cardiac silhouette as a result of displacement of the minor fissure inferiorly and major fissure superiorly.

Rounded Atelectasis

It is an unusual form of passive atelectasis that is thought to occur from pleural fibrosis as a result of chronic pleural effusion and/or asbestos-related disease. The pleural fibrosis causes folding of the adjacent lung parenchyma that appears as a focal, rounded opacity. On CT, a peripherally situated rounded opacity with associated pleural thickening, "comet-tail" sign, and volume loss of the affected lobe are noted.

Pulmonary Embolism

Pulmonary embolism (PE) is an important cause of morbidity and mortality, particularly in the postsurgical and hospitalized patients. Unfortunately, the diagnosis of acute PE is often delayed or unrecognized because of the nonspecific nature of its symptoms, signs, and laboratory test findings. The chest radiograph is often nonspecific or normal. Ventilation/perfusion scans have high sensitivity but low specificity, whereas pulmonary angiography is invasive, underused, and has considerable interobserver variability.

Pathophysiology of PE

PE refers to the transport of venous thrombus to the pulmonary artery circulation. Most thrombi arise from clots within the deep venous system of the lower extremities. Emboli are often multiple, and they have predilection for the lower lobes of the lung. This predilection is likely related to increased blood flow in the lower lobes.

CT Technique

In recent years, great advances have been made in the CT technology. Because of its ability to directly visualize PE noninvasively and with high accuracy, multirow detector CT scanners have become the imaging test of choice for the diagnosis of PE. One of the other potential advantages is the ability to diagnosis alternative diagnosis that may mimic PE clinically.

On multirow detector CT scanners, approximately 80 to 100 mL of iodinated IV contrast is injected at 4 mL/s after a fixed scan delay or a timing bolus of 20 mL. The patient is scanned in a single breath hold from the lung apices to the level of the diaphragm. Approximately 250 to 400 images per scan are obtained because the study is performed at 1.25-mm collimation. Thus, the CT interpretation is performed on computer workstation by actually scrolling through the images and altering the window width and level to optimally evaluate the pulmonary arteries.

CT Findings

The CT findings of acute PE are direct visualization of low-attenuation thrombus within the contrast-opacified pulmonary artery. Thrombus may be identified as partial or complete filling defect in the vascular lumen. Secondary signs of PE include oligemia of the affected segment and pulmonary infarcts.

Pitfalls in the diagnosis of PE can be classified into anatomic and technical etiologies. Common anatomic pitfalls include lymph nodes, pulmonary veins, impacted bronchi, and volume averaging of pulmonary arteries. On the computer workstation, if one scrolls in and out from the main pulmonary artery, following each of the lobar, segmental, and subsegmental arteries, it is impossible to mistake an artery for a vein, lymph node, or mucoid impacted bronchi for PE. Technical causes for suboptimal quality examinations are poor enhancement of pulmonary arteries, breathing motion artifact, and excessive noise in large patients. Bolus tracking software built into most CT scanners has significantly reduced nondiagnostic scans from poor enhancement. In addition, motion artifact is less of a problem with greater detector scanners because of the shorter breath holds needed.

Chronic Thromboembolism

Chronic thromboembolism is scarring of the pulmonary arteries after lysis of thrombi from either single or repeated bouts of PE. As a result, webs and occlusions are formed within the branches of the pulmonary arteries. The global effect of these is the overall increase of the pulmonary vascular resistance and subsequent pulmonary hypertension.

Characteristic CT findings can be classified into three categories: cardiac, pulmonary arteries, and parenchymal. The cardiac findings include right-sided chamber enlargement and right ventricular hypertrophy. Pulmonary artery findings include eccentric thrombus, abrupt vessel cut-off, webs, beaded vessels, and enlarged central arteries. Parenchymal findings include alternating hazy and lucent areas in lung called *mosaic attenuation* and enlarged bronchial arteries.

Mediastinum

The mediastinum is an anatomic region within the thoracic cavity that is bound laterally by the lungs, anteriorly by the sternum, and posteriorly by the vertebral bodies. A wide variety of focal and diffuse abnormalities occur within the mediastinum. To facilitate the differential diagnosis, the mediastinum has been divided into several compartments, primarily based on landmarks noted on the chest radiographs and CT rather than true anatomic fascial planes. They include the following: (1) anterior mediastinum, which includes the retrosternal clear space and cardiophrenic angle; (2) the middle mediastinum, which includes the retrosternal clear space, subcarinal region, and retrocardiac clear space; and (3) posterior mediastinum.

Retrosternal Clear Space

This is the region that is posterior to the sternum and anterior the aorta and great vessels. It corresponds to the region of the anterior junction line noted on the frontal chest radiographs. Normal structures that are present in this location include the thymus gland, lymph nodes, and fat. The differential diagnoses of lesions in this space include lesions of thymic origin (thymoma, thymic cyst); lymphoma; teratoma; aortic aneurysm; lipomatosis; and sternal lesions. In adults, thymomas account for the majority of the lesions in this space. On CT, they appear as round or lobulated soft-tissue density lesions. Most of them enhance homogeneously after IV contrast administration and may contain calcification. Most of the thymomas are encapsulated and considered benign, but roughly 30% demonstrate invasion through the fibrous capsule and are considered malignant. Imaging features that support malignancy include the following: (1) invasion of mediastinal structures, including the superior vena cava and great vessels; (2) chest wall invasion; and (3) contiguous spread along pleural surfaces.

Cardiophrenic Angle

This region is situated anterior and to the right of the heart. Typically, this region contains fat and lymph nodes. Most of the lesions occurring in this space are benign and include prominent fat, lipoma, pericardial cyst, and Morgagni hernia. Occasionally, they may contain lymph nodes from lymphoma or metastasis.

Retrotracheal Clear Space

This region is posterior to the trachea, anterior to the thoracic spine, and superior to the posterior portion of the aortic arch. It corresponds to the region of the posterior junction line as noted on the frontal chest radiograph. Normal structures that are present in this space include esophagus and lymph nodes. The differential diagnosis of lesions in this region includes abnormalities of the esophagus (tumor, achalasia, Zenker's diverticulum). However, a large percentage of lesions in this region are vascular (aberrant right subclavian artery) or thyroid in origin. The majority of the thyroid masses represent goiters, which almost always extend inferiorly from the thyroid gland into this space.

Subcarinal Region

This region is inferior to the carina and superior to the left atrium. Fat, lymph nodes, and the esophagus are normal structures that live in this space. Differential diagnoses of lesions in this region include lymphadenopathy, bronchogenic cyst, esophageal diverticula, and esophageal tumors. Lymphadenopathy is the most common lesion in this space. It may be neoplastic, inflammatory, or infectious in nature. CT is very helpful in detecting and characterizing the lymph nodes. On imaging, the nodes may demonstrate homogeneous enhancement, hyperenhancement, calcification or low-density (fat or necrosis) center. When present, these lymph node characteristics significantly help shorten very lengthy differential diagnosis of subcarinal adenopathy.

Retrocardiac Clear Space

This region is posterior to the heart and anterior the thoracic spine. The esophagus, aorta, azygos vein, fat, and lymph nodes are present in this region. Differential diagnoses include esophageal lesions (duplication cyst, varices, hiatal hernia, tumor); aortic aneurysm; and lymphadenopathy.

Posterior Mediastinum

It is defined as the area posterior to the anterior margin of the vertebral bodies. Normal structures that are present in this location include the vertebral column, fat, and nerves. The majority of the lesions occurring in this space are neurogenic (congenital, malignant, infection) in nature. MRI is the preferred imaging modality of choice for evaluation of posterior mediastinal lesions because of its ability to demonstrate intraspinal extension of tumor and detect spinal cord abnormalities.

Solitary Pulmonary Nodule

A solitary pulmonary nodule (SPN) is defined as a well-circumscribed round lesion that is surrounded by lung parenchyma measuring <3 cm. A larger lesion with the same characteristics is called a mass. A SPN can be solid, ground glass, or part solid (containing both ground-glass and solid components). The differential diagnoses are many, including benign and malignant neoplasms, granuloma, infection, vascular abnormalities, and intrapulmonary lymph nodes.

Once a nodule is detected on plain chest radiographs, comparison with previous films, if available, is recommended. If none are available, then HRCT scans at 1- to 2-mm thick sections through the nodule should be obtained. This scanning is helpful in detecting calcification, fat, and in defining the morphology of the nodule.

Morphologic characteristics of SPN often are nonspecific. For example, malignant lesions can be round and well-defined, whereas benign lesions can be irregular and speculated. However, some lesions have morphologic characteristics typical enough to allow a diagnosis to be made on CT. These include arteriovenous fistula, pulmonary artery pseudoaneurysms, mycetomas, and mucous plugs.

Demonstration of specific types of calcification or fat is the only reliable sign that a SPN is benign. "Benign" types of calcification include those with a central nidus, "popcorn," and laminated. Eccentric calcification can be identified in a small percentage of lung carcinomas that may incorporate adjacent calcified granulomas, or they may themselves calcify. In these instances, the calcification is often stippled or punctuate. Presence of fat within a nodule suggests the lesion as being a hamartoma.

Nodules <8 mm in size and present at the lung bases and in the peripheral aspect of the lung may be classified as intrapulmonary lymph nodes if they fulfill the following criteria: (1) a triangular shape and situated on the fissure and/or peripheral subpleural location or (2) be well-defined, smooth, round[,] or elliptical in contour, situated on a interlobular septa, and adjacent to a draining pulmonary vein. Nodules that fulfill the aforementioned criteria are benign and do not require further workup.

If the nodule is found to be indeterminate, further evaluation should be performed with: (1) nodule enhancement; (2) transthoracic percutaneous needle (TTPN) biopsy, bronchoscopy, and surgery; (3) PET scan; or (4) periodic follow-up.

Nodule Enhancement

After noncontrast images, sections through the nodule are obtained after IV contrast administration for up to 4 min at 1-min intervals. Attenuation of the nodule is measured before and at the peak of contrast enhancement. Those nodules that enhanced <15 Hounsfield units (HU) are strongly predictive of benign lesions. Lesions that enhanced >15 HU are indeterminate because carcinomas, active granulomas, inflammatory lesions, and hamartomas all can demonstrate enhancement.

TTPN Biopsy

TTPN biopsy can be performed on most CT-visible lesions. It has a high sensitivity for the diagnosis of malignant cells (79%) but is less accurate for benign processes.

PET Imaging

PET is a physiologic imaging technique in which 2-[fluorine-18]-fluoro-2-deoxy-D-glucose (FDG), a D-glucose analog, is labeled with a positron emitter (^{18}F). Increased glucose metabolism in lesions result in increased uptake and accumulation of FDG. Thus, metabolically active lesions will demonstrate increased FDG uptake. The degree of FDG accumulation is measured by the use of the standardized uptake ratio. Typically, lung cancers demonstrate standardized uptake ratio of >2.5. For nodules >1 cm, FDG-PET has sensitivity of about 95%. However, its role in evaluation of SPN should be approached with caution. The reason is infectious and inflammatory SPN can demonstrate increased FDG uptake and thus may give false-positive results. False-negative results may occur with carcinoid and bronchioloalveolar carcinomas. Those nodules that are too small for the resolution of PET imaging, are not approachable by biopsy, and do not qualify as intrapulmonary lymph nodes need periodic follow-up CT scans to ensure their stability or to assess for interval growth.

In summary, SPN is a common radiologic finding that may require extensive workup to establish a definitive diagnosis. There is no one correct management approach. The objective is to use a logical approach using clinical history and radiologic findings.

HRCT Features of Diffuse Lung Disease

HRCT scans provide detailed visualization of the lung parenchyma. Indications for HRCT scans include the following: (1) suspected diffuse lung disease, (2) for possible prebiopsy workup, and (3) assessment of disease activity. Knowledge of the secondary pulmonary lobule and the flow of lymphatics within the pulmonary interstitium are absolutely necessary for interpretation of HRCT scans. The secondary lobule is the smallest unit of the lung visible on HRCT. It is polyhedral in shape and measures about 1 to 2.5 cm. The core structures of the lobule include central pulmonary artery and terminal bronchiole. The septal structures include venules, lymphatics, and fibrous septa. The pulmonary lymphatic channels flow from the subpleural interstitium that is loculated beneath the visceral pleura into the interlobular septa of the secondary pulmonary nodule. It then flows to the intralobular interstitium and into the peribronchovascular interstitium before reaching the mediastinal lymph nodes.

HRCT Patterns

Several basic patterns of diffuse lung disease are characterized on HRCT scans. They include the following: (1) linear, (2) reticular, (3) nodular, (4) ground-glass opacity (GGO), (5) consolidation, and (6) cysts. Recognition of these basic patterns along with their distribution (central or peripheral, upper, or lower) on HRCT scans can help narrow the differential diagnosis in large majority of cases.

Linear pattern is defined by the presence of Kerley's lines and represents thickening of the interlobular septa. This pattern has a long differential diagnosis but is commonly seen in patients with pulmonary edema and lymphangitic spread of carcinoma.

Reticular pattern consists of interlacing line shadows that appear as a mesh or net-like. Visualization of this pattern suggests that the patient has pulmonary fibrosis and "honeycombing." It is seen in patients with usual interstitial pneumonia, asbestosis, collagen vascular disease, and drug toxicity.

Nodular pattern refers to multiple round opacities that are <1 cm in diameter. They are further classified based on their distribution within the lung. They can be present in the perilymphatic space, centrilobular location, or random distribution. Perilymphatic nodules occur at the pleural surfaces, on the interlobular septa, and in the peribronchovascular interstitium. Nodules in perilymphatic distribution are caused by diseases such as sarcoidosis and lymphangitic spread of carcinoma. Random nodules are evenly distributed throughout both lungs and suggest hematogenous spread of disease. Entities include metastasis and infections such as military tuberculosis. Centrilobular nodules occur in the center of the secondary pulmonary lobule. They are seen in patients with hypersensitivity pneumonitis and infection. Tree-in-bud opacities are a form of centrilobular nodules and represent dilated and impacted distal terminal bronchioles. Their presence is almost always indicative of endobronchial spread of infection.

GGO represents hazy increased attenuation of lung with preservation of the underlying bronchovascular margins while consolidation represents increased attenuation of lung with complete obscuration of underlying bronchovascular margins. GGO represents partial filling, whereas consolidation represents complete filling of the air spaces by transudative fluid, infectious material, blood, or malignancy. Both have a very long differential diagnosis. The presence of GGO with superimposed interlobular septal thickening has been termed a *crazy-paving pattern*. It has classically been described in cases of alveolar proteinosis; however, it can be seen in a number of entities. Most common etiologies in everyday practice include pulmonary edema and *Pneumocystis jiroveci* pneumonia. Other causes include hemorrhage, malignancy (such as bronchioloalveolar carcinoma), and lipoid pneumonia.

Cystic pattern refers to thin-walled, well-defined air lesions that are <1 cm in diameter. Entities manifesting a cystic pattern include lymphangioleiomyomatosis and Langerhans cell histiocytosis. In summary, knowledge of the pulmonary anatomy, recognition of HRCT patterns and their distribution are prerequisites in the proper interpretation of diffuse lung disease on HRCT scans.

Bibliography

General References

Felson B. Chest roentgenology. Philadelphia, PA: W. B. Saunders, 1973

Fraser RS, Pare PD. Diagnosis of diseases of the chest. 4th ed. Philadelphia, PA: W. B. Saunders, 1999

Webb WR, Muller NL, Naidich DP. High resolution CT of the lung. 3rd ed. Philadelphia, PA: Lippincott, Williams and Wilkins, 2001

Tracheobronchial Tree

Gamsu G, Webb WR. Computed tomography of the trachea and mainstem bronchi. Semin Roentgenol 1983; 18:51–60

Grillo HC, Donahue DM. Postintubation tracheal stenosis. Chest Surg Clin N Am 1996; 6:725–731

Kwong JS, Muller NL, Miller RR. Diseases of the trachea and main stem bronchi: correlation of CT with pathologic findings. Radiographics 1992; 12:647–657

Mariotta S, Pallone G, Pedicelli G, et al. Spiral CT and endoscopic findings in a case of tracheobronchopathia osteochondroplastica. J Comput Asst Tomogr 1997; 21:418–420

Pickford HA, Swenson SJ, Utz JP. Thoracic cross-sectional imaging of amyloidosis. AJR Am J Roentgenol 1997; 168:351–355

Screaton NJ, Sivasothy P, Flower CD, et al. Tracheal involvement in Wegner's granulomatosis: evaluation using spiral CT. Clin Radiol 1998; 53:809–815

Shin MS, Jackson RM, Ho KJ. Tracheobronchomegaly (Mounier-Kuhn syndrome): CT diagnosis. AJR Am J Roentgenol 1988; 150:777–779

Stark P. Radiology of the trachea. New York, NY: Thieme, 1991

Webb EM, Elicker BM, Webb WR. Using CT to diagnose nonneoplastic tracheal abnormalities: appearance of the tracheal wall. AJR Am J Roentgenol 2000; 174:1315–1321

Atelectasis

Batra P, Brown K, Hayashi K, et al. Rounded atelectasis. J Thorac Imaging 1996; 11:187–197

Blankerbaker DG. The Luftsichel sign. Radiology 1998; 208:319–320

Naidich DP, Ettinger N, Leitman BS, et al. CT of lobar collapse. Semin Roentgenol 1984; 19:222–235

Woodring JH, Reed JC. Types and mechanisms of pulmonary atelectasis. J Thorac Imaging 1996; 11:92–108

Woodring JH, Reed JC. Radiographic manifestations of lobar atelectasis. J Thorac Imaging 1996; 11:109–144

Mediastinum

Brown LR, Aughenbaugh GL. Masses of the anterior mediastinum: CT and MR imaging. AJR Am J Roentgenol 1991; 157:1171–1180

Franquet T, Erasmus JJ, Gimenez A, et al. The reterotracheal space: normal anatomic and pathologic appearances. Radiographics 2002; 22:S231–S246

Jeung M, Gasser B, Gangi A, et al. Imaging of cystic masses of the mediastinum. Radiographics 2002; 22: S79–S93

Nishino M, Ashiku SK, Kocher ON, et al. The thymus: a comprehensive review. Radiographics 2006; 26:335–348

Teece PM, Fishman EK, Kuhlman JE. CT evaluation of the anterior mediastinum. Radiographics 1994; 14:973–990

Whitten CR, Khan S, Munneke GJ, et al. A diagnostic approach to mediastinal abnormalities. Radiographics 2007; 27:657–671

Pulmonary Embolism

Castaner C, Gallardo X, Ballesteros E, et al. CT diagnosis of chronic pulmonary thromboembolism. Radiographics 2009; 29:31–50

Garg K, Sieler H, Welsh CH, et al. Clinical validity of helical CT being interpreted as negative for pulmonary embolism: implications for patient treatment. AJR Am J Roentgenol 1999; 172:1627–1631

Kavanagh EC, O'Hare A, Hargaden G, et al. Risk of pulmonary embolism after negative MDCT pulmonary angiography findings. AJR Am J Roentgenol 2004; 182:499–504

Kuzo RS, Goodman LR. CT evaluation of pulmonary embolism: technique and interpretation. AJR Am J Roentgenol 1997; 169:959–965

Patel S, Kazerooni EA. Helical CT for the evaluation of acute pulmonary embolism. AJR Am J Roentgenol 2005; 185:135–149

Remy-Jardin M, Remy J, Deschildre F, et al. Diagnosis of pulmonary embolism with spiral CT: comparison with pulmonary angiography. Radiology 1996; 200:699–706

Schoepf UJ, Costello P. CT angiography for diagnosis of pulmonary embolism: state of the art. Radiology 2004; 230:329–337

Schoepf UJ, Holzknecht N, Helmberger TK, et al. Subsegmental pulmonary emboli: improved detection with thin collimation multi-detector row spiral CT. Radiology 2002; 222:483–490

Wittram C, Maher MM, Yoo AJ, et al. CT angiography of pulmonary embolism: diagnostic criteria and causes of misdiagnosis. Radiographics 2004; 24:1219–1238

Solitary Pulmonary Nodule

Asad S, Aquino SL, Piyavisetpat N, et al. False-positive FDG positron emission tomography uptake in nonmalignant chest abnormalities. AJR Am J Roentgenol 2004; 182:983–989

Cheran SK, Nielsen ND, Patz EF. False-negative findings for primary lung tumors on FDG positron emission tomography: staging and prognostic implications. AJR Am J Roentgenol 2004; 182:1129–1132

Erasmus JJ, Connolly JE, McAdams HP, et al. Solitary pulmonary nodules: Part I. Morphologic evaluation for differentiation of benign and malignant lesion. Radiographics 2000; 20:43–58

Erasmus JJ, Connolly JE, McAdams HP, et al. Solitary pulmonary nodules: Part II. Evaluation of the indeterminate nodule. Radiographics 2000; 20:59–66

Erasmus JJ, McAdams HP, Patz EF, et al. Thoracic FDG PET: state of the art. Radiographics 1998; 18:5–20

Hiroyuki I, Naoya K, Tetsuro M, et al. Ultrasmall intrapulmonary lymph node: usual high resolution computed tomographic findings with histopathologic correlation. J Comput Assist Tomogr 2007; 31:409–413

Khouri NF, Stitik FP, Erozan YS, et al. Transthoracic needle aspiration biopsy of benign and malignant lesions. AJR Am J Roentgenol 1985; 144:281–288

MacMahon H, Austin JHM, Gamsu G, et al. Guidelines for management of small pulmonary nodules detected on CT scans: a statement from the Fleischner Society. Radiology 2005; 237:395–400

Matsuki M, Satoshi N, Yasumasa K, et al. Thin section CT features of intrapulmonary lymph nodes. J Comput Assist Tomogr 2001; 25:753–756

Ost D, Fein AM, Feinsilver SH. The solitary pulmonary nodule. N Engl J Med 2003; 348:2535–2542

Swensen SJ, Viggiano RW, Midthun DE, et al. Lung nodule enhancement at CT: multi-center study. Radiology 2000; 214:73–80

Tan BB, Flaherty KR, Kazerooni EA, et al. The solitary pulmonary nodule. Chest 2003; 123:89S–96S

Westcott JL. Direct percutaneous needle aspiration of localized pulmonary lesions: results in 422 patients. Radiology 1980; 137:31–35

Diffuse Lung Disease

Austin JH, Muller NL, Friedman PJ, et al. Glossary of terms for CT of the lung: recommendations of the nomenclature committee of the Fleischner Society. Radiology 1988; 167:327–331

Bergin CJ, Muller NL. CT of interstitial lung disease: a diagnostic approach. AJR Am J Roentgenol 1987; 148:8–15

Bergin C, Roggli V, Coblentz C, et al. The secondary pulmonary lobule: normal and abnormal CT appearances. AJR Am J Roentgenol 1988; 15:21–25

Hansell DM, Bankier AA, MacMahon H, et al. Fleischer society: glossary of terms for thoracic imaging. Radiology 2008; 246:697–722

Mueller-Mang C, Grosse C, Schmid K, et al. What every radiologist should know about idiopathic interstitial pneumonias. Radiographics 2007; 27:595–615

Raoof S, Amchentsev A, Vlahos I, et al. Pictorial essay: multidetector disease; a high resolution CT scan diagnostic algorithm. Chest 2006; 129:805–815

Swenson SJ, Aughenbaugh GL, Myers JL. Diffuse lung disease: diagnostic accuracy of CT in patients undergoing surgical biopsy of the lung. Radiology 1997; 205:229–234

Wittram C, Mark EJ, McLoud TC. CT-Histologic correlation of the ATS/ERS 2002 classification of idiopathic interstitial pneumonias. Radiographics 2003; 23:1057–1071

Notes

Ethics in Pulmonary and Critical Care Medicine

Mark J. Rosen, MD, FCCP

Objectives:

- Discuss the basic principles of bioethics as they apply to the practice of medicine (the Georgetown mantra)
- Summarize the common ethical issues that apply to all physicians
- Focus on issues that are most pertinent to pulmonary and critical care physicians, especially regarding ethical issues at the end of life

Key words: autonomy; end-of-life care; ethics; futility; preferences

---

When caring for patients, decisions about what is a "right" or "wrong" course of action are not always based on randomized clinical trials or even science. The complex and at times competing interests of patients, families, the care setting, the payor, society, the law, and physicians often complicate patient care, and these issues cannot be resolved by the use of scientific methods. Pulmonary and critical care physicians are on the front lines of these dilemmas, but few have formal training in bioethics, communication, conflict resolution, and related disciplines. Therefore, we often improvise based on past experience or a "see one, do one" training pathway. At the same time, physicians as a group (like the rest of humanity), including pulmonary and critical care physicians, may not want to confront difficult problems and choices.

This reticence was demonstrated by the landmark Study to Understand Prognosis and Preferences for Outcomes and Risks of Treatments, in which the authors attempted to improve end-of-life decision making and to reduce the frequency of prolonged and potentially unwanted and painful care at the end of life. Despite interventions that included providing physicians with prediction models and decision-making tools, together with timely reports by trained nurses of patient and surrogate preferences, there was no improvement in physician communication, knowledge of patients' preferences not to be resuscitated, control of pain, or duration of ICU stay and mechanical ventilation. This section will review the general principles of bioethics as they apply to patient care and will focus on the issues most pertinent to pulmonary and critical care physicians.

Basic Principles

Most medical ethics discussions can be framed in terms of the following four principles, which often are referred to as the *Georgetown mantra*. Some ethicists criticize the wide application of these principles as being simplistic and sometimes irrelevant, but their simplicity and clarity have stood the test of decades of use by frontline clinicians who lack formal training. The four principles are as follows:

- Autonomy: The patient has the right to accept or refuse every treatment;
- Beneficence: The clinician should act in the best interest of the patient;
- Nonmaleficence: "First, do no harm"; and
- Justice: The distribution of limited resources must be fair.

Many (or most) bedside ethical dilemmas arise when two or more of these values are in conflict. However, other conflicts are believed to arise from ethical concerns as a consequence of a lack of communication among patients, families, and the health-care team. With open communication (which may require the presence of a mediator when communications have broken down), the ethical issues often disappear.

In addition, two other core values are also commonly applied to the analysis of ethical issues, as follows:

- Dignity: Both the patient and the caregiver have a right to dignity; and
- Truthfulness and honesty: Clinicians should tell the truth.

Some criticize the term *medical ethics* as having a physician focus and prefer to use the term *health-care ethics* to make it more comprehensive. That physician focus is obvious in the American Medical Association preamble to their "Principles of Medical Ethics" (Table 1). Despite the focus on physicians, these principles are generally accepted.

Autonomy

The patient's right to make an informed and uncoerced decision regarding treatment generally overrides the other values, but autonomy has its limits. First, a decision must be legal; a request for euthanasia must be denied, even if it comes from an informed patient because it is against the law. Second, the patient must be competent, which is defined here as having the capacity to make decisions about the care (see the section "Informed Consent"). If patients with severe illness do not have this capacity, then we depend on surrogate decision makers. Autonomy depends on the proper process of informed consent, where the risks, benefits, and alternatives are explained honestly.

Beneficence and Nonmaleficence

A physician is not obligated to provide care that would not benefit the patient. However, conflicts arise when the patient or surrogate perceives of a benefit that is different from the clinician's view of their duty to beneficence and nonmaleficence. The obvious example is the common conflict between a family who wants "everything" despite all evidence that "everything" will not be effective and the clinician's view that such care will not lead to a benefit, may cause harm, and wastes resources. In most cases, patient autonomy dictates that the benefit must be judged by the patient's and surrogate's preferences, not by those of the team. Frustrating as this often is, it also provides a check against other pressures that may influence care (*eg*, need for an ICU bed or a perceived waste of money).

Justice

Although justice is one of the four basic tents of the Georgetown mantra, this should enter bedside decision making rarely, if ever, at least in the United States. All physicians are obligated to use resources in an appropriate and efficient manner, but the primary role of the physician is as a patient advocate. Therefore, we are not charged with rationing health-care resources at the bedside. Rather, this is a policy issue. The perennial exercise of "who gets the last bed in the medical ICU?" followed by a list of candidates often is amusing but usually specious because there are probably other ICU beds in the institution that could receive a critically ill patient temporarily. Unless there is a shortage of beds, physicians must allocate ICUs

Table 1. *The American Medical Association Principles of Medical Ethics**

1. A physician shall be dedicated to providing competent medical care, with compassion and respect for human dignity and rights.
2. A physician shall uphold the standards of professionalism, be honest in all professional interactions, and strive to report physicians deficient in character or competence, or engaging in fraud or deception, to appropriate entities.
3. A physician shall respect the law and also recognize a responsibility to seek changes in those requirements that are contrary to the best interests of the patient.
4. A physician shall respect the rights of patients, colleagues, and other health professionals and shall safeguard patient confidences and privacy within the constraints of the law.
5. A physician shall continue to study, apply, and advance scientific knowledge; maintain a commitment to medical education; make relevant information available to patients, colleagues, and the public; obtain consultation; and use the talents of other health professionals when indicated.
6. A physician shall, in the provision of appropriate patient care, except in emergencies, be free to choose whom to serve, with whom to associate, and the environment in which to provide medical care.
7. A physician shall recognize a responsibility to participate in activities contributing to the improvement of the community and the betterment of public health.
8. A physician shall, while caring for a patient, regard responsibility to the patient as paramount.
9. A physician shall support access to medical care for all people. Adopted by the AMA's House of Delegates June 17, 2001.

*Available at www.ama-assn.org/ama/pub/physician-resources/medical-ethics/code-medical-ethics/principles-medical-ethics.shtml. Accessed June 22, 2009.

beds, dialysis slots, bags of packed RBCs, and any other unit of resource fairly to all who would qualify to receive it. At the same time, we should advocate vigorously for rational health policies that would provide proper care to those who need it while educating the public about the limits of what such care can provide.

Ethical Decision Making

Ideally, medical decisions should be based on empiric information like the results of randomized trials. However, ethical dilemmas usually involve subjective considerations, including the preferences of patients, their surrogates, and clinicians, which in turn are often influenced by their experiences. These considerations defy a standard "evidence-based" approach to decision making. There is an emerging and contentious literature on "evidence-based ethics" that attempts to apply principles of evidence-based medicine to ethical dilemmas in clinical medicine.

Regardless of the outcome of this controversy, some basic principles apply. One potentially useful method includes first framing the ethical dilemma in the dimensions of autonomy, beneficence, nonmaleficence, and justice. The next step would be to evaluate potential decisions in terms of patient preferences, the medical benefits and harms, and how they impact on access to care and societal costs.

Specific Issues

Informed Consent

Physicians are required to obtain informed consent from patients before initiating treatment, and informed consent is valid only when a patient is competent to make voluntary choices among treatment options. This consent requires that the patient is capable of understanding the relevant information and the consequences of treatment options, can rationally process this information, and can communicate a choice.

Competent patients may refuse any treatment, even if that decision is contrary to the physician's recommendation. Studies of competency in patients with unstable angina, diabetes mellitus, and HIV infection failed to show an increased likelihood of incapacity to make medical decisions. However, impairment in the capacity for making medical decisions was found in outpatients with cancer, the elderly, and patients with dementia. Even patients with psychiatric illnesses are not necessarily incompetent to make treatment decisions; rather, they should be assessed by use of the same criteria as used for other patients.

Often, the great majority of patients in an ICU are deemed to lack the capacity to make decisions; therefore, the determination of capacity is an important part of ICU management. Obviously, critically ill patients who are deeply sedated or obviously delirious do not have decisional capacity, and their treating clinicians can determine incapacity. Other patients may lack capacity because they have cognitive impairments caused by preexisting disease, acute illness, or the effects of analgesics. Standardized assessment tools for these conditions may be helpful in assessing delirium, which is usually underestimated in hospitalized patients. Psychiatric consultation is not necessary to determine whether a patient is incompetent; rather, consultations should be reserved for cases in which the clinician believes that the patient is making an irrational decision, when there is associated mental illness, or in other situations that pose uncertainty.

Problems often arise in patients who lack the capacity to make decisions and also lack a surrogate. In most situations, physicians use the principle of "substituted judgment" and proceed with a course that most patients with capacity would choose. Often, hospitals have policies that require consultation and approval by an independent practitioner or an ethics committee. Withdrawing life support in a patient without capacity and with no surrogate presents a special issue. In one study surveying seven medical centers, 5.5% of all deaths occurred among patients in this category; in most cases, decisions were made by physicians with no institutional or judicial review, contrary to their institution's policies.

Informed consent for research also presents unique issues, especially when it involves subjects who are critically ill and incapable of providing consent because of their illness or medications that impair cognition. US Federal regulations permit consent by the subject's "legally authorized representative," which is defined as "an individual or judicial or other body authorized under applicable law to consent on behalf of a prospective subject to the subject's participation in the procedure(s) involved in the research." This requirement may be waived if an institutional review board determines that the research poses minimal risk, defined in U.S. Federal guidelines as "the probability and magnitude of harm or discomfort anticipated in the research are not greater in and of themselves than those ordinarily encountered in daily life or during the performance of routine physical or psychological examinations or tests." However, state laws vary widely in permitting surrogates to consent for participation in clinical research, and critical care research is generally not conducted in some states unless there is a court-appointed guardian. Others permit "emergency research" in situations such as after cardiopulmonary resuscitation.

Withdrawal of Life Support

It is widely accepted in modern societies that patients and their surrogates have the authority to decline or withdraw any medical intervention, as long as the decision maker is intellectually and psychologically competent to make such a decision. Withdrawing ventilatory support is generally deemed the moral and ethical equivalent of withholding it, but many families and physicians cannot help but think and act otherwise. Although it is ethically and legally prohibited to withdraw care with the specific intent of hastening death, the principle of "double effect" supports the use of medications intended to prevent or relieve suffering even if it incidentally hastens death.

The withdrawal of mechanical ventilatory support may be undertaken in most locations if there is an oral advance directive by the patient or with the agreement of the clinical team and family; the requirement for a written advance directive is unusual. The process should begin only after there is a consensus of both the medical team and the patient and family that this treatment is both unwanted and not likely to lead to a desired patient outcome. When the decision to limit or withdraw treatment is reached, the clinician is still responsible for treating the patient throughout the dying process and being attentive to the needs of the patient, family, and the clinical team. The ICU team needs to attend the family almost as much as the patient because they are often under great emotional stress. This process should be planned and communicated to the team and the family, preferably with an organized protocol including the administration of analgesics and sedatives titrated to maintain the comfort of the patient.

Whether to simply extubate the patient after administering and maintaining sedatives (called *terminal extubation*) or to gradually reduce support (*ie*, respiratory rate and fraction of inspired oxygen) with the endotracheal tube in place (called *terminal wean*) is a topic of ongoing controversy. Prompt extubation has the advantages of not prolonging the dying process, and the goals of care are clear and morally transparent. Gradual withdrawal of support with the endotracheal tube in place reduces the likelihood that visible distress will develop in patients from stridor and oral secretions, often promoting their own comfort and that of their family by reducing anxiety. However, this approach may prolong the dying process, and some family members may misinterpret this process as an attempt to extubate the patient successfully. No randomized trials have compared these two approaches from a patient-centered or family-centered perspective, and there is no consensus among clinicians and ethicists on which method is preferable. Rather, decisions on how to extubate patients who are expected to die depend on the preferences of the ICU team in consultation with the family.

Neuromuscular blocking agents have no sedative or analgesic properties, would mask signs of discomfort after the withdrawal of ventilatory support, and should almost always be discontinued before withdrawing ventilatory support. In addition, some patients survive to be discharged from the hospital despite predictions that the withdrawal of support will lead to death; this would be impossible in the presence of neuromuscular blockade. Unusual situations in which continuing therapy with these agents are warranted during the withdrawal of mechanical ventilator support would include patients who are certain not to survive more than a short interval after the withdrawal of support even without this treatment, or if the benefits of waiting for the return of neuromuscular function do not outweigh the burdens.

Regardless of the process of extubation, there is no evidence that increasing the dose of benzodiazepines and opiates before extubation with the goal of maintaining patient comfort is associated with a shorter time to death after extubation. Indeed, one study showed no relationship between narcotic dose and the time to death, and a direct relationship between the dose of benzodiazepines and the time to death after extubation. Therefore, a judicious use of sedation and analgesics does not appear to hasten death in these patients and should be part of any standard protocol.

Brain Death

It is now almost universally accepted that a person is considered to be dead when the whole brain (including the brainstem) is dead; therefore, establishing a precise diagnosis of brain death is often crucial in decisions about terminating life support and organ donation. Although the criteria for diagnosing brain death have evolved, the current guidelines and the laws in most countries require a detailed clinical assessment that includes the presence of coma and the absence of brainstem reflexes and apnea over the course of two successive examinations. These criteria must also be fulfilled in the absence of a complicating condition that may render clinical examination unreliable, including severe hypothermia, hypotension, severe metabolic disturbances, drug intoxication, and the use of neuromuscular blocking agents. A disorder that would preclude performing an apnea test (*eg*, high cervical cord injury, in which a patient may be incapable of breathing spontaneously) would also make clinical assessment impossible. In these cases, confirmatory tests of the cessation of brain function are needed.

Although EEG is frequently used because it can be performed at the bedside, the interpretation of the findings is subject to interobserver variability, as well as the possibility of false-positive findings (*eg*, as a result of the use of barbiturates or anesthetics, or undetectable subcortical neuronal activity) and false-negative results (*eg*, as a result of electrical artifacts in an ICU environment or agonal electrical activity). Tests of brain flow are more reliable for confirming the diagnosis. Cerebral angiography with findings that show a cessation of blood flow to the brain is considered to be the "gold standard," and technetium nuclear imaging is also reliable. CT scanning and magnetic resonance angiography are probably as accurate but are less well validated. Transcranial Doppler examinations of cerebral blood flow are safe, noninvasive, and can be performed at the bedside, although performing them requires a high level of skill. The determination of a complete absence of flow using this examination is unreliable in the diagnosis of brain death because false-positive results may occur in 10 to 15% of cases as the result of technical factors, which are often related to poor image acquisition.

Annotated Bibliography

General and Basic Topics

Aulisio MP, Arnold RM, Youngner SJ. Health care ethics consultation: nature, goals, and competencies—a position paper from the Society for Health and Human Values-Society for Bioethics Consultation Task Force on Standards for Bioethics Consultation. Ann Intern Med 2000; 133:59–69

Summary of a task force report delineating the role of ethics committees and consultative services, with recommendations on policies, competencies, and processes.

Beauchamp T, Childress J. Principles of biomedical ethics. Oxford, UK: Oxford University Press, 2001

Late edition of an influential textbook from the authors of the Georgetown mantra.

Snyder L, Leffler C, Ethics and Human Rights Committee, American College of Physicians. Ethics manual, fifth edition. Ann Intern Med 2005; 142:560–582

Concise overview of issues related to medicine, law, and social values that covers issues related to patient care, the practice of medicine, and the impact of economics and the government.

Strech D. Evidence-based ethics: what it should be and what it shouldn't. BMC Med Ethics 2008; 9:16

Discussion of the "evidence-based ethics," a new concept that attempts to synthesize evidence-based medicine principles with ethical decision making.

SUPPORT Principal Investigators. A controlled trial to improve care for seriously ill hospitalized patients: the Study to Understand Prognosis and Preferences for Outcomes and Risks of Treatments (SUPPORT). JAMA 1995; 274:1591–1598

Two-year study that shows that physicians in critical care units are not likely to know patient preferences about end-of-life care, nor are they likely to change their practice even with intensive intervention.

Informed Consent and Competence

Applebaum PS. Assessment of patients' competence to consent to treatment. N Engl J Med 2007; 357:1834–1840

Carrese JA. Refusal of care: patients' well-being and physicians' ethical obligations; "but doctor, I want to go home." JAMA 2006; 296:691–695

Detailed case-based discussion, with some useful recommendations.

Cohen LM, McCue JD, Green GM. Do clinical and formal assessments of the capacity of patients in the intensive care unit to make decisions agree? Arch Intern Med 1993; 153:2481–2485

Issues and methods to determine competence to make medical decisions.

Fan E, Shahid S, Kondreddi VP, et al. Informed consent in the critically ill: a two-step approach incorporating delirium screening. Crit Care Med 2008; 36:94–99

Luce JM. Informed consent for clinical research involving patients with chest disease in the United States. Chest 2009; 135:1061–1068

This is a thorough and thoughtful review of laws and issues surrounding performing clinical research, especially in potential subjects who lack decision-making capacity.

White DB, Curtis JR, Wolf LE, et al. Life support for patients without a surrogate decision maker: who decides? Ann Intern Med 2007; 147:34–40

In most cases of withdrawal of life support in patients without capacity and without a surrogate, physicians made the decision despite institutional policies that call for outside review.

Withdrawing Life Support

Campbell ML, Bizek K, Thill M. Patient responses during rapid terminal weaning from mechanical ventilation: a prospective study. Crit Care Med 1999; 27:73–77

Chan JD, Treece PD, Engelberg RA, et al. Narcotic and benzodiazepine use after withdrawal of life support: association with time to death? Chest 2004; 126:286–293

These two studies deal with the processes of withdrawing mechanical ventilatory support, indicating that the appropriate use of sedatives and narcotics is associated with minimal patient discomfort and does not hasten the time to death after extubation.

Rubenfeld GC. Principles and practice of withdrawing life-sustaining treatments. Crit Care Clin 2004; 20:435–451

Truog RS, Cist AF, Brackett SE, et al. Recommendations for end-of-life care in the intensive care unit: the Ethics Committee of the Society of Critical Care Medicine. Crit Care Med 2001; 29:2332–2348

These articles review ethical and practical aspects of withdrawing life-sustaining treatments.

Brain Death

Wijdicks EFM. Current concepts: the diagnosis of brain death. N Engl J Med 2001; 344:1215–1221

Young GB, Shemie SD, Doig CJ, et al. Brief review: the role of ancillary tests in the neurological determination of death. Can J Anesth 2006; 53:620–627

Chronic Obstructive Pulmonary Disease

Sidney S. Braman, MD, FCCP

Objectives:

- Review the definition of COPD that describes this disease as an airway and systemic inflammatory condition
- Explore the impact of COPD, including rates of morbidity and mortality
- Review the risk factors for COPD
- Explore the natural history of COPD from its earlier asymptomatic stages to the late stages associated with morbidity and mortality
- Explore the current understanding of the pathophysiology of COPD: the pathologic consequences of airway inflammation and parenchymal lung destruction.
- Explore the systemic consequences of the disease and the comorbidities associated with COPD
- Review the current state of pharmacologic and non-pharmacologic therapy for COPD, including preventive measures such as smoking cessation.

Key words: chronic bronchitis; COPD; emphysema; natural history; risk factors; treatment

Definition and Epidemiology

Internationally, the accepted definition of COPD is as a disease state characterized by chronic airflow limitation attributable to chronic bronchitis and emphysema. Chronic bronchitis has been defined in clinical terms: the presence of chronic productive cough for at least three consecutive months in two consecutive years. Other causes of chronic productive cough must been ruled out. Emphysema, on the other hand, has been defined by its pathologic description: an abnormal enlargement of the air spaces distal to the terminal bronchioles accompanied by destruction of their walls and without obvious fibrosis. Contrary to this traditional view, recent data have shown that this destructive process is accompanied by a net increase in the amount of collagen, suggesting there is indeed active fibrosis associated with the breakdown of the elastic framework of the lung.

During the past decade, as it became recognized that the disease was having a major worldwide impact, there has been increasing interest in the pathogenesis and management of COPD. It has been calculated that COPD ranks as the twelfth-largest disease burden in the world, with projections that it will rank as the fifth by the year 2020. In the United States, estimates from national interviews taken by the National Center for Health Statistics showed that >16 million people are afflicted with COPD; about 14 million are thought to have chronic bronchitis, whereas 2 million have emphysema. It is likely that these statistics underestimate the prevalence of COPD by as much as 50% because many patients underreport their symptoms and remain undiagnosed.

In the National Health and Nutrition Examination Survey (NHANES) III the prevalence of COPD in the United States was found to be 23.6 million adults (13.9% of the adult population). These statistics were derived using telephone surveys and physical examinations as well as pulmonary function testing of randomly selected subjects. The average number of days of restricted activities reported by patients with COPD is very high, ranking this condition among the highest chronic conditions for this measure of morbidity in the nation. In 1996, COPD was listed as the eighth-leading cause of disability-adjusted life-years in men and the seventh-leading cause of disability-adjusted life-years among women.

COPD is a leading cause of hospitalizations in the United States. In 1998, nearly 2% of all hospitalizations were attributed to COPD, and 7% of patients had COPD as a contributing cause of hospitalization. From 1995 to 2000, the trend in COPD hospitalization rates was about the same for men and women. However, the rates were slightly greater among black than white patients during this same period. In 2000, the COPD hospitalization rates were 31.5 and 36.0 per 10,000 persons for white and black subjects, respectively. More striking are COPD statistics regarding the elderly. Nearly 20% of all hospitalizations in patients >65 years had COPD as a primary or contributing cause.

Perhaps even more striking and ominous are the magnitude and trend of the mortality rates for COPD. During the past few decades, the mortality rates associated with other common diseases such as cardiovascular disease and stroke were decreasing. During the same time period, the mortality rate for COPD was increasing at an alarming rate. For example, the US death rate for COPD rose almost 33% during the years 1979 to 1991, resulting in COPD becoming the fourth-leading cause of death in this country. Although the death rate for men has reached a plateau in recent years, among women it has continued to increase. In 1998, 54,615 men and 51,377 women died from COPD. From 1995 to 1998, the death rate for COPD increased 9% for US women. In the year 2000, for the first time more women died from COPD than men.

The cost of COPD has also increased dramatically. In 2002, it was estimated to be $32.1 billion. Direct medical services accounted for $18.0 billion, and the indirect cost of morbidity and premature mortality was $14.1 billion. Medicare expenses for COPD beneficiaries were nearly 2.5 times that of the expenditures for all other patients. The cost per patient in other countries around the world varies depending on how health-care is provided and paid. There is a striking direct relationship between the severity of COPD and the cost of care.

As a result of the impact of COPD on morbidity, mortality, and health-care utilization and finances, a number of thoracic and respiratory disease societies offered consensus statements regarding the assessment and management of COPD. The dawn of the twenty-first century brings another guideline, the Global Initiative on Chronic Obstructive Lung Disease (GOLD) initiative sponsored by the World Health Organization and the National Heart, Lung, and Blood Institute (NHLBI). GOLD presents an evidenced-based approach that can be followed by all health-care systems throughout the world.

The term COPD defined by GOLD differs from previous consensus statements. It does not incorporate the terms chronic bronchitis and emphysema into the definition. Instead, it defines COPD as a disease state characterized by airflow obstruction that is no longer fully reversible and is usually progressive. The disease is caused by the interaction of noxious inhaled agents such as cigarette smoke, industrial, and other environmental pollutants and host factors (genetic, respiratory infections, etc) that result in chronic inflammation in the walls and lumen of the airways. The pathology of COPD, as well as the symptoms, the pulmonary function abnormalities, and complications all can be explained on the basis of the underlying inflammation.

In the 2006 GOLD definition of COPD, the phrase "preventable and treatable" was added, similar to recent American Thoracic Society/European Respiratory Society (ATS/ERS) recommendations. This was done to encourage a positive outlook for patients and the healthcare community toward COPD and to stimulate effective management programs to treat those with the disease.

Although the GOLD document does not specifically include chronic bronchitis and emphysema in the definition of COPD, it is clear that they are considered the predominant causes of COPD. In the past, asthma was also included under the umbrella term COPD. As asthma became recognized as an inflammatory disease with a different cellular and inflammatory mediator profile compared with smoking-induced chronic bronchitis and emphysema, it was no longer considered under the term COPD. This was also justified by the fact that asthma is thought to be distinct: airflow obstruction is predominantly reversible, and the airways of asthmatic subjects are markedly hyperresponsive to a variety of specific (aeroallergens) and nonspecific (methacholine, histamine, cold air) inhaled substances. Although it is still clinically useful to distinguish asthma from COPD (chronic bronchitis and emphysema), it is important to recognize three problems with this nosology:

- Remission rates for adults with asthma are much less than those observed in children, and if remission does occur, the probability of relapse increases with increasing age. As a result, most asthmatics, even those who have never smoked, who are at the age when COPD is most often recognized (>60 years), have evidence of poorly reversible airflow obstruction on pulmonary function testing. This statement is supported by data from longitudinal studies that the average FEV_1 in asthmatics decrease over a period of years. Despite these findings, there are many patients who show no correlation between their FEV_1 and the duration of their disease.

- Bronchial hyperresponsiveness, the exaggerated bronchoconstrictive response to nonspecific agonists such as methacholine, is a constant feature in asthmatics and is so important to its pathogenesis it has been incorporated into the definition of asthma. However, increased responsiveness to constrictors such as methacholine and histamine (but not indirect bronchoconstrictors such as cold air and bradykinin) is found in most middle-aged smokers with COPD and has even been shown to be a strong predictor of progression of airway obstruction in those who continue to smoke. In asthma, bronchial hyperresponsiveness is not related to baseline airway caliber, whereas in COPD the increased responsiveness to bronchoconstrictors can be explained entirely by the geometric effect of fixed airway narrowing.
- Unfortunately, many adult patients with asthma are current or former smokers. It is likely that such patients have more than one pathologic process with several pathways of inflammation. Although studies on the effects of smoking on the rate of decrease of FEV_1 in asthma have given conflicting results, most smoking asthmatics will present with some degree of fixed airflow obstruction. This finding has raised a complexity of semantic issues that have not been solved. One attempt has been to combine two of the major pathologic processes and describe such patients using the term *asthmatic bronchitis*, but this definition does not have widespread acceptance.

Risk Factors for COPD

The major risk factors for the development of COPD are listed in Table 1. All of these factors have one thing in common: they are associated with an accelerated decrease in FEV_1 over time. Cigarette smoking leads the list and in most countries is the responsible agent in at least 85 to 90% of cases. Because the basic cellular and molecular mechanisms of disease are still poorly understood, the reasons why only certain individuals with a positive exposure history become affected are not known. For example, it is common to see pulmonary function abnormalities reflecting obstruction

Table 1. *Risk Factors for COPD*

Risk	Comment
External factors	
Cigarette smoking: the most important risk factor in 85 to 90% of cases; 15 to 20% of one pack per-day smokers and 25% of two pack per-day smokers develop COPD	
Pipe and cigars	High risk but lower than cigarette smokers
Passive smoking	Children of smoking parents have more respiratory symptoms and lower airway function; unknown significance for adult COPD
Occupational exposure: risk in certain professions such as coal miners, gold miners, grain handlers, cement and cotton workers; interacts with smoking	
Environmental pollution: indoor use of biomass fuels for cooking and heating in underdeveloped countries; unknown particulate matter from urban pollution	
Host factors	
Genetic factor	AAT deficiency, >90% caused by homozygous ZZ phenotype. Gender: men are more at risk than women
Socioeconomic	More common with low socioeconomic status
Bronchial hyperresponsiveness	A strong predictor of progressive airway obstruction in smokers
Atopy and asthma	Many adult nonsmoking asthmatics develop fixed airway obstruction; atopy alone not a factor
Childhood illnesses	Low birth weight, respiratory infections, and symptomatic childhood asthma
Dietary influences	Vitamin C and E (tocopherol) deficiencies

in the small airways and nonuniform distribution of ventilation in young adults who smoke. These changes are not predictive, because only 15 to 20% of these heavy smokers will develop an accelerated decrease of their FEV_1 over time and clinically evident COPD. The differences in susceptibility to tobacco smoke injury are likely to be related to genetic factors.

It has been more difficult to demonstrate the association between COPD and occupational exposures than with cigarette smoking. There have been several reasons offered but perhaps the most compelling is that many exposed workers are also cigarette smokers or have been exposed to secondhand smoke. An increasing body of literature is providing longitudinal evidence that coal workers, hard rock miners, tunnel workers, concrete manufacturing workers, and other non-mining industrial workers (exposures to dusts, gases and/or fumes) have an excess annual loss of FEV_1 of 8 mL/yr compared with 9 to 11 mL/yr attributable to smoking. Some workers have been shown to have acute airflow obstruction when exposed to organic and inorganic dusts, isocyanates, and irritant gases. Such events appear to predict later findings of chronic, fixed obstructive lung disease. Recent estimates by the ATS suggest that for COPD, a population-attributable risk of approximately 15 to 20% is caused by occupational exposures.

Genetic Risk Factors for COPD

α_1-Antitrypsin Deficiency: One genetic abnormality that has been known and well studied is α_1-antitrypsin (AAT) deficiency. Also called *α_1 antiprotease deficiency*, this disorder accounts for <1% of COPD in the United States. AAT is a serum protein made in the liver that is capable of inhibiting the activity of specific proteolytic enzymes such as trypsin, chymotrypsin, and neutrophil elastase. If not inactivated by AAT, neutrophil elastase destroys lung connective tissue, particularly elastin, which leads to the development of emphysema.

AAT is coded for by a single gene on chromosome 14. The serum protease inhibitor phenotype (Pi type) is determined by the independent expression of two independent alleles. More than 90% of severely deficient patients are homozygous for the Z allele. Such patients are designated PiZZ and have a reduced serum AAT level to approximately 20% of the normal level. Other rarely observed phenotypes associated with very low levels of AAT are Pi SZ, Pi null-null, and Pi null-Z. The normal M allele phenotype is designated Pi MM. Individuals with this phenotype have AAT levels of 150 to 350 mg/dL reported from most commercial laboratories. Often the true laboratory standard values are reported. Normal levels are 20 to 48 μmol/L.

Most patients homozygous with the Z allele are of northern European descent. Asian and African Americans are rarely affected. Cigarette smoking is the most important risk factor for in the development of COPD in patients with AAT deficiency. Symptoms begin early in adult life (usually by age 40), and COPD leads to an early death. However, it is rare that PiZZ lifetime nonsmokers ever develop COPD. Most never develop any pulmonary symptoms, have a normal life expectancy, and remain undetected unless they are found through family screening. Heterozygotes that are Pi MZ have intermediate levels of [propto]-1 antitrypsin deficiency. Epidemiologic evidence suggests that they are not at increased risk for developing COPD when compared with Pi MM phenotypes. It is important to screen patients for AAT deficiency (Table 2) for family counseling and because multivariate analyses from the National Institutes of Health Registry suggest that severely deficient patients who receive augmentation therapy (IV infusions of human AAT) had decreased rates of mortality. In addition, those who were treated who had an FEV_1 percentage

Table 2. *Diagnosis of AAT Deficiency*

Features that prompt suspicion for screening

1. Onset of COPD in patients <50 years
2. COPD without a smoking history or other risk factor
3. Family history of AAT deficiency
4. Family history of COPD, bronchiectasis, panniculitis
5. Young adult asthmatic unresponsive to therapy
6. Patient with predominant lower-lobe emphysema
7. Necrotizing panniculitis
8. C-ANCA vasculitis
9. Unexplained liver disease

Laboratory testing for diagnosis

1. Protein electrophoresis reveals absence of α_1 peak
2. Serum AAT levels 2.5 to 7 μmol/L (normal 20 to 48 μmol/L)
3. Phenotyping by isoelectric focus; >90% PiZZ

predicted of 35 to 49% had a slowing in their decline in lung function compared with an untreated group. In addition to developing advanced emphysema, hepatitis and cirrhosis, AAT deficiency patients are at a 70 to 100% increased risk of developing lung cancer.

Other Genetic Factors: It is likely that a number of other genetically determined abnormal protective mechanisms against protease, oxidant, and toxic peptide injury are important in the pathogenesis of COPD. Multiple association studies have been performed for COPD using case-control and population- and family-based studies. Unfortunately, these studies have often yielded inconsistent results. Candidate genes that have been studied in COPD are those regulating proteases and antiproteases. For example, polymorphisms of the [propto]-1 antitrypsin gene not associated with deficiency of the protein predispose to the development of COPD. These abnormalities are located at the *Taq*I and *Hind*III sites of the [propto]-1 antitrypsin gene. There is speculation that abnormalities at these sites of the gene may not be normally responsive to inflammatory cytokines, which may lead to inappropriate synthesis and, hence, a relative deficiency of the protein during times of stress.

Antioxidant genes have also been of interest. Polymorphisms in the gene that controls glutathione S-transferases have also recently been linked to the development of COPD. This family of metabolic enzymes may play an important part in cellular defense by detoxifying various substances in tobacco smoke. There is recent evidence that genetic polymorphisms of cytochrome p450 and microsomal epoxide hydrolase may also be associated with the development of COPD, and also variants in the gene *ADAM33* have been significantly associated with COPD. Finally, genes regulating mucociliary clearance (*eg*, cystic fibrosis transmembrane regulator and mucins) and genes that regulate inflammatory mediators (tumor necrosis factor [TNF]-[propto], vitamin D-binding protein, and transforming growth factor-β1) have been of interest.

Natural History of COPD

The natural history of COPD includes a prolonged preclinical period of approximately 20 to 40 years. During this asymptomatic period, there is deterioration of lung function in marked excess of the normal age-related decline. This was first shown in population studies on London working men and reported in the 1970s. It was discovered that the FEV_1 decreases continuously and evenly during an individual's life. Nonsmokers without respiratory disease can expect to lose 25 to 30 mL/yr of lung function after age 35. The rate of decrease appears to accelerate slightly with aging, but sudden large irreversible decreases are very rare. Although nonsmokers lose FEV_1 slowly, they never develop significant airflow obstruction; this is also true of most smokers.

Susceptible smokers, on the other hand, develop varying degrees of airflow obstruction, as they often demonstrate a decrease in lung function of 60 mL/yr and more. This ultimately causes exertional dyspnea when the FEV_1 is 40 to 59% of its predicted value and becomes disabling when the FEV_1 decreases by approximately 70%. Such an inexorable decrease may lead to fatality; when the FEV_1 decrease to <1 L, the 5-year mortality is approximately 50%. Smoking cessation in the susceptible smoker will not result in recovery of lost FEV_1 but will slow the rate of decrease to normal (Fig 1). Smoking cessation in the patient with early changes of COPD at age 45 can make the difference between a normal life span and premature death.

A prospective multicenter longitudinal study of the effects of smoking cessation in patients identified with mild-to-moderate airflow obstruction has been conducted in this country and supported by the NHLBI. This Lung Health Study showed

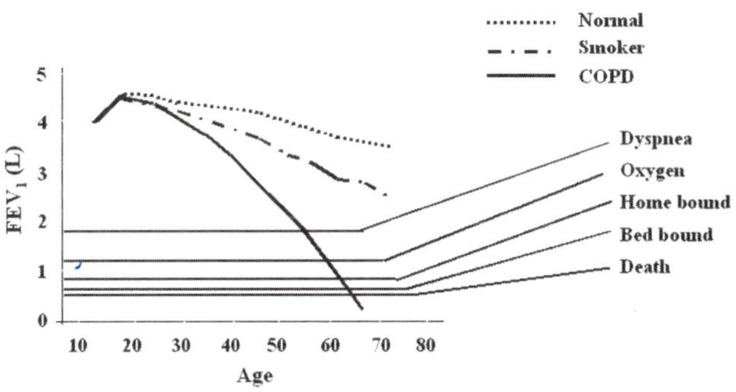

Figure 1. Natural history of COPD. Accelerated decline in lung function (FEV_1) in smoker and "susceptible" smoker in whom the progressive disability of COPD develops.

that smokers who stopped smoking with the help of an aggressive smoking-intervention program significantly reduced the decrease in their FEV_1 during a 5-year study period when compared with those who continued to smoke. The inhaled bronchodilator ipratropium did not slow the decline of lung function when given over the same time period.

The slowly progressive course of COPD is often interrupted by a sudden change in symptoms and lung function. These acute respiratory illnesses or exacerbations are usually caused by viral or bacterial infections and are heralded by an increase in symptoms. Patients with milder stages of COPD will often develop one to two exacerbations per year; those with more severe disease are likely to have many more. The exacerbations cause a decrease in lung function for up to 90 days. There is evidence that more frequent exacerbations play a causal role in accelerating the development of chronic airflow obstruction.

Pathology and Pathophysiology

The pathologic changes in COPD are found in the large and small (<2 mm) airways and in the lung parenchyma (Fig 2). In advanced stages, there are also changes in the pulmonary circulation, the heart, and the respiratory muscles. Alveolar hypoxia causes medial hypertrophy of vascular smooth muscle with extension of the muscularis layer into distal vessels that do not ordinarily contain smooth muscle. Intimal hyperplasia also occurs in advanced stages. These latter changes are associated with the development of pulmonary hypertension and its consequences: right ventricular hypertrophy and dilation. Loss of vascular bed also occurs with emphysema in association with the destructive alveolar processes. In some patients with advanced COPD, there is atrophy of diaphragmatic muscle, loss of skeletal muscle, and wasting of limb muscles.

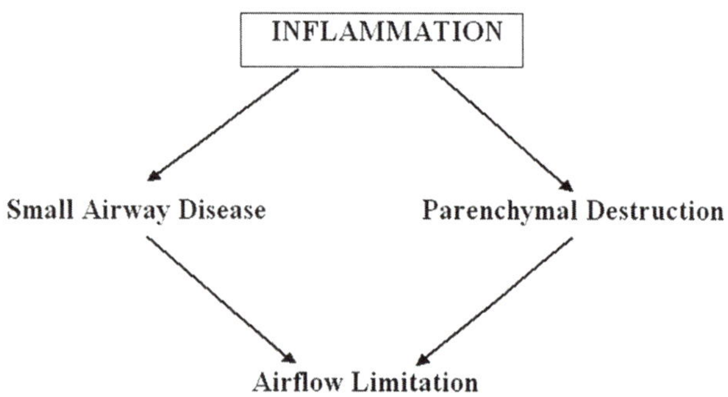

NIH/NHLBI. Global Initiative for Chronic Obstructive Lung Disease. NHLBI/WHO Workshop Report 2001.

Figure 2. Mechanisms underlying airflow limitation in COPD. Inflammation caused by cigarette smoke and other irritants causes inflammation in the large and mainly small airways (chronic bronchitis) and parenchymal destruction (emphysema).

Changes in the Airways of Smokers

Early structural changes have been described in otherwise-healthy smokers even as young as 20 to 30 years of age. These changes are attributed to the toxic effects of cigarette smoke and possibly the added effects of environmental pollution. Cigarettes contain a complex mixture of particles and gases and thousands of chemicals. The smoke that is inhaled contains many free radicals and reactive oxygen species that are injurious to the lungs. The burden of gases and particles that are inhaled into the lungs results in inflammatory and immune responses that are both innate and adaptive. The innate respiratory defense system includes an epithelial cell barrier and mucociliary transport system. When they are overwhelmed, foreign particles may penetrate the airway, and the epithelial disruption initiates an immune response. Inflammatory cells migrate into the epithelial layer, including polymorphonuclear cells, eosinophils, macrophages, natural killer cells, and mast cells. Uncommitted B cells and CD4 and CD8 lymphocytes also participate in the innate response. Antigens that are deposited on the epithelium are transported within the airway by antigen-presenting cells, the specialized epithelial M cells, and the dendritic cells. The antigens are transported to the bronchial-associated lymphatic tissue layer and to regional lymph nodes, where B and T lymphocytes initiate the cellular and humoral components of the adaptive immune response. This response assists in the destruction of microbes that may penetrate the airway as the innate immune system is overwhelmed and in the neutralization extracellular microbial toxins that are released by these microorganisms.

BAL studies in cigarette smokers have shown an increase in the number of neutrophils and macrophages. Macrophages likely play an important role in perpetuating the inflammatory process of COPD and are increased 5- to 10-fold in the BAL when the disease is present. They may release neutrophil chemotactic factors as well as proteolytic enzymes, such as matrix metalloproteinases, that damage the epithelial barrier. Neutrophils are also thought to be important in causing the tissue damage of COPD. They release a number of mediators, including proteases such as neutrophil elastase and matrix metalloproteinases, oxidants such as the oxygen free radical H_2O_2, and toxic peptides such as defensins. Proteases and free radicals can damage the epithelium as well as the basement membrane. The repair process that ensues includes the secretion of antiproteases, such as secretory leukocyte protease inhibitor and tissue inhibitor of metalloproteinases, by epithelial cells to regulate the proteolytic process.

The process of repair may be impaired in patients with COPD. In patients with more advanced airflow obstruction, T lymphocytes and neutrophils are found in the epithelium, and T lymphocytes and macrophages are found in the subepithelium of centriacinar airways where emphysema is most marked. Although $CD4^+$ lymphocytes are found in the airways of atopic asthmatics, the T lymphocytes of patients with cigarette-induced COPD are $CD8^+$ cells. These cells are also thought to cause cell damage. Eosinophilic inflammation of the airways is also a hallmark of asthma and not usually seen in chronic bronchitis, although there is an increase in eosinophilic basic proteins (eosinophil cationic proteins and eosinophil peroxidase) in induced sputum. This may indicate that eosinophils had been present in the sputum but were destroyed, possibly by neutrophil elastase. During attacks of acute bronchitis, to the contrary, the number of tissue and sputum eosinophils is markedly increased. Bronchial biopsies from former smokers show similar inflammatory changes as the active smoker, suggesting that inflammation may persist in the airway once established. The inflammatory cells involved in the pathogenesis of COPD are listed in Table 3.

A number of extracellular-signaling proteins called *cytokines* are important in the pathogenesis of COPD because they are thought to mediate the tissue damage and repair induced by cigarette

Table 3. *The Inflammatory Cells of COPD*

Neutrophils
- Potent chemokines (IL-8) and leukotriene B_4 attract neutrophils to airways
- Increased numbers in sputum and BAL fluid, few in airways
- Neutrophil numbers correlate with degree of airflow obstruction
- Secrete proteases: neutrophil elastase, cathepsin, and proteinase-3
- A causative link to mucus hypersecretion
- Phagocytic ability of neutrophils impaired by cigarette smoke (by suppression of caspase-3–like activity) predisposing to respiratory infection

Macrophages
- Activated by cigarette smoke
- Increased numbers found in sputum, BAL fluid, and bronchial submucosa
- Release inflammatory mediators: TNF-α, leukotriene B_4, IL-8, reactive oxygen species
- Release increased amounts of metalloproteinase-1 and metalloproteinase-9
- Have defective phagocytic function against apoptotic epithelial cells
- Numbers of macrophages increase with increasing COPD severity

T lymphocytes
- Increased numbers in lung parenchyma and airways
- Greatest number are $CD8^+$ cells
- T-cell numbers correlate with amount of alveolar destruction
- T-cell numbers also correlate with severity of airflow obstruction
- $CD8^+$ cells shown to cause cytolysis and apoptosis of alveolar epithelial cells

Eosinophils
- Usually not in sputum in COPD, but eosinophil basic protein is found
- Hence, they may have been present and degranulated by sputum elastase
- Increased numbers predict corticosteroid responsiveness and also asthma
- Increased in BAL fluid and airway biopsy in acute exacerbation of COPD

Epithelial cells
- Likely an important source of inflammatory mediators as in asthma
- Activated by cigarette smoke to produce IL-1 and IL-8, TNF-α, and granulocyte colony-stimulating factor
- Airway epithelial cells important source of transforming growth factor-β
- Transforming growth factor-β may the cause of airway fibrosis in COPD
- VEGF important
- VEGF receptor blockade causes alveolar cell destruction (emphysema)

Dendritic cells and B cells
- Found in increased numbers in lymphoid follicles in bronchial wall
- May reflect an adaptive immune response to infection
- May reflect a role for autoimmunity in COPD

smoking. Increased quantities of certain proinflammatory cytokines, including interleukin (IL)-8, IL-1, IL-6, and TNF-α, and the antiinflammatory cytokine IL-10 have been found in the sputum of smokers and even further increased during an acute exacerbation. Mediators found to be elevated during a COPD exacerbation are listed in Table 4. Exposure of bronchial epithelial cells to cigarette smoke causes a release of neutrophilic and monocytic chemotactic factors, with IL-8 and granulocyte colony stimulating factor accounting for increased neutrophilic activity and monocyte chemotactic protein-1 causing increased monocytic activity.

Cytokines may also be involved with tissue remodeling in COPD. There are distinct pathologic features of airway remodeling seen with COPD, including inflammatory cell proliferation, epithelial damage, subepithelial fibrosis, myofibroblast proliferation, increased collagen deposition in the lung parenchyma, smooth muscle hypertrophy, and neovascularization. Increased expression of transforming growth factor-β and epidermal growth factor (EGF) may activate fibroblastic proliferation in the airways of patients with COPD. Patients with COPD have increased levels of total collagen and collagen I, III, and IV in the lungs, and levels of collagen I and III, fibronectin, and laminin have been inversely related to FEV_1, suggesting that the deposition of extracellular matrix proteins contribute to the airflow obstruction observed with COPD. Vascular endothelial growth factor (VEGF), which is expressed in airway smooth muscle cells, plays a key role in neovascularization and vascular permeability and the in the expression of fibroblast growth factors. Vascular remodeling changes have also been inversely related to measures of lung function (FEV_1).

Table 4. *Inflammatory Mediators Elevated in Acute Exacerbations of COPD*

C-reactive peptide
Copeptin
IL-8
IL-6
TNF-α
Leptin
Eosinophilic cationic protein
Myeloperoxidase
α_1-Antitrypsin
Leukotrienes E_4 and B_4
Fibrinogen
Myeloid progenitor inhibitory factor-1
Pulmonary and activation–regulated chemokine
Soluble intercellular adhesion molecule-1
Adiponectin (ACRP-30)

Other structural changes in the airways of smokers include mucus hyperplasia, bronchiolar edema and smooth muscle hypertrophy, and peribronchiolar fibrosis. These changes result in narrowing of the small airways (<2 mm). Recent studies suggest that the inflammatory cellular infiltrate, fibrosis, and muscle in the airway wall show a progression worsening of pathologic changes when nonsmokers, smokers with mild COPD, and smokers with more severe disease are compared, and there is a progression of the number of airways <400 μm in diameter as the disease worsens.

Because the total cross-sectional area of these small airways is so much larger than the cross-sectional area of the central conducting airways (and hence they contribute so little to total airway resistance), dyspnea and changes in the FEV_1 are usually absent until the disease is quite advanced. This zone of the lungs is often referred to as the "silent zone" because these pathologic abnormalities usually go undetected by symptom assessment and routine spirometry. In some smokers, the inflammation and peribronchiolar fibrosis progress, and the pulmonary functional abnormalities associated with the small airway changes and the symptoms of COPD become progressively worse. However, the presence of chronic bronchitis (cough and sputum production) in cigarette smokers is not useful in predicting the future development of airflow obstruction. Progression from GOLD stages 0 to 4 has been correlated with the following: (1) the thickness of the airway walls; (2) degree to which the airway lumen is filled with mucous exudates; and (3) the extent of the inflammatory response measured by the number of airways containing polymorphonuclear leukocytes, macrophages, and lymphocytes (CD8 cells, CD4 cells, and B cells).

In addition to the structural abnormalities seen in the small airways, there is also a loss of alveolar attachments to the airway perimeter, which impairs elastic recoil and favors increased tortuosity and early closure of the small airways during expiration. Several tests, such as frequency dependence of compliance, nitrogen slope of the alveolar plateau, the closing volume and $\dot{V}$MAX at low lung volume (*eg*, $\dot{V}$MAX75) are thought to reflect small airway narrowing. These pathophysiologic abnormalities in airways ≤2 mm have been referred to as "small airway disease," implying that it is a distinct clinical entity. It is more important instead to think of the early inflammatory changes in the small airways as the first stage in a protracted process that eventually leads to persistent airflow obstruction and progressive decrease in the FEV_1. The pathogenesis of COPD that targets the airways (chronic bronchitis) and lung parenchyma (emphysema) is thought to occur because of a complex interaction between extracellular signaling proteins, oxidative stress, and proteolytic digestion of connective tissue (Fig 3).

Pathology of Chronic Bronchitis

The presence of a gel-like mucous in the airways of healthy people is essential for normal mucociliary clearance. This mucous is swallowed and rarely noticed. Smokers with chronic bronchitis produce larger amounts of sputum each day, averaging about 20 to 30 mL/d and even as high as 100 mL/d. This production occurs as a result of an increase in the size and number of the submucosal glands and an increase in the number of goblet cells on the surface epithelium. Mucous gland enlargement and hyperplasia of the goblet cells are therefore the hallmark of chronic bronchitis. Goblet cells are normally absent in the small airways, and their presence there (often referred to as mucous metaplasia) is important to the development of COPD. In the larger airways in chronic bronchitis, there is a reduction in serous acini of the submucosal glands. This depresses local defenses to bacterial adherence because these glands are known to produce deterrents such as lactoferrin, antiproteases, and lysozyme. Other epithelial alterations are seen in chronic bronchitis are a decrease in the number and length of the cilia and squamous metaplasia. The mucociliary abnormalities of chronic bronchitis cause a continuous sheet or blanket of mucous lining the airways instead of discreet deposits of mucous seen on normal airways. Pooling of secretions also may occur. This provides additional cause for bacterial growth, which, in turn, causes a release of toxins that are further damaging to the cilia and epithelial cells. Bacterial exoproducts are known to stimulate mucous production, slow ciliary beating, impair immune effector cell function, and destroy local immunoglobulins. This cycle is especially seen in current as opposed to former smokers.

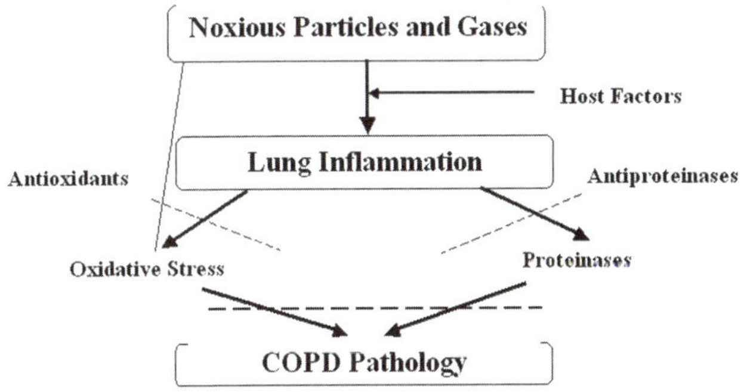

NIH/NHLBI. Global Initiative for Chronic Obstructive Lung Disease. NHLBI/WHO Workshop Report 2001.

Figure 3. Pathogenesis of COPD. COPD is caused by oxidative stress and proteolytic breakdown of connective tissue seen in this schema.

Pathology of Emphysema

Emphysema is a destructive process that occurs in the gas-exchanging airspaces: the respiratory bronchioles, alveolar ducts, and alveoli. It results in perforations (fenestrae), obliteration of airspace walls, and coalescence of small distinct air spaces into much larger ones. There is permanent enlargement of the gas-exchanging units of the lungs (acini). These pathologic changes cause loss of elastic recoil of the lungs and abnormal gas exchange. Recent studies have shown good correlation between physiologic measurements of lung elastic recoil and diffusing capacity and microscopic measures of airspace wall per unit of alveolar volume and alveolar surface area.

Two morphologic forms of emphysema have been described (Table 5). It should be recognized that most smoking-related emphysema has features of both and the clinical relevance is limited. The mechanisms by which emphysema and chronic bronchitis cause airflow obstruction are shown in Table 6. The release of large amounts of neutrophil elastase and metalloproteinases from inflammatory cells that overwhelm the antiprotease defenses of the lung are the most likely cause of the alveolar destruction of emphysema. In addition, lung repair is inhibited by cigarette smoke.

Table 5. *Pathologic Types of Emphysema*

Centriacinar (centrilobular): focal destruction of respiratory bronchioles; surrounded by normal lung parenchyma
- More severe in upper lobes
- Type most frequently associated with smoking

Panacinar (panlobular): uniform destruction of all airspaces beyond the respiratory bronchioles
- More lower-lobe distribution
- Occurs in smokers earlier in life
- Associated with AAT deficiency

Pathophysiology

The physiologic hallmark of COPD is the limitation of expiratory flow with relative preservation of inspiratory flow. Reductions in the FEV_1 and FEV_1/FVC percent are characteristic, whereas the maximal inspiratory flow rate is normal or near normal. The degree of reversibility in COPD is seldom brisk as it is in asthma. Differences in the degree of reversibility in COPD and asthma may be explained by the fact that in the latter disease, many inflammatory mediators have been implicated, including potent bronchoconstrictors such as histamine, kinins, and prostaglandins. In contrast, there are few bronchoconstrictor mediators released in COPD. One important inflammatory mediator found in the sputum of patients with COPD is leukotriene B_4. It is a potent chemoattractant for neutrophils. The term "partial reversibility" has been used in COPD, although this term has not been adequately defined. Reversibility in COPD patients can be acute, in response to bronchodilator drugs, mainly as the result of the release of cholinergic tone. It also may be in response to oral or inhaled corticosteroids, presumably as a result of decreased inflammation. Studies have shown that most patients with COPD will have a small but significant degree of reversibility of airflow obstruction (defined as a 12% and at least a 200-mL improvement in the FEV_1). Some longitudinal studies have suggested that increased reversibility is associated with a greater risk of dying from COPD, whereas others have suggested that the presence of reversibility coupled with close clinical treatment and follow-up is associated with better survival rates.

Table 6. *Mechanisms of Airflow Obstruction in COPD*

Emphysema
- Loss of elastic recoil
  1. Less driving pressure from alveoli to proximal airways
  2. As patency in smaller airways depends on elastic recoil, intraluminal pressure is reduced, and airways collapse during forced expiration

Chronic bronchitis
- Airway inflammation and hypersecretion of mucous
  1. Peribronchiolar fibrosis results in narrowing of peripheral airways, loss of alveolar attachments, and loss of elastic recoil
  2. Intraluminal mucous may contribute to airflow obstruction

Early in the course of COPD, the expiratory flow-volume curve shows a scooped out lower part of the expiratory limb as a result of abnormal flow at low lung volume. In later stages there is decreased expiratory flow at all lung volumes. Nonuniform ventilation of the lungs is seen even in the earlier stages of COPD and can be demonstrated with the N2 washout test. The multiple inert gas test has been used to quantify the ventilation/perfusion ($\dot{V}/\dot{Q}$) mismatch in the lungs of patients with COPD and has also shown these abnormalities in early stages of COPD. The predominant abnormalities detected by this test are low $\dot{V}/\dot{Q}$ regions. This type of mismatch causes arterial hypoxemia. There is little right-to-left shunting in COPD. Lung and thoracic wall hyperinflation are another consequence of the loss of elastic recoil. This favors expiratory flow. As lung volume increases, elastic recoil pressure also increases and causes the airways to enlarge, which in turn reduces the airway resistance. The hyperinflation may also have a deleterious effect. As the chest wall volume expands, the thoracic cage and diaphragm are placed at a mechanical disadvantage. This disadvantage increases the work of breathing and contributes to the sensation of dyspnea.

Systemic Inflammation and COPD

There is growing evidence that the inflammatory response of COPD is not limited to the lungs. Table 7 lists a number of systemic consequences of the disease that are considered related to systemic inflammation. Individuals with stable COPD have significantly increased blood levels of C-reactive protein (CRP), fibrinogen, TNF-α,

Table 7. *Systemic Consequences of COPD*

Cardiovascular disease
Osteoporosis
Metabolic disease (diabetes mellitus)
Gastrointestinal disease
Anorexia
Weight loss
Skeletal muscle dysfunction
Anemia of chronic disease
Generalized fatigue
Depression
Altered sleep
Cor pulmonale

endothelin-1, IL-6, and circulating leukocytes compared with normal subjects. Levels of VEGF, known to be involved in angiogenesis and inflammation, also have been shown to be increased in patients with COPD. Elevated levels of inflammatory cytokines in the blood of COPD patients suggests that there is a persistent level of systemic inflammation, possibly caused by a "spill over" of inflammatory from the inflammation that is occurring in the airways, the lung parenchyma, and the pulmonary vasculature. This latter theory has not been proven. There is some evidence that individuals with increased inflammatory markers such as fibrinogen and CRP are at risk for an accelerated decrease in FEV_1, greater rates of hospitalization, and death.

An analysis of the relative risk for systemic disease in patients with COPD followed by general practitioners has shown that patients with COPD are at increased risk for glaucoma, angina, fractures, myocardial infarction, osteoporosis, and respiratory infection when compared with control subjects without COPD. Anemia may occur in 10 to 15% of patients with severe COPD. Reduced hemoglobin in patients on long-term oxygen therapy has proven to be a strong predictor of survival and is associated with a greater hospitalization rate and a longer cumulative duration of hospitalization. In a nationally representative sample of 47 million hospitalizations from 1979 to 2001, hospital discharges with a diagnosis of COPD were more likely to be hospitalized with pneumonia, hypertension, heart failure, ischemic heart disease, pulmonary vascular disease, thoracic malignancies, and ventilatory failure when compared with age-adjusted discharges without COPD. Further, a diagnosis of COPD was associated with greater age-adjusted in-hospital rates of mortality for pneumonia, hypertension, heart failure, ventilatory failure, and thoracic malignancies when compared with hospital discharges with these comorbidities who did not have a diagnosis COPD. These results suggest that the burden of disease associated with COPD is largely underestimated because having a diagnosis of COPD is associated with increase risk for hospitalization and in-hospital mortality from other common diagnoses.

Another marker of inflammation, surfactant protein D (SP-D), has been recently studied. SP-D is a glycoprotein produced in the lungs. In addition to regulating surfactant homeostasis, SP-D also has a role in innate immunity and host defense responses to microorganisms and inhaled particles. Lung injury has been shown to increase levels of lung and systemic SP-D and systemic SP-D may be harmful. It has been associated with an increased risk of atherosclerosis and poor clinical outcomes with a variety of conditions. There is some evidence that treatment with an inhaled corticosteroid and long-acting β-agonist can reduce systemic SP-D levels. Attenuating lung inflammation may result in less leakage of SP-D into the systemic circulation. Further research on this mechanism of inflammation is needed.

The relationship of COPD, systemic inflammation, and cardiovascular disease has gained a great deal of attention because the presence of airflow obstruction doubles the risk of cardiovascular mortality irrespective of current smoking status. Ischemic heart disease, stroke, and sudden cardiac death rates can each be increased by the presence of COPD. Because systemic low-grade inflammation is implicated in affecting clot formation and subsequent cardiovascular events, the findings of systemic inflammation in COPD has a putative link. The direct effects of inflammatory markers of inflammation such as the CRP on the pathogenesis of clot formation and discovery of increased CRP levels in the blood of patients with COPD has provided a possible mechanism. Using the NHANES III population database, investigators have found that an increased CRP score coupled with moderate-to-severe airflow obstruction was associated with an increased occurrence of ischemic changes on the electrocardiograms of participants. The effects of inhaled corticosteroids, newer antiinflammatory agents such as phosphodiesterase-4 inhibitors, and statins on the cardiovascular and overall rate of mortality of COPD patients are under active investigation.

The prevalence of the metabolic syndrome has also been investigated in patients with COPD. Nearly half of all COPD patients in a pulmonary rehabilitation program were shown to have three or more features of the metabolic syndrome, including abdominal obesity, elevated triglyceride levels, elevated high-density lipoprotein cholesterol levels, elevated BP, and high fasting blood glucose levels. COPD patients with diabetes who have been hospitalized for an acute exacerbation have a greater rate of mortality than those without diabetes mellitus.

Patients with COPD have an increased risk for osteoporosis. This risk may be attributable to lifestyle, genetics, treatment with corticosteroids, endocrine abnormalities, or the impairment of the body composition and peripheral skeletal muscles. Some specifically identified risk factors for osteoporosis in patients with COPD are smoking, increased alchohol intake, reduced vitamin D levels, genetic factors, treatment with corticosteroids, reduced skeletal muscle mass and strength, low BMI and changes in body composition, hypogonadism, reduced levels of insulin-like growth factors, and chronic systemic inflammation.

Clinical Aspects of COPD

Symptoms of COPD

The symptoms that are associated with COPD are usually not present until the patient has been smoking a pack of cigarettes a day for at least 20 years. The patient usually presents in the fifth decade with a chronic cough that often is worsened after a viral respiratory infection. The second major symptom is dyspnea. It usually does not present until the sixth or seventh decade. Dynamic hyperinflation during exercise is recognized as an important factor in exercise limitation in COPD. The extent of dynamic hyperinflation during exercise in COPD correlates with a reduced resting inspiratory capacity. This limits the tidal volume response to exercise. This inability to expand the tidal volume in response to increasing metabolic demand is an important contributor to exercise intolerance in patients with COPD.

Dyspnea is a common symptom in the older population, and often it is difficult to distinguish whether heart disease or pulmonary disease is the cause or when both are present. High levels of brain natruretic protein (BNP) in the blood have been very helpful in differentiating cardiac and pulmonary causes of dyspnea in the acute setting. Natruretic peptides are the major hormones of the natruretic peptide system, which is highly activated in patients with both left and right heart failure. BNP is predominantly secreted by the cardiac ventricles, and in both acute and chronic left heart failure serum levels are increased. BNP levels can be increased in patients with COPD, but the levels are not nearly as high as those found with CHF.

In a large clinical trial called the Breathing Not Properly trial, a subgroup analysis of those with pulmonary disease (asthma or COPD) showed that BNP had a negative predictive value of 97.7% at a cut-off of 100 pg/mL. BNP levels have been shown to be associated with diminished exercise tolerance and a poor prognosis in patients with chronic left heart disease. In addition, BNP levels have been found to be increased in patients with pulmonary arterial hypertension and reflect the clinical and hemodynamic status in this patient population. Elevated BNP levels resulting from pulmonary hypertension secondary to end-stage lung disease have been reported in the absence of left ventricular failure. They have been shown to be a risk factor for death, independent of lung functional impairment or hypoxemia. Serum BNP can be used as a prognostic marker as well as a screening tool for significant pulmonary hypertension in patients with chronic obstructive lung disease.

The diagnosis of acute pulmonary embolism (PE) in patients with COPD is also often difficult to make, especially during an acute exacerbation of COPD when symptoms of the two conditions may be indistinguishable. In fact, the diagnosis may not be possible on clinical grounds. The prevalence of PE in postmortem series of patients with COPD is extremely high, ranging from 28 to 51%. In the Prospective Investigation of Pulmonary Embolism Diagnosis study, in a subgroup of patients with COPD and suspected PE, 19% received a diagnosis of PE on pulmonary angiography. Risk factors and symptoms were similar to those with and without pulmonary embolus. Recent studies have reported a 25% prevalence of PE in a group of patients admitted to the hospital for a severe exacerbation of COPD, but the study results may not be generalized to most occurrences of COPD because some patients in this study were excluded if they had evidence of a potential infection.

More recent evidence, which excluded the diagnosis of PE on the basis of a normal (<500 μg/mL) d-dimer test and negative diagnostic imaging studies, showed a much lower prevalence of pulmonary embolism. Only 6.2% of patients who had a clinical suspicion of pulmonary embolism and only 1.3% who had no clinical suspicion, judged by emergency department physicians, were discovered to have PE. This study showed that the prevalence of suspected PE in patients presenting with a COPD exacerbation is very low, and routine investigation for PE in this group is not warranted. There are some important lessons from these recent studies. When there is no suspicion of infection, either viral or bacterial, suspicion for PE in patients with a COPD exacerbation should be greater, especially in those patients who are sick enough require hospitalization as they my have more severe and debilitating disease that predisposes them to PE. Other clues that should increase clinical suspicion of pulmonary embolism in COPD patients are a previous history of malignancy and a decrease in the $Paco_2$ compared with baseline values. PE is a serious comorbid condition in patients with COPD, and a high clinical suspicion should be maintained in the appropriate clinical setting.

During the last two decades, as a result of an intense antismoking campaign, the rate of smoking in the United States has been reduced from approximately one third of the adult population to its current level of approximately 22%. In many susceptible smokers who stopped smoking in midlife, the onset of COPD symptoms is delayed until late in life. It is not unusual to see a patient with COPD present for the first time with symptoms at ≥75 years. The main symptoms and various stages of disease severity are presented in Table 8.

Table 8. *GOLD Guidelines: Classification of Severity of COPD, 2006*

Stage/characteristics
I: Mild COPD
$FEV_1 \geq 80\%$ of predicted
With or without chronic symptoms (cough, sputum production)
$FEV_1/FVC < 70\%$
II: Moderate COPD
$FEV_1/FVC < 70\%$
$50\% \leq FEV_1 < 80\%$ of predicted
Dyspnea worsens; ± cough sputum
III: Severe COPD
$FEV_1/FVC < 70\%$
$30\% \leq FEV_1 < 50\%$ of predicted
Dyspnea worsens; ± cough sputum
IV: Very severe COPD
$FEV_1/FVC < 70\%$
$FEV_1 < 30\%$ of predicted or respiratory/heart failure
Weight loss and anorexia
Hemoptysis
Cough syncope
Coughing spells
Depression and or anxiety
Cor pulmonale

Physical Examination and Laboratory Tests

The signs of COPD are well known: slow and prolonged expiration, wheezing, chest wall hyperinflation, limited diaphragmatic motion on auscultation, distant breath sounds, and heart sounds and often coarse early inspiratory crackles. The accessory muscles of respiration may be in use, and the patient may be using pursed-lip breathing. Signs of cor pulmonale include pedal edema, a tender congested liver, and neck vein distention. Cyanosis may be present as well as asterixis, which is associated with severe hypercapnia. The roentgenographic signs of COPD include a low flat diaphragm, increased retrosternal airspace, and a teardrop-shaped heart. Pruning of the pulmonary arterial vessels and bullae are seen in emphysema. The high-resolution CT scan has a much better sensitivity and specificity but is not recommended for routine use. It may be helpful when surgery for large bullae is contemplated.

Pulmonary function studies are important for the diagnosis and staging of COPD. Because the best correlate with rates of morbidity and mortality is the FEV_1, proposals for staging have used this test. The 1995 ATS standards suggested a severity scoring on the basis of the severity of airflow obstruction: stage I is $FEV_1 \geq 50\%$ of predicted; stage II is FEV_1 35 to 49% of predicted, and stage II is FEV_1 of $<35\%$ of predicted. Patients with stage I disease usually have little impairment in their quality of life. Patients with stage II COPD have a significant impairment in the quality of their lives, which results in a large per-capita health-care cost. Patients with stage III disease are profoundly impaired, are often hospitalized with severe exacerbations of disease, and therefore are frequent users of health-care resources.

A new severity scoring system was introduced by the GOLD guidelines (Table 8). It began staging with an "at-risk" group, stage 0, to emphasize the point that patients with risk factors (cigarette smoking, occupations) who have symptoms cough and sputum need to be counseled about COPD even though their screening spirometry is normal. The GOLD guidelines were updated in 2006 (www.goldcopd.com). The spirometric classification of severity of COPD now includes only four stages: stage I, mild; stage II, moderate; stage III, severe; stage IV, very severe. The category stage 0, at risk, is no longer included as a stage of COPD. The GOLD committee believed that there was incomplete evidence that the individuals who meet the criteria for this stage (chronic cough and sputum production, normal spirometry) necessarily progress on to stage I. Other GOLD stages are modifications of the previous (1995) ATS criteria now adopted in the new ATS/ERS Statement.

Although the measurement of lung function remains the best way to diagnose COPD, the routine use of spirometry for case finding in adults with exposure to risk factors (such as cigarette smoking) or for those with persistent respiratory symptoms remains controversial. This controversy is, in part, because no randomized clinical trial has demonstrated that early detection of COPD changes the course of disease or increases the rate of smoking cessation. A conclusion not to recommend spirometry screening was reached through a systematic review of the evidence by a task force of the Agency for Health-Care Research and Quality. The Agency for Health-Care Research and Quality conclusion was that the evidence does not justify recommending spirometry as a routine tool in the practice of primary care.

Differentiation From Asthma

Table 9 lists the most common distinguishing features between asthma and COPD. Epidemiologic studies have shown that as many as 30% of patients with fixed airflow obstruction have a history of asthma. Differentiating asthma from COPD may be difficult and at times not possible, especially in older patients. The most useful discriminator, the response to an inhaled short-acting β-agonist bronchodilator, may not differentiate asthma from COPD. When the postbronchodilator FEV_1 returns to normal, the diagnosis is asthma (no fixed airflow obstruction). On the one hand, many asthmatics, especially those with long-standing disease, may not show any response, and some patients with COPD will show a brisk bronchodilator response. On the other hand, asthmatics with fixed airflow obstruction show other features that are distinct from COPD caused by cigarette smoking.

When compared with patients with COPD of comparable age, patients with asthma have significantly more eosinophils in the peripheral blood, sputum, and BAL fluid on bronchial biopsy, have greater numbers of neutrophils in the sputum and BAL fluid, have greater ratios of $CD4^+/CD8^+$ T cells infiltrating the airway, and have greater thickness of the airway basement membrane than patients with COPD. Other distinguishing features include greater levels of exhaled nitric oxide, lower emphysema scores on high-resolution CT scans, and greater diffusing capacities. Because many of these tests are impractical, not available for widespread use, or not discriminatory enough for clinical use, the most recent ATS/ERS Statement

Table 9. *Distinguishing Features of COPD and Asthma*

COPD	Asthma
Onset in midlife	Onset early in life (often childhood)
Symptoms slowly progressive	Symptoms vary from day to day
Long history of tobacco smoking	Allergic rhinitis and/or eczema history
Dyspnea during exercise	Sudden dyspnea after acute exposure
Largely irreversible airflow limitation	Largely reversible airflow limitation

on COPD stated: "Some patients with asthma cannot be distinguished from COPD with the current diagnostic tests. The management of these patients should be similar to that of asthma."

COPD: Outpatient Management

Once the diagnosis of COPD is established, pulmonary function testing can be helpful by staging the disease. Pharmacologic intervention is offered according to disease severity and the patient's tolerance for specific drugs (Fig 4). The goals of therapy are to induce bronchodilation, decrease airway inflammation, and improve mucociliary transport. Because COPD is basically an irreversible condition, disease management of daily symptoms and other impacts on quality of life are most essential. The patient who still smokes should be encouraged to quit. Preventive therapy with a pneumococcal vaccine and a yearly influenza vaccine is recommended. Vaccination with the flu shot has been shown to result in 52% fewer hospitalizations for pneumonia and influenza in patients with COPD. Vaccinated patients also have fewer outpatient visits for respiratory symptoms.

Smoking Cessation

Cigarette smoking compromises airway function by damaging airway epithelial cells, increasing mucous viscosity, and slowing mucociliary clearance. There is a greater bacterial adherence to oropharyngeal epithelial cells in smokers compared with nonsmokers. Smokers are prone to

0: At Risk	I: Mild	II:Moderate	III: Severe	IV: Very Severe
•Chronic symptoms •Exposure to risk factors •Normal spirometry	•FEV_1/FVC <70% •FEV_1 ≥80% •With or without symptoms	•FEV_1/FVC <70% •50% ≤FEV_1≤80% •With or without symptoms	•FEV_1/FVC <70% •30% ≤FEV_1 ≤80% •With or without symptoms	•FEV_1/FVC <70% •FEV_1 <30% or presence of chronic respiratory failure or right heart failure
Avoidance of risk factor(s); influenza vaccination				
	Add short-acting bronchodilator when needed			
		Add regular treatment with one or more long-acting bronchodilators Add rehabilitation		
			Add ICS if repeated exacerbations	
				Oxygen for chronic respiratory failure Consider surgical treatments

Figure 4. Treatment plan from the GOLD guidelines.

attacks of acute bronchitis. As a result, they show increased rates of acute exacerbations, visits to the emergency department, work absences, and frequency of medication use. Smokers also show greater decrease in lung function, worsening of respiratory symptoms, and lower quality of life scores than a comparable group of nonsmoking patients. The presence of respiratory illness such as COPD is not a motivator for smoking cessation. Physician-delivered smoking cessation interventions can significantly increase smoking abstinence rates. Smoking cessation interventions for COPD should include the following: (1) physician intervention (set a quit date), (2) group smoking cessation clinics, and (3) pharmacologic therapy with nicotine replacement is needed in highly dependent smokers. These patients can be identified as those who smoke a pack a day or more, require their first cigarette within 30 min of arising in the morning, and find it difficult refraining from smoking in places where it is forbidden. Therapy with the antidepressant bupropion hydrochloride has also been shown to be effective. The Lung Health Study showed that despite intensive antismoking efforts, middle-age smokers with COPD are not likely to quit. Only 22% were sustained quitters after a 5-year follow-up.

Pharmacologic Therapy

Short-Acting β_2-Agonists: Short-acting β_2-agonists can be used for the following:

- Achieve variable degrees of bronchodilatation, *ie,* rapid onset of action with duration of 4 to 6 h;
- Improve symptoms and, in most studies, exercise capacity; and
- Metered-dose inhaler use of β_2-selective agents is safe tid or qid; greater doses may cause hypokalemia, cardiac arrhythmia, and reduced arterial oxygen tension.

Long-Acting β_2-Agonists: Long-acting β_2-agonists have the following advantages:

- Maximal effect comparable with short-acting β_2-agonists with longer duration of action (12 h) for agents such as salmeterol and formoterol;
- Improved symptoms and quality-of-life measures; no tachyphylaxis found, and

- Good safety profile with recommended doses: occasional tremor is noted that improves after several days of use.

Anticholinergic Therapy

Short-acting agents (*ie*, ipratropium) afford bronchodilatation and relieve of symptoms for 4 to 6 h. The long-acting anticholinergic tiotropium offers improved bronchodilatation for 24 h and therefore can be given once a day. No tachyphylaxis is noted with these agents, but their effects on long-term prognosis of COPD are being studied. Tiotropium has been shown to reduce exacerbation rates and hospitalizations caused by exacerbations. Finally, they have mild side-effects, such as occasional dry mouth.

β_2-Agonists Plus Anticholinergic Drugs: Combining both agents provides a small additional benefit to either drug alone, and no additional side effects from combination therapy are noted.

Theophylline: Theophylline causes small changes in FEV_1 with chronic use and an improvement in symptoms and exercise capacity. Frequent adverse effects, including nausea, diarrhea, headache, and irritability, are noted with therapeutic blood levels. Seizures and cardiac arrhythmias are considerably (*ie*, 10 to 15 times) more common in elderly with toxic blood levels.

Systemic Corticosteroids: Twenty to thirty percent of patients with chronic COPD symptoms improve if administered oral steroid therapy. Responders have more eosinophils in induced sputum and bronchial biopsies and likely have concomitant asthma. Long-term treatment with oral corticosteroids is not recommended for patients with COPD. The treatment of hospitalized patients with high doses results in fewer treatment failures and shorter stays; 2 weeks of therapy is sufficient after hospital discharge. Complications include cataracts, osteoporosis, secondary infection, and diabetes and skin damage.

Inhaled Corticosteroids: No significant benefit in long-term decline in FEV_1 has been noted for inhaled corticosteroids. They may provide small but significant improvements in lung function and 6-min walk test results. Studies have also demonstrated fewer exacerbations of COPD and improved quality of life indexes. Benefits are enhanced when coupled with long-acting β-agonist treatment. Guidelines recommend with FEV_1 <50% predicted and frequent exacerbations.

Mucolytic Drugs: The use of mucolytic drugs has a variable effect in patients with COPD. Randomized controlled trials suggest that they are ineffective at shortening the course or improving outcomes of patients with acute exacerbations.

Antibiotics: The results of multiple trials favor the use of antibiotics for acute exacerbations of COPD that include worsening dyspnea, increased sputum volume, and sputum purulence. However, there is little evidence to support their prophylactic use.

Oxygen Therapy: Several controlled studies have been completed: oxygen vs no oxygen (Medical Research Council [MRC]) and continuous vs nocturnal oxygen (Nocturnal Oxygen Therapy Trial). In patients with hypoxemia and congestive heart failure, death rates are significantly lower and quality of life indexes are improved when oxygen is in chronic use. Patients who used oxygen for at least 15 h/d had a significant decrease in their pulmonary artery pressures and an increase in cardiac output.

Oxygen should be prescribed when the following occur: (1) the arterial PaO_2 is <55 mm Hg or arterial oxygen saturation <88%, and (2) PaO_2 is 56 to 59 mm Hg with ECG evidence of P pulmonale, pedal edema, and/or secondary erythrocytosis. Long-term oxygen therapy does not improve survival in patients with moderate hypoxemia (PaO_2 56 to 65 mm Hg) or in patients with only nocturnal hypoxemia. Supplemental oxygen during exercise training may improve dyspnea and allow patients with COPD to tolerate greater levels of exercise. However, studies evaluating quality of life in patients who show hypoxemia during exercise have not supported oxygen use for this indication.

Pulmonary Rehabilitation: Pulmonary rehabilitation (PR) is a multidisciplinary program that attempts to return the patient with COPD to the highest functional capacity possible. PR addresses deconditioning, social isolation, anxiety and depression, muscle wasting, and weight loss. Evidence supports the use of lower-extremity exercise training because it improves exercise tolerance, and upper-extremity strength and endurance training is recommended as well.

PR improves dyspnea, improves quality of life scores, and reduces the number of hospitalizations and days in the hospital; however, the effects on survival are not definite. PR has been shown to help patients requiring long-term mechanical ventilation by improving overall strength, weaning outcomes, and functional status.

Nutrition and COPD

Malnutrition occurs in one quarter to one third of patients with moderate-to-severe COPD and is an independent risk factor for mortality. Both fat mass and fat-free mass are depleted, the latter caused by depressed protein synthesis. Because the proinflammatory cytokines IL-6 and TNF-α have been shown to be elevated, tt is believed that weight loss, particularly skeletal muscle mass loss, is associated with a systemic inflammatory response in malnourished patients with COPD. Skeletal muscle loss in COPD is probably multifactorial in origin. There is a link to systemic inflammation even without weight loss.

Studies have shown that leptin, an adipocyte-derived hormone involved in the control of body weight, is decreased in patients with COPD. Serum leptin levels have been correlated with TNF-α levels, thus creating a link between nutritional status and systemic inflammation in COPD. Resting energy expenditure is elevated and contributes to the negative energy balance. Nutritional supplements alone do not reverse the loss; results with anabolic steroids, growth hormone, and the progestational agent megestrol acetate show some effect on appetite and body weight; however, improved exercise tolerance and respiratory muscle function do not always follow. A combination of nutritional support and exercise as an anabolic stimulus appears to be the best approach to obtaining marked functional improvement

Noninvasive Positive Pressure Ventilation

A theoretical advantage has been shown to resting chronically fatigued muscles at night. Patients with COPD have a high prevalence of sleep apnea and hypoxemia and hypercarbia at night. They have less REM sleep and shorter sleep times than normal subjects. It has been theorized that noninvasive positive pressure ventilation (NPPV) would help. However, trials have shown conflicting conclusions. Patients without CO_2 retention show little gain; patients with severe CO_2 retention, especially those that have severe nocturnal O_2 desaturation, appear to respond most favorably.

The most recent Cochrane evidenced-based review on this topic concluded that nocturnal NIPPV for at least 3 months in hypercapnic patients with stable COPD had no consistent clinically or statistically significant effect on lung function, gas exchange, respiratory muscle strength, sleep efficiency, or exercise tolerance. However, the small sample sizes of these studies precluded a definite conclusion regarding the effects of NPPV in patients COPD.

Surgery for COPD

Lung volume reduction surgery (LVRS) has emerged as a treatment for far advanced COPD caused by emphysema. LVRS involves resection of functionless areas of emphysematous lung to improve lung elastic recoil and lung and chest wall hyperinflation. The overall rate of mortality with the procedure is 0 to 6% within 30 days of surgery and 0 to 8% at 6 months, although in patients with very severe degrees of obstruction the rates are much greater. The range of FEV_1 improvement before and after surgery is approximately 250 to 350 mL. Borg scale dyspnea scores on the 6-min walk test show improvement as do the distances walked. Sixteen percent to 42% of patients no longer require oxygen after surgery.

The recently completed National Emphysema Treatment Trial (NETT) defined a subgroup of patients a very high risk for mortality. Interim analysis showed that if the FEV_1 was $\leq 20\%$ predicted and the CT scan of the lungs showed homogeneous emphysema or the carbon monoxide diffusing capacity was $< 20\%$, there was a high risk of death after surgery and little chance of functional improvement. Among those not in the high-risk group, there was a 2.2% mortality with surgery at 30 days compared with a 0.2% mortality in the medically treated group. After 1 month, 28% of the surgery group were hospitalized, living in a nursing home or rehabilitation facility, or unavailable for interview. Changes in exercise capacity, pulmonary function, quality of life measures, and dyspnea at 6 to 24 months all favored surgery. Further subgroup analysis showed that those with upper-lobe emphysema on CT scans and with low exercise capacity at the beginning of the trial had the most favorable outcomes.

Given the potential risks of median sternotomy and thoracoscopy, the usual surgical approaches to LVRS, less-invasive procedures are being studied, including bronchoscopic LVRS, which is performed with the placement of endobronchial one-way valves. Preliminary studies have shown improvement in exercise capacity and dynamic hyperinflation with this procedure.

Resection of large bullae is occasionally necessary for dyspnea, chest pain, or recurrent pneumothorax. Other complications that can occur with large bullae are bleeding and infection. The best results occur when the bullae occupy more than one third of the hemithorax. Factors that do not favor surgical resection are the presence of multiple small bullae and diffuse emphysema in the remainder of the lungs. No prospective clinical trials have been performed. Case series have shown improvement in dyspnea and even reversal of respiratory failure after bullectomy. However, in those with underlying emphysema there is a progressive decline in the FEV_1 over time and return of crippling dyspnea in many. Bullectomy can be performed by thoracoscopic surgery in selected patients.

Lung transplantation can be life-saving for patients with very advanced disease complicated by respiratory failure and secondary pulmonary hypertension. Patients are considered for single or double lung transplantation when the FEV_1 is $<25\%$, and/or the $Paco_2$ is >55 mm. Hg. The procedure is costly, limited by lack of organs, and requires prolonged immunosuppression. Recent studies have suggested that unlike patients with cystic fibrosis and idiopathic pulmonary fibrosis, patients with COPD do not fair well after transplantation, with limited exercise capacity because of skeletal muscle dysfunction. In January 2008, The International Society for Heart and Lung Transplantation has reported survival figures for COPD of 85% at 1 year and 68% at 3 years.

Acute Exacerbation of COPD

Unfortunately, many definitions of the acute exacerbation or "flare" of COPD exist, and many authors use substantially different criteria. A widely quoted description of a COPD exacerbation includes "the Winnipeg criteria," which have also included a staging proposal. Patients with COPD exacerbation have the following three changes in their clinical condition: (1) worsening of dyspnea, (2) an increase in sputum volume, and (3) sputum purulence. Patients with type I exacerbations have all of the aforementioned symptoms. Patients with type II exacerbations have two of the three symptoms. Type III exacerbations are characterized by at least one of these symptoms and also one of the following clinical criteria: upper respiratory infection in the past 5 days, fever without other apparent cause, increased wheezing, increased cough, and increased respiratory rate or heart rate by 20% above baseline. A more simple and practical definition has been offered by the ATS as "an event in the natural course of the disease characterized by a change in the patient's baseline dyspnea, cough and/or sputum beyond day-to-day variability sufficient to warrant a change in management." The classification of severity offered with this definition ranks the clinical relevance of the episode and its outcome: level I, treatment at home; level II, requiring hospitalization; and level III, respiratory failure.

Before the onset of an exacerbation of COPD, there is usually a prodromal period of up to 7 days when symptoms of increased dyspnea, cough, sore throat, and the common cold occur. These symptoms are not accompanied with a decrease in lung function. On the day of the exacerbation, there is a small but significant decrease in lung function, including peak flow rates, FEV_1, and FVC. Peak flow rate recovery to baseline values is complete in 75% of patients by 1 month. Approximately 7% of patients with a COPD exacerbation do not return their peak flow rates to baseline by 3 months. This finding suggests that a substantial proportion of exacerbations of COPD are associated with a permanent loss of lung function. If this were to occur repeatedly, it could lead to an accelerated decrease in FEV_1 over years. Whether repeated respiratory infections or exacerbations of COPD do lead to a more rapid decrease of lung function over time has not been proven.

The most frequent cause of an acute exacerbation of COPD is thought to be respiratory infection. Sputum cultures in patients with mild to moderately severe COPD often show nonpathogenic bacteria (Gram-negative and Gram-positive such as *Streptococcus viridans*, *Neisseria* sp, or *Corynebacterium* sp). Pathogenic bacteria include *Haemophilus influenzae* (22%), *Pseudomonas aeruginosa* (15%), *Streptococcus pneumoniae* (10%), and *Moraxella catarrhalis* (9%). Sputum samples may have limited validity considering the possible contamination from oropharyngeal secretions.

Techniques that potentially preclude contamination include transtracheal aspirates, BAL, and protected brush sampling during bronchoscopy. Studies in which the authors used these techniques have shown that patients requiring hospitalization compared with those treated as outpatients for an exacerbation of COPD and those outpatients with the most severe degree of airflow obstruction are more likely to harbor Gram-negative enteric organisms. The presence of bacterial colonization in the stable state is associated with an increased exacerbation frequency, and patients colonized with *H influenzae* have an increased total symptom count and more sputum purulence at the time of exacerbation. When molecular typing is used, it has also been shown that the acquisition of new strains of bacteria such as *H influenzae*, *M catarrhalis*, and *S pneumoniae* are associated with an exacerbation of COPD in as many as one third of cases.

The role of viral infection has been recently revisited with the use of sophisticated methods such as polymerase chain reaction viral detection as well as more standard methods such as serologic testing and culture. Viruses may be detected in nearly 40% of COPD exacerbations when these techniques are used, including rhinovirus, respiratory syncytial virus, coronavirus, influenza, and parainfluenza. Evidence for Mycoplasma infection has been found in up to one third of the acute exacerbations of chronic bronchitis in some studies; however, in most patients Mycoplasma and Chlamydia pneumonia are seen in $<10\%$ of cases. A COPD exacerbation associated with a virus is likely to produce more severe symptoms, and the exacerbation is likely to last longer (13 days). There is also more laboratory evidence of an acute-phase response (*eg*, elevated levels of IL-6 and fibrinogen) with an associated viral infection.

Clearly, environmental factors are also important. Hospital admissions for COPD appear to be high when air pollution levels in the ambient environment are high. Small increases in SO_2 and airborne particles have been shown to cause increases in emergency room visits for COPD during winter and summer seasons by 6% and 9%, respectively. Whatever the cause of an acute exacerbation of COPD, it is clear that bronchial inflammation is enhanced during this event. Increased levels of myeloperoxidase have been found in the sputum, indicating neutrophilic activity, and high levels of IL-8 and leukotriene B_4, well-known neutrophil chemoattractants, are also seen. During recovery, levels of sputum chemoattractants and inflammatory markers rapidly decrease. Risk factors associated with COPD exacerbations are listed in Table 10.

Table 10. *Factors Associated With Increased Risk for Exacerbations*

Increased age
Severity of airway obstruction (FEV_1 impairment)
Chronic bronchial mucus hypersecretion
Frequent past exacerbations
Daily cough and wheeze
Persistent symptoms of chronic bronchitis
Hypercapnia
Hypoxia
Comorbid heart disease
Right ventricular failure
Low serum albumin
Single nucleotide polymorphism in *CCL1* gene

Diagnostic and Therapeutic Approaches

Often, patients present to a local emergency department or hospital with an acute exacerbation of COPD. It is useful to do a chest roentgenogram. The chest roentgenogram may be positive in approximately 15% of cases, and in 25% of such patients there is a change of management prompted by the chest roentgenogram result. Spirometry, on the other hand, has not been helpful in decision-making for patients with an acute exacerbation of COPD. There is poor correlation between arterial blood gases and the FEV_1 at the time of presentation. The FEV_1 has not been helpful in predicting need for hospital admission. Although severe abnormalities of arterial blood gases and history of previous relapses are helpful, there are no predictive models of adequate sensitivity and specificity on which to rely. The best indicators for the need for mechanical ventilation include the blood gas values on admission and the degree of change in pH after initial oxygen therapy. Significant predictors of hospital mortality include older age, lower body mass index, poor functional status before admission, lower ratio of arterial partial pressure of oxygen (Pao_2) over the fraction of inspired oxygen ratio, history of congestive heart failure, low serum albumin, and presence of cor pulmonale.

Most therapeutic interventions for the treatment of the acute exacerbation of COPD have been studied through randomized controlled trials. In general, mucolytic agents are ineffective in shortening the course and improving the outcome of patients. Chest physiotherapy and mechanical percussion of the chest are also ineffective and may be potentially harmful. β_2-agonists and anticholinergic agents appear to be equivalent in their usefulness and are superior to all parenterally administered bronchodilators, including methylxanthines. The addition of a methylxanthine to inhaled bronchodilators has also been carefully examined. One study showed a statistical trend toward lower hospitalization rates for patients given IV aminophylline in the emergency department, whereas two other studies showed no significant advantage. The effect of adding two inhaled bronchodilators has also been carefully studied. There appears to be only marginal improvement to the use of both agents. The side-effects of anticholinergic therapy are generally fewer and mild. The adverse effects of albuterol in the acute setting include tremors, headache, and palpitations. Changes in heart rate, BP, and ECG tracings are also possible.

The use of systemic steroids for patients with an acute exacerbation of COPD who require hospitalization is helpful. A change to po therapy continues to have a positive effect, but only for 2 weeks after hospitalization. The most common adverse effect was hyperglycemia. Antibiotic therapy has been a controversial issue. Patients with more severe exacerbations are more likely to benefit. For instance, antibiotics appear to be effective when two of the three symptoms of increased dyspnea, sputum volume, and purulence are present. However, there is still some controversy concerning the role of antibiotics for COPD exacerbations, especially in studies performed in primary care, where generally patients with milder disease are treated. Treatment with antibiotics in addition to oral corticosteroids has been associated with a longer time to the next exacerbation and a decreased risk of developing a new exacerbation. The most consistently measured end point with a positive result is an improvement in peak expiratory flow rate that improves a mean of 11 L/min, more in patients with the antibiotic treatment.

Arterial blood gas measurements should be done if a patient does not show prompt improvement with initial measures. The initiation of mechanical ventilation should be considered when, despite optimal medical therapy and oxygen administration, there is acidosis (pH <7.35) and hypercapnia ($Paco_2$ 45–60 mm Hg) and a persistently elevated respiratory rate >24 breaths/min. Mechanical ventilation can be administered via invasive ventilation (use of an endotracheal tube) or noninvasive (nasal or face masks). NPPV is beneficial for patients who have a high likelihood of respiratory failure and who may require invasive mechanical ventilation. In the first hours, NPPV requires the same level of supervision as conventional mechanical ventilation. The use of NPPV provides a statistically significant difference in the need for intubation reported in several clinical trials. Arterial blood gases improve because of an increase in alveolar ventilation without significant modifications in the alveolar $\dot{V}/\dot{Q}$ mismatching and gas exchange in the lungs.

The addition of NPPV to standard care in patients with an acute exacerbation of COPD have decreased the rate of endotracheal intubation 28%, length of hospital stay 4.57 days, and in-hospital mortality rate 10%. Subgroup analyses have shown that these beneficial effects occurred only in patients with severe exacerbations (pH <7.30), not in those with milder exacerbations. Optimal NPPV delivery methods, optimal duration of treatment, and appropriate delivery pressures are additional questions that need to be addressed in the literature. In general, a bilevel ventilatory support with continuous positive airway pressure of 4 to 8 cmH_2O and pressure support ventilation of 10 to 15 cmH_2O provides the most effective mode of NPPV.

Contraindications for NPPV include the following: respiratory arrest; cardiovascular instability (hypotension, arrhythmias, myocardial infarction);

impaired mental status causing an inability to cooperate, copious and/or viscous secretions with high aspiration risk, recent facial or gastroesophageal surgery, craniofacial trauma and/or fixed nasopharyngeal abnormality, burns, and extreme obesity. Patients meeting these exclusion criteria should be considered for immediate intubation.

Patients who are hospitalized with an acute exacerbation of COPD have a mortality rate of approximately 3%. Almost half of all patients admitted with hypercarbic respiratory failure will be readmitted to the hospital within the next 6 months. There is a significant decrement in functional status and quality of life and the likelihood in such patients. Mortality for those patients who require treatment in an ICU may be close to 50%.

Outcomes of COPD

COPD is the only major cause of mortality with an increasing incidence worldwide, and it is expected to become the third-leading cause of death by 2020. Traditionally, clinical staging of severity and risk of mortality has relied on the measurement of FEV_1. Staging criteria for COPD with use of the percentage of predicted FEV_1 can be useful in predicting impairment in health-related quality of life. Even patients with mild disease show substantially compromised health-related quality of life. Comorbid conditions are common, and they also negatively influence health-related quality of life.

Other measures of COPD such as the BMI and dyspnea scores have proved useful in predicting outcomes such as survival. BMI is easily obtained by dividing weight (in kilograms) over height (in m^2). Values $<21\ kg \cdot m^{-2}$ are associated with increased rates of mortality. Functional dyspnea can be assessed by the MRC dyspnea scale as follows: 0, not troubled with breathlessness except with strenuous exercise; 1, troubled by shortness of breath when hurrying or walking up a slight hill; 2, walks slower than people of the same age because of breathlessness or has to stop for breath when walking at own pace on the level; 3, stops for breath after walking approximately 100 m or after a few minutes on the level; and 4, too breathless to leave the house or breathless when dressing or undressing. A simple grading index, the BODE index, has been proposed as a useful tool to grade COPD severity and predict outcomes. The system uses the body mass index (B), the degree of airflow obstruction measured as the FEV_1 as percent predicted (O), dyspnea measured by the MRC dyspnea scale (D), and exercise capacity measured by the six-minute walk test (E). Patients with greater BODE scores were at greater risk for death. The score proved to be a better discriminator than lung function alone. A summary of indexes of COPD outcomes is listed in Table 11.

Table 11. *Outcome Measures for COPD (Morbidity/Mortality)*

FEV_1
Dyspnea (MRC scale)
BMI
Exercise capacity
BODE index
Arterial blood gases
COPD exacerbations
Quality of life health status

Summary

In the United States, >16 million adults have COPD. As the United States population ages, the prevalence for this disease will increase even more. COPD currently accounts for approximately 110,000 deaths per year. There are >500,000 hospitalizations in this country for COPD and >16 million office visits to physicians. The direct health costs are $18 billion/yr. It is likely that the care of patients with COPD will consume a growing proportion of the pulmonologist's time in the years to come. Differentiation from another chronic airway disease, asthma, is often difficult.

Annotated Bibliography

Agusti AG, Gari PG, Sauleda J, et al. Weight loss in chronic obstructive pulmonary disease: mechanisms and implications. Pulm Pharmacol Ther 2002; 15:425–432

Weight loss is a common occurrence in COPD, and when severe, it is labeled the pulmonary cachexia syndrome. It is a prognostic indicator of poor outcome. The mechanism is not entirely understood, but loss of skeletal muscle mass is them main cause of weight loss. Loss of fat is also contributory.

Poor nutritional intake, high metabolic rate, sedentary lifestyle, tissue hypoxia, and a systemic inflammatory response from high levels of TNF have all been proposed as causative. It is likely that oxidative stress also enhances muscle proteolysis.

Alsaeedi A, Sin DD, McAlister FA. The effects of inhaled corticosteroids in chronic obstructive pulmonary disease: a systematic review of randomized placebo-controlled trials. Am J Med 2002; 113:59–65

This article presents a systematic review of inhaled corticosteroids relating to the exacerbation rate with COPD. It reviews nine randomized trials and concludes that inhaled corticosteroids do reduce the exacerbation rate in COPD. It reminds us that side-effect profiles are also increased. Oropharyngeal candidiasis and skin bruising were more likely to occur. No effects on overall mortality were observed in these trials.

American Thoracic Society/European Respiratory Society statement. Standards for the diagnosis and management of individuals with alpha-1 antitrypsin deficiency. Am J Respir Crit Care Med 2003; 168:818–900

This is an updated comprehensive review of the many aspects of AAT deficiency and COPD. Augmentation therapy with purified human AAT concentrate is supported by two large observational studies suggesting that the progression of emphysema may be slowed in patients with moderate emphysema (FEV_1 *31 to 65% predicted). The rate of mortality may be decreased in patients with a lower* FEV_1*. Adverse reactions to the concentrate are rare occurrences.*

Anthonisen NR, Connett JE, Kiley JP, et al. Effects of smoking intervention and the use of an inhaled anticholinergic bronchodilator on the rate of decline of FEV_1: the lung health study. JAMA 1994; 272:1497–1505

This is a landmark study by a lung health study research group. This lung health study, in a prospective way, substantiated what had been learned from the Fletcher and Peto study of the 1970s. An aggressive smoking-intervention program significantly reduced the age-related decrease in FEV_1 *in middle-age smokers with COPD. Unfortunately, the use of the inhaled anticholinergic bronchodilator ipratropium did not show similar improvement. Of importance in this study is that with intense smoking intervention, only about 20% of the group compromised sustained smokers during the 5-year study.*

Balmes J, Becklake M, Blanc P, et al. Occupational contribution to the burden of airway disease: an official statement of the American Thoracic Society. Am J Respir Crit Care Med 2003; 167:787–797

This statement reviewed the evidence implicating occupational factors in the pathogenesis of obstructive airway diseases (asthma and COPD) and quantified the contribution of work-related risk to the burden of these diseases in the general population. The review demonstrated that approximately 15% of both asthma and COPD is likely to be work related, and a conservative estimate of the annual costs of this occupational asthma and COPD is nearly $7 billion in the United States alone.

Balmes JR. Occupational contribution to the burden of chronic obstructive pulmonary disease. J Occup Environ Med 2005; 47:154–160

This is an excellent review of the contribution of occupational exposures to the occurrence of COPD. Mechanisms, diagnosis, and management are each discussed.

Barnes PJ. Emerging pharmacotherapies for COPD. Chest 2008; 134:1278–1286

With better understanding of the inflammatory and destructive processes in the pathophysiology of COPD, the author argues that several new targets have been identified to treat the disease. Although mediator antagonists tested in patients with COPD have so far been disappointing, CXC receptor-2 antagonists that block pulmonary neutrophil and monocyte recruitment may be more promising. Broad-spectrum antiinflammatory drugs, including inhibitors of the enzymes phosphodiesterase 4, p38 mitogen-activated protein kinase, nuclear factor-kappaB, and phosphoinositide-3-kinase-gamma, may be more effective. The author argues that the most promising approach is the reversal of corticosteroid resistance through increasing histone deacetylase-2 activity. This might be achieved by theophylline-like drugs, more effective antioxidants, and nonantibiotic macrolide agents.

Barnes PJ. Mediators of chronic obstructive pulmonary disease. Pharmacol Rev 2004; 56:515–548

This is a very long and comprehensive review of the inflammatory cascade of COPD. For those who are interested in a more in-depth review of this topic, this comprehensive discussion will be most helpful.

Berry JK, Baum C. Reversal of chronic obstructive pulmonary disease-associated weight loss: are there pharmacological treatment options? Drugs 2004; 64:1041–1052

This is a review of the current approaches to weight loss in COPD. To date, interventional studies that have looked at newer pharmacotherapy such as growth hormone and anabolic steroids have been disappointments. Currently, early identification of patients at risk, aggressive nutritional supplementation, and a vigorous exercise program has demonstrated the greatest benefit.

Bhowmik A, Seemungal TAR, Sapsford RJ, et al. Relation of sputum inflammatory markers to symptoms and lung function changes in COPD exacerbations. Thorax 2000; 55:114–120

Patients with multiple exacerbations of COPD have higher mean stable sputum levels of IL-6 and IL-8 than those with few exacerbations. During acute exacerbations, cytokine levels correlate with sputum cells counts of inflammatory cells. The cell counts and cytokine levels do not predict the size and duration of lung function changes in the exacerbation.

Biskobing DM. COPD and osteoporosis. Chest 2002; 121:609–620

This review discusses the problem of osteoporosis in advanced COPD. Bone loss factors are diverse and include smoking, vitamin D deficiency, low mass index, hypogonadism, sedentary lifestyle, and the use of corticosteroids. Effective strategies to prevent bone loss including calcium and vitamin D are discussed. The use of calcitonin and bisphosphonate administration is also reviewed. Because up to 60% of patients with advanced COPD have osteoporosis, the causes and approaches to osteoporosis in COPD are extremely important.

Calverley PM, Anderson JA, Celli B, et al. Salmeterol and fluticasone propionate and survival in chronic obstructive pulmonary disease. N Engl J Med 2007; 22:775–789

The results of the Towards a Revolution in COPD *Health (TORCH) trial were published in early 2007. This was a randomized, double-blind trial comparing salmeterol plus fluticasone propionate at a dose of 500 μg twice daily (combination regimen), administered with a single inhaler, compared with placebo, salmeterol alone, or fluticasone propionate alone for a period of 3 years. The reduction in death from all causes (the primary outcome) among patients with COPD in the combination-therapy group did not reach the predetermined level of statistical significance. There were significant benefits in all other outcomes among these patients. When compared with placebo, the combination regimen reduced the annual rate of exacerbations from 1.13 to 0.85 and improved health status and spirometric values ($p < 0.001$ for all comparisons with placebo). There was no difference in the incidence of ocular or bone side effects.*

Celli BR, Cote CG, Marin JM, et al. The body-mass index, airflow obstruction, dyspnea, and exercise capacity index in chronic obstructive pulmonary disease. N Engl J Med 2004; 350:1005–1012

Traditionally the FEV_1 has been used as the main indicator of clinical outcomes including rate of mortality in COPD. This article explores other predictors for the risk of death in COPD. These predictors, BMI (B), the degree of airflow obstruction (O), dyspnea (D), and exercise capacity (E), offer an index of severity, the BODE index, that offers a superior grading system for COPD mortality.

Celli BR, MacNee W, Agusti A, et al. Standards for the diagnosis and treatment of patients with COPD: a summary of the ATS/ERS position paper. Eur Respir J 2004; 23:932–946

This is the latest American Thoracic Society statement and position paper on COPD. It is a comprehensive review of all aspects of the disease and a follow-up to the 1995 statement. Classification of disease and recommendations are similar to the GOLD international guidelines.

Celli BR, Thomas NE, Anderson JA, et al. Effect of pharmacotherapy on rate of decline of lung function in chronic obstructive pulmonary disease: results from the TORCH study. Am J Respir Crit Care Med 2008; 178:322–323

The primary outcome of the TORCH trial, death from any cause, did not reach statistical significance ($p = 0.052$; see aforementioned Calverley PM, et al. N Engl J Med 2007; 356:775). Before treatment unblinding of the TORCH data, the authors of this Celli study tested the hypothesis that pharmacotherapy would modify the rate of decline of postbronchodilator FEV_1 compared with placebo and explored factors that could affect this decline. The primary outcome was the rate of postbronchodilator FEV_1 decline. The rate of decline of FEV_1 was slowest in patients on combination therapy (39 mL/yr), fastest in those randomized to the placebo arm (55 mL/yr) and intermediate (42 mL/yr) in both single treatment arms. A slower rate of decrease in absolute milliliters per year was observed in former smokers, females, patients ≥ 65 years, and those with $FEV_1 < 30\%$ predicted and patients with a BMI ≥ 25.

The decline in FEV_1 has been accepted as a key marker for progression of COPD. The decline in postbronchodilator FEV_1 in this study was 55 mL/yr, similar to that seen in the Lung Health Study 1 (−52 mL), Lung Health Study 2 (−47 mL), Bronchitis Randomized on NAC Cost-Utility (−54 mL), and Inhaled Steroids in Obstructive Lung Disease studies (−59 mL). Before this study, smoking cessation was the only intervention conclusively shown to alter the rate of decline in FEV_1 with COPD. In this study, there was an association between exacerbation frequency and FEV_1 decline, supporting previous observations. However, in patients who had no exacerbations during the study, the rate of decline was significantly faster in the placebo group compared with active treatments (56 mL/yr vs 27−31 mL/yr), which suggests that the effect of treatment on exacerbations was not the sole mechanism responsible for the reduced rate of decline with active treatment. The authors suggest that maintenance of airway patency and reduction in hyperinflation, improvements in mucociliary clearance, or decreases in airway inflammation may contribute singly or together to *produce the observed functional changes. Further studies are needed to determine the mechanisms for the lung function improvements shown by TORCH.*

Chung KF, Adcock IM. Multifaceted mechanisms in COPD: inflammation, immunity, and tissue repair and destruction. Eur Respir J 2008; 31:1334–1356

The mechanisms of COPD are numerous and complex. They are discussed in the excellent review. The authors suggest that COPD severity and clinical phenotyping needs to be correlated with cellular and pathological processes. Small airways obstruction and emphysema are associated with cellular inflammation and structural remodeling. Other features include apoptosis as well as proliferation of cells and both tissue repair and lack of tissue repair. Metalloprotease release, together with that of apoptotic factors, may underlie the emphysema and, conversely, fibrosis of the small airways may be accounted for by the effects of growth factor activation. In advanced disease, they suggest that influential factors include the development of autoimmunity, with activation of dendritic cells and T-helper cells. An inability of macrophages to ingest apoptosed cells and bacteria may exacerbate inflammatory responses. A discussion of how systemic inflammation may reflect the effect of cigarette smoke on nonpulmonary cells.

Clini EM, Ambrosino, N. Nonpharmacologic treatment and relief of symptoms in COPD. Eur Respir J 2008; 31:1114–1124

An excellent review of the nonpharmacologic therapies available to the COPD patient, including pulmonary rehabilitation, long-term oxygen therapy, surgery, and noninvasive ventilation strategies.

Connors AF Jr, Dawson NV, Thomas C, et al. Outcomes following acute exacerbation of severe chronic obstructive lung disease. Am J Respir Crit Care Med 1996; 154:959–967

This is another landmark study from the Study to Understand Prognoses and Preferences for Outcomes and Risks of Treatments (SUPPORT) group. This five-center study described the outcomes of patients hospitalized with an acute exacerbation of hypercarbic (>55 mm Hg) COPD. The report shows that only 11% of the patients died during their hospital stay; however, the 60-day, 180-day, 1-year, and 2-year rates of mortality were extremely high (20%, 33%, 43%, and 49%, respectively). The mean cost of hospital stay was $7,100. After discharge, there was a considerably high readmission rate. During the next 6 months, almost half the patients were readmitted at least once. Some of the patients were readmitted several times. At 6 months, only 26% were both alive and well and able to report a good, very good, or excellent quality of life.

Eller J, Ede A, Schaberg T, et al. Infective exacerbations of chronic bronchitis: relation between bacteriologic etiology and lung function. Chest 1998; 113:1542–1548

This important paper looked at colonization of the airways of patients with severe COPD. It determined that there was a correlation between deterioration of lung function (FEV_1) and the bacteria isolated from patients with infected exacerbations of COPD. During an acute exacerbation, Enterobacteriaceae and Pseudomonas sp were the predominant bacteria in patients with an FEV_1 <35% of the predicted value.

Fabbri LM, Romagnoli M, Corbetta L, et al. Differences in airway inflammation in patients with fixed airflow obstruction due to asthma or chronic obstructive pulmonary disease. Am J Respir Crit Care Med 2003; 167:418–424

This article explores the differences in airway inflammation in a cohort of older patients (age 65) with fixed airflow obstruction caused by asthma vs COPD. Subjects with asthma had significantly more eosinophils in peripheral blood, sputum, BAL, and airway mucosa. There were also greater $CD4^+/CD8^+$ ratios of T cells in the airway mucosa and a thicker basement membrane in the asthmatic subjects. Asthmatics had greater diffusing capacities, residual volumes, and exhaled nitric oxide levels. High-resolution CT scan also differentiates the two conditions because patients with COPD had a greater emphysema score. The authors believe that older subjects with fixed airway obstruction should be differentiated into those with a history of asthma and those with distinct features of COPD. Although these distinctions are important from a research point of view, the differentiation may, at times, be impractical because of the high expense of the testing, lack of availability of these tests, and finally the fact that the tests are not always discriminatory between the two diseases.

Ferguson GT, Funck-Brentano C, Fischer T, et al. Cardiovascular safety of salmeterol in COPD. Chest 2003; 123:1817–1824

This study evaluated the cardiovascular safety of salmeterol from a pooled analysis of safety data from 17 studies. The incidence of adverse cardiovascular events was no different from placebo. The incidence increased with age and concurrent cardiovascular condition. There were no episodes of sustained ventricular tachycardia.

Fletcher C, Peto R. The natural history of chronic airflow obstruction. BMJ 1977; 1:1645–1648

This is a classic article. It is a study of London working men showing that the FEV_1 gradually decrease over the course of a lifetime in all nonsmokers. The same occurs in most smokers. Nonsmokers and most smokers never develop clinically significant airflow obstruction. In susceptible smoking people, *irreversible obstructive changes occur. These changes may lead to a rapid rate of loss of* FEV_1 *and high rates of morbidity and mortality. If the susceptible group stopped smoking, their rate of decrease returned to the normal decrease seen with aging.*

Gan WQ, Man SFP, Senthilselvan A, et al. Association between chronic obstructive pulmonary disease and systemic inflammation: a systematic review and a meta-analysis. Thorax 2004; 59:574–580

This review examines the association between COPD and systemic inflammation. Markers of systemic inflammation including C-reactive protein, fibrinogen levels, circulating leukocytes, and TNF-α levels are elevated in patients with COPD.

Garcia-Aymerich J, Monso E, Marrades RM, et al. Risk factors for hospitalization for a chronic obstructive pulmonary disease exacerbation. Am J Respir Crit Care Med 2001; 164:1002–1007

This group measured the risk factors for exacerbations of COPD by using a case-control approach. Multivariate logistic regression showed that low FEV_1*, underprescription of oxygen therapy, and current smoking were all factors that would predict frequent exacerbation rates.*

Hanania NA, Darken P, Horstman D, et al. The efficacy and safety of fluticasone propionate (250 μg)/salmeterol (50 μg) combined in the diskus inhaler for the treatment of COPD. Chest 2003; 124:834–843

These investigators show that treatment with fluticasone and salmeterol delivered by the diskus device and given twice daily improved lung function when compared with either of these two components alone. Similar studies have also shown improvements in quality of life indices and dyspnea score.

Hogg JC, Chu F, Utokaparch S, et al. The nature of small-airway obstruction in chronic obstructive pulmonary disease. N Engl J Med 2004; 350:2645–2653

Tissue from surgically resected lung specimens from patients with COPD was evaluated for signs of inflammation. Patients were categorized into GOLD stages of COPD. The progression of COPD from GOLD stage 0 to GOLD stage 4 was strongly associated with an increase in the volume of the tissue in the wall and the accumulation of inflammatory mucus exudates in the lumen of the small airways. As COPD severity progressed, the percentage of the airways that contained polymorphonuclear neutrophils, macrophages, CD4 cells, CD8 cells, B cells, and lymphoid aggregate increased.

Hogg JC, Senior RM. Chronic obstructive pulmonary disease 2: pathology and biochemistry of emphysema. Thorax 2002; 57:830–834

This article offers an excellent review of the pathogenesis of emphysema and particularly factors responsible for alveolar septal destruction in emphysema.

Hogg JC. Pathophysiology of airflow limitation in chronic obstructive pulmonary disease. Lancet 2004; 364:709–721

This review article introduces the topic of innate and adaptive immune responses to inhaled irritants such as cigarette smoke. There is an excellent discussion of the pathology of COPD with specific reference to the changes of emphysema and chronic bronchitis. This is an excellent tutorial on the pathophysiology of COPD.

Ionescu AA, Schoon E. Osteoporosis in chronic obstructive pulmonary disease. Eur Respir J Suppl. 2003; 46:64s–75s

Osteoporosis is one of the systemic effects associated with COPD. Potential risk factors of osteoporosis may be attributable to lifestyle, genetics, treatment with corticosteroids, endocrine abnormalities, or the impairment of the body composition and peripheral skeletal muscles. Evidence for the possible contribution of such factors is reviewed in this article.

Johnson M, Rennard S. Alternative mechanisms for long-acting (beta)2-adrenergic agonists in COPD. Chest 2001; 120:258–270

This is a review of the nonbronchodilating effects of long-acting agonists. These agents have important effects on the adherence of bacteria to the epithelium, capillary leak, mucus clearance, and inflammatory mediator release. It offers a reason for use of long-acting beta agonists in addition to their bronchodilating properties.

Jones AP, Rowe BH. Bronchopulmonary hygiene physical therapy for chronic obstructive pulmonary disease and bronchiectasis. Cochrane Database Syst Rev 2002; (2):CD000045

This review showed that there is not enough evidence to support or refute the use of bronchial hygiene physical therapy in people with COPD. The evidence-based report on acute exacerbation of COPD presented in Chest in 2001 clearly demonstrated that chest physiotherapy has no role in the acute exacerbation of COPD.

Kanner RE, Anthonisen NR, Connett JE. Lower respiratory illnesses promote FEV_1 decline in current smokers but not ex-smokers with mild chronic obstructive pulmonary disease. Am J Respir Crit Care Med 2001; 164:358–364

This important work is from the Lung Health Study showing that patients with lower-respiratory tract infections who are continuous smokers had greater decreases of lung function than the smokers who had no lower-respiratory tract infections.

Keenan SP, Sinuff T, Cook DJ, et al. Which patients with acute exacerbation of chronic obstructive pulmonary disease benefit from noninvasive positive-pressure ventilation? A systematic review of the literature. Ann Intern Med 2003; 138:861–870

This study examined selected randomized control trials examining the effects of noninvasive NPPV in patients with an acute exacerbation of COPD. The addition of this modality to standard care was shown in this systematic review to decrease the rate of endotracheal intubation by 28%, length of hospital stay 4.5 days, and reduce mortality rate by 10%. The subgroup analysis shows that the beneficial effects occurred only in patients with severe exacerbations (pH < 7.30) and not in those with milder exacerbation).

Kierszniewska-Stepien D, Pietras T, Gorski P, et al. Serum vascular endothelial growth factor and its receptor level in patients with chronic obstructive pulmonary disease. Eur Cytokine Netw 2006; 17:75–79

The authors investigated a cytokine VEGF known to be involved in angiogenesis in the serum of 20 patients with mild COPD and 10 patients with very severe COPD. They found that the concentration of VEGF and its soluble receptor (sVEGF R1) in the serum of patients with mild COPD was significantly greater (665.31 ± 102.20 pg/mL) in comparison to the control group (318.94 ± 51.40 pg/mL; $p < 0.05$), and there was a strong negative correlation with FEV1 ($r = -0.859$; $p < 0.001$). These results suggest that VEGF and sVEGF R1 receptor are involved in the development of abnormal pulmonary vascular remodeling in patients with COPD.

Kolodziej MA, Jensen L, Rowe B, et al. Systematic review of noninvasive positive pressure ventilation in severe stable COPD. Eur Respir J 2007; 30:293–306

The authors present a systematic review of the effectiveness of bilevel NPPV in the management of chronic respiratory failure attributable to severe stable COPD. Randomized controlled trials did not find improved gas exchange; lung hyperinflation and diaphragmatic work of breathing were reduced in a nonrandomized subset of patients. There is little evidence to support the use of NPPV in the management of stable hypercarbic patients with COPD.

Lacasse Y, Goldstein R, Lasserson TJ, et al. Pulmonary rehabilitation for chronic obstructive pulmonary disease. Cochrane Database Syst Rev 2006; (4):CD003793

This evidence-based review concludes that pulmonary rehabilitation relieves dyspnea and fatigue, improves emotional function, and enhances patients' sense of control over their condition. These improvements are moderately large and clinically significant.

Leuchte HH, Baumgartner RA, El Nounou M, et al. Brain natriuretic peptide is a prognostic parameter in chronic lung disease. Am J Respir Crit Care Med 2006; 173:744–750

Natruretic peptides are the major hormones of the natruretic peptide system that is highly activated in patients with both left and right heart failure. This study evaluated circulating BNP levels as a parameter for the presence and severity of pulmonary hypertension in patients with chronic lung disease. Patients with significant pulmonary hypertension had elevated BNP levels and a lower 6-min walk distance. The authors showed that an elevated BNP is a risk factor for death that is independent of lung functional impairment or hypoxemia in patients with COPD. Serum BNP can be used as a prognostic marker as well as a screening tool for significant pulmonary hypertension in patients with chronic obstructive lung disease.

Liesching T, Kwok H, Hill NS. Acute applications of noninvasive positive pressure ventilation. Chest 2003; 124:699–713

This is an excellent review of the use of NPPV to treat the acute exacerbation of COPD.

Mallia P, Johnston SL. How viral infections cause exacerbation of airway diseases. Chest 2006; 130:1203–1210

During the last decade, studies have established that respiratory viruses are a major cause of exacerbations of asthma and COPD and considerably create an impact on rates of morbidity, mortality, and health-care costs. The most prevalent viruses detected during exacerbations are the rhinoviruses. This article discusses the mechanisms of virus-induced exacerbations of airway diseases. Exacerbations are associated with increased airway inflammation in patients with both asthma and COPD. The authors conclude that identifying the key inflammatory mediators involved in exacerbations holds the promise of developing diagnostic and prognostic markers of exacerbation. In addition, such studies can identify new therapeutic targets for the development of novel drugs for the prevention and treatment of exacerbations.

Mannino DM, Gagnon RC, Petty TL, et al. Obstructive lung disease and low lung function in adults in the United States: data from the National Health and Nutrition Examination Survey, 1988–1994. Arch Intern Med 2000; 160:1683–1689

This NHANES III data suggests that 12.5% of current smokers and 9.4% of former smokers had evidence of obstructive lung disease. Sixty-three percent of patients with low lung function had no previous or current reported diagnosis of any obstructive lung disease.

McEvoy CE, Ensrud KE, Bender E, et al. Association between corticosteroid use and vertebral fractures in older men with chronic obstructive pulmonary disease. Am J Respir Crit Care Med 1998; 157:704–709

This is an important reminder that vertebral fractures are common in older men with COPD, and the likelihood of these fractures is greatest in men who continuously use systemic steroids.

McKay SE, Howie CA, Thomson AH, et al. Value of theophylline treatment in patients handicapped by chronic obstructive lung disease. Thorax 1993; 48:227–232

This older article reminds us of the advantages of using theophylline for COPD, including improvements in peak flow, trapped gas volumes, vital capacity, distance walk, breathlessness in everyday activities, and fatigue.

Meyers BF, Patterson GA. Chronic obstructive pulmonary disease 10: bullectomy, lung volume reduction surgery, and transplantation for patients with chronic obstructive pulmonary disease. Thorax 2003; 58:634–638

This is an excellent review of current surgical procedures for COPD, giving the indications for bullectomy and transplantation. The American view of lung volume reduction surgery is reported in other articles related to the NETT trial.

National Emphysema Treatment Trial Research Group. Patients at high risk of death after lung volume-reduction surgery. N Engl J Med 2001; 345:1075–1083

This is an early report from the NETT Research Group warning that lung volume-reduction surgery in patients who have a very low FEV_1*, homogenous emphysema, or a very low carbon monoxide diffusing capacity are at very high risk of death after surgery.*

National Emphysema Treatment Trial Research Group. A randomized trial comparing lung-volume-reduction surgery with medical therapy for severe emphysema. N Engl J Med 2003; 348:2059–2073

These are the long-awaited results of the NETT. It identified those patients that were most likely to benefit from lung volume-reduction surgery. Patients with upper-lobe emphysema and very poor exercise tolerance are those who had the best outcomes. After surgery, rate of mortality was lower, exercise capacity higher, and overall quality of life improved compared withthe medically treated group.

NHLBI/WHO workshop report. Global strategy for the diagnosis, management, and prevention of chronic obstructive pulmonary disease. Available at: http://www.goldcopd.com. Accessed May 7, 2009

This is the World Health Organization/NHLBI internal standard guideline for the prevention, recognition, and treatment of COPD.

Niewoehner DE, Erbland ML, Deupree RH, et al. Effect of systemic glucocorticoids on exacerbations of chronic obstructive pulmonary disease. N Engl J Med 1999; 340:1941–1947

This article received a great deal of press. It showed that treatment with systemic corticosteroids results in moderate improvement in clinical outcomes among patients hospitalized for exacerbations of COPD. The maximum benefit of corticosteroids, however, was seen only in the first 2 weeks after hospitalization. Hyperglycemia was a common problem.

Nonoyama ML, Brooks D, Guyatt GH, et al. Effect of oxygen on health quality of life in patients with chronic obstructive pulmonary disease. Am J Respir Crit Care Med 2007; 176:343–349

Long-term use of supplemental oxygen has been shown to be beneficial in patients with COPD and resting hypoxemia, and it is now standard of care. Short-term ambulatory oxygen for COPD patients who meet the hypoxemia criteria only during exercise has offered some improvement in exercise performance, but it is not clear whether the long-term use of oxygen in such patients would be clinically beneficial and worth the expense. Previous randomized controlled trials to answer this question have produced mixed results. The current study was performed as a series of individual randomized controlled trials (n-of-1) to measure the effect of oxygen in patients with COPD who do not meet the criteria of resting hypoxemia. The use of oxygen improved patients' 5-min walk test results (427 vs 412 steps, $p = 0.04$*), but quality of life questionnaires did not show any difference between the oxygen and placebo. However, 2 of the 27 patients showed consistent improvement of dyspnea measured on the Chronic Respiratory Questionnaire. This study does not support the long-term application of oxygen to patients with exercise-induced hypoxemia and normal resting oxygen levels. The costs of such therapy are great to the health-care system, and the therapy results in an imposition and discomfort to the patient. These are compelling reasons why this practice should be discouraged for most patients.*

O'Donnell DE, Hernandez P, Aaron S, et al. Canadian Thoracic Society COPD guidelines: summary of highlights for family doctors. Can Respir J 2003; 10: 183–185

This is a review of the Canadian guidelines for COPD.

O'Donnell DE, Revill SM, Webb KA. Dynamic hyperinflation and exercise intolerance in chronic obstructive pulmonary disease. Am J Respir Crit Care Med 2001; 164:770–777

This article looked at the role of dynamic hyperinflation and exercise limitation in COPD. During exercise, 80% of the patients showed significant dynamic hyperinflation above resting values. The extent of dynamic hyperinflation correlated best with the resting inspiratory capacity. Because dynamic hyperinflation curtails the tidal volume response to exercise, it was thought that this was an important factor in exercise limitation in response to increasing metabolic demands.

Patel IS, Seemungal TAR, Wilks M, et al. Relationship between bacterial colonisation and the frequency, character, and severity of COPD exacerbations. Thorax 2002; 57:759–764

This study shows a relationship between lower bacterial colonization and exacerbation frequency in COPD.

Plant PK, Owen JL, Elliott MW. Early use of non-invasive ventilation for acute exacerbations of chronic obstructive pulmonary disease on general respiratory wards: a multicentre randomised controlled trial. Lancet 2000; 355:1931–1935

This large trial of BiPAP for the treatment of the acute exacerbation of COPD was performed on a general respiratory ward. Patients were mild-to-moderately acidotic (pH 7.25 to 7.25) and were received standard therapy or the addition of NPPV. The use of NPPV significantly reduced the need for intubation (27% vs 15%) and inpatient rate of mortality (20% vs 10%). NPPV led to more rapid improvement of pH during the first hour and a greater decrease in the respiratory rate and the duration of breathlessness.

Puhan MA, Vollenweider D, Latshang T, et al. Exacerbations of chronic obstructive pulmonary disease: when are antibiotics indicated? A systematic review. Respir Res 2007; 8:30

This review discusses the unresolved debate about adequate prescription of antibiotics for patients suffering from exacerbations of COPD. The study analyzed randomized controlled trials investigating the clinical benefit of antibiotics for COPD exacerbation. Antibiotics did not reduce treatment failures in outpatients with mild to moderate exacerbations (pooled OR 1.09, 95% CI 0.75 to 1.59, I2 = 18%). Inpatients with severe exacerbations had a substantial benefit on treatment failure rates (pooled OR of 0.25, 95% CI 0.16 to 0.39, I2 = 0%; number-needed to treat of 4, 95% CI 3 to 5) and on mortality (pooled OR of 0.20, 95% CI 0.06 to 0.62, I2 = 0%; number needed to treat of 14, 95% CI 12 to 30). The authors concluded that antibiotics effectively reduce treatment failure and mortality rates in COPD patients with severe exacerbations. For patients with mild-to-moderate exacerbations, antibiotics may not be generally indicated and the authors felt that further research is needed to guide antibiotic prescription in these patients.

Qui Y, Zhu J, Bandi V, et al. Biopsy neutrophilia, neutrophil chemokine and receptor gene expression in severe exacerbations of chronic obstructive pulmonary disease. Am J Respir Crit Care Med 2003; 168:968–975

In this study, bronchial biopsies were performed on patients intubated for an acute exacerbation of COPD and those with stable COPD. The acute exacerbation is associated with an increase in IL-8 and marked airway neutrophilia.

Rana JS, Mittleman MA, Sheikh J, et al. Chronic obstructive pulmonary disease, asthma, and risk of type 2 diabetes in women. Diabetes Care 2004; 27:2478–2484

Inflammation plays a key role in COPD and asthma. Increasing evidence points toward a role of inflammation in the pathogenesis of type 2 diabetes The authors investigated the incidence of type 2 diabetes in patients with COPD by using data from the The Nurses' Health Study. The risk of type 2 diabetes was significantly greater for patients with COPD than those without (multivariate relative risk 1.8, 95% confidence interval [95% CI] 1.1 to 2.8). By contrast, the risk of type 2 diabetes among asthmatic patients was not increased (1.0, 0.8 to 1.2).

Reed CE. The natural history of asthma in adults: the problem of irreversibility. J Allergy Clin Immunol 1999; 103:539–547

This is an important article because it documents how many elderly asthmatic patients develop irreversible obstructive changes on their spirogram despite apparently adequate therapy. It suggests that chronic asthma does lead to chronic nonreversible airflow obstruction (COPD).

Rennard SI. Clinical approach to patients with chronic obstructive pulmonary disease and cardiovascular disease. Proc Am Thorac Soc 2005; 2:94–100

This review discusses the interactions between cardiac and pulmonary disease.

Ries AL, Bauldoff GL, Carlin BW, et al. Pulmonary rehabilitation: joint ACCP/AACVPR evidence-based clinical practice guidelines [review]. Chest 2007; (5 Suppl)131:4S–42S

This document provides a systematic, evidence-based review of the pulmonary rehabilitation literature that updates the 1997 guidelines published by the American College of Chest Physicians and the American Association of Cardiovascular and Pulmonary Rehabilitation. The new evidence strengthens the previous recommendations supporting the benefits of lower- and upper-extremity exercise training and improvements in dyspnea and health-related quality-of-life outcomes of pulmonary rehabilitation. Additional evidence supports improvements in health-care utilization and psychosocial outcomes. There are few additional data about survival. Some new evidence indicates that longer term rehabilitation, maintenance strategies following rehabilitation, and the incorporation of education and strength training in pulmonary rehabilitation are beneficial. Current evidence does not support the routine use of inspiratory muscle training, anabolic drugs, or nutritional supplementation in pulmonary rehabilitation. Evidence does support the use of supplemental oxygen therapy for patients with severe hypoxemia at rest or with exercise. Noninvasive ventilation may be helpful for selected patients with advanced COPD. Finally, pulmonary rehabilitation appears to benefit patients with chronic lung diseases other than COPD.

Roede BM, Bresser P, Bindels PJ, et al Antibiotic treatment is associated with reduced risk of a subsequent exacerbation in obstructive lung disease: an historical population based cohort study. Thorax 2008; 63:968–973

The risk of a subsequent exacerbation after treatment of an exacerbation with oral corticosteroids without (OS) or with (OSA) antibiotics was evaluated in a historical population based cohort study comprising patients using maintenance medication for obstructive lung disease. Treatment with antibiotics in addition to oral corticosteroids was associated with a longer time to the next exacerbation, and a decreased risk of developing a new exacerbation.

Rutschmann OT, Cornuz J, Poletti PA, et al. Should pulmonary embolism be suspected in exacerbation of chronic obstructive pulmonary disease. Thorax 2007; 62:121–125

The diagnosis of acute PE in patients with COPD is often difficult to make especially during an acute exacerbation of COPD when symptoms of the two conditions may be indistinguishable. The prevalence of PE in postmortem series of patients with COPD is extremely high, ranging from 28 to 51%, and one recent study (Ann Intern Med 2006; 144:390−396) showed a 25% prevalence of PE in a group of patients admitted to the hospital for a severe exacerbation of COPD, may not be generalized as patients in this study were excluded if they had a potential infection. This study by Rutschmann et al included consecutive patients admitted to the emergency department with a COPD exacerbation. Pulmonary embolism was excluded on the basis of a normal (< 500 μg/mL) d-dimer test and negative diagnostic imaging studies. 6.2% of the 48 patients who had a clinical suspicion of pulmonary embolism were discovered to have PE and in only 1.3% of the remaining patients who had no clinical suspicion. This study showed that the prevalence of suspected pulmonary embolism in patients presenting with a COPD exacerbation is very low and routine investigation for PE in this group is not warranted.

Saetta M, Turato G, Maestrelli P, et al. Cellular and structural bases of chronic obstructive pulmonary disease. Am J Respir Crit Care Med 2001; 163:1304–1309

This review article discusses the two pathological hallmarks of COPD: (1) inflammation of the peripheral airways and (2) destruction of the lung parenchyma (emphysema). In "normal" smokers, studies have shown that T lymphocytes and macrophages infiltrate the airway wall of the central airways, and that neutrophils in the airway wall are increased in the airway lumen. In the peripheral airways, the cellular infiltrate in the airway consists of mononuclear cells and macrophages. The peripheral airways are the major site of increased airway resistance. In "normal" smokers there is no sign of parenchymal destruction. In smokers with established COPD, there is a further increase in macrophages and T lymphocytes in the airway walls. Peripheral airways show more inflammatory changes of all cells, including neutrophils in severe disease. There is evidence of centriacinar and panacinar emphysema and some fibrosis in the lung parenchyma. In severe COPD, airflow limitation progressively worsens, and neutrophils in the bronchial wall increase. Their increase is correlated with the degree of airflow limitation. Data indicate that when emphysema is severe, loss of elastic recoil assumes overwhelming importance as a mechanism of airflow limitation, thus masking the effects of peripheral airway abnormalities.

Seemungal T, Harper-Owen R, Bhowmik A, et al. Respiratory viruses, symptoms, and inflammatory markers in acute exacerbations of stable acute exacerbations of chronic obstructive pulmonary disease. Am J Respir Crit Care Med 2001; 164:1618–1623

This study prospectively investigated the association of the exacerbation of COPD in viral infection. Polymerase chain reaction methodology was used to detect viral infection. The authors found that 64% of exacerbations were associated with a cold occurring up to 18 days before the exacerbation. The authors found that respiratory virus infections are associated with more severe and frequent exacerbations and may cause chronic infection in COPD.

Seemungal TA, Wilkinson TM, Hurst JR, et al. Long-term erythromycin therapy is associated with decreased chronic obstructive pulmonary disease exacerbations. Am J Respir Crit Care Med 2008; 178:1139–1147

Long-term erythromycin therapy is associated with decreased exacerbations of COPD. There has been much interest in the use of prophylactic antibiotics for the prevention of exacerbations of COPD. The results of a number of older studies were disappointing, but this study is more optimistic. Macrolides have airway antiinflammatory actions as well as antimicrobial properties, and erythromycin was chosen to determine whether regular therapy with macrolides reduces exacerbation frequency. Erythromycin was administered at 250 mg bid to patients with COPD over the course of 12 months, with the primary outcome variable being the number of moderate and/or severe exacerbations (treated with systemic steroids, treated with antibiotics, or hospitalized). The rate ratio for exacerbations for the macrolide-treated patients compared with placebo-treated patients was 0.648 (95% CI 0.489 to 0.859; p = 0.003), and these *patients had shorter-duration exacerbations compared with placebo-treated patients. There were no differences between the macrolide and placebo arms in terms of stable FEV_1, sputum IL-6, IL-8, myeloperoxidase, bacterial flora, serum C-reactive protein, or serum IL-6 or in changes in these parameters from baseline. The authors concluded that macrolide therapy was associated with a significant reduction in exacerbations compared with placebo.*

Seemungal TAR, Donaldson GC, Bhowmik A, et al. Time course and recovery of exacerbations in patients with chronic obstructive pulmonary disease. Am J Respir Crit Care Med 2000; 161:1608–1618

This group of authors studied a cohort 101 patients with moderately severe COPD (mean FEV_1 42%) during a 2.5-year period. Patients recorded daily morning peak flow rates and changes in respiratory symptoms. Exacerbation rates were followed. Before the onset of exacerbation there was deterioration in symptoms of dyspnea, sore throat, cough, and symptoms of the common cold but not a worsening of lung function. On the day of the attack, peak flow rates did decrease by a mean of 8.6 L/min. The FEV_1 decreased by 24 mL. Recovery of peak flow rates to baseline values was complete in only 72% of exacerbations at day 35. In 7% of exacerbations peak flow rate had not returned to baseline even at 3 months. The authors conclude that symptom changes during an exacerbation of COPD do not closely reflect those of lung function study, but their increase may predict an exacerbation. Recovery is incomplete in a significant proportion of COPD exacerbations.

Seersholm N, Kok-Jensen A. Clinical features and prognosis of lifetime non-smokers with severe α_1-antitrypsin deficiency. Thorax 1998; 53:265–268

This study documented that it is rare for homozygote ZZ AAT--deficient patients to develop COPD if they do not smoke.

Sethi S, Evans N, Grant BJB, et al. New strains of bacteria and exacerbations of chronic obstructive pulmonary disease. N Engl J Med 2002; 347:465–471

These investigators have shown an association between an exacerbation of COPD and the isolation of a new strain of bacterial pathogen. This supports a causative role of bacteria in exacerbations of COPD.

Sethi S. Infectious etiology of acute exacerbations of chronic bronchitis. Chest 2000; 117:3808–3858

This review discusses the role of infection in exacerbations of COPD. Respiratory viruses are associated with approximately 30% of exacerbations of COPD. A typical bacterium, mostly Chlamydia and Mycoplasma sp, have been implicated in <10% of cases. There is emerging evidence that supports the role of bacteria in the exacerbation of COPD. Concomitant infections by more than one infectious pathogen occur in 10 to 20% of patients.

Sevenoaks MJ, Stockley RA. Chronic obstructive pulmonary disease, inflammation and co-morbidity: a common inflammatory phenotype? Respir Res 2006; 7:70–78

A link has been identified between COPD and other systemic diseases such as cardiovascular disease, diabetes, and osteoporosis. These authors discuss how proinflammatory cytokines, in particular TNF-α, may be the driving force behind the disease process. The roles of inflammation and these proinflammatory cytokines may extend beyond the lungs and play a part in the systemic effects of the disease and associated co-morbidities. This article describes the mechanisms involved and proposes a common inflammatory TNF-a phenotype that may, in part, account for the associations.

Sin DD, Anthonisen NR, Soriano JB, et al. Mortality in COPD: role of comorbidities. Eur Respir J 2006; 28:1245–1257

This article reviews the role of comorbidities in the rate of COPD mortality, the putative underlying pathogenic link between chronic obstructive pulmonary disease and comorbid conditions (ie, inflammation), and the tools used to predict the rate of COPD mortality.

Sin DD, Man SF, Marciniuk DD, et al. The effects of fluticasone with or without salmeterol on systemic biomarkers of inflammation in chronic obstructive pulmonary disease. Am J Respir Crit Care Med 2008; 177:1207:1207–1214

The cause of systemic inflammation (as evidenced by biomarkers) is not known, but it has been suggested that it is the result of a "spillover" from inflammation in the lungs. Whether treating lung inflammation can reduce systemic inflammation has not been established. The aim of this randomized, double-blind, multicenter study was to determine whether the inhaled corticosteroid (fluticasone) with or without a long-acting beta agonist (salmeterol) could reduce blood inflammatory markers such as C-reactive protein, the primary outcome, and also IL-6 and SP-D. In this 4-week trial (mean FEV_1 = 48% predicted), neither fluticasone nor the combination therapy caused a significant reduction in C-reactive protein or IL-6, but it did significantly reduce SP-D levels compared with placebo ($p < 0.002$). Health status scores and lung function tests during the trial improved significantly and were related to circulating SP-D levels. The authors concluded that these treatments improved lung-specific but not generalized biomarkers of systemic inflammation.

Sin DD, Man SFP. Why are patients with chronic obstructive pulmonary disease at increased risk of cardiovascular diseases? The potential role of systemic inflammation in chronic obstructive pulmonary disease. Circulation 2003; 107:1514–1519

The NHANES III database was used by these investigators to determine whether C-reactive protein and other systemic inflammatory markers are present in patients with COPD and are associated with cardiac injury. Participants with severe airflow obstruction had a significant increase in markers of inflammation, including circulating leukocyte, platelet, and fibrinogen levels, as well as levels of C-reactive protein. Moderate airflow obstruction had similar but smaller increases. Both moderate and severe airflow obstruction were associated with an increased occurrence of ischemic changes on the electrocardiograms of participants.

Sin DD, McAlister FA, Man SF, et al. Contemporary management of chronic obstructive pulmonary disease: scientific review. JAMA 2003; 290:2301–2312

This is a careful review of the current evidence for the management of outpatients with COPD.

Singh SMD, Amin A, Yoon K, et al Long-term use of inhaled corticosteroids and the risk of pneumonia in chronic obstructive pulmonary disease. Arch Intern Med 2009; 169:219–229

Recent studies have suggested a possible association between pneumonia and the use of inhaled corticosteroids. The authors performed a systematic search to ascertain the risk of pneumonia with long-term inhaled corticosteroid use among patients with COPD. They included randomized controlled trials of any inhaled corticosteroid with at least 24 weeks of follow-up and reporting of pneumonia as an adverse event. Eighteen randomized controlled trials showed that inhaled corticosteroids were associated with a significantly increased risk of any pneumonia (relative risk [RR] 1.60; 95% CI 1.33 to 1.92, $p<.001$m $I^2 = 16\%$) and serious pneumonia (1.71; 1.46 to 1.99, $p<.001$, $I^2 = 0\%$) but without a significantly increased risk of pneumonia-related mortality (1.27, 0.80 to 2.03, $p = .31$, $I^2 = 0\%$) or overall mortality (0.96, 0.86−1.08, $p = 0.51$],$I^2 = 0\%$). The authors concluded that patients with COPD and inhaled corticosteroid use for at least 24 weeks have a significantly increased risk of serious pneumonia without a significantly increased risk of death.

Sobieraj DM, White CM, Coleman CI. Benefits and risks of adjunctive inhaled corticosteroids in chronic obstructive pulmonary disease: a meta-analysis. Clin Ther 2008; 30:1416–1425

The authors of this article conducted a metaanalysis to examine the benefits and risks associated with adjunctive inhaled corticosteroids treatment in patients with severe or very severe COPD. The authors found that the addition of an inhaled corticosteroid to a long-acting β-agonist was associated with a reduced risk for exacerbations but an increased risk for pneumonia and oral candidiasis compared with long-acting bronchodilator monotherapy in this metaanalysis of 9 randomized controlled trials. Although measured patient-perceived health and well-being increased to a statistically significant level, this did not translate into a clinically meaningful level for all patients with combination treatment. A lower risk of study withdrawal was observed in patients administered adjuvant inhaled corticosteroids.

Soriano JB, Visick GT, Muellerova H, et al. Patterns of comorbidities in newly diagnosed COPD and asthma in primary care. Chest 2005; 128:2099–2107

The authors quantified baseline rates of comorbidities in COPD patients and compared them with the risks in the general population. The authors showed that COPD patients are at increased risk for glaucoma, angina, fractures, myocardial infarction, osteoporosis, and respiratory infection when compared with control patients without COPD.

Studer SM, Levy RD, McNeil K, et al. Lung transplant outcomes: a review of survival, graft function, physiology, health-related quality of life and cost-effectiveness. Eur Respir J 2004; 24:674–685

This article reports on the success of lung transplantation that improved over time. There are better long-term survivals and functional outcomes. Despite this success, there are numerous problems and complications that may develop over the life of a lung transplant recipient. Significant improvement for the overall outcomes of lung transplantation will only occur when better methods exist to prevent or effectively treat chronic rejection.

Tashkin DP, Celli B, Senn S, et al; UPLIFT study investigators. A 4-year trial of tiotropium in chronic obstructive pulmonary disease. N Engl J Med 2008; 359:1543–1554

This study was a randomized, double-blind trial comparing 4 years of therapy with either tiotropium or placebo in patients with COPD who were permitted to use all respiratory medications except inhaled anticholinergic drugs. Therapy with tiotropium was associated with improvements in lung function, quality of life, and exacerbations during a 4-year period but did not significantly reduce the rate of decrease in FEV_1.

The α_1-Antitrypsin Deficiency Registry Study Group. Survival and FEV_1 decline in individuals with severe deficiency of α_1-antitrypsin. Am J Respir Crit Care Med 1998; 158:49–59

This is a report from the NHLBI Registry showing that subjects who received augmentation therapy had a lower *rate of mortality. Those with an FEV_1 between 35% and 49% predicted also showed a slowing of the FEV_1 decline.*

van Gestel YR, Hoeks SE, Sin DD, et al. Effect of statin therapy on mortality in patients with peripheral arterial disease and comparison of those with versus without associated chronic obstructive pulmonary disease. Am J Cardiol 2008; 102:192–196

The role of statin therapy in addition to standard treatment for COPD in a topic of intense interest, and the answer to this question will likely be forthcoming in the near future. Statins are widely used therapies to control elevated blood lipids and may show other benefits in patients with greater levels of inflammation, as measured by blood inflammatory markers such as CRP. Systemic inflammation is increased in COPD and has been linked to a number of comorbidities such as peripheral muscle wasting, which in turn plays a role in exercise intolerance. The purpose of this study was to determine whether the administration of a statin, pravastatin, 40 mg per day, was effective in improving exercise capacity in a group of patients with stable COPD and whether baseline levels or changes in CRP levels (measures as high sensitivity-CRP) predicted clinical outcomes. Previous studies have shown an inverse relationship between CRP levels and exercise capacity in patients with COPD. This is the first randomized controlled trial to show that treatment with statin therapy can improve exercise tolerance in patients with COPD, regardless of the cholesterol level attained. The improvement in exercise time and degree of breathlessness was observed in those patients who showed greater levels of inflammation at baseline, evidenced by high hs-CRP levels and also elevated IL-6 levels, and in those with a greater decrease in levels of these inflammatory markers after statin treatment. In this study, as in previous studies, the individual responses of CRP to statin therapy were highly variable. The mechanism proposed for improved exercise tolerance in these COPD patients is that the statins reduced muscle inflammation and hence exercise capacity.

Wedzicha JA, Calverley PMA, Seemungal TA, et al. The prevention of chronic obstructive pulmonary disease exacerbations by salmeterol/fluticasone propionate or tiotropium bromide. Am J Respir Crit Care Med 2008; 177:19–26

Investigating New Standards for Prophylaxis in Reducing Exacerbations is the first large-scale trial to compare the clinical outcomes of two frequently used treatments for COPD. The authors of this study made this comparison during a 2-year treatment period in a multicenter study patients with COPD and an FEV_1 $<50\%$ predicted and reversibility $<10\%$. They found no difference between the two study groups in the primary efficacy end point, exacerbation rates that required treatment with oral corticosteroids and/or antibiotics, or required hospitalization. More patients failed to complete the study with tiotropium (TIO); salmeterol/fluticasone propionate (SFC)—treated patients had a small statistically significant benefit with quality of life scores, an unexpectedly lower death rate (3% vs 6%), and a greater rate of pneumonia. However, exacerbations requiring antibiotics occurred more frequently in patients treated with SFC (SFC, 0.97 per year; TIO, 0.82 per year; $p = 0.028$), but those requiring systemic corticosteroids were less frequent than in the TIO-treated patients (SFC, 0.69 per year; TIO, 0.85 per year; $p = 0.039$). Mortality was significantly lower in the SFC treatment ($p = 0.032$), with an estimated 52% reduction in the risk of on-therapy all-cause mortality. However, because more patients who were administered TIO withdrew from the study, this difference may have led to a healthy survivor effect. A clinical diagnosis of pneumonia was reported in 8% of patients administered SFC and 4% of patients administered TIO, and the hazard ratio for time to reported pneumonia was 1.94 (95% CI 1.19 to 3.17, $p = 0.008$) for SFC compared with TIO over the 2 years.

Wijkstra PJ, Lacasse Y, Guyatt GH, et al. A meta-analysis of nocturnal noninvasive positive pressure ventilation in patients with stable COPD. Chest 2003; 124:337–343

A metaanalysis was conducted to determine whether nocturnal NPPV was helpful to patients with COPD and stable respiratory failure. The authors concluded that this type of ventilatory support did not improve lung function, gas exchange, or sleep efficiency in such patients. Some patients do improve their 6-min walk test results.

Wijkstra PJ, Lacasse Y, Guyatt GH, et al. Nocturnal non-invasive positive pressure ventilation for stable chronic obstructive pulmonary disease. Cochrane Database Syst Rev 2002; (3):CD002878

This evidence-based review by the Cochrane group concludes that randomized controlled trials in stable patients with COPD have not convincingly proven the benefits of NPPV. There was no consistent clinically or statistically significant effect on lung function, gas exchange, respiratory muscle strength, sleep efficiency, or exercise tolerance with this modality. Larger clinical trials would be necessary in the future to approve its usefulness conclusively.

Zielinski J, Tobiasz M, Hawrytkiewicz I, et al. Effects of long-term oxygen therapy on pulmonary hemodynamics in COPD patients: a 6-year prospective study. Chest 1998; 113:65–70
This important article looks at the effects of long-term oxygen therapy in patients with COPD and pulmonary hypertension. It followed patients over the course of 6 years. Pulmonary hypertension showed a small reduction after the first 2 years, followed by a return to initial values and subsequent stabilization over 6 years. The article concluded that long-term stabilization of pulmonary hypertension occurs despite progression of the airflow limitation and room air hypoxemia in these patients.

Notes

Pulmonary Function Testing

Darcy D. Marciniuk, MD, FCCP

Objectives:

- Review the indications, conduct, and interpretation of pulmonary function testing
- Highlight the limitation(s) of various testing methods, and emphasize the value of both laboratory and testing standardization and quality assurance
- Review characteristic pulmonary function test results associated with common respiratory disorders

Key words: interpretation; pulmonary function laboratory; pulmonary function testing; quality assurance; spirometry

The performance and interpretation of pulmonary function testing (PFT) is a defining competency of our specialty, and the PFT laboratory is a fundamental and indispensable resource for the pulmonologist. A thorough understanding of the indications, conduct, interpretation, and limitations of testing is essential. In addition, because our colleagues and patients are dependent on and trust the results derived from the laboratories we supervise, pulmonologists must also be experts in issues related to quality assurance, standardization, and testing procedures in the PFT laboratory. Although these two roles are related, the independent importance of each must be emphasized. In this regard, increasing attention is being focused on mastery of the technical aspects of testing and the laboratory, which will be reviewed in this chapter. A complete review of this topic is beyond the intent of this course and syllabus. Readers wanting more complete information are asked to review the referenced source documents listed at the end of this chapter.

Clinical Indications for PFT

The indications for pulmonary function testing are varied, and they depend on the clinical setting and question(s) to be addressed. Generally accepted clinical indications are listed in Table 1.

Important Considerations for Testing

The Patient

Testing is demanding, and results will be less meaningful in patients who are not physically capable of providing consistent, optimal effort. It is recommended that testing not be performed within 1 month of an acute coronary syndrome or myocardial infarction.[1] Similarly, patients with acute chest, abdominal, or facial pain, as well as in those with confusion or significant dementia, are likely to generate suboptimal test results.

Patient weight (in street clothes and without shoes) and height (without shoes) should be accurately measured and recorded. In patients with kyphoscoliosis or lower-limb amputations, arm span from fingertip to fingertip should be used as an estimate of height (regression equations are available).[2] Alternatively, knee height also can be used for handicapped individuals where arm span is difficult to assess.[3]

Dentures are often best left in place during testing unless they are loose or poorly fitting. It would be prudent for patients to refrain from smoking or undergoing vigorous exercise for 1 h, eating a large meal for 2 h, or consuming alcohol for 4 h before testing.[1]

Table 1. *Clinical Indications for PFT*

- Evaluate symptoms, signs, or abnormal investigations
- Assess and monitor the effect of disease/intervention/exposure on pulmonary function and respiratory symptoms
- Early detection of individuals at risk of pulmonary disease or impairment
- Assess preoperative risk
- Objectively assess impairment
- Understand severity and prognosis

The Laboratory and Equipment

It is essential that unintended factors do not contaminate the results and subsequently lead to misinterpretation regarding the patient, disease, or therapy. These factors are the most overlooked considerations in clinical PFT laboratories today, and a thorough understanding of these issues is especially necessary for PFT laboratory directors. Although specific important issues will be discussed in sections to follow and a number of overall principles deserve highlight, the topic is reviewed in detail elsewhere.[4]

Measurements of temperature and barometric pressure must be actually recorded, and it is also important to ensure accuracy of the instrument used to make those measurements. The time of day should be noted, and serial testing should ideally be made at similar times of the day to minimize variation.

Although the order of testing is not necessarily rigid, the order in a specific laboratory should be kept constant. Consideration should also be given to the effects of bronchodilator administration on lung volume determination, or factors influencing the diffusing capacity (discussed in Table 7). A suggested order for performing lung function tests is noted in Table 2.

Laboratory safety is important. Issues relating to building and general facilities; accident, fire, and evacuation procedures; compressed gas storage and use; electrical safety; and procedures and practices for tending to patient urgencies and emergencies must be addressed. Appropriate procedures must be established, understood, and practiced by all staff.

Infection control measures are also necessary for the protection of patients and staff. Although the risk of infection is small, the potential is real, and the consequences are serious. These risks can be minimized by the following steps:

Table 2. *Suggested Order for Conducting Lung Function Tests**

- Spirometry and flow-volume curves
- Lung volumes
- Bronchodilator administration
- Diffusing capacity
- Repeat spirometry and flow-volume curves

*Adapted from Miller et al.[1]

1. Proper hand-washing should be performed and barrier devices such as gloves should be used.
2. Reuseable mouthpieces, valves, mouthpieces, and manifolds must be appropriately disinfected or sterilized.
3. Disposable equipment, sensors, and devices should be discarded, never reused, even if disinfected or sterilized.
4. Sterilizing and disinfecting techniques should be strictly adhered to and should be established in consultation with the manufacturer's recommendations and local or hospital infection-control divisions.
5. In patients with known or suspected transmissible infectious diseases, additional precautions should be undertaken. These would include:
   (a) the use of equipment solely reserved for use in this clinical setting;
   (b) testing patients at the end of the day to allow for complete spirometry disassembly and disinfection; and
   (c) testing patients in their own rooms or in rooms with enhanced capabilities (*ie*, negative pressure ventilation, etc).

The use of inline disposable filters is controversial. Although some significant differences between measurements with and without filters have been demonstrated, the effects are not considered to be clinically significant, and they do not lead to misinterpretation.[5,6] However, because the benefits of filters have not been clearly identified, their use is not mandatory, particularly if all other precautions are strictly followed. Overall, most laboratories use inline filters, perhaps to reassure patients and staff that their safety and protection are a high priority. It deserves emphasis that the use of inline filters should not be viewed as a shortcut for appropriate infection control, and their use does not eliminate the need for regular cleaning and decontamination of lung function equipment.

Laboratory Personnel

All staff must be appropriately trained to understand the fundamentals of testing, to be familiar with signs and symptoms of common respiratory disease, and to properly execute all aspects of testing. Training requirements vary across regions, and many available opportunities

Table 3. *Evaluation and Feedback for Pulmonary Function Laboratory Technicians**

- Information regarding acceptable maneuvers and nonreproducible tests
- Specific corrective actions the technicians can undertake to improve the quality and number of acceptable maneuvers
- Positive feedback for excellence and good performance
- Feedback regarding system setup and reporting results
- Asking the technician to comment on current laboratory procedures and testing, specifically inquiring about opportunities for improvement.

*Adapted from Miller et al.[1]

for training courses are available. A period of mentorship in the laboratory under the experience of seasoned technicians is a crucial one for new staff. Opportunities for ongoing professional development should be availed to staff, ensuring that training and skills remain current, and upgraded when appropriate. This development is particularly important with alterations to equipment or changes in pulmonary function testing standards. Although manufacturers frequently provide training for new equipment or significant upgrades, laboratories should not solely rely on these methods as a guarantee that technician skills are up-to-date.

The value of continuous in-house feedback and evaluation of laboratory technicians has been validated.[7] This feedback helps to promote the collection of high-quality data, and it also works to ensure that staff remains well motivated and enthusiastic. Appropriate content for regular and formalized feedback to technicians is noted in Table 3.

Medical directors of PFT laboratories require all of the aforementioned attributes and skills, but they are also responsible for all aspects of quality assurance, selection of reference values, and practical operational issues relating to the day-to-day conduct of the laboratory.

Reference Values

The interpretation of PFTs is based on comparisons of data measured in an individual patient with reference values derived from a representative population of healthy subjects. Unlike many physiologic variables, normal values of pulmonary function vary with age, height, sex, and race. Moreover, because the range of normal is considerable (for example 80 to 120% of the predicted value), significant changes in pulmonary function can occur while values still remain within the normal range. These factors serve to complicate the choice of the most appropriate reference value regression equations to use in the clinical laboratory.

In general, a number of observations regarding lung function measurements in the population are known, and include the following:

1. Male patients have larger lung function than female patients.
2. Lung function values plateau when patients are 20 to 35 years of age.[8]
3. FEV_1 decreases approximately 30 mL/yr.
4. Vital capacity decreases, whereas the residual volume increases with age, leaving total lung capacity the same. The diffusing capacity decreases with age.
5. Taller individuals have larger lung volumes and greater maximal flow rates.
6. African-American patients have spirometric values that are lower than white patients of the same age, height, and sex. If predicted values for a healthy population of the same ethnic background are not available, predicted values for white patients should be corrected by 0.88 for African-American, Asian, and East-Indian patients. The FEV_1/FVC ratio should not be corrected for race.

Throughout the years, various reference values have been both developed and recommended, which this has led to uneasiness and, frequently, inappropriate reference value selection. However, a new coordinated recommendation has recently been put forth for the Third National Health and Nutrition Examination Survey reference equations to be used for spirometry in the United States.[9] Specific recommendations for lung volume and diffusing capacity reference values are less pointed (Table 4).[10] From a practical point of view, it is apparent that the discussions and debate regarding reference equations in the pulmonary function laboratory will not end soon. However, there is agreement that the reference equation chosen should reflect a similar age range, sex, and ethnic background of patients in the laboratory, and that all spirometric data should use the same source for reference values.

Although reference values are crucial for the correct first-time interpretation of pulmonary

Table 4. *Reference Values in the PFT Laboratory**

General comments
Predicted values should be obtained from normal subjects with the same anthropometric and ethnic characteristics of the patient being tested
Height and weight should be measured for each patient at each testing
All parameters should be taken from the same reference source when possible
Extrapolation beyond the size and age of the reference population should be avoided when possible
Values below the 5th percentile of the frequency distribution of values from the reference population should be considered as below the lower limit of normal.
Spirometry
In the United States, ethnically appropriate NHANES III reference equations published in 1999 for those patients 8 to 80 years of age are recommended.[10]
Lung volumes
No specific set of reference equations is recommended, however a list of potentially suitable reference equations is available.[9]
Diffusing capacity
No specific set of reference equations is recommended, however a list of potentially suitable reference equations is available.[9]

*Adapted from Pelligrino et al.[9] NHANES III = Third National Health and Nutrition Examination Survey.

function test results, if serial testing is undertaken, comparison with the patient's previous values is more appropriate and meaningful.

Specific values for "normalcy" are controversial, but in general, there is a move toward reporting the normal range in terms of a *lower limit of normal* (LLN; spirometry, lung volumes, diffusing capacity) and an *upper limit of normal* (lung volumes and diffusing capacity). The use of values such as the 80% of predicted as the lower range of normal is useful in some instances, but it does result in many false-positive and false-negative results. It is recommended that the LLN be determined from the fifth percentile (*ie,* mean, 1.96 SD; two-tailed *t* test, $p < 0.05$). In addition, categorizing results as borderline abnormal, if they encroach on the ULN or LLN, is an acceptable clinical concept. Although software is available to readily supply these values, clinical comfort and acceptance with these recommended changes in reporting and interpretation is still evolving. Overall guiding principles for the use of reference values in the PFT laboratory are listed in Table 4.

Spirometry

Spirometry is the most commonly performed pulmonary function test. It is used to measure the exhaled volume of air vs time. Volume or flow may be directly measured, and in many instances, both inhaled and exhaled maneuvers are undertaken. The basic variables of interest are the FVC and FEV_1, which both are expressed at body temperature, ambient pressure saturated with water vapor (BTPS).

Equipment

Basic equipment requirements are a spirometer capable of measuring volume for at least 15 s and at least 8 L, with an accuracy of ±3% or ±0.05 L, whichever is greater, with flows between 0 and 14.0 L/s.[11] Total resistance to airflow, at up to 14 L/s, should be < 1.5 cm H_2O/L/s, including all tubing, filters, and valves. Real-time display of flow vs volume is useful for assessing the magnitude of effort during the initial portion of the maneuver, whereas a volume vs time display provides information during the remainder of the maneuver for determining a satisfactory end of test. The spirometer must be appropriately calibrated at least daily, which establishes the relationship between sensor-determined values for flow or volume and the actual flow or volume. Calibration syringes must have an accuracy of ±0.5% of the full scale (*ie,* ±15 mL for a 3-L syringe). It is also important to ensure that the calibration syringe functions appropriately, and that monthly leak tests are conducted. The syringes themselves should be serviced, recalibrated, and verified on a regular basis. Finally, regular daily checks for system leaks must be undertaken and are easily performed.

More detailed instructions regarding calibration are discussed elsewhere.[4,11]

Testing Procedure

A detailed review of testing procedures is beyond the scope of this Board Review, but in-depth information on the subject is available elsewhere.[4,11] A number of important fundamentals will be highlighted here. There is significant unfamiliarity with assessing the "acceptability" and "repeatability" of spirometry. Inherent in optimal quality control is the acceptability of each individual spirogram, as well as the repeatability of a number of acceptable spirograms, recognizing that an adequate test requires at least three acceptable maneuvers.

Acceptability criteria are met if efforts are free from artifacts (cough, glottis closure, early termination, submaximal effort, leak, or obstructed mouthpiece); they have good starts (extrapolated volume is $<5\%$ of the FVC or 0.15 L, whichever is greater); and they show satisfactory exhalation duration of >6 s (or a plateau in the curve is noted). Within maneuver acceptability criteria are listed in Table 5.

Repeatability criteria are only applied after the acceptability of individual spirograms has been met, as outlined previously. The two largest values (from three acceptable individual spirograms) for both the FEV$_1$ and FVC must be within 0.15 L of each other to achieve repeatability criteria. If FEV$_1$ and FVC repeatability criteria are not achieved, testing may be terminated after a total of eight "acceptable" individual maneuvers have been performed (Table 5) or if the patient cannot or should not continue. Between-maneuver criteria are listed in Table 6.

The largest FVC and the largest FEV$_1$ should be reported after examining all acceptable curves, even if they do not come from the same curve. The "best test" curve should be from the trial with the largest sum of the FEV$_1$ and FVC, and other flow parameters should be derived from this best test curve. These procedures are summarized in Figure 1.

Table 5. *Within-Maneuver Acceptability Criteria for Spirometry**

- Individual spirograms are acceptable if they are free from artifacts (cough during first second of exhalation, glottis closures, early termination, submaximal effort, leak, obstructed mouthpiece)
- Efforts have good starts (extrapolated volume $>5\%$ of FVC or 0.15 L, whichever is greater)
- Efforts show satisfactory exhalation (duration of <6 s, or a plateau in the volume-time curve, or subject cannot/should not continue)

*Adapted from Miller et al.[11]

Table 6. *Between-Maneuver Reproducibility Criteria for Spirometry**

- After three acceptable spirograms have been achieved, testing can be concluded if the two largest values for both the FEV$_1$ and the FVC are within 0.15 L of each other
- After three acceptable spirograms have been achieved, testing is still continued if the two largest values for both the FEV$_1$ and the FVC are not within 0.15 L of each other, until both criteria are met with analysis of additional acceptable spirograms; or until a total of eight tests have been performed; or until the patient cannot/should not continue.
- All satisfactory maneuvers should be saved

*Adapted from Miller et al.[11]

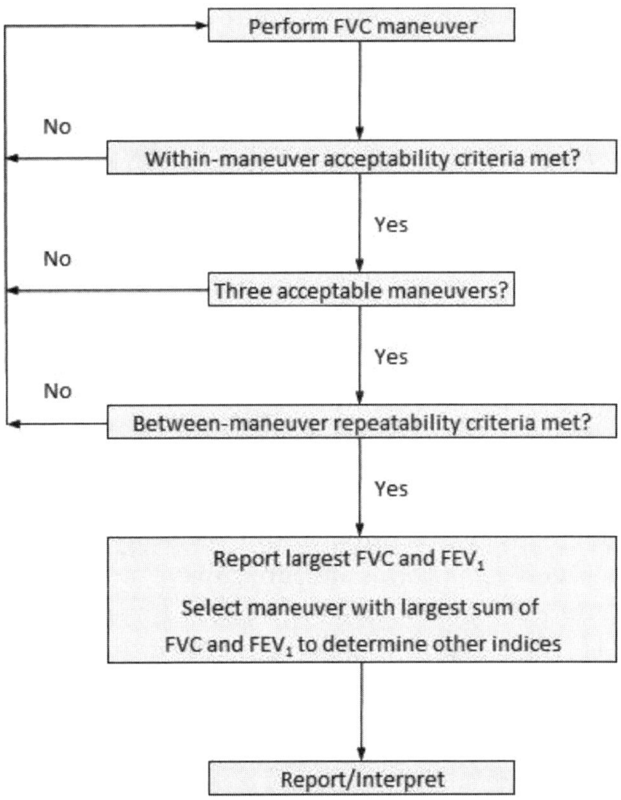

Figure 1. Required steps for performing spirometry.

Maximal Flow-Volume Curve

The maximal flow-volume curve is helpful in quality assurance, in detecting mild airflow obstruction, and in detecting central airway obstruction. For best results, both inspiratory and expiratory loops are obtained. The subject, while tidal breathing at rest, is typically asked to inspire to total lung capacity (TLC) and then expire with maximal force until empty, down to residual volume (RV), followed by a maximum inspiration back up to TLC. Evaluation of the efforts is the same as noted previously, although the inspiratory portion of the curve is often assessed only qualitatively. A volume vs time plot and a flow vs volume plot for the same maneuver are shown in Figure 2. Other measurements also are possible (volume vs time plot shown in Fig. 3, where measured volumes are shown in clear bars and summed capacities are shown in shaded bars).

The vital capacity (VC) is the volume of gas that can be expelled from full inspiration to complete expiration, whereas the FVC is the same measurement when the patient exhales with maximal speed and effort. The VC is occasionally greater than the FVC, the difference being related to the degree of obstruction. The inspiratory capacity (IC) is the volume from a position of passive resting end-tidal expiration (end-expiratory lung volume [EELV]) to full inspiration. The IC has been demonstrated to correlate with lung hyperinflation at rest, and it is responsive to changes in EELV with activity and pharmacologic interventions. These measurements are not forced, but at the same time, exhalation or inspiration should not be unduly slow. To provide absolute placement of these volumes and capacities (and to estimate RV), actual measurement of functional residual capacity (FRC) must be undertaken (see "Lung Volumes" in this chapter for further discussion). As always, a tight seal between the lips and mouthpiece and a comfortable, constant seated position with appropriate height adjustment of the mouthpiece is necessary to ensure validity and repeatability. Unlike other measurements, for IC should be reported as the average of at least 3 maneuvers. The mean coefficient of variation for the IC in COPD is estimated to be 5 ± 3%.

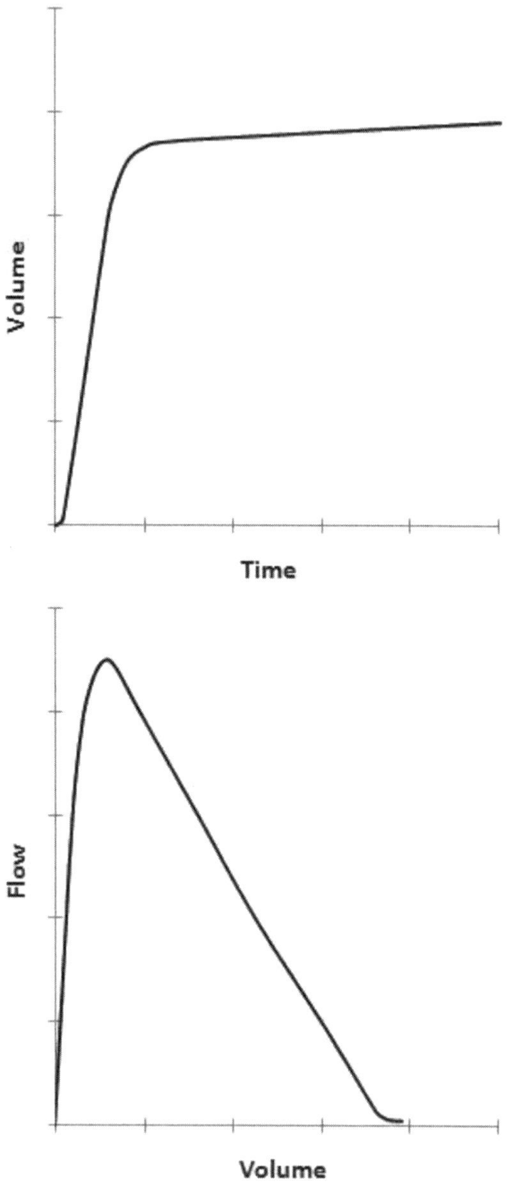

Figure 2. Volume vs time and flow vs volume plots.

Reversibility Testing

Reversibility testing after administration of a bronchodilator is frequently undertaken in the PFT laboratory. Baseline testing is followed by administration of a short-acting bronchodilator, after which repeat testing is repeated. Either a short-acting β_2-agonist (*ie*, salbutamol, 400 μg, with repeat testing at least 10 min afterward) or anticholinergic (*ie*, ipratropium, 160 μg, with repeat testing at least 30 min afterward) can be used.[11] Current recommendations are for increased doses of the bronchodilator (four puffs vs two puffs) as noted previously, unless there is concern for the patient's

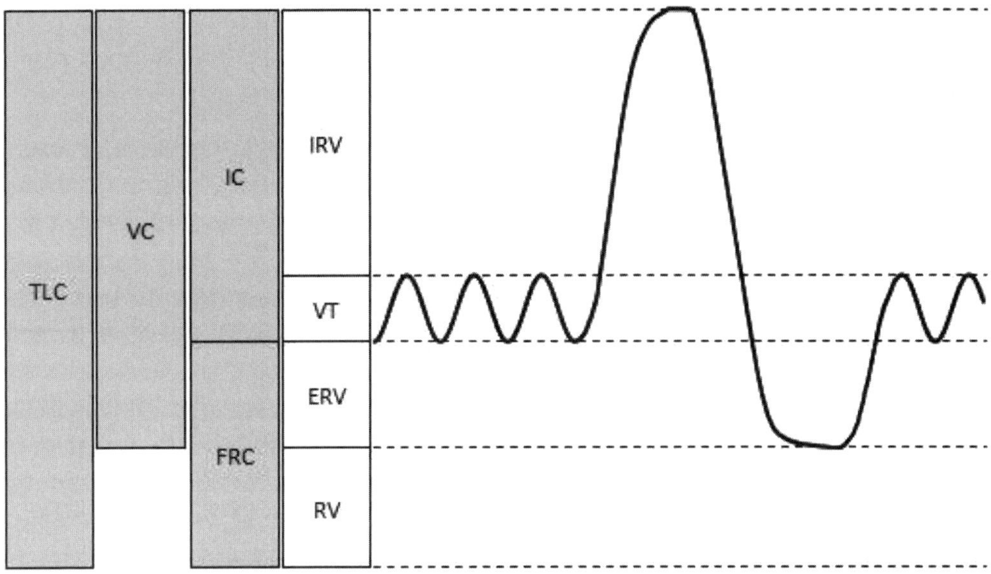

Figure 3. Lung volumes and capacities.

heart rate or tremor. An increase in either the FEV_1 or the FVC of ≥12% and ≥200 mL is now considered a "positive" bronchodilator response.[9] It should be recognized that the utility of a bronchodilator response is dependent on the clinical setting, and over-reliance on the result often leads to inappropriate clinical decision making. For example, a lack of a bronchodilator response does not necessarily predict lack of a therapeutic response. In this regard, it is important to know when the patient last received any medication that might affect the response. It is recommended that patients withhold taking short-acting bronchodilators for at least 4 h before testing and any long-acting or sustained-release bronchodilators for at least 12 h before testing.

Peak Expiratory Flows

Peak expiratory flow (PEF) is the highest flow achieved from a maximal forced expiratory maneuver from TLC. When obtained from a spirometer, PEF is normally expressed at BTPS in L/s, whereas most portable monitoring instruments display results in L/min. The measurement (and derived/related variables) is highly dependent on lung volume and effort. After achieving full inflation, the patient should deliver the blow without hesitation. A delay of as little as 2 s can alter tracheal viscoelastic properties enough to cause a reduction in the PEF by as much as 10%.[12]

Work on the measurement and clinical utility of the PEF are ongoing. These measurements are now embedded in asthma management strategies, but difficulties have been experienced with too much trust in the measurement. There are many other related and derived variables from the PEF (Fig. 4), but they have not been proven to be equal or superior to spirometry in the individual clinical setting.[11]

Maximum Voluntary Ventilation

The maximum voluntary ventilation is the maximum volume of air a subject can breathe over a period of time (typically 12 to 15 s), and it is expressed in L/min at BTPS. Its clinical contribution has largely been superseded by the FEV_1 and FVC and is now rarely measured. It may be useful in some clinical settings in which ventilatory capacity may be impaired by mechanisms different than those directly affecting the FEV_1, for example, neuromuscular disorders and central airway obstruction. Although it has been used as an estimate of maximal ventilation during exercise, there are significant limitations with this approach. (This will be discussed in further detail in the chapter "Cardiopulmonary Exercise Testing.")

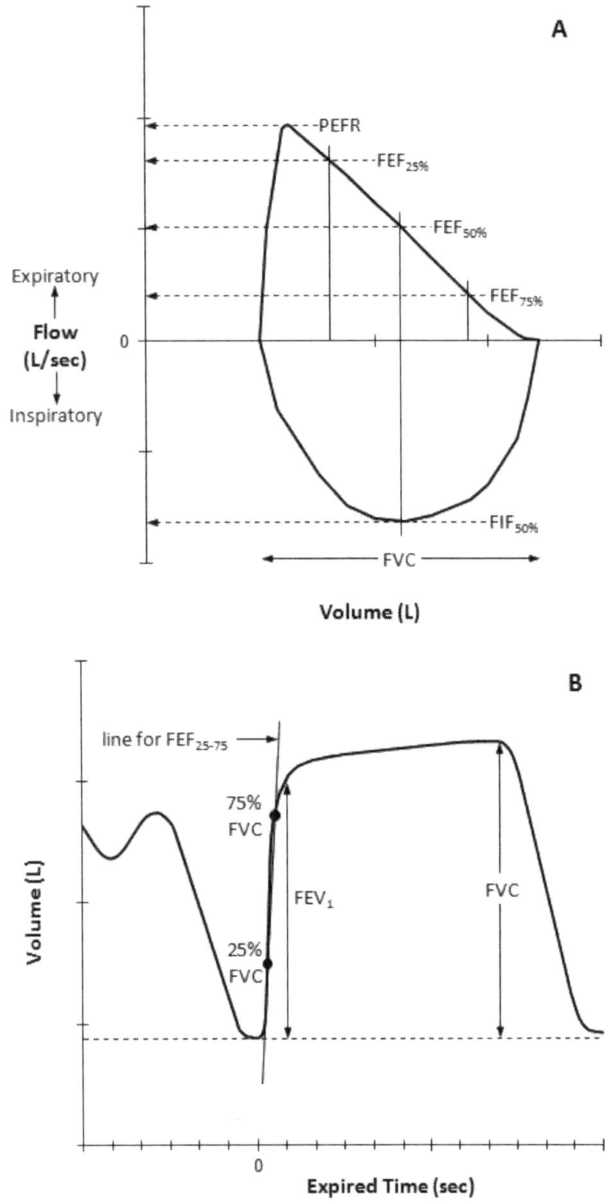

Figure 4. Peak expiratory flow and derived variables in flow vs volume [A] and volume vs time [B] plots.

Lung Volumes

Measurement of absolute lung volumes is more challenging and less available than assessing basic lung volumes by spirometry. However, although their utility in a variety of clinical settings continues to be studied, their measurement remains the gold standard for establishing a restrictive abnormality. There are a variety of available techniques in the pulmonary function laboratory that may be used to measure absolute lung volumes, including body plethysmography, nitrogen washout, and inhaled inert gas dilution. The lung volumes of interest are noted in Figure 3. In addition to the VC and IC (discussed and defined previously), other measurements are as follows:

- FRC is the volume of gas present in the lung at end-expiration during tidal breathing and is the absolute volume measured in the PFT laboratory.
- Expiratory reserve volume (ERV) is the volume of gas maximally exhaled from EELV during tidal breathing.
- Inspiratory reserve volume is the volume of gas that can be maximally inhaled from the end-inspiratory lung volume during tidal breathing.
- Tidal volume is the volume of gas inhaled or exhaled at rest with each breath.
- Total lung capacity (TLC) is the volume of gas in the lungs after maximal inspiration (the sum of all volumes).

The determination of FRC is the key component in the measurement of lung volumes. Regardless of the technique used to measure FRC, TLC and RV will be estimated from the FRC and the measurements of IC and ERV. Although opinion varies on the best technique, the preferred method is to measure ERV immediately after the FRC measurement, followed by a slow inspiratory vital capacity (IVC) maneuver, all performed with the patient remaining on the mouthpiece until the completion of the maneuver (Fig. 5).

Assuming technically satisfactory measurements, the reported value for FRC is the mean of FRC measurements associated with the ERV and IVC maneuvers used to calculate the RV and TLC. The reported value for the RV is the reported FRC minus the ERV linked to the acceptable FRC. The reported value for the TLC is the reported RV plus the largest of the IVCs. [13] An alternative recommended method involves determination of IC immediately after the measurement of FRC to estimate TLC. The VC measurement can then either linked to this maneuver, or it can be performed separately after an ERV maneuver as described previously.

Body Plethysmography Technique

The term thoracic gas volume refers to the plethysmographic measurement of intrathoracic gas volume at the time of airflow occlusion, *ie*, the

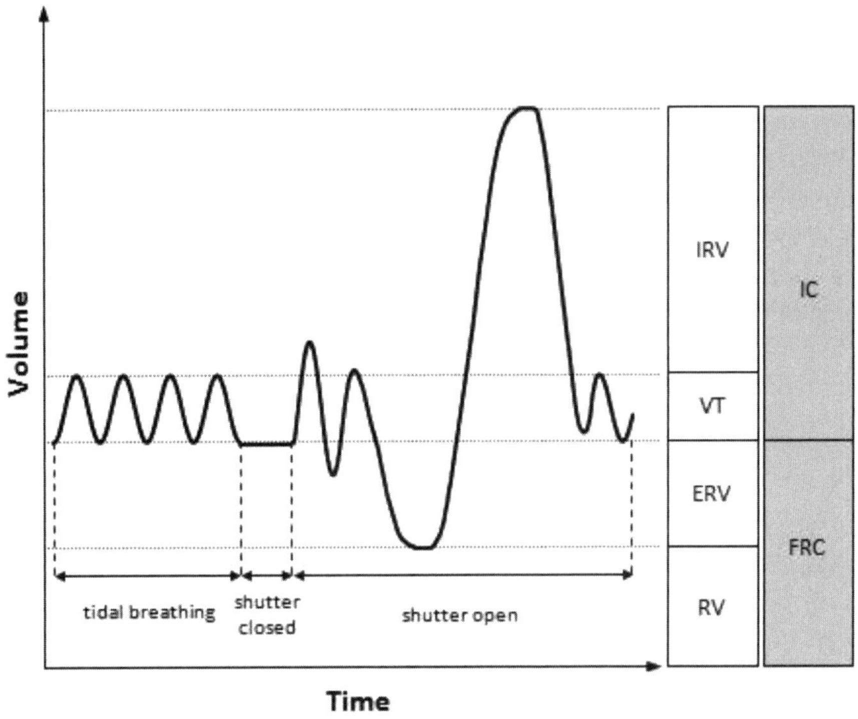

Figure 5. Recommended method for measuring lung volumes.

compressible gas within the thorax. In normal individuals, FRC measured by plethysmograph and gas dilution techniques yield similar results. In patients with obstructive lung disease and gas-trapping, FRC determined by plethysmography is typically greater than measured by gas dilution techniques.

Plethysmographic testing is performed by having the patient sit in a sealed box and pant against a closed shutter. During the inspiratory phase of the pant, thoracic volume increases slightly, decompressing the volume of air in the lungs while slightly compressing the volume of air in the box. Conversely, during the expiratory phase of the pant, thoracic volume decreases slightly, compressing the volume of air in the lungs while slightly decompressing the volume of air in the box. Using Boyle's law, where at a given temperature, the product of gas volume and pressure is constant:

(1) $V_1 \times P_1 = V_2 \times P_2$

where the initial pressure and volume at FRC are P_1 and V_1. Pressure and volume at the end of the inspiratory phase of the pant are P_2 ($P_1 + \Delta P$) and V_2 ($V_1 + \Delta V$). Thus:

(2) $V_1 \times P_1 = (V_1 + \Delta V) \times (P_1 + \Delta P)$

$P_1 + \Delta P$ are measured at the mouth, assuming that mouth and alveolar pressures are equal, and ΔV is measured using the change in box pressure, thus allowing for V_1 to be solved.

Body plethysmography measured lung volumes are considered the gold standard, but strict attention to testing methods, equipment upkeep and quality control, and panting technique and frequency is essential.

Gas Dilution Techniques

Gas dilution techniques measure the gas volume in the lungs that communicates via the airways by use of a mass balance approach. A mass balance equation uses both the initial volume and tracer gas concentration and the final tracer concentration to calculate the volume in the patient's lungs at the moment the tracer gas breathing began. The assumption that the tracer gas is largely insoluble, inert, and is well mixed in the lung is fundamental. For example, incomplete gas mixing would cause lung volumes to be underestimated, whereas use of a soluble gas would lead cause lung volumes to be overestimated. Either helium (He) rebreathing or nitrogen (N_2) washout techniques may be used, although both tend to underestimate lung volume when airway obstruction is present. For nitrogen washout, the washout is satisfactory when the N_2 concentration is $<1.5\%$ for at least 3 successive breaths.[13] For He rebreathing, a typical 10% He concentration with 25 to 30% oxygen (O_2) gas mixture inspirate is breathed until equilibration is reached, when the change in He concentration is $<0.02\%$ for at least 30 s.[13] If only room air is added to the 10% He gas mixture, it is important to ensure adequate O_2 replacement during the test. Both measurements must be corrected to BTPS, and the volume of the equipment dead space should be subtracted.

Diffusing Capacity

The carbon monoxide diffusing capacity of the lung (DLCO) assesses gas exchange by measuring the rate of carbon monoxide (CO) transfer from the lungs to the blood, with values reported in mL/min/mm Hg (standard temperature [0°C], pressure [760 mm Hg], dry). A number of both structural and functional properties influence the capacity of the lung to exchange gas across the alveolar-capillary border. These include the volume and distribution of ventilation, mixing and diffusion, the composition of the gas, characteristics of the alveolar membrane and lung parenchyma, the volume of alveolar capillary plasma, the concentration and binding properties of hemoglobin (Hgb), and the gas tensions in blood entering the alveolar capillaries.

As a test of gas transfer, CO uptake by the lung can be measured by a number of techniques (*ie*, steady-state, intrabreath, rebreathing, and single-breath techniques), but the most commonly used methodology is the single-breath technique. Testing begins with the patient exhaling down to RV, at which time a valve opens and the patient rapidly inhales the test gas to TLC. The patient holds his or her breath for 10 s and then breathes out rapidly while the exhaled gas is collected.

The gas inspirate usually consists of a mixture of N_2, 0.3% CO, an inert tracer gas such as He, and 19 to 21% O_2. An alveolar sample of the exhaled gas is considered after anatomic and mechanical dead space gas is discarded from the collected gas (~0.75 to 1.0 L, but as little as 0.5 L if the patient's vital capacity is <2.0 L). A submaximal inspired volume (V_I) can affect CO uptake. Therefore, it is important that the V_I be as close to the known VC as possible. Because a reduction in V_I of $>15\%$ may significantly reduce the measured DLCO, a V_I target of 85% of the largest VC is suggested.[14] To minimize variability in the measurement, inspiration should be rapid (<4 s), breath-hold should be 10 ± 2 s, and expiration should ideally also be <4 s in duration. At least 4 min should transpire between repeat testing to allow for adequate elimination of the test gas from the lungs. This time period should be extended (~10 min) in patients with significant obstruction.

Conditions affecting the DLCO are listed in Table 7. Other factors known to affect the DLCO are diurnal variation (increased in the morning, and reported to decrease 1 to 2%/h throughout the day),[15] menstrual cycle (up to 13% change, increased premenses), alcohol consumption (increased after ingestion), and bronchodilator administration (increased up to 6% after use).

Adjusting the DLCO Measurement

The DLCO measurement is dependent on a number of physiologic conditions, specifically

Table 7. *Factors Affecting DLCO**

Conditions that reduce DLCO
Submaximal inspiration or respiratory muscle weakness
Anemia
Valsalva maneuver
COHgb
Increased fraction of inspired O_2
Lung resection
Chronic COPD
Interstitial lung diseases
Pulmonary vascular disease, *ie*, emboli, pulmonary hypertension, vasculitis
Conditions that increase DLCO
Polycythemia
Left-to-right shunt
Asthma
Pulmonary hemorrhage
Muller maneuver
Exercise
Supine position
Obesity
Decreased fraction of inspired O_2

*Adapted from MacIntyre et al.[14]

changes with Hgb, lung volume, carboxyhemoglobin (COHgb), fraction of inspired oxygen, exercise and body position, in addition to age, sex, height, and possibly race.[14] Specific adjustments should be made for Hgb, COHgb, and fraction of inspired oxygen before interpretation.

Adjusting for Hemoglobin

Because COHgb binding is fundamental to the measurement of DLCO, Hgb concentration can substantially affect its measurement. Expressing Hgb in g/dL, the recommended equation for adjusting the predicted DLCO in adolescents and adult men is as follows[14]:

(3) DLCO (adjusted) = DLCO (predicted) × (1.7 Hgb/[10.22 + Hgb])

The recommended equation for adjusting the predicted DLCO in women is as follows[14]:

(4) DLCO (adjusted) = DLCO (predicted) × (1.7 Hgb/[9.38 + Hgb])

Adjusting for P_{AO_2}

P_{AO_2} also affects the measurement of DLCO either because of supplemental O_2 (higher F_{IO_2}) or because of testing at altitude (lower F_{IO_2}). The DLCO will change by ~0.35% per mm Hg increase change in P_{AO_2}, or by ~0.31% per mm Hg decrease change. The recommended equation for adjusting the predicted DLCO in a subject on supplemental O_2, and assuming a room air P_{AO_2} at sea level of 100 mm Hg is:

(5) DLCO (adjusted) = DLCO (predicted)/(1.0 + 0.0035[P_{AO_2} − 100])

The recommended equation for adjusting the predicted DLCO for altitude, and assuming a P_IO_2 at sea level of 150 mm Hg is:

(6) DLCO (adjusted) = DLCO (predicted)/(1.0 + 0.0031[P_IO_2 − 150])

Adjusting for COHgb Concentration and CO Back Pressure

COHgb may acutely reduce the DLCO[16] by occupying Hgb binding sites and by reducing driving pressure for CO transport from alveolar gas to capillary blood. Typical exposure to environmental CO and endogenous production results in measured COHgb of 1 to 2%, which is already incorporated into reference values based on healthy nonsmoking subjects. Cigarette smoke and other environmental sources of CO can lead to further appreciable increases in measured CO back pressure and COHgb that should be considered. Increases in COHgb also occur with repeated measurements because CO is inspired in the DLCO test. For example, five tests will increase COHgb by ~3.5%, which will decrease the measured DLCO by 3.0 to 3.5%. It is therefore recommended that no more than five repeated measurements be undertaken at any sitting.

Accounting for both the back pressure and COHgb effects, a 1% increase in COHgb reduces the measured DLCO by 0.8 to 1% from both known effects. This is represented by the following equation[14]:

(7) DLCO (adjusted) = DLCO (predicted) × (102% − COHgb %)

Adjusting for Lung Volume

Adjusting the DLCO for lung volume is both complex and confusing. It is complex because the reason(s) responsible for a reduced lung volume vary, as do the effects of the specific underlying reason on the resultant measured DLCO. Adjusting the DLCO for lung volume is also confusing because in some instances the relationship is proportional, whereas in other settings it is unpredictable and varied. In view of these realities, drawing definitive clinical conclusions based on a volume-corrected DLCO should be made with caution. As recommended in international guidelines,[14] further study and understanding is required before more specific volume-adjustment recommendations for the DLCO can be made and uniformly adopted.

The average of at least two acceptable tests should be reported for interpretation of the DLCO. Reporting should include the unadjusted DLCO, predicted and percent predicted DLCO, predicted and percent predicted DLCO/ alveolar volume, and a list of any adjustments made to the value because of corrections (*ie*, Hgb, COHgb, P_{AO_2}, or lung volume). As always, technician comments regarding the quality of the measurements should be noted.

Respiratory Muscle Pressures

Respiratory muscle strength can be assessed by determining the maximal inspiratory pressure (MIP) and the maximal expiratory pressure (MEP). The MIP reflects the strength of the diaphragm and other inspiratory muscles, whereas the MEP reflects the strength of the abdominal and other expiratory muscles. Clinical indications for assessing respiratory muscle strength are varied, but they relate to any clinical setting in which respiratory muscle weakness or neuromuscular disorders affecting respiratory status are suspected. Testing can be helpful in the diagnosis of respiratory muscle weakness, in assessing the severity of respiratory muscle weakness, in predicting clinical outcomes, and in the longitudinal follow-up of patients diagnosed with respiratory muscle weakness.

The equipment necessary for measuring the MIP and MEP is simple, and similar techniques are used in both measurements. A pressure gauge connected to a mouthpiece can be readily assembled or, alternatively, commercially available systems may be used. In either case, there must be a small hole of approximately 1 mm in the system to allow for an air leak, which minimizes the likelihood of the patient generating pressure with the use of their cheek muscles.

The MIP measurement is performed with the patient maintaining a tight seal between the lips and the mouthpiece, exhaling down to RV, and then breathing in as hard and fast as they can. The patient should keep up the maximal inspiratory pressure for ~2 s, with the largest negative pressure sustained for 1 s being recorded. A longer continuous inspiratory effort is not required nor recommended. After resting for ~1 min, the procedure is repeated for a total of at least three times, with the intent of obtaining repeat measurements with a variability of < 10 cm H_2O. It must be emphasized that testing is very dependent on a patient's effort and cooperation, which may be enhanced by the technician initially demonstrating the maneuver to the patient and by the use of a practice test. Other potential sources of error in the measurements include pressure gauge accuracy, the patient-device interface, and leaks.

The MEP measurement is similarly performed except that the patient is instructed to inhale to TLC and then blow out as hard and fast as he or she can. In similar fashion to the MIP, the largest positive pressure sustained for 1 s is recorded. After resting for ~1 min, the procedure is repeated for a total of at least three times, with the intent of obtaining repeat measurements with a variability of < 10 cm H_2O.

In both instances, the maximum value obtained from the three suitable maneuvers should be reported. Definitive reference ranges for the MIP and MEP have not been agreed on, although many are available.[17,18] In general, a number of key remarks are appropriate:

1. Values decrease with age, and are approximately one third lower in women when compared with men.
2. In adults 18 to 65 years of age, the MIP should exceed −90 cm H_2O in men and −70 cm H_2O in women. In adults > 65 years, the MIP should generally exceed −65 cm H_2O in men and −45 cm H_2O for women.
3. In adults, the MEP should exceed 140 cm H_2O in men and 90 cm H_2O in women.
4. A MIP less than on third of normal predicts hypercarbic respiratory failure.[19]
5. A MEP < 60 cm H_2O predicts a weak cough and difficulty clearing secretions.[20]

A normal MIP reliably excludes inspiratory muscle weakness (*ie*, good negative predictive value), but a low MIP does not reliably confirm inspiratory muscle weakness. The poor positive predictive value reflects the high frequency of falsely low MIP measurements caused by unrecognized poor effort or technique.[21] In normal healthy individuals, 95% of the test-to-test variation has a magnitude of < 25 cm H_2O.[22] Moreover, it has been demonstrated that improvements in the MIP of –13 cm H_2O and MEP of 24 cm H_2O do not necessarily correlate with symptomatic improvement.[23]

The VC or the FVC often are used as alternatives or complimentary measurements to the MIP and MEP in clinical practice. Comparisons of the MIP and the VC demonstrate similar sensitivity and specificity for detecting hypercarbic respiratory failure. In the upright position, a reduced FVC seems to be less specific for detecting respiratory muscle abnormalities than the MIP. However, a decrease in the FVC from upright to the supine position appears to detect inspiratory muscle weakness more reliably than the MIP.[24]

Airway Challenges

Assessing airway responsiveness is most commonly undertaken to either confirm or exclude a suspected diagnosis of asthma, recognizing that airway hyperresponsiveness (AHR) to exogenous stimuli is a characteristic feature of the disease. Testing can be performed by the use of a number of various techniques, using either selective (typically specific allergens, but uncommonly used outside of the research laboratory) or nonselective agents. Nonselective stimuli can be either direct (for example, methacholine and histamine) or indirect (for example, exercise, eucapnic voluntary hyperventilation, cold air and mannitol).

Methacholine is the most commonly performed direct challenge. It is typically undertaken with two different techniques: the tidal breathing method or the dosimeter method. Recent studies have questioned the sensitivity of the dosimeter method using TLC inhalations in patients with mild airway hyperresponsiveness. Thus, the use of the tidal breathing method or a modified dosimeter method is now recommended.[25] A more detailed description of the testing methods is available elsewhere.[26,27]

Methacholine responsiveness is usually reported as the provocation concentration (or dose) causing a 20% decrease in the FEV_1 (*ie*, PC_{20} or PD_{20}). The PC_{20} is log-normally distributed in the population, can be measured into the normal range, and is a relatively imprecise measurement with a repeatability of ± 1 doubling concentration. The results are typically interpreted as follows[26]: normal $PC_{20} > 16$ mg/mL; borderline $PC_{20} = 4$ to 16 mg/mL; mild AHR PC_{20} = 1 to 4 mg/mL; moderate AHR PC_{20} = 0.25 to 1 mg/mL; and marked AHR PC_{20} < 0.25 mg/mL. An example of results consistent with moderate AHR is demonstrated in Figure 6.

From a diagnostic point of view, the test has a strong negative predictive value, and therefore functions best when normal to rule out current asthma. Several caveats should be remembered. First, methacholine challenges should not be performed with TLC inhalations to maintain diagnostic sensitivity. Second, it is critical that symptoms be current (*ie*, within the past few days). It follows that a normal ("negative") methacholine challenge test in a currently asymptomatic patient cannot rule out asthma.

Most patients with exercise-associated bronchoconstriction (which when clinically occurring in isolation is frequently a manifestation of mild asthma) will have a positive direct inhalational challenge. However, it is now recognized that some patients, in particular high-performance athletes, may have positive exercise challenges but a negative direct (*ie*, methacholine) challenge. The

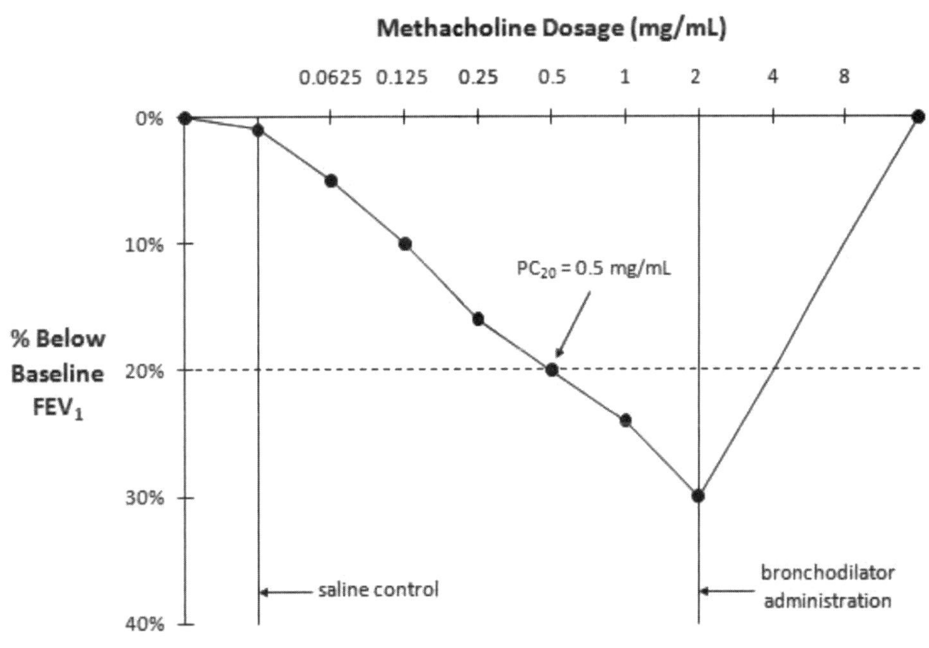

Figure 6. Methacholine challenge test study results.

implication is that a negative methacholine challenge will not completely rule out exercise-associated bronchoconstriction in this population. Exercise challenge testing will be discussed in further detail in the chapter "Cardiopulmonary Exercise Testing."

Another important and more frequent cause of a false-negative methacholine challenge is recent exposure to bronchodilating agents, including both β_2-agonists and anticholinergics. The suggested time periods these agents should be withheld before testing are listed in Table 8. The specificity of direct (*ie*, methacholine and histamine) challenge testing is affected by underlying airflow obstruction, which reflects resting airway geometry and not asthma.[28] Airflow obstruction is a clinical feature that reduces the specificity of the methacholine challenge, but it does not directly influence the sensitivity.

In summary, the clinical utility of the methacholine challenge test is primarily to exclude current asthma in a symptomatic patient when the tidal breathing methacholine $PC_{20} > 16$ mg/mL. A positive methacholine challenge test is not synonymous with a diagnosis of asthma, particularly in the presence of significant airflow obstruction (*ie*, $FEV_1 < 70\%$ predicted). It is also suggested that 5 to 15% of normal individuals and 20 to 40% of patients with rhinitis may also have a false-positive methacholine challenge test.[27]

General Considerations in Interpreting PFTs

Pulmonary function testing requires appropriate equipment, calibration, testing procedures, assessment of acceptability and repeatability, interpretation, and integration with the patient's clinical presentation. Interpretation of PFT results should be meaningful, *ie*, a rendition of only which results are normal or abnormal can readily be provided by a machine. Requisition forms for PFTs should be designed to encourage the requesting physician to provide as much clinical information as is reasonable to enable the interpretation to be valuable. The key principles for diagnosing common abnormal ventilatory disorders are listed in Table 9. Typical examples of commonly encountered flow-volume curves are shown in Figure 7.

Early evidence of airflow obstruction is qualitatively demonstrated by a concave shape of the expiratory flow-volume curve. Quantitative evidence is often inferred by a reduction in expiratory flows at mid-lung volumes (*ie*, FEF^{25-75} and others). However, a reduction in the mid-volume expiratory flows is not specific and not necessarily diagnostic for small airways disease in an individual patient. As airways disease becomes more pronounced, a disproportionate reduction in the FEV_1 compared with the FVC becomes evident and, as noted, this is more certain for a diagnosis of airway obstruction.

Pneumothoraces and bullae are clinical situations often characterized by a normal FEV_1/FVC and TLC measured in a body plethysmograph, but reduced FEV_1 and FVC values. In this instance,

Table 8. *Common Medications That Decrease Bronchial Responsiveness**

	Suggested Time Interval to Withhold Administration
Short-acting β_2 agonists	8 h
Short-acting anticholinergics	24 h
Long-acting β_2 agonists	48 h
Long-acting anticholinergics	Up to 7 d
Short-acting theophyllines	24 h
Sustained-release theophyllines	48 h

*Adapted from Crapo et al.[26]

Table 9. *Diagnosing Common Respiratory Disorders**

Obstruction
- FEV_1/VC > 5th percentile of predicted
- Reduced flows at low lung volumes are not specific for small airways disease in individual patients.
- A combined reduction in both FEV_1 and VC is most commonly related to suboptimal effort. This pattern may occasionally indicate airflow obstruction, but confirmation requires absolute lung volume measurement.
- Measurement of absolute lung volume measurement may assist in diagnosing and assessing COPD and asthma.

Restriction
- TLC > 5th percentile of predicted
- Spirometry can not accurately diagnose restriction.
- A reduced TLC from a single-breath technique should not be used to diagnosis restriction.

Mixed obstruction/restriction
- FEV_1/VC and TLC > 5th percentile of predicted.

*Adapted from Pelligrino et al.[9]

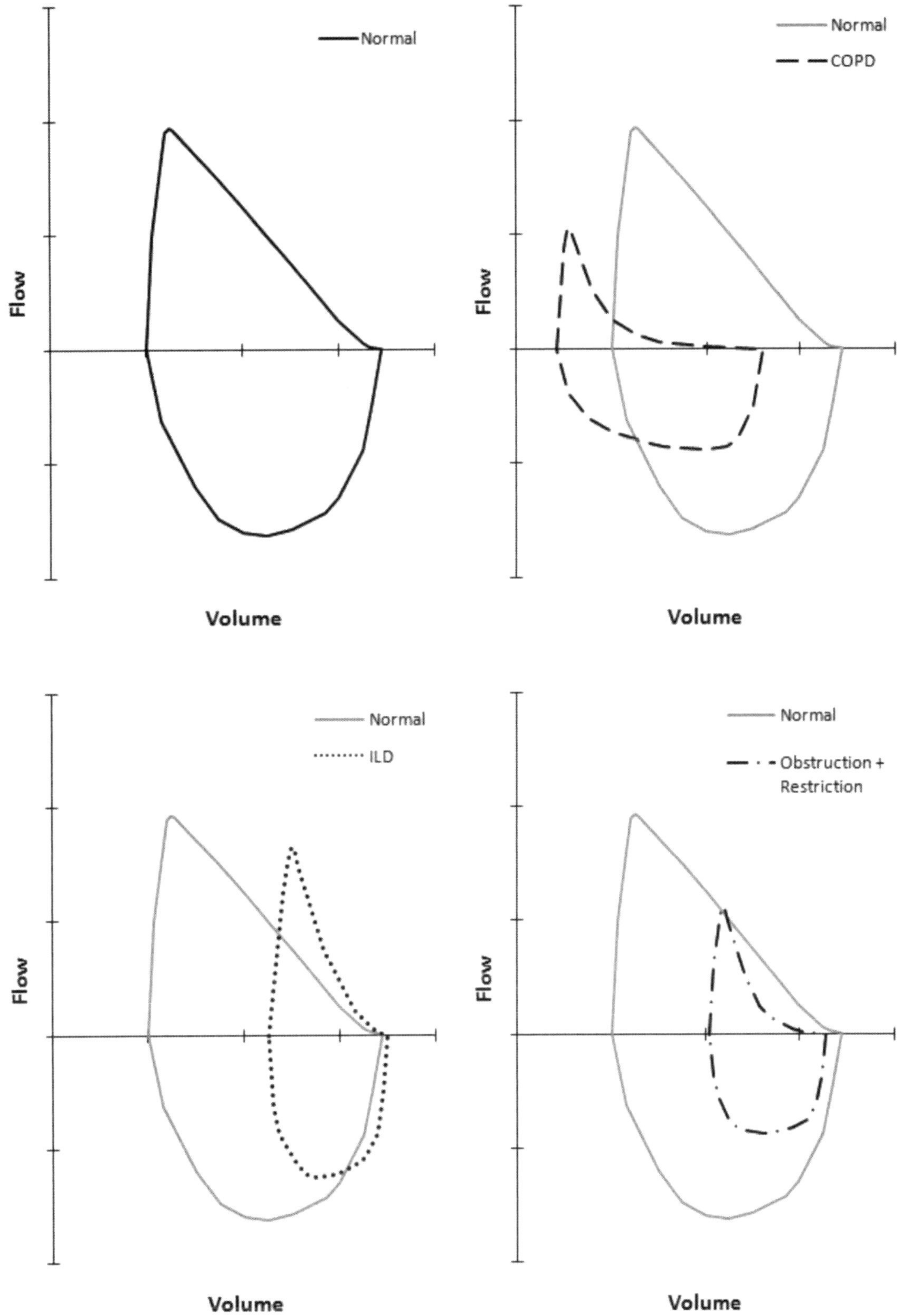

Figure 7. Flow-volume curves in common respiratory disorders.

TLC assessed by gas dilution techniques will be low. This difference between TLC measured in a body plethysmograph vs by gas dilution is also seen in patients with significant airflow obstruction, often accompanied by a significantly increased RV.

Although the FVC is often used in place of the VC, it is suggested to use the largest measured VC, whether it is the IVC, the slow expiratory vital capacity, or the FVC. The forced expiratory volume in 6 s may be substituted for the FVC, if appropriate reference equations are used.

Attention should always be paid to possible technical issues or problems, as well as to the comments from the performing technicians. In addition to common obstructive, restrictive, and mixed disorders, suspicion of possible neuromuscular disorders and central airway obstruction should always be present. Although they infrequently are found, these conditions should be actively excluded.

Typical flow-volume plots observed with differing types of physiologic central airway obstruction are shown in Figure 8. Poor or submaximal efforts should always be considered in this setting. It is important that repeated flow-volume maneuvers are maximal and reproducible, and the technician should confirm this in the report. In this setting, a printout of each individual maneuver can be very helpful.

Serial testing is routinely undertaken in clinical practice to monitor results over time, and to evaluate change following intervention(s). An understanding of test variability is required before one can conclude that any observed change relates to the underlying process or to an intervention. The reproducibility of variables can be presented in many different ways, and there is ongoing debate about which method is best. For example, the American Thoracic Society/European Respiratory Society recommends that in normal individuals, the year-to-year change in the FEV_1 should exceed 15% before confidence can be given that a meaningful clinical change has occurred.[9] The coefficient of variation (CV) is also commonly used for this purpose, and is calculated as:

$$CV (\%) = SD \text{ divided by the mean} \times 100$$

It is assumed that a difference of 2 × CV% is required to conclude a clinically significant change. Under ideal conditions, the mean CV for commonly measured lung function tests is as follows:[29,30] FEV_1 = 3.2 to 7.5%, FVC = 4.5 to 7.9%, TLC (plethysmography) = 2.2 to 4.3%, TLC (He) = 1.5 to 3.7%, FRC (plethysmography) = 3.5 to 6.8%, FRC (He) = 4.9 to 10.4%, RV (plethysmography) = 8.9 to 12.4%, RV (He) = 2.4 to 14.0%, and DLCO 4.1 to 4.5%.

The use of severity classification systems is currently fraught with difficulty and frustration for the practicing clinician. First, none have been specifically validated—as stated by others, "the number of categories and exact cut-off points are arbitrary."[9] Second, conflicting classifications

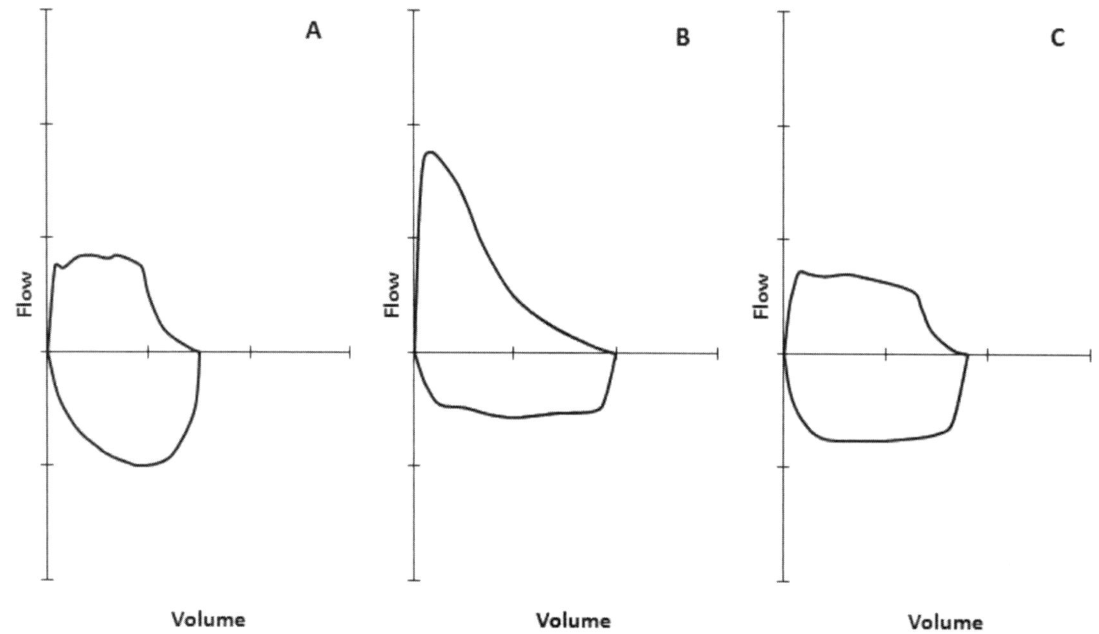

Figure 8. Flow-volume curves in physiologic central airway obstructions. A = variable intrathoracic obstruction; B = variable extrathoracic obstruction; C = physiologically fixed central airway obstruction.

Table 10. *Classifying Severity of Airflow Obstruction**

	ATS/ERS Standardization of Lung Function Testing[9]	ATS/ERS COPD Guidelines,[31] Canadian Thoracic Society,[32] and GOLD[33]
Degree of severity	(FEV_1 % predicted)	(FEV_1 % predicted)
Mild	<70	<80
Moderate	60–69	50-9
Moderately severe	50–59	—
Severe	35–49	30-49
Very severe	>35	>30

*ATS/ERS = American Thoracic Society/European Respiratory Society; GOLD = Global Initiative for Chronic Obstructive Lung Disease.

schemas exist (see Table 10).[31–33] It is therefore recommended that clinicians choosing to use a specific classification system should recognize these limitations, and make note of the specific schema utilized in their interpretation.

Similarly, a severity classification scheme has been proposed for the DLCO (mild >60% and <LLN; moderate 40 to 60%; severe <40% predicted). As mentioned previously, the relationship between DLCO and lung volume is not linear. Therefore, the DLCO/alveolar volume is not an appropriate method to normalize DLCO for lung volume.[9] Other methods to adjust the DLCO for lung volume have not been validated.

The author is grateful to Mr. R. Clemens for his assistance in the preparation of the figures and the manuscript.

References

1. Miller MR, Crapo R, Hankinson J, et al. Series ATS/ERS Task Force: standardization of lung function testing. General considerations for lung function testing. Eur Respir J 2005; 26:153–161
2. Parker JM, Dillard TA, Phillips YY. Arm span-height relationships in patients referred for spirometry. Am J Respir Crit Care Med 1996; 154:533–536
3. Chumlea WC, Guo SS, Steinbaugh ML. Prediction of stature from knee height for black and white adults and children with application to mobility-impaired or handicapped persons. J Am Dietetic Assoc 1994; 94:1385–1388
4. Wanger J, ed. American Thoracic Society pulmonary function laboratory management and procedure manual. 2nd ed. New York, NY: American Thoracic Society, 2005
5. Johns DP, Ingram C, Booth H, et al. Effect of a microaerosol barrier filter on the measurement of lung function. Chest 1995; 107:1045–1048
6. Fuso L, Accardo D, Bevignani C, et al. Effects of a filter at the mouth on pulmonary function tests. Eur Resp J 1995; 8:314–317
7. Enright PL, Johnson LR, Connett JE, et al. Spirometry in the Lung Health Study: 1. Methods and quality control. Am Rev Respir Dis 1991; 143:1215–1223
8. Robbins DR, Enright PL, Sherrill DL. Lung function development in young adults: is there a plateau phase? Eur Respir J 1995; 8:768–772
9. Pelligrino R, Viegi G, Brusasco V, et al. Series ATS/ERS Task Force: standardization of lung function testing. Interpretative strategies for lung function tests. Eur Respir J 2005; 26:948–968
10. Hankinson JL, Odencratz JR, Fedan KB. Spirometric reference values from a sample of the general US population. Am J Respir Crit Care Med 1999; 159:179–187
11. Miller MR, Hankinson J, Brusasco V, et al. Series ATS/ERS Task Force: standardization of lung function testing. Standardization of spirometry. Eur Respir J 2005; 26:319–338
12. Kano S, Burton DL, Lanteri CJ, et al. Determination of peak expiratory flow. Eur Respir J 1993; 6:1347–1352
13. Wanger J, Clausen JL, Coates A, et al. Series ATS/ERS Task Force: standardization of lung function testing. Standardization of the measurement of lung volumes. Eur Respir J 2005; 26:511–522
14. MacIntyre N, Crapo RO, Viegi G, et al. Series ATS/ERS Task Force: standardization of lung function

testing. Standardization of the single-breath determination of carbon monoxide uptake in the lung. Eur Respir J 2005; 26:720–735
15. Cinkotai FF, Thomson ML. Diurnal variation in pulmonary diffusing capacity for carbon monoxide. J Appl Physiol 1966; 21:539–542
16. Graham BL, Mink JT, Cotton DJ. Effects of increasing carboxyhemoglobin on the single breath carbon monoxide diffusing capacity. Am J Respir Crit Care Med 2002; 165:1504–1510
17. Harik-Khan RI, Wise RA, Fozard JL. Determinants of maximal inspiratory pressure: the Baltimore Longitudinal Study of Aging. Am J Respir Crit Care Med 1998; 158:1459–1464
18. Enright PL, Kronmal RA, Manolino TA, et al. Respiratory muscle strength in the elderly. Correlates and reference values. Am J Respir Crit Care Med 1994; 149:430–438
19. Lyall RA, Donaldson N, Polkey MI, et al. Respiratory muscle strength and ventilatory failure in amyotrophic lateral sclerosis. Brain 2001; 124:2000–2013
20. Man WD, Kyroussis D, Fleming TA, et al. Cough gastric pressure and maximum expiratory mouth pressure in humans. Am J Respir Crit Care Med 2003; 168:714–717
21. Aldrich TK, Spiro P. Maximal inspiratory pressure: does reproducibility indicate full effort? Thorax 1995; 50:40–43
22. Maillard JO, Burdet L, van Melle G, et al. Reproducibility of twitch mouth pressure, sniff nasal inspiratory pressure, and maximal inspiratory pressure. Eur Respir J 1998; 11:901–905
23. Goswami R, Guleria R, Gupta AK, et al. Prevalence of diaphragmatic muscle weakness and dyspnoea in Grave's disease and their reversibility with carbimazole therapy. Eur J Endocrinol 2002; 147:299–303
24. Lechtzin N, Wiener CM, Shade DM, et al. Spirometry in the supine position improves the detection of diaphragmatic weakness in patients with amyotrophic lateral sclerosis. Chest 2002; 121:436–442
25. Cockcroft DW, Davis BE, Todd DC, et al. Methacholine challenge: comparison of two methods. Chest 2005; 127:839–844
26. Crapo RO, Casaburi R, Coates AL, et al. Guidelines for methacholine and exercise challenge testing—1999. Am J Respir Crit Care Med 2000; 161:309–329
27. Cockcroft DW. Bronchial challenge testing. In: Adkinson NF, Bochner BS, Busse WW, et al, eds. Middleton's allergy. 7th ed. Philadelphia, PA: Elsevier Inc., 2009; 1295–1308
28. Verma VK, Cockcroft DW, Dosman JA. Airway hyperresponsiveness to inhaled histamine in chronic obstructive airways disease: chronic bronchitis vs emphysema. Chest 1988; 94:456–461
29. Punjabi NM, Shade D, Patel AM, et al. Measurement variability in single-breath diffusing capacity of the lung. Chest 2003; 123:1082–1089
30. Hankinson JL, Stocks J, Peslin R. Reproducibility of lung volume measurements. Eur Respir J 1998; 11:787–790
31. Celli B, MacNee W. ATS/ERS Task Force. Standards for the diagnosis and treatment of patients with COPD: a summary of the ATS/ERS position paper. Eur Respir J 2004; 23:932–946
32. O'Donnell DE, Aaron S, Bourbeau J, et al. Canadian thoracic society recommendations for management of chronic obstructive pulmonary disease—2007 update. Can Respir J 2007; 14(suppl B):5B–32B.
33. Rabe KF, Hurd S, Anzueto A, et al. Global strategy for the diagnosis, management, and prevention of chronic obstructive pulmonary disease: GOLD executive summary. Am J Respir Crit Care Med 2007; 176:532–555

Bronchoscopy and Interventional Pulmonology

David Feller-Kopman, MD, FCCP

Objectives:

- Review the indications for flexible and rigid bronchoscopy
- Review the diagnostic yield from various bronchoscopic procedures
- Review the procedures available to the interventional pulmonologist
- Stress the need for specific training in advanced procedures

Key words: airway obstruction; bronchoscopy; hemoptysis; interventional pulmonology; laser; lung cancer; pleuroscopy; stent; thoracoscopy

Gustav Killian has been described as the father of bronchoscopy.[1] Using a metallic tube, electric light, and topical cocaine anesthesia, Killian removed a pork bone from a farmer's airway in 1897.[2] Before the development of rigid bronchoscopy, more than one half of the patients who aspirated foreign bodies died as the result of pneumonia. Rigid bronchoscopy with foreign body removal quickly evolved into the treatment of choice in these patients, with a clinical success rate >98%.[3] Over the subsequent years, Killian published extensively and lectured throughout Europe and the United States. He went on to develop bronchoscopes, laryngoscopes, and endoscopes, and he described techniques such as the use of fluoroscopy and x-ray to define endobronchial anatomy and endoluminal radiotherapy (brachytherapy).

Chevalier Jackson, an otolaryngologist who practiced in Philadelphia, is credited with advancing the field of bronchoscopy and airway interventions in the United States. During the next 150 years, bronchoscopic techniques and instruments continued to be refined. In 1966, Shigeto Ikeda presented the first prototype flexible fiberoptic bronchoscope at the Ninth International Congress on Diseases of the Chest in Copenhagen. In 1968, Machita and Olympus both introduced commercially available fiberoptic bronchoscopes.[4] In 1980, Dumon presented his use of the Nd:YAG laser via the fiberoptic bronchoscope, and since that time, the flexible bronchoscope has been widely used as both a diagnostic and therapeutic tool for both diseases of the parenchyma and central airways. With the miniaturization of electronic devices, the first video bronchoscope was introduced in 1987. This development allowed endoscopic pictures to be printed out and shared and, even more importantly, physicians no longer needed to look through an eyepiece. Instead, the endoscopic image could be projected onto monitors, allowing everyone in the room to see what was happening in the airway.

Little has changed in the appearance of bronchoscopes since 1968. The external diameter of the flexible bronchoscope ranges from 2.8 to 6.3 mm in diameter. The diameter of the working channel ranges from 1.2 to 3.2 mm. A working channel ≥2.8 mm is recommended for more therapeutic flexible bronchoscopy because it allows for better suction and the passage of larger instruments. It is important to note the relative anatomy at the tip of the bronchoscope. By convention, as viewed from the operator's perspective, the camera is at 9:00, suction at 6:00, and the working channel at 3:00. These landmarks play a role when navigating the airways because the bronchoscope may need to be rotated to visualize or sample the intended target. There are several outstanding texts and review articles in which the authors summarize the current state of the art for bronchoscopy and interventional pulmonology.[5–9] This chapter will review some of the key factors associated with these fields.

Thoracic Anatomy

It is crucial that the bronchoscopist become an expert in airway and thoracic anatomy, including knowledge of the nasopharnyx and oropharynx in addition to the bronchial tree and mediastinal structures. Several excellent chapters/texts[10,11] are available to assist one with this process. The segmental anatomy of the lungs from both an external and internal perspective are required, and one should become familiar with the name (*ie*, superior segment of the right lower lobe), as well as the number system (*ie*, RB6) as initially proposed by Jackson and Huber[12] and Boyden.[13] It is also important to appreciate mediastinal anatomy, including intrathoracic vessels and lymph nodes, as well as their relationship to endobronchial landmarks. These will serve as reference points for transbronchial needle aspiration (TBNA) and endobronchial ultrasound (EBUS) and help avoid injury to the patient should the bronchoscopist use therapy such as the Nd:YAG laser or brachytherapy. The use of endoscopic simulators has been associated with a more rapid acquisition of bronchoscopic expertise.[14]

Diagnostic Bronchoscopy

There are many indications for diagnostic bronchoscopy. The most common indication is for the diagnosis of suspected lung cancer. Other indications include evaluation of diffuse lung disease, infiltrates in the immunocompromised host, hemoptysis, and cough. Additionally, bronchoscopy with bronchoalveolar lavage (BAL) and/or brushing may be useful for the diagnosis of ventilator-associated pneumonia.[15,16]

Cancer Diagnosis and Staging

Lung cancer is the leading cause of cancer deaths in the United States, and it will account for approximately 161,840 deaths in 2008, more than colon, breast, and prostate cancers combined.[17] It is estimated that there were 215,020 new cases of lung cancer in 2008, and the incidence and number of lung cancer deaths continues to increase among women in the United States.[18] Bronchoscopy provides a minimally invasive approach for the diagnosis tumors in the central airways. Although the yield is somewhat lower for solitary parenchymal lesions, advances in navigation such as CT fluoroscopy and electromagnetic and virtual bronchoscopic navigation have significantly improved the yield for peripheral tumors. Several comprehensive reviews discussing the diagnosis and staging of lung cancer, as well as the role of bronchoscopy, are available.[19–23]

The bronchoscopic evaluation of patients with suspected malignancy is guided by clinical symptoms as well as radiographic findings. Depending on the history and chest CT/PET-CT findings, bronchoscopy may be the diagnostic modality of choice because it can be used to make the diagnosis and stage the patient at the same sitting. If appropriate staging is to be performed, biopsy of the lesion that will place the patient in the highest clinical stage should occur before other biopsies. For example, if a patient presents with a left lower lobe mass and an enlarged subcarinal (station 7) and right paratracheal (station 4R) lymph node, the appropriate procedure would be a bronchoscopy with TBNA of the 4R node because this procedure would stage the patient with N3 disease, making the patient unresectable. If a diagnosis was not obtained from 4R, station 7 should be sampled next because this would be considered an N2 node if involved with cancer. Only if sampling of this node is nondiagnostic would one need to proceed with addressing the left lower lobe mass. Initial biopsy of the mass could contaminate the working channel and make the TBNA a false-positive finding, precluding the patient from curative surgery.

There are several available tools by which to obtain specimens during bronchoscopy, including forceps biopsy, brushing, bronchial wash/lavage, and TBNA. Electrocautery snare forceps is an excellent tool for the removal of a pedunculated airway lesion because it can open the airway and also provide excellent tissue for the pathologist.[24] The choice of the aforementioned modalities is primarily determined by the location of the pathology. However, data support the use of the combination of techniques to improve diagnostic yield, as opposed to using them in isolation.[19,20,25,26] Additionally, endobronchial needle aspiration should be used with all visible lesions because its use in combination with conventional techniques has been associated with an improvement in the yield from 65 to 96%.[27]

If the lesion is not visible endoscopically, BAL can be performed.[28–30] In brief, the bronchoscope is wedged in the target segmental or subsegmental bronchus leading to the lesion. Aliquots of normal saline solution are instilled and then aspirated. Ideally, the return should be 40 to 60% of the instilled volume; however, this result is dependent on the segment lavaged, with better return coming from less-dependent locations.[31] BAL is thought to sample approximately 1 million alveoli, and the cellular and noncellular contents of the lavage fluid have been shown to closely correlate with the inflammatory nature of the entire lower respiratory tract.[30,32–34] Transbronchial biopsy (TBBx), brushing, and TBNA can also be performed for peripheral lesions.

The diagnostic yield of BAL for peripheral cancer ranges from 4 to 68%.[35–37] Without advanced guidance (discussed in the next paragraph), the yield for TBBx ranges from 49 to 77%; for brushing, it is 26 to 57%. However, again, the combination of all three increases the yield to 68%.[35] TBNA of peripheral nodules has been shown to have a greater diagnostic yield than other sampling techniques, and it should be used for the biopsy of peripheral lesions.[38,39] Kawaraya et al[37] recommend washing the tools used to obtain samples and sending the wash for cytologic analysis, with a combined diagnostic yield of 93%.

As for peripheral nodules and masses, despite TBNA being introduced > 25 years ago, it remains an underused technique, with only 12% of pulmonologists reporting its routine use for the evaluation of patients with suspected lung cancer.[40,41] The technique, however, is incredibly useful. A study of 365 patients with documented malignancy found that the use of standard TBNA (without EBUS) would preclude further invasive surgery in 29% of patients and was able to establish exclusively a diagnosis in 18% of cases.[42,43] The yield with TBNA has been associated with tumor cell type (small cell > non-small cell > lymphoma), lymph node size, and lymph node location.[44]

The use of CT fluoroscopy to guide TBNA and TBBx has several advantages over standard fluoroscopy. As opposed to standard fluoroscopy, which is typically only used in two dimensions, CT provides the ability to visualize the target in three dimensions. With standard fluoroscopy, either the patient or the C-arm needs to be rotated to confirm the biopsy tool is not anterior or posterior to the target. CT fluoroscopy provides real-time three-dimensional confirmation of the appropriate and inappropriate biopsy sites. The use of CT fluoroscopy has been associated with an accuracy of 88%, including patients who have previously undergone a nondiagnostic bronchoscopy with standard TBNA.[45] The one frustration that can occur with CT-guided bronchoscopy is that one may be able to see the lesion but be unable to steer the bronchoscope/catheter into the correct airway.

EBUS is another important modality used to help improve the accuracy of sampling peripheral nodules, as well as in guiding TBNA. The earliest EBUS system used a radial probe with a 20-MHz transducer that could be inserted via a 2.8-mm working channel. Despite not allowing for real-time guidance, early studies[46–48] with radial-probe EBUS found significant improvements in the yield of TBNA, sampling of peripheral nodules, and distinguishing tumor invasion vs compression in the central airways. The sonographic characteristics of peripheral nodules also have been shown to correlate well with histology findings.[49,50]

More recently, a bronchoscope with a dedicated convex 7.5-MHz linear array transducer and a distinct working channel has been developed and has the major benefit of providing real-time guidance for TBNA of mediastinal and hilar lymph nodes, with excellent results.[51–53] Despite the high sensitivity and specificity of EBUS-TBNA, it is crucial to understand that a nondiagnostic result is not equivalent to a negative result. The false-negative rate for EBUS-TBNA can be as high as 20%. Therefore, it is mandatory for the physician to follow all nondiagnostic procedures with a confirmatory surgical biopsy or appropriate clinical follow-up before concluding that the test produced a true-negative result.[54]

Autofluoresence bronchoscopy can be used for the early detection of cancer in the central airways, primarily carcinoma *in situ* (CIS), and squamous cell carcinoma. When exposed to light in the violet-blue spectrum (400 to 450 nm), the normal airway fluoresces green. As submucosal disease progresses from normal, to metaplasia, to dysplasia, to CIS, there is a progressive loss of the green autofluoresence, causing a red-brown appearance of the airway wall. Several studies[54a-b] have shown that the use of autofluoresence increases the detection of early-stage lung cancer by up to sixfold when compared with white light bronchoscopy. The major limitation of autofluoresence lies in its low specificity, and one study[55] suggests that only one case of CIS is identified per 100 bronchoscopies. Other new technologies such as narrow-band imaging, optical coherence tomography, and confocal imaging may also help in the diagnosis of early-stage lung cancer, although definitive data are still pending.

Diffuse Parenchymal Lung Disease

Diffuse parenchymal lung disease describes a group of infectious and inflammatory and fibrotic disorders that may involve the interstitial, alveolar, bronchial, and vascular structures of the tracheobronchial tree. The most commonly used sampling techniques for patients with diffuse disease include BAL bronchial brushing, TBBx and, occasionally, endobronchial biopsy and TBNA.

Although associated with a low morbidity and mortality, TBBx should be used only when the potential results will have an impact on treatment decisions. Diseases in which TBBx can prove diagnostic or when it has been shown to significantly increase the diagnostic yield as compared with less-invasive means include lymphangitic carcinomatosis, sarcoidosis, rejection after lung transplantation, hypersensitivity pneumonitis and, sometimes, mycobacterial and invasive fungal infection.[29,56,57] The overall diagnostic yield for TBBx clearly depends on the disease entity as well as severity. For example, the yield for sarcoidosis can approach 90% in patients who have stage II and III disease.[58]

Aside from providing a specific diagnosis in cases of cancer or infection, the results of BAL can serve to limit the differential diagnosis considerably.[56] For example, BAL findings with lymphocyte predominance suggest granulomatous disease such as sarcoidosis, berylliosis, or a lymphoproliferative disorder. Neutrophil predominance suggests bacterial infection, acute interstitial pneumonia, and may also be found in patients with asbestosis or usual interstitial pneumonitis. Eosinophils are seen in patients with eosinophilic pneumonias, hypereosinophilic syndromes, or Churg-Strauss syndrome. The BAL fluid of patients with pulmonary alveolar proteinosis has a unique appearance that is described as milky or opaque. The alveolar macrophages are filled with pulmonary alveolar proteinosis-positive material, and lamellar bodies can be seen with electron microscopy.

Infectious Diseases

Community-Acquired Pneumonia

The role of bronchoscopy in community-acquired pneumonia remains controversial.[59] When used, BAL and protected brush are the main diagnostic procedures, and the specimens should ideally be sent for quantitative culture, with a threshold of 10^4 cfu in the BAL and 10^3 cfu in the protected brush. A study by van der Eerden and colleagues[60] found bronchoscopy to be of additive diagnostic value in 49% of patients who were unable to raise sputum for Gram stain and culture and in 52% of patients for whom treatment failed. As expected, pretreatment with antibiotics may significantly reduce the yield,[61] although Feinsilver et al[62] found an 86% yield in patients with nonresolving pneumonia who had already received antibiotics. Another important indication for bronchoscopy in patients with community-acquired pneumonia is the ruling out of an obstructing endobronchial lesion. Obviously, it is crucial to avoid contamination with upper airway secretions when performing bronchoscopy in patients with pneumonia. Key procedural aspects include minimizing suctioning, as well as minimizing the instillation of saline solution or lidocaine, because secretions in the working channel will be flushed back into the airways, and high concentrations of lidocaine can be bacteriostatic. Baselski and Wunderink[59] reviewed the indications, procedural details, mechanisms for specimen transport/handling, and interpretation of results.

Health Care and Ventilator-Associated Pneumonia

By using the techniques of evidence-based medicine to guide their recommendations, the American Thoracic Society and Infectious Diseases Society of America have recently reviewed these topics in great detail.[63] Some major points included the collection of a lower respiratory tract culture before the initiation of antibiotics, the use of semiquantitative or quantitative culture data, and the use of negative culture data to discontinue antibiotics in patients who have not had changes in their antibiotic regimen within the last 72 h.[63] Additionally, the use of a bronchoscopic strategy was supported as a way to reduce 14-day mortality.[15,63] More recently, an invasive strategy was found to have no impact on mortality.[16] A major criticism of this study was the fact that the authors excluded patients with pseudomonas and *Staphylococcus pneumoniae*.

The early diagnosis and initiation of the appropriate antibiotic administration is the cornerstone of successful treatment of the immunocompromised patient with pneumonia. Additionally, it is important to note that multiple diagnoses often can be present simultaneously in these patients[64] and that noninfectious conditions may have a similar presentation of cough, dyspnea, fever, and an infiltrate on imaging. Bronchoscopy is an excellent method of evaluating these patients because the use of less-invasive techniques can miss the diagnosis in approximately 30% of patients.[34] In addition, earlier diagnoses may improve rates of mortality.[65]

Helmers and Pisani[30] suggest three broad categories of immunocompromised patients: those who are pharmacologically immunosuppressed, those with hematologic malignancy/malfunction, and those with immunodeficiency. The reason for these categories is because each type of immunodeficiency predisposes the patient to distinct infections. For example, infection with *S pneumoniae* and *Haemophilus influenzae* is common in patients with hypogammaglobulinemia, whereas Aspergillus sp is more likely to cause disease in patients with neutropenia. Cryptococcus sp, Histoplasma sp, and viruses such as cytomegalovirus are seen in patients with defects in cell-mediated immunity.[66]

BAL, which has an overall diagnostic yield of approximately 60 to 70%, is the most commonly used bronchoscopic technique used to obtain a diagnosis in immunocompromised patients.[66] In comparative studies, the sensitivity of TBBx has been shown to be roughly the same,[67,68] although the combined use of both techniques may increase the yield.[69] The results of BAL have been shown to change disease management in up to 84% of cases.[70] Unfortunately, although bronchoscopy changed disease management in patients who have undergone bone marrow transplantation, the rate of mortality has remained extremely high.[64,71] Bronchoscopy with BAL remains a safe procedure, even in the immunocompromised host. Brushing and TBBx have been associated with a greater incidence of bleeding complications in patients who are thrombocytopenic.[72] The "gold standard" remains open-lung biopsy, which can yield a specific diagnosis in 62% of patients and result in a significant increase in survival.[73]

Hemoptysis

There are many causes of hemoptysis, including infectious and inflammatory, vascular, and neoplastic processes.[74] Although one would think that the use of bronchoscopy can often aid in the diagnosis of a radiographic occult neoplasm in a patient who presents with hemoptysis, a bronchoscopic diagnosis of malignancy is made in $<5\%$. The incidence of cancer is increased in patients who present with hemoptysis and normal chest imaging if they are >40 years of age, are male, and have a >40 pack-year smoking history.[75–77] As such, bronchoscopy is recommended in this patient population. Although the appropriate timing for bronchoscopy is controversial, there is a greater likelihood of identifying the bleeding source when performed within the first 48 h of symptoms.[78] The combined use of bronchoscopy and CT is also recommended.[74] If patients are clinically stable, I would recommend performing the CT first because it can serve as a road map to guide bronchoscopy.[79]

Therapeutic Bronchoscopy

Although many advanced techniques can be performed with flexible bronchoscopy, the rigid bronchoscope is the preferred tool in many situations.[80,81] The rigid bronchoscope provides an airway in which to oxygenate/ventilate the patient as well as pass multiple devices, including large-bore suction catheters, laser/argon plasma coagulation/electrocautery fibers, the microdebrider blade, and larger biopsy instruments. The rigid bronchoscope itself can also be used to achieve relative lung isolation, dilate stenosis, and "core-out" tumor tissue from the central airways. Unfortunately, only approximately 4% of pulmonologists currently perform rigid bronchoscopy,[82] and its use is typically not taught in pulmonary and critical care fellowship programs.[83]

Massive Hemoptysis

The definition of massive hemoptysis ranges from 100 to 1,000 mL expectorated during a 24-h period.[84,85] Because the majority of patients with massive hemoptysis die from asphyxia, not exsanguination, and because the anatomic dead space is approximately 150 mL, I consider any amount >100 mL in 24-h period as massive. By using a definition of 500 mL/24 h, Hirshberg et al[74] found that 14% of 208 patients presenting with hemoptysis had massive hemoptysis.

In addition to identifying the source and cause of bleeding, bronchoscopy clearly plays an important therapeutic role in patients with massive hemoptysis. If available, rigid bronchoscopy is generally considered the airway procedure of choice in these patients. If rigid bronchoscopy is not available, the options include intubation with a single-lumen endotracheal tube, a double-lumen tube, or placement of a bronchial blocker. Because double-lumen endotracheal tubes, or specialized tubes that come with an endobronchial blocker (*ie*, Univent; Vitaid; Williamsville, NY), can be more difficult to place, especially in the setting of massive hemoptysis, my practice is to place a larger single-lumen tube.

The main role of flexible bronchoscopy in the patient with massive hemoptysis lies in helping to obtaining lung isolation by guiding the endotracheal tube or bronchial blocker and providing some therapeutic aspiration to protect the "good" lung. All bronchoscopists should become familiar with bronchial blockers (*ie*, Arndt Bronchial Blocker; Cook Critical Care; Bloomington, IN), which can be passed in parallel to the bronchoscope. These catheters are guided to the culprit segmental, lobar, or mainstem bronchus, and the balloon is inflated to the recommended volume/pressure. After a maximum of 24 h, the balloon should be deflated under bronchoscopic visualization.[86–88] Other bronchoscopic techniques used to control hemoptysis include the topical application of iced saline, epinephrine (1:20,000), and thrombin/thrombin-fibrinogen/or cyanoacrylate solutions, although the data supporting these techniques are extremely limited.[89–91]

Advanced Bronchoscopic Techniques

Argon Plasma Coagulation

Argon plasma coagulation (APC) is a noncontact method that uses ionized argon gas (plasma) to achieve tissue coagulation and hemostasis. Because the plasma is directed to the closest grounded source, APC has the ability to treat lesions lateral to the probe. The depth of penetration for APC is approximately 2 to 3 mm and, hence, the risk of airway perforation is less when compared with lasers. Gas flow through the APC fiber should be kept to the lowest setting possible (*ie*, 0.5 L/min) to avoid the potential of gas emboli formation.[92]

Laser Therapy

The Nd:YAG laser is the most widely used laser in the lower respiratory system and has been used for both benign and malignant disease.[93] The primary advantage of laser photoresection is that it provides rapid destruction/vaporization of tissue. Care must be taken because the depth of penetration can approach 10 mm, and airway perforation with resultant pneumothorax, pneumomediastinum, and vascular injury has been reported. As such, it should be used only by experienced interventional bronchoscopists. Despite this caveat, the safety record of laser bronchoscopy is excellent, with an overall complication rate of <1%.[93] Lesions most amenable to laser therapy are central, intrinsic, and short (<4 cm), with a visible distal endobronchial lumen.[94] When lesions meet these criteria, patency can be reestablished in >90% of cases. Of note, the tissue destruction obtained with laser therapy is often more than that is visually appreciated at the time of the procedure.

Cryotherapy

Cryotherapy is a safe and effective tool for a variety of airway problems.[95,96] By releasing nitrous oxide or carbon dioxide stored under pressure, the tip of the cryoprobe rapidly cools to -89°C. Cryotherapy is especially useful for the removal of organic foreign bodies with high water content, such as grapes and vegetable matter, in addition to facilitating the removal of tenacious mucus or blood clots when performing flexible bronchoscopy. Compared with other techniques for tumor destruction, cryotherapy has a delayed effect and, thus, requires a repeat bronchoscopy to remove the necrotic tissue. The distinct advantage of cryotherapy lies in the fact that the normal airway tissue is relatively cryoresistant. Additionally, unlike "hot" thermal techniques, cryotherapy is not associated with a risk of airway fires.

Electrocautery

Electrocautery uses alternating current at high frequency to generate heat, which cuts, vaporizes, or coagulates tissue depending on the power. Electrocautery is a contact mode of tissue destruction, and a variety of cautery probes are available, including blunt tip probes, knifes, and snares. The snare is an ideal tool for pedunculated lesions because the stalk can be cut and coagulated while preserving the majority of the tissue for pathologic interpretation.[97] The knife is also an excellent tool for producing radial incisions before dilation of web-like tracheal stenosis. As with laser therapy, the risks of electrocautery include airway perforation, airway fires, and damage to the bronchoscope.

Photodynamic Therapy

Photodynamic therapy (PDT) involves the IV injection of a photosensitizing agent, and then activating the drug with a nonthermal laser to produce a phototoxic reaction and cell death. Because the laser is not a heat source, airway fires are not an issue. Because tumor cells retain the drug longer than other tissues, waiting approximately 48 h after drug injection will lead to preferential tumor cell death as compared with normal tissue injury. Similar to cryotherapy, maximal effects are delayed, and a repeat, "clean-out" bronchoscopy should be performed 24 to 48 h after drug activation. The primary side effect from PDT is systemic phototoxicity, which can last up to 6 weeks after injection. Newer drugs are being developed with the hope of increasing tumor selectivity and reducing the duration of skin phototoxicity. PDT has been shown to be curative for early-stage lung cancer of the airways and is an especially attractive option for patients with endobronchial CIS are not surgical candidates as the result of other comorbidities.[98,99]

Brachytherapy

Brachytherapy refers to endobronchial radiation, primarily used for the treatment of endobronchial malignant airway obstruction.[100,101] The most commonly used source of radiation is ^{192}Ir, which is delivered through a catheter inserted bronchoscopically. Brachytherapy may be delivered by either low-dose rate, intermediate-dose rate, or high-dose rate (HDR) methods, with most authors currently recommending the afterloading HDR technique. This technique allows the bronchoscopist to place the catheter in the desired location and the radiation oncologist to deliver the radiation in a protected environment. The main advantage of HDR is patient convenience because each session lasts <30 min; however, multiple bronchoscopies are required to achieve the recommended total 1,500 cGy dose. The low-dose rate technique may be appropriate for patients who live far from the hospital or who are otherwise hospitalized because it only requires one bronchoscopy; however, the catheter has to stay in place for 20 to 60 h, which is often poorly tolerated by the patient. The main advantage of brachytherapy as compared with external-beam radiation is the fact that less normal tissue is exposed to the toxic effects of radiation. The most common side effects include intolerance of the catheter, radiation bronchitis, airway perforation and, occasionally, massive hemorrhage. The greatest incidence of hemorrhage occurs during the treatment of tumors in the right and left upper lobes because they are located near the great vessels.

Airway Stents

Montgomery is credited as initiating the widespread use of airway stents after his development of a silicone T tube in 1965 for use in patients with tracheal stenosis.[102] Dumon, however, introduced the first completely endoluminal airway stent in 1990.[103] Airway stents are the only technology that can alleviate extrinsic airway compression. They are commonly used in conjunction with the other modalities for patients with intrinsic or mixed disease.

During the last 15 years, there has been an explosion in both stent design and in the number of endoscopists who place airway stents. As with any procedure, it is crucial to understand the indications and contraindications of the procedure as well as be able to anticipate, prevent, and manage the associated complications. Unfortunately, the ideal stent has not yet been developed. This stent would be easy to insert and remove, yet not migrate; of sufficient strength to support the airway, yet be flexible enough to mimic normal airway physiology and promote secretion clearance; biologically inert to minimize the formation of granulation tissue; and available in a variety of sizes.

There are currently two main types of stents: metal, which generally is composed of Nitinol Super-Elastic Archwire (3M Unitek; Monrova, CA), and silicone. Although metal stents are easy to place, they can be extremely difficult to extract. They are available in covered (typically with silicone or polyurethane) and uncovered varieties. For malignant airway obstruction, the only appropriate metal stents are covered models, which minimize tumor in-growth. Some authors believe that there is no indication for an uncovered metal stent. The overuse of metallic stents in patients with nonmalignant airway obstruction has led to the US Food and Drug Administration creating a black-box warning recommending their use as a modality of last resort in these patients.[104] The main advantage of metal stents is their larger internal/external diameter ratio as compared with silicone stents. Although silicone stents require rigid bronchoscopy for placement, they are more easily removed and are significantly less expensive.

In addition to malignant airway obstruction, airway stents can be helpful in patients with tracheobronchomalacia and tracheoesophageal fistula. In patient with tracheoesophageal fistula, double stenting of the esophagus and airway is recommend to maximally prevent aspiration.[105]

Future Directions in Bronchoscopy

Bronchoscopic Lung Volume Reduction

In the patient with upper lobe predominant disease and low exercise capacity, lung volume reduction surgery has been shown to improve both quality and length of life.[106] The major drawback to surgical lung volume reduction is its invasiveness and cost. As such, several techniques to achieve lung volume reduction bronchoscopically are currently under investigation, although no such device has been approved by the US Food and Drug Administration.

Bronchial Thermoplasty

Bronchoscopic thermoplasty is a technique in which controlled thermal energy (radiofrequency energy at 65°C) is applied directly to visible airways through the bronchoscope. The goal is to achieve ablation of the airway smooth muscle without causing scarring and stenosis. In a preliminary study,[107] the use of this technique in the treatment of patients with mild-to-moderate asthma led to reduction in airway hyperresponsiveness, which was associated with improvements in daily symptoms and peak expiratory flow for a period of 2 years. In a study[108] of 112 subjects in whom asthma control was impaired, bronchial thermoplasty reduced the rate of mild exacerbations, and at 12 months, there were significantly greater improvements in the bronchial-thermoplasty group than in the control group. Widespread clinical application of this technique requires validation by other ongoing multicenter studies.

Enhanced Navigation

The use of electromagnetic navigation, especially when used in conjunction with radial-probe EBUS, is a novel technology that has been shown to allow accurate sampling of peripheral solitary pulmonary nodules <2 cm in diameter.[109,110] In brief, a virtual bronchoscopy is generated from the patient's CT scan. Anatomic landmarks that are easily identified, such as the carina, are marked, as is the target. At the time of bronchoscopy, the patient lies in an electromagnetic field and a steerable, locatable guide is placed through an extended working channel of the bronchoscope. The location of the guide in the electromagnetic field is accurate to <5 mm in the x, y, and z axes, as well as yaw, pitch, and roll. The points previously identified in the virtual bronchoscopy are then marked with the locatable guide that in essence fuses the CT scan with the patient's anatomy.

Navigation is then performed by examining the CT in the axial, saggital, and coronal planes, and the guide is steered toward the target. Once found, the guide is removed, and standard bronchoscopic tools such as TBNA needles, forceps, and brushes are placed through the extended working channel. This technology can be used for both diagnostic bronchoscopy as well as therapeutic modalities. For example, if a patient with a 2.5-cm, stage Ia non-small cell cancer is not an operative candidate, this technology may allow for bronchoscopic treatment by either radiofrequency ablation or the implantation of fiducials to allow stereotactic radiosurgery.[111] Other techniques of virtual bronchoscopic navigation are also being developed that do not require the presence of an electromagnetic field and rely on high-definition virtual bronchoscopic road maps with ultrathin bronchoscopes.[112–114]

Other Interventional Pulmonary Procedures

Pleural Interventions

Ultrasound has revolutionized the evaluation and management of patients with pleural disease.[115] Although randomized trials have not been performed, the use of ultrasound appears to be associated with an increased success as well as a reduction in the pneumothorax rate for patients undergoing thoracentesis. Ultrasound allows for the precise placement of small-bore chest tubes in loculated effusions and has been shown to be extremely accurate in ruling out pneumothorax.[116]

Medical thoracoscopy describes the insertion of a semirigid or rigid thoracoscope with the intent of draining pleural fluid, obtaining biopsies of the parietal pleura, and/or instilling an agent to achieve pleurodesis.[66,117,118] Whereas video-assisted thoracic surgery is typically performed in the operating room with general anesthesia and lung isolation with two or three ports, medical thoracoscopy is commonly performed in an endoscopy suite with moderate sedation on a spontaneously breathing patient with one access port. Common indications for medical thoracoscopy include a recurrent exudative effusion with no clear diagnosis or a known malignant effusion requiring pleurodesis.

Indwelling, tunneled pleural catheters are an excellent treatment option for patients with dyspnea caused by a recurrent malignant pleural effusion. Although the treatment of choice for patients with lung entrapment, they may also be used for patients with expandable lung. Pleural palliation can be achieved in close to 90% of patients, and side effects are relatively few.[119]

Additional Airway Procedures

Many interventional pulmonologists routinely perform percutaneous dilational tracheostomy. As compared with open tracheostomy, percutaneous tracheostomy is at least as safe, and it may be associated with reduced infectious and bleeding complications. It is also less expensive and does not require transport of a critically ill patient to the operating room.[120]

Complications

Bronchoscopy is generally considered a relatively safe procedure.[5] However, it is common that patients in whom bronchoscopy is performed can have multiple comorbidities, and therefore, the bronchoscopist needs to be aware of the patient's medical history, including medications and allergies. Additionally, the bronchoscopist needs to have a thorough understanding of the effects and side effects of the medications he or she will use to achieve adequate topical anesthesia and moderate sedation and to be skilled in airway management should the patient experience hypoxemia/hypercapnia.

Transient fever is the most common adverse event after BAL is performed, and it can be seen in up to one-third of patients. Major adverse events including hypoxemia, pneumothorax, bleeding, and death may also occur, and both patient and procedure-related factors are important determinants. The British Thoracic Society has published their recommendations concerning the performance of diagnostic flexible bronchoscopy. These recommendations include steps that should be taken to minimize complications.[5] Although still relatively safe, complications associated with the more advanced procedures including rigid bronchoscopy, pleuroscopy/thoracoscopy, indwelling pleural catheters, and percutaneous tracheostomy are slightly greater as a result of the increased acuity of the patient population as well as the invasiveness of the interventions.[8,9]

Training

Flexible bronchoscopy is one of the most commonly performed procedures by the pulmonologist. Although 96% of fellowship programs offer the recommended number of diagnostic flexible bronchoscopies, the percentage of programs achieving the recommended number was only 69% for TBNA and decreased dramatically for more advanced procedures.[83] As such, recommendations are forthcoming that a year of advanced training should be required for the majority of procedures considered essential to the interventional pulmonologists. Clearly, it is not necessary to obtain a formal additional year of training to become an expert in any one technique, such as EBUS. To fully understand the diagnostic approach and available therapeutic modalities as well as obtain the necessary skills to anticipate, prevent, and manage complications in patients with complex central airway or pleural disease, it is best to obtain formal training in the subspecialty of interventional pulmonology.

References

1. Zollner F. Gustav Killian, father of bronchoscopy. Arch Otolaryngol 1965; 82:656–659
2. Killian G. Ueber direkte Bronchoskopie. Muench Med Wochen 1898; 27:844–847
3. Becker HD, Marsh BR. History of the rigid bronchoscope. In: Bolliger CT, Mathur PN, eds. Interventional bronchoscopy. Basel: Karger, 2000; 2–15
4. Miyazawa T. History of the flexible bronchoscope. In: Bolliger CT, Mathur PN, eds. Interventional bronchoscopy. Basel: Karger, 2000; 16–21
5. British Thoracic Society guidelines on diagnostic flexible bronchoscopy. Thorax 2001; 56:i1–i21
6. Ernst A, Feller-Kopman D, Becker HD, et al. Central airway obstruction. Am J Respir Crit Care Med 2004; 169:1278–1297
7. Wahidi MM, Herth FJF, Ernst A. State of the art: interventional pulmonology. Chest 2007; 131:261–274
8. Bolliger CT, Mathur PN, Beamis JF, et al. ERS/ATS statement on interventional pulmonology: European Respiratory Society/American Thoracic Society. Eur Respir J 2002; 19:356–373
9. Ernst A, Silvestri GA, Johnstone D. Interventional pulmonary procedures: guidelines from the American College of Chest Physicians. Chest 2003; 123:1693–1717
10. Cortese DA, Prakash UBS. Anatomy for the bronchoscopist. In: Prakash UBS, ed. Bronchoscopy. New York: Raven Press, 1994; 13–42
11. Becker HD. Atlas of bronchoscopy: technique, diagnosis, differential diagnosis, therapy. Philadelphia; BC Decker, 1991
12. Jackson CL, Huber JF. Correlated anatomy of the bronchial tree and lungs with a system of nomenclature. Dis Chest 1943; 9:319–326
13. Boyden EA. Segmental anatomy of the lung. New York, McGraw Hill, 1955
14. Ost D, DeRosiers A, Britt EJ, et al. Assessment of a bronchoscopy simulator. Am J Respir Crit Care Med 2001; 164:2248–2255
15. Fagon JY, Chastre J, Wolff M, et al. Invasive and noninvasive strategies for management of suspected ventilator-associated pneumonia: a randomized trial. Ann Intern Med 2000; 132:621–630
16. Heyland D, Cook D, Dodek P, et al. A randomized trial of diagnostic techniques for ventilator-associated pneumonia. N Engl J Med 2006; 355:2619–2630
17. American Cancer Society. Cancer facts and figures 2008. Available at: http://www.cancer.org/downloads/STT/2008CAFFfinalsecured.pdf. Accessed April 22, 2009
18. National Cancer Institute. SEER cancer statistics review 1975–2005. Available at: http://seer.cancer.gov/csr/1975_2005/results_merged/sect_15_lung_bronchus.pdf. Accessed April 22, 2009
19. Mazzone P, Jain P, Arroliga AC, et al. Bronchoscopy and needle biopsy techniques for diagnosis and staging of lung cancer. Clin Chest Med 2002; 23:137–58, ix.
20. Arroliga AC, Matthay RA. The role of bronchoscopy in lung cancer. Clin Chest Med 1993; 14:87–98
21. Hyer JD, Silvestri G. Diagnosis and staging of lung cancer. Clin Chest Med 2000; 21:95-ix
22. Rafanan AL, Mehta A. Role of bronchoscopy in lung cancer. Semin Respir Crit Care Med 2000; 21:405–420
23. Wang KP. Staging of bronchogenic carcinoma by bronchoscopy. Chest 1994; 106:588–593
24. Hooper RG, Jackson FN. Endobronchial electrocautery. Chest 1985; 87:712–714
25. Saita S, Tanzillo A, Riscica C, et al. Bronchial brushing and biopsy: a comparative evaluation in diagnosing visible bronchial lesions. Eur J Cardiothorac Surg 1990; 4:270–272
26. Mak VH, Johnston ID, Hetzel MR, et al. Value of washings and brushings at fibreoptic bronchoscopy in the diagnosis of lung cancer. Thorax 1990; 45:373–376

27. Dasgupta A, Jain P, Minai OA, et al. Utility of transbronchial needle aspiration in the diagnosis of endobronchial lesions. Chest 1999; 115:1237–1241
28. Anzueto A, Levine SM, Jenkinson SG. The technique of bronchoalveolar lavage: a guide to sampling the terminal airways and alveolar space. J Crit Illn 1992; 7:1817–1824
29. Kvale PA. Bronchoscopic biopsies and bronchoalveolar lavage. Chest Surg Clin N Am 1996; 6:205–222
30. Helmers RA, Pisani RJ. Bronchoalveolar lavage. In: Prakash UB, ed. Bronchoscopy. New York, NY: Raven Press, 1994; 155–182
31. Baughman RP. Technical aspects of bronchoalveolar lavage: recommendations for a standard procedure. Semin Respir Crit Care Med 2007; 28:475–485
32. Hunninghake GW, Gadek JE, Kawanami O, et al. Inflammatory and immune processes in the human lung in health and disease: evaluation by bronchoalveolar lavage. Am J Pathol 1979; 97:149–206
33. Goldstein RA, Rohatgi PK, Bergofsky EH, et al. Clinical role of bronchoalveolar lavage in adults with pulmonary disease. Am Rev Respir Dis 1990; 142:481–486
34. Reynolds HY. Bronchoalveolar lavage. Am Rev Respir Dis 1987; 135:250–263
35. Bilaceroglu S, Kumcuoglu Z, Alper H, et al. CT bronchus sign-guided bronchoscopic multiple diagnostic procedures in carcinomatous solitary pulmonary nodules and masses. Respiration 1998; 65:49–55
36. Shiner RJ, Rosenman J, Katz I, et al. Bronchoscopic evaluation of peripheral lung tumours. Thorax 1988; 43:887–889
37. Kawaraya M, Gemba K, Ueoka H, et al. Evaluation of various cytological examinations by bronchoscopy in the diagnosis of peripheral lung cancer. Br J Cancer 2003; 89:1885–1888
38. Katis K, Inglesos E, Zachariadis E, et al. The role of transbronchial needle aspiration in the diagnosis of peripheral lung masses or nodules. Eur Respir J 1995; 8:963–966
39. Shure D, Fedullo PF. Transbronchial needle aspiration of peripheral masses. Am Rev Respir Dis 1983; 128:1090–1092
40. Prakash UB, Offord KP, Stubbs SE. Bronchoscopy in North America: the ACCP survey. Chest 1991; 100:1668–1675
41. Haponik EF, Shure D. Underutilization of transbronchial needle aspiration: experiences of current pulmonary fellows. Chest 1997; 112:251–253
42. Harrow EM, Abi-Saleh W, Blum J, et al. The utility of transbronchial needle aspiration in the staging of bronchogenic carcinoma. Am J Respir Crit Care Med 2000; 161:601–607
43. Salathe M, Soler M, Bolliger CT, et al. Transbronchial needle aspiration in routine fiberoptic bronchoscopy. Respiration 1992; 59:5–8
44. Sharafkhaneh A, Baaklini W, Gorin AB, et al. Yield of transbronchial needle aspiration in diagnosis of mediastinal lesions. Chest 2003; 124:2131–2135
45. Garpestad E, Goldberg SN, Herth F, et al. CT fluoroscopy guidance for transbronchial needle aspiration: an experience in 35 patients. Chest 2001; 119:329–332
46. Herth FJ, Becker HD, Ernst A. Ultrasound-guided transbronchial needle aspiration: an experience in 242 patients. Chest 2003; 123:604–607
47. Herth F, Becker HD, Ernst A. Conventional vs endobronchial ultrasound-guided transbronchial needle aspiration: a randomized trial. Chest 2004; 125:322–325
48. Herth F, Ernst A, Schulz M, et al. Endobronchial ultrasound reliably differentiates between airway infiltration and compression by tumor. Chest 2003; 123:458–462
49. Kurimoto N, Murayama M, Yoshioka S, et al. Analysis of the internal structure of peripheral pulmonary lesions using endobronchial ultrasonography. Chest 2002; 122:1887–1894
50. Herth FJ, Ernst A, Becker HD. Endobronchial ultrasound-guided transbronchial lung biopsy in solitary pulmonary nodules and peripheral lesions. Eur Respir J 2002; 20:972–974
51. Yasufuku K, Chiyo M, Sekine Y, et al. Real-time endobronchial ultrasound-guided transbronchial needle aspiration of mediastinal and hilar lymph nodes. Chest 2004; 126:122–128
52. Yasufuku K, Nakajima T, Motoori K, et al. Comparison of endobronchial ultrasound, positron emission tomography, and CT for lymph node staging of lung cancer. Chest 2006; 130:710–718
53. Herth FJ, Eberhardt R, Vilmann P, et al. Real-time endobronchial ultrasound guided transbronchial needle aspiration for sampling mediastinal lymph nodes. Thorax 2006; 61:795–798

54. Detterbeck FC, Jantz MA, Wallace M, et al. Invasive mediastinal staging of lung cancer: ACCP evidence-based clinical practice guidelines (2nd edition). Chest 2007; 132(3 suppl):202S–220S

54a. Lam S, Kennedy T, Unger M, Miller YE, Gelmont D, Rusch V et al. Localization of bronchial intraepithelial neoplastic lesions by fluorescence bronchoscopy. Chest 1998;113(3):696–702

55b. Weigel TL, Yousem S, Dacic S, Kosco PJ, Siegfried J, Luketich JD. Fluorescence bronchoscopic surveillance after curative surgical resection for non-small-cell lung cancer. Ann Surg Oncol 2000;7(3):176–180

55. Haussinger K, Becker H, Stanzel F, et al. Autofluorescence bronchoscopy with white light bronchoscopy compared with white light bronchoscopy alone for the detection of precancerous lesions: a European randomised controlled multicentre trial. Thorax 2005; 60:496–503

56. Poletti V, Chilosi M, Olivieri D. Diagnostic invasive procedures in diffuse infiltrative lung diseases. Respiration 2004; 71:107–119

57. Ensminger SA, Prakash UB. Is bronchoscopic lung biopsy helpful in the management of patients with diffuse lung disease? Eur Respir J 2006; 28:1081–1084

58. Gilman MJ, Wang KP. Transbronchial lung biopsy in sarcoidosis: an approach to determine the optimal number of biopsies. Am Rev Respir Dis 1980; 122:721–724

59. Baselski VS, Wunderink RG. Bronchoscopic diagnosis of pneumonia. Clin Microbiol Rev 1994; 7:533–558

60. van der Eerden MM, Vlaspolder F, de Graaff CS, et al. Value of intensive diagnostic microbiological investigation in low- and high-risk patients with community-acquired pneumonia. Eur J Clin Microbiol Infect Dis 2005; 24:241–249

61. Hohenthal U, Sipila J, Vainionpaa R, et al. Diagnostic value of bronchoalveolar lavage in community-acquired pneumonia in a routine setting: a study on patients treated in a Finnish university hospital. Scand J Infect Dis 2004; 36:198–203

62. Feinsilver SH, Fein AM, Niederman MS, et al. Utility of fiberoptic bronchoscopy in nonresolving pneumonia. Chest 1990; 98:1322–1326

63. Guidelines for the management of adults with hospital-acquired, ventilator-associated, and healthcare-associated pneumonia. Am J Respir Crit Care Med 2005; 171:388–416

64. Campbell JH, Blessing N, Burnett AK, et al. Investigation and management of pulmonary infiltrates following bone marrow transplantation: an eight year review. Thorax 1993; 48:1248–1251

65. Rano A, Agusti C, Jimenez P, et al. Pulmonary infiltrates in non-HIV immunocompromised patients: a diagnostic approach using non-invasive and bronchoscopic procedures. Thorax 2001; 56:379–387

66. Hersh CP, Feller-Kopman D, Wahidi M, et al. Ultrasound guidance for medical thoracoscopy: a novel approach. Respiration 2003; 70:299–301

67. Abramson MJ, Stone CA, Holmes PW, et al. The role of bronchoalveolar lavage in the diagnosis of suspected opportunistic pneumonia. Aust N Z J Med 1987; 17:407–412

68. Stover DE, Zaman MB, Hajdu SI, et al. Bronchoalveolar lavage in the diagnosis of diffuse pulmonary infiltrates in the immunosuppressed host. Ann Intern Med 1984; 101:1–7

69. Hsu AA, Allen DM, Yeo CT, et al. Bronchoscopy in immunocompromised host with pulmonary infiltrates. Ann Acad Med Singapore 1996; 25:797–803

70. Hohenadel IA, Kiworr M, Genitsariotis R, et al. Role of bronchoalveolar lavage in immunocompromised patients with pneumonia treated with a broad spectrum antibiotic and antifungal regimen. Thorax 2001; 56:115–120

71. White P, Bonacum JT, Miller CB. Utility of fiberoptic bronchoscopy in bone marrow transplant patients. Bone Marrow Transplant 1997; 20:681–687

72. Dunagan DP, Baker AM, Hurd DD, et al. Bronchoscopic evaluation of pulmonary infiltrates following bone marrow transplantation. Chest 1997; 111:135–141

73. White DA, Wong PW, Downey R. The utility of open lung biopsy in patients with hematologic malignancies. Am J Respir Crit Care Med 2000; 161:723–729

74. Hirshberg B, Biran I, Glazer M, et al. Hemoptysis: etiology, evaluation, and outcome in a tertiary referral hospital. Chest 1997; 112:440–444

75. Jackson CV, Savage PJ, Quinn DL. Role of fiberoptic bronchoscopy in patients with hemoptysis and a normal chest roentgenogram. Chest 1985; 87:142–144

76. Poe RH, Israel RH, Marin MG, et al. Utility of fiberoptic bronchoscopy in patients with hemoptysis and a nonlocalizing chest roentgenogram. Chest 1988; 93:70–75

77. Freimanis AS. Ultrasound and thoracentesis [letter]. JAMA 1977; 238:1631
78. Gong H Jr., Salvatierra C. Clinical efficacy of early and delayed fiberoptic bronchoscopy in patients with hemoptysis. Am Rev Respir Dis 1981; 124:221–225
79. McGuinness G, Beacher JR, Harkin TJ, et al. Hemoptysis: prospective high-resolution CT/bronchoscopic correlation. Chest 1994; 105:1155–1162
80. Ayers ML, Beamis JF Jr. Rigid bronchoscopy in the twenty-first century. Clin Chest Med 2001; 22:355–364
81. Helmers RA, Sanderson DR. Rigid bronchoscopy: the forgotten art. Clin Chest Med 1995; 16:393–399
82. Colt HG, Prakash UBS, Offord KP. Bronchoscopy in North America: survey by the American Association for Bronchology, 1999. J Bronchol 2000; 7:8–25
83. Pastis NJ, Nietert PJ, Silvestri GA. Variation in training for interventional pulmonary procedures among US pulmonary/critical care fellowships: a survey of fellowship directors. Chest 2005; 127:1614–1621
84. Dweik RA, Stoller JK. Role of bronchoscopy in massive hemoptysis. Clin Chest Med 1999; 20:89–105
85. Cahill BC, Ingbar DH. Massive hemoptysis: assessment and management. Clin Chest Med 1994; 15:147–167
86. Jean-Baptiste E. Clinical assessment and management of massive hemoptysis. Crit Care Med 2000; 28:1642–1647
87. Jougon J, Ballester M, Delcambre F, et al. Massive hemoptysis: what place for medical and surgical treatment. Eur J Cardiothorac Surg 2002; 22:345–351
88. Karmy-Jones R, Cuschieri J, Vallieres E. Role of bronchoscopy in massive hemoptysis. Chest Surg Clin N Am 2001; 11:873–906
89. Bhattacharyya P, Dutta A, Samanta AN, et al. New procedure: bronchoscopic endobronchial sealing: a new mode of managing hemoptysis. Chest 2002; 121:2066–2069
90. Conlan AA, Hurwitz SS. Management of massive haemoptysis with the rigid bronchoscope and cold saline lavage. Thorax 1980; 35:901–904
91. Dupree HJ, Lewejohann JC, Gleiss J, et al. Fiberoptic bronchoscopy of intubated patients with life-threatening hemoptysis. World J Surg 2001; 25:104–107
92. Feller-Kopman D, Lukanich JM, Shapira G, et al. Gas flow during bronchoscopic ablation therapy causes gas emboli to the heart: a comparative animal study. Chest 2008; 133:892–896
93. Cavaliere S, Foccoli PO, Toninelli C, et al. Nd: YAG laser in lung cancer: an 11 year experience with 2,253 applications in 1,585 patients. J Bronchol 1994; 1:105–111
94. Mehta AC, Lee F, DeBoer G. Flexible bronchoscopy and the use of lasers. In: Wang KP, Mehta AC, eds. Flexible bronchoscopy. Oxford, MA: Blackwell Science, 1995; 247–274
95. Maiwand MO, Mathur PN. Endobronchial cryotherapy. Semin Respir Crit Care Med 1997; 18:545–554
96. Maiwand MO, Homasson JP. Cryotherapy for tracheobronchial disorders. Clin Chest Med 1995; 16:427–443
97. Hooper RG, Jackson FN. Endobronchial electrocautery. Chest 1988; 94:595–598
98. Moghissi K, Dixon K, Stringer M, et al. The place of bronchoscopic photodynamic therapy in advanced unresectable lung cancer: experience of 100 cases. Eur J Cardiothorac Surg 1999; 15:1–6
99. Cortese DA, Edell ES, Kinsey JH. Photodynamic therapy for early stage squamous cell carcinoma of the lung. Mayo Clin Proc 1997; 72:595–602
100. Macha HN, Wahlers B, Reichle C, et al. Endobronchial radiation therapy for obstructing malignancies: ten years' experience with iridium-192 high-dose radiation brachytherapy afterloading technique in 365 patients. Lung 1995; 173:271–280
101. Kelly JF, Delclos ME, Morice RC, et al. High-dose-rate endobronchial brachytherapy effectively palliates symptoms due to airway tumors: the 10-year M. D. Anderson Cancer Center experience. Int J Radiat Oncol Biol Phys 2000; 48:697–702
102. Montgomery WW. T-tube tracheal stent. Arch Otolaryngol 1965; 82:320–321
103. Dumon JF. A dedicated tracheobronchial stent. Chest 1990; 97:328–332
104. FDA public health notification: complications from metallic tracheal stents in patients with benign airway disorders. Available at: www.fda.gov/cdrh/safety/072905-tracheal.html. Accessed April 22, 2009
105. Freitag L, Tekolf E, Steveling H, et al. Management of malignant esophagotracheal fistulas with airway stenting and double stenting. Chest 1996; 110:1155–1160

106. Fishman A, Martinez F, Naunheim K, et al. A randomized trial comparing lung-volume-reduction surgery with medical therapy for severe emphysema. N Engl J Med 2003; 348:2059–2073
107. Cox G, Miller JD, McWilliams A, et al. Bronchial thermoplasty for asthma. Am J Respir Crit Care Med 2006; 173:965–969
108. Cox G, Thomson NC, Rubin AS, et al. Asthma control during the tear after bronchial thermoplasty. N Engl J Med 2007; 356:1327–1337
109. Eberhardt R, Anantham D, Herth F, et al. Electromagnetic navigation diagnostic bronchoscopy in peripheral lung lesions. Chest 2007; 132:930–935
110. Eberhardt R, Anantham D, Ernst A, et al. Multimodality bronchoscopic diagnosis of peripheral lung lesions: a randomized controlled trial. Am J Respir Crit Care Med 2007; 176:36–41
111. Anantham D, Feller-Kopman D, Shanmugham LN, et al. Electromagnetic navigation bronchoscopy-guided fiducial placement for robotic stereotactic radiosurgery of lung tumors: a feasibility study. Chest 2007; 132:930–935
112. Hofmeister CC, Czerlanis C, Forsythe S, et al. Retrospective utility of bronchoscopy after hematopoietic stem cell transplant. Bone Marrow Transplant 2006; 38:693–698
113. Asano F, Matsuno Y, Tsuzuku A, et al. Diagnosis of peripheral pulmonary lesions using a bronchoscope insertion guidance system combined with endobronchial ultrasonography with a guide sheath. Lung Cancer 2008; 60:366–373
114. Shinagawa N, Yamazaki K, Onodera Y, et al. Virtual bronchoscopic navigation system shortens the examination time: feasibility study of virtual bronchoscopic navigation system. Lung Cancer 2007; 56:201–206
115. Feller-Kopman D. Ultrasound-guided thoracentesis. Chest 2006; 129:1709–1714
116. Lichtenstein D, Meziere G, Biderman P, et al. The comet-tail artifact: an ultrasound sign ruling out pneumothorax. Intensive Care Med 1999; 25:383–388
117. Colt HG. Therapeutic thoracoscopy. Clin Chest Med 1998; 19:383–394
118. Lee P, Colt HG. State of the art: pleuroscopy. J Thorac Oncol 2007; 2:663–670
119. Tremblay A, Michaud G. Single-center experience with 250 tunnelled pleural catheter insertions for malignant pleural effusion. Chest 2006; 129:362–368
120. De LP, Bedert L, Delcroix M, et al. Tracheotomy: clinical review and guidelines. Eur J Cardiothorac Surg 2007; 32:412–421

Pulmonary Complications of HIV Infection

Mark J. Rosen, MD, FCCP

Objectives:

- Review the types of pulmonary disorders that occur in patients with HIV infection
- Understand how demographic factors, the degree of immunosuppression, and the application of anti-Pneumocystis prophylaxis and antiretroviral therapy influence the risk of the development of different types of pulmonary disorders
- Summarize the clinical, radiographic, and laboratory features of infections, neoplasms, and other pulmonary disorders in patients with HIV infection
- Discuss the diagnostic evaluation and treatment of HIV-associated pulmonary disorders

Key words: bacterial pneumonia; cytomegalovirus; fungi; HIV; Kaposi sarcoma; mycobacteria; *Pneumocystis jiroveci* pneumonia; pulmonary diseases

For the last two decades, the AIDS pandemic has remained the most serious infectious global health problem. In 2007, every day, >7,400 persons become infected with HIV, and >5,400 die from AIDS; an estimated 33.2 million people are living with HIV infection worldwide. Around the world, the pandemic seems to have leveled off as the result of intensive public health efforts at prevention; in developed nations, the rates of opportunistic infections and death in persons with AIDS have decreased dramatically since 1995 because of advances in the treatment of HIV. There is now a general perception that AIDS may be considered to be not uniformly fatal but a chronic and controllable disorder. By the end of 2007, >1 million cases of AIDS had been reported in the United States, of whom approximately 583,000 have died. Approximately 56,000 Americans are infected with HIV each year; in 2006, persons 13 to 29 years of age accounted for approximately one third of new HIV infections. African Americans comprised approximately half of the new cases in the past few years. At the end of 2007, an estimated 732,000 people in the United States were living with HIV infection, of whom 468,000 had AIDS. However, the US death rate in persons with AIDS decreased 17% from 2004 to 2007. In many urban communities, AIDS-related diseases are still the leading causes of death among young adults.

The lung is a frequent site of opportunistic infection in immunocompromised patients, and noninfectious pulmonary disorders associated with HIV infection and antiretroviral treatments are increasingly common. Table 1 lists the infectious, neoplastic, and inflammatory diseases that

Table 1. *HIV-Associated Respiratory Disorders*

Bacterial pneumonia
S pneumoniae
H influenzae
P aeruginosa
Staphylococcus aureus
Moraxella catarrhalis
R equi
M tuberculosis
MAC
Other nontuberculous mycobacteria
Fungal infections
P jiroveci
C neoformans
H capsulatum
Aspergillus fumigatus
Coccidioides immitis
Blastomyces dermatitidis
Protozoal infections
Strongyloides stercoralis
Toxoplasma gondii
Viral infections
CMV
Adenovirus
Herpes simplex
Malignancies
KS
Non-Hodgkin lymphoma (NHL)
Primary effusion lymphoma (PEL)
Carcinoma of the lung
Other disorders
Sinusitis
Bronchitis
Bronchiectasis
Emphysema
Lymphocytic interstitial pneumonia
Nonspecific interstitial pneumonia
Cryptogenic organizing pneumonia
Primary pulmonary hypertension
Immune reconstitution inflammatory syndrome

occur in patients with HIV infection, and their typical radiographic patterns are summarized in Table 2.

HIV-Associated Pulmonary Disorders

The pulmonary disorders associated with HIV infection range from asymptomatic and mild abnormalities in pulmonary function to fulminating opportunistic infections. The risk for the development of each of these disorders is strongly influenced by the severity of immunosuppression, the patient's demographic characteristics, the place of current or previous residence, and whether the patient is using prophylaxis against common HIV-associated infections. Genetic factors probably also are important but have been less precisely defined.

Influence of Immune Function

The severity of the abnormality in host defense is the primary determinant of the risk of the development of specific pulmonary disorders. Early in the course of HIV infection, when the immune system is not severely compromised, respiratory disorders occur that are generally similar to those found in the general population. Opportunistic infections occur only with severe immunodeficiency.

The CD4$^+$ lymphocyte count is still the most reliable surrogate marker for immune function, the risk of opportunistic infection, and the risk of progression of HIV disease. The measurement of HIV activity with serum HIV RNA (called the *viral load)* is used routinely to assess the response to treatment with antiretroviral agents and to stratify patients by risk of the progression of disease. However, it is a less reliable predictor than CD4$^+$ count in determining the risk of the development of specific HIV-related diseases. In a survey of the medical records of $>$18,000 HIV-infected subjects who received care in $>$100 sites in 10 US cities, common disorders such as sinusitis, bronchitis, and pharyngitis occurred at all strata of CD4$^+$ cell counts (Table 3). With lower counts, different pulmonary infections occurred with increasing frequency. Some opportunistic infections tend to occur only

Table 2. *HIV Infection: Chest Radiographic Patterns and Common Etiologies*

Radiographic Patterns	Etiologies
Focal opacities	Mediastinal lymphadenopathy
Bacteria	*M tuberculosis*
M tuberculosis	MAC
P jiroveci	KS
Fungi	Lymphoma
	Fungi
	Immune reconstitution
Diffuse opacities	Pleural effusion
P jiroveci	Bacteria
M tuberculosis	*M tuberculosis*
KS	KS
Bacteria	Lymphoma (including primary effusion lymphoma)
Fungi	
CMV	Cardiomyopathy
Immune reconstitution	Hypoproteinemia
	Immune reconstitution
Diffuse nodules/cavities	
KS (large nodules)	*M tuberculosis* (high CD4$^+$ count)
M tuberculosis (miliary)	*P jiroveci* (low CD4$^+$ count)
Fungi (small nodules)	*P aeruginosa* (low CD4$^+$ count)
P jiroveci (small nodules)	Fungi
	R equi
Pneumothorax	
P jiroveci	

Table 3. *Select Disease Conditions Listed by Usual CD4$^+$ at Time of Diagnosis**

Condition
CD4$^+$ > 500 cells/µL
Sinusitis/mastoiditis/otitis
Bronchitis
Pharyngitis
Lung cancer
CD4$^+$ < 400 cells/µL
Bacterial pneumonia
Pulmonary *M tuberculosis*
Cardiomyopathy
CD4$^+$ < 200 cells/µL
PCP
KS
Bacterial sepsis
Disseminated *M tuberculosis*
CD4$^+$ < 100 cells/µL
Disseminated MAC
CMV disease
Disseminated fungal infections

*Adapted from Hanson et al.

with severe immunodeficiency (*ie*, CD4$^+$ count, < 100 cells/µL), including disseminated nontuberculous mycobacterioses, disseminated fungal infections, CNS toxoplasmosis, and cytomegalovirus (CMV) disease. Therefore, common respiratory problems such as sinusitis and bronchitis may occur at any CD4$^+$ count, and bacterial pneumonia and tuberculosis (TB) often occur before AIDS-defining opportunistic infections and neoplasms. Decreasing immune function increases the risk for all HIV-associated respiratory diseases.

Demographic Factors

The increasing proportion of injection drug users in the HIV-infected population was accompanied by the recognition of bacterial pneumonia and TB as important HIV-associated infections. Bacterial pneumonia occurs more frequently than *Pneumocystis* pneumonia (PCP) in all HIV-infected groups, and the risk of bacterial pneumonia is significantly greater in injection drug users than in other persons with HIV infection. Race and ethnicity may also influence the risk of the development of bacterial pneumonia and TB, but these associations are confounded by differences in access to health care, the greater prevalence of TB in minority communities, and the disproportionately high numbers of injection drug users who are black or Hispanic.

Residence

The place of residence strongly influences the risk of the development of specific infections. The high incidence of PCP in the United States and Europe contrasts sharply with that in Africa, where it is much less common. It is likely that both genetic and environmental factors account for the lower incidence of PCP in Africa. In the United States, the incidence of HIV-associated TB is greatest in the Northeast. The geographic distribution of endemic fungi is a strong determinant of the risk of those infections developing; disseminated histoplasmosis and coccidioidomycosis are common in patients with AIDS who live in endemic areas. These infections also may occur as a reactivation disease after HIV-infected persons move to other areas and immunocompromise develops.

Use of Prophylaxis and Antiretroviral Therapy

The risk of specific opportunistic infections decreases with the use of prophylaxis. Even before the availability of combination active antiretroviral therapy (ART), the incidence of PCP and TB, along with their attendant mortality rates, was decreasing, partly attributable to the use of prophylaxis by susceptible persons. After the widespread use of ART, beginning around 1996, the incidence of opportunistic infections and death among HIV-infected persons decreased dramatically because successful ART inhibits viral replication and restores immune function. However, immune reconstitution is associated with the occurrence of other clinical syndromes.

Bacterial Pneumonia

HIV infection impairs humoral immunity through quantitative and functional defects in CD4$^+$ lymphocytes, which in turn increases the risk of bacterial infection, including sinusitis and pneumonia, and the risk of pneumonia developing increases as the CD4$^+$ lymphocyte count decreases. Injection drug users are at a greater risk than other groups, and neutropenia is an independent risk factor. Anti-Pneumocystis prophylaxis with trimethoprim (TMP)-sulfamethoxazole (SMX) appears to reduce the risk of bacterial pneumonia. Bacterial pneumonia also may accelerate the course of HIV disease because it is an independent predictor of progression to AIDS and mortality.

Streptococcus pneumoniae and *Haemophilus influenzae* are the most frequent bacterial pathogens (Table 1). Pneumonia caused by Mycoplasma, Legionella, and Chlamydia is described but seems to be relatively uncommon, especially in patients with severe immunosuppression. *Rhodococcus equi*, an aerobic Gram-positive acid-fast bacillus, may cause focal consolidation, endobronchial disease, and cavitation, usually in patients with advanced HIV disease. Pneumonia caused by *Pseudomonas aeruginosa* may develop in patients with very low $CD4^+$ lymphocyte counts (typically <50 cells/μL), even in the absence of risk factors such as neutropenia, corticosteroid use, and hospital-acquired infection. *Nocardia asteroides* may cause nodules, consolidation, cavitation, pleural effusions, empyema, and intrathoracic lymphadenopathy in HIV-infected persons.

The diagnosis and treatment of bacterial pneumonia in persons with HIV infection is in almost all respects the same as that for patients who are not infected. Patients usually present with fever, chills, productive cough, and localized areas of consolidation on chest radiographs. Although this clinical picture strongly suggests bacterial pneumonia, it may also occur with TB and fungal infection. Conversely, patients with bacterial pneumonia may have diffuse pulmonary opacities that resemble PCP.

Polyvalent pneumococcal vaccine is recommended for all HIV-infected people, although those with low $CD4^+$ counts are less likely to mount an adequate antibody response. A vaccine against *H influenzae* type B is available, but its use in patients with HIV infection is limited because most infections are caused by other strains. Although administration of the influenza vaccine is also recommended, there are no data indicating that patients with HIV infection are at an increased risk of contracting influenza or that the illness is more severe than in the general population.

Pneumocystis jiroveci *Pneumonia*

Pneumonia caused by *P jiroveci* (formerly classified as *P carinii)* was the first opportunistic infection described in patients with AIDS and has always been a major cause of illness and death. The term PCP has been used for decades, and rather than changing our terminology to PJP to reflect the new nomenclature, a consensus exists that PCP be used to refer to the term PCP. Once thought to be a parasite, genomic analysis revealed that *P jiroveci* is in fact a fungus that infects only humans, whereas *P carinii* is pathogenic only in immunodeficient rats. The organism cannot be cultured reliably outside the lung, and its source is still not identified; therefore, the precise route of transmission is elusive.

Although ART and effective prophylaxis for PCP have existed for years, this infection still occurs frequently for the following reasons: many patients do not know that they have HIV infection until an opportunistic infection develops, other patients know that they have HIV but are not receiving medical care, and some patients are receiving care and are not prescribed PCP prophylaxis or ART. Adherence to complex regimens with intolerable side effects often is problematic, and the development of resistant strains of HIV is common. Some patients receive prophylaxis for PCP but are still so profoundly immunocompromised that it is ineffective.

Diagnosis

Patients with PCP usually present with fever and gradually increasing cough and dyspnea for a few weeks, but the disease sometimes presents as an acute illness with rapid deterioration over the course of a few days. The chest radiograph usually shows diffuse granular opacities, which strongly suggest the diagnosis. Some patients with PCP have nodular densities, lobar consolidation, or normal radiographic findings. Cystic abnormalities and spontaneous pneumothoraces in patients with known or suspected HIV infection are usually caused by PCP.

Adjunctive testing may support the diagnosis but by themselves do not establish a diagnosis. PCP is unlikely in a patient who had a $CD4^+$ cell count of >200 cells/μL in the preceding 2 months in the absence of other HIV-associated symptoms. Approximately 90% of patients with PCP have an elevated serum lactate dehydrogenase level, but this increase may occur in the presence of other pulmonary diseases, especially mycobacterial and fungal infections. Oxygen desaturation with exercise is a relatively sensitive and specific test in patients who are suspected to have PCP, but it is not diagnostic. ^{67}Ga and ^{111}In lung scans are highly sensitive indicators of PCP, but isotope uptake also occurs in other pulmonary infections and therefore they seldom are useful.

Microbiological Diagnosis

P jiroveci cannot be cultured *in vitro*; therefore, the diagnosis of PCP can be confirmed only by demonstrating organisms in a lung-derived specimen, either in sputum induced by the inhalation of hypertonic saline solution or by bronchoscopy. Although establishing a diagnosis is not difficult, many clinicians treat patients with suspected PCP empirically, reserving bronchoscopy for patients who do not respond to treatment. The examination of BAL fluid establishes the diagnosis in > 90% of cases, and some centers have reported that bronchoscopic lung biopsy increases the diagnostic yield not only for PCP but also for other infections (especially *Mycobacterium tuberculosis)* and noninfectious disorders. The optimal approach to the diagnosis of HIV-associated pulmonary disorders (including PCP) can be determined only by a prospective randomized clinical trial with outcome measures that include economic and survival analyses, but no trial has yet been performed, nor is such a trial likely as the incidence of PCP is now low compared with earlier in the AIDS epidemic.

Treatment

Antimicrobial Agents: TMP-SMX is the preferred treatment for PCP in patients who have not had an adverse reaction to this drug, regardless of the severity of disease, and even in patients in whom PCP develops despite TMP-SMX prophylaxis. It is consistently the most effective in comparative studies and is also inexpensive and available in both oral and IV preparations. Patients with severe PCP who do not respond to or who do not tolerate TMP-SMX usually are given pentamidine, but this drug is associated with adverse reactions that are more serious than the adverse reactions associated with TMP-SMX. Trimetrexate-leucovorin is not as effective as TMP-SMX but is better tolerated than pentamidine. Mild-to-moderate PCP can be treated in the outpatient setting with dapsone/TMP, clindamycin/primaquine, or atovaquone. The optimal duration of treatment is unknown, but most clinicians treat the patient for 21 days, followed by prophylaxis.

Adjunctive Corticosteroids: Animal models of PCP have shown that the clinical severity of infection correlates more closely with markers of inflammation than with the burden of organisms, suggesting that the immune response and its attendant inflammation account for the clinical manifestations of pneumonia. Respiratory compromise is associated with the presence of activated CD8$^+$ cells and neutrophils in the lung, and corticosteroids are thought to attenuate these effects. The administration of corticosteroids at the start of antipneumocystis treatment reduces the likelihood of respiratory failure, the deterioration of oxygenation, and death in patients with moderate-to-severe pneumonia. Patients who are likely to benefit from therapy have a Pao_2 of < 70 mm Hg or an arterial-alveolar oxygen pressure difference of > 35 mm Hg. No benefits have been shown with less severe gas exchange abnormalities at the start of therapy or in patients to whom corticosteroids were administered > 72 h after antipneumocystis treatment was started. Adverse reactions to adjunctive corticosteroid therapy occur infrequently; life-threatening superinfections have been described, but they are uncommon. Patients in whom pulmonary symptoms with diffuse radiographic opacities develop shortly after apparently successful treatment of PCP should be evaluated for the presence of another opportunistic infection, especially CMV.

Respiratory Failure

Because the incidence of PCP decreased in the last decade, fewer patients with PCP have been admitted to the ICU. Nevertheless, when the treatment of PCP is delayed or ineffective, hypoxemic respiratory failure may develop; the clinical and radiographic features of severe PCP resemble those of ARDS, and the supportive treatment is similar, including intubation, mechanical ventilation with low tidal volume (6 mL/kg ideal body weight), and the application of positive end-expiratory pressure. Survival after respiratory failure in PCP seems to have improved since the early days of the AIDS epidemic and is perhaps related to improved strategies for mechanical ventilation. However, the development of respiratory failure in patients after several days of appropriate therapy for PCP or of a pneumothorax while receiving mechanical ventilation portend a poorer prognosis.

Prevention

Prophylaxis can be discontinued safely in patients who achieve a sustained increase in CD4$^+$ lymphocyte count to >200 cells/µL after starting ART. In those patients who have a suboptimal response to ART, lifelong anti-Pneumocystis therapy is recommended for all HIV-infected patients with CD4$^+$ cell counts of <200 cells/µL or for patients with HIV-related symptoms, including unexplained persistent fever (temperature, >100°F [37.8°C]) for 2 weeks, oropharyngeal candidiasis that is unrelated to antibiotic or corticosteroid therapy, and unexplained weight loss. Prophylaxis with TMP-SMX is most effective but is associated with more adverse events requiring the discontinuation of therapy with aerosolized pentamidine and dapsone. Therapy with TMP-SMX is also inexpensive and prevents other infections, including cerebral toxoplasmosis and infection with some strains of pathogenic bacteria. Current expert opinion recommends the administration of one double-strength tablet (160 mg of TMP/800 mg of SMX) daily or a single-strength tablet daily if the former is not tolerated. A lack of response to TMP-SMX prophylaxis is associated with nonadherence to treatment and with severe immunosuppression, as measured by very low CD4$^+$ lymphocyte counts.

TB

Coinfection with HIV and *M tuberculosis* is discussed in detail in another section. Modest reductions in cell-mediated immunity increase the risk of the reactivation of latent TB, and the risk increases as the CD4$^+$ cell counts decrease. In HIV-infected persons, TB often occurs before the occurrence of opportunistic infections, probably because *M tuberculosis* is more virulent. In patients with mild immunodeficiency, the clinical presentation is similar to TB in HIV-negative patients. Atypical pulmonary presentations, including the presence of diffuse infiltrates, miliary patterns, intrathoracic lymphadenopathy, or normal chest radiograph findings occur more frequently in patients with advanced immunosuppression (Table 2). These patients also have a high incidence of extrapulmonary infection, including infections in the pleura, lymph nodes, GI tract, bone marrow, and blood.

The diagnosis of TB may be difficult in HIV-infected persons. Cutaneous anergy is more prevalent as CD4$^+$ cell counts decrease, making tuberculin skin tests less useful. Radiographic clues to the diagnosis include cavitation, hilar and mediastinal lymphadenopathy, and pleural effusions. When there is cavitation, acid-fast smears and cultures of sputum usually are positive. In patients who do not expectorate spontaneously, sputum may be induced with hypertonic saline solution. Bronchoscopy with BAL fluid, transbronchial biopsy, and postbronchoscopy sputum often are diagnostic. Biopsy specimens enhance the immediate diagnostic yield of bronchoscopy in the diagnosis of pulmonary TB compared with BAL fluid alone.

Despite an appropriate evaluation, acid-fast smears of sputum and bronchoscopic specimens maybe negative, and cultures may not be positive for several weeks. The early treatment of TB improves the outcome and reduces the transmission of the disease to others; therefore, initial empiric therapy is warranted for patients with radiographic abnormalities that *are* consistent with TB, unless another disorder is identified.

Atypical Mycobacteria

Mycobacterium avium complex (MAC) causes devastating complications and death in patients with severe immunosuppression. Patients may have persistent fever, wasting, and diarrhea. However, MAC is rarely a pulmonary pathogen in patients with AIDS. Its isolation in patients with symptomatic pulmonary disease usually occurs in association with that of another pathogen, such as Pneumocystis. Other nontuberculous mycobacteria also cause pulmonary infections in patients with HIV infection. However, if acid-fast bacilli are identified from sputum or bronchoscopic specimens, patients should be treated presumptively for *M tuberculosis* until the mycobacterial species is identified, mainly because TB is more common, has a better response to treatment, and the early treatment of active TB is an essential public health measure.

CMV

In patients with $CD4^+$ lymphocyte counts of <50 cells/μL, CMV commonly causes retinitis, esophagitis, gastritis, colitis, hepatitis, encephalitis, pneumonia, and death. Curiously, CMV pneumonitis is uncommon in patients with AIDS. Although the virus often is isolated in cultures of BAL fluid, it is not usually pathogenic. Pulmonary infection can be inferred when typical intranuclear or intracytoplasmic inclusions are found in BAL fluid or biopsy material. The likelihood that CMV is a pulmonary pathogen is also greater when CMV infection is found at other sites. It also seems to be relatively common in patients whose conditions deteriorate after receiving corticosteroid treatment for PCP.

CMV pneumonitis usually occurs in patients who have had previous AIDS-defining illnesses. They present with a clinical syndrome similar to PCP, with dyspnea, nonproductive cough, fever, and diffuse pulmonary opacities noted on chest radiographs. Unilobar radiographic involvement, cavitation, nodules, and pleural effusions also have been described. CMV pneumonitis is treated in the same way as infection in other sites, with IV ganciclovir or foscarnet, and the responses to therapy are similar to those of patients with CMV retinitis or GI disease. Because CMV infection occurs only in patients with very severe immunosuppression, the long-term prognosis is very poor.

Fungal Pneumonias

Fungal infections have been discussed in detail elsewhere. Life-threatening fungal disease may occur in HIV-infected patients, either by new infection or the reactivation of latent disease. The types of fungal infections depend on the severity of immunodeficiency and whether the patient has lived in endemic areas.

Cryptococcosis

Cryptococcus neoformans is distributed throughout the world and is the most common fungus causing life-threatening illness in patients with AIDS. The meninges are the most common site of infection, and cryptococcal meningitis is often the first manifestation of AIDS. With cryptococcal pneumonia, the chest radiograph usually shows diffuse infiltrates, similar to PCP, but localized infiltrates, nodules, cavitation, pleural effusions, miliary patterns, and lymphadenopathy also are seen. Most patients with cryptococcal pneumonia have meningitis and disseminated disease, and $CD4^+$ lymphocyte counts typically are <100 cells/μL. The diagnosis is established by the identification of the organism from sputum, BAL fluid, pleural fluid, or lung biopsy specimens. A high titer of cryptococcal antigen in serum is strongly suggestive of and an antigen titer of $>1:8$ in BAL fluid is diagnostic of cryptococcal pneumonia.

Histoplasmosis

Histoplasma capsulatum is endemic in the Ohio and Mississippi river valleys, Central and South America, and the Caribbean islands. Disseminated disease may develop in patients with HIV infection who come from endemic areas when immunodeficiency permits the reactivation of latent infection. The clinical presentation is usually subacute, and the chest radiograph typically shows a diffuse or miliary pattern, although localized infiltrates may occur. The diagnosis is established by the identification or culture of the organism from blood, lung-derived specimens, bone marrow, or liver.

Amphotericin B is the treatment of choice for most cases of HIV-associated histoplasmosis. The liposomal form is less toxic and more effective than the standard deoxycholate formulation. Itraconazole maybe used for patients who cannot tolerate amphotericin B or have milder disease and should be used as a long-term suppressive therapy for the life of the patient after the primary infection is controlled. Voriconazole is not recommended in treatment or prevention of histoplasmosis.

Aspergillosis

Life-threatening pulmonary aspergillosis may develop in patients with advanced immunosuppression. The following two common patterns of disease have been identified: an invasive parenchymal infection, which is usually fatal, and a predominantly bronchial disease presenting with dyspnea and airway obstruction. The classic risks for Aspergillus infection, namely, prolonged neutropenia and treatment with high-dose corticosteroids, often are absent. Aspergillosis probably occurs in patients with advanced AIDS because of defects in neutrophil or alveolar macrophage function. The CD4+ lymphocyte count is typically <30 cells/µL, and the previous use of corticosteroids and neutrophil counts of <500 cells/µL increase the risk. Disseminated disease is common, especially in the brain.

Clues to the diagnosis of invasive pulmonary aspergillosis include upper-lobe disease with cavitation and hemoptysis. This diagnosis has traditionally required histologic proof, because Aspergillus is ubiquitous, and its presence in nasopharyngeal secretions, sputum, and BAL fluid may represent contamination or colonization. However, studies in patients with severe immunosuppression, including AIDS, have indicated that the isolation of Aspergillus in BAL fluid correlates strongly with histologic proof of tissue invasion. Although voriconazole has not been studied for the treatment of invasive aspergillosis in AIDS patients, the Centers for Disease Control and Prevention recommend it as the first choice for therapy, with amphotericin B (liposomal or deoxycholate) as an alternative. Caspofungin has been approved for patients who cannot tolerate standard therapy, but it has not been studied in patients with HIV infection.

Other Fungal Infections

In endemic areas, disseminated coccidioidomycosis and blastomycosis may occur in patients with AIDS, usually as a complication of advanced immunosuppression. The reactivation of a previous infection may develop in some patients after moving from an endemic area. These infections usually involve the lung; patients present with cough, fever, dyspnea, and the appearance of nodular, focal, cavitary, or diffuse disease. The diagnosis is established by demonstrating the presence of the organism by microscopy or culture in respiratory specimens.

Neoplastic Diseases of the Lungs

Kaposi Sarcoma

Kaposi sarcoma (KS) is the most common malignancy in persons with HIV infection, and the skin is the major site of involvement. KS is caused by human herpesvirus (HHV)-8. This virus infects many healthy adults and can be isolated commonly in saliva, prostate tissue, and semen. It is probably transmitted by sexual contact and causes disease when activated by HIV-associated immunosuppression. This hypothesis helps to explain why KS is much more common among HIV-infected gay men than in other transmission groups.

Visceral involvement with KS is common in patients with advanced disease and may involve the airways, lungs tissue, mediastinal lymph nodes, and pleura. Patients with thoracic KS usually have obvious mucocutaneous lesions, but the lung may be the only site of disease in up to 15% of cases. The involvement of the airways, parenchyma, pleura, and intrathoracic lymph nodes causes a diverse range of symptoms and radiographic findings. The majority of patients with pulmonary KS that was diagnosed antemortem had cough, dyspnea, and fever. In the airways, KS lesions usually are asymptomatic but sometimes cause obstruction or hemoptysis. The finding of typical lesions on inspection of the airways is usually considered to be diagnostic. A histologic diagnosis may be difficult because the yield of the forceps biopsy is low. Some clinicians believe that a forceps biopsy of KS lesions places the patient at significant risk of bleeding, but this notion is controversial.

Parenchymal involvement with KS is suggested by bronchial wall thickening, nodules, Kerley B lines, and coexisting pleural effusions, especially in patients with cutaneous disease. The use of bronchoscopy can determine whether diffuse radiographic opacities are caused by KS or an opportunistic infection. The yield of bronchoscopic lung biopsies in the diagnosis of KS is low, and even open-lung biopsy is nondiagnostic in approximately 10% of cases because of the focal distribution of the lesions. Therefore, the diagnosis of pulmonary parenchymal KS is usually inferred in patients with cutaneous disease, chest radiograph findings, or CT scan findings that suggest this disorder; visual confirmation of airway lesions; and no evidence of opportunistic infection in BAL fluid or bronchoscopic lung biopsy specimens. Patients with parenchymal opacities who have typical lesions in the airways and no identified pulmonary infection are assumed to have parenchymal KS.

When KS involves the pleura, effusions are usually exudative and sanguineous, but the cytologic examination is nondiagnostic. Closed pleural biopsy specimens are rarely positive for KS due to the focality of the pleural lesions and the predominant involvement of the visceral pleura, rather than the parietal pleura. Because establishing a diagnosis usually necessitates a thoracoscopic or open pleural biopsy, the presence of pleural involvement with KS is usually inferred in a patient with cutaneous disease and a serosanguineous effusion without a reasonable alternative explanation.

Patients with disseminated disease may benefit from cytotoxic chemotherapy. The most promising approach may be the use of ART, which may lead to the regression of KS lesions. In many cases, ART leads to a reduction in HHV-8 load, which is associated with regression inhibition of angiogenesis and of KS tumor growth.

Lymphoma

Non-Hodgkin B-cell lymphoma is associated with HIV infection and, unlike most other HIV-related disorders, it continues to occur despite the use of highly active ART (*ie*, HAART). Although pulmonary involvement is usually clinically innocuous, the lung is a common site of extranodal disease. HIV-associated primary pulmonary lymphoma is usually a high-grade B-cell tumor occurring in the setting of advanced HIV infection. If symptoms occur, they usually do so late in the course of HIV disease and simulate common opportunistic infections. Even in patients with lymphoma, lung involvement is usually a late feature of HIV disease. It may present with lobar consolidation, nodules, reticular opacities, and masses. The biopsy is established by bronchoscopic or open biopsy; BAL fluid has a very low diagnostic yield. In contrast to non-AIDS patients, mediastinal and hilar lymphadenopathy are generally not prominent in patients with non-Hodgkin B-cell lymphoma and HIV infection. Pleural involvement is characterized by effusions and pleural thickening and the airway involvement by atelectasis. The diagnosis is established by biopsy or cytologic analyses of pleural fluid.

Primary effusion lymphoma or "body cavity lymphoma" is a disorder characterized by pleural, pericardial, or peritoneal growth of malignant lymphoma cells, usually in the absence of solid tumors. In almost all cases, tumor DNA shows HHV-8, which is also the etiologic agent of KS and multicentric Castleman disease, a dysplastic lymphoid disorder that may progress to plasmablastic lymphoma. The virus has a strong tropism for B cells, and in some patients HHV-8-infected clones proliferate and transform into a large cell "liquid lymphoma" within serous cavities. In HIV-seropositive persons, the prognosis of primary effusion lymphoma is no better, and is probably worse, than in most other forms of lymphoma.

Carcinoma of the Lung

The incidence of lung cancer is now recognized to be increased in persons with HIV infection, especially in the years after the use of ART as the standard of care. Although persons in most populations with HIV infection are current or former smokers, their risk of the development of lung cancer appears to be increased even when incidence ratios are adjusted for smoking. The prevalence of microsatellite alternations reflecting genomic instability also occurs with greatly increased frequency in HIV-associated lung cancers, possibly playing a role in their pathogenesis. Patients with lung cancer in the setting of HIV infection tend to be relatively young at presentation (mean age, 45 years) and have mild or moderate immunosuppression. Similar to age-matched control subjects, 75 to 90% of patients present with stage III or IV disease. Adenocarcinoma is the most common histologic type, and the prognosis appears to be worse in patients with HIV infection. Until further studies are performed, the diagnostic and therapeutic approaches to patients with HIV-associated lung cancer are the same as for other patients, although the efficacy and toxicity of chemotherapy and radiotherapy may be different.

Other Pulmonary Disorders

Obstructive Lung Disease

There is a propensity for the development of chronic bronchitis and bronchiectasis in patients with advanced HIV infection, even if they do not smoke. The $CD4^+$ count is usually low (<100 cells/μL). Therapy with standard antimicrobial agents is usually effective, but symptoms are likely to recur, especially when *P aeruginosa* is isolated from the sputum. The role and efficacy of therapy with bronchodilators and antiinflammatory agents in patients with HIV-associated airway disease have not been studied.

HIV infection also appears to accelerate the onset of smoking-related emphysema, possibly through cytotoxic lymphocyte activity, lung capillary endothelial injury, and increased oxidative stress. The incidence of emphysema appears to be increased in patients with HIV infection independent of smoking status.

Idiopathic Inflammatory Disorders

Pulmonary disorders without a defined infectious or neoplastic etiology occur in HIV-infected persons. Lymphocytic interstitial pneumonitis (LIP) and nonspecific interstitial pneumonitis (NIP) are believed to comprise a spectrum of inflammatory changes in response to HIV infection in the lung itself. LIP is most common in HIV-infected children and persons of African descent. It may occur as part of a systemic $CD8^+$ lymphoproliferative syndrome, with lymphadenopathy, blood lymphocytosis, and the involvement of other organs. NIP is very common in persons with low $CD4^+$ counts but is rarely diagnosed because it usually causes no symptoms. When symptomatic, both LIP and NIP are treated with corticosteroids. Bronchiolitis obliterans organizing pneumonia has a similar clinical presentation in patients with and without HIV infection. Lung biopsy, either transbronchial or open, is necessary for the diagnosis. This disorder often improves dramatically with corticosteroid therapy.

Pulmonary Hypertension

Pulmonary hypertension occurs more commonly in HIV-infected patients than in the general population. It may eventually lead to cor pulmonale and death. Some evidence links HHV-8 (the etiologic agent of KS) with pulmonary hypertension in patients without HIV infection, perhaps through the dysregulation of endothelial cell growth or growth-factor signaling. An alternative explanation is that the presence of HIV antigens in the pulmonary endothelium may stimulate apoptosis, growth, and proliferation. HIV-associated pulmonary hypertension appears to occur at all stages of HIV infection, and the approach to diagnosis and treatment is the same as that for idiopathic pulmonary arterial hypertension in HIV-uninfected persons. The effects of starting ART during a course of treatment for pulmonary hypertension are not known.

Immune Restoration Syndromes

The effectiveness of ART in restoring immune function has given rise to a new disorder, the immune reconstitution inflammatory syndrome (IRIS), which is defined as a paradoxical deterioration in clinical status that is attributable to the recovery of the immune system during ART. When treatment with ART is successful, the number of blood $CD4^+$ lymphocytes increases, as does their activity. Increased immune function then leads to inflammation that may have been otherwise clinically silent, leading to overt clinical illness. The diagnostic criteria for IRIS include the diagnosis of AIDS, treatment with anti-HIV medications that lead to a reduction in HIV viremia (followed by an increase in the $CD4^+$ lymphocyte count), symptoms consistent with an infectious or inflammatory condition that appeared while the subject was receiving ART, and symptoms that cannot be explained by a newly acquired infection, by the expected clinical course of the disease, or by the side effects of therapy.

Paradoxical worsening of TB was described in patients in whom transient worsening of TB-related symptoms developed after ART. The presence of fever that worsened or the emergence of cervical intrathoracic lymphadenopathy, pulmonary infiltrates, pleural effusions, or other tuberculous lesions develop in these patients shortly after starting ART, which is associated with the restoration of cutaneous reactivity to skin test antigens. Respiratory failure caused by IRIS was reported in several cases after the introduction of ART after the successful treatment of PCP. Other patients had apparent exacerbations of disease after the introduction of ART after or during infection with MAC, cryptococcosis, CMV, herpes zoster, hepatitis B and C viruses, and the agent that causes progressive multifocal leukoencephalopathy.

IRIS is a diagnosis of exclusion, which is suggested by a compatible clinical syndrome in a patient who is recovering from an infection and has begun receiving ART in the prior several months. The plasma HIV load and CD4$^+$ lymphocyte counts usually are improved compared with prior measurements, but the circulating CD4$^+$ count may be unchanged because these cells are compartmentalized to sites of active inflammation. Opportunistic infection is usually a diagnostic consideration but, in the absence of a severe illness and in the proper clinical setting, invasive procedures can usually be avoided and the patient observed. If bronchoscopy is performed, the mean CD4/CD8 ratio is significantly greater (0.54) than in HIV-infected patients who are undergoing bronchoscopy for other respiratory complaints (0.07). Most patients should just receive palliative therapy for symptoms, such as antipyretic agents for fever. Systemic corticosteroids have been used successfully in the treatment of severe inflammatory disease causing significant end-organ damage.

It is not known when to start therapy with antiretroviral agents in patients with active opportunistic infection. However, there is a consensus that in patients who have an HIV-associated disorder for whom there is no alternative treatment (such as cryptosporidiosis and progressive multifocal leukoencephalopathy), the benefits of ART would outweigh the risks. However, many (but not all) experts would defer starting ART in patients with active treatable disorders like PCP and tuberculosis until there is a response to the infection.

Annotated Bibliography

General

Centers for Disease Control and Prevention. HIV/AIDS surveillance report: 2007. (Vol 19). Atlanta: U.S. Department of Health and Human Services, Centers for Disease Control and Prevention, 2009; 1–63. Available at: http://www.cdc.gov/hiv/topics/surveillance/resources/reports/. Accessed April 4, 2009

An updated report describing the epidemiology of AIDS in the United States. It documents the decreasing rates of opportunistic infections and death in addition to the trends in the incidence of AIDS in different risk groups. It is troubling that the estimated number of newly diagnosed cases of HIV/AIDS increased 15% from 2004 to 2007, with 15% of all of these cases among persons 40 to 44 years of age.

Centers for Disease Control and Prevention. Guidelines for prevention and treatment of opportunistic infections in HIV-infected adults and adolescents: recommendations from CDC, the National Institutes of Health, and the HIV Medicine Association of the Infectious Diseases Society of America. Available at: http://www.cdc.gov/mmwr/preview/mmwrhtml/rr58e324a1.htm?s_cid=rr58e324a1_e. Accessed April 5, 2009

Latest version of comprehensive guidelines for the prevention of opportunistic infections in persons with HIV infection. They emphasize the prevention of PCP, TB, toxoplasmosis, and MAC.

Hanson DL, Chu SY, Farizo KM, et al. Distribution of CD4$^+$ T lymphocytes at diagnosis of acquired immunodeficiency syndrome-defining and other human immunodeficiency virus-related illnesses. Arch Intern Med 1995; 155:1537–1542

Stratifies risk of developing HIV disorders by CD4$^+$ lymphocyte count.

Palella FJ, Delaney KM, Moorman AC, et al. Declining morbidity and mortality among patients with advanced human immunodeficiency virus infection. N Engl J Med 1998; 38:853–860

Mortality rate in a cohort of 1,255 patients with advanced HIV infection decreased from 29.4 per 100 person-years in 1995 to 8.8 per 100 person-years in 1997, with a corresponding dramatic decrease in opportunistic infections, although the rate of use of prophylaxis against PCP and MAC disease remained similar. This study demonstrated that combination ART in an outpatient cohort dramatically reduced morbidity and mortality related to HIV infection.

UNAIDS. 2007 AIDS epidemic update. Available at: http://data.unaids.org/pub/EPISlides/2007/2007_epiupdate_en.pdf. Accessed April 30,2008 *Provides a detailed summary of the HIV/AIDS pandemic around the world.*

Wallace JM, Rao AV, Glassroth J, et al. Respiratory illness in persons with human immunodeficiency virus infection. Am Rev Respir Dis 1993; 148:1523–1529
Multicenter prospective study of HIV-infected subjects who did not have AIDS (1987 definition) at the time of study enrollment showed that the most frequent respiratory diagnoses were also common in the general population (ie, upper respiratory tract infections, acute bronchitis, and sinusitis). Bacterial pneumonia and PCP occurred significantly more frequently in subjects whose CD4+ count at study enrollment was < 250 cells/µL, and bacterial pneumonia was more common in injection drug users compared with others.

Bacterial Pneumonia

Baron AD, Hollander H. *Pseudomonas aeruginosa* broncho-pulmonary infection in late human immunodeficiency virus infection. Am Rev Respir Dis 1993; 148:992–996
Reviews the clinical features and risks for the development of P aeruginosa *lower respiratory tract infection in HIV-infected persons.*

Hirschtick RE, Glassroth J, Jordan MC, et al. Bacterial pneumonia in patients infected with human immunodeficiency virus. N Engl J Med 1995; 333:845–851
Describes the risk factors and bacteriology in a prospective cohort study. Mortality during the follow-up period was almost fourfold greater in subjects who had an episode of bacterial pneumonia than in others. Prophylaxis with TMP-SMX was associated with a significant reduction in the incidence of bacterial pneumonia.

PCP

Huang L, Morris A, Limper AH, et al. Proc Am Thorac Soc 2006; 3:655–664
Review of the biology, host defense mechanisms, epidemiology and clinical features, diagnosis, and treatment of Pneumocystis, recommending directions for future investigations.

Morris A, Lundgren JD, Masur H, et al. Current epidemiology of Pneumocystis pneumonia. Emerg Infect Dis 2004; 110:1713–1720
Trends in the epidemiology and clinical features of PCP in the era of ART.

National Institutes of Health, University of California. Consensus statement on the use of corticosteroid as adjunctive therapy for Pneumocystis pneumonia in the acquired immunodeficiency syndrome: National Institutes of Health-University of California Expert Panel for Corticosteroid as Adjunctive Therapy for Pneumocystis Pneumonia. N Engl J Med 1990; 323:1500–1504
Review of studies of adjunctive corticosteroid therapy for PCP, with recommendations for clinical use.

Rosen MJ. Intensive care of patients with HIV infection: time to take another look. J Intensive Care Med 2005; 20:312–315
Review of trends in critical care of patients with HIV infection, including the declining incidence of PCP and the increase in mortality from non-HIV-associated disorders.

Viral and Fungal Pneumonia

Lortholary O, Meyohas MC, Dupont B, et al. Invasive aspergillosis in patients with acquired immunodeficiency syndrome: report of 33 cases. Am J Med 1993; 95:177–187
A large series of patients is the basis of this description of the clinical features of invasive aspergillosis in AIDS patients demonstrating that a positive culture finding in BAL fluid is diagnostic of the disease.

Rodriguez-Barradas MC, Stool E, Musher D. Diagnosing and treating cytomegalovirus pneumonia in patients with AIDS. Clin Infect Dis 1996; 23:76–81
The diagnosis of CMV pneumonia is difficult to establish with certainty because it is commonly found in association with other pathogens and may be isolated from lung-derived specimens without histologic evidence of disease. This study describes the clinical and laboratory features of patients with confirmed CMV pneumonia.

Noninfectious Pulmonary Diseases

Ascoli V, Lo-Coco F. Body cavity lymphoma. Curr Opin Pulm Med 2002; 8:317–322
Reviews the pathogenesis and clinical features of primary effusional lymphoma.

Barnett CF, Hsue PY, Machado RF. Pulmonary hypertension: an increasingly recognized complication of hereditary hemolytic anemias and HIV infection. JAMA 2008; 299:324–331
Concise case-based review of epidemiology, mechanisms, diagnosis, and treatment.

Engels EA, Brock MV, Chen J, et al. Elevated incidence of lung cancer among HIV-infected individuals. J Clin Oncol 2006; 24:1383–1388

Herida M, Mary-Krause M, Kaphan R, et al. Incidence of non-AIDS defining cancers before and during the highly active antiretroviral therapy era in a cohort of human immunodeficiency virus-infected patients. J Clin Oncol 2003; 21:3447-3453

The incidence of lung cancer is increasing in the era of ART. It is unknown whether this is simply related to increased longevity leading to increased cancer rates, is an effect of HIV or ART on oncogenesis, or is a failure of immune surveillance.

Huang L, Schnapp LM, Gruden J, et al. Presentation of AIDS-related Kaposi's sarcoma diagnosed by bronchoscopy. Am J Respir Crit Care Med 1996; 153:1385–1390

The clinical, laboratory, radiographic, and bronchoscopic features of pulmonary KS are described in a large series of patients.

Petrache I, Diab K, Knox KS, et al. HIV associated pulmonary emphysema: a review of the literature and inquiry into its mechanism. Thorax 2008;63:463–469

Recent review of clinical features and mechanisms.

Travis WD, Fox CH, Devaney KO, et al. Lymphocytic pneumonitis in 50 adult HIV-infected patients: lymphocytic interstitial pneumonitis versus nonspecific interstitial pneumonitis. Hum Pathol 1992; 23:529–541

The clinical and pathologic features of these inflammatory disorders were studied. They probably represent different manifestations of HIV infection of the lung.

Wistuba II, Behrens C, Milchgrub S, et al. Comparison of molecular changes in lung cancers in HIV-positive and HIV-indeterminate subjects. JAMA 1998; 279:1554–1559

Lung cancers in patients with HIV infection have a greater increased incidence of microsatellite alterations than in other patients with lung cancer. These differences reflect genomic instability and provide evidence for a link between HIV infection and lung cancer.

Immune Restoration Syndromes

Naccache JM, Antoine M, Wislez M, et al. Sarcoid-like pulmonary disorder in human immunodeficiency virus-infected patients receiving antiretroviral therapy. Am J Respir Crit Care Med 1999; 159:2009–2013

Narita M, Ashkin D, Hollender ES, et al. Paradoxical worsening of tuberculosis following antiretroviral therapy in patients with AIDS. Am J Respir Crit Care Med 1998; 158:157–161

Shelburne SA, Montes M, Hamill R. Immune reconstitution inflammatory syndrome: more answers, more questions. J Antimicrob Chemother 2006;57:167–170.

Reviews the definition and mechanisms of IRIS.

Wislez M, Bergot E, Antoine M, et al. Acute respiratory failure following HAART introduction in patients treated for Pneumocystis pneumonia. Am J Respir Crit Care Med 2001; 164:847–851

Notes

Pulmonary Complications of Cardiothoracic Surgery and Trauma

Bruce P. Krieger, MD, FCCP

Objectives:

- Apply physiologic parameters preoperatively to predict postoperative pulmonary complications following thoracic resection or cardiac surgery
- Explain the pathophysiology of hypoxemia in patients following cardiac surgery and chest trauma
- Describe the initial assessment of the patient who has suffered blunt chest trauma
- Recognize and treat the most common causes of postcardiac surgery respiratory failure

Key words: diaphragm dysfunction; exercise testing; sternotomy; thoracic surgery; thoracic trauma; thoracoscopy

Many recently trained chest surgeons have more experience in cardiac surgery than in thoracic surgery. For the pulmonologist, a surgeon with expertise in thoracic surgery is essential for patients undergoing complicated pulmonary procedures. Thoracocardiac surgery encompasses procedures involving the lungs, chest wall, mediastinum, thoracic aorta, and heart (Table 1). This article will concentrate on those problems most frequently encountered by a practicing pulmonologist, including preoperative evaluation prior to lung resection surgery, pulmonary complications following thoracic and cardiac surgery, diagnostic thoracoscopy, and pulmocardiac complications following chest trauma. Lung transplantation and lung volume reduction surgery (LVRS) are discussed elsewhere in this course.

Pulmonary Complications Following Lung Resection Surgery

Lung resection surgery is performed in the United States at least 30,000 times annually, usually in an attempt to cure bronchogenic carcinoma. The pulmonologist is often consulted preoperatively to evaluate the advisability of lung resection. There are two general aspects to this evaluation, the first being whether the cancer can be fully resected and cured (resectability), and the second being whether the patient will survive the operation and be able to function in a "reasonable manner" afterwards (operability). A large number of thoracic surgery patients have underlying lung diseases that are associated with an increase in the morbidity and mortality from surgery, especially in the elderly. Therefore, preoperative evaluation is critical before deciding on the advisability of thoracic surgery.

Table 1. *Thoracic Surgical Procedures*

Indication	Approach	Procedures
Resectional	Thoracotomy	Pneumonectomy, lobectomy, segmentectomy, wedge resection, rib and chest wall resection
	Thoracoscopy	Wedge resection, lobectomy
Diagnostic	Thoracotomy	Biopsy of lung, pleura, pericardium, mediastinal structures, adenopathy
	Thoracoscopy	Biopsy of lung, pleura, pericardium, mediastinal structures, nodes; diagnose diaphragmatic injury
Therapeutic	Thoracotomy	Control hemorrhage/pneumothorax/pleual effusion/empyemas/granulomatous infections; lung transplanats; LVRS; others*
	Thoracoscopy	Control pneumothoraxpleural effusion/empyema, granulomatous lung infection; LVRS; others*

*Others = pericardial window, ligation of thoracic duct, esophageal surgery, vagotomy.

The decreases in lung function that occur after thoracic surgery are more complicated than the changes that occur following upper-abdominal or cardiac surgery because a functional lung is removed. Following laparotomy, there is an approximately 50% decrease in FVC for the first few postoperative days. There are similar predictable decreases in lung function following cardiac surgery, as described later in this article. The effect of thoracic surgery on postoperative pulmonary function is not only permanent but also more difficult to predict since it depends on the amount of viable lung parenchyma that remains following surgery. If the patient has limited pulmonary reserve preoperatively, further worsening following lung resection can result in postoperative atelectasis, pneumonia, prolonged mechanical ventilator support (MVS), or even death. Over the past 5 decades, various pulmonary function tests have been utilized to predict postresection pulmonary function and thus screen for patients who are at increased risk for postoperative complications.

Bronchospirometry

Sixty years ago, thoracic surgery was most commonly performed to control tuberculosis. During that time, bronchospirometry was introduced as a means of predicting postoperative pulmonary function. Bronchospirometry measures minute ventilation ($\dot{V}E$) and oxygen uptake ($\dot{V}O_2$) from each individual lung. This is accomplished by placing a double-lumen endotracheal tube (under conscious sedation) that essentially isolates the right from the left lung, therefore allowing measurements to be made unilaterally. Predicted postpneumonectomy function is calculated by multiplying the total preoperative pulmonary function by the percentage of lung that will remain postoperatively.

Unilateral Pulmonary Artery Occlusion

Unilateral pulmonary artery occlusion was used 50 years ago as a means of assessing whether a patient could withstand a pneumonectomy. A catheter was placed into the pulmonary artery of the lung that was going to be resected, and a large (50 mL) balloon was then inflated, thus directing all blood flow to the contralateral lung. If the mean pulmonary artery pressure increased to > 35 mm Hg or the Pao_2 decreased to < 45 mm Hg, the candidate was deemed inoperable because of the risk of postoperative death. However, this technique is difficult to perform (26% technical failure), and pulmonary artery catheters are no longer equipped with large balloons. Given the improvement in other less invasive testing techniques for predicting postoperative pulmonary function, the temporary unilateral pulmonary artery occlusion is rarely used in modern times.

Standard Pulmonary Function Testing

The history of using pulmonary function testing (PFT) as a predictor of postoperative morbidity and mortality dates back to 1955, when the combination of a preoperative maximal breathing capacity (maximal voluntary ventilation [MVV]) < 50% of predicted combined with a FVC < 50% of normal predicted a 40% mortality rate in patients undergoing resection surgery or thoracoplasty for tuberculosis. Over the next 50 years, other parameters were proposed to be more accurate prognostic indicators of postoperative pulmonary failure. These included FEV_1 < 2 L for pneumonectomy or < 1 L for lobectomy, and FEV_1/FVC ratio < 50%. In the 1980s, diffusing capacity of the lung for carbon monoxide (DLCO) was proposed to be a reliable predictor of mortality when < 50% of predicted. In the early 1980s, the accepted criteria for pneumonectomy included an FEV_1 > 2 L along with a MVV > 55%, and for a lobectomy a MVV > 40% of predicted with an FEV_1 > 1 L. However, most of these parameters were derived from studies that included mainly men in their sixth to eighth decades. As such, an FEV_1 of 2 L would be distinctly abnormal for a man but not necessarily for a small, female octogenarian. In addition, these parameters lacked sufficient specificity for the individual patient, and therefore attention was directed to more accurate predictors of postoperative pulmonary function based on the amount of predicted lung parenchyma that would remain following resection. Radionuclide quantitative lung scanning coupled with preoperative pulmonary function testing was introduced as a way of refining postoperative lung function by coupling anatomic and physiologic relationships. The postpneumonectomy or postlobectomy FEV_1 and FVC are predicted by multiplying the percentage of total radioactivity that would remain after lung resection surgery by the preoperative FEV_1 and

FVC. Initially, an absolute lower limit of acceptable postoperative lung function was established to be <0.8 L based on an accepted dictum that hypercarbia frequently occurred in patients with COPD when the FEV_1 was <0.8 L. However, Olsen and associates suggested that further accuracy could be obtained by this technique if the predicted postoperative FEV_1 was corrected for the patient's age, height, and sex (*ie*, based on percentage of predicted rather than an absolute number).

Markos and coworkers prospectively studied 55 consecutive patients utilizing quantitative lung scanning, PFT based on percentage of predicted, and incremental load cycle ergometry. Three deaths occurred, all in patients with postoperative predicted FEV_1 and DLCO $<35\%$. Based on these data and other studies, "acceptable" criteria in the 1990s included either a postoperative predicted $FEV_1 > 40\%$ or a combination of an FEV_1 postoperative predicted $> 30\%$ along with a postoperative predicted DLCO $\geq 40\%$. This combined approach is applicable to pneumonectomy or lobectomy. Combining LVRS with small resections has extended the limits of thoracic surgery, since postoperative pulmonary function may actually improve after LVRS while successfully removing small bronchogenic carcinomas.

Exercise Testing as a Predictor of Postoperative Morbidity and Mortality

The history of establishing a global assessment of pulmonary reserve utilizing exercise testing dates back to simple walking and stair-climbing protocols. Refinement that utilized incremental exercise testing has shown that a preoperative maximum $\dot{V}O_2$ ($\dot{V}O_2$max) <10 mL/kg/min or 40% of predicted was associated with a high percentage of fatal postoperative pulmonary complications, whereas few postpneumonectomy complications occurred when the $\dot{V}O_2$ max was >20 mL/kg/min or 75% of predicted. Lobectomy is considered to be relatively safe when the $\dot{V}O_2$ max is >15mL/kg/min. Some algorithms for assessing the operability of a lung resection patient suggest utilizing formal exercise testing before undergoing quantitative lung scanning when either the preoperative FEV_1 or DLCO are $<80\%$ of predicted. Recent studies have correlated symptom-limited stair climbing with $\dot{V}O_2$ in patients with COPD. The inability to climb two flights of stairs preoperatively had an 82% positive predictive value for the development of a postoperative cardiopulmonary complication. However, the simple shuttle (6 min) walk test was not useful in distinguishing lung cancer surgical outcome.

Cardiac Risk Factors

Cardiac complications are the second-most-common difficulty encountered after thoracotomy. Therefore, exercise testing is theoretically desirable since it stresses the combined cardiopulmonary systems. Recently, a "risk index" that combines cardiac and pulmonary signs and tests has been advocated as a guide to reliably predict postoperative risks.

From these studies, it is apparent that no single parameter can be used to exclude surgery in the individual patient. Rather, a combination of parameters can be helpful in predicting a statistically high risk of postoperative morbidity and mortality so that the patient, with the counseling of their physicians, can make an informed decision as to whether to proceed with potentially curative lung resection surgery. For many patients, the relatively high likelihood of a poor quality of life postoperatively may be a more important concern than a limited chance of surviving for 5 years following resection of a pulmonary carcinoma. For other patients, an "acceptable" postoperative mortality is worth the risk if the alternative is close to 100% mortality. A guide to help the prediction of postoperative pulmonary function and thus quality of life is shown in Figure 1.

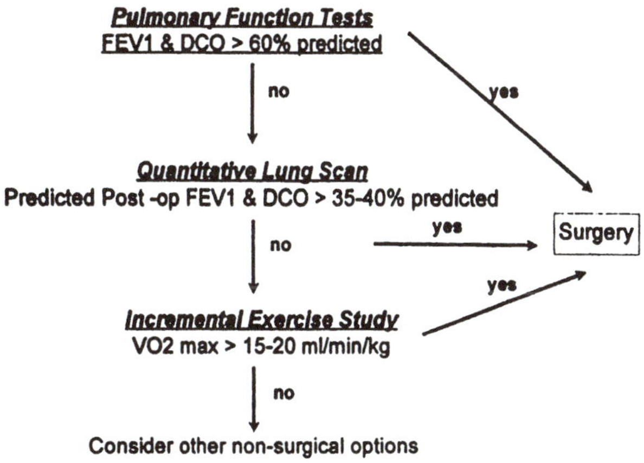

Figure 1. Stepwise approach for evaluating whether a patient has the pulmonary reserve to undergo thoracic resectional surgery.

Pulmonary Complications Following Cardiac Surgery

Pulmonologists are frequently asked to participate in the postoperative management of patients following median sternotomy for cardiac surgery. Respiratory failure is one of the most feared complications following this surgery. Ryan et al reported that patients who required ICU care for > 14 days following cardiac surgery had a 43.5% in-hospital mortality, especially if the requirement for mechanical ventilation was due to a nonpulmonary cause. As noted in Table 2, there are some causes of poststernotomy pulmonary complications that are unique to this surgical approach. These include diaphragmatic dysfunction, chest wall (sternal instability), and various forms of noncardiogenic pulmonary edema. In addition, there is a predictable decline in pulmonary function following cardiac surgery that in some respects is more severe than the changes that occur following upper-abdominal laparotomy (Table 3). Despite this, preoperative PFT has not been as accurate in predicting postoperative complications as it has in thoracic procedures, probably because lung volumes are decreased by pulmonary edema. Rady and Ryan analyzed the hospital outcome of 11,330 patients and reported the following predictors of extubation failure: age ≥ 65 years; the presence of COPD, pulmonary hypertension, severe left ventricular dysfunction, or cardiac shock; requirement for hospitalization preoperatively; surgical parameters (multiple transfusions, prolonged cardiopulmonary bypass time, redo operations, and procedures involving thoracic aorta); and various laboratory values (hematocrit $\leq 34\%$, elevated BUN, lower albumin concentrations, and systemic oxygen delivery ≤ 320 mL/min/m^2). Although abnormal PFT results did not predict extubation failure in this study, they quantitated the patient's physiologic pulmonary reserve and thus helped to determine the patient's ability to mount an appropriate response to postoperative processes that increase carbon dioxide production and $\dot{V}_E$ requirements. In an analysis of 1,112 patients, reduced FEV_1 was a statistically significant risk factor for prolonged intubation following coronary artery bypass grafting (CABG). Another retrospective multivariate survival analysis of 4,863 consecutive patients who underwent CABG also identified preoperative respiratory or cardiac instability as a risk factor

Table 2. *Causes of Pulmonary Complications Following Cardiac Surgery**

Category	Causes
Parenchymal lung injury	Pulmonary edema (cardiogenic and noncardiogenic) Atelectasis Pneumonia Hemorrhage
Airways disease	COPD, asthma Bronchorrhea (bronchitis, infectious, recurrent aspiration)
Chest bellows disease	Diaphragm weakness, paresis, paralysis or flutter Sternal instability Morbid obesity Prolonged effect of muscle relaxants Pain and chest tubes
Depressed respiratory drive	Drugs Neurological complications
Pleural disease	Pleural effusions and hemithorax Pneumothorax
Pulmonary vascular disease	Pulmonary emboli Pulmonary hypertension (valvular surgery)
Nonpulmonary disease	SIRS (increased metabolic demands) Cardiac dysfunction Neurogenic hyperventilation Psychosis Postlaparotomy

*SIRS = systemic inflammatory response syndrome, which includes sepsis, septic syndrome, bacteremia, and septic shock.

Table 3. *Postcardiac Surgery Pulmonary Function**

	POD 2	POD 4	POD 50
VC (% preop)			
IMA	36	56	74
SVG	45	63	84
FRC (% preop)			
IMA	59	69	
SVG	66	72	88

*POD = postoperative day; VC (% preop) = vital capacity expressed as a percent of the preoperative value; FRC (% preop) = functional residual capacity expressed as a percent of the preoperative; value; IMA = internal mammary artery graft; SVG = saphenous vein graft.

for MVS. Preoperative renal failure or mechanical ventilation for > 24 h after CABG identified patients at risk for readmission to the ICU.

Yende et al prospectively studied 400 patients and identified tumor necrosis factor (TNF) gene polymorphisms and angiotensin-converting enzyme gene polymorphisms preoperatively and showed that the presence of specific haplotypes was associated with prolonged mechanical ventilation after CABG. Another recent study involving 325 consecutive patients noted that an elevated lactate level (> 3 mmol/L) was associated with a significantly elevated risk for morbidity and mortality after cardiac surgery.

As noted in Table 3, postoperative declines in lung volume are more marked when the internal mammary artery is utilized rather than saphenous veins for grafts. Adverse effects may be even more severe when patients have pulmonary diseases such as COPD or pulmonary fibrosis. Oxygenation decreases by approximately 12 mm Hg postoperatively due to a combination of shunting and low ventilation/perfusion units. These effects have been shown to be secondary to bibasilar atelectasis that can be imaged on CT scanning postoperatively. Hypoxemia is exaggerated when pulmonary edema (cardiogenic or noncardiogenic) or pneumonia are present. In addition, thoracoabdominal discoordination has been shown to contribute to the physiologic changes that occur poststernotomy.

Pulmonary Edema Following Cardiac Surgery

The most common cause of postoperative pulmonary edema is poor left ventricular function that sometimes is exaggerated by the negative inotropic effects of anesthesia. In addition, diastolic dysfunction may occur, which can be difficult to recognize. It is underappreciated that the pulmonary artery occlusion pressure may not necessarily reflect the propensity for cardiogenic edema to develop unless other factors, such as hypoalbuminemia, left ventricular compliance, and elevated intrathoracic pressure from positive pressure ventilation, are considered. In addition, alveolar-capillary membrane permeability is often altered by cardiopulmonary bypass, and therefore capillaries may "leak" without an exceptionally high wedge pressure reading. Poststernotomy noncardiogenic pulmonary edema has been recognized since the 1960s, when it was called "pump lung." Most of the theories that have been proposed to explain this form of ARDS revolve around the effect of extracorporeal membrane oxygenation (ECMO) on neutrophils and alveolar epithelial cells. The occurrence of ARDS following cardiac surgery carries a 15% mortality risk and has been linearly correlated with the length of cardiopulmonary bypass. Studies in animals and humans have shown activation of polymorphonuclear leukocytes (PMNs) that results in an increase in markers of toxic oxygen radical production and adherence of PMNs to pulmonary endothelium. The sequestration of PMNs activates the complement and coagulation systems as well as other proteolytic enzymes, resulting in injury to pulmonary endothelial cells. Proinflammatory cytokines (TNF, interleukins-6 and -8) and intracellular and vascular cell adhesion molecules measured in the plasma or on platelets and PMNs have been demonstrated to be increased in pulmonary venous blood compared to right-atrial and preoperative blood. In addition, it has been hypothesized that surfactant production may be depressed during bypass because of inadequate blood supply to the alveolar epithelium that results in atelectasis and ARDS. Despite these effects, ARDS has been reported in < 2% of patients undergoing cardiopulmonary bypass. Previous cardiac surgery, shock, and the need for blood products were associated with the development of ARDS.

Atelectasis and Diaphragmatic Dysfunction

Partial atelectasis of the left lung has been reported in up to 88% of all patients who have undergone CABG. In addition, partial atelectasis of the right lung has also been reported in a high percentage (61%) of patients following CABG. In the 1980s, the term *frostbite injury* to the left phrenic nerve was introduced to describe the phrenic nerve palsy that was associated with the use of cold (specifically, ice slush) cardioplegic solutions intraoperatively. However, phrenic nerve conduction studies subsequently showed that only 20% of patients with left-lower-lobe atelectasis following sternotomy had evidence for phrenic neuropathy. Even so, most surgeons use a protective insulation blanket prior to the insertion of cold cardioplegic solutions to minimize any physical effects on the phrenic nerve. If the phrenic nerve is severely demyelinated, axonal repair requires up to 9 months before diaphragm function is restored. Mild demyelination repair may occur within 6 to 28 days. Other possible explanations for the frequent occurrence of left-lower-lobe atelectasis include intraoperative compression of lung tissue, pulmonary endothelial damage with resultant loss of surfactant, ischemia during ECMO, and possibly decreased ventilation of the left lower lobe due to a combination of cardiomegaly and the supine operating position. Atelectasis of the left lung has been associated with the number of coronary grafts, the length of surgery, the use of the left anterior mammary artery for a graft, and low body temperatures. However, the presence of atelectasis does not appear to increase the length of hospital stay.

Diaphragmatic flutter has been described in a small number of patients following sternotomy. This is defined as an involuntary contraction of the diaphragm at rates >40 times per minute that is not associated with contraction of other respiratory muscles. Diaphragmatic flutter is not suppressible voluntarily or by mechanical hyperventilation. It appears to be associated with sternal complications, and it can be an unrecognized cause for prolonged MVS. It is important to distinguish the rapid-shallow breathing of diaphragmatic flutter from a similar pattern that occurs when patients have increased $\dot{V}_E$ requirements (such as during sepsis or neurogenic hyperventilation). Since flutter is an involuntary diaphragmatic contraction, it will be associated with discoordination of the thoracic cage and therefore thoracoabdominal asynchrony that can be detected on physical examination or with respiratory inductive plethysmography or magnetometry.

The adverse effect of median sternotomy on the chest bellows is often underappreciated. A study by Locke et al using magnetometers correlated the uncoordinated rib cage expansion that occurred following sternotomy with the restrictive ventilatory changes seen on PFT. Although air flow and abdominal wall motion remained coordinated, there was a delay in rib cage expansion. If increased ventilatory demands are required, this delay would act as a significant preload to inspiration with resulting increase in work of breathing. Postoperative bone scans have detected occult rib fractures or costochondral dislocations in two-thirds of patients undergoing sternotomy. The worst postoperative lung function is noted in patients undergoing internal mammary artery grafting that is believed to be due to loss of blood flow to the sternum. However, detailed studies show that a significant decrease in blood supply occurs in only approximately 5% of patients.

The combination of diaphragmatic dysfunction and chest bellows disease results in global respiratory muscle strength deterioration following median sternotomy. This amounts to an approximately 17% drop in the maximal inspiratory pressure measured at the mouth and a decrease of the maximal expiratory pressure of 47%, which reverses when measured 6 weeks postoperatively.

Other Pulmonary Complications Following Cardiac Surgery

Left-sided pleural effusions occur in >50 to 80% of patients undergoing left internal mammary artery grafting and in >35% receiving only saphenous vein grafting. These effusions are bilateral in approximately 10% of all CABG patients. The effusions are characterized by having a marked lymphocytosis (>82%) and a potential to have a trapped lung due to fibrosis. The effusions occur less frequently when valvular surgery alone is performed. Usually, pleural effusions are small to moderate in volume but contribute to a more marked reduction in FVC in patients following CABG then when effusions are not present (38% decrease compared to 26%). Because pleurotomy is required when internal mammary artery grafting is used, the occurrence of pleural effusions >3 weeks after CABG is more common in these patients. Delayed massive effusions have also been reported.

Etiologies for these effusions include perioperative hemorrhage or contusion, pulmonary thromboemboli, and postcardiac injury syndrome. Postcardiac injury syndrome (Dressler syndrome) usually occurs 1 to 12 weeks after surgery and is associated with a combination of pleuritis, pericarditis, and pneumonitis, along with fever, leukocytosis, and elevation of the sedimentation rate. The diagnosis is one of exclusion but is important to establish since this syndrome requires treatment with nonsteroidal antiinflammatory drugs or systemic corticosteroids. The incidence of this syndrome appears to be declining.

Deep venous thrombosis and pulmonary emboli occur less commonly following cardiac surgery than after other major surgical procedures. It is believed that the use of anticoagulants during ECMO may protect the patient from the development of a nidus for clot formation intraoperatively. The incidence of pulmonary emboli reported after CABG is approximately 1%, although when pulmonary embolism occurs there is a significant (> 30%) postoperative mortality. This may reflect the finding that when pulmonary thromboembolic disease occurs in patients after CABG, it usually is in the setting of other postoperative complications.

Infections significantly affect pulmonary function after sternotomy and thus contribute to morbidity and mortality. Postoperative pneumonia has been associated with preexisting pulmonary dysfunction and older patients. However, wound infections occur more commonly than postoperative pneumonias. When sternal infections occur, significant thoracic instability results in deleterious effects reflected in decreased lung volumes and respiratory muscle endurance.

Respiratory Management Following Cardiac Surgery

The most important aspect of treating patients with respiratory failure following cardiac surgery is to determine the etiology or etiologies for their inability to support their required $\dot{V}_E$ postoperatively. Astute assessment of the patient for diaphragmatic dysfunction, thoracic instability, pulmonary edema (which may be radiographically masked by the use of high-level positive pressure ventilation) and nonpulmonary sources of increased ventilatory requirements is important. Often, the most important approach to "weaning" the patient postoperatively is to place the patient back on full MVS while improving their mechanics, decreasing their $\dot{V}_E$ requirements, and controlling their pain. The need for reintubation after CABG is associated with prolonged hospitalization, infectious complications, and increased mortality. Risk factors for prolonged MVS include a reduced FEV_1, renal failure, a positive fluid balance 24 h postoperatively, and the presence of specific polymorphisms in the promoter region of the TNF gene.

Thoracoscopy

Technological advances, such as thoracoscopy, have allowed access to body cavities without the need for traditional surgery. By using fiberoptic technology and miniaturized cameras, diagnostic and therapeutic procedures are now commonly performed without requiring large incisions and prolonged recovery time. This type of surgery has been termed *minimally invasive*, and when performed by thoracic surgeons usually utilizes video assistance (video-assisted thoracic surgery [VATS]). Proponents of VATS consider this procedure to have potentially revolutionary effects on the fields of pulmonology and cardiothoracic surgery.

The history of thoracoscopy dates back to 1910, when Jacobaeus diagnosed two cases of tuberculous pleuritis. Thoracoscopy was used during the first half of the 20th century exclusively for the lysis of pleural adhesions by means of cautery. "Medical" thoracoscopy, performed under conscious sedation using nondisposable rigid instruments, is still commonly used in Europe as a means of diagnosing pleural disease. However, in North America, VATS is more commonly utilized, not only for diagnosis but also for resection and therapeutic procedures.

The advantage of VATS over thoracotomy is the ability to access the thoracic cavity without rib spreading or rib resection, resulting in less postthoracotomy pain, neuralgia, and delayed recovery. The procedure still requires general anesthesia, unilateral lung ventilation, and lack of significant pleural adhesions that would prevent safe insertion of instruments through small (2 cm) intercostal incisions. With perfection of the technique, complications are rare. This has become the diagnostic procedure of choice for patients with diffuse interstitial lung disease who require lung biopsy and the therapeutic treatment of choice for pleural diseases such as persistent pneumothorax or empyema. In addition, as discussed elsewhere in the syllabus, it has become one of the most common approaches to LVRS.

Chest Trauma

Trauma remains the major cause of accidental death in the United States. Thoracic injuries account for approximately 37,000 deaths per year and significantly contribute to another 37,000 trauma-related deaths. Fatal hemorrhage or an inability to secure an adequate airway are the major causes of death in one third of these injuries. Other life-threatening conditions associated with chest trauma are listed in Table 4. The severity of the injury relates to the magnitude and duration of the applied force, the velocity and contact area of that force, body compression that occurs in blast injuries and falls, and the hyperdynamic stress response that follows trauma. This stress response is manifested by an increase in cardiac output, $\dot{V}o_2$, and carbon dioxide production, along with a decrease in systemic vascular resistance and oxygen extraction relative to oxygen delivery. It is believed that the posttraumatic "stress" results from cytokine release from macrophages that stimulates increased toxic oxygen radical production, PMN activation, and the release of endotoxin from ischemic tissues. The pulmonologist is often involved after the initial resuscitation to deal with problems such as hypoxemia (Fig 2) associated with fractures, flail chest, and pulmonary contusions. In addition, the pulmonologist/intensivist may also be asked to evaluate the patient for myocardial injuries or tracheobronchial tears.

Tracheobronchial Tears

Although uncommon, tracheobronchial tears may be life threatening and are frequently overlooked. The diagnosis is suspected when persistent barotrauma and air leaks persist following blunt chest trauma. Hemoptysis is usually, but not always, present along with concomitant fracture of the first and second ribs. The tear is usually within 2.5 cm of the carina and often involves the membranous trachea.

Table 4. *Life-Threatening Chest Trauma*

Acutely	Potentially
Airway obstruction	Tracheobronchial tear
Tension pneumothorax	Lung contusion
Open pneumothorax	Multiple rib fractures
Flail chest	Cardiac tamponade
Massive hemothorax	Aortic rupture

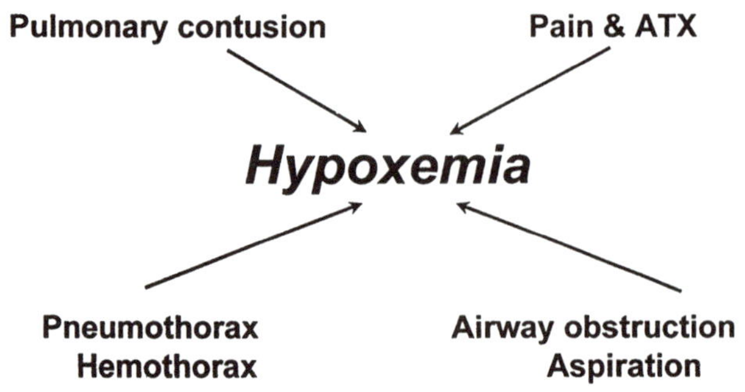

Figure 2. Factors that contribute to hypoxemia after chest trauma.

Bronchoscopic findings include lacerations, transections, and bared cartilage that may be hidden below "heaped-up" mucosa. Early surgical repair is usually required except for small tears (less than one third the circumference of the bronchus or trachea). Stabilization often requires placement of a double-lumen tube or use of high-frequency jet ventilation prior to repair.

Barotrauma

Pneumothorax and hemothorax are potentially life-threatening complications of chest trauma. Pneumomediastinum is reported in 5 to 10% of blunt chest trauma victims. This form of barotrauma can result from tracheobronchial tears, pneumothorax with or without associated rib fractures, or the Macklin effect. The Macklin effect involves alveolar rupture that results in dissection of air along the bronchovascular sheath (pulmonary interstitial emphysema) and then into a mediastinum. The Macklin effect has been identified by chest CT scanning as the cause of the pneumomediastinum in approximately 40% of blunt trauma cases and was associated with a significantly prolonged stay in the ICU.

Flail Chest

Rib or sternal fractures are caused by sudden decompression forces. Children's ribs are more

Table 5. *Treatment of Rib Fractures**

	CPAP Mask (n = 36)	CPAP via ETT (n = 33)
Age (yrs)	46	58
CPAP (cm H_2O)	5.4	6.6
Barotrauma	3	3
Pneumonia	5	16†
Septicemia	0	3
Death	0	2
LOS (days)	8.8	14.6

*CPAP = continuous positive airway pressure; ETT = endotracheal tube; LOS = length of stay. Adapted from Bollegir and van Eeden (Chest 1990; 97:943–948)
†$p < 0.05$ compared with CPAP mask group.

flexible and therefore are less frequently fractured by the same degree of force compared to older victims' ribs. When first or second ribs are fractured, suspicion is raised for injury to great vessels or to the tracheobronchial tree. Prior to 1960, various methods were used to try to stabilize these fractures. After 1960, "internal stabilization" using positive pressure mechanical ventilation with an endotracheal tube was the treatment of choice. Presently, internal stabilization via continuous positive airway pressure (CPAP) mask is the desired approach if the patient's ventilatory status does not require MVS (Table 5). For a flail chest to occur, two or more contiguous ribs need to be fractured in two or more places that results in an unstable segment of the chest wall that paradoxes inward during inspiration because of negative intrathoracic pressure. However, diagnosis of a flail chest can be delayed if the patient is only examined while receiving ventilation with positive pressure. The hypoxemia that frequently accompanied a flail chest was thought to be due to "internal rebreathing" (Pendelluft). However, in a canine model of flail chest that specifically avoided any underlying pulmonary contusion, no significant changes in rib cage distortion or oxygenation occurred in the experimental animals vs controls despite multiple rib fractures. Therefore, it was concluded that the hypoxemia that accompanies a flail chest is due to underlying pulmonary contusion and other associated injuries and not to internal rebreathing (Fig 2).

Pulmonary Contusion From Blunt Chest Trauma

External forces applied to the pulmonary parenchyma during blunt chest trauma, such as acceleration/deceleration during motor vehicle accidents, or blast injury from explosions, can result in disruption of the lung parenchyma. This disruption is amplified if the glottis is closed at the time that airway pressure is suddenly increased. It causes disruption of alveolar-capillary membranes, intraparenchymal hemorrhage, an increase in ventilation/perfusion mismatch, shunt, and dead space as well as increased permeability and extravascular lung water. Pulmonary edema following terrorist incidents is often complicated by other tertiary effects, such as crush, shrapnel, or inhalational injuries. Nosocomial pneumonia and ARDS can occur early or late. The treatment for pulmonary contusion is similar to treating other forms of ARDS except that concomitant injuries, such as barotrauma and neurological injuries, may require modification of ventilatory strategies (such as having to avoid permissive hypercarbia) that would otherwise be used. If the patient survives his or her injuries, lung recovery is usually complete except if there has been significant permanent chest wall damage.

Nonpulmonary Effects of Blunt Chest Trauma

Disruption of the esophagus, diaphragm, or great vessels can also occur. However, myocardial injuries are more frequent. At the present time, the most accurate test for the diagnosis of myocardial injury is either surface or transesophageal echocardiography. Other modalities, such as cardiac enzymes, are too nonspecific to be diagnostic. An echocardiogram is able to image wall motion as well as diagnose potentially life-threatening pericardial effusion and valvular damage.

The pulmonologist's role in the ICU has dramatically expanded over the past decade. Therefore, familiarity with traditional surgical fields, such as trauma, cardiac surgery, and thoracic surgery is essential for the care of our patients.

Annotated Bibliography

Postthoracotomy Pulmonary Function

Datta D, Lahiri B. Preoperative evaluation for patients undergoing lung resection surgery. Chest 2003; 123: 2096–2103

Outlines the basis for the recommended preoperative physiologic assessment of a patient prior to undergoing thoracotomy as outlined in Figure 1.

Girish M, Trayner E, Dammann O, et al. Symptom-limited stair climbing as a predictor of postoperative cardiopulmonary complications after high-risk surgery. Chest 2001; 120:1147–1151

The inability to climb two flights of stairs was associated with an 82% positive predictive value for the development of a postoperative cardiopulmonary complication.

Markos J, Mullan BP, Hillman DR, et al. Preoperative assessment as a predictor of mortality and morbidity after lung resection. Am Rev Respir Dis 1989; 139:902–910

Used combination of postoperative predicted $FEV_1 < 35\%$ and DLCO < 35% to predict an unacceptably high risk of mortality following lung resection.

Marshall MC, Olsen GN. The physiologic evaluation of the lung resection candidate. Clin Chest Med 1993; 14:305–320

Review of the history and scientific data of how to determine post-thoracic surgery pulmonary complications by one of the pioneers in this field (Dr. Olsen).

Reilly JJ. Evidence-based preoperative evaluation of candidates for thoracotomy. Chest 1999; 116:474S–476S

Summary of criteria that can be used to predict postoperative morbidity and mortality, including combined cardiac-pulmonary risk index.

Weisman IM. Cardiopulmonary exercise testing in preoperative assessment for lung resection surgery. Semin Thorac Cardiovasc Surg 2001; 13:116–125

Concise review of how to use exercise testing to help determine the advisability of allowing borderline candidates to undergo lung resection. $\dot{V}O_2$ max <40% of predicted or <10 mL/kg/min precludes resection surgery.

Win T, Groves AM, Wells FC, et al. Relationship of shuttle walk test and lung cancer surgical outcome. Eur J Cardiothorac Surg 2004; 26:1216–1219

The shuttle (6 min) walk distance was not predictive of a poor surgical outcome.

Zeihar BG, Gross TJ, Kern JA, et al. Predicting postoperative pulmonary function in patients undergoing lung resection. Chest 1995; 108:68–72

Reports an underestimation of postoperative FEV_1 when the number of segments (times 5.2% per segment) to be removed are used to predict postoperative lung function.

Chest Trauma

Bolliger CT, van Eeden SF. Treatment of multiple rib fractures: randomized trial comparing ventilatory with nonventilatory management. Chest 1990; 97:943–948

Patients who did not have concomitant severe pulmonary contusion or did not require associated laparotomies recovered better when CPAP was delivered noninvasively.

Cappello M, Yuehua C, de Troyer A. Rib cage distortion in a canine model of flail chest. Am J Respir Crit Care Med 1995; 151:1481–1485

In a canine model of flail chest without underlying pulmonary contusion, there were no significant harmful effects on breathing pattern, ventilation, or oxygenation.

Demling RH, Pomfret EA. Blunt chest trauma. New Horiz 1993; 1:402–421

Review article with multiple references.

DePalma RG, Burris DG, Champion HR, et al. Blast injuries. N Engl J Med 2005; 352:1335–1342

The onslaught of terrorism acts has made this review article all too relevant.

Hirshberg B, Oppenheim-Eden A, Pizoo R, et al. Recovery from blast lung injury: one-year follow-up. Chest 1999; 116:1683–1688

Despite requiring mechanical ventilation because of severe lung injury, victims of blast injuries frequently recovered to normal lung function.

Kshettry VR, Bolman RM III. Chest trauma: assessment, diagnosis, and management. Clin Chest Med 1994; 15:137–153

Review article.

Newman PG, Feliciano DV. Blunt cardiac injury. New Horiz 1999; 7:26–34

Review article.

Pretre R, Chilcott M. Blunt trauma to the heart and great vessels. N Engl J Med 1997; 336:626–632

Reviews myocardial and great vessel injuries.

Shaker KG, Hollingworth HM, Irwin RS, et al. Tracheobronchial injuries caused by blunt trauma. J Intensive Care Med 1995; 10:226–233

Comprehensive review with illustrative chest radiographs.

Wintermark M, Schnyder P. The Macklin effect: a frequent etiology for pneumomediastinum in severe blunt chest trauma. Chest 2001; 120:543–547

The Macklin effect was identified by chest CT scans as the cause of pneumomediastinum in 39% of 51 patients, and was associated with prolonged ICU stays.

Postcardiac Surgery Pulmonary Complications

Baisden CE, Greenwald LV, Symbas PN. Occult rib fractures and brachial plexus injury following median sternotomy for open-heart operation. Ann Thorac Surg 1984; 38:192–194

Two-thirds of the patients studied had positive bone scans.

Bardell T, Legare JF, Buth KC, et al. ICU readmission after cardiac surgery. Eur J Cardiothorac Surg 2003; 23: 354–359

Preoperative renal failure and prolonged mechanical ventilation (> 24 h) postoperatively predicted a higher incidence of ICU readmission.

Branca P, McGaw P, Light RW, et al. Factors associated with prolonged mechanical ventilation following coronary artery bypass surgery. Chest 2001: 119:537–546

Fewer than 5% of patients required mechanical ventilation for > 3 days after CABG. Preoperative cardiac or respiratory instability are predictive of prolonged MVS.

Cohen AJ, Katz MG, Frenkel G, et al. Morbid results of prolonged intubation after coronary artery bypass surgery. Chest 2000: 118:1724–1731

Sixty-six of 1,112 patient undergoing CABG required MVS for > 48 h or reintubation. Multivariate regression analysis identified three factors that were associated with prolonged intubation: elevated creatinine level, lower FEV_1*, and a positive fluid balance at 24 h postoperatively. Prolonged intubation significantly increased hospital stay and mortality rates.*

Dimopoulou I, Daganou M, Dafni U, et al. Phrenic nerve dysfunction after cardiac operations: electrophysiologic evaluation of risk factors. Chest 1998; 113:8–14

Thirteen of 63 surgery patients had delayed phrenic nerve conduction latency times postoperatively compared to preoperative testing. The only risk factor that was significantly associated with this complication by logistic regression analysis was the use of cardioplegic ice slush.

El-Chemaly S, Abreu A, Krieger B. What are the risks of pulmonary complications after cardiac surgery? J Crit Illness 2003; 18:266–273

General review with 39 references.

Hoffman R, Yahr W, Krieger B. Diaphragmatic flutter resulting in failure to wean from mechanical ventilator support after coronary artery bypass surgery. Crit Care Med 1990; 18:499–501

Report of four patients who had diaphragmatic flutter after cardiac surgery.

Lee YC, Vaz MAC, Ely KA, et al. Symptomatic persistent postcoronary artery bypass graft pleural effusions requiring operative treatment: clinical and histologic features. Chest 2001; 119:795–800

The effusions were lymphocytic (> 80% lymphocytes) and often resulted in fibrosis and occasional trapped lungs.

Locke TJ, Griffith TL, Mould H, et al. Rib cage mechanics after median sternotomy. Thorax 1990; 45:465–468

Thoracic wall discoordination was documented by magnetometers in 9 of 16 patients 1 week postoperatively.

Massoudy P, Zahler S, Becker BF, et al. Evidence for inflammatory responses of the lungs during coronary artery bypass grafting with cardiopulmonary bypass. Chest 2001; 119:31–36

Proinflammatory cytokines (interleukin-6 and -8) increased in pulmonary venous blood after bypass. In addition, adhesion molecule counts on platelets and PMNs also became elevated.

Maillet JM, Besnerais P, Cantoni M, et al. Frequency, risk factors and outcome of hyperlactatemia after cardiac surgery. Chest 2003; 123:1361–1366

A lactate level > 3 mmol/L measured within 4 h after surgery was associated with increased mortality.

Milot J, Perron J, Lacasse Y, et al. Incidence and predictors of ARDS after cardiac surgery. Chest 2001; 119: 884–888

The incidence of ARDS in a retrospective analysis of 3,278 patients was 0.4% but carried a 15% mortality rate. Risk factors identified by multivariate analysis included previous cardiac surgery, shock, and number of blood products received.

Ng CSH, Wan S, Yim APC, et al. Pulmonary dysfunction after cardiac surgery. Chest 2002; 121:1269–1277

This article reviews the associated physiologic, biochemical, and histologic changes associated with the pulmonary dysfunction following cardiac surgery with particular attention to PMN activation, free radicals, and cytokines.

Rady MY, Ryan T. Perioperative predictors of extubation failure and the effect on clinical outcome after cardiac surgery. Crit Care Med 1999; 27:340–347

Clinical predictors of extubation failure included age > 65 years; inpatient hospitalization; COPD; pulmonary hypertension; severe left ventricular dysfunction; redo operation; thoracic aorta procedures; and bypass time ≥ 120 min.

Wynne R, Botti M. Postoperative pulmonary dysfunction in adults after cardiac surgery with cardiopulmonary bypass: clinical significance and implications for practice. Am J Crit Care 2004; 13:384–393

A nursing review that is worth reading with 159 references.

Yende S, Quasney M, Tolley E, et al. Association of tumor necrosis factor gene polymorphisms and prolonged mechanical ventilation after coronary artery bypass surgery. Crit Care Med 2003; 31:133–140

Yende S, Quasney M, Tolley E, et al. Clinical relevance of angiotensin-converting enzyme gene polymorphisms to predict risk of mechanical ventilation after coronary artery bypass graft surgery. Crit Care Med 2004; 32: 922–927

The presence of a specific haplotype in the promoter region of the TNF gene site and angiotensin-converting enzyme gene polymorphisms were associated with a significantly higher rate of prolonged MVS following a CABG procedure.

Thoracoscopy

Colt HG. Thoracoscopy: window to the pleural space. Chest 1999; 116:1409–1415

Reviews the indications for VATS and quotes a procedure-related mortality rate of 0.24% "in experienced hands."

Loddenkemper R. Thoracoscopy: state of the art. Eur Respir J 1998; 11:218–221

Comprehensive review of the diagnostic utility of "medical" thoracoscopy as performed by pulmonologists in Europe.

Sleep Physiology

Teofilo L. Lee-Chiong, Jr., MD, FCCP

Objectives:

- Understand the various neural processes that control sleep and wakefulness
- Describe the physiologic changes that occur during sleep
- Identify the consequences of sleep deprivation
- Review the rules related to the scoring of sleep stages and respiratory events in adults

Key words: circadian rhythm; polysomnography; sleep; sleep deprivation; sleep homeostasis; sleep physiology

---

Sleep is a complex reversible state characterized by both behavioral quiescence and diminished responsiveness to external stimuli. Sleep is generated and maintained by CNS networks using specific neurotransmitters localized in specific areas of the brain.

Neuroscience of Sleep

Neural systems generating wakefulness include the ascending reticular formation in the medulla, pons, and midbrain; basal forebrain (neurotransmitter: acetylcholine); hypothalamus (hypocretin); locus ceruleus (norepinephrine); tuberomammillary nucleus (histamine); and ventral tegmental area and substantia nigra (dopamine). Neural systems generating non-rapid eye movement (NREM) sleep consist of the hypothalamus (gamma aminobutyric acid [GABA]), basal forebrain (GABA and adenosine), and thalamus, which is where sleep spindles are generated. Finally, neural systems generating rapid eye movement (REM) sleep include the pons and basal forebrain. REM sleep is associated with activation of "REM-on" neurons (cholinergic) and inhibition of "REM-off" neurons (noradrenergic, serotonergic, and histaminergic).

Sleep and wake neurotransmitters consist of the following: (1) acetylcholine, the main REM sleep neurotransmitter; (2) adenosine, which is responsible for homeostatic sleep drive; (3) glutamate, the main CNS excitatory neurotransmitter; (4) GABA, the main CNS inhibitory neurotransmitter and the main NREM sleep neurotransmitter; (5) glycine, the main inhibitory neurotransmitter in the spinal cord and is responsible for REM sleep-related muscle atonia/hypotonia; and (6) hypocretin, the dysfunction of which is responsible for narcolepsy.

Sleep-Wake Regulation

Two basic intrinsic components interact to regulate the timing and consolidation of sleep and wake: sleep homeostasis, which is dependent on the sleep-wake cycle, and circadian rhythm, which is independent of the sleep-wake cycle.[1] These two processes influence sleep latency, duration, and quality. In addition, the timing of sleep is also determined by behavioral influences, such as social activities and work schedules.

Sleep homeostasis is defined as increasing sleep pressure related to the duration of previous wakefulness: the longer a person is awake, the sleepier one becomes. This sleep pressure then decreases after a sufficient duration of sleep.

The circadian system consists of biological rhythms that are ubiquitous and genetically determined. Natural circadian rhythms free-run at slightly $>$24 h ($\approx$24.2 h [referred to as "*tau*"]). The process of entrainment adjusts the circadian rhythm to the external 24-h period by the use of environmental cues called *zeitgebers.* Zeitgebers can be photic or nonphotic (*eg*, mealtimes and social schedules) and cause either a phase advance, a shift of the circadian period to an earlier time, or a phase delay, a shift of the circadian period to a later time.

The suprachiasmatic nucleus (SCN) in the anterior hypothalamus is the master circadian rhythm generator in mammals. Other anatomic sites also harbor endogenous clocks. SCN activity is greater during the daytime than at night. Actions of the SCN consist of promotion of wakefulness during the day as well as consolidation of sleep during the night. Ablation of the SCN results in both random distribution of sleep throughout the day and night and a reduction in the duration of waking periods (in some).

There are two circadian peaks in wakefulness (wake-maintenance zones), namely in the late morning and early evening; there are also two circadian troughs in alertness (increased sleep propensity) in the early morning and early midafternoon.

Several afferent pathways provide inputs, both photic and nonphotic, to the SCN. The main afferent connection involves the retinohypothalamic tract that relays photic stimuli from the photosensitive retina ganglion cells containing melanopsin to the SCN by the use of glutamate as its neurotransmitter. Retinal photoreceptors are most sensitive to shorter-wavelength light (450 to 500 nm [blue to blue-green]). An alternate afferent connection exists that relays stimuli via the thalamic lateral geniculate nuclei and geniculohypothalamic tract. Light entrainment is lost with disruption of the main pathway but not of the alternate pathway. The SCN, in turn, has widespread efferent projections to the basal forebrain, hypocretin neurons of the hypothalamus, locus ceruleus, thalamus, and pineal gland.

Melatonin is synthesized and released by the pineal gland, with greatest secretion at night. Secretion inhibited by light exposure. Actions of melatonin on the sleep-wake rhythm consist of a phase delay when administered in the morning and phase advance when given in the evening. Melatonin is less effective in phase shifting circadian rhythms than light exposure, but it possesses mild hypnotic properties.

Physiologic Processes During Sleep

Autonomic Nervous System

Compared with wakefulness, during NREM sleep there is a relative decrease in sympathetic activity, accompanied by an increase in parasympathetic activity. There is a further reduction in sympathetic activity and enhanced parasympathetic activity during REM sleep compared with NREM sleep. Transient increases in sympathetic activity occur during phasic REM sleep.

Respiratory System

Respiration is controlled by both metabolic and behavioral factors during the wake state. In contrast, only metabolic control is present during sleep. Compared with levels during wakefulness, there is a decrease in both Pao_2 and arterial oxygen saturation (Sao_2) and an increase in $Paco_2$ during sleep. Hypoxic and hypercapnic ventilatory responses, upper airway dilator muscle tone, and activity of the accessory muscles of respiration all diminish during NREM sleep, compared with wakefulness, and decrease further during REM sleep. The activity of the diaphragm remains intact during REM sleep. NREM stage N1 sleep is characterized by periodic breathing, with episodes of hypopnea and hyperpnea. Respiratory patterns become stable and regular during stage N3 sleep. During REM sleep, respiration is irregular, with variable respiratory rates and tidal volumes. Central apneas or periodic breathing may emerge during phasic REM sleep.

Cardiovascular System

Decreases in heart rate (HR), cardiac output (CO), and BP occur during NREM sleep compared with the wake state. Further reductions in HR, CO, and BP develop during tonic REM sleep compared with NREM sleep. Increases in HR, CO, and BP may occur during phasic REM sleep compared wih NREM and tonic REM sleep, as well as during awakenings. Nighttime systolic BP is commonly approximately 10% less than corresponding levels during the daytime (*ie*, "dipping" phenomenon).

GI System

Sleep is associated with decreased swallowing rate, salivary production, and esophageal and intestinal motility. Basal gastric acid secretion demonstrates a circadian pattern with peak levels generally between 10:00 PM and 2:00 AM and lowest levels from 5:00 AM to 11:00 AM.

Renal System

Urine output diminishes during sleep as a result of an increase in water reabsorption, decreased glomerular filtration, and increase in release of renin (during NREM sleep) and antidiuretic hormone. Obstructive sleep apnea (OSA) is associated with an increased risk of nocturia, with the latter improving with optimal positive airway pressure (PAP) therapy.

Endocrine System

Certain hormones exhibit increasing levels during sleep (*eg*, growth hormone, prolactin, parathyroid hormone, and testosterone), whereas levels of others decrease during sleep (*eg*, cortisol, insulin, and thyroid-stimulating hormone). Acromegaly is associated with a greater prevalence of OSA and central sleep apnea, and therapy of acromegaly with surgery or octreotide can improve sleep-related breathing disorders (SRBDs). OSA can result in lower levels of growth hormone and testosterone, both of which increase with PAP therapy. Finally, polycystic ovarian syndrome is associated with both increased testosterone levels and greater risk of OSA.

OSA also increases the risk of insulin resistance and type II diabetes mellitus, independent of body mass index. There is an increase in both leptin and ghrelin levels in OSA. Insulin sensitivity and levels of leptin and ghrelin improve with PAP therapy.

Musculoskeletal System

Skeletal muscle relaxation (hypotonia or atonia) and inhibition of deep tendon reflexes develop during sleep.

Immunity

Proinflammatory cytokines, such as interleukin (IL)-1β and tumor necrosis factor-α, generally enhance sleep, whereas antiinflammatory cytokines, including IL-4 and IL-10, suppress sleep. Viral and bacterial infections result in a reduction in NREM and increase in REM sleep. Changes in the immune system also develop in persons with OSA, namely increases in C-reactive protein, IL-6, and tumor necrosis factor-α; levels improve with PAP therapy.

Thermoregulation

Core body temperature follows a circadian rhythmicity that peaks in the late afternoon and early evening (from 6:00 PM to 8:00 PM) and decreases at the onset of sleep, with lowest levels at approximately 2 h before usual wake time (from 4:00 AM to 5:00 AM). Changes in thermoregulation during sleep include a decrease in core body temperature, decrease in thermal set point, reduced thermoregulatory responses to thermal challenges, and loss of heat production from shivering during REM sleep. Nocturnal sleep typically occurs during the decreasing phase of the temperature rhythm (after maximum core body temperature), whereas awakening occurs during the increasing phase of the temperature rhythm (after minimum core body temperature).

Metabolism

Metabolism decreases during NREM sleep compared with the wake state, and metabolic rate during REM sleep is either similar or higher than during NREM sleep.

Sleep Deprivation

Several physiologic parameters become increased during sleep deprivation, including subjective and objective sleepiness, sympathetic activity, insulin resistance, and levels of cortisol and ghrelin. Medical errors and motor vehicle accidents also increase. On the other hand, vigilance, cognition and attention, seizure threshold, resistance to infection, and levels of growth hormone and leptin activity decrease during sleep deprivation.[2]

Polysomnography

Polysomnography involves the continuous and simultaneous recording of several physiologic variables during sleep. These variables commonly consist of an electroencephalogram (EEG), electrooculogram (EOG), chin electromyogram (EMG), ECG, airflow, respiratory effort, oxygenation and ventilation, snoring, and anterior tibialis EMG.

Polysomnography is indicated for the following: (1) the diagnosis of SRBD; (2) PAP titration for

SRBD; (3) follow-up after upper airway surgery or dental devices for OSA; and (4) evaluation of narcolepsy, idiopathic hypersomnia, periodic limb movement disorder (PLMD), atypical or injurious parasomnias, and nocturnal seizures.

Diagnostic sleep studies can be classified into four levels: level 1 (attended laboratory full polysomnography), level 2 (unattended full polysomnography), level 3 (cardiorespiratory sleep studies including at least 4 bioparameters), and level 4 (limited sleep studies with one to two bioparameters).

A polygraph consists of a series of alternating current and direct current amplifiers and filters that are used to record physiologic variables during sleep. Alternating current amplifiers are commonly chosen for high-frequency (fast) physiologic variables, such as EEG, EOG, and EMG, whereas direct current amplifiers are used for low-frequency (slow) physiologic variables, such as oxygen saturation (*ie*, Sao_2). A derivation is defined as the difference in voltage between two electrodes and can either be bipolar, *ie*, when two standard electrodes are matched to each other, or referential, *ie*, when a standard electrode is matched to a reference electrode.

In EEG, electrodes are placed based on the International 10-20 system, wherein each electrode is provided with a letter, which represents a region of the brain (F [frontal], C [central], O [occipital], and M [mastoid]), and a numerical subscript, with odd numbers representing left-sided electrodes, even numbers representing right-sided electrodes, and the designation Z used for midline electrodes. Recommended electrode placements for EEG are F4M1, C4M1, and O2M1.[3] Additional EEG electrodes are required when one is evaluating suspected nocturnal seizures.

EEG voltage originates from the summed potential activity of cortical neurons. EEG waves can be differentiated based on frequency of EEG waves into delta waves (< 4 Hz), theta waves (4–7 Hz), alpha waves (8–13 Hz), and beta waves (> 13 Hz). Delta waves define the presence of stage N3 sleep. Theta waves are present in stages N1, N2, and R sleep. Alpha waves are seen during drowsiness with eyes closed. Beta waves are present during alert wakefulness. Stage N2 sleep is characterized by the presence of either K complexes or sleep spindles. A K complex consists of a high-amplitude, biphasic wave with duration of 0.5 s and an initial sharp negative deflection followed by positive high-voltage slow wave. Sleep spindles are oscillations with a frequency of 12 to 14 Hz lasting 0.5 to 1.5 s; their amplitude is generally < 50 µV.

EOG is used to record the difference in potentials, referred to as a *dipole*, between the cornea, which is positively charged, and the negatively charged retina. Recommended electrode placements for EOG are E1M2 and E2M2, with E1 representing an electrode below the left outer canthus, E2 an electrode above the right outer canthus, and M2 the right mastoid process.[3] The dipole changes with eye movements. Two patterns of eye movements can often be seen: slow rolling eye movements that occur during drowsiness when eyes are closed and REMs that occur during wakefulness (*ie*, eye blinks) or REM sleep.

Recording chin EMG involves the use of three electrodes that are located midline above the mandible, right of midline below the mandible, and left of midline below the mandible. Derivation consists of one electrode below and one electrode above the mandible. ECG uses a modified lead II electrode.

Airflow is measured by the use of either an oronasal thermal sensor, which is the recommended technique for identifying apneas, or a nasal air pressure transducer, which is recommend for identifying hypopnea. With nasal air pressure monitoring, inspiratory flow signals show a plateau (flattening) with obstructive events or reduced but rounded signal with central events.

Measuring respiratory effort involves esophageal manometry or inductance plethysmography, which are important in distinguishing obstructive, central, and mixed apneas.

Pulse oximetry is the recommended technique for measuring oxygenation, whereas transcutaneous ($Ptcco_2$) or end-tidal ($Petco_2$) monitoring is recommended for the measurement of alveolar hypoventilation, especially in children. A microphone is used to identify snoring.

EMG of the anterior tibialis is important in the detection of periodic limb movements during sleep. Additional EMG electrodes can be placed in the upper extremities to aid in the diagnosis of REM sleep behavior disorder.

Scoring Adult Sleep Stages

Polysomnographic data are divided into 30-s time periods, or epochs. Standard sleep study paper speed is 10 mm/s (30 cm per epoch page). Each epoch is assigned a sleep stage that comprises the greatest percentage of the epoch. Sleep among adults is typically composed of stage N1 (5%), N2 (45%), N3 (25%) and R (25%).

Stage wake is scored when >50% of the epoch has alpha EEG waves when eyes are closed. If alpha waves are absent, stage wake is defined by the presence of vertical eye blinks, reading eye movements, or voluntary rapid open eye movements. Chin EMG tone is generally high.[3] Stage N1 sleep is present if alpha waves are replaced by low amplitude, mixed frequency (4–7 Hz) waves that occupy >50% of the epoch. Slow eye movements may be present. Sleep spindles and K complexes are absent. Tonic chin EMG levels are lower than stage wake.[3]

Stage N2 sleep is defined by low amplitude, mixed frequency waves with the presence of K complexes (not associated with arousals) or sleep spindles during the first half of the epoch or during the last half of the previous epoch.[3] Stage N3 sleep is scored if at least 20% of the epoch is occupied by slow wave (0.5–2 Hz and >75 μV) EEG activity over the frontal regions.[3] Stage REM sleep is characterized by low amplitude, mixed frequency EEG activity, REMs, and low chin EMG tone.[3]

Scoring Respiratory and Movement Events

An apnea is defined by a decrease in peak thermal sensor amplitude by at least 90% of baseline for a duration of at least 10 s. Apneas can be either obstructive, when inspiratory effort is present throughout the entire event; central if inspiratory effort is absent throughout the entire event; or mixed when a central event is followed by an obstructive event.[3]

Hypopnea is a decrease in nasal pressure by at least 30% of baseline for duration of at least 10 s accompanied by oxygen desaturation of at least 4%.[3] A respiratory effort-related arousal is characterized by breaths associated with increasing respiratory efforts for at least 10 s and flattening of the nasal pressure waveform. Event precedes an arousal, and does not meet criteria for either apneas or hypopneas.

Hypoventilation is present when there is an increase in Pa_{CO_2} of at least 10 mm Hg during sleep compared to supine wake levels.[3] Cheyne-Stokes respiration (CSR) is characterized by a crescendo-decrescendo amplitude in respiration, with at least 5 central apneas/hypopneas per hour of sleep.[3]

Periodic limb movements during sleep are scored if there are at least 4 consecutive leg movements, each 0.5–10 s in duration, and if the movements are between 5 and 90 s apart.[3] REM sleep behavior disorder is suggested by sustained chin EMG muscle activity or the presence of excessive transient chin or limb EMG muscle activity during REM sleep.[3]

Definitions of Sleep Parameters

The time when a sleep recording is started is designated *lights out*, and the time when sleep recording ended is termed *lights on*. Time in bed (TIB) is the duration of monitoring between "lights out" and "lights on." Total sleep time (TST) is the sum of all sleep stages (*ie*, N1-3 sleep plus REM sleep). Time in bed and total sleep time are used to calculate sleep efficiency (SE), which is the ratio of TST to TIB [(TST × 100)/TIB]. Wake time after sleep onset (WASO) is the time spent awake from sleep onset to final awakening.

Sleep onset latency (SOL) is defined as the time from lights out to the onset of sleep (*ie*, the first epoch of any sleep stage). REM sleep latency is the time from sleep onset to the first epoch of REM sleep. REM sleep occurring within 10 to 15 min of sleep onset is referred to as a *sleep onset REM period* (SOREMP).

The apnea-hypopnea index (AHI) is the number of apneas plus hypopneas per hour of sleep. The number of arousals per hour of sleep is referred to as an *arousal index*. An oxygen desaturation index (ODI) refers to the number of oxygen desaturation events per hour of sleep. Finally, the periodic limb movement index (PLMI) is defined as the number of periodic limb movements per hour of sleep.

Sleep Architecture

Polysomnographic features of many primary sleep, medical, neurologic and psychiatric disorders can be differentiated into two general patterns of sleep architecture: a high sleep input pattern (short sleep latency, high sleep efficiency, increased total sleep time and reduced wake time after sleep onset) and a low sleep input pattern (prolonged sleep latency, reduced sleep efficiency and total sleep time, and increased wake time after sleep onset). The high sleep input pattern can be seen following sleep deprivation, in disorders presenting with excessive sleepiness, such as narcolepsy, and during administration of sedating medications, whereas the low sleep input pattern often accompanies disorders presenting with insomnia or use of stimulant medications.

Epworth Sleepiness Scale

The degree of sleepiness is often subjectively determined using an eight-item questionnaire that measures a person's propensity to fall asleep in specific situations in recent times, including the following: (a) sitting and reading, (b) watching television, (c) sitting and inactive in a public place, (d) riding as a passenger in a car for an hour without a break, (e) lying down to rest in the afternoon, (f) sitting and talking to someone, (g) sitting quietly after lunch without drinking alcohol, and (h) stopped in a car for a few minutes in traffic. The chances of dozing are rated as one of the following: 0 (never), 1 (slight chance), 2 (moderate chance) or 3 (high chance). An aggregate score between 0 and 9 is considered as representing a normal level of alertness. Scores of 10 and above suggest the presence of sleepiness that might require intervention.

The correlation between sleepiness measured subjectively by the Epworth sleepiness scale and objective measures using the multiple sleep latency test (MSLT) and the maintenance of wakefulness test (MWT) is poor. Epworth sleepiness scale scores are elevated in patients with OSA; scores improve following effective therapy for OSA.

Multiple Sleep Latency Test

The MSLT is an objective measure of a person's tendency to fall asleep in quiet situations, and is indicated for evaluation of unexplained sleepiness and suspected narcolepsy, and to distinguish between narcolepsy and idiopathic hypersomnia.[4] A regular sleep-wake schedule is required for at least 1 to 2 weeks prior to testing. Medications that affect sleep latency and REM sleep should be discontinued for at least 2 weeks before performing the test. Polysomnography (but not a split-night study) should be performed immediately before an MSLT to ensure at least 6 h of sleep and to exclude the presence of either OSA or PLMD that can affect the interpretation of study results. In persons with OSA, PAP therapy should be used during both polysomnography and MSLT. Smoking is not allowed prior to each nap trial, and persons should not drink caffeine or engage in vigorous physical activity on the day of the study. A urine drug screen may be performed on test day.

The multiple sleep latency test consists of 4 or 5 nap opportunities performed every 2 h, with each nap trial lasting 20 min in duration. The patient is asked to lie down in a comfortable position in a dark, quiet room, close his/her eyes and try to fall asleep, while EEG, EOG, chin EMG, and ECG are continuously monitored. Sleep onset latency and SOREMPs, if present, are determined for each nap trial. Sleep onset latency is recorded as 20 min if no sleep occurs during a nap trial. Each nap trial is terminated after 20 min if no sleep is recorded; if sleep is noted, the test is continued for another 15 min to allow REM sleep to occur. The test is stopped after the first epoch of REM sleep. The patient is asked to get out of bed and to remain awake between nap trials.

A short mean SOL, *ie*, <8 min, suggests the presence of excessive sleepiness. A short SOL is present in persons with narcolepsy, idiopathic hypersomnia, OSA and PLMD. It can also be seen during sleep deprivation, following acute withdrawal of stimulant agents, and in 15% to 30% of healthy individuals. Sleep onset REM periods are present in persons with narcolepsy or OSA, during sleep deprivation, after withdrawal from REM suppressants or alcohol, and in 1% to 3% of healthy individuals.

Maintenance of Wakefulness Test

The MWT is an objective measure of a person's ability to remain awake in quiet situations for a specified period of time.[4] An MWT is indicated to assess a person's ability to maintain wakefulness as well as to assess response to treatment for excessive sleepiness. This test is less sensitive than MSLT in measuring sleepiness.

The MWT consists of four nap opportunities, each 40 min in duration and performed at 2-h intervals. The first nap trial is started about 1.5 to 3 h after the person's customary wake time. Standard monitoring leads include EEG, EOG and chin EMG. The need for polysomnography prior to testing is not routinely indicated and should be determined by the clinician for each specific individual.

During testing, the person is asked to sit in bed in a semi-reclined position in a dark, quiet room, and asked to try to stay awake. Measures to stay awake (*eg*, singing) are not allowed, and no tobacco, caffeine, or stimulant agents are permitted during test day. The nap trial is stopped if either sleep occurs or after 40 min if no sleep is recorded.

Sleep onset latency is determined for each nap; it is recorded as 40 min if no sleep occurs during a nap trial. Mean SOL correlates with the ability to stay awake, with <8 min being abnormal; 8 or more minutes but <40 min is considered indeterminate, and 40 min is considered normal.

Sleep and Aging

Sleep requirements do not decline with aging. Older adults, however, have greater nocturnal sleep disturbance, more complaints of excessive sleepiness, and more frequent daytime napping. Older women are better able to maintain satisfactory sleep compared with older men. Causes of sleep disturbance in older adults include aging itself (rarely the sole cause); menopause; medical disorders, such as nocturia; neurologic disorders, including dementia and Parkinson disease; psychiatric disorders, such as depression; adverse effects of medications; and primary sleep disorders. Aging is associated with a greater prevalence of insomnia, OSA, central sleep apnea, PLMD, restless legs syndrome, REM sleep behavior disorder, and advanced sleep phase disorder. Compared with younger adults, there is poorer correlation between subjective sleep complaints and objective polysomnography findings in this population group.[5]

Among older adults, OSA remains more prevalent in men, but its risk increases with menopause among women. Hormonal replacement therapy (HRT) decreases the prevalence of OSA in postmenopausal women; nevertheless, data do not conclusively support the use of HRT as therapy for OSA among postmenopausal women. Compared with younger counterparts, OSA among older adults is associated with relatively less risk of cardiopulmonary diseases, and the AHI is less able to predict mortality risk.

References

1. Borbely AA, Achermann P. Sleep homeostasis and models of sleep regulation. J Biol Rhythms 1999; 14:557–568
2. Mullington JM, Haack M, Toth M, et al. Cardiovascular, inflammatory, and metabolic consequences of sleep deprivation. Prog Cardiovasc Dis 2009; 51:294–302
3. Iber C, Ancoli-Israel S, Chesson A, et al, for the American Academy of Sleep Medicine. The AASM manual for the scoring of sleep and associated events: rules, terminology and technical specifications. 1st ed. Westchester, IL: American Academy of Sleep Medicine, 2007
4. Standards of Practice Committee of the American Academy of Sleep Medicine. Practice parameters for clinical use of the multiple sleep latency test and the maintenance of wakefulness test. Sleep 2005; 28:113–121
5. Ancoli-Israel S, Ayalon L, Salzman C. Sleep in the elderly: normal variations and common sleep disorders. Harv Rev Psychiatry 2008; 16:279–286

Notes

Sleep-Related Breathing Disorders

Teofilo L. Lee-Chiong, Jr., MD, FCCP

Objectives:

- Differentiate the clinical and polysomnographic features of obstructive and central sleep apnea
- Describe the various effective therapies for OSA
- Distinguish the causes of hypercapnic vs nonhypercapnic CSA
- Identify the key features of the hypoventilation syndromes

Key words: central sleep apnea; hypoventilation; obstructive sleep apnea; positive airway pressure therapy

Obstructive Sleep Apnea

Obstructive sleep apnea (OSA) is characterized by repetitive reduction or cessation of airflow despite the presence of respiratory efforts caused by partial or complete upper-airway occlusion during sleep.[1]

Definitions

An apnea is defined as a reduction in peak thermal sensor amplitude by at least 90% of baseline for at least 10 s. Respiratory events can either be central (no respiratory effort), obstructive (respiratory efforts are present), or mixed (initial central apnea followed by obstructive apnea). A hypopnea is present if there is a decrease in nasal pressure by at least 30% of baseline for duration of at least 10 s accompanied by at least 4% oxygen desaturation. Complex sleep apnea is characterized by central apneas that develop or become more frequent during continuous positive airway pressure (CPAP) titration for OSA.

Demographics

OSA affects an estimated 24% of adult men and 9% of adult women if OSA is defined by an apnea-hypopnea index (AHI) of at least 5 events/ hour, or 4% of adult men and 2% of adult women if OSA is defined by an AHI of at least 5 events/h plus the presence of excessive sleepiness. It affects men more commonly than women, in whom prevalence increases with menopause.

Pathophysiology

The upper airway can be conceptualized as a collapsible cylinder, with airflow determined by both the difference in upstream (nasal) vs downstream pressure and airway resistance. Therefore, airflow is greater with the following: (1) greater upstream pressure, (2) lesser downstream pressure, and (3) reduced airway resistance. Upper-airway patency is dependent on the balance of factors that maintain airway opening (activation of dilator muscles) or promote airway closure (decrease in intraluminal pressure and Bernoulli forces). Airway size is also influenced by lung volume, which decreases during sleep. The critical closing pressure (PCRIT) is the intraluminal pressure at which the upper airway collapses; it becomes progressively less negative from nonsnorers and snorers to OSA. Activation of the upper-airway dilator muscles lowers PCRIT. Ventilatory loop gain is also important in the pathogenesis of OSA. Persons with OSA are more likely to have intrinsically unstable negative feedback ventilatory control system, with a high loop gain increasing the risk of periodic breathing.

Compared with persons without the disorder, those with OSA tend to have narrower airways that are more vulnerable to collapse. The most common sites of upper-airway obstruction are behind the palate (retropalatal), behind the tongue (retrolingual), or both. In OSA, repetitive upper-airway obstruction is associated with episodic decreases in arterial oxygen saturation (Sao_2); snoring that may alternate with periods of silence; arrhythmias, with a relative reduction in heart rate developing during upper-airway obstruction followed by a relative increase in heart rate during apnea termination; arousal at apnea termination; and increase in BP in the immediate postapneic period.

Several factors might worsen hypoxemia during obstructive respiratory events, including low awake supine and baseline sleep Sao_2, increased percentage of total sleep time with apneas or hypopneas, greater duration of apnea or hypopneas, decrease in functional residual capacity and expiratory reserved volume, comorbid lung disorders such as COPD, or stage of sleep (more severe oxygen desaturation during rapid eye movement [REM] sleep compared with non-rapid eye movement [NREM] sleep).

Classification Based on Severity

The severity of OSA can be measured based on the AHI as mild (5 to 15), moderate (16 to 30), or severe (>30). In addition to the AHI, other factors can influence the clinical severity of OSA, such as the degree of daytime sleepiness, nadir of Sao_2, severity of sleep fragmentation, presence of nocturnal arrhythmias, and the presence of comorbid cardiovascular or neurologic disorders.

Risk Factors

Risk factors for OSA include a positive family history of OSA, male gender (for adults), menopausal state in women, aging, excess body weight, snoring, smoking and alcohol use, medication use (*eg*, muscle relaxants), and primary disorders, such as untreated hypothyroidism (inconsistent data), acromegaly, neuromuscular disorders, and stroke. Androgen therapy has been shown to increase the risk of OSA. Central obesity, *ie*, waist-hip ratio, is more important than general obesity.

Specific craniofacial and oropharyngeal features predispose one to the development of OSA, including increased neck circumference, namely >17 inches in men and >16 inches in women; nasal narrowing or congestion; macroglossia; low-lying soft palate; enlarged tonsils and adenoids; mid-face hypoplasia; retrognathia or micrognathia; and mandibular hypoplasia. The prevalence of OSA is greater among African-Americans, Mexican Americans, and Asians and Pacific Islanders compared with white subjects. The apolipoprotein ε4 gene is associated with an increased risk and severity of OSA, and polymorphism in the angiotensin-converting enzyme gene is associated with the development of hypertension in persons with OSA.

Clinical Features

Persons with OSA most commonly present with complaints of daytime sleepiness. It is important to note that the severity of excessive sleepiness does not correlate closely with AHI. Other complaints include repeated awakenings with gasping or choking, snoring, witnessed apneas, attention deficit and/or hyperactivity (particularly in children), changes in mood such as treatment-resistant depression, and decline in work or school performance. It is not unusual for OSA to be encountered in persons complaining of a dry mouth/throat sensation on awakening, fatigue, gastroesophageal reflux, impaired memory and concentration, insomnia, morning headaches, nighttime diaphoresis, or nocturia.

Physical Examination

Physical examination may reveal the presence of excess body weight (*ie*, BMI >25 kg/m^2); large neck circumference; nasal septal deviation or turbinate hypertrophy; crowded posterior pharyngeal space; enlarged tonsils and adenoids (especially in children); high, narrow hard palate; large uvula; low-lying soft palate; macroglossia; or retrognathia or micrognathia. The physical examination results may be entirely normal.

Consequences

In addition to increased mortality rates, persons with OSA are more likely to have insulin resistance; parasomnias, including sleep-related eating disorder; ischemic heart disease; and stroke. Cardiac arrhythmias are frequently encountered, the most common of which is sinus arrhythmia that consists of relative bradycardia at the onset of the apneic episode and relative tachycardia after the termination of the event. There is also an increased likelihood of recurrence of atrial fibrillation after successful cardioversion in persons with untreated OSA.

Systemic hypertension can develop when systemic BP fails to decrease during sleep ("nondipping"). OSA can further worsen heart function in persons with congestive heart failure (CHF). Pulmonary hypertension and cor pulmonale can develop in persons with severe OSA, for whom the degree of oxygen desaturation may be predictive of the risk of pulmonary hypertension. There is a greater likelihood of pulmonary hypertension in persons with daytime hypoxemia and hypercapnia, morbid obesity, and comorbid COPD. Pulmonary hypertension secondary to OSA is generally mild. Other consequences of OSA include depression and anxiety, impaired cognition (decreased alertness, executive function, learning, and memory); erectile dysfunction; gastroesophageal reflux; nocturia; driving and work-related accidents; impaired school and work performance; and greater health-care utilization.

Evaluation

Evaluation of persons suspected of having OSA should consist of a thorough clinical history as well as physical examination, with particular emphasis on the upper airway and neck circumference. Laboratory testing should be individualized; routine screening for hypothyroidism is not indicated. Polysomnography is required for the diagnosis of OSA, the current standard of practice being an attended laboratory study. The latter can either be a full-night study with separate diagnostic and positive airway pressure (PAP) titration study nights, or a split-night study consisting of an initial diagnostic portion and a subsequent PAP titration on the same night. During polysomnography, respiratory events are more frequent, last longer, and are associated with more profound oxygen desaturation during REM sleep. Paradoxical breathing may be appreciated.

Therapy

Therapy for OSA requires a multidisciplinary approach, including general measures, PAP therapy, oral devices, and/or upper-airway surgery. The avoidance of alcohol, smoking, and muscle relaxants is important, as is proper sleep hygiene and safety counseling, such as not driving whenever drowsy. Optimal weight management is crucial for persons who are overweight. Positional therapy, with the avoidance of a supine sleep position, may be considered if respiratory events occur exclusively or predominantly during supine sleep and if polysomnography demonstrates a normal AHI in the lateral or prone sleep position. Oxygen therapy is not indicated as sole therapy for OSA but may be of benefit in persons with significant hypoxemia uncontrolled by PAP therapy alone. Topical nasal corticosteroids may be used as adjunct therapy for persons with concurrent rhinitis.[2]

Modafinil or armodafinil is indicated for the management of residual excessive sleepiness despite effective PAP therapy and if there is no other known cause for sleepiness. Hormone-replacement therapy has been suggested for postmenopausal women; however, data regarding its efficacy for this indication are inconsistent.

PAP Therapy: PAP therapy is the treatment of choice for most persons with OSA.[3] PAP functions as a pneumatic splint that maintains upper-airway patency and increases nasal pressure above P_{CRIT}. Greater pressures may be required to control respiratory events during REM sleep and supine sleep. PAP therapy is indicated for persons with an AHI of at least 15 events per hour; or if the AHI is at least 5 events/h but <14 events/h if there are complaints of excessive sleepiness, impaired cognition, mood disorder or insomnia, or documented hypertension or coronary artery disease, or history of stroke.

There are several PAP modalities that are currently available, including CPAP, which provides a single constant pressure throughout the respiratory cycle. With the use of CPAP with expiratory pressure relief technology, a single pressure is provided throughout the respiratory cycle, but a transient reduction in pressure during expiration and a subsequent return of pressure to baseline setting before next inspiration is allowed. Bilevel PAP provides two pressure levels during the respiratory cycle, namely: a higher level during inspiration (*ie,* inspiration PAP), and a lower pressure during expiration (*ie*, expiration PAP). With autotitrating PAP (APAP), variable pressures are provided based on device-specific diagnostic and therapeutic algorithms; thus, this device is able to automatically and continuously adjust delivered PAP to maintain upper-airway patency.[4] Adaptive servoventilation delivers pressure support (inspiration PAP minus expiration) that increases during periods of hypoventilation and decreases during hyperventilation. Finally, nocturnal noninvasive positive pressure ventilation provides two pressure levels at a set rate to assist ventilation.

Several methods have been developed to help determine a single optimal CPAP pressure for subsequent nightly use by the patient at home. A full-night attended laboratory polysomnography remains the preferred method, but a split-night polysomnography (*ie*, an initial diagnostic and subsequent PAP titration portions on the same night) is frequently used. Finally, titration using an APAP device is increasing in popularity, but there remains minimal data regarding its efficacy and applicability across different population groups.

PAP therapy has been shown to decrease mortality, reduce sleepiness (both subjective and objective), decrease or eliminate snoring, normalize AHI, and improve Sao_2. It also improves driving simulator steering performance, BP control, and left ventricular function in persons with CHF. Health-care utilization declines after initiation of PAP therapy. However, there have been inconsistent or inconclusive data on any benefits to sleep quality, quality of life, neurocognitive function, and mood. Persons initiating PAP therapy may experience nasal congestion, dryness, epistaxis, or rhinorrhea; sinus discomfort or pain; facial skin irritation, rash or abrasion; eye irritation; gastric distention as the result of aerophagia; or chest discomfort and tightness, many of which may result in the patient discontinuing therapy.

Adherence to PAP therapy should be monitored objectively. Most studies report an objective compliance (*ie*, use for >4 h per night for 70% of nights) of 50 to 80%, with an average nightly use of just 5 h. Only patient education and the use of heated humidification have been consistently demonstrated to enhance PAP adherence. Factors predicting the need for heated humidification include the following: (1) age >60 years, (2) use of drying medications, (3) presence of chronic mucosal disease, and (4) a history of uvulopalatopharyngoplasty. Other approaches that have been recom-mended to help improve a patient's adherence to PAP, such as the use of bilevel PAP, CPAP with expiratory pressure relief technology and ramping mechanism, and changing a poorly fitting nasal mask after therapy has started, have shown inconsistent benefits.

Bilevel PAP therapy may be considered for persons who complain of excessively high pressures with significant difficulty breathing out against these pressures, or of gastric distention caused by aerophagia. It may also be beneficial for persons with comorbid obstructive or restrictive lung disease, hypoventilation syndrome, or with persistent oxygen desaturation despite CPAP therapy.

APAP devices have been used for PAP titration to identify a single fixed pressure for subsequent treatment with a conventional CPAP device (this is not recommended for split-night PAP titration) or PAP treatment when used in a self-adjusting mode for nightly therapy of OSA. APAP devices are contraindicated for persons with CHF, significant respiratory disease (*eg*, COPD), daytime hypoxemia and respiratory failure, and nocturnal oxygen desaturation unrelated to OSA, such as in cases of obesity-hypoventilation syndrome.

Compared with conventional CPAP, there are no significant differences with APAP in reductions of AHI and arousal indexes, changes in sleep architecture, Sao_2 levels, or subsequent CPAP acceptance. Mean airway pressure tends to be lower and peak airway pressure tends to be greater (as the result of air leaks) with APAP compared with CPAP. Proper mask fitting is crucial before the patient uses APAP unattended. Finally, noninvasive positive pressure ventilation is indicated for cases of persistent sleep-related hypoventilation and CO_2 retention.

Oral Devices: Oral devices are effective therapies for selected persons with snoring, mild-to-moderate OSA, and severe OSA (in some). There are two general types of oral devices: mandibular repositioners, which displace the mandible and tongue anteriorly and are the most commonly used oral devices; and tongue-retaining devices which, by securing the tongue in a soft bulb located anterior to the teeth, hold the tongue in an anterior position.[5] Tongue-retaining devices are preferred for edentulous persons or for those with compromised dentition. As a class, oral devices have a reported efficacy of 40 to 80%. Compliance is greater than with PAP devices and ranges from 50 to 80%. A follow-up polysomnography is indicated after optimal fit has been attained. In addition, periodic assessments by a dentist and sleep physician are recommended to ensure continued effectiveness.

Contraindications to the use of oral devices include an inability to breathe nasally and sleep apnea that is primarily central in nature. The devices generally are not recommended for growing children. In addition, mandibular repositioners should not be used in persons with inadequate or compromised dentition or in those with significant temporomandibular joint dysfunction. Complications associated with the use of oral devices consist of a dry mouth sensation or excessive salivation, dental pain, undesirable dental movements with mandibular repositioners, and jaw or temporomandibular joint pain with mandibular repositioners.

Upper-Airway Surgery: Upper-airway surgery may be considered for persons with definitive craniofacial or upper-airway abnormalities that are responsible for OSA. Polysomnography is required after upper-airway surgery to determine therapeutic efficacy, and patients require long-term follow-up. Several types of upper-airway surgical procedures have been developed to address specific upper-airway abnormalities, including tonsillectomy and adenoidectomy, which are commonly used to treat childhood cases of OSA. Nasal septoplasty, polyp removal, and turbinectomy are used to increase the dimensions of the nasal airway. Uvulopalatopharyngoplasty increases the size of the retropalatal airspace, whereas genioglossal advancement, hyoid myotomy and suspension, and mandibular advancement enlarge the retrolingual airway. Uvulopalatopharyngoglossoplasty and maxillomandibular advancement increase the retrolingual, retropalatal, and transpalatal airway. Finally, tracheotomy can be used to bypass the narrow upper airway and is the only surgical procedure that is consistently effective as a sole procedure for OSA. In addition to tracheotomy, the most effective surgical procedures for the therapy of OSA are bariatric surgery for weight management and maxillomandibular advancement.

Medicolegal Considerations

Sleepy persons with OSA are at increased risk of car accidents; the risk is increased further with concurrent alcohol ingestion. A history of near-miss accidents predicts future risk of car accidents. Effective therapy of OSA decreases this risk. Patients with OSA should be instructed to avoid driving whenever drowsy. Adherence to PAP therapy must be assessed objectively in all patients, and periodic follow-up to identify adverse effects is recommended. A multiple sleep latency test should be considered whenever there is doubt about a person's degree of sleepiness. Modafinil and armodafinil, wake-promoting agents, may benefit persons who are excessively sleepy despite PAP therapy. Consider reporting patients with excessive sleepiness as the result of OSA to appropriate authorities if (1) there is a history of severe car accidents related to untreated sleepiness; (2) if prompt therapy for OSA cannot be provided; (3) if the patient refuses, or is consistently nonadherent with, therapy for OSA; (4) if the patient fails to restrict driving until OSA has been adequately controlled; or (5) if such situations are considered reportable based on local legislation.

Upper-Airway Resistance Syndrome

This syndrome is characterized by repetitive sleep-related episodes of decreased inspiratory airflow attributable to increasing upper-airway resistance accompanied by increased or constant respiratory effort and arousals from sleep.[6] Upper-airway resistance syndrome should be excluded in persons with unexplained sleepiness. Polysomnography demonstrates an AHI that is <5 events/h. With esophageal pressure monitoring, increasingly negative esophageal pressure excursions precede arousals and are followed by less negative esophageal pressure excursions as airflow increases during arousals. Nasal pressure monitoring demonstrates inspiratory flattening followed by a rounded contour during arousals.

Snoring

Risk factors for snoring include obesity; supine sleep position; nasal obstruction; medications, such as muscle relaxants, opioids or benzodiazepines; and alcohol use. Snoring is often loudest during stage N3 sleep and diminishes during REM sleep. OSA is present in an estimated 25 to 95% of snorers.

Central Sleep Apnea

Central sleep apnea (CSA) refers to repetitive cessation of airflow during sleep caused by the loss of ventilatory effort. Persons with CSA may present with insomnia or sleepiness or may be asymptomatic.[7]

Polysomnography

Polysomnography is necessary for the diagnosis of CSA and demonstrates cessation of respiration and ventilatory effort lasting at least 10 s, with at least five central apneas per hour of sleep. Respiratory events are most common during sleep onset and N1/N2 sleep. There is an absence of chest and abdominal movement. No respiratory muscle activity is present in diaphragmatic EMG, and no changes in pressure are noted in esophageal pressure monitoring.

Classification

CSA can be classified as either hypercapnic or nonhypercapnic. Hypercapnic CSA is characterized by high sleep $Paco_2$ and is often associated with high waking $Paco_2$. Persons with the hypercapnic form of CSA have decreased ventilatory responsiveness to hypercapnia. Causes of hypercapnic CSA include neuromuscular disorders and long-term use of long-acting opioids. Persons with nonhypercapnic CSA have normal or low waking $Paco_2$ and an increased ventilatory response to hypercapnia. In nonhypercapnic CSA, brief arousals during sleep trigger a hyperventilatory "overshoot" that lowers $Paco_2$ to less than its apneic threshold. Causes of nonhypercapnic CSA include idiopathic CSA, sleep-onset CSA, CSA caused by CHF, high-altitude periodic breathing, and complex sleep apnea (see the subheading "Complex Sleep Apnea" to follow).

Idiopathic CSA: The etiology of this rare condition is unknown. It affects men more commonly than women, and its prevalence is greatest in middle-aged and older adults.

Cheyne-Stokes Respiration (CSR): Periodic breathing in CSR consists of recurring periods of crescendo--decrescendo ventilation separated by central apneas or hypopneas. Periodic breathing develops during NREM sleep and improves or resolves during REM sleep. CSR may develop in persons with CHF or stroke. Risk factors for CSR in CHF include male gender, age >60 years, atrial fibrillation, and hypocapnia. There are several important differences between CSA and CSR. With CSA, the nadir of oxygen desaturation often follows the termination of apnea, arousals occur at the termination of apnea, cycle time is shorter (generally <45 s), and the period of hyperpnea is shorter. In contrast, CSR is associated with a more delayed nadir of oxygen desaturation, longer cycle time (>45 s), and longer period of hyperpnea. In addition, arousals associated with CSR commonly occur at the peak of hyperpnea.

High-Altitude Periodic Breathing: Cycles of central apneas and hyperpneas can develop on ascent to high altitude, usually at elevations $>4{,}000$ to 7,600 m. The likelihood of high-altitude periodic breathing is greater in persons with greater hypoxic ventilatory drive, at greater elevations, after faster speed of ascent, and among men. Central apneas occur primarily during NREM sleep, with respiratory patterns improving during REM sleep.

Medication-Induced CSA: CSA can develop during administration of long-acting opioids, such as methadone, as the result of depression of the hypercapnic respiratory drive.

CSA Caused by CHF: CSA or CSR can develop in persons with CHF, the prevalence and severity of which are correlated with left ventricular function. The rate of mortality is greater in CHF patients with CSR than in those without CSR.

Sleep-Onset CSA: Central apneas may occur if $Paco_2$ (greater during sleep and lower during wakefulness) fluctuates above or below the apneic threshold. This sleep-onset CSA is generally transient and resolves as sleep progresses.

Complex Sleep Apnea: Complex sleep apnea is defined as the development of CSA or CSR during acute application of CPAP in patients with predominantly OSA at baseline. This phenomenon occurs in an estimated 15% of persons with OSA titrated with CPAP.

Therapy for CSA

It is important to treat any known underlying cause of CSA, such as heart failure. Respiratory depressants should be avoided in persons with hypercapnic CSA. High-altitude periodic breathing may improve with oxygen therapy or after descent to lower altitudes. Effective pharmacologic therapies for CSA include acetazolamide for high-altitude periodic breathing and hypnotic agents for sleep-onset central apneas. Many persons with CSA benefit from PAP therapy. CPAP or bilevel PAP may be tried for patients with CSA or CSR attributable to CHF; this type of therapy might improve cardiac function but may have no benefit on mortality, making close monitoring of therapeutic efficacy crucial. Adaptive servo ventilation has been developed to manage persons with complex sleep apnea. Finally, nocturnal noninvasive ventilation may be considered for those with hypercapnic forms of CSA.

Hypoventilation Syndromes

The main features of sleep-related hypoventilation syndromes are oxygen desaturation and increased $Paco_2$ during sleep, with $Paco_2$ either >45 mm Hg or <45 mm Hg but abnormally increased relative to waking levels. Waking arterial blood gas levels may be normal or abnormal.

Several mechanisms may be responsible for hypoventilation developing during sleep, including a decrease in minute ventilation and/or tidal volume, abnormal ventilation/perfusion relationships, or changes in ventilatory chemosensitivity and respiratory load responsiveness. Therapy generally involves treating any underlying disorder/s and, if necessary, ventilatory assistance during sleep.

Congenital Central Alveolar Hypoventilation Syndrome

Failure of automatic control of breathing in this syndrome results in hypoxemia and hypercapnia. There is diminished responsiveness of central and peripheral chemoreceptors to hypoxemia and hypercapnia. Onset is usually in infancy. Hypoventilation is worse during sleep than wakefulness; during sleep, hypoventilation is more severe during NREM sleep than REM sleep. Congenital central alveolar hypoventilation syndrome may be associated with autonomic dysfunction, Hirschsprung disease and neural crest tumors. Many cases of congenital central alveolar hypoventilation syndrome involve *de novo* mutations in the *PHOX2B* gene.[8]

References

1. Olson EJ, Park JG, Morgenthaler TI. Obstructive sleep apnea-hypopnea syndrome. Prim Care 2005; 32:329–359
2. Morgenthaler TI, Kapen S, Lee-Chiong T, et al. Practice parameters for the medical therapy of obstructive sleep apnea. Sleep 2006; 29:1031–1035
3. Kushida CA, Littner MR, Hirshkowitz M, et al. Practice parameters for the use of continuous and bilevel positive airway pressure devices to treat adult patients with sleep-related breathing disorders. Sleep 2006; 29:375–380
4. Morgenthaler TI, Aurora RN, Brown T, et al. Standards of Practice Committee of the AASM. Practice parameters for the use of autotitrating continuous positive airway pressure devices for titrating pressures and treating adult patients with obstructive sleep apnea syndrome: An update for 2007. Sleep 2008; 31:141–147
5. Kushida CA, Morgenthaler TI, Littner MR, et al. Practice parameters for the treatment of snoring and obstructive sleep apnea with oral appliances: an Update for 2005. Sleep 2006; 29:240–243
6. Badr MS. Central sleep apnea. Prim Care 2005; 32:361–74
7. Bao G, Guilleminault C. Upper airway resistance syndrome—one decade later. Curr Opin Pulm Med 2004; 10:461–467
8. Amiel J, Laudier B, Attie-Bitach T, et al. Polyalanine expansion and frameshift mutations of the paired-like homeobox gene PHOX2B in congenital central hypoventilation syndrome. Nat Genet 2003; 33:459–461

Notes

Nonrespiratory Sleep Disorders

Teofilo L. Lee-Chiong, Jr., MD, FCCP

Objectives:

- Describe the different causes of insomnia and excessive sleepiness and the treatment options for each disorder
- Identify the key features of the various parasomnias
- Understand the clinical manifestations of restless legs syndrome
- Distinguish the main presenting symptoms of the different circadian rhythm sleep disorders

Key words: circadian rhythm sleep disorders; insomnia; narcolepsy; parasomnias; restless legs syndrome; sleepiness

The differential diagnoses of excessive sleepiness is extensive and include the following: (1) narcolepsy; (2) idiopathic hypersomnia; (3) circadian rhythm sleep disorders; (4) insufficient sleep syndrome; (5) obstructive sleep apnea (OSA); (6) periodic limb movement disorder (PLMD); (7) posttraumatic hypersomnia (head injury); (8) recurrent hypersomnia, including Kleine Levin syndrome; (9) medical, neurologic and psychiatric disorders; and (10) medication or substance use or withdrawal. Transient insomnia can be a result of the following: (1) acute stressors, (2) jet lag, (3) acute medication and substance use, and (4) shift work. Chronic insomnia can either present as sleep-onset sleep disturbance, sleep maintenance insomnia, or early morning awakenings. Causes of sleep-onset insomnia consist of the following: (1) idiopathic insomnia; (2) psychophysiologic insomnia; (3) restless legs syndrome (RLS); (4) delayed sleep phase disorder; (5) psychiatric disorders, such as anxiety, mood disorder, or posttraumatic stress disorder; (6) paradoxical insomnia; or (7) use of stimulants. Sleep-maintenance insomnia can result from the following: (1) alcohol withdrawal; (2) medical, neurologic and psychiatric disorders, such as asthma, COPD, congestive heart failure (CHF), and mood and panic disorders; (3) primary sleep disorders, including OSA and central sleep apnea (CSA), PLMD, psychophysiologic insomnia, and parasomnias; and (4) medication or substance use. Early morning awakenings can be caused by advanced sleep phase disorder, depression, or withdrawal from short-acting hypnotic agents. There are many causes of nocturnal oxygen desaturation, including OSA, CSA, asthma, COPD, alveolar hypoventilation syndromes, diaphragm paralysis, neuromuscular disorders, restrictive lung disease, CHF, and high altitude.

Insomnia

Insomnia is characterized by repeated difficulty with either falling or staying asleep that is associated with impairment of daytime function.[1] Sleep disturbance can present as difficulty falling asleep (sleep-onset insomnia), frequent or prolonged awakenings (sleep-maintenance insomnia), final morning awakening that is earlier than desired (terminal insomnia), and unrefreshed feeling on awakening (nonrestorative sleep). Polysomnographically, insomnia can be defined as prolonged sleep-onset latency (SOL), >30 min; increased wake time after sleep onset, >30 min; reduced sleep efficiency, <85%; and diminished total sleep time, <6 to 6.5 h.

Demographics

Insomnia is the most common sleep disorder, with 30 to 50% of adults complaining of occasional insomnia and 10 to 30% of adults describing chronic insomnia. Women are affected more frequently than men.

Risk Factors

Risk factors for insomnia include the following: (1) female sex; (2) advancing age; (3) lower socioeconomic status or unemployment; (4) marital status, either divorced or widowed; (5) poor health status and physical disability; and (6) medical, neurologic, and psychiatric disorders (*eg*, respiratory disorders).

Consequences

Persons with insomnia have an increased risk of psychiatric illness developing, such as major depression. Other consequences of insomnia include fatigue, cognitive impairment, impaired academic and occupational performance, diminished quality of life, and greater health-care utilization.

Classification

Forms of insomnia can be classified, based on duration of sleep disturbance, as transient if the insomnia lasts only a few days, or chronic if it persists > 1 to 3 months. Another useful distinction classifies the causes of sleep disturbance into primary or comorbid insomnia. Primary (idiopathic) insomnia includes idiopathic insomnia, paradoxical insomnia, and psychophysiologic insomnia.

Adjustment Insomnia

In this syndrome, sleep disturbance is a result of an identifiable acute stressor, such as a momentous life event, change in the sleep environment, or an acute illness. Sleep improves with resolution of acute stressor or when adaptation to the stressor develops.

Idiopathic Insomnia

This type of insomnia is not associated with any identifiable etiology. It has its onset during infancy or early childhood, and its course is generally chronic and life-long.

Inadequate Sleep Hygiene

Poor sleep hygiene consists of activities or behavior that increase arousal or decrease sleep propensity and that are primarily responsible for sleep disturbance. These activities and behavior are under a person's control and can be eliminated if the person desires to do so.

Paradoxical Insomnia

Also known as *sleep-state misperception,* persons report very minimal or no sleep during most nights, but polysomnography generally demonstrates normal sleep quality and architecture. Likewise, there is no daytime napping or impairment of daytime functioning.

Psychophysiologic Insomnia

Sleep disturbance is secondary to heightened cognitive and somatic arousal at bedtime. Causes consist of rumination and intrusive thoughts, increased agitation and muscle tone, and learned maladaptive sleep-preventing behavior, such as excessive anxiety about the inability to sleep. Conditioned arousal is typically limited to a person's own bed and bedroom, with better sleep being described when attempted in another room. Onset of sleep disturbance is generally during adolescence or early adulthood. Unlike generalized anxiety disorder, anxiety is limited to issues related to sleep in psychophysiologic insomnia.

Common Medications That Can Cause Insomnia

Many medications can cause insomnia; the most common include antidepressants such as fluoxetine or protriptyline, β-adrenergic blocking antihypertensive agents, bronchodilators, decongestants, corticosteroids, and stimulant agents.

Evaluation

The evaluation of insomnia relies primarily on a compatible history and sleep diary. Psychometric tests, including validated measures for depression and anxiety, may be considered for selected patients. Polysomnography, actigraphy, and laboratory tests are not routinely indicated; nevertheless, polysomnography may be helpful in person with suspected OSA, PLMD, or paradoxical insomnia.

Cognitive-Behavioral Therapy

In addition to instructions regarding proper sleep hygiene, persons with insomnia often benefit from cognitive-behavioral treatments (CBTs); short-term benefits of these interventions are comparable with pharmacologic therapy and, unlike the latter, beneficial effects are sustained over time. At long-term follow-up, CBT is more effective than pharmacotherapy. Effective CBT techniques consist of cognitive therapy, paradoxical intention, relaxation techniques, sleep restriction, and stimulus control.[2,3]

Cognitive therapy addresses dysfunctional beliefs accompanying insomnia, identifies irrational expectations and excessive worry related to the inability to sleep, challenges unrealistic concerns about poor sleep, and provides a more appropriate understanding of insomnia and its accompanying daytime impairment.

Paradoxical intention is designed to decrease performance anxieties related to efforts to fall asleep. Patients are instructed to go to bed and try to stay awake as long as they can. Relaxation techniques address both somatic and cognitive hyperarousal and reduce them by progressive muscle relaxation (*ie*, sequential tensing and relaxing of various muscle groups), biofeedback, or guided imagery.

With sleep restriction, time spent awake in bed is reduced to enhance homeostatic sleep drive, and time in bed is subsequently increased once sleep efficiency improves. In this technique, bedtime is advanced or delayed based on calculated sleep efficiency. An earlier bedtime is allowed if sleep efficiency is >90%. In contrast, bedtime is delayed if sleep efficiency is <80%. No change in bedtime is required if sleep efficiency is 80 to 90%. Patients are instructed to wake up at the same time each morning, and no daytime napping is permitted.

Stimulus control strengthens the association of bedroom and bedtime to a conditioned response for sleep. Patients are instructed to use the bed only for sleep or sex, lie down to sleep only when sleepy, get out of bed and go to another room if unable to fall asleep, engage in a restful activity, and return to bed only when sleepy.

Pharmacotherapy

Hypnotic agents may enhance sleep but often do not improve daytime performance. In addition, there is minimal long-term beneficial effects on sleep after drug discontinuation. Benzodiazepines and nonbenzodiazepine benzodiazepine receptor agonists are effective hypnotic agents. There is insufficient evidence regarding the efficacy of sedating antidepressants, sedating antipsychotic agents, antihistamines, and botanical compounds for the therapy of insomnia.

Hypnotic agents are indicated for the treatment of transient sleep disruption (*eg*, jet lag or adjustment sleep disorder), chronic primary insomnia that fails to respond to cognitive behavioral therapy, and chronic comorbid insomnia that does not improve with treatment of the underlying condition and cognitive behavioral therapy. Hypnotic agents can be classified based on elimination half-lives into short acting (<1 h; ramelteon, zaleplon); intermediate acting (2 to 5 h); eszopiclone, triazolam, and zolpidem; long acting (5 to 24 h; estazolam and temazepam); and extra-long acting (>40 h; flurazepam and quazepam). Short-acting agents are usually used for sleep-onset insomnia, intermediate-acting agents for concurrent sleep-onset and sleep-maintenance insomnia, and long-acting and extra-long-acting agents for early morning awakenings and daytime anxiety.

Benzodiazepine receptor agonists bind to the gamma-aminobutyric acid-benzodiazepine (GABA-BZ) receptor complex. Various GABA-BZ receptor subunits have different actions, namely BZ1 (hypnotic and amnesic actions) and BZ2 and BZ3 (muscle relaxation, antiseizure and antianxiety actions). Benzodiazepines bind nonselectively to the different GABA-BZ receptor subunits, BZ1, BZ2, and BZ3 and, thus, possess hypnotic, anxiolytic, myorelaxant, and anticonvulsant properties.

Many adverse effects are associated with the use of benzodiazepines, including (1) rebound daytime anxiety, especially with short-acting agents; (2) residual daytime sleepiness with long-acting agents; (3) cognitive and psychomotor impairment; (4) development of tolerance defined as the need for increasingly higher dosages to attain similar therapeutic benefit during chronic use; (5) withdrawal symptoms, such as anxiety, irritability and restlessness; (6) rebound insomnia; (7) respiratory depression and worsening of OSA; (8) increase risk of falls, particularly in some older adults; and (9) dependency and abuse liability (low risk). Benzodiazepines are contraindicated during pregnancy or lactation; in persons with significant renal or hepatic impairment, in whom dosage adjustments are required; in cases of untreated OSA; and in persons with severe obstructive and restrictive ventilatory impairment.

The nonbenzodiazepine benzodiazepine receptor agonists selectively bind to the BZ1 receptor subunit. Duration of action varies, with zaleplon having the shortest, zolpidem having an intermediate effect, and esopiclone having the longest duration of action. Compared with conventional benzodiazepines, this class of agents have a similar hypnotic action; possess no muscle relaxant, anticonvulsant, or anxiolytic properties; and are less likely to cause rebound insomnia, withdrawal symptoms or tolerance, or to alter sleep architecture.

Ramelteon is a melatonin receptor agonist with selectivity for the suprachiasmatic nucleus melatonin receptor. Because of its short half-life, it is primarily used for persons with sleep-onset insomnia. Ramelteon should not be used in persons on fluvoxamine therapy or those with hepatic impairment.

Other hypnotic agents include trazodone, tricyclic antidepressants, first-generation histamine antagonists, and melatonin. Trazodone is widely popular because of its lack of significant potential for tolerance or dependency; adverse effects associated with trazodone use consist of cardiac arrhythmias, orthostatic hypotension, and priapism. Tricyclic antidepressants also have numerous adverse effects, such as urinary retention, constipation, cardiac arrhythmias, orthostatic hypotension, and exacerbation of restless legs and periodic limb movements during sleep. The first-generation histamine antagonists, including diphenhydramine, constitute the majority of over-the-counter hypnotic agents. Adverse effects of first-generation histamine antagonists consist of rapid development of tolerance; residual daytime sedation as the result of long half-life; and anticholinergic effects (*eg*, confusion, delirium, dry mouth, and urinary retention). Melatonin is used primarily for insomnia associated with circadian rhythm sleep disorders. Melatonin has a short half-life of 20 to 30 min.

Excessive Sleepiness

Excessive daytime sleepiness (EDS) describes an inability to consistently achieve and sustain wakefulness and alertness to accomplish the tasks of daily living. Manifestations of EDS include frequent napping, sleep attacks, microsleep episodes, hyperactivity in children, and automatic behavior. Consequences of EDS consist of greater risk of accidents, impaired work and academic performance, and mood disorder. Disorders that can cause excessive sleepiness include narcolepsy, insufficient sleep syndrome, idiopathic hypersomnia, and recurrent hypersomnia. Sleepiness can also be caused by a variety of medical disorders or by drugs or substance use.[3,4]

Narcolepsy

Narcolepsy is a neurologic disorder characterized by the clinical tetrad of excessive sleepiness, cataplexy, sleep paralysis, and sleep hallucinations. However, only 10 to 15% of patients demonstrate this full tetrad. Excessive sleepiness is the first, primary, and most disabling symptom of narcolepsy. It can manifest as brief naps, each lasting about 10 to 20 min, that occur repeatedly throughout the day. Sleepiness transiently improves after naps. Sleep attacks can also occur.

Cataplexy consists of transient episodes of muscle atonia/hypotonia that are precipitated by intense emotion, such as laughter, anger, or excitement. There is sparing of respiratory and oculomotor muscles, and memory and consciousness are unaffected. Cataplexy is the only pathognomonic symptom of narcolepsy.

Patients with narcolepsy may experience sleep hallucinations that may be visual, auditory, tactile or kinetic, occurring at sleep onset (hypnagogic), or occurring on awakening (hypnopompic). Sleep hallucinations may be accompanied by sleep paralysis, which could also be either hypnagogic, hypnopompic, or both. Sleep paralysis generally lasts a few seconds or minutes, affects voluntary muscles, and spares the respiratory, oculomotor and sphincter muscles. Sensorium is unaffected. Sleep disturbance, manifesting as repetitive arousals and awakenings, are common in persons with narcolepsy who may complain of sleep-maintenance insomnia.

Other clinical features of narcolepsy are memory impairment, automatic behavior, and hyperactivity and learning disability (in children). Patients with narcolepsy have an increased risk of OSA and CSA, periodic limb movements during sleep, REM sleep behavior disorder, and depression.

Narcolepsy affects approximately 0.05% of the US population. It may affect men more commonly than women. Excessive sleepiness is usually the presenting symptom, with onset generally from 15 to 25 years of age. Clinical course is chronic with persistent sleepiness; the severity of cataplexy may decrease over time. Narcolepsy is believed to result from loss of hypothalamic hypocretin neurons; other pathogenetic mechanisms include defective cholinergic system regulating REM sleep and impairment of norepinephrine and dopamine systems.

Narcolepsy can also present without cataplexy. In this syndrome, cataplexy-like symptoms, such as prolonged episodes of tiredness or muscle weakness associated with atypical triggers, may be present. Narcolepsy without cataplexy accounts for 10 to 50% of cases of narcolepsy.

Narcolepsy with cataplexy can be diagnosed by history alone. Polysomnography followed by multiple sleep latency testing is required if cataplexy is absent, atypical, or equivocal. Polysomnography generally demonstrates a shortened SOL of ≤10 min, sleep-onset REM periods (SOREMPs) of ≤20 min in 25 to 50% of cases, and repetitive awakenings.

The multiple sleep latency test typically shows a mean SOL of ≤8 min and at least two SOREMPs. The combination of a shortened SOL and SOREMPs is present in 60 to 85% of cases of narcolepsy. The maintenance of wakefulness test may be used to monitor treatment response to stimulant medications used for excessive sleepiness.

Levels of cerebrospinal fluid hypocretin-1 are ≤110 pg/mL or less than one third of mean normal control values in persons with narcolepsy with cataplexy. Levels of cerebrospinal fluid hypocretin-1 are normal in many persons with narcolepsy without cataplexy. Human leukocyte antigen typing has limited diagnostic utility.

Every person with narcolepsy should be instructed on proper sleep hygiene, including maintaining regular sleep-wake schedules, obtaining sufficient nocturnal sleep duration, taking scheduled naps during the day, and avoiding driving until sleepiness is adequately managed. Excessive sleepiness can be managed pharmacologically with modafinil, armodafinil, dextroamphetamine, or methylphenidate. Sleep disturbance often improves with the use of hypnotic agents or γ-hydroxybutyrate (sodium oxybate). REM sleep-suppressant agents, such as serotonin reuptake inhibitors, tricyclic antidepressants, venlafaxine, and monoamine oxidase inhibitors, as well as γ-hydroxybutyrate, can be used to reduce attacks of cataplexy.

Insufficient Sleep Syndrome

Insufficient sleep is the most common cause of sleepiness in many industrialized countries, including the United States. In this syndrome, sleepiness is caused primarily by chronic voluntary, but unintentional, sleep deprivation or sleep restriction. Sleepiness generally improves with sleep extension, as is frequently noted during "sleep-ins" on weekends or holidays. Diagnosis is based on clinical history and sleep diaries, and polysomnography is not indicated. Therapy consists of sleep extension.

Idiopathic Hypersomnia

Persons with idiopathic hypersomnia complain of constant sleepiness despite sufficient, or even increased, amounts of nighttime sleep. They often describe frequent daytime napping which, unlike narcolepsy, are longer and less refreshing. Etiology for the sleepiness is unknown. Cataplexy is absent. Diagnosis requires polysomnography and Multiple Sleep Latency Test, the latter showing a shortened SOL and less than two SOREMPs. Cerebrospinal fluid hypocretin-1 levels are normal. Therapy includes sleep hygiene and stimulant agents.

Recurrent Hypersomnia

Both Kleine-Levin syndrome and menstrual-related sleep disorder can present as recurrent episodes of hypersomnia occurring weeks or months apart, with sleep and alertness normalizing between episodes. Kleine-Levin syndrome is characterized by sleepiness, hyperphagia, hypersexuality, aggressive behavior, and cognitive impairment. Cases mostly involve men. Etiology is unknown.

Hypersomnia Caused by Medical Disorders

Many medical disorders can give rise to excessive sleepiness, including hepatic encephalopathy, hypothyroidism, Prader-Willi syndrome, renal failure, CNS infections or tumors, head trauma, Parkinson disease, stroke, atypical depression, bipolar type II mood disorder, and seasonal affective disorder.

Hypersomnia Caused by Drugs or Substances

Excessive sleepiness may develop during use or abuse of sedative-hypnotic agents or after withdrawal from stimulants.

Evaluation of Sleepiness

Excessive sleepiness is often diagnosed with a comprehensive sleep history aided by sleep diaries and/or actigraphy. Subjective tests of sleepiness, such as the Epworth sleepiness scale, are commonly used. Polysomnography is necessary to exclude OSA and PLMD. Multiple sleep latency testing generally demonstrates a mean SOL of <8 min, and the Maintenance of Wakefulness Test may show a mean SOL of <40 min.

Therapy for Sleepiness

Sleep extension should be recommended for suspected insufficient sleep syndrome. Scheduled napping may be beneficial for some patients, as is caffeine intake, which has additive effects to napping. Many patients, especially those with moderate-to-severe sleepiness, will require stimulant agents.

Parasomnias

Parasomnias are physical or experiential phenomena that occur during sleep. They consist of activation of skeletal muscles or the autonomic nervous system. Parasomnias can occur primarily during non-REM (NREM) sleep, during REM sleep, or occur randomly throughout the sleep period. Parasomnias occurring during NREM sleep (*ie*, disorders of arousal) include confusional arousals, sleep terrors, and sleepwalking. Parasomnias occurring during REM sleep include nightmares and REM sleep behavior disorder.

NREM Parasomnias

The disorders of arousal occur predominantly during N3 sleep and mostly in the first third of the night. They are most commonly encountered in children, and cases generally resolve by adolescence. Risk factors for NREM parasomnias include sleep deprivation, OSA, and PLMD. They often respond to either proper sleep hygiene, such as avoidance of sleep deprivation, and scheduled awakenings. A trial of low-dose benzodiazepines may be considered for intractable cases.[5]

Confusional Arousals: In this disorder, episodes of confusion follow arousals from sleep, accompanied by inappropriate behavior, amnesia, inconsolability, and diminished responsiveness to external stimuli. There is minimal fear or autonomic hyperactivity. Most episodes last from 5 to 15 min.

Sleepwalking: Ambulation during sleep may be precipitated by sleep deprivation (which is the most important risk factor), febrile states, or OSA. If ambulation is significantly disruptive of the individual's sleep or if sleepwalking is potentially injurious, therapy, such as avoidance of sleep deprivation, scheduled awakenings, and medications (eg, low-dose benzodiazepines) can be tried.

Sleep Terrors: Sleep terrors consist of abrupt awakenings with profound fear and intense autonomic discharge, such as tachycardia, tachypnea, sweating, and mydriasis. Vocalization, including talking or screaming, may accompany frenzied activity and ambulation. Therapy is similar to that for sleepwalking.

REM Parasomnias

REM parasomnias tend to occur during the second half of the sleep period. Episodes are characterized by full alertness after awakening, good dream recall, and minimal tachycardia or tachypnea.[6]

Nightmare Disorder: Nightmares are unpleasant and frightening dreams that can suddenly awaken a person from sleep, followed by a delayed return to sleep. Nightmares can be precipitated by OSA, febrile illness, medications, or alcohol ingestion.

Medications that can cause nightmares include amphetamines, antidepressants, and β-blockers.

REM Sleep Behavior Disorder: REM sleep behavior disorder consists of abnormal "dream-enacting" behavior occurring during REM sleep accompanied by loss of REM-related muscle atonia. Men are affected more commonly than women, and prevalence is greatest in adults >50 years of age. Its course is chronic and progressive. REM sleep behavior disorder can result in injuries to the patient or bed partner. It often responds favorably to low-dose clonazepam at bedtime. Environmental precautions are essential to minimize injury.

Other Parasomnias

Catathrenia is characterized by expiratory groaning during sleep, particularly REM sleep. Hoarseness can be present on waking. Episodes are not associated with respiratory distress, oxygen desaturation, or cardiac arrhythmias, and an upper-airway examination is generally normal as is sleep architecture.

Persons experiencing exploding head syndrome may describe an awakening with a loud sound or sensation of explosion in the head. Exploding head syndrome may be a variant of sleep starts. Women are affected more commonly than men. Events are not associated with pain or neurologic complications.

In sleep enuresis, recurrent involuntary voiding may occur during sleep. Enuresis can be classified as either primary or secondary. Primary sleep enuresis affects a child <5 years of age who has never been consistently dry during sleep for 6 consecutive months. Secondary enuresis is present when the child or adult, who had previously been dry, begins bedwetting again. Risk factors for secondary sleep enuresis include CHF, diabetes, OSA, seizures, use of diuretics, and urinary tract infection or disease. Structural urinary tract pathology should be suspected if daytime enuresis is also present, if there are abnormalities in the initiation of urination, or if urinary flow is abnormal. Evaluation of sleep enuresis commonly consists of a urinalysis and urine culture. Urologic evaluation may be considered for intractable cases or if structural abnormalities are suspected.

Sleep-related eating disorder should be considered if a person presents with complaints of repetitive bouts of eating or drinking during arousals from sleep. There is often a lack of awareness of the abnormal behavior, with total or partial amnesia. Risk factors include OSA, sleepwalking, and medication use (*eg*, zolpidem).

RLS

Persons with RLS may describe an urge to move, or unpleasant sensations, in the legs (less commonly the arms) that (1) begin or worsen during periods of rest or inactivity; (2) are relieved transiently by movement; and (3) are worse, or occur only, at night.[7] RLS affects an estimated 3 to 15% of the general population, and prevalence is greater in those with anemia or uremia, during pregnancy, and with aging. Women are more commonly affected, as are middle-aged and older adults. Its course is chronic. An estimated 70 to 90% of persons have periodic limb movements during sleep; conversely, one third of persons with periodic limb movements during sleep have RLS.

Risk factors for RLS include the following: (1) iron deficiency anemia; (2) uremia; (3) pregnancy; (4) Parkinson disease; (5) diabetes mellitus; (6) alcohol or caffeine ingestion; (7) smoking; and (8) medication use (*eg*, selective serotonin reuptake inhibitors, tricyclic antidepressants, monoamine oxidase inhibitors, lithium, antihistamines, neuroleptics, and dopamine antagonists). RLS can give rise to either sleep-onset and sleep-maintenance insomnia or sleepiness caused by sleep fragmentation.

The diagnosis of RLS is usually arrived at by clinical history. Laboratory evaluation (CBC count, serum iron, ferritin, folate, electrolytes, thyroid function tests, fasting glucose, and renal panel) are recommended to exclude secondary causes of the disorder. Polysomnography is not routinely indicated; however, if performed, it often demonstrates a delayed SOL, diminished sleep efficiency, and increase in wake time after sleep onset. Periodic limb movements during wakefulness >15/h may be noted before sleep onset. As stated previously, periodic limb movements during sleep may be present. RLS has to be differentiated from akathisia related to the use of neuroleptic agents or dopamine receptor antagonists or from peripheral neuropathy.

Therapy for RLS should start with treatment of known underlying causes or precipitating factors. Iron supplementation may be considered if serum ferritin is < 50 μg/L. Dopaminergic agents, such as levodopa, pramipexole, or ropinirole, are the preferred first-line agents.[8,9] Adverse effects of dopaminergic agents include augmentation, or earlier onset or increased severity of symptoms, or involvement of other body parts such as the arms, which is more commonly encountered with levodopa. Use of pramipexole and ropinirole can give rise to nausea, sleepiness, orthostasis, and the development of compulsive disorder. The administration of pergolide has been associated with the development of pleuropulmonary and cardiac valve fibrosis. Another useful class of agents are the benzodiazepines, such as clonazepam, which provides symptomatic relief. Opioid agents may be necessary for severe symptoms refractory to other therapy. Finally, gabapentin may be considered for RLS accompanied by pain.

PLMD

In this disorder, recurrent leg movements, consisting of partial flexion of the ankle, knee, and hip with extension of the big toe, are accompanied by complaints of sleep disturbance or excessive sleepiness. Involvement of the upper extremity consists of flexion at the elbow. PLMD shares many of the risk factors of RLS. Polysomnography is required for diagnosis; periodic limb movement index is abnormal if it is > 5 in children or > 15 in adults. Therapy of PLMD is similar to that of RLS. Specific therapy is not indicated for asymptomatic periodic limb movements during sleep.

Circadian Rhythm Sleep Disorders

Circadian rhythm sleep disorders are caused by a recurrent or persistent misalignment between the desired sleep schedule and the circadian sleep-wake rhythm. They can present with either insomnia or sleepiness, or both.[10]

Advanced Sleep Phase Disorder

Persons with advanced sleep phase disorder (ASPD) are often referred to a *morning larks* that prefer an early bedtime, between 6:00 and 9:00 PM, and an equally early wake time, from 2:00 to 5:00 AM.[11] Sleep, itself, is normal for age. Sleep-related complaints include excessive sleepiness in the late afternoon or early evening, or morning awakening that is earlier than desired. Onset of ASPD is commonly during middle age. It is diagnosed by history and sleep diary or actigraphy. Therapy consists of early evening bright light therapy administered before minimum core body temperature.

Delayed Sleep Phase Disorder

This disorder is characterized by night owls that have a preferred late bedtime, between 1 and 6 AM, and a delayed wake time, from 10:00 AM to 2:00 PM.[11] There is generally no difficulty remaining asleep after the onset of sleep. Onset of delayed sleep phase disorder is commonly during adolescence. Clinical course is chronic, but severity of nighttime insomnia and daytime sleepiness may diminish with increasing age. Like ASPD, diagnosis if based on history and sleep diary or actigraphy. Persons with delayed sleep phase disorder often respond to timed early morning light exposure provided after the minimum core body temperature accompanied by evening avoidance of bright light. Chronotherapy can either involve a progressive phase delay or progressive phase advancement. Melatonin administered in the early evening is also helpful.

Free-Running Circadian Disorder

In this circadian rhythm disorder, there is a progressive daily delay in sleep-onset and wake times, with the major sleep period "marching" progressively throughout the day, afternoon, and evening.[11] This pattern of the major sleep period results in periodically recurring complaints of insomnia or excessive sleepiness. Free-running disorder is rare in the general population, and most affected patients are totally blind and lack photic entrainment. It has a chronic course. This disorder is diagnosed by a compatible history, often aided by sleep diaries or actigraphy. Polysomnography is not routinely indicated for diagnosis. Therapy consists of evening administration of melatonin. A regular sleep-wake and daytime activity schedule is important.

Irregular Sleep-Wake Rhythm

There are no stable circadian sleep-wake rhythms in this disorder. Rather, variable, inconsistent, and multiple sleep and wake periods occur throughout the day and from one day to another.[11] Nevertheless, aggregate sleep time during a 24-h period is normal. This disorder is most frequently seen in association with dementia or mental retardation. Diagnosis is arrived at by history and sleep diary or actigraphy. Evening administration of melatonin is useful in establishing a more consistent bedtime.

Jet Lag

Jet lag consists of either transient insomnia or sleepiness after rapid eastward or westward air travel across multiple time zones and is caused by the lack of synchrony to the new local time zone.[12] Thus, persons may complain of sleep-onset insomnia and/or difficulty awakening the next day after eastward flights. On the other hand, after westward flights, they may describe early evening sleepiness as well as early morning awakenings. Symptoms of jet lag remit spontaneously within about a day for every time zone change. If needed, therapy involves bright light therapy, with evening bright light exposure for westward travel, and morning bright light exposure after eastward travel. Short-acting hypnotic agents or melatonin may be used at bedtime for insomnia.

Shift Work Sleep Disorder

Shift work sleep disorder is defined by sleep disturbance related to nonstandard work schedules, with persons either complaining of sleepiness and decreased alertness during night shifts as well as insomnia during daytime sleep periods.[12] Clinical history and sleep diaries are helpful in the diagnosis of this disorder. Therapy, if required, consists of measures to increase nighttime alertness, such as bright light exposure in the workplace; napping before (or during) night work; psychostimulants (*eg*, caffeine, modafinil, or armodafinil); and measures to enhance daytime sleep, including hypnotic agents, melatonin, and restriction of daytime light exposure.

Medical Disorders

Hypertension

OSA is a risk factor for hypertension independent of known confounding factors; indeed, the odds of hypertension increase by approximately 1% for each additional apneic event per hour of sleep. There is often loss of the nocturnal decrease in BP ("dipping" phenomenon) in persons with OSA and improvement in BP control with positive airway pressure therapy.

Coronary Artery Disease

Risk of coronary artery disease is increased in middle-aged persons with OSA. Possible mechanisms include endothelial dysfunction, hypercoagulability, insulin resistance, oxidative stress, and increased sympathetic activity during sleep.

Congestive Heart Failure

The prevalence of OSA, CSA, and Cheyne-Stokes respiration is increased in CHF. Alternatively, OSA may contribute to worsening left ventricular dysfunction, and the rate of mortality is greater in CHF persons with worse apnea-hypopnea indexes.

Cardiac Arrhythmias

There is a decreased prevalence of premature ventricular contractions during sleep as the result of greater parasympathetic tone and an increase in ventricular arrhythmias during arousals from sleep.

Respiratory Disorders

Several respiratory disorders, including asthma, COPD, diaphragm paralysis, restrictive pulmonary diseases, and neuromuscular disorders are associated with significant sleep disturbance.

Asthma

Persons with asthma commonly complain of insomnia and sleep fragmentation. Nocturnal hypoxemia may develop as can nocturnal bronchoconstriction, the latter occurring as a result of either (1) circadian variability in airflow, which is lowest in the early morning; (2) sleep-related changes in autonomic nervous activity, *ie*, greater parasympathetic tone and decrease in sympathetic activity; (3) changes in lung capacity and inflammatory mediators; and (4) gastroesophageal reflux. Diagnosis is aided by showing a decrease in evening peak expiratory flow or FEV_1 compared with daytime values.

COPD

COPD may present at night with repetitive awakenings as the result of coughing or dyspnea. Nocturnal hypoxemia and hypercapnia may develop in advanced disease. Episodes of oxygen desaturation tend to be more frequent, of greater duration, and more severe during REM sleep compared with NREM sleep. There are several mechanisms that may be responsible for sleep-related oxygen desaturation, including hypoventilation (most important factor), ventilation/perfusion mismatching, and decrease in lung volumes. Overlap syndrome is defined by the presence of both COPD and OSA. Compared with isolated COPD, persons with the overlap syndrome tend to have lower Pao_2, greater $Paco_2$, and greater mean pulmonary artery pressures.

Diaphragm Paralysis

Nocturnal hypoxemia can develop in persons with diaphragm paralysis and is worse during REM sleep.

Restrictive Pulmonary Diseases

Restrictive pulmonary diseases are commonly associated with sleep disturbance and frequent awakenings. Both OSA and CSA can develop. Nocturnal oxygen desaturation can either be transient or sustained and is worse during REM sleep.

Neuromuscular Disorders

Neuromuscular disorders are associated with an increased risk of OSA and CSA as well as nocturnal dyspnea. Nocturnal oxygen desaturation primarily is caused by hypoventilation and occurs predominantly during REM sleep. Nocturnal hypoventilation can precede abnormalities during waking by months to years. The risk of nocturnal oxygen desaturation is greater in those with maximal inspiratory pressure < 60 cm H_2O, or if FVC is $< 50\%$ of predicted.

References

1. Schutte-Rodin S, Broch L, Buysse D, et al. Clinical guideline for the evaluation and management of chronic insomnia in adults. J Clin Sleep Med 2008; 4:487–504
2. Morin CM, Bootzin RR, Buysse DJ, et al. Psychological and behavioral treatment of insomnia: update of the recent evidence (1998–2004). Sleep 2006; 29:1398–1414
3. Morgenthaler TI, Kapur VK, Brown TM, et al. Standards of Practice Committee of the AASM. Practice parameters for the treatment of narcolepsy and other hypersomnias of central origin. Sleep 2007; 30:1705–1711
4. Wise MS, Arand DL, Auger RR, et al. Treatment of narcolepsy and other hypersomnias of central origin. Sleep 2007; 30:1712–1727
5. Mahowald MW, Schenck CH. Non-rapid eye movement sleep parasomnias [review]. Neurol Clin 2005; 23:1077–1106
6. Schenck CH, Mahowald MW. Rapid eye movement sleep parasomnias [review]. Neurol Clin 2005; 23:1107–1126
7. Itin I, Comella CL. Restless legs syndrome. Prim Care 2005; 32:435–448
8. Standards of Practice Committee of the American Academy of Sleep Medicine. Practice parameters for the dopaminergic treatment of restless legs syndrome and periodic limb movement disorder. Sleep 2004; 27:557–559
9. A Review by the Restless Legs Syndrome Task Force of the Standards of Practice Committee of the American Academy of Sleep Medicine. An update on the dopaminergic treatment of restless legs syndrome and periodic limb movement disorder. Sleep 2004; 27:560–583

10. Morgenthaler TI, Lee-Chiong T, Alessi C, et al. Standards of Practice Committee of the AASM. Practice parameters for the clinical evaluation and treatment of circadian rhythm sleep disorders. Sleep 2007; 30:1445–1459
11. Sack R, Auckley D, Auger RR, et al. Circadian rhythm sleep disorders: part II, advanced sleep phase disorder, delayed sleep phase disorder, free-running disorder, and irregular sleep-wake rhythm. Sleep 2007; 30:1484–1501
12. Sack RL, Auckley D, Auger RR, et al. Circadian rhythm sleep disorders: part I. Basic principles, shift work and jet lag disorders. Sleep 2007; 30:1460–1483

Notes

Pulmonary Fungal Infections

George A. Sarosi, MD, FCCP

Objectives:

- Describe the epidemiology of the endemic mycosis
- Describe the clinical syndromes of endemic mycosis
- Familiarize participants with the various diagnostic tests pertaining to pulmonary fungal infections
- Show the various manifestations of aspergillosis and candidiasis
- Show different therapeutic strategies pertaining to fungal diseases

Key words: aspergillosis; blastomycosis; candidiasis; coccidioidomycosis, cryptococcosis; histoplasmosis

Histoplasmosis

Histoplasmosis is the infection caused by the pathogenic, soil-dwelling fungus *Histoplasma capsulatum*. The organism is endemic throughout the south-central United States, especially along river valleys. Heavy concentrations of the fungus are found in excrement of chickens, pigeons, starlings, and bats. A pulmonary infection will occur when the mycelium is disturbed and aerosolized fungal spores are inhaled.

Clinical Features

Primary Pulmonary Histoplasmosis: The primary disease may have few or no symptoms. Even in the asymptomatic patient, a chest radiograph may show patchy areas of pneumonitis with or without ipsilateral hilar adenopathy. Patients become symptomatic around 14 days after exposure. In the event of a very large inoculum, the symptoms may begin sooner. The illness is an influenza-like disease with fever, chills, myalgia, and nonproductive cough. During the early nonimmune phase of the infection, the fungus disseminates widely throughout the body. With the advent of specific T-cell–mediated immunity, the infection is brought under control.

Patients who have been exposed to a very large infective inoculum will present with a potentially lethal illness. The main difficulty is with gas exchange, and the chest radiograph shows a picture similar to that of ARDS. After recovery, the chest radiograph may return to normal or may be left with residual abnormalities. The initial patchy infiltrate may become denser and smaller, leading to the formation of pulmonary nodules. Central necrosis within these nodules can result in calcification, leading to the development of the characteristic "target" lesion. Lymph node calcification alone or with a pulmonary nodule is common. These calcifications occur more frequently in younger patients.

Local complications may occur but, fortunately, not often. Extensive fibrosis (caused by exaggerated response by the host) in the mediastinum may cause vascular compression and result in the superior vena cava syndrome. Inflammatory masses adjacent to the esophagus may cause dysphagia. Calcified nodes may erode into various structures, leading to hemoptysis.

Chronic Cavitary Histoplasmosis: This disease closely resembles reinfection tuberculosis both in symptomatology and radiographic appearance. The mechanism of infection, unlike in tuberculosis, is that of a primary infection in a patient with a structurally abnormal lung, typically a middle-aged smoker who has centrilobular emphysema. The acute infection in such patients usually resolves, but occasionally (in up to 20%) it will go on to produce progressive upper-lobe fibrocavitary disease. Once the disease establishes itself and progresses under observation, treatment is necessary because of continuing pulmonary destruction.

Progressive Disseminated Histoplasmosis: Progressive disseminated histoplasmosis (PDH) is a progressive extrapulmonary infection. It may occur as part of an overwhelming postprimary spread (frequently seen in infants) with little or no tendency to granuloma formation despite the huge burden of organisms that are present in reticuloendothelial tissues. Symptoms include high fever accompanied by diffuse lymphadenopathy, hepatosplenomegaly, and severe pancytopenia.

Death may occur within weeks and is usually secondary to respiratory compromise.

Dissemination also occurs in nonimmunocompromised adults, in for whom the disease is a smoldering, subacute illness of many months in duration. Fever is low grade at most, and most of the symptoms relate to weight loss. Physical examination shows skin and mucous membrane lesions along with hepatosplenomegaly. Histopathologic examination shows well-formed granulomas and only rare organisms.

In recent years, PDH has occurred primarily in patients with significant T-cell dysfunction, including organ transplant recipients, patients receiving glucocorticoids and/or cytotoxic drug therapy for malignant neoplasms, and patients with HIV infection. In this latter group, PDH is frequently the AIDS-defining infection. The density of the organisms in biopsy material is greater than that in other immunosuppressed patients, helping materially with the laboratory diagnosis.

It is important to note that perhaps as many as one half of patients with PDH have no symptoms related to the lung. Especially in patients with AIDS, PDH is primarily a debilitating, febrile illness. Eventually, chest radiographic abnormalities develop in all patients.

The incidence of PDH complicating untreated HIV infections has resulted in the acknowledgment of parts of the world as being endemic for histoplasmosis that were not known to harbor the fungus. These areas include the entire Caribbean basin extending all the way to the northern coast of South America. In addition, many of the states of sub-Saharan Africa have identified patients with histoplasmosis. The extent of the disease in Europe is not known. Although in Europe most patients who present with PDH come from endemic areas, a handful of cases appear to have had no exposure outside of Europe.

The recent emergence of tumor necrosis factor (TNF)-α inhibitors has caused a clear-cut association with PDH. All anti-TNF-α agents may lead to PDH, but its occurrence is most frequent after the administration of infliximab. In fact, PDH is the second most common infectious complication after tuberculosis.

Diagnostic Tests

Histopathologic specimens reveal small yeasts that are highly suggestive of histoplasmosis either within macrophages or lying free in areas of necrosis. Although the organisms occasionally may be visualized in routine hematoxylin-eosin–stained sections, as a general rule they are difficult to visualize unless special stains are applied. Most experienced pathology laboratories will use one of the silver stains or the periodic acid-Schiff stain. The organism is best visualized from biopsies of the reticuloendothelial system, with the highest yield coming from bone marrow biopsy and from blood cultures.

Whenever skin lesions are present, biopsies should be performed. In patients with AIDS, the density of Histoplasma organisms is so high that they may be visible on Wright-stained smears of the buffy coat of the peripheral blood.

The organism is readily recovered from biological material, and whenever the disease is suspected, every attempt should be made to obtain adequate specimens for cultures. The availability of the lysis-centrifugation system has increased our ability to isolate the fungus from circulating blood, but standard radiometric tests also will grow the fungus readily. The main difficulty with culture identification is that it is time-consuming; whenever possible, histopathologic sections should be examined because they are less time-consuming. Intradermal skin testing with histoplasmin is a reliable epidemiologic tool, but it is useless for the diagnosis of individual cases. In addition, it is no longer available commercially.

Complement-fixing antibodies to mycelial and yeast phase antigens may be detected 4 to 6 weeks after exposure (2 to 4 weeks after onset of fever). The titers usually decrease gradually during the next 12 months, but in some patients they may remain positive at a very high dilution for many years. Titers against the yeast antigen of ≥1:32 in a patient with an appropriate clinical history should suggest histoplasmosis. Similarly, a documented fourfold increase of titer is diagnostic of acute Histoplasma infection. Unfortunately, complement-fixing antibody test results are negative in as many as 50% of immunocompromised patients with PDH; thus, a negative complement-fixing test result cannot be used to rule out the disease.

The currently available immunodiffusion test, although highly specific, is not sensitive enough for routine clinical use. Its main use is in patients whose serum is anticomplementary. The availability of the Histoplasma polysaccharide antigen is a major step forward. The test is extremely useful in diagnosing PDH, especially in immunocompromised patients. The test is able to detect excretion of this antigen in the urine and blood and can be used both for diagnosis and to follow the course of the disease, including prediction of relapses.

Treatment

Primary pulmonary histoplasmosis requires no treatment. In a rare incident of an individual with massive inhalation and ARDS, amphotericin B or a lipid formulation of amphotericin B(L-amphotericin) is the treatment of choice when gas exchange abnormalities threaten his or her life. A total dose of 500 to 1,500 mg may be sufficient, although this dose is based on purely anecdotal information.

Chronic cavitary histoplasmosis responds readily to itraconazole 200 mg bid for at least 6 months. Although the response to amphotericin is quicker, the reduction in side effects that accompanies itraconazole administration makes it the agent of choice. Occasional treatment failures and delayed relapses with itraconazole respond to a subsequent course of itraconazole or amphotericin. The newer azoles voriconazole and posaconazole both have excellent activity against the fungus, but their high cost makes them less attractive alternatives.

Itraconazole can also be used to treat PDH in the rare event of a patient whose illness is slow to progress. In most other patients, the drug of choice is amphotericin; the dose is rapidly accelerated to 50 mg/d and continues until clinical stability is reached, which may take 500 to 1,000 mg of amphotericin. After clinical stability is reached, patients should be treated with itraconazole for 6 to 12 months. Most nonimmunocompromised patients should respond well, with cure of the disease achieved. Immunocompromised patients whose immunosuppressive state cannot be improved and patients with AIDS who continue to have $CD4^+$ counts <200 μL require continued suppression.

Coccidioidomycosis

Coccidioidomycosis, or "cocci," is the infection by the fungus *Coccidioides immitis*. This organism is endemic in the desert southwestern United States and adjacent areas of Mexico and is responsible for approximately 100,000 new infections each year. Approximately 60% of infected patients have no symptoms, whereas the remaining 40% usually have only mild symptoms of a febrile, influenza-like illness that lasts 1 to 3 weeks. Patients usually have a nonproductive cough along with myalgias and arthralgias, headaches, and pleuritic chest pain. The pleuritic chest pain may be very severe. A chest radiograph may show localized alveolar infiltrate, a single nodular density, or a pleural effusion. Many patients with acute cocci have an illness that is indistinguishable from community-acquired pneumonia. In a recent small series from the endemic area, acute cocci were seen in approximately one third of the patients. In rare instances, the patient may present with a pneumothorax secondary to the rupture of a subpleural cavity. Fortunately, most patients recover without further problems. Approximately 5% may continue to show persistent chest radiographic abnormalities but remain in good health.

Disseminated disease will be present in $<1\%$ of patients, and it most commonly occurs among black, Filipino, and diabetic individuals, and in patients who are receiving cytotoxic therapy or glucocorticoids for other disease entities. Dissemination is also likely to occur in organ transplant recipients, patients receiving anti-TNF-α therapy, as well as in patients infected with HIV.

The so-called allergic manifestations of the illness, such as erythema multiforme or erythema nodosum, occur in up to 20% of patients, most often in young white women. These are thought to be favorable prognostic signs. In endemic areas, this manifestation of "valley fever" is readily recognized by all practitioners. A persistent thin-walled cavity or a single nodule is the most common radiographic residue of acute coccidioidomycosis. On occasion, a slowly progressive fibrocavitary disease may develop that resembles reinfection tuberculosis.

Disseminated Cocci

Fortunately, this most-dreaded form of the disease is uncommon. It may be a fulminant illness with development of meningitis along with bone and skin lesions. Other patients, especially severely immunocompromised patients, will present with a rapidly progressive extensive pulmonary infiltrate that leads to air exchange abnormalities and that may become fatal. For non-immunocompromised patients, the onset of dissemination is usually more leisurely, and it may follow the primary infection by several weeks to several months. In many instances, the primary infection was asymptomatic, and thus cannot be accurately dated.

Cocci meningitis is a frequent manifestation of extrapulmonary disease. Approximately one third of patients will have single organ dissemination to the meninges. The inflammatory process involves the base of the brain, where it obstructs the flow of cerebrospinal fluid (CSF) and entraps cranial nerves. Headache is common, and changes in mental acuity are frequently seen. Stiff neck and other meningeal signs are seldom seen. Examination of CSF reveals a mononuclear cell pleocytosis with depressed glucose and elevated protein levels. Other organs frequently involved in disseminated disease include the bones and the skin. Eventually, most patients with disseminated cocci will have cutaneous involvement.

Coccidioidomycosis is being recognized with increased frequency in patients with HIV infection. Depending on immune status, the disease may look no different from that found in non-HIV-infected patients; toward the end of the HIV infection, when the $CD4^+$ count is <250 μL, coccidioidomycosis is usually a rapidly progressive, hematogenously spread, and rapidly fatal illness. The characteristic radiograph in this form of coccidioidomycosis is a micronodular infiltrate throughout all lung fields.

Diagnostic Tests

The pathognomonic feature of cocci infection is the giant spherule. This form of the organism may range up to 100 μm and is filled with numerous small endospores. The spherule is sufficiently large and is readily seen on hematoxylin-eosin-stained sections. Giant spherules may also be seen by Papanicolaou stain-treated smears of sputum or pus, but less well as on potassium hydroxide-treated smears. The organism can readily be cultured in the laboratory, but great care must be exercised because this is a highly infectious organism.

Most experts believe skin tests are helpful. Unfortunately, a single skin test cannot date the onset of the illness and is therefore better thought of as an epidemiologic tool than as a useful test for the diagnosis of individual patients with cocci.

Serologic diagnosis is extremely useful in coccidioidomycosis. Serum IgM precipitants may be demonstrated by tube precipitations or by latex agglutination. These are first detected 2 to 3 weeks after the onset of symptoms of the primary infection and will eventually be noticed in 75% of patients. Positive precipitins will diminish within 4 to 6 months. Serum IgG antibodies, the so-called *complement-fixing antibodies*, occur later; and by 3 months after the onset of symptoms, nearly 90% of patients have such antibodies. High titers or rising titers can also be used to alert the clinician to the possibility of disseminating infection. Recently, immunodiffusion tests measuring both IgM and IgG antibodies came into use and are replacing other methods of measuring antibodies. Their sensitivity and specificity are very much the same, but they are much easier to perform.

The height of the titer will vary from laboratory to laboratory, and before a great deal of emphasis is placed on the relative height of a given titer, the origin of the titer needs to be determined. In approximately 70% of patients with cocci meningitis there are complement-fixing antibodies in the CSF. The presence of such antibodies is diagnostic of cocci meningitis. This is particularly important because the organism is seldom cultured initially from CSF. Recently, an antigen-based diagnostic test became available that requires the specimens of either urine or blood. Initial results have been promising, but more data are needed.

Treatment

Primary pulmonary cocci require no treatment. However, treatment is advised for immunocompromised patients or other patients who have a high risk of dissemination (*eg*, diabetic, black, or pregnant patients). Treatment may also be recommended for those with severe, persistent infection. The usual dose of amphotericin for primary infection under these circumstances is between 500 and

1,500 mg. Fluconazole, an orally administered azole, is frequently used by practitioners in the endemic area for the treatment of acute coccidioidomycosis despite the fact that the efficacy of this treatment has never been established.

Residual thin-walled cavities usually require no treatment. Resection with or without amphotericin may be needed if hemoptysis develops or if the cavities enlarge, move subpleurally, and threaten rupture. The chronic fibrocavitary form of pulmonary coccidioidomycosis requires treatment. Although some patients respond to itraconazole or fluconazole, more severely ill patients will require amphotericin for effective treatment. Although the results with amphotericin are better, the treatment is seldom curative.

Disseminated cocci have to be treated with amphotericin. An initial course of 2.5 g is recommended, but if a patient does not respond, the dose may be increased to greater levels. In all patients with disseminated cocci, a lumbar puncture must be performed to rule out meningeal dissemination.

Cocci meningitis always requires treatment. When amphotericin is chosen, both IV and intrathecal amphotericin therapy might be used. In many patients, prolonged intrathecal therapy is necessary for the meningeal disease in addition to the standard course of IV amphotericin. It is administered in doses ranging from 0.25 to 1 mg by cisternal puncture, by lumbar puncture, or via an intraventricular reservoir. Treatment may be given up to three times weekly and is usually continued until both the cell count and complement-fixing activity diminish. At that time, the interval of administration may be extended to twice per week, then to once per week, and eventually to biweekly or monthly as the patient improves. This form of treatment will need to be continued for the remainder of the patient's life. Recently, however, fluconazole replaced amphotericin as primary therapy and amphotericin, is used in when fluconazole therapy has failed. When fluconazole is used, it must be continued for the patient's life. The withdrawal of fluconazole leads to an unacceptable relapse rate.

Disseminated coccidioidomycosis involving skin, bone, and noncavitating pulmonary lesions may be treated with itraconazole, 200 mg bid, or fluconazole, 400 mg/d. Ttreatment of coccidioidomycosis in patients with HIV infection is a daunting challenge. Response is poor, and the eventual prognosis is grim. Treatment should begin with amphotericin to the maximum tolerated dose, and once the patient stabilizes, most investigators will switch to fluconazole. The exact dose needed is not determined.

Blastomycosis

Blastomycosis refers to an infection by the fungus *Blastomyces dermatitidis*. The organism is endemic in the Midwest, southwestern United States, and the Canadian provinces Ontario and Manitoba. Similar to histoplasmosis and coccidioidomycosis, blastomycosis is a soil fungus, existing in soil of high organic content in microfoci in the endemic area.

Clinical Features

Acute Pulmonary Blastomycosis: The infection may or may not be symptomatic. Radiography reveals patchy alveolar to lobar infiltrates. Hilar enlargement is common, but pleural disease and cavitation are infrequent. The clinical symptoms include an influenza-like illness with high fever, and a cough productive of mucopurulent sputum along with myalgias and arthralgias. Although symptomatic disease is usually short-lived, radiographic abnormalities may persist for several months. Progressive pulmonary infection with continued suppuration and eventual cavitation is an infrequent occurrence. An occasional patient may present with rapidly progressive bilateral macronodular illness, leading to ARDS.

Most cases of blastomycosis present in a chronic or subacute form. Patients usually have no antecedent history of an acute pulmonary illness but will complain of chronic respiratory symptoms of at least 2 months in duration. Symptoms include a chronic cough, low-grade fever, night sweats, and weight loss. The chest radiograph may reveal either a single mass or a lobar infiltrate. It is important to realize that in certain patients, the primary pulmonary process may well have healed before the infection develops in distant sites.

Diagnostic Tests

The fungus is readily visualized in expectorated sputum or other purulent material after digestion of 10% potassium hydroxide. The large, single-budding organism is characterized by its broad neck of attachment and its double refractile cell wall. The organism is difficult to see in standard hematoxylin-eosin-stained sections but is readily visualized with periodic acid-Schiff- or silver-stained sections. The organism is readily recovered in cultures, although it is a somewhat time-consuming process. Depending on inoculum size, cultures may take up to 3 weeks before they are recognizable.

There is no commercially available skin test, and the serologic diagnosis in blastomycosis is quite rudimentary. At present, even the presence of a positive serologic test (measuring antibody) result using one of the more recent ultrasensitive assays does not confirm the diagnosis of blastomycosis—it merely points one in the direction of the infection. The recently available urine antigen has performed well in preliminary studies.

Treatment

Acute pulmonary blastomycosis may not require treatment in some patients; most patients with acute pulmonary disease should be treated with itraconazole, 200 mg bid, for at least 6 months. In severely ill patients in whom gas exchange abnormality forces the issue, amphotericin is used until the patient reaches clinical, and this should be followed by a course of oral itraconazole, 200 mg bid, daily ≥6 months. All patients with blastomycotic meningitis should receive amphotericin; there is no evidence that intrathecal amphotericin administration improves prognosis. Because itraconazole reach high levels in CSF, high-dose fluconazole is used as step-down therapy after clinical stability is reached.

Cryptococcosis

Cryptococcosis is the infection caused by the encapsulated yeast *Cryptococcus neoformans*. In the normal host, primary pulmonary infection seldom produces a clinical illness. The organism exists worldwide and is frequently associated with bird droppings, especially from pigeons. Most patients with significant cryptococcal disease have an underlying immunocompromised state.

Clinical Features

Primary pulmonary cryptococcosis usually is discovered accidentally because most patients have no symptoms. When symptoms are present, fever is modest and a chest radiograph frequently shows a large, localized lobar infiltrate. The usual natural history of acute pulmonary cryptococcal infection in immunocompetent hosts is that of spontaneous recovery. Nevertheless, in some patients with an apparently normal immune system, progressive pulmonary or disseminated disease may develop; the current recommendation is to treat all such patients with a course of fluconazole. If the decision is to treat a patient with pulmonary disease, a lumbar puncture should be done to make sure the patient does not have meningeal involvement.

The vast majority of the patients with cryptococcal disease have cryptococcal meningitis. The symptoms frequently are trivial; change in mental acuity and the presence of headaches frequently are the only clue to the involvement of the meninges by the fungus. More definite signs of meningeal irritation are uncommon. CSF examination usually shows increased protein with a predominant mononuclear pleocytosis and depressed glucose levels. It is important to remember that the CSF formula may be completely normal in patients with HIV coinfection.

Diagnostic Tests

The organism is a single-budding yeast with a narrow-necked bud that may reach up to 12 µm in diameter. The character feature is the very large carbohydrate capsule. Histopathologic examination of involved tissue will frequently show the organism stained with mucicarmine and the various silver stains. Frequently, no inflammatory infiltrate surrounds the mass of organisms. The large carbohydrate capsule is the background behind the India ink test, which will demonstrate the organisms in up to 70% of the immunocompromised patients' lumbar puncture specimens.

The organism grows really readily in most standard laboratory media and lends itself to rapid laboratory diagnosis. Cultures findings in

CSF are positive in 80 to 90% of patients. A blood culture also should performed because it results frequently are positive in immunocompromised patients. However, interpretation of sputum cultures is very difficult because the organism may be a colonizer. There is no commercially available skin test.

Besides culture, serologic tests form the mainstay of diagnosis. Direct measure of the fungal antigen is possible with the widely available latex agglutination method. Results are positive in the CSF of 95% of patients with cryptococcal meningitis, and the method is more sensitive than the culture itself. It should also be determined in the blood since it frequently reaches very high titers, especially in patients with HIV infection.

Treatment

All immunocompetent patients with pulmonary cryptococcosis and a negative spinal tap result should be treated with a 6- to 12-week course of fluconazole, 400 mg/d. Pulmonary cryptococcosis in immunocompromised patients is a progressive illness, and all such patients should receive prompt treatment, even if the meninges are not involved. Most of the data dealing with treatment of cryptococcal disease were derived from large groups of patients with cryptococcal meningitis, and treatment of cryptococcal pulmonary disease is largely derivative of these studies.

All patients with cryptococcal meningitis should receive amphotericin, 0.7 mg/kg/d, plus flucytosine, 100 mg/kg/d divided into four equal doses, for 2 weeks. If at the end of 2 weeks the CSF is sterile, the patient should be switched to oral fluconazole, 400 mg/d, for 6 additional weeks. The addition of flucytosine is clearly beneficial, but great care must be exercised to maintain flucytosine levels <100 mg/mL to prevent bone marrow suppression. The combination of AIDS and cryptococcal meningitis is a particular problem to treat. Although many patients respond to treatment, substantial numbers will not and proceed to die. Relapse is extremely common once treatment is stopped; thus, it is necessary to treat all responding patients with suppressive doses of fluconazole, 200 mg/d, to decrease the frequency of relapse.

Aspergillosis

Epidemiology

Aspergillosis sp are soil fungi found everywhere there is decaying vegetation. There are >300 species of Aspergillus, but only a handful have been associated with human disease. By far the most common are *Aspergillus fumigatus*, followed by *Aspergillus flavus*, *Aspergillus clavatus*, and *Aspergillus nidulans*.

Pathogenesis

Aspergillus spores are inhaled regularly by all individuals. Colonization of the respiratory tree may occur, especially after heavy exposure. The same Aspergillus spores may cause colonization of any devitalized area of the lung. The most common and certainly the most characteristic feature of aspergillosis is colonization of previously formed cavities in the lung. Aspergillus growing in preformed cavities produces a characteristic lesion, the intracavitary fungus ball or aspergilloma. Although occasional symptoms such as hemoptysis are distressing to the patient, as a general rule the fungus does not invade surrounding lung tissue.

Inhaled Aspergillus spores may also colonize the mucus within the bronchi, especially when they are associated with moderately severe asthma and they are thick and tenacious in nature. In this clinical setting, invasion of the mucus plug occurs, exacerbating the underlying airways disease and leading to increased inflammation and eventual fibrosis. This disease entity is allergic bronchopulmonary aspergillosis.

A recently described form of aspergillosis involves colonization of previously abnormal lung substance. The involved patients usually have a minimal degree of immunosuppression and frequently have sarcoidosis or diabetes. Aspergillus spores may invade adjacent lung tissues and produce a gradually progressive and destructive process in lung containing centrilobular emphysema. Occasionally, fungus balls may form in these cavities. Although distant spread is rare, the disease may be locally invasive and destructive.

The most lethal form of aspergillosis is disseminated or pyemic aspergillosis. When spores are inhaled by an abnormal host with reduced or nonfunctional neutrophils and macrophages, dissemination of the infection will occur. Without appropriate inflammatory cell activity, the fungi will grow within the alveoli and invade adjacent vascular structures, leading to occlusion of these vessels. Necrosis follows occlusion of the vessels, leading to wedge-shaped areas of infarction. Metastatic abscesses in brain, lung, liver, heart, and other organs are common. When lesions involve the skin, they give rise to a characteristic skin lesion, with an area of central necrosis and a black eschar. This skin lesion is referred to as *ecthyma gangrenosum*. Occasionally, Aspergillus endocarditis may follow pyemic spread.

Clinical Manifestation

Hemoptysis is the major clinical feature of the fungus ball. Although rare, occasional exsanguinating hemorrhage has been noted. No drug therapy has proven to be effective. In patients whose pulmonary reserve warrants it, lung resection is an effective mode of therapy. The principal symptom of allergic bronchopulmonary aspergillosis is episodic dyspnea, largely because of the underlying reactive airways disease. The otherwise-severe course of underlying asthma is punctuated by episodes of worsening, when thick mucus plugs become inspissated in bronchi, causing an inflammatory process distal to the obstruction. This propensity to cause bronchial obstruction gives rise to the characteristic radiographic pattern of the disease, the so-called finger-in-glove appearance, in which multiple adjacent bronchi are distended with the mucus plug. Fever, cough, and pleuritic chest pain are common, and peripheral blood eosinophilia is seen. Between clinical exacerbations, patients tend to return to their baseline symptomatic state from their asthma. Eventually, however, because of the development of chronic fibrous changes, the restrictive lung function pattern is overlaid on top of the reactive airways disease.

Disseminated or pyemic aspergillosis occurs primarily in patients with profound bone marrow suppression. This danger is the greatest one in patients with acute leukemia or bone marrow transplantation. Characteristic clinical manifestations are all related to the vascular occlusive nature of the disease, leading to a syndrome mimicking multiple pulmonary emboli or stroke syndrome secondary to involvement of the intracranial blood vessels. Aspergillosis also complicates AIDS in a small number of patients. The same factors predisposing to aspergillosis are found in both patients with and without HIV infection.

Diagnosis

Aspergilloma is usually diagnosed by the characteristic radiographic pattern and confirmed by sputum culture. Diagnosis of allergic bronchopulmonary aspergillosis is made with the recovery of the fungus from sputum, the presence of increased IgE levels (especially specific IgE levels), peripheral blood eosinophilia, and the expectoration of bronchial plugs. Chronic necrotizing aspergillosis is diagnosed by the presence of a slowly progressive, usually upper-lobe disease that is also accompanied by repeated isolations of Aspergillus sp from sputum. The radiographic features of this disease frequently are indistinguishable from those of other chronic inflammatory lung infections, such as tuberculosis or other fungal infections.

Disseminated aspergillosis is frequently a diagnostic challenge. Blood culture results are almost always negative; unless a highly characteristic clinical picture develops, such as the development of ecthyma gangrenosum, the diagnosis can be made only by visualization in tissue or recovery in culture of the organism after either tissue biopsy or bronchoscopic specimen examination. Radiographic findings are variable, but the so-called *halo sign* surrounding an infiltrate is suggestive. Although frequently negative, a positive sputum culture result is extremely helpful in suggesting the diagnosis. Measurement of serum galactomannan has been shown to be the key in diagnosing early disease in stem-cell transplant patients.

Treatment

Aspergilloma usually responds to surgery. No antifungal agent has shown any consistent activity against the intracavitary fungus ball. Allergic bronchopulmonary aspergillosis responds quite well to administration of high-dose glucocorticoids. Improvement is hastened and enlarged on by the addition of itraconazole at a dose of 200 mg bid. Chronic necrotizing aspergillosis and disseminated or pyemic aspergillosis are treated with systemic antifungal therapy.

Amphotericin and L-amphotericin have been used with variable success. Itraconazole has good activity against aspergillosis, but voriconazole is favored. The new azole posaconazole is also active, but it exists only in oral form, precluding its use in critically ill patients. A new class of antifungal agent is the echinocandin. Although they all have activity against aspergillus, they are used primarily as rescue therapy. Combination therapy with two different classes of antifungal drugs has been used, but it is difficult to determine during which circumstances they should be used. Most reports are case series only.

Candidiasis

Candida sp are normal inhabitants of the microbiologic flora of people. Superficial Candida sp infections usually respond to simple measures. During the past 20 to 25 years, candidiasis became a common problem in severely immunocompromised patients and more recently in nonimmunocompromised critically ill patients. Candida sp bloodstream invasion is now the fourth-most-common nosocomial bloodstream invasion. In addition to Candida sepsis, other organs may become infected with the fungus. It is especially common as a central line-associated sepsis in critically ill antibiotic-treated patients.

Diagnosis requires recovery of the fungus in blood cultures or cultures from other sterile sites. Isolation of the fungus from other sites implies colonization. Measurement of β (1-3) glucan detects components of the fungal wall, and it may be positive in candidiasis as well as other fungal infections. Of the three classes of antifungal agents available, *ie*, polyenes, azoles, and echinocandins, the decision to pick one agent over another is left to the discretion of the attending physician

Annotated Bibliography

Baddley JW, Perfect JR, Oster RA, et al. Pulmonary cryptococcosis in patients without HIV infection: factors associated with disseminated disease. Eur J Clin Microbiol Infect Dis 2008; 27:937–943

A useful discussion of the primary infection and the potential for extrapulmonary spread.

Bergstom L, Yocum DE, Ampel NM, et al. Increased risk of coccidioidomycosis in patients treated with tumor necrosis factor alpha antagonists. Arthritis Rheum 2004; 50:1959–1966

Similar to histoplasmosis, the use of these agents often leads to secondary infections.

Bradsher RW Jr. Pulmonary blastomycosis. Semin Respir Crit Care Med 2008; 29:174–181

An excellent and current review of the most common form of blastomycosis.

Bradsher RW Jr., Chapman SW, Pappas PG. Blastomycosis. Infect Dis Clin North Am. 2003; 17:21–40

Comprehensive presentation of the infection.

Chapman SW, Dismukes WE, Proia LA, et al. Clinical practice guidelines for the management of blastomycosis: 2008 update by the infectious Diseases Society of America. Clin Infect Dis 2008; 46:1801–1812

The last word in treatment.

Chow JK, Golan Y, Ruthazer R, et al. Factors associated with candidemia caused by non-albicans *Candida* species versus *Candida albicans* in the intensive care unit. Clin Infect Dis 2008; 46:1206–1213

Discusses the fate on non-albicans Candida sp infections.

Davies SF, Khan M, Sarosi GA. Disseminated histoplasmosis in immunologically suppressed patients. Am J Med 1978; 64:94–100

Elaborates on the various immunosuppressive regimens that appear to predispose to the development of progressive dissemination.

Durkin M, Connolly P, Kuberski T. et al. Diagnosis of coccidioidomycosis with the use the Coccidiodes antigen enzyme immunoassay. Clin Infect Dis 2008; 47: e69–e73

An exciting and promising new development.

Eggiman P, Garbino J, Pittet D. Epidemiology of *Candida* species infections in critically ill non-immunosuppressed patients. Lancet Infect Dis 2003; 11:685–702

A very careful review of the pertinent literature on the subject.

Fish DG, Ampel NM, Galgiani JN, et al. Coccidioidomycosis during human immunodeficiency virus infection: a review of 77 patients. Medicine 1990; 69:384–391

The first large article chronicling the impact of coccidioidomycosis as an opportunistic infection in AIDS.

Galgiani JN, Ampel NM, Blair JE, et al. Coccidioidomycosis. Clin Infect Dis 2005; 41:1217–1223

The most recent guidelines for the treatment of coccidioidomycosis by the Infectious Diseases Society of America.
Goodwin RA Jr., Loyd JE, DesPrez RM. Histoplasmosis in normal hosts. Medicine 1981; 60:231–266
This article expands on the many faces of acute histoplasmosis. For clinicians living in an endemic area, this article is a "must read."
Goodwin RA Jr., Owens FT, Snell JD, et al. Chronic pulmonary histoplasmosis. Medicine 1976; 55:413–452
An excellent description of the chronic pulmonary form of histoplasmosis. Points out the seldom-appreciated fact that this form of histoplasmosis occurs only in individuals with abnormal lungs, usually smokers.
Goodwin RA Jr., Shapiro JL, Thurman GH, et al. Disseminated histoplasmosis: clinical and pathologic correlations. Medicine 1980; 59:1–33
The article elaborates in detail on the many varied clinical manifestations of PDH. It further enlarges on the observation that progression of the initial dissemination occurs mainly in abnormal hosts.
Green RE, Schlamm HT, Oestmann JW, et al. Imaging findings in acute invasive pulmonary aspergillosis: clinical significance of the halo sign. Clin Infect Dis 2007; 44:373–379
Discusses the prevalence and significance of the halo sign.
Judson MA. Noninvasive Aspergillus pulmonary disease. Semin Respir Crit Care Med 2004; 25:203–219
An excellent and comprehensive treatise on the subject.
Kerkering TM, Duma RD, Shadomy S. The evolution of pulmonary cryptococcosis. Ann Intern Med 1981; 94:611–616
This study looks at the fate of pulmonary cryptococcosis in both compromised and intact hosts. It documents that pulmonary cryptococcal disease in normal hosts is usually a self-limited disease, while in immunocompromised hosts it is only a single manifestation of disseminated cryptococcal disease.
Klein BS, Vergeront JM, Weeks RF, et al. Isolation of Blastomyces dermatitidis in soil associated with a large outbreak of blastomycosis in Wisconsin. N Engl J Med 1986; 314:529–534
The first successful investigation of a point source epidemic of blastomycosis. The authors succeeded where others repeatedly failed: they isolated the fungus from nature in association with the largest outbreak of blastomycosis to date.
Lortholary O, Fontanet A, Memain N, et al. Incidence and risk factors of immune reconstruction inflammatory syndrome complicating HIV-associated cryptococcosis in France. AIDS 2005; 19:1043–1049
The immune reconstitution inflammatory syndrome may occur after successful treatment in all the endemic fungal infections and in cryptococcosis.
Maertens J, Theunissen K, Verhoef G, et al. Galactomannan and computed tomography-based preemptive antifungal therapy in neutropenic patients at high risk for invasive fungal infections: a prospective feasibility study. Clin Infect Dis 2005; 41:1242–1250
Discusses in detail the value of this approach.
Marr KA. Fungal infections in hematopoietic stem cell transplant recipients. Med Mycol 2008; 46:293–302
An excellent summary of the diseases discussed.
Ostrosky-Zeichner L, Alexander BD, Kett DH, et al. multicenter clinical evaluation of the (1-3)beta-D-glucan assay as an aid to diagnosis of fungal infections in humans. Clin Infect Dis 2005; 41:654–669
An other diagnostic test of great promise.
Pappas PG, Kauffman CA, Andes D, et al. Clinical practice guidelines for the management of candidiasis: 2009 update by the Infectious Diseases Society of America. Clin Infect Dis 2009; 48:503–535
Comprehensive recommendations for the treatment of both albicans and non-albicans Candida.
Regnard JF, Icard P, Nicolosi M, et al. Aspergilloma: a series of 89 surgical cases. Ann Thorac Surg 2000; 69:898–903
A large contemporary series exploring the surgical option for an aspergilloma.
Saag MS, Graybill RJ, Larsen RA, et al. Practice guidelines for the management of cryptococcal disease Infectious Diseases Society of America. Clin Infect Dis 2000; 20:711–717
Although somewhat dated, this is still the official treatment guideline.
Saraceno JL, Phelps DTR, Ferro TJ, et al. Chronic necrotizing pulmonary aspergillosis: approach to management. 1997; 131:1435–1441
An excellent expose on this uncommon lung infection.
Saubolle MA. Laboratory aspects in the diagnosis of coccidioidomycosis. Ann N Y Acad Sci 2007; 1111:301–314
A comprehensive reference for the intricacies of diagnosis.
Valdivia L, Nix D, Lindberg E, et al. Coccidioidomycosis as a common cause of community-acquired pneumonia. Emerg Infect Dis 2006; 12:958–962
An important consideration for practitioners in the endemic area.
Walsh TY, Anaissie EJ, Denning DW, et al. Treatment of aspergillosis: clinical practice guidelines of the Infectious Diseases Society of America. Clin Infect Dis 2008; 46:327–360

The official treatment guide of a very complicated topic.

Wheat LJ. Histoplasmosis. Experience during outbreaks in Indianapolis and review of the literature. Medicine 1997; 76:339–354

A careful description of the largest outbreak ever studied.

Wheat LJ, Connolly-Stringfield P, Baker RL, et al. Disseminated histoplasmosis in the acquired immunodeficiency syndrome: clinical findings, diagnosis and treatment, and review of the literature. Medicine 1990; 69:361–374

An excellent review of PDH complicating AIDS. Since the advent of the AIDS epidemic, this form of histoplasmosis made its appearance in parts of the country where histoplasmosis previously was never recognized.

Wheat LJ, Freifeld AG, Kleiman MB, et al. Clinical practice guidelines for the management of patients with histoplasmosis: 2007 update by the Infectious Society of America. Clin Infect Dis 2007; 45:807–825

This report is the most up-to-date treatment guide.

Wheat LJ, Goldman M, Sarosi G. State-of-the-art review of pulmonary fungal infections. Semin Respir Infect 2002; 17:158–181

Description of the epidemiology and ecology of the major endemic mycoses.

Wood KL, Hage CE, Knox KS, et al. Histoplasmosis after treatment with anti-tumor necrosis factor-alpha therapy. Am J Respir Crit Care Med 2003; 167:1279–1282

Introduction of new agents have led to complicating infections by fungi, tuberculosis and other agents.

Notes

Other Pulmonary Disorders

Mark J. Rosen, MD, FCCP

Objectives:

- Discuss the pathogenesis, clinical features, and treatment of pulmonary disorders that occur in patients with sickle-cell hemoglobinopathies
- Review the pathogenesis, clinical features, and treatment of lung disease in patients with liver disease
- Review the pathogenesis and clinical features of pulmonary oxygen toxicity
- Discuss pulmonary injury caused by radiation therapy of malignancy
- Outline the pulmonary disorders that occur after thermal injury and smoke inhalation
- Review the causes and effects of methemoglobinemia

Key words: acute chest syndrome; carbon monoxide; hepatopulmonary syndrome; oxygen toxicity; pulmonary radiation injury; smoke inhalation

Pulmonary Disorders in Persons With Sickle-Cell Hemoglobinopathies

The sickle-cell (SC) hemoglobinopathies are characterized by a predominance of hemoglobin S. The most common is SC anemia (hemoglobin SS), which affects approximately 1 in 600 African Americans. Other disorders occur when hemoglobin S is associated with another abnormal hemoglobin. SC disease occurs predominantly in African Americans in the United States and in Hispanics from the Caribbean, Central America, and South America.

Pathogenesis

When deoxygenated hemoglobin SS polymerizes, the RBCs assume a rigid configuration and occlude the microvasculature, leading to ischemia or infarction of tissues. Compared with hemoglobin AA, hemoglobin SS has reduced affinity for oxygen, facilitating polymerization. Altered properties of these RBCs lead to hemolysis and vaso-occlusive episodes. SS RBCs also interact with the vascular endothelium, and the increased adherence of these cells to endothelial surfaces is an important feature of vasoocclusive crises. In addition, the release of arginase and free hemoglobin from hemolyzing RBCs leads to nitric oxide (NO) dysregulation, endothelial dysfunction, and pulmonary hypertension. SC disease also is associated with a hypercoagulable state as the result of thrombocytosis and the procoagulant effects of RBC membrane lipids, but the incidence of venous thromboembolism does not appear to be increased in these patients. The following three overlapping pulmonary syndromes are described in patients with SC hemoglobinopathies: acute chest syndrome (ACS), fat embolism syndrome, and chronic restrictive lung disease with pulmonary hypertension.

Acute Chest Syndrome

Patients with SC disease frequently present with a syndrome of chest pain, fever, and cough, usually shortly after the onset of a painful crisis. In adults, the radiograph typically shows multilobe or lower lobe pulmonary opacities; pleural effusion is present in approximately 15% of cases. When severe, ACS resembles ARDS. ACS is the leading cause of death in patients with SC disease, most commonly because of respiratory failure or vasoocclusive neurologic complications. The pathogenesis of ACS often is multifactorial, and it is usually impossible to demonstrate one specific cause for an episode. Disorders leading to ACS include infection, fat embolism from infarcted bone marrow, pulmonary microvascular occlusion, and *in situ* thrombosis. The most common pathogens identified in ACS are *Chlamydia pneumoniae*, *Mycoplasma pneumoniae*, and respiratory viruses. Other bacteria are less common causes of ACS but include *Streptococcus pneumoniae*, *Haemophilus influenzae*, and *Staphylococcus aureus*. Thoracic bone infarction occurs commonly during an acute painful crisis and may lead to atelectasis and pneumonia by causing splinting from pain.

Because the pathogenesis of ACS is multifactorial, each treatment is of uncertain benefit in a specific patient. Patients almost always are treated with analgesics, are hydrated to prevent hemoconcentration, and are given oxygen supplementation to reduce sickling. Most patients receive antibiotics empirically because it usually is impossible to determine whether or not they have pneumonia. Antibiotics should be directed against both "typical" and "atypical" pathogens. In severe cases, the transfusion of RBCs may improve ACS rapidly. Incentive spirometry was shown to prevent atelectasis and pulmonary infiltrates in patients with SC disease who were hospitalized with acute chest pain. The use of inhaled NO to inhibit microvascular adhesion of RBCs appears promising but cannot be recommended until large clinical trials determine its efficacy, safety, and proper dose.

Fat Embolization Syndrome

Besides being a common cause of ACS, fat embolization may cause a systemic disorder with neurologic changes, renal failure, petechiae, and multilobe opacities or ARDS. The syndrome usually occurs during an active painful crisis; the circulation of free fatty acids from necrotic bone marrow is implicated in the pathogenesis of diffuse vascular injury that may lead to ARDS and multiorgan failure. Fat globules may be detected in sputum and urine, and bone scan findings usually are positive. The systemic fat embolization syndrome appears to be especially common in patients with hemoglobin SC and in the postpartum period of pregnant women. Treatment is supportive.

Chronic Lung Disease and Pulmonary Hypertension

Progressive, irreversible, and profound lung disease may develop in patients with SC disease, especially in those with recurrent ACS. Undoubtedly, recurrent fat embolization, infarction, and infection all contribute to this syndrome. As the disease progresses, increasing hypoxemia, radiographic evidence of pulmonary fibrosis, and a predominantly restrictive functional impairment develop in patients.

Pulmonary hypertension (PH) is common in patients with SC disease. Mild PH, defined as a pulmonary arterial systolic pressure >35 mm Hg, occurs in approximately 20% of adult patients and severe disease (pulmonary arterial systolic pressure >45 mm Hg) in 10%. The presence of PH is also is associated with a high risk of death. Hemolysis and NO dysregulation play central roles in the development of PH. NO is a soluble gas molecule that is produced by the conversion of L-arginine to citrulline and mediates pulmonary vascular tone through the relaxation of smooth muscle and reduction of the expression of endothelin-1 and endothelin receptor. NO also reduces the endothelial expression of adhesion molecules, decreases platelet activation, and inactivates reactive oxygen species. Hemolysis releases arginase from RBCs, reducing the plasma availability of arginine for NO synthesis; free hemoglobin itself is also an NO scavenger.

Increasing severity of hemolysis, as determined by serum free hemoglobin, lactate dehydrogenase, indirect bilirubin, and blood reticulocyte count, correlates with the increasing risk of developing PH. PH is most often diagnosed by echocardiographic estimation of systolic pressure derived from measurements of the velocity of the tricuspid valvular regurgitant jet. In general, patients with PH should undergo cardiac catheterization both to confirm the diagnosis and to evaluate left ventricular pressures. New therapies under investigation include arginine supplementation and drugs used in the treatment of idiopathic pulmonary arterial hypertension (IPAH).

Liver-Lung Syndromes

Because venous blood flows from the liver to the lungs, these organs are in some ways interdependent. PH may cause hepatic congestion and ascites. Conversely, decreased hepatic synthetic and metabolic function may lead to deranged production and metabolism of vasoactive substances and other mediators that profoundly affect the lung. The major pulmonary complications of liver disease are the so-called *hepatopulmonary syndrome* (HPS), portopulmonary hypertension, α_1-antitrypsin deficiency, and hepatic hydrothorax.

HPS

Liver disease, hypoxemia, and pulmonary vascular abnormalities referred to as *intrapulmonary vascular dilations* constitute the hallmark of HPS. Hypoxemia is caused by precapillary and capillary dilation and pulmonary and pleural arteriovenous anastomoses. The most common presenting symptom is dyspnea, but the presence of stigmata of chronic liver disease (spider nevi, clubbing) and severe hypoxemia strongly suggest the diagnosis. Patients may note platypnea (*ie*, shortness of breath while upright) because of increased shunting of pulmonary blood to the systemic circulation through spider nevi in the lung bases. Arteriovenous shunts are the most important determinant of hypoxemia in patients with severe HPS; these patients may not respond well to the administration of supplemental oxygen. Vascular dilations probably cause hypoxemia by *diffusion-perfusion* impairment, in which oxygen may not diffuse all the way to the center of a dilated pulmonary capillary. Serum that streams through the center of that capillary is therefore unoxygenated. Intrapulmonary vascular dilations may be caused by dysregulated vasoactive mediators leaving the liver and entering the lungs, causing remodeling of the pulmonary vessels. NO is also implicated in the pathogenesis of this disorder. The lungs of patients with cirrhosis generate excessive NO, which in turn leads to vasodilation.

An estimated 15 to 20% of patients with cirrhosis have HPS. It is diagnosed by use of the following criteria: portal hypertension (with or without cirrhosis); arterial hypoxemia (alveolar-arterial oxygen difference, >15 mm Hg); and pulmonary vascular dilation demonstrated by the echocardiographic appearance of microbubbles in the left atrium within three to six cycles after the injection of hand-agitated circulation into a peripheral vein or abnormal brain uptake seen on radionuclide scanning. The most effective treatment for HPS is liver transplantation, which may lead to resolution of hypoxemia after several months.

Long-term oxygen therapy is recommended for patients with HPS, but its usefulness may be limited in the presence of significant shunts. Pharmacologic approaches have been disappointing, and liver transplantation is the only known effective treatment. However, HPS is associated with increased postoperative mortality. A $Pao_2 < 60$ mm Hg is considered to be an indication for transplantation, and patients with this disorder are given high priority on waiting lists.

Portopulmonary Hypertension

Up to 20% of patients with cirrhosis and portal hypertension have modestly increased pulmonary arterial systolic pressures (>25 mm Hg at rest or >30 mm Hg with exercise) that are caused by increased cardiac output despite reduced pulmonary vascular resistance. However, portopulmonary hypertension, with pulmonary vasoconstriction and pathologic changes indistinguishable from IPAH, develops in 1 to 2% of patients with cirrhosis. Criteria for this diagnosis include the presence of liver disease and portal hypertension, pulmonary artery systolic pressure >25 mm Hg, mean pulmonary arterial occlusion pressure <15 mm Hg, and pulmonary vascular resistance >250 dynes · s · cm^{-5}. The diagnostic and treatment strategies are similar to those for IPAH, but less well studied, although hepatotoxicity of some agents (such as bosentan) are of special concern. Unfortunately, and for unknown reasons, the response of patients with portopulmonary hypertension to liver transplantation is unpredictable, and many centers consider severe portopulmonary hypertension to be a contraindication for transplantation.

α_1-Antitrypsin Deficiency

The pulmonary manifestations of this genetic defect are actually the result of a primary hepatic abnormality. With a gene mutation, abnormal α_1-protein levels accumulate in hepatocytes and are not released from the liver. The resulting low circulating concentration of this protective protease inhibitor leads to excessive neutrophil elastase activity in the lungs and the destruction of pulmonary elastic tissue. The section on COPD discusses this disorder in detail.

Hepatic Hydrothorax

Some patients have congenital anatomic defects in the diaphragm. If ascites develops, the positive infradiaphragmatic pressure moves fluid through these defects into the negative-pressure pleural space, causing the accumulation of pleural fluid with the same characteristics as the ascites. This condition is referred to as *hepatic hydrothorax*. Pleural fluid is typically a transudate and occurs more often on the right side than the left. Spontaneous bacterial empyema may occur with or without spontaneous bacterial peritonitis. The initial treatment is directed at reducing the volume of ascites by the restriction if salt and the administration of diuretics. Thoracentesis may be helpful to relieve dyspnea and hypoxemia acutely; however, the fluid usually reaccumulates. Chest tube drainage is often hazardous because ascitic fluid translocates rapidly into the pleural space, leading to volume depletion and electrolyte abnormalities. Pleurodesis is generally unsuccessful because the fluid usually reaccumulates too rapidly for the pleural surfaces to come together and adhere. Surgical repair of diaphragmatic defects by videothoracoscopy can be attempted, but few centers are experienced in performing the procedure, and the results often are disappointing.

Peritoneovenous shunts usually are not successful in patients with hepatic hydrothorax because the pleural space has a lower pressure than the venous system and because fluid moves preferentially to the pleural space. The transjugular intrahepatic portosystemic shunt is an option in patients who have recurrent hydrothorax despite receiving diuretic therapy and undergoing repeated thoracenteses. The best treatment for refractory hepatic hydrothorax is liver transplantation.

Oxygen Toxicity

Oxygen is necessary for life, but it also has the potential to be toxic through the generation of free-radical intermediates. A balance of oxidative and antioxidant processes maintains life while maintaining organ function. Our knowledge of oxygen toxicity is largely inferred from experimental data obtained from other mammalian species and from clinical observations.

Mechanisms of Oxygen-Induced Injury

The stepwise reduction of oxygen to water produces free radicals that in turn are injurious to tissues. These include the superoxide anion ($-O_2^-$), hydrogen peroxide (H_2O_2), and hydroxyl radical species ($-OH^-$). The latter is among the most reactive biological molecules known and is capable of damaging almost any component of living cells. Oxygen radicals have a beneficial role because they are used by neutrophils during phagocytosis and the killing of bacteria and may be important mediators of vascular tone by interacting with NO. However, unopposed hyperoxia promotes the excessive production of these molecules (termed *oxidative stress*), leading to damage to cellular and lysosomal membranes and in turn increasing cell permeability, releasing lysosomal proteolytic enzymes, inactivating cellular enzymes, and damaging DNA. Thus, many cells that are exposed to sufficient oxidative stress stop dividing and die, some by entering apoptotic pathways and committing "suicide," others by oxidation-induced necrosis. This may be the case with ischemia-reperfusion injury in patients with myocardial infarction and stroke. The recruitment of neutrophils augments tissue injury by releasing radicals when activated.

Oxidant injury is opposed by antioxidant mechanisms. Intracellular enzymes that reduce oxidant activity include superoxide dismutase (eliminates superoxide anion), catalase (metabolizes H_2O_2), and glutathione peroxidases (reduces levels of H_2O_2 and lipid peroxides). Vitamin E inhibits lipid peroxidation in membranes, and deficiencies of vitamin E result in the increased susceptibility of cells to oxidant injury.

The lung and capillary endothelium are the only tissues that can be exposed to high concentrations of oxygen because other tissues consume more oxygen than is dissolved in the blood. Thus, lung cells may be exposed to a Po_2 of >600 mm Hg in a pure oxygen atmosphere under normobaric conditions, but other tissues are rarely exposed to oxygen tensions that are >10 mm Hg above normal because dissolved O_2 accounts for $<10\%$ of total O_2 content.

Other factors may influence the degree of injury on exposure to O_2. Previous exposure stimulates the production of antioxidant enzymes, conferring protection at the next exposure. In experimental models, endotoxin also induces antioxidant enzyme activity and increases tolerance to high concentrations of O_2. Conversely, drugs and toxins enhance lung injury caused by oxygen. Hyperoxia and bleomycin exert synergistic toxic effects on the lung, probably because bleomycin increases the generation of free O_2 radicals. Amiodarone, nitrofurantoin, mitomycin, and paraquat also potentiate hyperoxic injury. NO combines with O_2^- to form the peroxynitrite anion ONOO, which is potentially extremely toxic.

Clinical Manifestations of Pulmonary Oxygen Toxicity

Patients may notice retrosternal pain after inhaling pure oxygen for a few hours, and tracheobronchitis is found in biopsy specimens. Mucociliary velocity is impaired, possibly as the result of damage to ciliated airway epithelium. It is difficult to diagnose parenchymal oxygen toxicity in humans because the clinical picture is always obscured by the disease that prompted the need for oxygen therapy. In experimental models, damage to type I pneumocytes increases permeability and leads to the recruitment of inflammatory cells into capillaries and alveolar septae. The alveolar epithelium may undergo extensive necrosis with hyaline membrane formation and be replaced with proliferating type II cells. With ongoing injury, fibrosis ensues. These changes are morphologically indistinguishable from ARDS as the result of other causes.

What Is a "Safe" Concentration of Oxygen?

There is no treatment for oxygen-induced lung injury; therefore, the best strategy should be to prevent it by minimizing exposure. However, no safe threshold has been established in humans. The question is in some ways misguided because any concentration is potentially harmful in the absence of adequate antioxidant defenses. In studies of experimental lung injury, even 50% O_2 enhances lung damage, and that concentration is the threshold at which the replication of human pulmonary epithelial cells is inhibited. In patients who received bleomycin, any supplemental O_2 is deemed to be potentially hazardous. For general clinical management, most clinicians assume that a fraction of inspired oxygen of ≤ 0.5 is safe, even for prolonged periods, but this has not been established convincingly.

Pulmonary Radiation Injury

Radiation is intentionally given to the lung in the treatment of lung cancer and cannot be avoided in radiation therapy of cancers of the esophagus and breast. The lungs are exposed in mantle radiation of the mediastinum for lymphoma, and the lungs are the dose-limiting tissue for whole-body irradiation in preparation for bone marrow transplantation. Killing tumor cells is accompanied by the destruction of surrounding normal lung tissue, leading to the following two clinical syndromes: radiation pneumonitis and radiation fibrosis. Although many patients who receive radiotherapy have radiographic changes, symptoms develop only in approximately 5%. With advances in combined chemotherapy and radiation therapy for cancers, this disorder should become even less common.

Pathogenesis

Radiation causes the death of cells in mitosis. Type II pneumocytes and capillary endothelial cells have the greatest turnover rates and are, therefore, the most susceptible to radiation injury. Histopathologic changes include edema and increased permeability of small vessels and capillaries, followed by the obstruction by platelets, fibrin, and collagen. Damage to type II pneumocytes leads to the formation of hyaline membranes, followed by hyperplasia and interstitial fibrosis. Tissue injury also causes a cytokine response that recruits immune cells to perpetuate the inflammatory response and subsequent reparative fibrosing process.

Predisposing Factors

The magnitude of lung injury depends on several factors:

1. Irradiated volume of lung tissue: The risk of pneumonitis increases with the volume of exposed lung.
2. Total dose: The total dose of radiation predicts the development of radiation fibrosis better than pneumonitis. There is a steep dose–response relationship; <30 Gy is usually well tolerated, >40 Gy almost always causes radiographic changes, and >50 Gy almost always causes symptomatic lung injury.
3. Fraction size: Dividing the total dose over time reduces the risk of lung injury.

4. Previous irradiation increases the risk.
5. Chemotherapy may potentiate radiation damage. The classic example is bleomycin.
6. Withdrawal of therapy with corticosteroids may lead to overt pneumonitis when subclinical lung injury becomes overt.

Radiation Pneumonitis

After a latent period of up to 6 months, dyspnea (the most common symptom), dry cough, pleuritic chest pain, and fever may develop. The physical examination findings usually are normal. A progression of chest radiographic findings is typical, manifesting as ground-glass opacities that may progress to consolidation, coalescing to form a sharply demarcated opacity corresponding to the field of radiation. Radiographic changes may occur outside the radiation field, perhaps attributable to a lymphocyte-mediated hypersensitivity reaction. Pleural effusions are observed occasionally.

Most patients with radiation pneumonitis have mild symptoms and require no therapy. Although controlled studies in humans are lacking, animal data and clinical experience indicate that therapy with corticosteroids is an effective treatment in patients with more severe disease. The optimal dose is unknown; prednisone, approximately 60 mg/d, is recommended, followed by a gradually tapered dose. The disease may flare during a steroid taper. There is no effective treatment for radiation-induced fibrosis.

Radiation Fibrosis

When lung injury is chronic, fibrosis may occur. This fibrosis usually is not apparent until at least 6 months after exposure, may take up to 2 years to evolve, and generally remains stable thereafter. The symptoms depend on the extent and severity of fibrosis, ranging from no symptoms to severe dyspnea, hypoxemia, and death. Mediastinal fibrosis may cause superior vena cava syndrome or constrictive pericarditis, and exposure of the coronary arteries to the beam may cause obstruction. Severe fibrosis may occur in the absence of clinically apparent pneumonitis. The chest radiograph typically shows volume loss in the affected areas. Bronchiectasis and pleural thickening are common findings on CT scans. At times, confluent fibrosis may be difficult to distinguish from the recurrence of a tumor.

Smoke Inhalation

Smoke generated in a fire is a suspension of particles and toxic gases in hot air. Fire victims may experience a variety of inhalation injuries, including thermal injury to the airways and the effects of inhaling carbon monoxide (CO) and other products of combustion.

Thermal and Toxic Injury

The same high temperatures that burn the skin may injure the upper airways, and inhalation injury is an important predictor of mortality in burn victims. The peripheral airways and alveoli are not burned unless steam is inhaled because the heat is dissipated centrally. Along with hot air, soot and toxic gases also are inhaled. Upper airway obstruction caused by laryngeal edema or spasm may be severe, especially in patients with facial burns. Smoke inhalation is associated with bronchospasm, impaired mucociliary function, mucus hypersecretion, inflammation, and edema. The expectoration of soot with sputum reflects smoke inhalation but not necessarily airway injury.

The chest radiograph findings usually are normal at the time of presentation. Therefore, fiberoptic laryngoscopy and bronchoscopy should be performed to assess the degree and extent of airway damage in patients with suspected airway injury. Even if the airway is not grossly compromised at the time of the initial examination, inflammation and edema usually progress during the first 24 to 48 h. The presence of edema and blistering should prompt intubation, but if the airway appears uninjured, then the patient should be observed closely. In the absence of a significant airway burn, intubated patients can usually be extubated safely after a few days, when the edema subsides. Corticosteroid administration does not attenuate the course of pulmonary injury and increases the risk of infection and death.

With improvements in burn wound management, pneumonia is now the most common cause of infection in burn units and is a very common cause of death. Pathogens associated with nosocomial pneumonia, especially *Pseudomonas aeruginosa*, are also common in burn patients. Herpes simplex tracheobronchitis is common, perhaps due to direct extension from an oral source in patients who are immunocompromised due to severe burn injury.

CO Poisoning

The inhalation of CO is the most common cause of unintentional poisoning death in the United States. CO is produced by the incomplete combustion of carbonaceous materials in the presence of a decrease in ambient oxygen. Fires, automobile exhaust, and unvented coal, kerosene, and wood-burning stoves and fireplaces are the most common causes of CO poisoning.

CO competes with O_2 for hemoglobin binding sites. Its affinity is >200 times greater than that of O_2, and CO shifts on the oxyhemoglobin binding curve to the left. The result is decreased O_2 content of arterial blood and decreased O_2 release to the tissues, leading to tissue hypoxia. In addition, CO binds to proteins and increases production of free radicals that injure tissues and impair mitochondrial function and oxygen utilization. Pao_2 may be normal, and pulse oximetry overestimates arterial oxygen saturation because most devices do not reliably distinguish oxyhemoglobin from carboxyhemoglobin. However, direct measurement of arterial oxygen saturation and content are reduced. The major signs of CO poisoning are CNS and cardiac disturbances, and patients with severe CO poisoning (>40%) may have severe lactic acidosis.

CO measurements may be used to guide treatment, but they do not necessarily correlate with clinical abnormalities, especially when measured hours after exposure. In asymptomatic persons, levels up to 20% may require no treatment, but because normobaric oxygen is inexpensive, easily available, and generally considered to be safe, some authorities recommend its administration with a goal of lower CO levels to <5%. The use of 100% oxygen reduces the half-life of CO in the blood from around 5 hours to 80 minutes. The role of hyperbaric oxygen is controversial, but most experts recommend therapy with hyperbaric oxygen in severe cases (*ie*, CO >40%, coma or other CNS dysfunction, arrhythmia, or cardiac ischemia). Hyperbaric oxygen treatment hastens the resolution of acute symptoms, and there are some studies that support the notion that it protects the patient against the development of delayed neuropsychiatric dysfunction, although this issue remains a contentious one.

After apparent recovery from the initial intoxication, cognitive and personality changes, Parkinsonism, incontinence, dementia, or psychosis develop in approximately 25 to 50% of patients within the next few weeks. The delayed neuropsychiatric syndrome appears not to be directly related to cerebral ischemia alone; postischemic reperfusion injury, the effects of CO on vascular endothelium, and oxygen radical-mediated brain lipid peroxidation also may play a role. The lack of availability of hyperbaric chambers, concerns about the risks of transporting critically ill patients to hyperbaric facilities, and the lack of optimal patient selection criteria and treatment regimens still limit the use of this therapeutic modality.

Methemoglobinemia

Another effect of oxygen on metabolism comes through its interaction with iron; oxidizing agents convert the ferrous iron (Fe^{2+}) in hemoglobin to the ferric form (Fe^{3+}), creating methemoglobin. When oxidizing agents are administered in excess or to patients with deficiency in enzyme systems that convert methemoglobin to hemoglobin, toxic levels of methemoglobin may develop. This molecule has a much greater affinity for oxygen than oxyhemoglobin, reducing the oxygen content of arterial blood. The presence of methemoglobin also shifts the oxyhemoglobin curve to the left. Thus, both the decreased oxygen content of arterial blood and the increased affinity of oxygen for hemoglobin lead to reduced tissue oxygenation and the symptoms associated with methemoglobinemia. Cyanosis generally develops in patients at methemoglobin levels of approximately 15%, symptoms develop at levels of approximately 30%, and mental status changes at levels of approximately 50%. Methemoglobin levels <70% usually are fatal.

Commonly used drugs are oxidants, which include metoclopramide, chloroquine, dapsone, local anesthetics (*eg*, benzocaine and lidocaine), nitrates (*eg*, nitroglycerin, nitroprusside, and NO), and sulfonamides; however, their use may cause methemoglobinemia in susceptible patients. High levels of methemoglobin turn blood brown, and the blood does not turn red when exposed to air.

Pulse oximetry is inaccurate in the diagnosis because the peak absorbance of methemoglobin is at 631 nm, whereas pulse oximetry estimates oxygen saturations at wavelengths of 660 and 940 nm. Pulse oximeters may read falsely high oxyhemoglobin levels, and when methemoglobin levels of approximately 30% are detected, the oximeter tends to read the oxygen saturation at a value of approximately 85%. A clue to the diagnosis in this case is the finding of a high Pa_{O_2} at the same time that the pulse oximeter reads 85%. The diagnosis is established using cooximetry, which measures oxyhemoglobin, deoxyhemoglobin, carboxyhemoglobin, and methemoglobin as percentages of total hemoglobin.

Treatment usually is indicated for patients with methemoglobin levels of >30%. Methylene blue is a cofactor of nicotinamide adenine dinucleotide phosphate-methemoglobin-reductase and increases the capacity of that enzyme to reduce to ferric iron levels. The usual dose is 1 to 2 mg/kg for over 5 min; methylene blue may increase methemoglobin levels in doses of >15 mg/kg and in patients with glucose-6-diphosphate deficiency.

Annotated Bibliography

SC Pulmonary Syndromes

Bellet PS, Kalinyak KA, Shukla R, et al. Incentive spirometry to prevent acute pulmonary complications in sickle cell diseases. N Engl J Med 1995; 333:699–703
Forty percent of patients with SC disease and chest pain had thoracic bone infarction. Pulmonary complications (atelectasis and infiltrates) were much less frequent in a group randomized to be treated with incentive spirometry compared with those who were not. This finding suggests that atelectasis is an important factor in the development of ACS.

Gladwin MT, Sachdev V, Jison ML, et al. Pulmonary hypertension as a risk factor for death in patients with sickle cell disease. N Engl J Med 2004; 350:886–895
Describes the incidence and poor prognosis of PH complicating SC disease and its relationship to the severity of hemolysis.

Gladwin MT, Vichinsky E. Pulmonary complications of sickle cell disease. N Engl J Med 2008; 359:2254–2265
Recent and thorough review of mechanisms and clinical features of ACS and PH. The authors propose a model of pulmonary complications in SC disease as driven by either vaso-occlusion or the effects of intravascular hemolysis on endothelial cell and vascular function.

Morris CR, Kato GJ, Poljakovic M. Dysregulated arginine metabolism, hemolysis-associated pulmonary hypertension and mortality in sickle cell disease. JAMA 2005; 294:81–90
This investigation supports the hypothesis that hemolysis drives the development of PH in patients with SC disease by release of arginase and hemoglobin from RBCs.

Powars DR, Weidman JA, Odon-Maryon T, et al. Sickle cell chronic lung disease: prior morbidity and the risk of pulmonary failure. Medicine (Baltimore) 1988; 67:66–76
Describes a progressive syndrome of irreversible pulmonary disease that may lead to profound hypoxemia, PH, cor pulmonale, and death. The risk of the development of chronic lung disease increases with the number of episodes of ACS and painful crises.

Vichinsky EP, Neumayr LD, Earles AN, et al. Causes and outcomes of the acute chest syndrome in sickle cell disease. N Engl J Med 2000; 342:1855–1865
Multicenter study of 671 episodes of ACS in 583 patients that demonstrates the importance of fat embolism and pulmonary infection with atypical pathogens and shows that respiratory failure and neurologic disorders are common complications. Packed RBC transfusions and bronchodilators improve oxygenation.

Vichinsky EP, Styles LA, Colangelo LH, et al. Acute chest syndrome in sickle cell disease: Clinical presentation and course. Blood 1997; 89:1787–1792
Prospective study of >1,700 episodes of ACS. Adults are often afebrile and report dyspnea, chills, and severe pain, usually after a vaso-occlusive event. Cases are more common in winter; respiratory failure generally rapidly develops in patients with fatal cases of ACS, and one-third of fatal cases are bacteremic.

Liver–Lung Syndromes

de Campos JRM, Filho LOA, Werebe EC, et al. Thoracoscopy and talc poudrage in the management of hepatic hydrothorax. Chest 2000; 118:13–17
This procedure was effective in approximately 50% of cases and associated with a high 3-month mortality.

Deibert P, Allgaier HP, Loesch D, et al. Hepatopulmonary syndrome in patients with chronic liver disease: role of pulse oximetry. BMC Gastroenterol 2006; 6:15
An arterial oxygen saturation of ≤92% in the supine position and/or a decrease of ≥4% after a change to the

upright position correlated strongly with the presence of HPS.

Garcia N, Mihas AA. Hepatic hydrothorax: Pathophysiology, diagnosis and management. J Clin Gastroenterol 2004; 38:52–58

Useful review of current concepts.

Lazaridis KN, Frank JW, Krowka MJ, et al. Hepatic hydrothorax: Pathogenesis, diagnosis and management. Am J Med 1999; 107:262–267

A thorough review with useful algorithms for diagnosis and treatment.

Rodriguez-Roisin R, Krowka MJ. Hepatopulmonary syndrome—a liver-induced lung vascular disorder. N Engl J Med 2008; 358:2378–2387

Thorough review of the mechanisms, clinical features, diagnosis, and treatment.

Rodriguez-Roisin R, Krowka MJ. Herve P, et al. Pulmonary-hepatic vascular disorders. Eur Respir J 2004; 24:861–880

Reviews hepatopulmonary syndrome and portopulmonary hypertension, with recommendations for diagnosis and treatment by an expert task force.

Oxygen Toxicity

Crapo JD. Morphologic changes in pulmonary oxygen toxicity. Annu Rev Physiol 1986; 48:721–731

Review of the histopathology associated with oxygen pulmonary injury.

Gaston B, Drazen JM, Loscalzo J, et al. The biology of nitrogen oxides in the airways. Am J Respir Crit Care Med 1994; 149:538–551

NO may combine with oxygen radicals to form highly toxic compounds. Enthusiasm for NO therapy should be tempered until its efficacy and safety are established.

Heffner JE, Repine JE. State of the art: Pulmonary strategies of antioxidant defense. Am Rev Respir Dis 1989; 140:531–554

Review of antioxidant mechanisms that prevent hyperoxic injury.

Ingrassia TS 3rd, Ryu JH, Trastek VF, et al. Oxygen-exacerbated bleomycin pulmonary toxicity. Mayo Clin Proc 1991; 66:173–178

Even "acceptable" levels of O_2 supplementation potentiate bleomycin lung toxicity.

Pryor WA, Houk KN, Foote CS, et al. Free radical biology and medicine: It's a gas, man! Am J Physiol Regul Integr Comp Physiol 2006; 291:R491–R511

A thorough review of oxygen and the mechanisms of radical generation and oxidative stress.

Repine JE, Bast A, Lankhorst I, et al. Oxidative stress in chronic obstructive pulmonary disease. Am J Respir Crit Care Med 1997; 156:341–357

This "state of the art" article develops the hypothesis that oxidant-antioxidant disturbances are pivotal to the development of lung injury in patients with COPD.

Radiation Injury

Arbetter KR, Prakash UBS, Tazelaar HD, et al. Radiation-induced pneumonitis in the "nonirradiated" lung. Mayo Clin Proc 1999; 74:27–36

Six cases, with excellent radiographs. Patients had histology of bronchiolitis obliterans organizing pneumonia, suggesting an immunologic mechanism.

Choi YW, Munden RF, Erasmus JJ, et al. Effects of radiation therapy on the lung: radiographic appearances and differential diagnosis. Radiographics 2004; 24: 985–997

Review of radiation techniques and types of radiation-induced injury, with excellent images.

Roach M 3rd, Gandara DR, You HS, et al. Radiation pneumonitis following combined modality therapy for lung cancer: Analysis of prognostic factors. J Clin Oncol 1995; 13:2606–2612

Results of a retrospective analysis of almost 2,000 patients from 24 series. The daily fraction size, number of daily fractions, and total dose were associated with the risk of radiation pneumonitis.

Roberts CM, Foulcher E, Zaunders JJ, et al. Radiation pneumonitis: a possible lymphocyte-mediated hypersensitivity reaction. Ann Intern Med 1993; 118:696–700

After unilateral radiotherapy for breast carcinoma, patients with pneumonitis had similar increased BAL fluid lymphocyte counts and gallium uptake in both lungs. Treatment of a hypersensitivity reaction may account for the effectiveness of therapy with corticosteroids in radiation pneumonitis.

Smoke Inhalation and CO

Cobb N, Etzel RA. Unintentional carbon monoxide-related deaths in the United States, 1979 through 1988. JAMA 1991; 266:659–663

Improvements in the insulation of homes often lead to poor ventilation. Coupled with the use of coal, kerosene, and wood in stoves and fireplaces, the risk of CO poisoning increases.

Ernst A, Zibrak JD. Carbon monoxide poisoning. N Engl J Med 1998; 39:1603–1608

Excellent, concise review.

Hampson NB. Pulse oximetry in severe carbon monoxide poisoning. Chest 1998; 114:1036–1041

Pulse oximetry overestimates oxygen saturation in CO poisoning.

Hantson P, Butera R, Clemessy J, et al. Early complications and value of initial and paraclinical observations in victims of smoke inhalation without burns. Chest 1997; 111:671–675

Emphasizes the value of laryngoscopy in patients with smoke inhalation.

Masanes MJ, Legendre C, Lioret N, et al. Fiberoptic bronchoscopy for the early diagnosis of subglottal inhalation injury: comparative value in the assessment of prognosis. J Trauma 1994; 36:59–67

Bronchoscopy was more reliable in the immediate diagnosis of inhalational airway disorders than clinical, laboratory, and radiographic findings. It was also the strongest predictor of the development of ARDS and death.

Ryan CM, Schoenfeld DA, Thorpe WP, et al. Objective estimates of the probability of death from burn injuries. N Engl J Med 1998; 338:362–366

In a retrospective review of 1,665 patients with acute burn injuries, three risk factors for death were identified: age > 60 years, >40% of body surface area burned, and inhalation injury. When all three risk factors are present, the mortality rate was 90%.

Shirani KZ, Pruitt BA, Mason AD. The influence of inhalational injury and pneumonia on burn mortality. Ann Surg 1987; 205:82–87

In a US Army Institute of Surgical Research study, pneumonia was present in 55% of burn patients who died and was a major predictor of excess mortality.

Weaver LK. Carbon monoxide poisoning. N Engl J Med 2009; 360:1217–1225

Review of mechanisms, clinical features, and treatment, with helpful illustrations.

Weaver LK, Hopkins RO, Chan KJ, et al. Hyperbaric oxygen for acute carbon monoxide poisoning. N Engl J Med 2002; 347:1057–1067

Three hyperbaric oxygen treatments reduced the incidence of the delayed emergence of cognitive dysfunction by almost 50% compared with a control group. Optimal patient selection criteria and treatment regimens need more investigation.

Methemoglobinemia

Karim A, Ahmed S, Siddiqui R, et al. Methemoglobinemia complicating topical lidocaine used during endoscopic procedures. Am J Med 2001; 111:150–153

König MW, Dolinski SY. A 74-year-old woman with desaturation following surgery. Chest 2003; 123:613–616

Novaro GM, Aronow HD, Militello MA, et al. Benzocaine-induced methemoglobinemia: experience from a high-volume transesophageal echocardiography laboratory. J Am Soc Echocardiogr 2003; 16:170–175

These articles discuss the mechanisms of methemoglobinemia and common clinical situations in which they may occur.

Medical Statistics/Test-Taking Strategies

David W. Kamp, MD, FCCP

Objectives:

- Understand and analyze how well a clinical test "performs" in diagnosis
- Comprehend the "how" and "why" one test is better than another
- Review how we should use test results to help make medical decisions
- Summarize recommendations for successful test-taking strategies

Key words: medical statistics; probability; receiver operator curves

Introduction

A firm understanding of medical statistics is vitally important for interpreting the medical literature, yet it often is perceived as a mysterious science. This was nicely captured in Mark Twain's infamous remark regarding statistics: "There are lies; damn lies and statistics." Because many physicians lack the necessary skills in statistical analysis to adequately assess the quality and conclusions of studies, medical decisions may be impaired.[1] For example, only 18% of medical students, residents, and attending physicians at several teaching hospitals correctly answered a simple hypothetical problem that involved decision analysis. Berwick et al[2] administered a simple statistics test to medical students, residents, private attending physicians, and academic attending physicians and found that the percentages of correct answers were 73%, 70%, 55%, and 74%, respectively. A more recent study[3] found that 59% of 277 medical residents had trouble performing basic numerical tasks that translated into difficulty interpreting medical literature. Thus, physicians require a better understanding of the fundamentals of medical statistics. There are many detailed resources, including Web-based materials, which are available to enhance the understanding of medical statistics.[4,5] This chapter reviews the basic principles underlying medical statistics that are clinically relevant as well as important for taking pulmonary boards.

An important concept about statistics is that it does not define "truth" but rather, when used correctly, it allows a sense of what the truth is based on (*ie*, the data and assumptions that have been used). Every statistical test has important assumptions underlying its validity. Although some statistical tests are fairly rigorous (*ie*, insensitive to the violation of assumptions), the results will be questionable if an incorrect statistical test is used. Study design is the most important aspect of the science of statistics. Minor study flaws (*eg*, randomization, use of appropriate controls, and double blinding) will limit confidence in the results that have been analyzed, even those that use the proper statistical tests.

For example, an analysis[6] of 250 controlled trials found that studies with inadequate concealment had a 41% greater treatment effect compared with those in trials with adequately concealed treatment allocation and that studies that were not double-blinded had a 17% greater treatment effect compared with those in double-blinded studies. In an analysis of 32 studies, van Nieuwenhoven et al[7] found an inverse relationship between the quality of the methods and the benefit of the selective decontamination of the digestive tract on the incidence of ventilator-associated pneumonia. Thus, studies with the most appropriate methodologic design demonstrate the least benefit of selective decontamination of the gut on the incidence of ventilator-associated pneumonia and, as such, strongly argue against such a policy.

Another important example is illustrated in studies published in the 1980s and 1990s suggesting that there is a pathologic supply dependence of oxygen utilization in which, unlike the normal situation, oxygen uptake ($\dot{V}o_2$) increased as oxygen delivery (Do_2) increased. This finding led to a decade in which critical care physicians regularly used hemodynamic monitoring in patients with sepsis in an attempt to increase Do_2 to supranormal levels so as to improve $\dot{V}o_2$. However, these conclusions turned out to be incorrect based on an artifact derived from improper methodology in which Do_2 and $\dot{V}o_2$ were each calculated from measurements containing a common variable, cardiac output (CO) (*ie*, $Do_2 = CO \times Cao_2$; $\dot{V}o_2 = CO(Cao_2 - C\dot{V}o_2)$, where Cao_2 is the oxygen content or the arterial blood whereas $C\dot{V}o_2$ is the oxygen content or the venous blood.

Basic Terminology

The purpose of medical statistics is to understand the "true" effect in the general population on the basis of the results of a single experiment in a limited population sample (*eg*, the effect on FEV_1 of methacholine). The basic assumption of all studies is that the underlying truth can be "estimated" from a single, properly designed experiment. Because we cannot possibly measure the FEV_1 response to methacholine in the entire population, we must use statistics. Expressed another way, there would be no need for statistics if we could measure the end point of interest in the entire population. Because statistics must be used to evaluate study populations of interest, many important issues regarding study samples (*eg*, size and selection/exclusion criteria) must be carefully considered in determining how relevant the data are to the general population.

Any measured parameter has some distribution within a study population (*eg*, Gaussian, uniform, skewed right, skewed left, bimodal, u-shaped, exponential, and others). A Gaussian distribution is defined as a symmetric, unimodal, bell-shaped distribution with a size and shape in patients with and without disease that may be completely distinct or may nearly totally overlap (Fig 1). There are statistical tests for assessing whether a sampled variable has been drawn from a population with an underlying Gaussian distribution. Occasionally, a non-Gaussian distribution can be transformed to be Gaussian (*ie*, a logarithmic transformation of data skewed to the right, such as length of stay in the ICU), which facilitates parametric statistical tests on the data. The assumption that data have a particular distribution is important and prone to error, but when it is true, it greatly simplifies statistical testing.

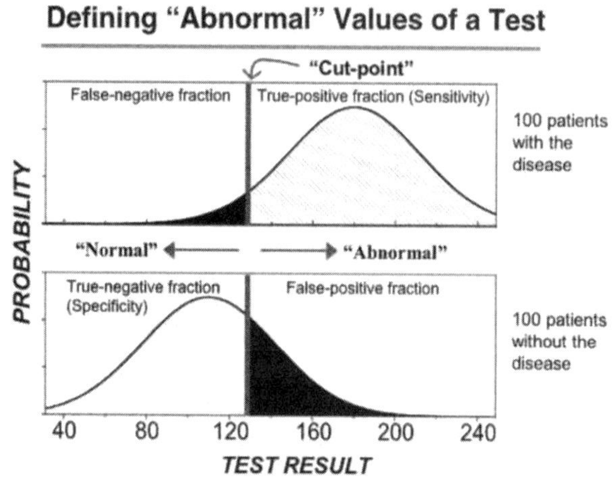

Figure 1. Defining "abnormal" values of a test.

The primary aim of most statistical analyses is the comparison of the central tendency between different groups. To do this, there are some fundamental statistical terms that physicians must understand, including the following:

- *Variable:* defined as the things that are measured or manipulated in research. Most research belongs to one of two general categories, correlational or experimental. In correlational research, the variables are not manipulated but are only measured to determine relations (correlations) between some set of variables (*eg*, FEV_1 and age). Correlational research does not enable causal relationships to be established. In experimental research, some variables are manipulated, and then the effects of this manipulation on other variables are assessed (*eg*, studies examining the effects of varying doses of methacholine on FEV_1). Experimental data are the only conclusive way to demonstrate causal relations between variables. For example, we can infer that "A influences B" if alterations in variable A result in predictable changes in variable B. Independent variables are those items that are manipulated in the experimental research, whereas dependent variables are those items that are only measured and are never manipulated experimentally.
- *Mean:* defined as the average $= (\Sigma X_1)/N$, where X_1 is a symbol referring to the N individual values of your distribution. Thus, the first value in the distribution would be X_1, the second would be X_2, and so on until the last value, X_N.

- *Median:* defined as the value of X such that 50% of the values are higher and 50% are lower. The advantage of using the median is that it is not as influenced by data outliers. For symmetric distributions (including Gaussian), mean equals median. For distributions that are skewed to the high side (*eg*, length of stay in the ICU) the mean is greater than the median (*eg*, a few patients with a very long length of stay will substantially move the mean upward but will have very little if any impact on the median, which gives us a more accurate indication of the length of stay for most patients).
- *Percentile:* defined such that of all the values under consideration, Z% are less than that, so that (100 – Z)% are greater than that. For example, the fact that your 2006 pulmonary board scores are in the 95th percentile indicates that 95% of all other scores are worse than your scores. In contrast, an extramural grant score of 150 that is in the 5th percentile indicates that only 5% of grants have lower scores that are better (similar to golf, in which low scores are better in grading grants). The median is the 50th percentile, whereas we often also look at the 25th and 75th percentiles.
- *Variance:* defined as a measure of the "spread" of the data distribution. It is determined numerically by $(\Sigma(X_i - \langle X \rangle)^2 / (N - 1)$, in which $\langle X \rangle$ is defined as the population mean.
- *SD:* defined as $(\text{variance})^{1/2}$. The SD is a commonly used measure of data variation. Only when a data set has a Gaussian distribution is it true that 95% of values in the sample fall with in ± 2 SDs of the mean. The SEM, which also often is used to express data variance, is the theoretical SD of all sample means of size n that are derived from a population.
- *Sensitivity:* defined as the fraction of those with the disease whose test result is positive (*ie*, greater than the cut point). It is also known as the *true-positive fraction*, which is defined numerically as (TP/ [TP + FN]), where TP is the *true-positive result* and FN is the *false-negative result* (Fig 1). It is also defined as (1 – FN fraction). For example, if 95 of 100 patients with asthma have a positive methacholine challenge result, then the sensitivity of the methacholine challenge in detecting patients with asthma is 95%. A high sensitivity means few FN results.
- *Specificity:* defined as the fraction of those persons without the disease who have a negative test result (*ie*, less than the cut point). It is also known as the *true negative fraction*, which is defined numerically as (TN/[TN + FP]) in which TN is the *true-negative result* and FP is the *false-positive* (Fig 1). It is also defined as (1 – FP fraction). For example, if 25 of 100 patients without asthma have a positive methacholine challenge result, then the specificity of the methacholine challenge is 75% (75/[75 + 25]). A high specificity means few FP results.
- *The null hypothesis:* the hypothesis states that the means of two data sets in the underlying population are identical (*ie*, difference between means = 0). Statistical testing is performed to either support or refute the null hypothesis. The *null hypothesis accepted* is the same as saying that there is "no statistically significant difference" between the two groups. The *null hypothesis rejected* is the same as saying that is highly likely that there is a "statistically significant difference" between the two groups.

In summary, when interpreting data sets, it is important to identify the central tendency as well as the spread of the distribution. For Gaussian distributions, the data typically are expressed as the mean ± SD. For most other distributions, the data are better expressed as the median and interquartile range (*ie*, 25th/50th/75th percentiles). For very small samples, the minimum and maximum values (range) should be listed. Sensitivity is used for ruling out disease, especially as a screening tool, whereas specificity is used to rule in disease. Some useful mnemonics include the following: "snout" for sensitivity (rules out disease), and "spin" for specificity (rules in disease). For example, the d-dimer test often is used to rule out the presence of pulmonary embolism (PE) in patients who have not undergone recent surgery or who have cancer or liver disease because of its high sensitivity, whereas, when the d-dimer test result is positive, the PE protocol chest CT scan or, less commonly pulmonary angiogram, is used because of the high specificity of the test. Finally, beware of data outliers since these grossly distort distributions and statistical test results that are based on the mean.

Hypothesis Testing

Statistics often are performed to assess samples or a set of samples that are taken from the study population to make assumptions about the entire population. For measuring a continuous variable (*eg*, FEV_1), one should determine whether the population has a Gaussian distribution. Statistical comparisons of means within samples is based on the principle that if you took the mean value of FEV_1 in a random sample of N members of the whole population and do this many times ($N > 50 - 100$), then the distribution of sampling means will be Gaussian regardless of the distribution in the underlying population (*ie*, the central limit theorem). Because we do not typically generate numerous samples but rather use one such sample for each arm of the study (*eg*, the FEV_1 response to methacholine in healthy patients vs patients with asthma) to compare the means of these samples and use statistical methods to make inferences about the truth in the underlying populations (*ie*, to identify patients who are healthy or who have asthma).

Hypothesis testing begins with the null hypothesis that the means of the two groups in the underlying population are identical. Statistical testing will either refute or confirm this hypothesis. Because these are independent samples from the population, even if the null hypothesis is true, it is not likely that the two samples will have identical means. Therefore, we use the sampling distribution to tell us how unlikely it is that two samples that are drawn from the same populations will have a difference in the size observed. This is done by picking some arbitrary threshold for believing that the likelihood that the two samples are from the same population is sufficiently small that we think it is acceptable to conclude that they are probably not. An arbitrary threshold of 5% ($p < 0.05$) is usually used (called the *type I error* or *α level error*). However, there may be circumstances in which one accepts as a relevant statistically significant difference a p value of >0.05 and others in which a clinically relevant effect may not be accepted unless the p value were much <0.05 (*ie*, $p < 0.01$, in which there is an arbitrary threshold of a 1% chance that the samples are identical). A study that fails to achieve statistical significance does not prove the null hypothesis but rather simply says that the data do not provide sufficient evidence to reject it.

Student t Test for Comparing Means

The Student *t* test is a parametric test that is used to compare a continuous, metric variable (*eg*, FEV_1) within two groups or the effect of two alternative treatments in a single group. This test assumes that either the underlying population distribution is Gaussian or that N is large enough that the distribution of sampling means is Gaussian. An unpaired *t* test should be used if there are different persons in the two groups (*eg*, separate groups of normal patients and asthma patients) to examine <FEV_1 normal> vs <FEV_1 asthma>, with the null hypothesis being <FEV_1 normal> = <FEV_1 asthma>. However, a paired *t* test should be used if instead the experiment gives placebo and albuterol to the *same* patients at different times (preferably in random order) to determine whether <FEV_1 placebo> – <FEV_1 albuterol> is zero (null hypothesis accepted). The specific question of interest determines whether differences between groups should be assessed in both directions (two-tailed tests) or only in one direction (one-tailed tests).

Power Analysis, Type II Errors, and Sample Size

To avoid erroneously concluding that there is not a true difference between two sample groups requires an adequately sized N value to ensure that the two group means are far enough apart to minimize overlap between the groups. An insufficient N value to address this possibility is called a *type II error.* If the chance of a type II error is β, then $1 - \beta$ defines the power of the study to detect a true difference between the groups. For example, if the chance of a type II error is 10%, then the power of the study to detect a real difference is 90%. Similar to type I errors, the threshold set for type II errors is arbitrary, but typically is 10% or 20% (90% or 80% power, respectively). An 80% power indicates that the sample size is large enough so that there is a <20% probability that there really is a difference but random fluctuation prevented detecting statistical significance (*eg*, $p > 0.05$). This highlights the importance of calculating sample size in the study design. Sample size is calculated by choosing a numerical value for α and β and by using some reasonable estimates from the available literature about the estimated difference one expects to find between the means of the two groups using standard published formulas. Sample size determination should always be performed before the study and not after the study to validate the results.

Nonparametric Tests

Nonparametric testing is used when the distribution of the variable of interest in the underlying population is non-Gaussian (*ie*, not bell-shaped). Nonparametric statistical testing uses ranks rather than the actual numerical values so that the average ranks rather than the means for the groups are compared. For example, FEV_1 values for the placebo group are 2.4 L, 2.8 L, and 3.0 L and those for the methacholine group are 2.1 L, 2.3 L, and 2.7 L. If we put these values in ascending rank order, it would look as follows: rank 3, 2.4 L; rank 5, 2.8 L; rank 6, 3.0 L; rank 1, 2.1 L; rank 2, 2.3 L; and rank 4, 2.7 L. Therefore, the average rank for placebo is 14/3 = 4.6, whereas that for methacholine is 7/3 = 2.3. The data are then analyzed with the test equivalent of *t* tests. For example, with unpaired data sets the use of the Wilcoxon rank sum test or Mann-Whitney *U* test would be appropriate, whereas for paired data use of the Wilcoxon signed rank test is appropriate. There are at least two reasons for not using nonparametric tests when the data set is Gaussian, including the following: nonparametric tests are a bit more inflexible for detecting differences and, thus are more prone to type II errors, and the confidence intervals (CIs) cannot be easily calculated.

Multiple Comparisons

Multiple statistical comparisons to a single control group can lead to spurious differences when none really exist. For × comparisons, the chance of finding one spurious "statistically significant" result is 1 – 0.95× (*ie*, for 10 comparisons, there is a 40.1% chance of getting at least one such type I error).

There are several approaches to prevent this problem, including the following: (1) make an adjustment for multiple comparisons by using a Bonferroni correction, which is a very rigorous way to maintain protection against type I errors and is calculated by dividing the chosen p value (0.05) by the number of comparisons, and to use this adjusted p value to reject any of the various null hypotheses (*ie*, if we do 10 pairwise comparisons, the adjusted p value would be calculated as $< 0.05/10$ or < 0.005 to be considered statistically significant). (2) Use a smaller p value (*eg*, 0.01 or 0.005). (3) Identify a primary outcome before the study if multiple outcomes will be assessed, with the understanding that the decision to accept or reject the null hypothesis will hinge on this single outcome. Although many studies identify a primary outcome, secondary outcomes with an unadjusted $p < 0.05$ often are reported, especially when the primary outcome is not statistically significant. Because the utility of such an approach is fraught with error, ideally the significance of any secondary end points should be addressed by an appropriately designed study with that new finding as the primary end point (*ie*, a second interferon for idiopathic pulmonary fibrosis trial that is underway to determine whether there is a survival benefit with active treatment, as suggested in the initial study as a secondary end point). (4) Combine the multiple end points into a single overall end point. (5) Use analysis of variance (ANOVA) with *post-hoc* testing, which is one of the most common approaches, as described in the section to follow.

ANOVA

The one-way ANOVA is the appropriate statistical approach to use when comparing two or more independent groups (*ie*, to assess whether the FEV_1 is different among groups that were randomized to receive five different treatment regimens compared with a single control group). ANOVA, which is subject to the same data distribution assumptions as is *t* testing (*ie*, Gaussian distribution), provides an overall measure of whether there are statistically significant differences among the groups overall ($p < 0.05$). Once a true difference is noted among the groups, there are a number of different *post-hoc* tests (*eg*, Dunnett, Duncan, Scheffé, least significant difference, Tukey, Student-Newman-Keuls, and others) one can perform that prevent type I errors that might result from performing all the separate pairwise comparisons that are possible in the five groups in our example. For nonparametric data, the Kruskal-Wallis test is a version of a one-way ANOVA but without *post-hoc* tests. A Bonferroni correction on the pairs of groups studied is often used in this situation.

Proportions or Counts

When comparing data that are categoric, rather than numerical, the number, fraction, or proportion of patients in each category is analyzed. Similar to a numerical continuous variable analysis, the observed proportions in the sample are used to approximate those in the entire population of interest, with inferences about the entire population made from the single sample. When the N is large, the distribution approaches a Gaussian curve. These studies use n × m tables, with the value in each cell being either the number or the fraction of patients, and then are analyzed with the use of a χ^2 or Fisher exact test. For example, patients in the ICU who experienced stress gastritis bleeding when they received prophylaxis with sucralfate, cimetidine, omeprazole, or placebo yield a 2 × 4 table such as that shown in Table 1.

Confidence Intervals: An Alternative to Hypothesis Testing

Hypothesis testing using p values is limited by simply addressing the null hypothesis based on a p value threshold with an arbitrary cutoff. A statistically significant difference may be technically correct but of limited clinical significance. For example, a large study may show that a bronchodilator raises the mean FEV_1 by 50 mL ($p < 0.01$) compared with placebo, but the magnitude of that increase probably will not be likely to generate any benefit for patients and, as such, is not clinically significant. In contrast, a small study that is not statistically significant may indeed provide a clinically relevant benefit of the new drug. CIs provide a way to more easily judge the clinical relevance of the findings while reporting the observed effect (*ie*, the *point estimate*) in the study along with the 95% CI. The CI provides the following two useful pieces of information: the point estimate, which is the single value, based on the study, that is most likely to represent the true difference between the drug and placebo, and the 95% CI, which is the plausible range of differences within which lies the true difference. No value within this 95% CI can be rejected as representing the true effect within a 5% significance level. The null hypothesis is accepted (*ie*, there is no difference between groups) if the 95% CI includes the value representing no effect (*ie*, 0% difference in FEV_1 or 1.0 for an odds ratio [OR; defined below] for death in a study with mortality as the end point), whereas the null hypothesis is rejected if the 95% CI does not cross this value.

The CI provides information beyond the "no-effect" value. With the use of a hypothetical example, the authors of a small study of survival time that used a new drug for the treatment of advanced small cell lung cancer (median survival time with standard therapy, 6 months) found that the 95% CI for median survival when using the new drug was 0.50 to 1.68. Although this range includes 1.00 (*ie*, it is a negative study because it crosses the no-effect line), the CI is very useful. The study shows that, at best, we can expect the new drug to increase the median survival time by only 4 months (0.68 × 6 months) and may reduce survival time to 3 months (0.5 × 6 months), which questions the utility of any future larger study.

Table 1. *Hypothetical Relationship Between Various GI Prophylactic Regimens and Stress Gastritis Bleeding in the ICU*

Type of Prophylaxis	Did Bleed, No. (%)	Did Not Bleed, No.
Sucralfate	8 (6.6)	114
Cimetidine	13 (10.8)	107
Omeprazole	16 (14.8)	92
Placebo	21 (14.9)	120

Relative Risks and ORs

Physicians who read the medical literature should be familiar with the fundamentals behind terms such as absolute risk (AR), relative risk (RR), AR reduction (ARR), RR reduction (RRR), and OR. The authors of a study reporting that a new drug gave a RRR for death of 25% sounds great, but if the risk of death in the control group is 4%, then the new drug reduced the death rate by just 1%. Physicians must then decide whether this difference is a clinically relevant one when factoring in other issues, such as the cost and side effects of the drug. Table 2 shows how AR is calculated from a hypothetical study in which the authors examined cough in patients who were randomized to receive enalapril or valsartan.

RR (also called the *risk ratio*) is defined as the ratio of the rates of cough occurrence. In Table 2, the risks for cough in the two groups are 44.6% and 28.1%, respectively, so the RR = 0.281/0.446 = 0.63, which translates into a 37% lower risk of the development of a cough while one is receiving therapy with valsartan compared with therapy with enalapril. Of note, RR cannot be calculated for case-control studies because the case group is chosen based on having the disease under study whereas the control subjects are selected because they do not have the disease.

ARR (also called *risk difference*) is defined as the absolute difference in rates of occurrence between the experimental and control patients in a trial. Using the data in Table 2, ARR is defined as 44.6% – 28.1% = 16.5% ARR for the development of a cough while one is receiving therapy with valsartan.

RRR is defined as the percentage difference in rates of occurrence of events (good or bad) between the experimental and control patients in a trial. RRR = 1 – RR, which in our hypothetical Table 2 would be 1 – 0.63 = 0.37. It is also calculated as follows: ARR/AR among the appropriate reference group = 0.165/0.446 = 0.37 or 37% RRR for the development of a cough while one is receiving therapy with valsartan compared with therapy with enalapril. A major limitation when using the RR and RRR is that they can be misleading. For example, if the RRR is 33%, this could result from the actual risk decreasing from 3 to 1% or by decreasing from 66 to 22%. Without knowing the ARs for each condition, the RR and RRR can have very different implications for the efficacy of a treatment or the incidence of a side effect.

LR (also called the *likelihood ratio*) summarizes information about the diagnostic test or treatment response by combining data about the sensitivity and specificity.[8,9] The LR informs how much a positive or negative result alters the likelihood that the patient would have the disease or treatment response of interest. The LR of a positive test result (LR+) is defined as follows: sensitivity / (1 – specificity). The LR of a negative test result (LR–) is defined as follows: (1 – sensitivity) / specificity. A useless test has a LR = 1.0, whereas a test is better the more it is further from 1.0; >1.0 for LR+ and lower than 1.0 for LR–. The LR can then be used to compare various test results to ascertain which has better discriminative power. An example of how LRs are calculated is illustrated in Figure 2

OR is defined as the ratio of the odds of a particular end point for each treatment. In our aforementioned example, the odds of a cough developing while one is receiving therapy with enalapril = a/b = 29/36 = 0.81, whereas the odds of a cough developing while one is receiving therapy with valsartan = c/d = 18/46 = 0.39. The OR of a cough developing while one is receiving therapy with enalapril compared with therapy with valsartan would be calculated as 0.81/0.39 = 2.07. The utility of ORs is that they are the natural measure arising from certain statistical approaches (*eg*, logistic regression, case-control studies, and meta-analyses). ORs are not an intuitive measure of risk. For example, the OR of 2.07 in this example does not mean that enalapril-treated patients had twice as much chance as valsartan-treated patients of having a cough develop (that is the RR, which is 1.59 = 0.446/0.281). As illustrated in Table 3, the RR approximates the OR only if the event (*eg*, outcome or complication) is rare, as may occur with the effect of an active drug (vs placebo).

The number needed to treat (NNT) is defined as the ratio of 1/ARR. The NNT represents the number of patients who would need to be treated with the better therapy to avoid a single case of the adverse outcome. For example, the ARR in the rate

Table 2. *Hypothetical Relationship Between Two Different Angiotensin-Converting Enzyme Inhibitors and Cough*

Drug	Cough	No Cough	Total No.	Patients with Cough, % (=AR)
Enalapril	29 = a	36 = b	a + b = 65	a/(a + b) = 44.6%
Valsartan	18 = c	46 = d	c + d = 64	c/(c + d) = 28.1%

Table 3. *Hypothetical Relationship Between Placebo and a Test Drug in Causing an Adverse Event*

Variables	No.	Events, No.	Without Event, No.	Odds	AR	RR	RRR, %	ARR, %	OR
Placebo	100	2	98	2/98	2/100	0.5	50	1	0.495
Drug	100	1	99	1/99	1/100				
Placebo	100	90	10	90/10	90/100	0.5	50	45	0.091
Drug	100	45	55	45/55	45/100				

of cough while one is receiving therapy with valsartan over therapy with enalapril is 0.165 (16.5%), and therefore, treating 1/0.165, or 6.1 patients, with valsartan instead of with enalapril will eliminate a single case of drug-induced cough. The best index to use in describing the data depends on that which you are examining. Typically, the one that most transparently reflects the actual difference in event rates is the ARR or the reciprocal of ARR, the NNT. The RR and RRR obscure the actual change in rates and may have widely different implications when the actual data are assessed. The OR reflects the actual change in rates but in a manner that is not always intuitive.

Medical Decision Making: Receiver Operator Characteristic Curves

Physicians must use tests that have some arbitrary cut point between normal and abnormal based on studies in patients with and without the disease of interest. Choosing a cut point involves inevitable trade-offs between sensitivity and specificity. The usual way this trade-off is examined is via the receiver operating characteristic (ROC) curve (Fig 3). Note that the ROC curve lives in a box with lengths and widths both equal to 1.0, with sensitivity on the *y*-axis and 1-specificity (otherwise known as the *FP rate*) on the *x*-axis. The

	Mesothelioma (D)		
Test (T)	**Positive**	**Negative**	**Total**
Positive	**160**	**120**	**280**
Negative	**40**	**680**	**720**
Total	**200**	**800**	**1000**

Sensitivity of T is the probability of a positive test result in people with (D) 160 / 200 = **0.80**

Specificity of T is the probability of a negative test result in people with D 680 / 800 = **0.85**

PPV of test result T is the probability of D in people with positive test result 160 / 280 = **0.57**

NPV of test result T is the probability of no D in people with negative test result 680 / 720 = **0.94**

The **likelihood ratio (LR)** of test result T is the probability of the test result T in people with D divided by the probability of T in people without D. A useless (non-discriminative) test has a LR = 1.0

LR + is defined as: (160 / 200) / (120 / 800) = 5.3

LR - is defined as: (40 / 200) / (680 / 800) = 0.23

The **odds ratio (OR)** summarizes the overall discrimination of a test T: (160 / 40) / (120 / 680) = **22.7**

A test is useless if the OR = 1.0 and is better the further the OR is from 1.0

Figure 2. Calculating measures of discrimination of a new serum test (T) to detect mesothelioma (D) in a group of asbestos workers with a mesothelioma prevalence of 20%.

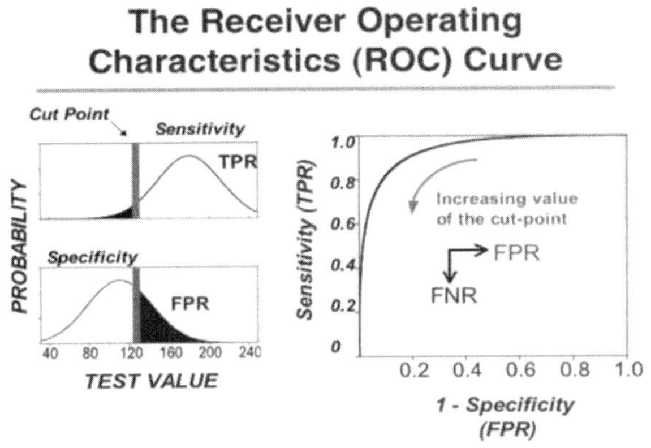

Figure 3. ROC curve.

ROC curve analysis provides a global sense of how well a test distinguishes patients with disease from disease-free individuals. This distinction is particularly helpful when there are multiple tests that exist for a given disease to decide which is superior. Inevitably, there is a trade-off between sensitivity and specificity at all possible values of the cut point. If a particular test result is no better than a flip of the coin (*ie*, a useless test), then the graph will show a diagonal line from the bottom left-hand corner to the upper right-hand corner. On the other hand, when the distributions of test results between those with and without the disease are widely separated (*ie*, a helpful test with little overlap), then the area under the curve is high (*ie*, approaches 1.0). In this instance, the best cut point for a test result is one that is located in the upper-most left-hand corner of the graph.

To illustrate how ROC curves are used to determine the best test cut point, the role of d-dimer testing is helpful. Clinicians use d-dimer testing as a strategy to rule out PE and avoid the use of expensive testing. For this purpose, the ideal d-dimer test cut point requires virtually everyone with PE to have a positive test result (*ie*, very high sensitivity and very small FN rate), but we can accept FP d-dimer test results (*ie*, low specificity) because we will confirm the presence of PE by imaging. Thus, a low value for the cut point with the highest specificity while maintaining a very low FN rate (*ie*, a d-dimer enzyme-linked immunosorbent assay value of >500 ng/mL) would be chosen based on data from the medical literature. The cut point chosen should maximize "utility" for the entire population under consideration. This requires assigning some measure of the costs that occur as a consequence of both FP and FN results (*eg*, money, morbidity, and mortality). The optimal operating point is where the slope of the ROC curve is defined as:

{Cost of FP misclassification} (1 – probability of disease)
= ——————————×——————————
{Cost of FN misclassification} (Probability of disease)

Thus, when the costs of FN misclassifications are large, you need a point at which the ROC slope is small (*ie*, the upper right of the ROC curve where sensitivity is sure to be high and FN results are minimized; Fig 2). However, when the costs associated with FP results are large, you need an operating point at which the ROC curve slope is large (*ie*, on the left side of the ROC curve where specificity is large and FP results are thus minimized). In a rare disease, there is typically a large ROC curve slope (*ie*, left side of the ROC curve where specificity is large and FP results are minimized). This is preferred because, in patients with rare diseases, even good test results have more FP results than TP results, and as a consequence, the cumulative adverse costs of FP results are magnified.

Bayes Theorem

Sensitivity and specificity alone are inadequate to meaningfully understand the implications of a test result in a real clinical practice. Clinicians require an understanding of Bayes theorem that involves determining the positive predictive value (PPV) and negative predictive value (NPV) of a test by calculating the posttest probability of disease based on a pretest probability of disease, sensitivity, and specificity, as follows: (1) the PPV is defined as the percentage of patients with a positive test result (*ie*, greater than the cut point) who really have the disease in question and is determined by the equation (TP)/(TP + FP); (2) the NPV is defined as the percentage of patients with a negative test result who are actually disease-free and is determined by the equation (TN)/(TN + FN); (3) posttest probability of disease is defined as 100% – NPV (this provides an estimate of the probability of the disease after calculating the PPV and NPV from the sensitivity and specificity); and (4) the likelihood ratio (LR) is defined as the ratio of the probability of a test result in patients with the particular disease in question to the probability of that same test in patients who are free of that disease. The LR for a positive test result (*ie*, LR +) is determined from the ratio of sensitivity/(1 – specificity). The LR of a negative test (*ie*, LR –) is determined from the ratio of (1 – sensitivity)/specificity. The posttest odds reflect the odds that the patient has the disease of interest after the test is conducted (*ie*, pretest odds × LR).

The best way to determine the PPV and NPV of a particular test is to set up a 2 × 2 table, as illustrated in Table 4. For hypothetical purposes, we will determine the PPV and NPV of d-dimer testing f or PE in which the pretest probability for PE in our patient population is 25%. The PPV reflects the posttest probability of disease after a positive test result. In the hypothetical case, the PPV of a positive d-dimer test result is only 62% (*ie*, not much better than the flip of a coin) and is of little clinical value in the diagnostic evaluation of PE. However, the value of d-dimer testing is in its NPV, which in our illustrative example is 98%, as calculated in Table 4. Thus, the posttest probability of disease after a negative d-dimer test result would be 2% (*ie*, 100 to 98%). The high NPV of d-dimer testing (98% in our hypothetical model) and the low posttest probability of PE (2%) is very attractive in excluding PE when the d-dimer test result is low in this patient population (PE estimate, 25%). Accordingly, this allows clinicians to confidently focus on other causes for the patient's complaints. Notably, however, if the PE disease prevalence is greater (*ie*, 75%), then the NPV decreases and the posttest probability of PE increase. For example, when the same sensitivity and specificity is used, the FN test result incidence is 4 of 24 negative test results; therefore, the NPV decreases to approximately 83% and the posttest probability of PE is 17%, which are values that

Table 4. *Calculating the PPV and NPV of d-Dimer Testing in a Population With an Estimated PE Prevalence of 25%*

Steps	Disease Present	Disease Absent	Total
1*			
Positive test result	TP	FP	
Negative test result	FN	TN	
PE prevalence	25	75	
2†			
Positive test result	24		
Negative test result	1		
PE prevalence	25	75	
3‡			
Positive test result	24	15	
Negative test result	1	60	
PE prevalence	25	75	
4§			
Positive test result	24	15	39
Negative test result	1	60	61
PE prevalence	25	75	100
5‖			
Positive test result	24	15	39 PPV = 24/39 = 62%
Negative test result	1	60	61 NPV = 60/61 = 98%
PE prevalence	25	75	100

*Presume a theoretical group of 100 patients with possible PE and fill in the columns.
†Sensitivity = 95%; therefore, of the 25 patients with disease, 24 have a positive test result, and 1 does not.
‡Specificity = 20%; therefore, of the 75 patients without disease, 60 have a negative test result, and 15 have positive test results.
§Add up across.
‖Compute the PPV and NPV from the rows.

may not be clinically reassuring in stopping the evaluation for PE. Indeed, this is precisely what limits the predictive value of d-dimer testing in patients who are deemed to be at very high risk for PE.

It is important to remember that no test is perfect (*ie*, 100% sensitivity and 100% specificity). Furthermore, even the "gold standard" test can be wrong in a small percentage of cases (*ie*, pulmonary angiogram to diagnose PE has both FP results [erroneous reading by a radiologist] and FN results [sampling error or erroneous reading by a radiologist]). Thus, the sensitivity and specificity are insufficient for informing clinicians about the utility of a particular test in medical decision making. It is essential to know or to make an estimate about the pretest probability of disease in the patient population of interest.

As illustrated previously in our example of d-dimer testing in patients with PE, in patients with a low pretest probability, even a test with high sensitivity will result in a very high percentage of the positive test results being false-positive ones, especially if the specificity is not very high. In contrast, in patients with a high pretest probability (*ie*, 75%), even a test with high sensitivity will result in enough FN results that one will be prevented from confidently ruling out PE even if the d-dimer test result is negative. Clinicians should use the Bayes theorem to determine the PPV, NPV, and posttest probability of disease to avoid important assumptions and conclusions about the test results. Calculation of the PPV and NPV before the test is performed, especially if it is expensive, dangerous, or invasive, will help in the assessment of whether the test result will be of much clinical benefit.

Metaanalysis

Metaanalysis involves a statistical analysis of two or more primary data sets that have been published or otherwise communicated to address a specific question or hypothesis. The methods, strengths, and weaknesses of this approach have recently been reviewed.[10] Compared with a single study, the major potential strength of a properly performed metaanalysis is that it enables better determination of whether a particular theory or finding is correct based on the accumulated findings of multiple data sets. The major limitation is that it is unable to correct for underpowered primary data sets that introduce sample bias as well as insensitivity to confounders.

In summary, there are some fundamental statistical principles that clinicians must be intimately familiar with to properly interpret the medical literature as well as to make logical medical decisions. In particular, an understanding of how basic statistical terms are calculated, how hypothesis testing occurs, as well as the concepts behind ROCs in medical decisions are all vitally important. Table 5 summarizes the appropriate statistical tests that are available to analyze data in a wide variety of situations, some of which are well beyond the scope of this review. The best statistical test is based on the nature of the dependent (Y) variable and the independent (X) variable.

Test-Taking Strategies

Test Preparation Tips

There are a number of common sense recommendations to optimize success on any test. First, confidence in your test taking begins with adequate test preparation beforehand. The principles behind successful test preparation include the following: (1) budget your time to be sure that you have sufficient time to study so that you are well prepared for the test; (2) go to a review course if possible (it is important to pay attention to hints that the instructor may give, as well as to take careful notes and to ask questions about areas that you find confusing; (3) review any material from, for example, old tests, sample problems, review material, or textbooks that might be on the test; (4) put the main ideas/information/formulas onto a sheet that can be quickly reviewed many times because this makes it easier to retain the key concepts that will be on the test; (5) review for several short periods rather than one long period, because you will find that you retain information better and be less fatigued; (6) avoid pulling an "all-nighter" before the test, and plan on getting at least 7 to 8 h of sleep the night before taking the test; (7) eat a healthy meal before a test to ensure that you will have the energy and focus necessary; (8) arrive at the testing site well before the start time (you may wish to set your alarm as well as a backup

Table 5. *Summary of the Most Appropriate Statistical Test Based on the Dependent and Independent Variables**

Nature of the Dependent Variable	Nature of the Independent Variables	Tests To Use
Continuous	Two independent groups	
That is Gaussian		Unpaired t test
With a large N		Unpaired t test
Neither Gaussian or large N		Wilcoxon rank-sum test Mann-Whitney U test
Categoric or ordinal		χ^2 test Fisher exact test (2 × 2 tables only)
Continuous	More than two independent groups	
That is Gaussian		ANOVA
That is not Gaussian		Kruskal-Wallis test
Categoric or ordinal		χ^2 test
Continuous, Gaussian with repeated/serial measurements for each individual		Repeated-measures ANOVA
Continuous	Paired (one population measured twice or two populations that are matched up)	
That is Gaussian		Paired t test
With a large N		Paired t test
Neither Gaussian or large N		Wilcoxon signed rank test
Categoric or ordinal		McNemar test
Continuous and Gaussian	A single continuous variable	Correlation Univariate linear regression
Binary		Univariate logistic regression
Continuous and Gaussian	Two or more variables, continuous and/or categoric	Multivariate linear regression ANCOVA
Binary		Multivariate logistic regression

*ANCOVA = analysis of covariance. From http://bama.ua.edu/~jleeper/627/choosestat.html.

alarm); and (9) go to the bathroom before walking into the examination room to avoid wasting any time worrying about your bodily needs during the test.

Test-Taking Tips

Once a test is underway, there are also a number of helpful recommendations to optimize success. (1) Read the directions carefully! Do not rush, but rather pace yourself by reading the entire question and finding the key words. Always read the whole question carefully and do not make assumptions about what the question might be. Simply not following directions can result is a loss of many easy points on questions to which you actually knew the answers. (2) When you first receive your test, do a quick survey of the entire test so that you know how to efficiently budget your time. (3) Bring a watch to the test with you so that you can better pace yourself. (4) Keep a positive attitude throughout the whole test and try to stay relaxed. If you feel nervous or overwhelmed, stop and take a few deep breaths to relax, then move to a portion of the test with which you are more comfortable. If you do not know an answer, skip it, go on with the rest of the test, and come back to it later. Perhaps on another part of the test there will be something that will help you out with that question. (5) Do the easiest problems first; do not stay on a problem on which you are stuck, especially when time is a factor. (6) Do not worry if others finish before you but rather focus on the test in front of you. If you have time left, look over your test, make sure that you have answered all the questions, and only change an answer if you misread or misinterpreted the question because the first answer that you put down is usually the correct one. Look for careless mistakes and make sure that you have not left out any answers or parts of answers.

Multiple Choice Test-Taking Strategies

There are a variety of useful recommendations to consider when answering multiple choice questions. (1) Read the question before you choose the answer after reading all the answers. Look for the central idea of each question. What is the main point? (2) Come up with the answer in your head before looking at the possible answers. In this way, the choices given on the test will not throw you off or trick you. (3) Eliminate the answers that you know are not right. (4) Avoid answers that begin with always, never, none, except, most, or least. Underline these or other key words on the test paper. (5) Because there is no guessing penalty on the pulmonary boards, always make an educated guess, and select an answer. If you have to guess, the following guidelines are helpful: (A) because the length of choices can be a clue, choose the longest; (B) if two choices are similar, choose neither; (C) if two choices are opposites, choose one of them; and the most general alternative is usually the right answer. (6) Do not keep on changing your answers because your first choice is usually the right one, unless you have incorrectly read the question. (7) In "all of the above" and "none of the above" choices, if you are certain one of the statements is true, do not choose "none of the above." Likewise, if one of the statements is false, do not choose "all of the above." (8) In a question with an "all of the above" choice, if you see at least two correct statements, then "all of the above" is probably the answer. (9) A positive choice is more likely to be true than a negative one. (10) If there is an "all of the above" option, and you know that at least two of the choices are correct, select the "all of the above" choice. (11) The correct answer is usually the choice with the most information.

True/False Test Tips

There are a number of common sense recommendations to consider when answering true/false questions. The basic ground rule for answering true/false items is that if any part of the statement is not true, then the student should select false as the answer. (1) Usually, there are more true answers than false answers because false statements often are more difficult to construct as looking correct. Thus, if you are guessing on a true/false question, there is a >50% chance of being right with a true answer. (2) As with multiple choice questions, read through each statement carefully and pay attention to the qualifiers and keywords. Qualifiers like "never," "always," and "every" mean that the statement must be true all of the time. Usually, these types of qualifiers lead to a false answer. Qualifiers like "usually," "sometimes," and "generally" mean that the statement can be considered true or false depending on the circumstances. Usually, these type of qualifiers lead to an answer of true. (3) If any part of the question is false, then the entire statement is false, but just because part of a statement is true does not necessarily make the entire statement true. (4) Every part of a true sentence must be true. (5) Negatives can be confusing. If the question contains negatives such as "no," "not," or "cannot," drop the negative and read what remains to decide whether that sentence is true or false. If it is then true, then its opposite, or negative, is usually false. Remember, double negatives make a positive (*ie*, not uncommon actually means common). (6) Questions that state a reason tend to be false. Words in the statement that cause justification or reason (*ie*, since, because, when, or if) tend to make the statement false. Pay close attention. The reason that is given maybe incorrect or incomplete.

Acknowledgment

The author is very appreciative of the materials and comments provided by Dr. Allan Garland (Case Western Reserve University School of Medicine, Cleveland, OH). This work was supported in part by a Merit Review grant from the Department of Veterans Affairs.

References

1. Casscells W, Schoenberger A, Graboys TB. Interpretation by physicians of clinical laboratory results. N Engl J Med 1978; 299:999–1001
2. Berwick DM, Fineberg HV, Weinstein MC. When doctors meet numbers. Am J Med 1981; 71:991–998
3. Windish DM, Huot SJ, Green ML. Medicine residents' understanding of the biostatistics and results of the medical literature. JAMA 2007; 298:1010–1022
4. Windish DM, Diener-West M. A clinician-educator's roadmap to choosing and interpreting statistical tests. J Gen Intern Med 2006; 21:656–660

A succinct overview of statistical terminology that also provides a logical approach for selecting the appropriate statistical test.

5. Guyatt GH, Haynes RB, Jaeschke RZ, et al. Users' guides to the medical literature: XXV. Evidence-based medicine: principles for applying the users' guides to patient care. JAMA 2000; 284:1290–1296
   This is the 25th installment of a superb multipart series reviewing various topics that practically illustrate how physicians should use medical statistics and evidenced-based medicine in their practice.
6. Schulz KF, Chalmers I, Hayes RJ, et al. Empirical evidence of bias: dimensions of methodological quality associated with estimates of treatment effects in controlled trials. JAMA 1995; 273:408–412
7. van Nieuwenhoven CA, Buskens E, van Tiel FH, et al. Relationship between methodological trial quality and the effects of selective digestive decontamination on pneumonia and mortality in critically ill patients. JAMA 2001; 286:335–340
8. Knottnerus JA, van Weel C, Muris JWM. Evaluation of diagnostic procedures. BMJ 2002; 324: 477–481
9. Perera R. Making sense of diagnostic test likelihood ratios. ACP Journal Club 2007; 146:A8–A9
10. Noble JH. Meta-analysis: methods, strengths, weak nesses, and political uses. J Lab Clin Med 2006; 147:7–20
    This is an excellent overview of a potentially powerful statistical tool that can be misused if not well understood. It contains 106 references.

Acid-Base Disorders

Janice L. Zimmerman, MD, FCCP

Objectives:

- Define terminology used in describing acid-base disturbances
- Diagnose simple and complex acid-base disorders
- Differentiate anion gap and non-anion gap metabolic acidoses
- Review appropriate treatment for major causes of acidosis and alkalosis

Key words: acid; acidemia; acidosis; alkalemia; alkalosis; anion gap; base; strong ion difference

Acid-base disturbances are common in the critically ill and result from a variety of clinical disorders. Appropriate diagnosis and management of acid-base disorders require accurate interpretation of simultaneous measurements of electrolytes, albumin (alb), and arterial blood gases, as well as knowledge of compensatory physiologic responses.

Acid-Base Physiology

The acidity of body fluids is measured in terms of hydrogen ion concentration, which is expressed as pH (the negative log of the hydrogen ion concentration). Hydrogen ion concentration and pH are inversely related. Changes in acidity can be stabilized although not totally corrected by endogenous buffers, molecules that accept or donate hydrogen ions. Important buffers include the following: bicarbonates ($HCO_3^- + H^+ \leftrightarrow H_2CO_3 \leftrightarrow H_2O + CO_2$); proteins ($protein^- + H^+ \leftrightarrow$ H-protein); hemoglobin ($hemoglobin^- + H^+ \leftrightarrow$ H-hemoglobin); and phosphates ($HPO_4^{2-} + H^+ \leftrightarrow H_2PO_4^-$).

The major buffering system in the body is the carbonic acid–bicarbonate pair. The relation of pH to this buffering system is expressed by the Henderson-Hasselbalch equation: $pH = pK + \log HCO_3/H_2CO_3 = 6.1 + \log HCO_3^-/0.03\ Paco_2$.

The interrelation of H^+, $Paco_2$, and HCO_3^- can also be illustrated by the Henderson equation. This equation is helpful as a bedside tool to predict or evaluate the accuracy of the three acid-base parameters: $H^+ = 24 \times Paco_2/HCO_3^-$. An estimation of H^+ can be made from pH. Between pH 7.2 and 7.5, H^+ changes by 1 mmol/L for each 0.01-U change in pH (Table 1).

Although acid-base status is typically characterized by H^+ and HCO_3^- for clinical problem solving, Stewart's physicochemical analysis more accurately describes the determinants of acid-base status in biological systems. Three independent variables determine acid-base changes: (1) $Paco_2$. (2) The strong ion difference (SID). This is the net electric charge on strong electrolytes. It is the sum of all strong cation concentrations minus the sum of all strong anion concentrations, or SID = ($Na^+ + K^+ + Ca^{2+} + Mg^{2+}$) − ($Cl^-$ + other strong anions). The normal value is 38 to 42 mmol/L. The SID is dependent primarily on renal function but may also be impacted by GI function and tissue metabolism. (3) The total concentrations of nonvolatile weak acids. The main weak acids are inorganic phosphate (Pi) and serum proteins, particularly albumin.

Other variables such as H^+ and HCO_3^- are dependent variables that change based on primary alterations in the independent variables above. Evaluation of acid-base status by Stewart's

Table 1. *Relationship Between pH and H^+*

pH	H^+, mmol/L
7.65	22
7.60	25
7.55	28
7.50	32
7.45	35
7.40	40
7.35	45
7.30	50
7.25	56
7.20	63
7.15	71
7.10	79
7.05	89
7.00	100

approach requires assessment of all the independent variables.

This chapter will primarily review the more traditional analysis of acid-base problems using formulas based on H^+ and HCO_3^-. However, some correlates of Stewart's approach will be mentioned and may help in understanding the limitations of traditional acid-base analysis.

Definitions

The following definitions are used: *acidemia*, an increase in H^+ and a decrease in arterial pH; *alkalemia*, a decrease in H^+ and elevation of arterial pH; *acidosis*, a process that, if unopposed, will lead to a decrease in pH; and *alkalosis*, a process that, if unopposed, will lead to an increase in pH.

Acid-Base Disturbances

The development of an acid-base disorder is traditionally identified by changes in the bicarbonate concentration (the metabolic or renal component) or by changes in $Paco_2$ (the respiratory component). A primary metabolic disturbance results from a primary alteration in bicarbonate concentration, whereas a primary respiratory disturbance results from a primary alteration in $Paco_2$. In Stewart's approach, metabolic disturbances result from changes in the strong ion difference and/or concentrations of weak acids.

Features of acid-base disturbances are noted in Table 2. Primary acid-base disturbances also initiate compensatory responses that are predictable. Compensatory processes help normalize the arterial pH but usually never return the pH fully to normal. Appropriate compensatory responses require normal functioning of lungs and kidneys, and failure to develop a compensatory response defines the presence of a second primary disorder.

Table 2. *Features of Acid-Base Disturbances*

Disorders	Primary Problem	pH	Compensation
Metabolic acidosis	$\downarrow HCO_3^-$, ↓SID, ↑alb, ↑Pi	↓	$\downarrow Paco_2$
Metabolic alkalosis	$\uparrow HCO_3^-$, ↑SID, ↓alb	↑	$\uparrow Paco_2$
Respiratory acidosis	$\uparrow Paco_2$	↓	$\uparrow HCO_3^-$
Respiratory alkalosis	$\downarrow Paco_2$	↑	$\downarrow HCO_3^-$

Metabolic Acidosis

In metabolic acidosis, the following are seen: (1) defect: increased acid accumulation or decreased extracellular HCO_3^-; decreased SID, increased concentration of alb, or increased Pi; (2) laboratory manifestation: decreased pH, decreased plasma HCO_3^-; and (3) compensation: increased ventilation leading to decreased $Paco_2$; exchange of intracellular Na^+ and K^+ for extracellular H^+; increased renal H^+ excretion with urinary buffers and regeneration of new bicarbonate (slower process).

The degree of respiratory compensation can be estimated by the following formulas: $Paco_2 = 1.5 \times HCO_3^- + 8 \pm 2$; and $\Delta Paco_2 = 1.2 \times \Delta HCO_3^-$. During prolonged acidosis, when respiratory compensation is complete, the last two digits of pH equal $Paco_2$ (if pH > 7). The lower limit of normal compensation is $Paco_2$ of 10 mm Hg.

Etiologies

Metabolic acidosis can result from an increase in endogenous acid production that overwhelms renal excretion (*eg*, ketoacidosis), exogenous acid input, excessive loss of bicarbonate (*eg*, diarrhea), or decreased renal excretion of endogenous acids (*eg*, chronic renal failure). Metabolic acidoses are usually further characterized by the anion gap (AG). Unmeasured anions (proteins, phosphates, sulfates, and organic acids) in healthy persons exceed the unmeasured cations (potassium, calcium, and magnesium), and this difference results in the AG. The AG can be estimated by the following formula: $AG = Na^+ - (Cl^- + HCO_3^-) = 10 \pm 4$.

The AG can be increased because of a decrease in unmeasured cations, an increase in unmeasured anions, or laboratory error in measurement. The classification of metabolic acidoses by the AG is shown in Table 3. In addition, lactic acidosis has been associated with drugs such as metformin, nucleoside reverse transcriptase inhibitors, linezolid, lorazepam, and propofol. Base deficit determined by measured plasma pH and $Paco_2$, and hemoglobin concentration using algorithms and nomograms of Siggard-Andersen, has also been

Table 3. *Classification of Metabolic Acidosis by AG*

Increased AG
Lactic acidosis
Type A (tissue ischemia)
Type B (altered cell metabolism)
Ketoacidosis
Diabetes
Alcohol induced
Starvation
Renal failure
Toxin ingestion
Salicylates
Methanol
Ethylene glycol
Paraldehyde
Normal AG (hyperchloremic)
GI loss of HCO_3^-
Ureteral diversion
Diarrhea
Ileostomy
Proximal colostomy
Renal loss of HCO_3^-
Proximal renal tubular acidosis
Carbonic anhydrase inhibitor
Renal tubular disease
Acute tubular necrosis
Chronic tubulointerstitial disease
Distal rental tubular acidosis (type 1 and 4)
Hypoaldosteronism, aldosterone inhibitors
Pharmacologic
Ammonium chloride
Hyperalimentation
Dilutional acidosis

used to evaluate metabolic acidosis. However, this approach is less reliable in critically ill patients.

The AG has several limitations as the sole indicator of a metabolic acidosis. An AG acidosis can exist even with a normal AG in patients who are severely hypoalbuminemic or have pathologic paraproteinemias. In such patients, the normal AG may be as low as 4 to 5 mmol/L. For every decrease of 1 g/dL in alb, a decrease of 2.5 to 3 mmol in AG will occur. Pathologic paraproteinemias lower the AG because Igs are largely cationic. Another exception can occur when an elevated AG does not reflect an underlying acidosis. In patients with significant alkalemia (usually pH >7.5), alb is more negatively charged, which increases unmeasured anions.

Normal AG acidoses can also be categorized by the potassium level. Hypokalemia (<3.5 mmol/L) is associated with ureteral diversion, diarrhea, proximal colostomy, ileostomy, proximal renal tubular acidosis (RTA), type 1 distal RTA, and hyperalimentation. Hyperkalemia (>4.5 mmol/L) can be found in hypoaldosterone states, ammonium chloride administration, and type 4 distal RTA.

A decreased AG implies an increase in unmeasured cations or a decrease in unmeasured anions. Possible etiologies include paraproteinemias, hypoalbuminemia, hyponatremia, lithium toxicity, profound hyperkalemia, hypercalcemia, or hypermagnesemia, and halide poisoning (bromide and iodide).

In an uncomplicated AG metabolic acidosis, every increase of 1 mmol/L in the AG should result in a concomitant decrease of 1 mmol/L in HCO_3^-. Deviation from this relation suggests a mixed acid-base disorder. The difference between these two values has been termed the *Δgap*, and can be expressed as follows: Δgap = (deviation of AG from normal) − (deviation of HCO_3^- from normal). If the normal AG is assumed to be 12 mmol/L and the normal HCO_3^- is 24 mmol/L, then the following equation results: $\Delta gap = (AG - 12) - (24 - HCO_3^-)$.

The normal value for Δgap should be zero. However, variance in measurements can result in a Δgap of 0 ± 6. If the Δgap is positive, then either a simultaneous metabolic alkalosis or a respiratory acidosis exists. If the decrease in HCO_3^- is greater than the increase in AG, which results in a negative Δgap, then a concomitant normal AG acidosis (hyperchloremic) or chronic respiratory alkalosis with compensating hyperchloremic acidosis may exist. Small deviations of the Δgap may not indicate mixed acid-base disorders, and clinical information must always be considered in the evaluation.

In Stewart's approach, a decreased SID in metabolic acidosis results from an elevated Cl^- or accumulation of unidentified anions analogous to a normal AG or increased AG acidosis described above. A simplified formula that can be used to estimate the SID takes into account changes in alb and phosphate: $SID = HCO_3^- + 0.28$ alb g/L + 1.8 Pi mmol/L.

Clinical Manifestations

The clinical features of metabolic acidosis depend primarily on the underlying disorder. Some effects of acidosis can be related to the change in pH. The effects of acidemia on the cardiovascular system have been questioned and may not be significant.

CNS: Increased cerebral blood flow; decreased mental status.

Pulmonary: Hyperventilation with rapid and/or deep respiration (Kussmaul respiration); increase in pulmonary vascular resistance.

Cardiovascular: Potential decreased myocardial contractility; arrhythmias; potential decreased responsiveness to catecholamines; arterial vasodilation.

Metabolic: Insulin resistance; hyperkalemia; hypercalcemia; increased protein catabolism; catecholamine stimulation. Metabolic acidosis shifts the oxyhemoglobin dissociation curve to the right, which promotes oxygen release at the tissue level.

Treatment

Treatment requires appropriate diagnosis of the etiology of metabolic acidosis and correction of the underlying disorder. Therapy for a non-AG metabolic acidosis requires replacing volume losses with a bicarbonate-containing solution that has a low chloride concentration. Treatment of most AG metabolic acidoses is well established (*ie*, insulin for ketoacidosis, dialysis for renal failure). Adjunctive therapy with sodium bicarbonate in this setting is usually not recommended. Treatment of lactic acidosis with bicarbonate does not improve survival. In circumstances when pH < 7.1 is associated with severe hemodynamic compromise, some studies show that bicarbonate may improve cardiovascular responsiveness. However, myocardial performance is often normal in the setting of metabolic acidosis. Potential complications of bicarbonate administration frequently outweigh possible benefits (Table 4). Other nonbicarbonate buffers, such as tris-hydroxymethyl aminomethane, dichloroacetate, and carbicarb, may avoid some of the complications, but clinical data do not support their use.

Table 4. *Potential Complications of Bicarbonate Administration*

Volume overload
Paradoxical CSF/intracellular acidosis
Respiratory acidosis
Impaired oxygen delivery (tissue hypoxia)
Hypokalemia
Hypocalcemia
Hypernatremia
Hyperosmolality
Overshoot alkalemia

Metabolic Alkalosis

In metabolic alkalosis, the following are seen: (1) defect: extracellular fluid increase in base or loss of acid; increased SID or decreased concentration of alb; (2) laboratory manifestation: increase in pH and increase in HCO_3^-; and (3) compensation: hypoventilation leading to increased $Paco_2$. $Paco_2$ may rise 6 to 7 mm Hg for every increase of 10 mmol/L in HCO_3^-. This response is limited by hypoxemia to a maximum $Paco_2$ of 50 to 55 mm Hg. A characteristic feature of metabolic alkalosis is that the kidneys contribute to the process by adding HCO_3^- to the circulation and hyperabsorbing filtered HCO_3^- rather than enhancing HCO_3^- excretion.

Etiologies

The etiologies of metabolic alkalosis can be divided into those characterized by chloride depletion (hypovolemic) and those characterized by chloride expansion (hypervolemic). These etiologies are also referred to as *chloride or saline responsive* and *chloride or saline resistant*, respectively (Table 5). In Stewart's approach, an increased SID in metabolic alkalosis is due to decreased Cl^-. Hypokalemia

Table 5. *Etiologies of Metabolic Alkalosis*

Hypovolemic, Cl^- depleted
GI loss of H^+
Vomiting
Gastric suction
Cl^- rich diarrhea
Villous adenoma
Renal loss of H^+
Diuretics
Posthypercapnia
Hypervolemic, Cl^- expanded
Renal loss of H^+
Primary hyperaldosteronism
Primary hypercortisolism
Adrenocorticotropic hormone excess
Pharmacologic hydrocortisone/mineralocorticoid excess
Renal artery stenosis with right ventricular hypertension
Renin secreting tumor
Hypokalemia
Bicarbonate overdose
Pharmacologic overdose of $NaHCO_3$
Milk-alkali syndrome
Massive blood transfusion

is common to both types of metabolic alkalosis. Measurement of urine chloride (UCl) is helpful in distinguishing the two categories: UCl < 20 mmol/L in chloride depletion, and UCl > 20 mmol/L in chloride expansion. In metabolic alkalosis, UCl is a more accurate reflection of intravascular volume than urine sodium because sodium must be excreted with excess HCO_3. Diuretic use alters the utility of UCl for assessing volume status.

Clinical Manifestations

Severe metabolic alkalosis is associated with a high mortality rate in hospitalized patients.

Cardiovascular: Tachycardia; arrhythmias; increased cardiac contractility.

CNS: Decreased cerebral blood flow; seizures; altered mental status.

Metabolic: Ionized hypocalcemia; hypokalemia; hypophosphatemia; impaired enzyme function. In contrast to metabolic acidosis, metabolic alkalosis shifts the oxyhemoglobin dissociation curve to the left, which increases oxygen affinity for hemoglobin and may impair oxygen release at the tissue level.

Treatment

The clinical setting along with measurement of UCl usually allows appropriate classification of the metabolic alkalosis. Etiologies associated with chloride depletion respond to volume replacement (saline responsive). Normal saline solution offers more chloride per liter (154 mmol/L) than lactated Ringer solution (104 to 109 mmol/L). Etiologies associated with chloride expansion usually indicate imbalances in the renal-adrenal axis. Potassium deficiencies should be corrected as appropriate. It is rarely necessary to consider hydrochloric acid (0.1 N solution) administration or deliberate hypoventilation to correct severe metabolic alkalosis. Acetazolamide, 250 to 375 mg qd or bid, will increase excretion of HCO_3^- but may result in acidemia and worsening hypokalemia because of kaliuresis. A single 500-mg dose of acetazolamide may be sufficient.

Respiratory Acidosis

In respiratory acidosis, the following are seen: (1) defect: ineffective alveolar ventilation; increase in carbon dioxide production; (2) laboratory manifestation: increased $Paco_2$; decreased pH; and (3) compensation: buffers (primarily intracellular proteins); increased respiratory rate; slow renal response (> 24 to 36 h) with increased bicarbonate reabsorption. The normal respiratory response to hypercapnia is an increase in alveolar ventilation. The stimulus to increase ventilation is mediated by changes in the H^+ of the cerebrospinal fluid (CSF), which affects chemoreceptors in the medulla. Because CSF is essentially devoid of nonbicarbonate buffers, carbon dioxide that diffuses readily across the blood-brain barrier results in a marked increase in CSF H^+. The CSF pH is corrected toward normal by a slower rise in CSF HCO_3^- that results from transfer of cerebral or blood HCO_3^-.

A very small increase in plasma HCO_3^- can be seen acutely because of titration of intracellular nonbicarbonate buffers. For each increase of 10 mm Hg in $Paco_2$, the HCO_3^- increases by 1 mmol/L. Acute increases in $Paco_2$ change the plasma HCO_3^- only 4 to 5 mmol/L to a maximum of 30 to 32 mmol/L. If the respiratory acidosis is acute, the pH should decrease by 0.08 for each increase of 10 mm Hg in $Paco_2$.

The renal reabsorption of HCO_3^- is slower and plays a minimal role in acute respiratory acidosis. Over hours to days, the kidneys compensate with proximal reabsorption of filtered bicarbonate and secretion of H^+ in the distal tubule, which is trapped by ammonia and excreted. Bicarbonate reabsorption is accompanied by loss of Cl^-. This mechanism provides adequate, although incomplete pH compensation for chronic respiratory acidosis. The transition from acute to chronic respiratory acidosis is defined by HCO_3^- retention due to renal compensation. In chronic respiratory acidosis, the HCO_3^- increases 3.5 mmol/L for each increase of 10 mm Hg in $Paco_2$. The limit of renal compensation in chronic respiratory acidosis is HCO_3^- of approximately 45 mmol/L. Higher values suggest an associated secondary metabolic alkalosis. In chronic respiratory acidosis, the pH decreases by 0.03 for each increase of 10 mm Hg in $Paco_2$.

Etiologies

Common causes of acute respiratory acidosis include airway obstruction, respiratory center depression, neuromuscular disorders, and pulmonary disorders (Table 6).

Table 6. *Etiologies of Respiratory Acidosis*

Airway obstruction
Foreign body
Tongue displacement
Laryngospasm
Obstructed endotracheal tube
Severe bronchospasm
Obstructive sleep apnea
Respiratory center depression
General anesthesia
Sedative, narcotic drugs
Cerebral injury, ischemia
Increased CO_2 production
Malignant hyperthermia
Shivering
Hypermetabolism
High carbohydrate diet
Neuromuscular disorders
Drugs or toxins
Electrolyte disorders
Spinal cord injury
Guillain-Barré syndrome
Myasthenia gravis
Polymyositis
Lung conditions
Restrictive disease
Obstructive disease
Hemothorax or pneumothorax
Flail chest
Acute lung injury
Obesity-hypoventilation syndrome
Inappropriate ventilator settings

Clinical Manifestations

The clinical manifestations of acute respiratory acidosis depend on the absolute increase in $Paco_2$, the rate of $Paco_2$ increase, and severity of associated hypoxemia. Intentional hypoventilation (permissive hypercapnia) is well tolerated and has little impact on hemodynamics.

Nervous System: Somnolence; anxiety or confusion; psychosis; tremors, myoclonus, or asterixis; headache; papilledema. (Cerebral vasodilation leads to increased intracranial pressure.)

Cardiovascular System: Tachycardia; hypertension; supraventricular/ventricular arrhythmias; peripheral vasodilation.

Treatment

Treatment involves the rapid identification of the etiology of respiratory acidosis and implementation of corrective action. In many circumstances, intubation and mechanical ventilation are necessary to support alveolar ventilation. Administration of $NaHCO_3$ for acute respiratory acidosis is not indicated. Remember that $NaHCO_3$ is metabolized to carbon dioxide, which may worsen acidosis. In addition, normally functioning kidneys excrete most of the bicarbonate in the acute setting.

A therapeutic pitfall to avoid in the treatment of respiratory acidosis is creation of a posthypercapnic alkalosis. This condition most commonly occurs when a patient with compensated chronic respiratory acidosis is overventilated to a normal or near-normal $Paco_2$. A high plasma HCO_3^- results in alkalemia. Appropriate ventilator management and goals should prevent this situation.

Respiratory Alkalosis

The following are seen in respiratory alkalosis: (1) defect: primary hyperventilation; (2) laboratory manifestation: decreased $Paco_2$; increased pH; and (3) compensation: protein or hemoglobin release of hydrogen ion; slow renal response with bicarbonate loss in urine. Alveolar ventilation is regulated by several factors: chemoreceptors in the medulla (sensitive to H^+) and great vessels (sensitive to oxygen), cortical input (voluntary control), and pulmonary chemoreceptors and stretch receptors. Any of these factors or a combination may lead to hyperventilation. The HCO_3^- decreases 2 mmol/L for each decrease of 10 mm Hg in $Paco_2$ in acute respiratory alkalosis.

Similar to changes noted in respiratory acidosis, pH increases 0.08 for every decrease of 10 mm Hg in $Paco_2$ in acute respiratory alkalosis, and pH increases 0.03 for each decrease of 10 mm Hg in $Paco_2$ in chronic respiratory alkalosis. However, chronic respiratory alkalosis is unique among acid-base disorders in that pH may return to normal if the condition is prolonged. Persistent hypocapnia results in decreased renal H^+ secretion. Plasma HCO_3^- decreases 5 mmol/L for each decrease of 10 mm Hg in $Paco_2$.

Etiologies

The etiologies of respiratory alkalosis are listed in Table 7.

Table 7. *Etiologies of Respiratory Alkalosis*

Hypoxemic drive
- Pulmonary disease with arterial-alveolar gradient
- Cardiac disease with right-to-left shunt
- Cardiac disease with pulmonary edema
- High altitude

Acute and chronic pulmonary disease
- Emphysema
- Pulmonary embolism
- Pulmonary edema

Mechanical overventilation

Stimulation of respiratory center
- Neurologic disorders
- Pain
- Psychogenic
- Liver failure with encephalopathy
- Sepsis/infection
- Salicylates
- Progesterone
- Pregnancy
- Fever

Clinical Manifestations

Acute respiratory alkalosis results in neurologic, cardiovascular, muscular, and metabolic abnormalities.

Nervous System: Confusion or dizziness; seizures; paresthesias; circumoral numbness.

Cardiovascular System: Tachycardia; arrhythmias (especially at pH >7.6).

Muscular System: Cramps; carpopedal spasms.

Metabolic Changes. Hypokalemia; hypophosphatemia; ionized hypocalcemia. In chronic respiratory alkalosis, mild hypokalemia (from intracellular shift) and hyperchloremia (from renal retention) result.

Treatment

Severe alkalemia is associated with high mortality and requires aggressive treatment. Therapy is directed at the underlying cause because pharmacologic agents are not available for the alkalemia.

Complex Acid-Base Disorders

When a single process, such as metabolic alkalosis, results in the acid-base disturbance, it is classified as simple. In many patients, multiple acid-base disturbances exist concurrently and are labeled complex acid-base disorders (Table 8). Triple acid-base disorders involve two metabolic disturbances with a superimposed primary respiratory disturbance. Such conditions may be seen in patients with a chronic acid-base disturbance who have a superimposed mixed disturbance. Clues to the presence of a complex disorder include a normal pH (with the exception of respiratory alkalosis), $Paco_2$ and HCO_3^- deviating in opposite directions, and a pH change in the opposite direction for a known primary disorder.

Complex disorders require an organized approach to interpretation of acid-base parameters for accurate diagnosis. The following

Table 8. *Mixed Acid-Base Disorders*

Acid-Base Disorders	Clinical Syndromes
Respiratory acidosis with metabolic acidosis	Cardiopulmonary arrest Intoxication with methanol, ethylene glycol COPD with lactic acidosis, diabetic ketoacidosis, etc. Severe hypophosphatemia Respiratory failure with renal failure, diarrhea, etc.
Respiratory alkalosis with metabolic alkalosis	Cirrhosis with diuretic use, vomiting Pregnancy with hyperemesis Overventilation in COPD patient
Respiratory acidosis with metabolic alkalosis	COPD with diuretic use, vomiting, gastric suction Severe hypokalemia
Respiratory alkalosis with metabolic acidosis	Sepsis Salicylate intoxication Renal insufficiency with congestive heart failure, pneumonia Advanced liver disease with lactic acidosis
Metabolic acidosis with metabolic alkalosis	Uremia or ketoacidosis with vomiting, gastric suction, diuretics, etc.

Table 9. *Acid-Base Calculations**

Acid-Base Disorder	Formula
Respiratory acidosis	
Acute	Decrease in pH = $0.08 \times \frac{(Paco_2 - 40)}{10}$
	Increase in $[HCO_3^-] = \frac{\Delta Paco_2}{10} \pm 3$
Chronic	Decrease in pH = $0.03 \times \frac{(Paco_2 - 40)}{10}$
	Increase in $[HCO_3^-] = 3.5 \times \frac{\Delta PaCO_2}{10}$
Respiratory alkalosis	
Acute	Increase in pH = $0.08 \times \frac{(40 - Paco_2)}{10}$
	Decrease in $[HCO_3^-] = 2 \times \frac{\Delta Paco_2}{10}$
Chronic	Increase in pH = $0.03 \times \frac{(40 - Paco_2)}{10}$
	Decrease in $[HCO_3^-] = 5 - 7 \times \frac{\Delta PaCO_2}{10}$
Metabolic acidosis	$AG = [Na] - ([Cl^-] + [HCO_3^-])$ $Paco_2 = 1.5 \times [HCO_3^-] + 8 \pm 2$ $\Delta gap = (AG - 12) - (24 - [HCO_3^-])$
Metabolic alkalosis	Increase in $Paco_2 = 0.6 - 0.7 \times \Delta[HCO_3^-]$

*AG = anion gap.

considerations are one system that may be useful in determining the disturbances present:

1. Determine the overall acid-base condition by measuring pH. Is acidemia or alkalemia present?
2. Determine if the primary process is metabolic (HCO_3^- deviation) or respiratory ($Paco_2$ deviation).
3. If a respiratory disturbance is present, determine if it is acute or chronic.
4. If a metabolic disturbance is present, determine if respiratory compensation is appropriate.
5. If a metabolic acidosis is present, calculate the AG.
6. If an AG metabolic acidosis is present, calculate the Δgap to determine if other metabolic disturbances are present.

A summary of useful calculations for acid-base evaluation is found in Table 9.

Annotated Bibliography

Adrogue HJ, Madias NE. Management of life-threatening acid-base disorders: first of two parts. N Engl J Med 1998; 338:26–34

Adrogue HJ, Madias NE. Management of life-threatening acid-base disorders: second of two parts. N Engl J Med 1998; 338:107–111

Review of adverse consequences and management of severe acid-base disorders.

Dubose TD. Acid-base disorders. In: Brenner BM, ed. Brenner and Rector's the kidney. 6th ed. Philadelphia, PA: WB Saunders, 2000; 925–997

A detailed review of all acid-base disorders

Fencl V, Jabor A, Kazda A, et al. Diagnosis of metabolic acid-base disturbances in critically ill patients. Am J Respir Crit Care Med 2000; 162:2246–2251

Use of the SID compared to the AG and base excess in analysis of acid-base status.

Forsythe SM, Schmidt GA. Sodium bicarbonate for the treatment of lactic acidosis. Chest 2000; 117:260–267

A review of the literature on the use of bicarbonate to correct lactic acidosis and its lack of benefit.

Kaufman D, Kitching AJ, Kellum JA. Acid-base balance. In: Hall JB, Schmidt GA, Wood LDH, eds. Principles of critical care. 3rd ed. New York: McGraw-Hill, 2005; 1201–1208

This chapter outlines an approach to acid-base disorders using SID.

Kellum JA. Disorders of acid-base balance. Crit Care Med 2007; 35:2630–2636
A review of quantitative and traditional approaches to acid-base analysis.
Levraut J, Grimaud D. Treatment of metabolic acidosis. Curr Opin Crit Care 2003; 9:260–265
A review of the effects of acidosis and treatment approaches.
Narins RG, Emmett M. Simple and mixed acid-base disorders: a practical approach. Medicine (Baltimore) 1980; 59:161–187
An old but classic review of all acid-base disorders.
Narins RG, Kupin W, Faber MD, et al. Pathophysiology, classification and therapy of acid-base disturbances. In: Arieff AI, DeFronzo RA, eds. Fluid, electrolyte, and acid-base disorders. New York: Churchill Livingstone, 1995; 105–198
A detailed review of pathophysiology and management of all acid-base disorders.
Paulson WD. How to interpret the anion gap. J Crit Illness 1997; 12:96–99
Brief review of the use of the AG and its limitations.
Salem MM, Mujais SK. Gaps in the anion gap. Arch Intern Med 1992; 152:1625–1629
A detailed review of limitations of the use of the AG in clinical practice.
Stewart PA. Modern quantitative acid-base chemistry. Can J Physiol Pharmacol 1983; 61:1444–1461
The original explanation of physicochemical analysis and use of SID in acid-base problems.
Wrenn K. The delta gap: an approach to mixed acid-base disorders. Ann Emerg Med 1990; 19:1310–1313
A concise review of the derivation, interpretation, and clinical application of the Δ*gap.*

Notes

Drug-Induced Lung Diseases

David W. Kamp, MD, FCCP

Objectives:

- Appreciate the diverse clinical syndromes of drug-induced pulmonary diseases
- Understand the general approach to the patient with suspected drug toxicity
- Review the common abnormalities associated with specific chemotherapeutic agents
- Comprehend the typical manifestations of pulmonary toxicity caused by nonchemotherapeutic agents

Key words: acute lung injury; drugs; hypersensitivity pneumonitis; pulmonary fibrosis

Drug-induced lung diseases have challenged clinicians since the dawn of modern medicine. In 1880, William Osler described a patient with pulmonary edema associated with opiate exposure and suggested that there was a pathophysiologic relationship. In 1972, Edward Rosenow[1] extensively reviewed this topic and identified 20 drugs that clearly caused pulmonary toxicity. A decade later, Cooper and colleagues[2] expanded the list to 37 drugs. Since then, >350 drugs have been implicated in causing a wide array of pulmonary manifestations that involve virtually all components of the respiratory system including the airways, parenchyma, pleura, pulmonary circulation, mediastinum, vocal cords, and respiratory muscles (Table 1). The number of drugs that cause lung disease will undoubtedly continue to grow as new agents and biological response modifiers are developed.

Although the clinical syndromes associated with certain drugs are well defined, the full scope of the epidemiology of drug-induced lung disease is not firmly established, partly because of the fact that the diagnosis is one of exclusion (*eg*, infection and tumor). Notably, there are no pathognomonic clinical, laboratory, physiologic, radiographic, or histologic findings. Also, most reactions are idiosyncratic, without any clear relationship to dose or time of exposure. Indeed, some drugs can cause toxicity years after exposure (*eg*, cyclophosphamide). With few exceptions, the risk factors for drug-induced lung diseases are poorly defined. Moreover, confounding variables such as the use of other drugs, oxygen, or radiation therapy, each of which can cause pulmonary injury or have interactive effects (*eg*, bleomycin and oxygen), often hamper the diagnosis. Rechallenge with the implicated drug is rarely performed because effective alternative agents are nearly always available. Thus, clinicians evaluating patients with possible drug-induced pulmonary symptoms must obtain a thorough drug exposure history, maintain a high index of suspicion, and use a systematic diagnostic approach that is reviewed herein.

The management of patients with drug-induced pulmonary side effects is largely supportive. Typically, therapy with the implicated drug is withdrawn, and a trial of corticosteroids is considered, particularly in the setting of significant symptoms and/or gas-exchange abnormalities. The scientific basis for using corticosteroids is, unfortunately,

Table 1. *Major Clinical Syndromes of Drug-Induced Pulmonary Disease*

1. Chronic pneumonitis/fibrosis*
2. Hypersensitivity-type lung disease*
3. Acute noncardiogenic pulmonary edema*
4. Bronchiolitis obliterans with organizing pneumonia
5. Alveolar hypoventilaton
6. Bronchospasm
7. Cough
8. Concentric bronchiolitis obliterans
9. Pleural effusions
10. Venous thromboembolism
11. Pulmonary vasculitis
12. Pulmonary hypertension
13. Drug-induced SLE
14. Alveolar hemorrhage
15. Pulmonary renal syndrome
16. Alveolar proteinosis
17. Mediastinal abnormalities (*eg*, adenopathy, lipomatosis, or mediastinitis)
18. Panlobular emphysema
19. Pulmonary calcinosis
20. Pseudosepsis syndrome

*Most common pulmonary manifestations.

supported by anecdotal reports rather than well-designed controlled studies.

Major Clinical Syndromes of Drug-Induced Pulmonary Disease

Chronic Pneumonitis/Fibrosis

A wide array of drugs has been implicated in causing chronic interstitial pneumonitis and/or fibrosis, making them the most common manifestations of drug-induced lung disease. Some of the agents implicated are listed in Table 2. There is a small increase in antidepressant use, especially tricyclic-related agents and selective serotonin receptor inhibitors, in patients with idiopathic pulmonary fibrosis (IPF; odds ratio [OR], 1.52; 95% confidence interval 1.24 to 1.86).[3] These patients commonly present with insidious onset of cough and dyspnea. Weight loss and clubbing may also be present, raising the possibility of an underlying malignancy or IPF, respectively. Chest radiography and high-resolution chest CT (HRCT) generally reveal reticular infiltrates beginning in the basilar subpleural regions and progressing to diffuse disease. The results of pulmonary function tests (PFTs) typically show reduced lung volumes (*eg*, restrictive physiology), a reduced diffusing capacity of the lung for carbon monoxide (DLCO), and arterial hypoxemia at rest or with exercise.

Table 2. *Some Drugs That Cause Chronic Pneumonitis/Fibrosis*

Chemotherapeutic Agents	Nonchemotherapeutic Agents
• Azathioprine	• Amiodarone*
• BCNU	• Anti-TNF-α-targeted therapy
• Bleomycin*	• Cocaine
• Busulfan	• Gold
• Chlorambucil	• Heroin
• Cyclophospamide	• Methysergide
• Fludarabine	• Nitrofurantoin
• Gemcitabine	• Penicillamine
• 6-Mercaptopurine	• Phenytoin
• Methotrexate	• Sirolimus
• Mitomycin C	• Statins
• Taxanes (paclitaxel/docetaxel)	• Sulfasalazine
• Tyrosine kinase inhibitors (imatinib)	• Tocainide

*Most commonly implicated.

Hypersensitivity-Type Lung Disease

Virtually any drug can cause a generalized hypersensitivity-type reaction with respiratory symptoms that are associated with pulmonary infiltrates and eosinophilia (PIE). The agents commonly implicated are listed in Table 3. Patients can present with Loeffler syndrome, consisting of an acute onset over several days of cough, dyspnea, fever, rash, myalgias, peripheral eosinophilia, and fleeting infiltrates. Alternatively, patients may present with chronic eosinophilic pneumonia consisting of a subacute onset over several months of low-grade fever, night sweats, nonproductive cough, and weight loss. Establishing a diagnosis may be challenging because not all findings, especially peripheral eosinophilia, are present in each patient. The diagnosis is often secured by bronchoscopy with BAL and biopsy and, in some instances, after a prompt response to therapy with corticosteroids. The prognosis is generally favorable with a mortality rate of $<1\%$.

Acute Noncardiogenic Pulmonary Edema

Noncardiogenic pulmonary edema can occur after exposure to a variety of drugs (Table 4). These patients generally present with acute dyspnea and a nonproductive cough that develops during a period of hours. A physical examination of the chest reveals inspiratory crackles, whereas arterial blood gas levels show hypoxemia. The chest radiograph generally demonstrates diffuse acinar and/or ground-glass infiltrates. The histopathology can

Table 3. *Some Drugs That Cause Hypersensitivity-Type Lung Disease*

Chemotherapeutic Agents	Nonchemotherapeutic Agents
• Azathioprine	• Antibiotics (β-lactam and sulfa-containing)*
• Bleomycin	
• Busulfan	• Anti-TNF-α-targeted therapy
• Imatinib	• Isoniazide
• Methotrexate*	• Nitrofurantoin
• Nitrogen mustards	• NSAIDs
• Procarbazine	Penicillamine
• Taxanes	• Phenytoin
	• Statins

*Most commonly implicated.

Table 4. *Some Drugs That Cause Acute Noncardiogenic Pulmonary Edema*

Chemotherapeutic Agents	Nonchemotherapeutic Agents
• Azathioprine • Cytosine arabinoside • Gemcitabine • G-CSF • IL-2 • Methotrexate • Mitomycin C • Nitrogen mustards • Retinoic Acid • TNF • Vinblastine (with mitomycin)	• Amiodarone • Aspirin and NSAID overdose • Cocaine • Opiate overdose (*eg*, heroin) • Sedative/hypnotic drug overdose • Sulfasalazine • Tocolytic therapy (*eg*, terbutaline, ritodrine) • IFN-γ1b

Table 5. *Some Drugs That Cause Bronchilolitis Obliterans With Organizing Pneumonia (BOOP) / Cryptogenic Organizing Pneumonia (COP)*

Chemotherapeutic Agents	Nonchemotherapeutic Agents
• Bleomycin • Cyclophosphamide • Methotrexate • Mitomycin C	• Amiodarone • Amphotericin B • Carbamazepine • Cocaine • Nitrofurantoin • Penicillamine • Phenytoin • Sirolimus • Sulfasalazine • Ticlodipine

be similar to ARDS. Several mechanisms have been implicated in causing drug-induced noncardiogenic pulmonary edema. First, some drugs increase the filtration coefficient of the respiratory membrane, making it more permeable (*eg*, overdose of narcotics/sedatives). Second, certain agents depress the CNS, resulting in neurogenic pulmonary edema. Finally, some drugs cause an idiosyncratic reaction resulting in noncardiogenic pulmonary edema within hours of absorption. The prognosis varies depending on the offending agent. For example, pulmonary edema associated with an overdose of salicylates is potentially reversible with appropriate management, whereas patients with carmustine-induced pulmonary edema generally have a poor prognosis.

Cryptogenic Organizing Pneumonia

A variety of drugs cause bronchiolitis obliterans with organizing pneumonia (BOOP), which is preferentially now called *cryptogenic organizing pneumonia* (COP; Table 5). Thus, any new diagnosis of COP requires a careful review of their drug exposure before concluding that COP is "cryptogenic." These patients typically present with cough, dyspnea, crackles on physical examination, and patchy airspace infiltrates seen on the chest radiograph. PFT results reveal a mixed obstructive and restrictive defect. Gold and penicillamine, the two best-characterized etiologic agents, are often used in the management of rheumatoid arthritis (RA), a disease that can also cause COP. Thus, it may be difficult to distinguish drug-induced COP from the patient's underlying collagen vascular disorder. Management requires a high clinical suspicion, lung biopsy, prompt withdrawal of therapy with the implicated drug, and the administration of corticosteroids. The outcome is generally favorable, as it is with idiopathic COP.

Alveolar Hypoventilation

Alveolar hypoventilation is caused by drugs that induce respiratory depression or block respiratory muscle function. Patients with underlying pulmonary or neuromuscular disorders are particularly prone to the development of acute hypercarbic respiratory failure. Some of the agents implicated in causing neuromuscular blockade or motor neuropathies/myopathies are listed in Table 6. Aminoglycoside-induced neuromuscular blockade is a rare but potentially life-threatening adverse effect that has been described in patients who have been exposed to neomycin, streptomycin, tobramycin, gentamicin, amikacin, kanamycin, and netilmicin.[4] The risk of aminoglycoside-induced neuromuscular blockade is increased in the presence of a disease or drug that promotes neuromuscular blockade, increasing aminoglycoside drug levels, hypomagnesemia, and hypocalcemia. The management of these disorders requires a high clinical suspicion to identify the offending drug and withdrawal of therapy with the agent to avoid further respiratory failure.

Table 6. *Some Drugs That Cause Alveolar Hypoventilation*

Neuromuscular blockade	
• Aminoglycosides	• Opiates (*eg*, heroin)
• Cocaine	• Polymixins
• Gamma-hydroxybutyrate (GHB)	• Sedative/hypnotic drugs
Motor neuropathies or myopathies	
• Amiodarone	• Isoniazid
• Captopril	• Phenytoin
• Corticosteroids	• Procainamide
• Diuretics	

Bronchospasm

Drug-induced bronchospasm is caused by various agents (Table 7). Patients generally present with wheezing, cough, and/or dyspnea. Spirometry typically shows airways obstruction. The mechanism of drug-induced bronchospasm varies with the particular agent. In patients with asthma, unlike healthy individuals, β-adrenergic blockers induce bronchospasm within minutes by mechanisms involving the inhibition of adrenergic bronchodilator tone. Virtually any route of administration (*eg*, oral, IV, or ophthalmic) can induce bronchospasm. Aspirin-induced bronchospasm is mediated by an enhanced 5-lipoxygenase pathway, resulting in the production of bronchoconstricting cysteinyl-leukotrienes and, to a lesser extent, by a reduction in bronchodilating prostaglandins (*eg*, prostaglandin E_2). Dipyridamole causes bronchospasm by augmenting the levels of adenosine, a bronchoconstricting agent. Gold and penicillamine cause irreversible airways obstruction due to concentric bronchiolitis obliterans.

Table 7. *Some Drugs That Cause Bronchospasm*

Chemotherapeutic Agents	Nonchemotherapeutic Agents
• IL-2	• Aspirin and NSAIDs
• Methotrexate	• β-blockers
• Vinblastine	• Contrast media
• Vinca alkaloids plus mitomycin	• Corticosteroids
	• Dipyridamole
	• Gold
	• Nitrofurantoin (acute)
	• Opiates (cocaine, heroin)
	• Penicillamine
	• Protamine

Isolated Cough

Cough, which is one of the most common manifestations of drug-induced lung disease, is a vagus nerve-mediated reflex caused by various chemical and mechanical stimuli virtually anywhere within the upper and lower respiratory tracts. Cough often occurs in patients with drug-induced bronchospasm or drug-induced interstitial lung disease. However, angiotensin-converting enzyme (ACE) inhibitors induce an isolated nonproductive cough without associated bronchospasm or parenchymal lung disease in nearly 10% of patients receiving any type of ACE inhibitor.[5]

Pleural Effusions

Although a number of drugs can cause a pleural effusion (Table 8; see also Dr. Sahn's chapter on pleural disease in this book), the number is much less than those that involve the lung parenchyma.[6] Pleural effusions occur with acute onset as part of a hypersensitivity reaction after exposure to amiodarone, methotrexate, and nitrofurantoin, as well as a systemic lupus erythematosus (SLE)-like reaction that is described below. Anticoagulants can induce an acute bloody effusion. Chronic pleural effusion may occur after long-term exposure to drugs that induce a delayed hypersensitivity-type response (*eg*, methotrexate or procarbazine) or in association with the development of interstitial pulmonary inflammation/fibrosis (*eg*, busulfan and methotrexate). A variety of chemotherapeutic agents, including some of the newer antineoplastic agents, are associated with an increased risk of pleural fluid formation.[7]

Table 8. *Some Drugs That Cause Pleural Effusions*

Chemotherapeutic Agents	Nonchemotherapeutic Agents
Bleomycin	Amiodarone
Busulfan	Anticoagulants
Etoposide	Bromocriptine
Gemcitabine	Dantrolene
Methotrexate	Esophageal sclerosing agents
Mitomycin	Methysergide
Procarbazine	Nitrofurantoin
Taxanes	
Tyrosine kinase inhibitors	

Pulmonary Vascular Disease

Drugs that affect the pulmonary vascular circulation by causing venous thromboembolism (VTE), pulmonary hypertension, vasculitis, or pulmonary venoocclusive disease are listed in Table 9. Oral contraceptives and other estrogen-containing agents can induce VTE. The VTE risks are relatively small in patients using second-generation and third-generation oral contraceptives compared with nonusers (15, 30, and 5 per 100,000 patients treated, respectively).[8] There is an important synergistic interaction between hypercoagulable conditions (*eg*, factor V Leiden deficiency) and the risks of VTE from hormonal replacement therapy.[9] Thus, the risk from hormonal replacement in the absence of other VTE risk factors appears too small to recommend against using these agents.

Drug-induced pulmonary hypertension can occur after exposure to a variety of drugs by mechanisms that are unclear. A case-control study[10] showed that appetite suppressants (*eg*, amphetamines, fenfluramine, and dexfenfluramine) are associated with an increased risk of primary pulmonary hypertension (OR: overall, 6.3; if the drugs were used for >3 months, >20). Although fenfluramine and dexfenfluramine have been withdrawn from the market worldwide, clinicians should remain vigilant for drug-induced pulmonary hypertension because an estimated 5 million adults in the United States continue to use appetite suppressants. Oral contraceptives and other estrogen-containing agents have also been associated with an increased risk of pulmonary hypertension.

An inflammatory vasculitis has been noted in conjunction with a generalized hypersensitivity reaction in patients exposed to busulfan, nitrofurantoin, or illicit drugs such as cocaine and heroin. However, it is uncertain whether the vascular response represents a primary or secondary effect of drug exposure. Leukotriene receptor antagonists (LTRAs), such as zafirlukast and montelukast, rarely (*ie*, 1 case per 15,000 to 20,000 patient-years treated) induce an idiosyncratic syndrome similar to Churg-Strauss vasculitis with peripheral eosinophilia, eosinophilic vasculitis, peripheral neuropathy, and cardiac failure.[11] Because most of the patients were receiving either high-dose inhaled or systemic corticosteroids, a preexisting vasculitis may have accounted for their symptoms. However, a review of the literature through 2007 identified 62 cases from 40 publications, 7 of whom were entirely steroid naïve (*eg*, not receiving any form of inhaled or oral steroids when symptoms developed), suggesting that there may be a causal relationship.[12] An accompanying editorial reviewing this study as well as another case-control study involving 78 patients concluded that Churg-Strauss vasculitis can occur in association with exposure to LTRA in three settings: (1) use for worsening asthma, (2) use resulting in clinical improvement leading to a reduction in steroids and an unmasking

Table 9. *Some Drugs That Cause Pulmonary Vascular Disease*

Complication	Chemotherapeutic Agents	Nonchemotherapeutic Agents
Thromboembolic disease		Estrogens/hormonal treatment Phenytoin Steroids
Pulmonary hypertension	Mitomycin IL-2	Aminorex (recalled) Amphetamines Dexfenfluramine (recalled) Fenfluramine (recalled) L-tryptophan (recalled) Oral contraceptives
Vasculitis	Busulfan	Cocaine/heroin Nitrofurantoin Zafirlukast/montelukast
Veno-occlusive disease	Bleomycin Busulfan BCNU Mitomycin	Oral contraceptives

of the vasculitis, and (3) use in steroid-naïve patients.[13] Pulmonary venoocclusive disease is a very rare adverse effect reported after exposure to various agents (Table 9).

Miscellaneous Drug-Induced Pulmonary Reactions

There are a variety of less common drug-induced adverse pulmonary effects (Table 10). SLE is associated with the use of a wide variety of drugs, although five agents are involved in >90% of the cases (Table 10). More recently, anti-tumor necrosis factor (TNF)-α–targeted therapy (*eg*, etanercept, infliximab, and adalimumab) has also been associated with drug-induced SLE reactions. Five to twelve percent of all cases of SLE are caused by drugs. It is unclear whether these agents cause or unmask a latent case of SLE. Hydralazine-induced and isoniazid-induced SLE occur more frequently in patients who are slow acetylators of these drugs. Hydralazine-induced SLE occurs in up to 20% of patients receiving doses of ≥400 mg/d but can be found in patients receiving low-dose therapy. Procainamide-induced SLE is time related rather than dose related in that positivity for antinuclear antibodies (ANAs) develops in approximately 50% of patients after 3 months of therapy and in nearly all patients by 1 year. Notably, patients with drug-induced SLE, unlike other patients with SLE, are usually negative for double-stranded DNA ANA. Typically, pleurisy and dyspnea, in conjunction with systemic complaints of fever and arthralgias, develop in an insidious manner after using the drug for several months or even years. Chest radiograph abnormalities include pleural effusions, atelectasis, diffuse interstitial infiltrates, and alveolar infiltrates. The withdrawal of therapy with the offending agent generally results in the prompt resolution of symptoms within days, but occasionally, corticosteroids are required for symptomatic relief.

Alveolar hemorrhage and hemoptysis can occur after exposure to certain drugs (Table 10). Drug-induced hemoptysis is most commonly caused by pulmonary embolism with infarction. Penicillamine can cause a pulmonary-renal syndrome similar to Goodpasture syndrome. Therapy with oral anticoagulants can induce spontaneous pulmonary hemorrhage days to years after the onset of therapy. Abciximab, a chimeric monoclonal antibody directed against platelet glycoprotein IIb/IIIa receptor that reduces restenosis after angioplasty and stent placement, can cause severe alveolar hemorrhage.[14] This relatively rare complication (7 of 2,533 patients [0.3%] vs 0 of 5,412 control subjects) should be suspected in patients presenting with hemoptysis, hypoxemic respiratory

Table 10. *Miscellaneous Drug-Induced Pulmonary Reactions*

Condition	Implicated Drugs	
Drug-Induced SLE	Hydralazine	Procainamide
	Isoniazid	Penicillamine
	Anti-TNF-α-targeted therapy	Quinidine
Alveolar hemorrhage	Abciximab	Cocaine
	Bevacizumab	Amphotericin B
	Alemtuzumab	Mitomycin C
	Amiodarone	Nitrofurantoin
	Anticoagulants	Penicillamine
Alveolar proteinosis	Busulfan	
Churg-Strauss vasculitis	Zafirlukast	Montelukast
Mediastinal abnormalities	Methotrexate	Phenytoin
Lipomatosis	Corticosteroids	
Mediastinitis	Esophageal sclerosing agents	
Panlobular emphysema	Methylphenidate	
Pulmonary calcification	Antacids	High-dose vitamin D
	Calcium	
Pseudosepsis syndrome	Chronic salicylate intoxication	

failure, diffuse alveolar infiltrates, and progressive decline in hemoglobin levels within hours to 2 days after the first dose of abciximab. Bevacizumab, a monoclonal antibody against vascular endothelial growth factor that is used to treat a variety of cancers, including lung and colon cancer, can result in fatal pulmonary hemorrhage.[15]

Mediastinal abnormalities can be a manifestation of an adverse drug effect (Table 10). Phenytoin can induce a pseudolymphoma syndrome that is associated with peripheral adenopathy and, rarely, mediastinal adenopathy. Methotrexate may cause transient hilar adenopathy during a hypersensitivity-type response. Typically, the adenopathy regresses 1 to 2 weeks after drug withdrawal. Mediastinal fullness caused by lipomatosis is an unusual manifestation of an adverse effect of corticosteroids. Although mediastinal widening in patients receiving corticosteroids may raise the suspicion of adenopathy, the diagnosis of lipomatosis is suggested by the characteristic chest radiograph appearance of a straight mediastinal border without the lumpy features of adenopathy and the typical CT scan findings of lipid-containing tissue. Mediastinitis associated with fever and chest pain is a relatively rare adverse effect of esophageal variceal sclerotherapy.

Other rare pulmonary adverse drug effects reported in the literature include busulfan-induced alveolar proteinosis, methylphenidate-induced panlobular emphysema, and pulmonary parenchymal calcium deposition associated with hypercalcemic conditions or drugs such as antacids, calcium, and high-dose vitamin D. Long-term salicylate ingestion can cause a pseudosepsis syndrome (reviewed in the section "Antiinflammatory Drugs").

Approach to the Patient With Suspected Drug-Induced Lung Disease

Differential Diagnosis

As mentioned previously, the diagnosis of drug-induced lung disease is one of exclusion because there are no pathognomonic criteria. The differential diagnosis is broad, especially in cancer patients receiving therapy with multiple drugs, often including immunosuppressive agents. However, the differential diagnosis can be narrowed based on the presenting clinical syndrome reviewed above as well as by the presence of localized or diffuse infiltrates (Table 11). In some instances, the patient may have minimal or absent symptoms and findings but demonstrate abnormalities on the chest radiograph or PFT results. A high level of clinical suspicion is required because drug-induced disease may occur years after initial exposure and the radiographic abnormalities may be subtle.

Diagnostic Approach

Because drug-induced pulmonary toxicity has a profound impact on patient management, it is important to establish a firm diagnosis as soon as possible. This begins with an understanding of the clinical syndromes caused by various agents combined with the prudent use of noninvasive studies and invasive procedures. Evaluation of the chest radiograph, PFT results and, on occasion, chest CT scan help narrow the differential diagnosis. Noninvasive studies that may be useful include the following: (1) an echocardiogram to assess cardiac function; (2) sputum studies to identify an infectious pathogen (*eg*, Gram stain, culture, direct fluorescent antibody for *Pneumocystis carinii* or Legionella, and acid-fast bacteria stain and culture); and (3) immunologic studies to exclude collagen vascular disorders and vasculitis.

If a firm diagnosis is not established, then the judicious use of invasive diagnostic procedures is warranted. Typically, fiberoptic bronchoscopy with BAL and transbronchial lung biopsy is the next step in the evaluation of patients with localized or diffuse pulmonary disease of unclear etiology.

Table 11. *Differential Diagnosis of Radiographic Abnormalities*

Diffuse Disease	Localized Disease
Infection	Infection
Malignancy	Malignancy
Lymphangitic metastasis	Pulmonary emboli
Pulmonary edema	Radiation pneumonitis
Pulmonary fibrosis	Drug toxicity
Radiation pneumonitis/fibrosis	
Leukoagglutinin reaction	
ARDS	
Hypersensitivity pneumonitis	
Pulmonary hemorrhage	
Drug toxicity	

Although this procedure has an excellent diagnostic yield for infections and malignant lesions (approximately 70 to 90%), it has a lower diagnostic yield for interstitial inflammatory lesions, including those caused by drug-induced toxicity. In the proper clinical setting, a nondiagnostic bronchoscopy may be sufficient to suggest the diagnosis of drug-induced injury. A thoracoscopic biopsy or, less commonly, an open-lung biopsy is recommended in patients for whom the diagnosis remains unclear and the differential diagnosis includes other pulmonary abnormalities, especially interstitial lung disease.

These procedures have the greatest diagnostic yield and a relatively low complication rate, even in critically ill patients. The histopathologic changes associated with drug toxicity are nonspecific, revealing elements of diffuse alveolar damage, fibrinous exudate, atypical or reactive alveolar type II cells, inflammatory cells, and fibrotic foci. One study[14] showed that up to 20% of patients with diffuse infiltrates undergoing an open-lung biopsy had histologic changes that could be attributed to a drug reaction.

PFTs

The role of PFTs for detecting adverse drug-induced pulmonary effects has been extensively investigated. The majority of the studies have focused on bleomycin, busulfan, and amiodarone. The most common PFT result abnormalities are diminished lung volumes and a reduced DLCO. However, it is controversial whether these abnormalities accurately predict that clinically overt disease will develop.[17,18] Overt drug-induced disease can develop in patients in the absence of PFT result abnormalities and, conversely, patients can have abnormal PFT results in the absence of drug-induced lung disease. Patient effort and anemia are important confounding variables that affect PFT results. For most drugs, well-designed clinical studies validating the role of PFTs to detect adverse pulmonary effects are not available. Until definitive data are available, it is reasonable for clinicians to continue using PFTs in select settings with the goal of identifying subclinical disease as long as the physiologic interpretation is made in the context of the entire clinical situation.

Chemotherapy-Associated Pulmonary Toxicity

Azathioprine/Mercaptopurine

Azathioprine, a purine analog that inhibits DNA synthesis, is an immunosuppressive agent used in the treatment of nonmalignant disease (*eg*, IPF and organ transplantation). Mercaptopurine, the active metabolite of azathioprine, is an antineoplastic agent. Azathioprine rarely (<1%) causes pulmonary fibrosis, hypersensitivity-type reactions/PIE, or diffuse alveolar damage.

BCNU

Carmustine, or *bis*-chloronitrosourea (BCNU), is the best-known and extensively studied member of the nitrosourea family of drugs that includes lomustine (chloroethylnitrosourea), semustine (methyl-chloroethylnitrosourea), and chlorozotocin. These cytotoxic agents, which are unique in their ability to cross the blood-brain barrier, are active against a variety of neoplasms, including CNS malignancies. BCNU causes interstitial pulmonary fibrosis and granulomatous inflammation that can progress after drug withdrawal. The pathogenesis of BCNU-induced pulmonary toxicity is unclear. BCNU promotes oxidant-induced lung injury by inhibiting glutathione reductase, thereby reducing glutathione stores, which is an important antioxidant defense. BCNU causes cytotoxic changes characterized by alveolar type II cell hyperplasia and dysplasia, fibroblastic foci of proliferation, and interstitial fibrosis.

Patients presenting with BCNU-induced pulmonary toxicity will typically note an insidious onset of a nonproductive cough and dyspnea associated with reticular nodular interstitial infiltrates on the chest radiograph. However, the onset of symptoms is highly variable, appearing within days to as many as 17 years after beginning therapy BCNU.[19] Risk factors include the total dose, other agents, and preexisting lung disease. In terms of dose, the incidence of pulmonary toxicity with high-dose BCNU (>1,500 mg/m^2) varies from 20 to 50%, whereas with low-dose BCNU the incidence is on the order of 1 to 5%, primarily when administered concurrently with other agents. Other agents such as cyclophosphamide and radiation increase the risk of BCNU-induced lung injury; however, a synergistic interaction has not been documented. In regard to preexisting lung disease, patients with preexisting symptomatic pulmonary disorders, especially with a reduced vital capacity or DLCO, are typically excluded from receiving BCNU. A reduced DLCO without chest radiographic abnormalities occurs in patients receiving BCNU.

Although there are no prospective studies to guide the timing of PFT monitoring, PFTs are typically performed during BCNU therapy to monitor for subclinical disease as well as intermittently for the long term, given the extended latency period between treatment and pulmonary toxicity. This approach is supported in part by the poor outcomes of patients in whom BCNU-induced pulmonary fibrosis develops. BCNU-induced lung injury is associated with a mortality rate of nearly 90%. Corticosteroid therapy has little impact in preventing or treating BCNU-induced lung injury. The primary treatment is to withdraw BCNU promptly and provide supportive care. Although there is less information about the frequency of pulmonary injury caused by the other nitrosoureas, each has been reported to have effects similar to those of BCNU.

Bleomycin

Bleomycin, which is a cytotoxic antibiotic that is isolated from *Streptomyces verticillus*, is very useful in treating patients with head and neck carcinomas, germ-cell tumors, and Hodgkin and non-Hodgkin lymphomas. Bleomycin accumulates in the skin and lung, resulting in skin ulcerations and pulmonary fibrosis. Bleomycin-induced pulmonary damage, which is the major dose-limiting side effect, was first recognized in 1972.[20] The overall incidence of pulmonary toxicity is 10% (range, 3 to 40%) and is fatal in 1 to 2% of patients.

The pathogenesis of bleomycin-induced lung injury has not been firmly established.[18] Because bleomycin reproducibly causes interstitial pneumonitis and fibrosis in animal models, it has become a paradigm for the study of the pathogenic mechanisms underlying pulmonary fibrosis. Early bleomycin-induced pulmonary injury shows acute and organizing diffuse alveolar damage that is similar to the fibroproliferative phase of ARDS. Bleomycin binds to intracellular iron in alveolar epithelial and vascular endothelial cells and, in the presence of oxygen, generates highly reactive oxygen species (ROS), such as hydroxyl radicals.

ROS alter important cellular components (*eg*, DNA, lipids, and proteins), resulting in damage to the respiratory membrane. Intratracheal or IV bleomycin increases cytokine levels within the lung in animal models. The important cytokines implicated in the pathogenesis of bleomycin-induced pulmonary toxicity include transforming growth factor (TGF)-β, TNF-α, interleukin (IL)-1, and others. Pathogenic roles for ROS and certain cytokines are supported by the protective effects of various agents, including antioxidants, iron chelators, IL-1 receptor antagonists, IL-12, keratinocyte growth factor, CD36 peptides (binds TGF-β_1), or antibodies against TGF-β, TNF-α, or CD3 receptors.[18]

A crucial role for alveolar epithelial cell injury is supported by the finding that transgenic mice deficient in the epithelial cell-restricted integrin αvβ6 do not exhibit bleomycin-induced pulmonary inflammation or fibrosis because they are unable to activate latent TGF-β.[21] Bleomycin lung toxicity can also be prevented by blocking excessive alveolar epithelial cell apoptosis or DNA damage, by enhancing DNA repair, and by augmenting fibrinolysis.[22–25] Notably, the expression of the bleomycin-resistant *Streptoalloteichus hindustanus* gene, which encodes a protein that binds bleomycin and blocks DNA damage, can prevent bleomycin-induced fibrosis.[24] Recently, increased expression of epithelial cell-derived integrin αvβ6 was noted[26] in the distal alveoli of patients with IPF and antibodies against αvβ6 blocked bleomycin-induced fibrosis in mice, even when administered after the development of fibrosis. A disease-specific gene expression-profiling study in which the authors used multiple murine models of lung disease identified 12 unique transcripts characteristic of bleomycin-induced pulmonary fibrosis that were not evident in the other models.[27] Although the pathogenic mechanisms underlying bleomycin toxicity are better understood and lead to potentially novel antifibrotic therapies, it is unclear why certain patients are predisposed to pulmonary fibrosis.

There are three major clinical manifestations of bleomycin-induced lung toxicity: (1) chronic interstitial fibrosis, (2) hypersensitivity-type disease, and (3) COP. Interstitial fibrosis is by far the most common, occurring in approximately 11% of those patients treated. Patients typically present with a subacute onset of a nonproductive cough and dyspnea within a few weeks to 6 months after treatment.[15] Pleuritic substernal chest pain occurs in approximately 3% of patients. However, nearly 20% of patients with bleomycin-induced lung injury will be asymptomatic. Physical examination findings may show tachypnea, bibasilar crackles, and hyperpigmented skin lesions. Chest radiographs typically reveal basilar, predominant reticular, or fine nodular infiltrates that often originate from the costophrenic angles. Other less common radiographic patterns include patchy alveolar infiltrates, lobar consolidation, and lung nodules. PFT results generally show reduced lung volumes and DLCO. Patients with bleomycin-induced hypersensitivity-type disease may have similar symptoms but often with an associated fever, malaise, and chest radiographic changes of chronic pneumonitis and ground glass-appearing parenchyma with little fibrosis. The radiographic and pathologic distinctions between fibrosis and pneumonitis are not always clear.

Risk factors for the development of bleomycin-induced pulmonary toxicity include the following. (1) Total dose: a dose relationship has been described with an incidence of 3 to 5% when the total dose is < 300 U but > 20% when the total dose is > 500 U[18]; however, pulmonary toxicity can occur after receiving only 20 U. (2) Oxygen: bleomycin, more than any other drug, has a well-known synergistic toxic interaction with oxygen that can occur years after bleomycin exposure. Although this reaction does not develop in all patients, the inspired oxygen concentration for patients who have ever received bleomycin should be kept < 25%, if possible. (3) Radiation: radiation therapy, even years after bleomycin exposure, increases the risk. (4) Age: persons > 70 years of age are at an increased risk of lung injury. (5) Abnormal renal function: patients with reduced renal function are more susceptible to bleomycin-induced pulmonary toxicity because of the fact that the kidneys primarily excrete bleomycin. (6) Concurrent use of other cytotoxic agents: some drugs may increase the risk of bleomycin-related injury, including cyclophosphamide, doxorubicin, granulocyte colony-stimulating factor (G-CSF), methotrexate, and vincristine.

The management of patients with bleomycin-induced pulmonary toxicity centers on withdrawing the drug and limiting exposure to exogenous oxygen, as noted previously. Although the overall mortality rate is approximately 1 to 2%, the mortality rate varies from 10 to 83% in patients with pulmonary disease. Corticosteroids (60 to 100 mg/d) are generally administered to all patients with clinically significant toxicity and then slowly tapered according to the patient's clinical response. Clinical improvement typically occurs within weeks and may take 2 years to completely resolve. Select patients will be left with residual radiographic and abnormalities on the PFT results.

Busulfan

Busulfan, an alkylating agent that is used in the management of chronic myeloproliferative disorders, was the first chemotherapeutic agent implicated in causing chronic pneumonitis/pulmonary fibrosis. In general, alkylating agents (*eg*, busulfan, cyclophosphamide, chlorambucil, and melphalan) have a lower frequency of inducing lung injury than other cytotoxic agents. Like bleomycin, these agents can induce synergistic pulmonary damage when a patient is exposed to oxygen, radiation, or other cytotoxic chemotherapeutic agents. The incidence of symptomatic busulfan-induced pulmonary fibrosis is approximately 4 to 5%. However, histologically evident fibrosis and cytotoxic changes (hyperplastic and dysplastic type II cells) occur in up to 46% of busulfan-treated patients, most of whom are asymptomatic.[28] A threshold dose has not been established.

The clinical presentation is an insidious onset, often > 3 years after initiating therapy, of cough, dyspnea, fever, malaise, and weight loss. The PFT results show restrictive lung volumes, a reduced DLCO, and hypoxemia. The chest radiograph typically shows diffuse interstitial and alveolar infiltrates with a basilar predominance. Occasionally, pleural effusions, nodular densities, or normal chest radiograph findings are noted. Management centers on drug withdrawal and the administration of corticosteroids. The prognosis is poor, with the mortality rate ranging from 50 to 80%. Alveolar proteinosis has also been reported after exposure to busulfan. Unlike primary alveolar proteinosis, it does not respond to therapeutic BAL.

Cyclophosphamide

Cyclophosphamide, an alkylating agent that causes pulmonary toxicity less frequently than busulfan, is widely used to treat malignant diseases (*eg*, lymphomas, breast carcinoma, and ovarian carcinoma) and nonmalignant diseases (*eg*, collagen vascular disorders, IPF, and Wegener granulomatosis). The incidence of adverse pulmonary effects is <1%. The extensive clinical indications for cyclophosphamide and its frequent use in conjunction with other cytotoxic drugs increases the likelihood that lung toxicity will be seen by pulmonologists. Although cyclophosphamide alone induces pulmonary toxicity in humans relatively infrequently,[29] it clearly does so in animals.[30] The pathogenesis of pulmonary toxicity has not been established but likely involves oxidant-mediated mechanisms. Cyclophosphamide is metabolized into two active agents, phosphoramide mustard and acrolein, both of which reduce hepatic glutathione stores.

Chronic pneumonitis and/or fibrosis are the most common clinical manifestations of pulmonary toxicity. Symptoms develop as soon as 2 weeks to as long as 13 years after the initiation of therapy, without any clear dose relationship. Patients present with cough, dyspnea, fever, and bibasilar interstitial infiltrates seen on chest radiographs. Synergistic toxicity has been described in patients receiving radiation therapy or other cytotoxic agents.[31] Cyclophosphamide-induced pulmonary fibrosis, unlike IPF, may present with bilateral pleural thickening typically without clubbing and "Velcro" crackles.[29] The prognosis is generally poor, with a mortality rate approaching 50%. Most patients are treated with corticosteroids based on anecdotal reports of benefit.

Methotrexate

Methotrexate is a folic acid antagonist that is used in the management of malignant and nonmalignant inflammatory diseases. The incidence of pulmonary toxicity is nearly 7% for high-dose methotrexate, as used to treat malignancies, but 2 to 3% with low-dose methotrexate regimens used to treat chronic inflammatory conditions such as RA. Methotrexate-induced pulmonary toxicity does not have a clear dose relationship because it occurs over a broad range of doses (40 to 6,500 mg).

Clinical manifestations include the following: (1) hypersensitivity-type disease, the most common form; (2) chronic pneumonitis/fibrosis; (3) COP; (4) acute chest pain; (5) noncardiogenic pulmonary edema; (6) acute pleurisy/pleural effusions; and (7) bronchospasm.[32] Methotrexate-induced hypersensitivity-type reactions typically occur within 10 days to 4 months after initiating therapy but can occur up to 1 month after therapy with methotrexate ceases.[32] Patients may complain of fever, cough, dyspnea, arthralgias and, less commonly, skin rash (approximately 17%). Chest radiographs reveal diffuse interstitial infiltrates with ground-glass changes seen on HRCT scans. Other radiographic abnormalities that are occasionally seen include nodular infiltrates, hilar/mediastinal adenopathy, and pleural effusions. Blood eosinophilia is present in nearly 40% of patients. BAL fluid findings typically reveal a predominance of lymphocytes, especially T-suppressor cells, which are characteristic of a hypersensitivity reaction.[33]

The diagnosis of methotrexate-induced pulmonary toxicity requires the following three major criteria: (1) hypersensitivity pneumonitis by histopathology, (2) radiographic evidence of interstitial and/or alveolar infiltrates, and (3) blood cultures (if febrile) and sputum cultures (if available) that are negative for microbes. Patients must also have three of the following five minor criteria: (1) dyspnea of <8 weeks in duration, (2) nonproductive cough, (3) room air oxygen saturation of ≤90%, (4) DLCO of ≤70% of predicted, and (5) leukocyte count of ≤15,000 cells/μL.[34]

Risk factors for the development of methotrexate-induced pulmonary toxicity include the following: (1) appearance of symptoms within the first 32 weeks of therapy, (2) multidrug regimens (synergy with cyclophosphamide has been reported), (3) diabetes mellitus, (4) age ≥50 years, (5) rheumatoid pleuropulmonary disease, and (6) hypoalbuminemia.[35] Dose, frequency, smoking status, previous lung disease, and route of administration route (*eg*, oral, IV, intrathecal, and IM) do not consistently affect the frequency of methotrexate-induced adverse pulmonary effects. Notably, PFT results have not been helpful in identifying patients with RA who are at risk for the development of pulmonary toxicity while receiving long-term low-dose methotrexate.[36] Chronic pneumonitis/fibrosis, which occurs less commonly as the result of methotrexate than other chemotherapeutic agents, typically presents 4 months to >3 years after the initiation of therapy. Management centers on the withdrawal of therapy with the drug and the administration of corticosteroids. Chronic fibrosis will develop in approximately 7% of patients with methotrexate-induced hypersensitivity reactions, and 8% will die of progressive respiratory failure.

Mitomycin

Mitomycin is an alkylating cytotoxic antibiotic that is used in the treatment of breast, GI, gynecologic, and lung carcinomas. The incidence of pulmonary cytotoxicity is approximately 5% (range, 3 to 39%).[37] However, the full scope is difficult to assess because mitomycin is typically administered concurrently with other agents and is also a cotoxin with oxygen and radiation. The presenting features as well as the radiographic and physiologic changes are similar to those seen with bleomycin-induced interstitial pneumonitis/fibrosis. Of note, this reaction seems to occur most frequently after the third cycle of treatment. Although serial monitoring of the DLCO to detect clinically occult disease is unproven, it is generally recommended and widely used for this purpose. Prednisone can rapidly resolve the symptoms and interstitial infiltrates. A unique reaction of mitomycin is the induction of microangiopathic hemolytic anemia concurrently with noncardiogenic pulmonary edema and renal failure. The mortality rate associated with this uncommon reaction is >90%.

The combination of mitomycin with vinca alkaloids (*eg*, vinblastine and vincristine) induces an acute onset (<3 h after receiving the vinca alkaloid) of bronchospasm that is associated with focal or diffuse interstitial infiltrates seen on chest radiographs and hypoxemia.[38] Vinca alkaloids alone do not cause this adverse side effect. Chronic respiratory symptoms that respond to corticosteroids develop in approximately two thirds of the patients.

Retinoic Acid

All-*trans*-retinoic acid (ATRA) is a highly effective biological response modifier that induces clinical remission in patients with acute promyelocytic leukemia by augmenting the differentiation of malignant stem cells into mature neutrophils. An ARDS-like picture, termed *retinoic acid syndrome*, developed in nearly 25% of patients who were initially treated with ATRA. Prednisolone therapy (75 mg/d) reduces the incidence of ATRA to approximately 8%.[39] The syndrome is characterized by the sudden onset of fever, dyspnea, effusions (pleural and pericardial), diffuse alveolar infiltrates seen on chest radiographs, and hypoxemic respiratory failure. Before the efficacy of steroid therapy was recognized, more than half of the patients required mechanical ventilation, and the mortality rate was 33%.

The pathogenesis has not been established but likely relates partly to the rapid increase in mature leukocytes. Autopsy studies[39] reveal diffuse alveolar damage with edema and hemorrhage as well as leukemic cells in the interstitium. Mechanisms implicated in ATRA-induced capillary leak syndrome include the release of vasoactive cytokines, oxidants, and lipid mediators from inflammatory cells, as well as enhanced expression of leukocyte adhesion molecules that impair leukocyte transit through the pulmonary microcirculation. Some patients in whom retinoic acid syndrome develops while they are receiving prednisolone have responded to therapy with dexamethasone. Management is otherwise largely supportive, similar to patients with ARDS.

Other Chemotherapeutic Agents/Newer Antineoplastic Drugs

Other chemotherapeutic drugs are less commonly associated with adverse pulmonary effects, which are seen more often than with the agents reviewed earlier. Chlorambucil, which is an alkylating agent similar to cyclophosphamide, is used in the treatment of lymphoproliferative disorders as well as nonmalignant diseases. Pulmonary toxicity is relatively rare, but chronic pneumonitis/fibrosis has been reported. Cytosine arabinoside, which is an antimetabolite used to treat acute leukemia, causes noncardiogenic pulmonary edema in 13 to 20% of patients.[40] The mortality rate varies from 2 to 50%. Corticosteroids may improve outcome, but this finding remains uncertain. Fludarabine, an antimetabolite that is used in the management of patients with chronic lymphoproliferative disorders, can cause chronic pneumonitis/fibrosis as well as a hypersensitivity-type reaction in nearly 9% of patients that is often responsive to therapy with corticosteroids.[41]

Although older chemotherapeutic agents induce a wide array of pulmonary toxicity in nearly 10% of patients, there is less information concerning the frequency as well as the clinical manifestations resulting from exposure to the newer agents.[7,42] Gemcitabine, an agent that is increasingly being used in the management of a variety of solid tumors, can induce an ARDS-like condition that is potentially fatal.[42] The estimated frequency of gemcitabine-induced pulmonary toxicity ranges from <1 to 1.4% and, in addition to ARDS, includes nonspecific interstitial pneumonitis (NSIP), pulmonary fibrosis, and pleural effusions.[7,42]

Taxanes (*eg*, paclitaxel and docetaxel) are used in the management of solid tumors (*eg*, breast, lung, gastric, and ovarian). Paclitaxel induces bronchospasm and a type 1 hypersensitivity reaction in up to 30% of patients.[7,42] Other much less common taxane-induced pulmonary manifestations include NSIP, hypersensitivity pneumonitis, pulmonary fibrosis, ARDS, and pleural effusion. Topoisomerase I inhibitors (*eg*, irinotecan and topotecan), which are used in the management of various solid tumors, cause pulmonary toxicity that includes NSIP and bronchiolitis obliterans.[7,42] Synergy between irinotecan and paclitaxel or radiation increases the frequency of pulmonary toxicity from 1.8 to 13% or 56%, respectively. Tyrosine kinase inhibitors (*eg*, gefitinib and imatinib) uncommonly cause pulmonary toxicity (approximately 2%), consisting of NSIP, hypersensitivity pneumonitis, pulmonary fibrosis, COP, alveolar hemorrhage, ARDS, and pleural effusions.[7,42]

Biological response modifiers, such as IL-2 and TNF-α, are used in experimental protocols to treat various malignancies. Each can induce noncardiogenic pulmonary edema which, in the case of IL-2, is also associated with massive fluid retention. Granulocyte-macrophage CSF and G-CSF can cause a hypersensitivity-type pneumonitis when administered in conjunction with other cytotoxic agents. Also, G-CSF, especially in the presence of other cytotoxic agents, can induce ARDS.[43] Although it is beyond the scope of this review, immunosuppressive agents can promote the development of opportunistic pulmonary infections.

Nonchemotherapy-Associated Pulmonary Toxicity

Antiinflammatory Drugs

Aspirin: Aspirin (acetylsalicylic acid), which is the most commonly prescribed drug worldwide, causes the following two forms of pulmonary toxicity: bronchospasm and noncardiogenic pulmonary edema. Aspirin-induced asthma (AIA) occurs in <1% of healthy individuals and in up to 20% of asthmatic individuals. However, aspirin sensitivity occurs in a larger proportion of asthmatic patients with nasal polyps, which is a clinical triad that was first identified by Samter and Beers.[44]

Symptoms of AIA occur within minutes to hours after ingestion and may be associated with facial flushing, rhinorrhea, angioedema, and conjunctivitis. The pathogenesis of AIA is mediated by the enhanced production of cysteinyl leukotrienes via the 5-lipoxygenase pathway and, to a lesser extent, by a reduction in bronchodilating prostaglandins secondary to cyclooxygenase inhibition. Aspirin-sensitive asthmatic patients who are challenged with aspirin have increased levels of urinary leukotriene E_4, which is a general marker of serum leukotriene levels, because of the increased activity of leukotriene C synthase, the rate-limiting step in leukotriene synthesis.[45] As expected, they exhibit symptomatic and spirometric improvement in the presence of 5-lipoxygenase inhibition and cysteinyl leukotriene receptor antagonism.[45] An increased risk of AIA is also associated with several single nucleotide polymorphisms in the promoters of prostaglandin-E_2 receptor subtype 2, cysteinyl leukotriene receptor 1, cysteinyl leukotriene receptor 2, and T-cell T box.[46] A similar syndrome occurs with other nonsteroidal antiinflammatory drugs (NSAIDs). Agents that do not block the cyclooxygenase pathway, such as acetaminophen and salicylate, can be safely used in patients with aspirin-induced or NSAID-induced bronchospasm.[45]

Aspirin-induced noncardiogenic pulmonary edema occurs in 10 to 15% of patients with a severe salicylate overdose. This can occur inadvertently in long-term aspirin users, typically elderly patients with multiple medical problems, or intentionally in individuals attempting suicide. These patients will often present with dyspnea, tachypnea, altered mental status, and a chest radiograph revealing diffuse alveolar infiltrates. Most patients will manifest with a simple respiratory alkalosis or a mixed anion gap metabolic acidosis plus a respiratory alkalosis. The constellation of findings can mimic a pseudo-sepsis syndrome.[47] The diagnosis is made by first considering aspirin ingestion in the differential diagnosis of patients presenting with noncardiogenic pulmonary edema or a sepsis-like picture and then determining the serum salicylate level. Respiratory alkalosis is typically seen with serum salicylate levels of 35 mg/dL (therapeutic range, 10 to 20 mg/dL), whereas noncardiogenic pulmonary edema occurs at serum levels of ≥45 mg/dL. Although the pathogenesis of aspirin-induced noncardiogenic pulmonary edema is unclear, it likely results from increased capillary permeability resulting from toxic levels of salicylates. Management is based on drug withdrawal and supportive care, often in the ICU with the patient receiving mechanical ventilation. Alkaline diuresis should be performed as soon as the diagnosis is suspected to enhance renal clearance and thereby reduce the serum salicylate level. Hemodialysis is reserved for patients with aspirin-associated seizures, refractory acidosis, coma, or very high salicylate levels (80 to 100 mg/dL). Outcome is generally favorable in young patients with an acute salicylate overdose. However, there is a high mortality rate in older patients who have multiple medical problems and a long-term history of the ingestion of salicylates, and they have a more subtle presentation.

Gold: Gold has been widely used for decades in the management of chronic inflammatory conditions, most notably RA but also pemphigus, psoriatic arthritis, bronchial asthma, and ankylosing spondylitis. Both the oral (auranofin) and the IM (gold sodium thiomalate) preparations can induce chronic pneumonitis/interstitial fibrosis. Bronchiolitis obliterans, in the presence or absence of organizing pneumonia, occurs less frequently. Interstitial lung disease caused by gold therapy can be distinguished from the patient's underlying rheumatoid lung disease by the following: (1) an acute onset of dyspnea and a nonproductive cough; (2) fever (*ie*, temperature >38°C); (3) skin rash; (4) crackles on chest examination; (5) absence of finger clubbing or subcutaneous nodules; (6) the presence of blood eosinophilia, proteinuria, or liver dysfunction; (7) BAL fluid lymphocytosis with a predominance of CD8 (suppressor) cells typical of a hypersensitivity-type reaction; (8) alveolar opacities in a nonbasilar distribution; and (9) an HRCT scan that shows bronchovascular infiltrates, rather than peripheral infiltrates.[48] A favorable clinical response typically occurs after drug withdrawal and a course of corticosteroids. Recurrent disease has been documented following retreatment, which is not warranted.

NSAIDs: NSAIDs are among the most commonly prescribed drugs because they are widely used in the management of an array of rheumatologic disorders as well as for minor musculoskeletal pain in healthy individuals. Similar to salicylates, NSAIDs can precipitate asthma as well as noncardiogenic pulmonary edema in aspirin-sensitive individuals. Ophthalmic NSAIDs also can trigger bronchospasm. Nearly every type of NSAID can induce a hypersensitivity-type reaction that may be associated with PIE. In general, prompt resolution occurs with drug withdrawal, and rarely, a course of corticosteroids is required.

Methotrexate: See the section "Chemotherapy-Associated Pulmonary Toxicity" for a discussion.

Penicillamine: Penicillamine is an antiinflammatory, antifibrotic, and copper-chelating agent that is used in the treatment of RA, scleroderma, primary biliary cirrhosis, and Wilson disease. The manifestations of penicillamine-induced pulmonary toxicity include the following: (1) interstitial pneumonitis/fibrosis; (2) bronchiolitis obliterans, in the presence or absence of organizing pneumonia; (3) drug-induced SLE; and (4) alveolar hemorrhage due to a pulmonary-renal syndrome.

Patients with penicillamine-induced interstitial pneumonitis/fibrosis generally present with the insidious onset of dyspnea and cough associated with restricted lung volumes and a reduced DLCO. A subset of patients present with a hypersensitivity-type reaction associated with peripheral blood eosinophilia and increased serum IgE levels. As with gold therapy, it can be challenging to distinguish drug-induced pulmonary toxicity from the patient's underlying collagen vascular disorder.

The incidence of penicillamine-induced bronchiolitis obliterans is unknown but is estimated to occur in <1% of patients with RA receiving this therapy. There are no clear risk factors. Patients present with a subacute onset of dyspnea, cough, and wheeze. The chest radiograph reveals hyperinflation in the absence of infiltrates, whereas PFT results are used to confirm the presence of increased lung volumes as well as airflow limitation without a bronchodilator effect. Lung biopsy specimens from these patients reveal bronchiolar constriction caused by mononuclear inflammation and fibrosis. Management centers on drug withdrawal, supportive therapy, and the consideration of a trial of corticosteroids, azathioprine, or cyclophosphamide. However, there are no data demonstrating the value of immunosuppressive therapy. The prognosis for patients with penicillamine-induced bronchiolitis obliterans is poor; nearly 50% of patients die, whereas the remainder have very poor quality of life due to a severe permanent residual obstructive impairment.

Penicillamine rarely induces Goodpasture syndrome, which consists of diffuse alveolar hemorrhage and rapidly progressive glomerulonephritis caused by autoantibodies directed against components of the alveolar and glomerular basement membranes. There are case reports of this syndrome occurring after penicillamine was used to treat RA as well as Wilson disease, demonstrating that it is not simply attributable to the patient's underlying collagen vascular disease. Typically, the serum ANA level is increased, but the double-stranded DNA antibodies seen in classic SLE are not apparent. However, it is important to consider SLE or an antineutrophil cytoplasmic antibody-related vasculitis in the differential diagnosis because a number of these patients will not have serum and tissue antiglomerular basement membrane antibodies. Despite drug withdrawal and corticosteroids, the mortality rate is nearly 50%, and there is a high incidence of progression to chronic renal failure necessitating long-term dialysis.

TNF-α–Targeted Therapy: Anti–TNF-α antibodies (*eg*, etanercept, infliximab, and adalimumab) are increasingly being used to block the effects of TNF-α in autoimmune diseases such as RA and Crohn disease. Because TNF-α has a critical role in host defense against infections, not surprisingly its utility is complicated by pulmonary infections, most prominently the reactivation of tuberculosis as well as fungal infections.[49,50] It is recommended that all patients receiving anti-TNF-α-targeted therapy be screened and treated for latent tuberculosis before the drug is used. Further, these agents, especially etanercept and infliximab, can also cause various noninfectious pulmonary manifestations such as NSIP, pulmonary fibrosis, loosely formed granulomatous inflammation, pleural effusions, increased size of RA nodules, and SLE-like reactions.[50,51]

Antimicrobial Drugs

Antibiotic-Induced Hypersensitivity-Type Disease: The most common antibiotics causing a hypersensitivity-type lung reaction in the presence of PIE include β-lactam and sulfa antibiotics. Less commonly, fluoroquinolones, tetracycline, erythromycin, nitrofurantoin, isoniazid, paraaminosalicylic acid, and ethambutol cause this type of a reaction. There are no known risk factors, and most reactions are idiosyncratic. Typically, the patients present during a period of 1 to 4 weeks (can be delayed up to 1 year) with minimal, nonspecific respiratory complaints. Prompt resolution occurs with drug withdrawal perhaps with a short course of corticosteroids and antihistamines.

Nitrofurantoin: Nitrofurantoin has been used for decades in the management of acute urinary tract infections and as long-term suppressive therapy for patients with asymptomatic bacteruria. Nitrofurantoin has the following two main distinct adverse pulmonary manifestations: (1) acute hypersensitivity-type reaction and (2) chronic pneumonitis/fibrosis that mimics IPF. Alveolar hemorrhage and noncardiogenic pulmonary edema have also been described but are less common. The incidence of nitrofurantoin-induced adverse pulmonary effects is not firmly established. One study[52] has shown that the nitrofurantoin-induced acute hypersensitivity-type reaction that was severe enough to warrant hospitalization occurred in 1 in 5,000 new drug administrations, whereas the chronic form occurred in 1 in 50,000 new drug administrations.

Acute nitrofurantoin pulmonary toxicity is a very rare (<0.1%) side effect that occurs within 1 month of the first dose in 86% of patients.

Symptoms consist of dyspnea, cough, fever, chest pain, and a macular/papular skin rash . There is an elevated erythrocyte sedimentation rate (ESR) and peripheral blood eosinophilia in most patients. The chest radiograph shows a mixed alveolar/interstitial infiltrative pattern but is normal in 18% of patients. One third of patients have a small pleural effusion. PFT results typically reveal a restrictive pattern with a reduced DLCO. Although the diagnosis is generally made clinically, a lung biopsy specimen and BAL fluid should be obtained in any patient in whom infection, metastatic tumor, and/or an inflammatory condition are in the differential diagnosis. Histopathologic findings include interstitial inflammation with lymphocytes and plasma cells and, in the more severe cases, alveolar edema, hyaline membranes, and hemorrhage. The prognosis is generally favorable with drug withdrawal and, occasionally, therapy with corticosteroids. Although ARDS develops in some situations, the overall mortality rate is $< 1\%$.[53]

Chronic nitrofurantoin pulmonary toxicity occurs in elderly patients who have been treated with long-term suppressive therapy for asymptomatic bacteruria. Although much less common than the acute form, it is similar to the acute form in that patients present with dyspnea and cough, but, in contrast, fever and rash are uncommon. Unlike the acute form, patients with the chronic form of the disease have systemic complaints of fatigue and weight loss. Infrequently, they have an increased ESR and peripheral blood eosinophilia. Low-level elevations of the serum ANA and rheumatoid factor can be seen that are similar to those in patients with IPF. The chest radiograph shows a bilateral interstitial infiltrative pattern typically without pleural effusions. PFT results generally reveal a restrictive pattern with a reduced DLCO. As with the acute form, the diagnosis is usually made on clinical grounds. However, lung biopsy and BAL fluid are indicated in any patient who might have an infection, a metastatic tumor, and/or an inflammatory condition. The characteristic histopathologic findings include lymphocytic interstitial inflammation along with interstitial and alveolar fibrosis that can be indistinguishable from the usual interstitial pneumonitis form of IPF. Unlike the generally reversible acute form of the disease, three fourth of patients with chronic nitrofurantoin pulmonary toxicity do not improve at all or are left with substantial residual disease despite drug withdrawal and a trial of corticosteroids. The overall mortality rate is nearly 8%.[53]

Sulfasalazine/Mesalamine: Sulfasalazine, which is an antibiotic used in the management of inflammatory bowel disease, can cause COP, PIE, pulmonary fibrosis, and bronchospasm. Sulfapyridine, which is the carrier component of sulfasalazine, is responsible for the majority of the side effects. However, mesalamine, the clinically active component, can also induce pulmonary adverse side effects.

Pentamidine: Pentamidine can cause bronchospasm when administered IV or via nebulizer. The adverse effect can be prevented by pretreatment with β-agonists or ipratropium.

Cardiovascular Drugs

Amiodarone: Amiodarone is an effective agent for treating ventricular and supraventricular arrhythmias that are refractory to other drugs. However, the utility of this drug is limited by adverse pulmonary effects that can occur in 5 to 10% of patients, as well as toxicity to the eyes, thyroid gland, liver, GI tract, and nervous system. The adverse effects of amiodarone are typically associated with a high daily dose ($>$400 mg/d) and a prolonged duration of therapy ($>$12 months). A metaanalysis[54] of randomized, placebo-controlled, low-dose amiodarone efficacy trials involving 1,465 patients receiving $<$400 mg/d amiodarone for a minimum of 12 months demonstrated a trend toward increased pulmonary toxicity compared with those patients receiving placebo (OR, 2.0; 95% confidence interval, 0.9 to 5.3; $p = 0.07$), but this difference did not reach statistical significance. In contrast, compared with placebo, the use of low-dose amiodarone did increase pulmonary toxicity (1.2% vs 3.8%, respectively) in the Canadian Myocardial Infarction Amiodarone Trial.[55] An analysis of 237 patients with amiodarone-induced pulmonary toxicity demonstrated that only patient age ($>$60 years; OR, 3; 95% confidence interval, 1.3 to 7) and duration of therapy ($>$6 at 12 months; OR, 18; 95% confidence interval, 6 to 52) significantly impacted the risk.[56]

The mechanisms underlying amiodarone-induced pulmonary toxicity are not firmly established. As reviewed elsewhere,[57] several theories that are not mutually exclusive have been implicated, including the following: (1) direct cellular damage in part due to alveolar epithelial-cell apoptosis, (2) enhanced phospholipidosis, (3) immunologic injury, (4) ROS-induced damage, (5) alterations in membrane properties, (6) increased intracellular calcium in vascular endothelial cells, (7) activation of G proteins, and (8) inhibition of pulmonary epithelial cell sodium-potassium adenosine triphosphatase. More recent studies show that amiodarone causes lung epithelial-cell mitochondrial dysfunction, ROS production, and mitochondria-regulated apoptosis that can be blocked with the administration of angiotensin system antagonists.[58,59] Amiodarone has a large volume of distribution with a very long half-life of 30 to 60 days. Thus, the antiarrhythmic effects as well as the adverse effects of amiodarone will persist for weeks to months after the drug is withdrawn from therapy. Amiodarone is an iodine-containing phospholipase inhibitor that causes lipid accumulation in nearly all tissues, especially the lungs, skin, and liver. This blockade results in the accumulation of undigested surfactant phospholipids in the lung, a feature that is seen in virtually all patients receiving the drug.

The histologic features of amiodarone-induced pulmonary toxicity include the following: (1) accumulation of foamy macrophages with characteristic lamellated inclusions in the interstitium and alveolar spaces; (2) hyperplasia of alveolar type II cells; and (3) widening of the alveolar septa with infiltration of lymphocytes, plasma cells, eosinophils, and neutrophils. Edema, intraalveolar fibrin exudation, lamellar inclusions in pulmonary endothelial cells, bronchiolar epithelial cells and type II cells, and fibrosis can also occur.

The clinical and laboratory manifestations of amiodarone-induced pulmonary toxicity include the following: (1) interstitial pneumonitis/fibrosis, (2) ARDS, (3) COP, (4) mass lesions that can cavitate, (5) eosinophilic pneumonia, (6) diffuse alveolar hemorrhage, and (7) pleural effusions. Uncommon reactions include hypersensitivity pneumonitis, alveolar hypoventilation, and bronchospasm. The patients typically present with an insidious onset of a nonproductive cough and dyspnea with radiographic evidence of asymmetric chronic pneumonitis/fibrosis and an elevated ESR. Occasionally, ill-defined alveolar infiltrates, a lung mass, or pleural effusions may be seen. Risk factors for amiodarone-induced adverse pulmonary side effects are not firmly established, but some that have been implicated include the following: (1) maintenance dose of >400 mg/d, (2) age >60 years, (3) duration >6 to 12 months, (4) angiography/acute lung injury, and (5) cardiothoracic surgery/ARDS. The total cumulative dose or serum levels of amiodarone are not useful. Further, a reduction in the DLCO and increased gallium uptake may support a clinical diagnosis, but they are not reliable predictors of pulmonary toxicity in the absence of clinical and radiographic abnormalities.

The diagnosis of amiodarone-induced pulmonary toxicity is one of exclusion, especially heart failure, pulmonary embolism, infection, and other inflammatory interstitial diseases (*eg*, COP and chronic eosinophilic pneumonia). Chest CT scans may reveal high-attenuation areas caused by the iodine present in amiodarone. However, this finding is a nonspecific one that may be present in healthy subjects. The typical PFT abnormalities include a reduction in the DLCO and reduced lung volumes. Although a decreased DLCO is a nonspecific finding that is seen in all patients with amiodarone-induced disease, a normal DLCO suggests that heart failure, rather than amiodarone, may account for the respiratory symptoms. Bronchoscopy may be necessary to exclude infection. KL-6, a high-molecular-weight glycoprotein secreted by alveolar type II cells, is a potentially useful serum marker that is increased (>500 U/mL) in patients with interstitial lung disease caused by IPF, radiation, and amiodarone.[60,61] Serum KL-6 levels are typically <500 U/mL in patients with congestive heart failure and pneumonia. Although further studies are necessary to corroborate the findings of these small observational studies, the sensitivity and specificity of an increased serum KL-6 level in identifying interstitial disease approaches 94% and 96%, respectively.[60,61]

The management of amiodarone-induced pulmonary toxicity includes drug withdrawal and the initiation of a new antiarrhythmic agent or implantation of an automatic cardioverter/defibrillator if required. A trial of corticosteroids is often used in symptomatic patients, but the efficacy of steroids has not been established. Radiographic resolution generally occurs over 2 months, and patients are treated for at least 6 months to reduce the likelihood of relapse. Recurrent amiodarone pulmonary toxicity can also occur. If amiodarone is the only effective agent in a patient with life-threatening arrhythmias, the dose must be reduced to the minimum that is effective (ideally <400 mg/d) and corticosteroids added to therapy.

ACE Inhibitors: Cough occurs in up to 5 to 15% of patients receiving any type of ACE inhibitor.[5] The cough generally appears from 1 to 2 months up to 1 year after initiating therapy. Patients without asthma in whom ACE inhibitor-induced cough develops, compared with those patients without cough, are slightly more sensitive to methacholine. However, ACE inhibitors do not consistently cause airways obstruction, nor are patients with asthma at an increased risk.[62] Although the mechanism of ACE inhibitor-induced cough has not been firmly established, it likely involves blocking the metabolism of cough-inducing neuropeptides such as substance P and bradykinin. Before extensive testing is performed to evaluate the source of a cough in a patient receiving ACE inhibitors, therapy with the drug should be discontinued. Patients with an ACE inhibitor-induced cough will generally show resolution within 1 to 4 days. Management is simple: avoid all ACE inhibitors. Patients can be switched to an angiotensin II receptor antagonist (*eg*, losartan), which rarely induces cough.[63] However, losartan can induce angioedema in a manner similar to that of ACE inhibitors.[64] If ACE inhibitors are required for the management of a patient's cardiovascular disease and there are no alternative agents, there are reports that the cough can be partly controlled with oral theophylline or nebulized cromolyn or lidocaine.[65,66]

Angioneurotic edema is a rare adverse effect of ACE inhibitors (0.1 to 0.2% of patients) that is potentially life threatening.[67] It is manifested by swelling of the tongue, lips, and mucous membranes within hours or at most 1 week after initiating treatment, and can rapidly evolve into acute respiratory distress, upper airway obstruction, and death. Patients with a history of idiopathic angioneurotic edema should avoid using ACE inhibitors because they may be at increased risk. The mechanism underlying this serious adverse effect is unknown, but immune pathways, increased tissue levels of bradykinin or histamine, and/or a deficiency of complement 1-esterase inactivator have all been implicated. The management of ACE inhibitor-induced angioedema includes drug withdrawal, attention to airway patency and, if severe, the subcutaneous injection of epinephrine (0.01 mL/kg body weight of a 1:1,000 solution) every 15 to 20 min along with IV saline solution to correct hypotension. Diphenhydramine (1 to 2 mg/kg up to 50 mg IV or IM) and steroids are also useful.

β-Blockers: β-Adrenergic receptor blockers administered by any route (*eg*, oral, IV, or ophthalmic solutions) can precipitate bronchospasm, especially in patients with asthma or COPD. Propranolol, a nonselective β-blocker, causes dose-dependent reductions in airflows and should be avoided in patients with asthma or COPD.[68] Timolol, a nonselective β-blocker used in ophthalmic solutions, has predictable adverse effects on these patients, similar to propranolol, and should also be avoided. Severe bronchospasm and sporadic deaths have been reported with nonselective β-blocker ophthalmic solutions. Physicians should specifically inquire about ophthalmic solutions in patients with glaucoma presenting with respiratory complaints since most patients do not consider these to be "drugs." Selective β_1-blockers (*eg*, atenolol and betaxolol ophthalmic solution) are better tolerated in patients with airflow obstruction.

A 2002 metaanalysis[69] showed that selective β_1-blockers are well tolerated in patients with asthma and COPD and result in minimal reductions in FEV_1 when used over the long term. A recent study showed that cardioselective β-blockers reduce the rate of mortality in patients with COPD undergoing vascular surgery.[70] Thus, in carefully selected patients with COPD, the use of a cardioselective β-blocker can be safely used. However, caution is warranted: β_1-selectivity is relative because β_1-selective inhibitors, especially in high doses, can block β_2-adrenergic receptors and trigger bronchospasm. Esmolol is the drug of choice in critically ill patients with asthma or COPD who require a β-blocker (*eg*, unstable angina) because it is an IV selective β_1-blocker in doses of <300 μg/kg/min and has an extremely short half-life (approximately 9 min).

Statins: Statins are the most widely prescribed lipid-lowering drug primarily because of their well-documented beneficial effect on cardiovascular morbidity and mortality. Statins inhibit cholesterol formation by blocking 3-hydroxy-3-methylglutamyl reductase. There have been several case reports[71,72] of statin-induced hypersensitivity pneumonitis and NSIP resulting from exposure to pravastatin, lovastatin, or simvastatin. The chest radiographic abnormalities include bilateral patchy ground-glass opacities and interstitial infiltrates. Although the mechanism of lung injury is unknown, increased alveolar CD8$^+$ suppressor T lymphocytes, hyperplastic type II pneumocytes, peripheral blood eosinophilia, and clinical deterioration accompanying statin reintroduction support hypersensitivity in the pathogenesis. Statin-induced pneumonitis may become more commonly observed when used at the higher doses advocated in some reports for the prevention of cardiovascular diseases.

Illicit Drugs

The use of illicit drugs continues to be a significant health-care problem of epidemic proportions worldwide. Respiratory symptoms in patients using illicit drugs may be caused by a wide array of pulmonary disorders, including the following: (1) alveolar hypoventilation (hypercarbic respiratory failure); (2) aspiration; (3) noncardiogenic pulmonary edema; (4) barotrauma (*eg*, pneumothorax, pneumomediastinum, and pneumoperitoneum); (5) endocarditis/septic emboli; (6) foreign-body granulomatosis; (7) PIE; (8) COP; (9) alveolar hemorrhage; (10) bronchospasm; (11) interstitial pneumonitis/fibrosis; and (12) HIV-associated infections. Knowledge about the drugs used, the route of administration, and the presenting clinical syndrome helps to narrow the broad differential diagnosis in these patients.

Noncardiac Pulmonary Edema: Noncardiac pulmonary edema is an infrequent complication of heroin, cocaine, or methadone abuse, but heroin abuse is by far the most common cause.[73] Naloxone, an opiate antagonist, also causes a similar syndrome. There are no known risk factors for opiate-induced pulmonary edema. Although the pathogenesis is not established, several mechanisms have been proposed, including the following: (1) altered alveolar/capillary permeability; (2) neurogenic pulmonary edema; (3) direct opiate cytotoxicity; (4) drug hypersensitivity; and (5) hypoxemic alveolar injury. However, none of these mechanisms have been adequately tested in animal models or human studies. Typically, patients present within minutes to hours (at most 24 h) after use with dyspnea, reduced respirations and mental status, miotic pupils, and a chest radiograph demonstrating perihilar alveolar infiltrates in a "batwing" distribution. Pathologic studies from autopsies have revealed changes similar to ARDS, such as the following: (1) alveolar edema and hemorrhage, (2) diffuse alveolar damage, (3) hyaline membranes, (4) interstitial inflammatory cell infiltrates, and (5) type II cell hyperplasia. Management centers on supportive care including mechanical ventilation, which is needed in 40%.[73] Unlike other causes of ARDS, the prognosis in opiate-induced noncardiogenic pulmonary edema is good, with resolution of pulmonary edema >48 to 72 h, and nearly all patients survive.

Cocaine: Cocaine, which is an alkaloid extracted from the leaves of *Erythroxylon coca*, is a sympathomimetic agent that causes topical anesthesia and CNS stimulation. In 1995, an estimated 1.5 million people in the United States regularly used cocaine.[74] Cocaine hydrochloride, the salt form that can be injected IV or rapidly absorbed across the nasal mucosa, causes pulmonary manifestations similar to those of IV opiates (*eg*, heroin). A unique feature of cocaine is that it causes nasal mucosal vasoconstriction that can result in ischemic necrosis and the perforation of the nasal septum. Free-base cocaine, which is derived from the alkaline crystallization of the salt, vaporizes when heated and is rapidly absorbed across the respiratory membranes. The term *crack* refers to the popping sound that occurs when cocaine crystals are heated.

Free-base crack cocaine smoking causes a distinct set of pulmonary abnormalities that are termed *crack lung*.[75] These patients typically present with cough, chest pain, dyspnea, hemoptysis, and wheezing. Chest pain from either a pulmonary or cardiac origin occurs in approximately 20 to 40% of cocaine users. Cocaine can induce direct coronary artery vasoconstriction. Unlike IV crack users, patients with crack lung from inhalation may have a cough productive of black, soot-like material (approximately 10 to 33% of patients), bronchospasm (approximately 50% of patients), and thermal burns to the upper and lower airways. Other pulmonary complications of crack cocaine use include PIE; COP; pulmonary hypertension; and alveolar hemorrhage/hemoptysis, and barotrauma (*eg*, pneumothorax, pneumomediastinum, and pneumoperitoneum). Barotrauma is likely caused by the Valsalva maneuver that is performed to enhance alveolar-capillary cocaine absorption. The DLCO is either normal or mildly reduced within weeks to months after using crack cocaine.[75,76] The reason for the reduction in DLCO is unclear, but it may reflect a loss of alveolar-capillary surface area.[75–77] Some evidence[78] has demonstrated that crack users have increased lower respiratory tract iron and ferritin levels that may contribute to lung injury via oxidant-induced mechanisms.

Foreign-Body Granulomatosis: Foreign-body granulomatosis is caused by the IV injection of insoluble particulate contaminants used to "cut" street heroin or from talc or cellulose in crushed tablets (*eg*, amphetamines, methadone, or hydromorphine). Initially, patients may be asymptomatic despite abnormal chest radiograph findings showing reticular nodular interstitial infiltrates. However, relentless progression of the infiltrates generally occurs accompanied by increasing dyspnea. The nodules may coalesce in a manner similar to that seen in silicosis, resulting in progressive massive pulmonary fibrosis with surrounding cysts and bullae. Notably, PFT results reveal airways obstruction, rather than restriction, that progresses to severe disease with a reduced DLCO.[79] The lungs demonstrate vascular and interstitial noncaseating giant-cell granulomatous infiltrates containing birefringent talc crystals. As the disease progresses, parenchymal destruction and pulmonary hypertension occur, leading to respiratory failure/cor pulmonale. The poor outcome noted in most patients is generally not altered by therapy with corticosteroids.

Miscellaneous Agents

Contrast Media: Both the ionic and nonionic forms of contrast media can induce bronchospasm and a reduction in airflow. Typically, this occurs within 5 min of infusion and resolves within 30 min after infusion. Contrast media rarely induces potentially fatal leukostasis in the pulmonary arterioles and capillaries.[80] This occurs within minutes to an hour after injection, resulting in dyspnea and hypoxemic respiratory failure caused by noncardiogenic pulmonary edema. Although the mechanism is unclear, a complement-mediated pathway has been implicated. Management centers on supportive care, and therapy with high-dose corticosteroids, IV diphenhydramine, and heparin.

Interferon-γ1b: Although there are no proven treatments for IPF, some studies[81] have suggested a possible role for interferon (IFN)-γ1b based on its antifibrotic actions (*eg*, decreases fibroblast proliferation and collagen synthesis, augments fibroblast apoptosis, and inhibits profibrotic cytokine production) and its protective effect in animal models of pulmonary fibrosis. Acute respiratory failure developed in four patients with severe IPF (total lung capacity, 38 to 59% of predicted; DLCO, 20 to 37% of predicted) after 2 to 35 doses of IFN-γlb.[81] In two patients who underwent a lung biopsy, pathologic studies revealed diffuse alveolar damage. To date, there is no clear beneficial role for IFN-γlb in the management of IPF, yet serious adverse pulmonary toxicity can occur, especially in patients with severe disease.

Tocolytic Agents: Tocolytic agents, such as albuterol, terbutaline, ritodrine, isoxuprine, and salbutamol, are β-adrenergic$_3$ agents that are used to inhibit uterine contractions during premature labor. Although acute pulmonary edema reportedly occurs in 0.5 to 5% of patients, in one study[82] of 8,700 patients there was an incidence of only 0.32%. The mechanism of pulmonary edema has not been established but is believed to be caused by β-adrenergic–induced peripheral vasodilation and increased intravascular volume. After the tocolytic drug is discontinued, the vascular tone normalizes, thereby promoting fluid movement into the extravascular spaces, including the alveoli. Left ventricular function and pulmonary wedge pressure are usually normal. Patients typically present during or within 12 h of delivery (rarely beyond 12 h postpartum) with an acute onset of dyspnea, cough productive of pink-tinged sputum, chest pain, tachycardia, tachypnea, hypoxemic respiratory failure, and diffuse alveolar infiltrates seen on a chest radiograph. The differential diagnosis includes the following: gastric acid aspiration, cardiac pulmonary edema, pulmonary embolism, amniotic fluid embolism, and peripartum cardiomyopathy. The transthoracic echocardiogram findings generally are normal. Management involves supportive care and diuresis. The prognosis is generally favorable, with intubation/mechanical ventilation required in < 10% of patients and a mortality rate of nearly 3%.[83]

Sirolimus (Rapamycin): Sirolimus is an immunosuppressive agent that is used in organ-transplant patients in the presence or absence of cyclosporine. The frequency of pulmonary toxicity varies from "rare" to approximately 11%.[84,85] Of 24 patients with sirolimus-associated pneumonitis, symptoms occurred within 5 months of initiating therapy and consisted of cough (96%), fatigue (83%), fever (67%), and dyspnea (33%).[84,85] The HRCT scan/pathologic patterns include COP (79%), ground-glass attenuation (17%), and, less commonly, interstitial fibrosis, alveolar proteinosis, necrotizing vasculitis, and pleural effusions.[84,85] BAL findings show a lymphocyte predominance (CD4 > CD8) with occasional eosinophils and rarely (8%) diffuse alveolar hemorrhage. Sirolimus withdrawal results in complete recovery within weeks to 6 months.

References

1. Rosenow EC III. The spectrum of drug-induced pulmonary disease. Ann Intern Med 1972; 77:977–991
2. Cooper JA Jr, White DA, Matthay RA. Drug-induced pulmonary disease: part 1. Cytotoxic drugs. Am Rev Respir Dis 1986; 133:321–340
3. Hubbard R, Venn A, Britton J. Exposure to antidepressants and the risk of cryptogenic fibrosing alveolitis: a case-control study. Eur Respir J 2000; 16:409–413
4. Snavely SR, Hodges GR. The neurotoxicity of antibacterial agents. Ann Intern Med 1984; 101:92–104
5. Howard PA, Dunn MI. Is your patient's cough caused by an ACE inhibitor? J Respir Dis 1997; 18:762–768
6. Morelock SY, Sahn SA. Drugs and the pleura. Chest 1999; 116:212–221
7. Dimopoulou I, Bamias A, Lyberopoulos P, et al. Pulmonary toxicity from novel antineoplastic agents. Ann Oncol 2006; 17:372–379
8. Poulter NR, Chang CL, Farley TMM, et al. Venous thromboembolic disease and combined oral contraceptives: results of international multicentre case control study. Lancet 1995; 346:1575–1582
9. Vandenbroucke JP, Rosing J, Bloemenkamp KWM, et al. Oral contraceptives and the risk of venous thrombosis. N Engl J Med 2001; 344:1527–1535
10. Abenhaim L, Moride Y, Brenot F, et al. Appetite-suppressant drugs and the risk of primary pulmonary hypertension. N Engl J Med 1996; 335:609–616
11. Drazen JM, Israel E, O'Byrne PM. Drug therapy: treatment of asthma with drugs modifying the leukotriene pathway. N Engl J Med 1999; 340:197–206
12. Nathani N, Little MA, Kunst H, et al. Churg-Strauss syndrome and leukotriene antagonists use: a respiratory perspective. Thorax 2008; 63:883–888
13. Beasley R, Bibby S, Weatherall M. Leukotriene receptor antagonist therapy and Churg--Strauss syndrome: culprit or innocent bystander. Thorax 2008; 63:847–848
14. Kalra S, Bell MR, Rihal CS. Alveolar hemorrhage as a complication of treatment with abciximab. Chest 2001; 120:126–131
15. Sandler A, Gray R, Perry MC, et al. Paclitaxel carboplatin alone or with bevacizumab for non-small cell lung cancer. N Engl J Med 2006; 355:2542–2550
16. Cockerill FR III, Wilson WR, Carpenter HA, et al. Open lung biopsy in immunocompromised patients. Arch Intern Med 1985; 145:1398–1404
17. Mason JW. Prediction of amiodarone-induced pulmonary toxicity [editorial]. Am J Med 1989; 86:2–3
18. Sleifer S. Bleomycin-induced pneumonitis. Chest 2001; 120:617–624
19. O'Driscoll BR, Hasleton PS, Taylor PM, et al. Active lung fibrosis up to 17 years after chemotherapy with carmustine (BCNU) in childhood. N Engl J Med 1990; 323. 378–382
20. Yagoda A, Mukherji B, Young C, et al. Bleomycin, an antitumor antibiotic: clinical experience in 274 patients. Ann Intern Med 1972; 77:861–870
21. Munger JS, Huang X, Kawakatsu H, et al. The integrin αvβ6 binds and activates latent $TGF\beta_1$ a mechanism for regulating pulmonary inflammation and fibrosis. Cell 1999; 96:319–328
22. Eitzman DT, McCoy RD, Zheng X, et al. Bleomycin induced pulmonary fibrosis in transgenic mice that either lack or overexpress the murine plasminogen activator inhibitor-1 gene. J Clin Invest 1996; 97:232–237
23. Wang R, Ibarra-Sunga O, Pick R, et al. Abrogation of bleomycin-induced epithelial cell apoptosis and lung fibrosis by captopril or by a caspase inhibitor. Am J Physiol Lung Cell Mol Physiol 2000; 279: L143–L151

24. Tran PL, Weinbach J, Opolon P, et al. Prevention of bleomycin-induced pulmonary fibrosis after adenovirus-mediated transfer of the bacterial bleomycin resistance gene. J Clin Invest 1997; 99:608–617
25. He Y-H, Wu M, Kobune M, et al. Expression of yeast apurinic/apyrimidinic endonuclease (APN1) protects lung epithelial cells from bleomycin toxicity. Am J Respir Cell Mol Biol 2001; 25:692–698
26. Horan GS, Wood S, Ona V, et al. Partial inhibition of integrin αvβ6 prevents pulmonary fibrosis without exacerbating inflammation. Am J Respir Crit Care Med 2008; 177:56–65
27. Lewis CC, Yang JTH, Huang X, et al. Disease-specific gene expression profiling in multiple models of lung disease. Am J Respir Crit Care 2008; 177:376–387
28. Heard BE, Cooke RA. Busulphan lung. Thorax 1958; 23:187–193
29. Malik SW, Myers JL, DeRemee RA, et al. Lung toxicity associated with cyclophosphamide use. two distinct patterns. Am J Respir Crit Care Med 1996; 154:1851–1856
30. Cooper JAJr, Merrill WW, Reynolds HY. Cyclophosphamide modulation of bronchoalveolar cellular populations and macrophage oxidative metabolism: possible mechanisms of pulmonary pharmacotoxicity. Am Rev Respir Dis 1986; 134:108–114
31. Trask CW, Joannides T, Harper PG, et al. Radiation-induced lung fibrosis after treatment of small cell carcinoma of the lung with very high-dose cyclophosphamide. Cancer 1985; 55:57–60
32. Imokawa S, Colby TV, Leslie KO, et al. Methotrexate pneumonitis: review of the literature and histopathological findings in 9 patients. Eur Respir J 2000; 15:373–381
33. White DA, Rankin JA, Stover DE, et al. Methotrexate pneumonitis: bronchoalveolar lavage findings suggest an immunologic disorder. Am Rev Respir Dis 1989; 139:18–21
34. Searles G, McKendry RJ. Methotrexate pneumonitis in rheumatoid arthritis: potential risk factors; four case reports and a review of the literature. J Rheumatol 1987; 14:1164–1171
35. Alarcon GS, Kremer JM, Macaluso M, et al. Risk factors for methotrexate-induced lung injury in patients with rheumatoid arthritis: A multicenter, case-control study; methotrexate-Lung Study Group. Ann Intern Med 1997; 127:356–364
36. Cottin V, Tebib J, Massonnet B, et al. Pulmonary function in patients receiving long-term low-dose methotrexate. Chest 1996; 109:933–938
37. Linette DC, McGee KH, McFarland JA. Mitomycin-induced pulmonary toxicity: case report and review of the literature. Ann Pharmacother 1992; 26:481–484
38. Raderer CM, Kornek M, Hejna F, et al. Acute pulmonary toxicity associated with high-dose vinorelbine and mitomycin. Ann Oncol 1996; 7:973–975
39. Wiley JS, Firkin FC. Reduction of pulmonary toxicity by prednisolone prophylaxis during all-trans retinoic acid treatment of acute promyelocytic leukemia: Australian Leukaemia Study Group. Leukemia 1995; 9:774–778
40. Andersson BS, Cogan BM, Keating MJ, et al. Subacute pulmonary failure complicating therapy with high-dose Ara-C in acute leukemia. Cancer 1985; 56:2181–2184
41. Helman DL, Byrd JC, Ales NC, et al. Fludarabine related pulmonary toxicity. Chest 2002; 122:785–790
42. Vahid B, Marik PE. Pulmonary complications of novel antineoplastic agents for solid tumors. Chest 2008; 133:528–538
43. Azoulay E, Attalah H, Hauf A, et al. Granulocyte colony stimulating factor or neutrophil-induced pulmonary toxicity: myth or reality? Chest 2001; 120:1695–1701
44. Samter M, Beers RF Jr. Concerning the nature of intolerance to aspirin. J Allergy 1967; 40:281–293
45. Babu KS, Salvi SS. Aspirin and asthma. Chest 2000; 118:1470–1476
46. Kim S-H, Park H-S. Pathogenesis of nonsteroidal anti-inflammatory drug-induced asthma. Curr Opin Allergy Clin Immunol 2006; 6:617–622
47. Leatherman JW, Schmitz PG. Fever, hyperdynamic shock, and multiple-system organ failure: A pseudosepsis syndrome associated with chronic salicylate intoxication. Chest 1991; 100:1391–1396
48. Tomioka R, King TE Jr. Gold-induced pulmonary disease: clinical features, outcome, and differentiation from rheumatoid lung disease. Am J Respir Crit Care Med 1997; 155:1011–1020
49. Keane J, Gershon S, Wise RP, et al. Tuberculosis associated with infliximab, a tumor necrosis factor α neutralizing agent. N Engl J Med 2001; 345:1098–1104
50. Mutlu GM, Mutlu EA, Bellmeyer A, et al. Pulmonary adverse events of anti TNF-α antibody therapy. Am J Med 2006; 119:639–646

51. Thavarajah K, Wu P, Rhew EJ, et al. Pulmonary complications of tumor necrosis factor-targeted therapy. Respir Med 2009; 103:661–669
52. Jick SS, Jick H, Walker AM, et al. Hospitalizations for pulmonary reactions following nitrofurantoin use. Chest 1989; 96:512–515
53. Holmberg L, Boman G. Pulmonary reactions to nitrofurantoin: 447 cases reported to the Swedish Adverse Drug Reaction Committee 1966–1976. Eur J Respir Dis 1981; 62:180–189
54. Vorperian VR, Havighurst TC, Miller S, et al. Adverse effects of low-dose amiodarone: a meta-analysis. J Am Coll Cardiol 1997; 30:791–798
55. Cairns JA, Connolly SJ, Roberts R, et al. Randomized trial of outcome after myocardial infarction in patients with frequent or repetitive ventricular premature depolarisations: CAMIAT. Lancet 1997; 349:675–682
56. Ernawati DK, Stafford L, Hughes JD. Amiodarone-induced pulmonary toxicity. Br J Clin Pharmacol 2008; 66:82–87
57. Reasor MJ, Kacew S. An evaluation of possible mechanisms underlying amiodarone-induced pulmonary toxicity. Proc Soc Exp Biol Med 1996; 212:297–304
58. Nicolescu AC, Ji Y, Comeau JL, et al. Direct mitochondrial dysfunction precedes reactive oxygen species production in amiodarone-induced toxicity in human peripheral lung epithelial HPL1A cells. Toxicol Appl Pharmacol 2008; 227:370–379
59. Nikaido A, Tada T, Nakamura K, et al. Clinical features of and effects of angiotensin system antagonists on amiodarone-induced pulmonary toxicity. Int J Cardiol 2008 Dec 22. [Epub ahead of print]
60. Yasuhiro E, Ritsuko H, Kenta U, et al. KL-6 as a potential new marker for amiodarone-induced pulmonary toxicity. Am J Cardiol 2000; 86:229–231
61. Ohnishi H, Yokoyama A, Kondo K, et al. Comparative study of KL-6, surfactant protein A, surfactant protein D, and monocyte chemoattractant protein-1 as serum markers for interstitial lung disease. Am J Respir Crit Care Med 2002; 165:378–381
62. Kaufman J, Casanova JE, Riendl P, et al. Bronchial hyperreactivity and cough due to angiotensin converting enzyme inhibitors. Chest 1989; 95:544–548
63. Conigliaro RL. Gleason PP. Losartan-induced cough after lisinopril therapy [letter]. Am J Health Syst Pharm 1999; 56:914–915
64. Acker CG, Greenberg A. Angioedema induced by the angiotensin II blocker losartan [letter]. N Engl J Med 1995; 333:1572
65. Aldis WL. Cromolyn for cough due to angiotensin-converting enzyme inhibitor therapy: preliminary observations [letter]. Chest 1991; 100:1741–1742
66. Fogari R, Zoppi A, Tettamanti F, et al. Effects of nifedipine and indomethacin on cough induced by angiotensin-converting enzyme inhibitors: a double-blind, randomized, cross-over study. J Cardiovasc Pharmacol 1992; 19:670–673
67. Zafar H, Hall WD. Cough and angioneurotic edema associated with angiotensin-converting enzyme inhibitor therapy. Ann Intern Med 1992; 117:234–242
68. Chester EH, Schwartz HJ, Fleming GM. Adverse effect of propranolol on airway function in non-asthmatic chronic obstructive lung disease. Chest 1981; 79:540–544
69. Salpeter SR, Ormiston TM, Salpeter EE. Cardioselective 3-blockers in patients with reactive airway disease: a meta-analysis. Ann Intern Med 2002; 137:715–725
70. van Gestel YRBM, Hoeks SE, Sin DD, et al. Impact of cardioselective 3-blockers on mortality in patients with chronic obstructive pulmonary disease and atherosclerosis. Am J Respir Crit Care Med 2008; 178:695–700
71. Liebhaber MI, Wright RS, Gelberg HJ, et al. Polymyalgia, hypersensitivity pneumonitis and other reactions in patients receiving HMG-CoA reductase inhibitors: a report of 10 cases. Chest 1999; 115:886–889
72. Lantuejoul S, Brambilla E, Brambilla C, et al. Statin-induced fibrotic nonspecific interstitial pneumonia. Eur Respir J 2002; 19:577–580
73. Sporer KA, Dorn E. Heroin-related noncardiogenic pulmonary edema. Chest 2001; 120:1628–1632
74. Albertson TE, Walby WF. Respiratory toxicities from stimulant use. Clin Rev Allergy Immunol 1997; 15:221–241
75. Haim DY, Lippmann ML, Goldberg SK, et al. The pulmonary complications of crack cocaine: a comprehensive review. Chest 1995; 107:233–240
76. Itkonen J, Schnoll S, Glassroth J. Pulmonary dysfunction in "freebase" cocaine users. Arch Intern Med 1984; 144:2195–2197
77. Kleerup EC, Koyal SN, Marques-Magallanes JA, et al. Chronic and acute effects of "crack" cocaine on diffusing capacity: membrane diffusion, and

pulmonary capillary blood volume in the lung. Chest 2002; 122:629–638

78. Janjua TM, Bohan AE, Wesselius LJ. Increased lower respiratory tract iron concentrations in alkaloidal ("crack") cocaine users. Chest 2001; 119:422–427
79. Pare JP, Cote G, Fraser RS. Long-term follow-up of drug abusers with intravenous talcosis. Am Rev Respir Dis 1989; 139:233–241
80. Hauggaard A. Non-cardiogenic pulmonary oedema after intravenous administration of non-ionic contrast media. Acta Radiol 1996; 37:823–825
81. Honore I, Nunes H, Groussard O, et al. Acute respiratory failure after interferon γ1b therapy of end-stag pulmonary fibrosis. Am J Respir Crit Care Med 2003; 167:953–957
82. Perry KG Jr., Morrison JC, Rust OA, et al. Incidence of adverse cardiopulmonary effects with low-dose continuous terbutaline infusion. Am J Obstet Gynecol 1995; 173:1273–1277
83. Pisani RJ, Rosenow EC III. Pulmonary edema associated with tocolytic therapy. Ann Intern Med 1989; 110:714–718
84. Champion L, Stern M, Israel-Biet D, et al. Sirolimus associated pneumonitis: 24 cases in renal trans plant recipients. Ann Intern Med 2006; 144:505–509
85. Roberts RJ, Wells AC, Unitt E, et al. Sirolimus induced pneumonitis following liver transplantation. Liver Transpl 2007; 13:853–855

Annotated Bibliography

Internet Site

Foucher P, Camus P, the GEPPI. Pneumotox on line. Available at: http://www.pneumotox.com. Accessed March 28, 2009

This is an excellent resource for a complete up-to-date listing of all the drugs reported to cause adverse pulmonary effects. It includes a detailed reference list, starting with the initial description and including the most current reports, for >350 agents organized alphabetically and by chest radiographic pattern.

General Reviews

Cleverley JR, Screaton NJ, Hiorns MP, et al. Drug-induced lung disease: high resolution CT and histologic findings. Clin Radiol 2002; 57:292–299

A study comparing HRCT scan appearances with histologic findings in 20 patients with drug-induced lung disease that found concordance in only nine patients (45%). The most common HRCT scan findings included ground-glass opacities (85%), consolidation (70%), interlobar septal thickening (75%), and central lobular nodules (40%). The HRCT scan findings are of limited value in determining the histologic picture and prognosis in such patients.

Cooper JAD Jr. Drug-induced lung disease. Adv Intern Med 1997; 42:231–268

An excellent overview of the area emphasizing the pulmonary clinical syndromes and diagnostic approach (149 references).

Limper AH. Drug-induced pulmonary disease. In: Mason RJ, Murray JF, Broaddus VC, et al, eds. Murray & Nadel's textbook of respiratory medicine. 4th ed. Philadelphia, PA: WB Saunders Co., 2005; 1888–1908

An excellent overview of the topic that includes 167 references.

Meyers JL. Diagnosis of drug reactions in the lung. Monogr Pathol 1993; 32–53

A detailed analysis of the characteristic pathologic changes associated with drug-induced adverse pulmonary effects that includes 121 references.

Chemotherapeutic Agents

Alarcon GS, Kremer JM, Macaluso M, et al. Risk factors for methotrexate-induced lung injury in patients with rheumatoid arthritis. Ann Intern Med 1997; 127:356–364

A multicenter, case-control study demonstrating the strongest clinical predictors for lung injury.

Castro M, Veeder MH, Mailliard JA, et al. A prospective study of pulmonary function in patients receiving mitomycin. Chest 1996; 109:939–944

A prospective study of the role of PFTs in 133 patients showing that serial changes in the Dlco did not predict clinical toxicity.

Cherniak RM, Abrams J, Kalica AR. NHLBI Workshop summary: pulmonary disease associated with breast cancer therapy. Am J Respir Crit Care Med 1994; 150:1169–1173

A concise summary of lung toxicity due to chemotherapeutic agents used to treat breast cancer.

Cottin V, Tebib J, Massonnet B, et al. Pulmonary function in patients receiving long-term low-dose methotrexate. Chest 1996; 109:933–938

This prospective study of 124 patients receiving low-dose methotrexate shows that pneumonitis developed in 3.2% of patients and that PFTs did not detect abnormalities prior to clinical presentation.

Dimopoulou I, Bamias A, Lyberopoulos P, et al. Pulmonary toxicity from novel antineoplastic agents. Ann Oncol 2006; 17:372–379

A thorough review of adverse pulmonary effects from novel chemotherapeutic agents that includes 127 references.

Limper AH. Chemotherapy-induced lung disease. Clin Chest Med 2004; 25:53–64

A succinct review of adverse pulmonary effects from new and old chemotherapeutic agents that includes 79 references.

Sleifer S. Bleomycin-induced pneumonitis. Chest 2001; 120:617–624

A nice overview of the area with 96 references.

Nonchemotherapeutic Agents

Evans RB, Ettensohn DB, Fawaz-Estrup F, et al. Gold lung: recent developments in the pathogenesis, diagnosis, and therapy. Semin Arthritis Rheum 1987; 16:196–205

A review of 60 patients with gold-induced pulmonary toxicity and an extensive review of the literature.

Everitt DE, Avorn J. Systemic effects of medications used to treat glaucoma. Ann Intern Med 1990; 112:120–125

A concise summary of the adverse effects from commonly used ophthalmic solutions.

Hunt LW, Rosenow EC III. Asthma-producing drugs. Ann Allergy 1992; 68:453–462

An extensive review of all the drugs that induce bronchospasm as well as the mechanisms implicated.

Israili ZH, Hall WD. Cough and angioneurotic edema associated with angiotensin-converting enzyme inhibitor therapy: a review of the literature and pathophysiology. Ann Intern Med 1992; 117:234–242

A concise summary of ACE inhibitor-induced cough and angioneurotic pulmonary edema clinical presentation, pathogenesis, and management.

Kennedy JI Jr. Clinical aspects of amiodarone pulmonary toxicity. Clin Chest Med 1990; 11:119–129

A good overview of the clinical, radiographic, and histologic features as well as management of amiodarone-induced lung disease.

Leatherman JW, Scmitz PG. Fever, hemodynamic shock and multiple organ failure: a pseudosepsis syndrome associated with chronic salicylate intoxication. Chest 1991; 100:1391–1396

A concise review of acute and chronic salicylate toxicity.

Pisani RJ, Rosenow EC III. Pulmonary edema associated with tocolytic therapy. Ann Intern Med 1989; 110:714–718

An overview of the clinical presentation and management of 58 patients with tocolytic therapy-induced pulmonary edema.

Reasor MJ, Kacew S. An evaluation of possible mechanisms underlying amiodarone-induced pulmonary toxicity. Proc Soc Exp Biol Med 1996; 212:297–304

A detailed review of how amiodarone may injure the lungs with 89 references.

Tomioka H, King TE Jr. Gold-induced pulmonary diseases: clinical features, outcome, and differentiation from rheumatoid arthritis. Am J Respir Crit Care Med 1997; 155:1011–1020

A thorough review of the topic with 137 references.

Illicit Drugs

Albertson TE, Walby WF. Respiratory toxicities from stimulant use. Clin Rev Allergy Immunol 1997; 15:221–241

A concise update of the topic with 178 references.

Haim DY, Lippmann ML, Goldberg SK, et al. The pulmonary complications of crack cocaine: a comprehensive review. Chest 1995; 107:233–240

A succinct review of the pulmonary adverse effects of crack cocaine.

Notes

Hemodynamic Monitoring and Shock

Janice L. Zimmerman, MD, FCCP

Objectives:

- Understand the indications, complications, and use of pulmonary artery catheterization
- Apply hemodynamic information to determine appropriate clinical management
- Review techniques of estimating cardiac output
- Outline types, characteristic hemodynamic patterns, and management of shock

Key words: cardiac output; hemodynamics; monitoring; pulmonary artery catheter; sepsis; shock

Pulmonary artery catheterization (PAC) with a flow-directed, balloon flotation catheter was introduced into clinical practice in 1970. Many physicians believe that the ability to assess cardiac function and left ventricular filling pressure with PAC is helpful in diagnosis and therapy. Because PAC is a monitor, its clinical utility depends on appropriate interpretation of data and institution of effective therapeutic measures. Observational studies found that use of PAC was associated with either no reduction in complication rates or increased mortality and use of resources, in comparison with patients who did not undergo PAC. Randomized studies of PAC use in high-risk surgical patients, patients with shock and ARDS, patients with heart failure, and patients admitted to the ICU have found no difference in mortality between groups managed with and without PAC. The first part of this chapter will concentrate on reviewing the principles of PAC and correct interpretation of data rather than on the definitive benefit of the PAC. More detailed information on aspects of PAC use, including waveform analysis, is available through the Pulmonary Artery Catheterization Education Project, available at www.pacep.org.

Indications and Complications

PAC is without therapeutic purpose with the rare exception of emergency cardiac pacing. PAC should be considered for use when hemodynamic information is needed for optimum care of the patient that that cannot be supplied by clinical evaluation or other noninvasive modalities. Studies have demonstrated that PAC data are more accurate than clinical assessment in determining hemodynamic variables in complicated cases. Common indications for PAC monitoring are listed in Table 1. Many of the diagnostic uses of PAC have been supplanted by the use of echocardiography. The most common diagnostic uses of PAC are to determine intravascular volume status and cardiac function, which allow assessment of the type of shock and cause of pulmonary edema.

Various complications are associated with PAC, but dysrhythmias such as premature ventricular depolarizations or conduction abnormalities that occur during passage of the catheter are most common (Table 2). Dysrhythmias have been described in 13 to 78% of patients, and the risk is increased in the presence of cardiac ischemia, hypotension, hypokalemia, hypocalcemia, hypoxemia, and acidosis. When possible, metabolic abnormalities should be corrected before PAC. In patients with preexisting left bundle-branch block, the potential for development of complete heart block exists. This rare occurrence is more likely when the left bundle-branch block is new and associated with a recent myocardial infarction. Other complications occur at an overall rate of 4 to 7%, but the frequency of data misinterpretation or misapplication is unknown.

Use of the PAC

Insertion

The basic multilumen, 110-cm pulmonary artery (PA) catheter is depicted in Figure 1. The distal lumen opens at the catheter tip, and the proximal lumen (right atrial lumen) opens approximately 30 cm from the tip. A thermistor is located 3 to 5 cm from the tip. Adaptations that allow

Table 1. *Indications for PAC Monitoring*

Diagnostic
Evaluate volume status
Evaluate cardiac function
Determine type of shock
Determine cause of pulmonary edema
Diagnose cardiac tamponade
Diagnose ventricular septal rupture
Diagnose acute mitral regurgitation
Diagnose constrictive pericarditis
Therapeutic/preventive
Guide therapy
Monitor response to fluids, diuretics, vasoactive drugs, and positive pressure ventilation
Monitor high-risk patients perioperatively

Table 2. *Complications of PAC*

Establishment of central venous access
Arterial puncture/damage
Pneumothorax
Bleeding
Air embolism
Neuropathy
Catheterization procedure
Dysrhythmias
Right bundle-branch block
Catheter knotting
Catheter presence
Thrombosis
Infection
PA rupture
Balloon rupture
Endocardial damage
Pulmonary embolism/infarction
Misinterpretation of data

continuous venous oximetry and right ventricular cardiac output measurements are available. A PA catheter (usually 7F or 7.5F) is preferably inserted aseptically into the subclavian vein or internal jugular vein using a modified Seldinger technique. However, clinical circumstances of an individual patient dictate the appropriate selection of the site. Insertion through the femoral vein may require fluoroscopic assistance. Fluoroscopic guidance may also be necessary in patients with low cardiac output states, dilated right-heart chambers, severe tricuspid regurgitation, or PA hypertension. Ideally, PAC should be performed by a physician who is skilled in the insertion technique, knowledgeable of complications, and capable of appropriately interpreting and utilizing the data obtained.

The catheter should be advanced with continuous ECG and pressure monitoring. Once the catheter has passed into an intrathoracic vein as noted by respiratory fluctuation in pressures, the balloon should be inflated with 1.3 to 1.5 mL of air to facilitate passage through the right heart and into the PA. In the average patient, the distance from insertion to the right atrium is approximately 10 cm from a subclavian approach, 10 to 15 cm from the right internal jugular, and 35 to 45 cm from the femoral site. The PA is usually reached within 50 to 55 cm from the internal jugular or subclavian vein and within 65 to 70 cm from the femoral vein. Greater insertion lengths may indicate coiling in the right atrium or right ventricle. Characteristic waveforms and pressures are obtained during passage through the right atrium, right ventricle, and PA (Table 3, Fig 2). Atrial pressure waves can usually be recorded from the right atrium and the PA occlusion position. The a-wave is absent in atrial fibrillation.

If particular waveforms are not seen, placement of the catheter may be incorrect. The clinician must always be alert for the possibility of dysrhythmias and abnormal waveform patterns. The balloon should be deflated after a PA occlusion pressure (PAOP) waveform is verified. With

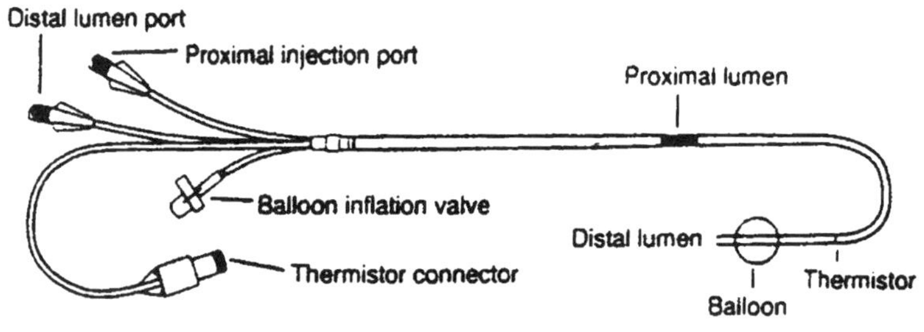

Figure 1. PAC (Swan-Ganz catheter).

Table 3. *Components of Hemodynamic Waveforms*

Waveform	Description
Atrial pressure and PAOP	
a-wave	Atrial contraction; follows P-wave (within PR interval) on ECG in right atrial tracing; near end of or after QRS in PAOP tracing.
c-wave	Sudden motion of mitral and tricuspid valve rings toward right and left atria at onset of ventricular systole; follows a-wave but not always present in right atrial tracing and not visible in PAOP tracing.
v-wave	Venous filling of left and right atria during ventricular systole when mitral and tricuspid valves closed; near end of T-wave on ECG in right atrial tracing, after T-wave in PAOP tracing.
x-descent	Atrial relaxation and sudden downward motion of the atrioventricular junction during early ventricular systole; follows a-wave.
y-descent	Rapid atrial emptying following opening of mitral and tricuspid valves; follows v-wave
Right ventricular	Systolic peak with rapid downstroke to end-diastolic pressure; peak systolic wave occurs after the QRS on ECG but before the T-wave with end-diastole in the T-QRS period.
PA	Systolic peak and diastolic trough with dicrotic notch due to closure of pulmonic valve; peak systolic wave occurs after the QRS but before the peak of T-wave on ECG; end-diastolic trough near end of QRS.

deflation, a characteristic PA pressure waveform should be apparent. If a PA pressure tracing is not present, continued occlusion of the pulmonary vessel ("overwedging") is possible and requires repositioning of the PAC to prevent pulmonary infarction. A chest radiograph should be obtained after the procedure to evaluate proper positioning. Daily chest radiographs should be inspected for distal migration of the catheter tip.

Measurements

The PAC allows measurement of right atrial pressure, right ventricular pressure (during passage through the chamber), PA pressure, and PAOP ("wedge" pressure). In addition, cardiac output and mixed venous oxyhemoglobin saturation (Svo_2) can be directly measured. Normal values for these measurements are listed in Table 4. In general, trends in these measurements over time are more useful clinically than single values. From these primary measurements, other physiologic variables that may be useful in evaluation and management of patients can be calculated. These equations and values are listed in Table 5.

Large variations in intrathoracic pressure due to labored spontaneous respiration (*eg*, severe bronchospasm) or mechanical ventilation, especially with positive end-expiratory pressure (PEEP), can cause difficulty in interpreting measurement of vascular pressures. To minimize these effects, vascular pressures are measured at end-expiration. Digital readouts of mean PAOP are not adequate in patients with rapid or labored breathing because

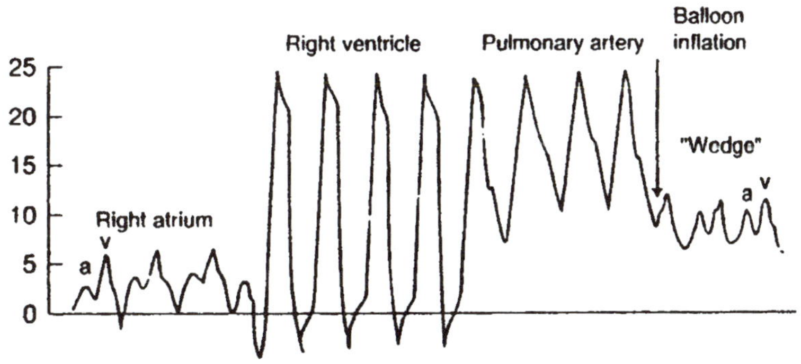

Figure 2. Characteristic waveforms and pressures seen during insertion of a PAC. A valid wedge pressure is not a straight line but has a-waves and v-waves indicative of transmitted left atrial pressure.

Table 4. *Normal Values Obtained From PAC*

Variables	Normal Range
Right atrial pressure, mm Hg	2–8
Right ventricular pressure, mm Hg	
Systolic	20–30
Diastolic	Same as right atrial pressure
PA pressure, mm Hg	
Systolic	20–30
Diastolic	5–15
PAOP, mm Hg	6–12 (must be less than diastolic PA pressure)
Svo_2, %	65–75

more than end-expiration will be averaged. Visual assessment of the pressure tracing allows more accurate determination of PAOP. Disconnection of patients from the ventilator or decrease in PEEP in order to measure hemodynamic variables are not recommended. Either of these actions alters hemodynamic conditions and may result in deterioration of clinical status.

PAOP

The measurement of PAOP is a major reason for PAC. Accurate measurement is essential for correct physiologic interpretation of data. The correct position of the catheter for determination of PAOP can be confirmed using the following criteria: (1) Mean PAOP should be less than or equal to the PA diastolic pressure, and lower than the mean PA pressure. (2) The waveform should be characteristic of left atrial pressures with an a-wave and v-wave. A damped waveform, straight line, or waveform deflections only related to respiratory changes are not acceptable. Balloon inflation and deflation should consistently result in disappearance and reappearance of the PA pressure tracing. (3) A free-flowing column of fluid or continuous flush excludes catheter obstruction. (4) Blood gas analysis of a sample withdrawn from the presumed PAOP position should usually have an oxygen saturation greater than or equal to systemic arterial blood.

The correct catheter position is necessary to interpret the PAOP as a reflection of left atrial

Table 5. *Physiologic Data Derived From Invasive Monitoring**

Cardiac index:
CO/BSA (normal range, 2.4 to 4.4 L/min/m^2)
Systemic vascular resistance:
(MAP − CVP)/CO × 79.9 (normal range, 900 to 1,400 dyne•s•cm^{-5})
Pulmonary vascular resistance
(MPAP − PAOP)/CO × 79.9 (normal range, 150 to 250 dyne•s•cm^{-5})
Stroke volume index
CI/HR × 1,000 (normal range, 36 to 48 mL/beat/m^2)
Stroke volume index
SV/BSA = CI/HR (normal range, 30 to 65 mL/min/m^2)
Left ventricular stroke work index
SVI × (MAP − PAOP) × 0.0136 (normal range, 43 to 61 g•m/m^2)
Right ventricular stroke work index
SVI × (MPAP − CVP) × 0.0136 (normal range, 7 to 12 g•m/m^2)
O_2 content
Hb × arterial O_2 saturation × 1.36 + (Po_2 × 0.003) [normal approximately 19.5 mL/dL]
Arteriovenous oxygen content difference
$Cao_2 = Cvo_2$ (normal range, 3 to 5 mL/dL)
Oxygen delivery
CO × Cao_2 × 10 (normal range, 800 to 1,200 mL/min)
Oxygen consumption
CO × ($Cao_2 - Cvo_2$) × 10 (normal range, 180 to 280 mL/min)
Pulmonary shunt (veno-arterial admixture)
($Cco_2 - Cao_2$)/($Cco_2 - Cvo_2$) [normal range, < 3 to 5%]

*BSA = body surface area; Cao_2 = arterial O_2 content; Cco_2 = pulmonary capillary O_2 content (assumed equal to alveolar Po_2); CI = cardiac index; CO = cardiac output; Cvo_2 = mixed venous oxygen content; CVP = central venous pressure; Hb = hemoglobin concentration; HR = heart rate; MPAP = mean pulmonary artery pressure; SV = stroke volume; SVI = stroke volume index.

pressure. The pulmonary vascular system distal to the catheter tip must be patent and provide a blood-filled connection with the left atrium. Left atrial pressures cannot be estimated in the upper lung (zone 1), where alveolar pressure usually exceeds PA and venous pressures (Fig 3). These conditions close pulmonary capillaries, and blood flow does not occur. In the central lung area (zone 2), flow is determined by the PA pressure and alveolar pressure with alveolar pressure exceeding pulmonary venous pressure. Balloon inflation converts zone 2 to zone 1 conditions by stopping blood flow and allowing collapse of the vessel distal to the balloon. Thus, PAOP reflects alveolar pressure rather than left atrial pressure in these zones. In zone 3, PA and venous pressures exceed alveolar pressures and capillaries remain open providing the necessary connection between the catheter tip and left atrium. With supine positioning, most of the lung is in zone 3, and flow-directed catheters usually enter these areas. Placement in non-zone 3 areas or conversion of zone 3 to other zones can occur with hypovolemia, change in patient position, or application of positive pressure ventilation. It has been estimated that if the PAOP changes > 50% of the change in PEEP, the catheter tip is likely to be in a non-zone 3 position.

The PA diastolic pressure is sometimes used to estimate the PAOP if wedging is unsuccessful. The PAOP is usually only 1 to 3 mm Hg less than the PA diastolic pressure in individuals with a normal heart rate and pulmonary vasculature. With tachycardia (> 120 to 130 beats/min) or pulmonary hypertension (*eg*, chronic lung disease or hypoxemia), the difference in the two measurements may be large and vary over time.

Appropriate interpretation of the measurements obtained with a PAC requires an understanding of the physiologic assumptions. The PAOP is a common measurement that is obtained to reflect left ventricular filling pressure (left ventricular end-diastolic pressure). Balloon occlusion of a branch of the PA interrupts flow and allows transmission of pressure back from the pulmonary veins and, ultimately, the left atrium. In general, the PAOP approximates left atrial pressure in the absence of any mechanical disruption of the large pulmonary veins. Pressures within the left atrium are a reflection of the pressure within the left ventricle at end-diastole. Left ventricular end-diastolic pressure is a major determinant of left ventricular end-diastolic volume, or preload. However, preload is also determined by compliance of the ventricle (pressure-volume relationship) and transmural ventricular distending pressure (intracavitary pressure less juxtacardiac pressure). Figure 4 illustrates these principles. Changes in juxtacardiac pressure, as with PEEP therapy (or auto-PEEP), or changes in ventricular compliance, as with ischemia or vasoactive agents, alter the interpretation of the PAOP as a reflection of myocardial function. The effect of PEEP on juxtacardiac pressure depends

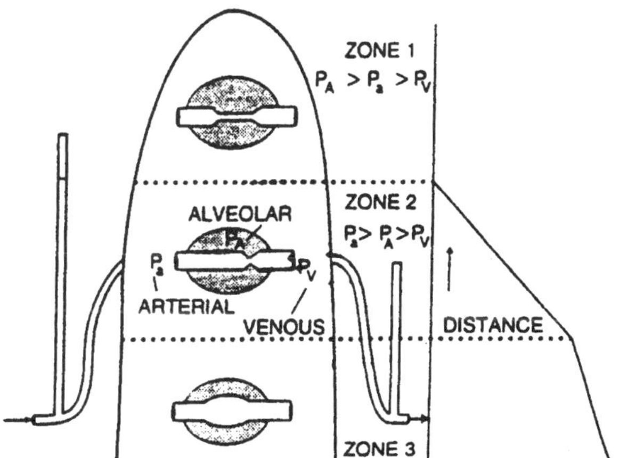

Figure 3. Catheter tip placement can occur in various west zones of the lung. PA = alveolar pressure; Pa = arterial pressure; Pv = venous pressure.

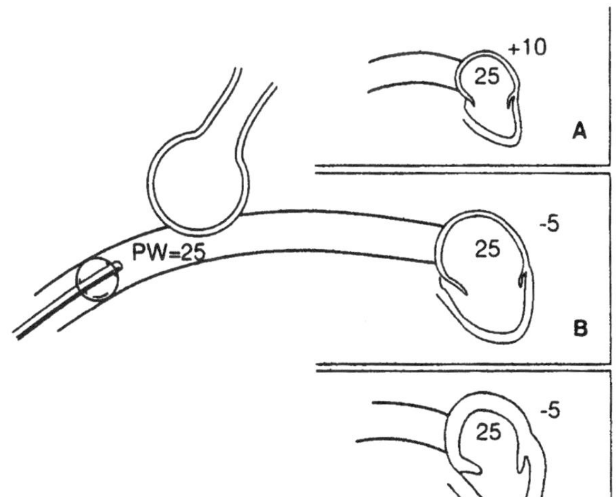

Figure 4. Wedge pressure (PW) may be associated with different ventricular volumes, or preload, depending on whether juxtacardiac pressure is elevated (*top, A*), as may occur with PEEP therapy, or whether ventricular compliance is decreased (*bottom, C*), as may occur with ischemia. *B* illustrates a normal heart and juxtacardiac pressure.

Table 6. *Conditions That Alter Pressure and Volume Relationships**

PAOP overestimates LVEDP
Mitral valve obstruction
Atrial myxoma
Mitral valve regurgitation
Pulmonary venous obstruction/vasoconstriction
Intracardiac shunt (left to right)
Non-zone 3 catheter position
Tachycardia
PAOP underestimates LVEDP
Aortic regurgitation
Decreased left ventricular compliance
PAOP and LVEDP do not reflect preload (LVEDV)
Positive pressure ventilation
Abnormal left ventricular compliance
Vasoactive drugs
Dilated right ventricle

*LVEDP = left ventricular end-diastolic pressure; LVEDV = left ventricular end-diastolic volume.

on lung and chest wall compliance. Usually, PEEP causes a decrease in left ventricular transmural pressure despite an increase in measured PAOP. Overall, measured PAOP will overestimate left ventricular end-diastolic pressure with PEEP, but the extent is difficult to determine precisely. In addition, mitral or aortic valve dysfunction alter the association of PAOP with left ventricular end-diastolic pressure (Table 6). The PAOP as a measure of preload does not reliably predict fluid responsiveness.

The PAOP is an indirect assessment of pulmonary capillary pressure but does not equal pulmonary capillary pressure. The pulmonary capillary pressure exceeds left atrial pressure and PAOP by a variable degree depending on vascular resistance in the pulmonary venous system. A normal PAOP may be present despite high pulmonary capillary pressures if marked resistance exists. Physiologic (*eg*, pulmonary embolism and hypoxia) and pharmacologic alterations (*eg*, prostaglandin administration and sympathetic stimulation) affect the pulmonary venous resistance. In such cases, the PAOP may underestimate the degree to which elevated pulmonary capillary pressure contributes to the development of pulmonary edema.

Thermodilution Cardiac Output

Determination of cardiac output by thermodilution involves the injection of an indicator through the proximal port (right atrium) with detection of a temperature change by a thermistor at the distal end of the catheter. The volume and temperature of injectate and the area under the thermodilution curve enable the cardiac output to be calculated. Thermodilution cardiac output generally has a good correlation with the Fick or dye dilution technique. However, even under the best circumstances, this measurement has a reliability of ± 10%. To ensure the best accuracy, the following steps should be taken: (1) temperature and volume of the injectate must be carefully measured; (2) average of three separate measurements obtained at least 1 min apart; (3) inject the solution over 2 s at the same phase of respiration, which preferentially is end-expiration; (4) use of room temperature injectate except for patients who are severely hypothermic ($<30°C$) who require iced injectate; a temperature difference of 10°C is necessary for accurate measurements; and (5) inspect graphic display of cardiac output thermodilution curve for rapid upstroke and gradual, smooth return to baseline.

Falsely low measurements may be obtained in the presence of tricuspid regurgitation and falsely elevated results in the presence of intracardic shunts or distal catheter position. Measurements may be unreliable in the presence of atrial fibrillation because of poor reproducibility. Other noninvasive and semiinvasive measurements of cardiac output that are used include the following:

Transesophageal Doppler Ultrasonography

This technique determines the velocity of blood in the descending thoracic aorta during ventricular systole. Stroke volume is estimated from this velocity using a nomogram and measurement of aortic diameter. Proper positioning is necessary for accurate measurements, and requires training and experience.

CO_2 Partial Rebreathing

Monitors using this technique are based on the Fick principle applied to CO_2. Determinations are made of CO_2 production and arterial CO_2 content during normal and rebreathing conditions. Patients must be receiving controlled mechanical ventilation because an increase in minute ventilation during the rebreathing period in spontaneously breathing patients reduces the accuracy of the cardiac output estimation. Inaccurate measurements also result with low minute ventilation, high shunt fraction, and high cardiac output.

Pulse Contour Analysis

Analysis of the arterial pressure waveform is used to compute stroke volume with or without initial calibration of cardiac output by transpulmonary thermodilution or indicator dilution (*eg*, lithium chloride). The pulse contour methodology is based on changes in the pulse pressure waveform. The pulse pressure varies with the stroke volume and changes in vascular compliance. An elevated pulse pressure variation may predict fluid responsiveness in critically ill patients. These techniques are not reliable when the arterial waveform is poorly defined or arrhythmias are present.

Studies of the reliability, validity, and clinical utility of the less invasive techniques report variable results. The advantages, disadvantages, and limitations of the various techniques suggest that a single method may not be applicable to all patients. Further clinical investigations are needed to determine the optimal method of assessing the hemodynamic status of critically ill patients.

Mixed Venous Blood Measurements

Measurements of Svo_2 are obtained by withdrawing blood from the distal port of the catheter with the balloon deflated. At least 2.5 to 3 mL of blood must be eliminated to allow for catheter dead space before removal of blood for analysis. Blood should be removed slowly in patients receiving high fraction of inspired oxygen levels or PEEP to avoid contamination with oxygenated capillary blood. Inaccurate measurements also occur in the presence of severe mitral regurgitation, left-to-right cardiac shunts, and distal tip placement. PA catheters and special central venous catheters that provide continuous measurement of Svo_2 make use of fiberoptic reflectance oximetry.

The Svo_2 reflects the balance between tissue O_2 delivery and O_2 consumption. The four variables that determine Svo_2 are cardiac output, arterial oxygen saturation, hemoglobin, and tissue oxygen consumption.

Although this measurement is often used to reflect changes in cardiac output, decreases in arterial oxygen saturation (hypoxemic lung disease) or hemoglobin as well as increased tissue oxygen consumption (fever, hypermetabolism, shivering, seizures, pain, or work of breathing) can result in decreases in Svo_2. A normal Svo_2 in a stable patient usually indicates that tissue oxygen needs are being met. An exception to this rule is in sepsis and certain poisonings (*eg*, cyanide), in which tissue hypoxia may exist with normal or elevated Svo_2.

In many critically ill patients without PAC, central venous catheterization allows measurement of central venous oxyhemoglobin saturation ($Scvo_2$). The $Scvo_2$ is usually 2 to 3% less than Svo_2 because the lower body extracts less oxygen. However, in patients with shock, this relationship is altered due to increased oxygen consumption by the GI tract. Under such conditions, the $Scvo_2$ is 5 to 7% higher than Svo_2, but both values change in parallel.

Clinical Indications for Hemodynamic Monitoring

Myocardial Infarction and Heart Failure

The first use of PAC was in patients with myocardial infarction complicated by shock. Estimation of preload by PAOP, measurement of cardiac output, and calculation of systemic vascular resistance (SVR) allow institution and titration of fluids and inotropic or vasopressor agents. Newer less invasive techniques may also provide similar information. The recognition of ischemic right ventricular dysfunction has implications for treatment different from that of left ventricular dysfunction. The characteristic hemodynamic findings in acute right ventricular dysfunction include an elevated right atrial pressure that equals or exceeds PAOP, a steep y descent, and a right ventricular pressure tracing with a diastolic dip and plateau (square root sign). The right atrial pressure may increase during inspiration (Kussmaul sign) or with the hepatojugular reflux maneuver.

PAC has been utilized in patients with heart failure to optimize inotropic and vasodilator therapy. The randomized trial of PAC use in patients with severe symptomatic heart failure (ejection fraction $< 30\%$) failed to show any benefit but was associated with a greater incidence of in-hospital adverse events. The benefit of PAC in cardiogenic shock has not been evaluated in clinical trials.

Shock

PAC or less invasive techniques may be helpful in the diagnosis of shock not due to myocardial infarction. Characteristic hemodynamic patterns that use filling pressures, cardiac output, and/or SVR are usually sufficient to distinguish cardiogenic, distributive, hypovolemic, and obstructive shock.

Mitral Regurgitation

Chronic mitral regurgitation is best diagnosed by noninvasive echocardiography. In acute decompensation, as may occur in myocardial infarction, PAC information will often distinguish mitral regurgitation from other complications if echocardiography is not readily available. Elevated left atrial pressure and PAOP are noted, and tall, peaked v-waves are seen in the PAOP tracing. A bifid PA waveform composed of the PA systolic wave and the v-wave may be seen. Regurgitant flow makes accurate assessment of the PAOP difficult if not impossible. In such circumstances, the a-wave on the PAOP tracing can be used to estimate left ventricular end-diastolic pressure. The pressure tracing should be examined together with a simultaneous ECG tracing. The v-wave occurs at the end of the T-wave on ECG, with the PA waveform occurring earlier in the cardiac cycle. Prominent v-waves can also be noted when the left atrium is distended and noncompliant due to left ventricular failure from any cause.

Tricuspid Regurgitation

Tricuspid regurgitation usually occurs in the setting of pulmonary hypertension and right ventricular dilatation. Tricuspid regurgitation is associated with elevated right atrial and right ventricular end-diastolic pressures. A prominent early v-wave is seen in the right atrial pressure tracing with PAC, and the x-descent may be absent or diminished. A steep y-descent is present. In severe tricuspid regurgitation, the right atrial pressure tracing may resemble the right ventricular pressure tracing.

Intracardiac Shunt

The presence of an intracardiac shunt may be determined using PAC to obtain blood samples for oxygen content in the right atrium, right ventricle, and PA, or by using PAC with oximetry. This assessment may be helpful in distinguishing acute ventricular septal defect from acute mitral regurgitation in myocardial infarction. A step-up in oxygen content (≥ 10%) between the right ventricle and right atrium indicates a ventricular septal defect. With development of an acute ventricular septal defect, the right atrial pressure, PA pressure, and PAOP are elevated.

Pulmonary Edema

The clinical differentiation of noncardiac and cardiac pulmonary edema may be difficult, particularly in critically ill patients. The differentiation of the two types of pulmonary edema is important because therapeutic interventions and prognosis differ significantly. Patients with noncardiac pulmonary edema have normal or near-normal PAOP in contrast to the elevated PAOP noted in myocardial dysfunction.

Acute Massive Pulmonary Embolism

Massive pulmonary embolism can produce a clinical presentation similar to cardiogenic shock. Although rarely needed as a diagnostic tool, PAC will demonstrate elevated systolic and diastolic PA pressures in massive pulmonary embolism but no elevation in PAOP. The mean PA pressure rarely exceeds 40 mm Hg unless there is a chronic component of pulmonary hypertension.

Acute Cardiac Tamponade

Echocardiography is most commonly used to diagnose pericardial effusion and its hemodynamic effects on myocardial function. In those instances in which echocardiography is not available, or when there is a question of hemodynamic impact of pericardial effusion, PAC may be helpful particularly with focal effusions. The characteristic hemodynamic pattern of acute cardiac tamponade includes elevation and equalization of right-sided and left-sided filling pressures (right atrium and PAOP) and a prominent systolic x-descent and blunted y-descent on the right atrial pressure tracing. The right atrial pressure declines in inspiration in contrast to right ventricular infarction and constrictive pericarditis.

Constrictive Pericarditis

Constrictive pericarditis produces equalization and elevation of right-sided and left-sided filling pressures similar to cardiac tamponade. In addition, constrictive pericarditis usually produces an early diastolic dip followed by a pressure plateau in the right and left ventricular pressure tracings. An inspiratory increase in pressure (Kussmaul sign) can often be seen in the right atrial tracing along with a systolic x-descent and prominent early diastolic y-descent.

Restrictive Cardiomyopathy

The hemodynamic pattern in restrictive cardiomyopathy is similar to constrictive pericarditis. Differentiation of the two conditions may be very difficult. Left-sided filling pressures tend to be higher than right-sided filling pressures in restrictive cardiomyopathy. In addition, the diastolic pressure plateau is usually less than one third of the right ventricular systolic pressure.

Shock

Shock is a syndrome of impaired tissue oxygenation and perfusion that results from one of the following mechanisms: an absolute or relative decrease in oxygen delivery; ineffective tissue perfusion; or impaired utilization of delivered oxygen. Shock results when the oxygen balance is disturbed and oxygen demands exceed supply. Although hypotension is often present in shock states, BP may be normal or even slightly increased due to compensatory vasoconstriction. Additional clinical manifestations in shock are related to tissue hypoperfusion, the compensatory responses initiated by shock, and the underlying etiology of shock.

Shock is usually classified into the following four categories: hypovolemic; distributive; cardiogenic; and obstructive (Table 7). However, most patients with shock demonstrate features of more than one type of shock (*ie*, mixed shock). For example, a patient who is in septic shock will likely have a hypovolemic component before resuscitation in addition to the decreased SVR that is characteristic of distributive shock.

The different types of shock are characterized by hemodynamic patterns (Table 8) that assist

Table 7. *Classification of Shock*

- Hypovolemic
  - Hemorrhagic (trauma and GI bleed)
  - Nonhemorrhagic (*eg*, external loss, interstitial fluid redistribution)
- Distributive
  - Sepsis
  - Adrenal crisis
  - Neurogenic (spinal shock)
  - Anaphylaxis
  - Thyroid storm
- Cardiogenic
  - Myopathic (*eg*, ischemia, cardiomyopathy)
  - Mechanical (*eg*, valvular lesions, septal defects)
  - Arrhythmias
- Obstructive
  - Massive pulmonary embolism
  - Tension pneumothorax
  - Cardiac tamponade
  - Constrictive pericarditis

Table 8. *Hemodynamic Patterns of Shock**

Type of Shock	SVR	CO	CVP	PAOP	SvO_2 or $ScvO_2$
Distributive					
Septic	↓	↑ or N* (rarely↓)	↓ or N	↓ or N	↓ or N
Neurogenic	↓	↑ or ↓	↓	↓	↑ or N
Hypovolemic	↑	↓	↓	↓	↓
Cardiogenic	↑	↓	↑	↑	↓
Obstructive					
Cardiac tamponade	↑	↓	↑	↑	↓
Pulmonary embolism	↑	↓	↑	↓ or N	↓

*N = Normal; CO = cardiac output; CVP = central venous pressure; ↑ = increase; ↓ = decrease.

with diagnosis and the determination of appropriate management. Specific measurements may not always be available, and clinical findings in a specific patient may be variable due to the specific etiology of shock, the underlying cardiac function, the duration of shock, and degree of resuscitation.

Management Principles of Shock

The management of shock requires treatment of the underlying etiology, and the restoration of adequate oxygen delivery and tissue perfusion. Oxygen delivery is optimized with interventions to achieve an appropriate BP, cardiac output, and oxygen content of arterial blood (see Table 5). The first goal is a minimum BP to maintain blood flow to the heart and vital organs while other components of oxygen delivery are addressed. An initial mean arterial pressure (MAP) of ≥65 mm Hg is usually recommended, but the specific goal for an individual patient should aim to optimize tissue perfusion without increasing myocardial oxygen demand. Once a minimum BP is achieved, oxygen delivery is improved by increasing cardiac output, hemoglobin concentration, or oxyhemoglobin saturation. Hemoglobin concentration can be increased by blood transfusion and oxyhemoglobin saturation by the administration of supplemental oxygen and/or mechanical ventilation. Therapeutic intervention with fluids, vasopressor agents, inotropic agents, and, rarely, vasodilators (cardiogenic shock) is utilized to optimize BP and cardiac output.

Fluids

Most types of shock benefit from initial volume resuscitation. Even patients with cardiogenic shock may require fluids to increase ventricular filling pressures in order to optimize myocardial performance (the Frank Starling principle). Isotonic crystalloid solutions or colloid solutions are equivalent as long as an appropriate quantity is administered to achieve hemodynamic goals. Although some studies have suggested that specific groups of patients may benefit more from a specific type of fluid, further study is needed to confirm these hypotheses. In general, crystalloids require two to three times greater volume than colloids to achieve similar goals. Hypotonic crystalloids should not be used for volume resuscitation. Colloid solutions have the potential advantage of achieving adequate volume resuscitation more quickly and with smaller volumes. Some studies have suggested that hetastarch solutions may be associated with more renal dysfunction and increased mortality, but the different properties of these hetastarch solutions preclude extrapolation of the results to the entire class of fluids. Therapy with titrated boluses of fluids (500 to 1,000 mL of crystalloid and 300 to 500 mL of colloid) is recommended in patients who are in shock, with close monitoring of the response until the hemodynamic goals are achieved.

Vasoactive Agents

Vasoactive medications for the treatment of shock include agents with vasopressor, intropic, and/or vasodilator effects. Some agents have combined effects (vasopressor and inotropic), and effects may vary with the dose. An agent should be selected based on the physiology of the type of shock, the effect desired, and the specific assessment of the patient. There have been no clinical trials that have established the superiority of a single agent or combination of agents in treating shock. Common vasoactive agents, dosing ranges, and adrenergic effects are listed in Table 9. In general, agents with predominantly α-adrenergic properties will have greater vasopressor effects, and agents with greater β-adrenergic properties will have more inotropic and chronotropic effects. Therapy with potent vasopressor agents will generally result in increases in afterload, MAP, and preload, with decreases in cardiac output and relative bradycardia. Agents with potent inotropic effects increase myocardial contractility, cardiac output, and heart rate, and may decrease BP.

Severe Sepsis and Septic Shock

Consensus guidelines have been developed for the management of severe sepsis and septic shock. The clinician should be familiar with these recommendations and the evidence supporting the interventions. A recent revision of the international guidelines resulted in a total of 73 recommendations, as follows: initial resuscitation

Table 9. *Vasoactive Agents in Shock: Adrenergic Effects*

Drug	Usual IV Dose	α	β_1	β_2	Dopaminergic
Dopamine	1–2 µg/kg/min	1+	0–1+	0–1+	3+
	2–10 µg/kg/min	2+	1–2+	0–1+	3+
	10–30 µg/kg/min	3+	1–2+	0–1+	3+
Dobutamine	2–30 µg/kg/min	0–1+	3+	1+	0
Norepinephrine	0.5–80 µg/min	3+	2+	0	0
Epinephrine	Low: 0.005–0.02 µg/kg/min	0	3+	2+	0
	High: >0.02 µg/kg/min	2+	3+	1–2+	0
Phenylephrine	20–200 µg/min	3+	0	0	0
Vasopressin	0.01– 0.04 U/kg/min	0	0	0	0

(3 recommendations); infection issues (15 recommendations); hemodynamic support (13 recommendations); adjunctive therapy (9 recommendations); and supportive therapy (33 recommendations). Recommendations of particular interest are listed below. Recommendations with a grade of 1 are strong recommendations, and those with a rating of 2 are suggested recommendations. The letter designations refer to the quality of the evidence behind them. Additional information on the guidelines can be found at www.survivingsepsis.org or in the published article.

Initial Resuscitation

- Initiate resuscitation immediately in patients with hypotension or lactate concentration of >4 mmol/L. Grade of recommendation, 1C
- Resuscitation goals are central venous pressure of 8 to 12 mm Hg, MAP of ≥65 mm Hg, urine output of ≥0.5 mL/kg/h, $Scvo_2$ of ≥70% or Svo_2 of ≥65%. Grade of recommendation, 1C
- If the goals for $Scvo_2$ and Svo_2 are not achieved, consider therapy with additional fluid, transfusion to a hematocrit of ≥30%, or dobutamine infusion to a maximum of 20 µg/kg/min. Grade of recommendation, 2C

Infection Issues

- Begin therapy with IV antibiotics as soon as possible but always within 1 h of recognizing the presence of severe sepsis (grade of recommendation, 1D) and septic shock (grade of recommendation, 1B)
- Reassess the antibiotic regimen daily to optimize efficacy, prevent resistance, avoid toxicity, and decrease costs. Grade of recommendation, 1C
- Consider using combination therapy for ≤3 to 5 days and deescalate therapy when susceptibilities are known. Grade of recommendation, 2D
- Implement source control measures as soon as possible after initial resuscitation. Grade of recommendation, 1C

Hemodynamic Support

- Use crystalloids or colloids for fluid resuscitation. Grade of recommendation, 1B
- Maintain MAP at ≥65 mm Hg. Grade of recommendation, 1C
- Norepinephrine and dopamine are the initial vasopressors of choice. Grade of recommendation, 1C
- Epinephrine, phenylephrine, or vasopressin should not be the initial vasopressor. Grade of recommendation, 2C
- Epinephrine is the first alternative therapeutic agent to be used when BP is poorly responsive to norepinephrine or dopamine. Grade of recommendation, 2B

Adjunctive Therapy

- Consider therapy with IV hydrocortisone when hypotension responds poorly to adequate fluid resuscitation and vasopressors. Grade of recommendation, 2C
- An adrenocorticotropic hormone stimulation test is not recommended to identify patients who

should receive hydrocortisone. Grade of recommendation, 2B

- Consider therapy with activated protein C in patients with sepsis-induced organ dysfunction and a clinical assessment of the high risk of death (APACHE [acute physiology and chronic health evaluation] II score of ≥25 or multiple organ failure) if there are no contraindications. Grade of recommendation, 2B
- Patients with severe sepsis and a low risk of death (APACHE II score of < 20 or single organ failure) should not receive activated protein C. Grade of recommendation, 1A

Supportive Care

- After initial resuscitation, transfuse RBCs when hemoglobin concentration decreases to < 7 g/dL to target a hemoglobin concentration of 7 to 9 g/dL. Grade of recommendation, 1B
- Use IV insulin to control hyperglycemia following stabilization. Grade of recommendation, 1B
- Control glucose concentration to a target value of < 150 mg/dL using a protocol for insulin adjustment. Grade of recommendation, 2C

Annotated Bibliography

American Society of Anesthesiologists Task Force on Pulmonary Artery Catheterization. Practice guidelines for pulmonary artery catheter. Anesthesiology 2003; 99:888–1014

An updated guideline with recommendations and rationale for the role of PAC in the perioperative setting.

Botero M, Kirby D, Lobato EB, et al. Measurement of cardiac output before and after cardiopulmonary bypass: comparison among aortic transit-time ultrasound, thermodilution, and noninvasive partial CO_2 rebreathing. J Cardiothoracic Vasc Anesth 2004; 18:563–572

A study comparing three methods of determining cardiac output in cardiopulmonary bypass patients.

Brunkhorst F, Engel C, Bloos F, et al. Intensive insulin therapy and pentastarch resuscitation in severe sepsis. N Engl J Med 2008; 358:125–139

A randomized, controlled trial demonstrating no benefit of tight glucose control in patients with severe sepsis and an association of renal dysfunction with the use of pentastarch.

Cohen MG, Kelly RV, Kong DF, et al. Pulmonary artery catheterization in acute coronary syndromes: insights from the GUSTO IIb and GUSTO III trials. Am J Med 2005; 118:482–488

A retrospective analysis of randomized international trials in acute coronary syndromes showing increased mortality associated with PAC use except in patients in cardiogenic shock.

Connors AF Jr, Speroff T, Dawson NV, et al. The effectiveness of right heart catheterization in the initial care of critically ill patients. JAMA 1996; 276:889–897

This article, which revived the controversy of benefit of PAC, reports a retrospective study with extensive matching that found a higher mortality and use of resources in patients with a PA catheter.

Cruz K, Franklin C. The pulmonary artery catheter: uses and controversies. Crit Care Clinics 2001; 17:271–291

A review of the principles and interpretation of hemodynamic data as well as discussion of controversies on use of PAC.

Dark PM, Singer M. The validity of trans-esophageal Doppler ultrasonography as a measure of cardiac output in critically ill adults. Intensive Care Med 2004; 30:2060–2066

A systematic review of clinical studies to evaluate the validity of transesophageal Doppler ultrasonography.

Dellinger RP, Levy MM, Carlet JM, et al. Surviving sepsis campaign: international guidelines for management of severe sepsis and septic shock: 2008. Crit Care Med 2008; 36:296–327

A revision of the 2004 guidelines for severe sepsis and septic shock based on new evidence and consensus.

ESCAPE investigators and ESCAPE study coordinators. Evaluation study of congestive heart failure and pulmonary artery catheterization effectiveness. JAMA 2005; 294:1625–1633

Randomized controlled trial of PAC in patients with heart failure (ejection fraction < 30%) found no benefit on mortality and hospitalization, and PAC use increased adverse events.

Harvey S, Stevens K, Harrison D, et al. An evaluation of the clinical and cost-effectiveness of pulmonary artery catheters in patient management in intensive care: a systematic review and a randomised controlled trial. Health Technol Assess 2006; 10:iii-iv, ix-xi, 1–133

An extensive review of PAC clinical trials and detailed findings of the PAC-Man trial that concludes that withdrawal of PAC from the United Kingdom would save money.

Harvey S, Young D, Brampton W, et al. Pulmonary artery catheters for adult patients in intensive care (review). Cochrane Database of Systematic Reviews (database online). Issue 3, 2006

A comprehensive review of the quality and outcomes of clinical trials of PAC use.

Hollenberg S. Vasopressor support in septic shock. Chest 2007; 132:1678–1687

A review of the evidence and experience with specific vasopressors in treating patients with septic shock.

Marik PE, Baram M. Noninvasive hemodynamic monitoring in the intensive care unit. Crit Care Clin 2007; 23:383–400

A review of newer noninvasive monitoring techniques and global indicators of perfusion.

Marx G, Reinhart K. Venous oximetry. Curr Opin Crit Care 2006; 12:263–268

A review of the applications and limitations of Svo_2 *and* $Scvo_2$ *as indicators of tissue oxygenation.*

Michard F, Teboul J. Predicting fluids responsiveness in ICU patients. Chest 2002; 121:2000-2008

A review of studies predicting response to fluids that suggests that dynamic rather than static parameters are more useful.

National Heart, Lung, and Blood Institute Acute Respiratory Distress Syndrome (ARDS) Clinical Trials Network. Pulmonary artery versus central venous catheter to guide treatment of acute lung injury. N Engl J Med 2006; 354:2213–2224

A randomized clinical trial of 1,000 patients with ARDS showing that PAC-guided therapy did not improve outcomes but was associated with complications as compared to therapy guided by a central venous catheter.

PACEP Collaborative. Pulmonary Artery Catheter Education Project. Available at: www.pacep.org. Accessed April 2, 2008

A self-paced educational program on basic principles of hemodynamics, correct analysis of waveforms, and interpretation of data developed by several critical care organizations.

Polanczk CA, Rohde LE, Goldman L, et al. Right heart catheterization and cardiac complications in patients undergoing noncardiac surgery: an observational study. JAMA 2001; 286:309–314

This study found more postoperative major cardiac and noncardiac events in patients undergoing right-heart catheterization even when matched for multiple variables.

Rhodes A, Cusack RJ, Newman PJ. A randomized, controlled trial of the pulmonary artery catheter in critically ill patients. Intensive Care Med 2002; 28:256–264

This study found no difference in mortality in patients managed with or without PAC.

Richard C, Warszawski J, Anguel N, et al. Early use of the PAC and outcomes in patients with shock and acute respiratory distress syndrome. JAMA 2003; 290:2713–2720

This randomized trial in France found no harm but also no mortality or morbidity benefit from PAC.

Russell JA, Walley KR, Singer J, et al. Vasopressin versus norepinephrine infusion in patients with septic shock. N Engl J Med 2008; 358:877–887

Randomized, controlled trial demonstrating the equivalence of therapy with norepinephrine and therapy with vasopressin plus norepinephrine in treating patients with septic shock.

Sakr Y, Vincent J-L, Reinhart K, et al. Use of the pulmonary artery catheter is not associated with worse outcome in the ICU. Chest 2005; 128:2722–2731

An observational study in European ICUs showing that PAC use was not associated with increased mortality.

Sandham JD, Hull RD, Brant RF, et al. A randomized, controlled trial of the use of pulmonary-artery catheters in high-risk surgical patients. N Engl J Med 2003; 348:5–14

This Canadian randomized trial of PAC use with goal-directed therapy found no difference in mortality but a higher rate of pulmonary embolism in the PAC group.

Shah MR, Hasselblad V, Stevenson LW, et al. Impact of the pulmonary artery catheter in critically ill patients. JAMA 2005; 294:1664–1670

A metaanalysis of randomized trials of PAC use showing PAC use did not increase mortality or benefit patients.

Sharkey SW. Beyond the wedge: clinical physiology and the Swan-Ganz catheter. Am J Med 1987; 83:111–122

An older article with a good review and illustrations of hemodynamic waveforms in a variety of clinical conditions.

Sprung CL, Annane D, Keh D, et al. Hydrocortisone therapy for patients with septic shock. N Engl J Med 2008; 358:111–124

Randomized, controlled trial of hydrocortisone therapy in the treatment of patients with septic shock showing no benefit, even in nonresponders to an adrenocorticotropic hormone stimulation test.

Tuman KJ, Carroll GC, Ivankovich AD. Pitfalls in interpretation of pulmonary artery catheter data. J Cardiothoracic Anesth 1989; 3:625–641

A thorough review of conditions that affect and sometimes invalidate interpretation of PAC data.

Uchino S, Bellomo R, Morimatsu H, et al. Pulmonary artery catheter versus pulse contour analysis: a prospective epidemiological study. Crit Care 2006; 10:R174; available at: http://ccforum.com/content/10/6/R174. Accessed May 19, 2007

An observational study showing that the choice of monitoring did not influence major outcomes in critically ill patients.

Wiedemann HP, Matthay MA, Matthay RA. Cardiovascular-pulmonary monitoring in the intensive care unit: part 1. Chest 1984; 85:537–549

Wiedemann HP, Matthay MA, Matthay RA. Cardiovascular-pulmonary monitoring in the intensive care unit: part 2. Chest 1984; 85:656–658

Still a classic series covering PAC technique, complications, and physiologic correlates of measurements.

Weiniger CF, Ginosar Y, Sprung C, et al. Arterial and pulmonary artery catheters. In: Parrillo JE, Dellinger RP, eds. Critical care medicine: principles of diagnosis and management in the adult. 2nd ed. St. Louis, MO: Mosby, 2001; 36–63

A good textbook chapter on PAC use, including insertion, complications, and interpretation of data.

Yu DT, Platt R, Lanken PN, et al. Relationship of pulmonary artery catheter use to mortality and resource utilization in patients with severe sepsis. Crit Care Med 2003; 31:2734–2741

A case-control study finding that use of a PAC was not associated with a change in mortality rate or resource utilization.

Community-Acquired Pneumonia: Advances in Management

Ronald R. Grossman, MD, FCCP

Objectives:

- Identify the common pathogens causing community-acquired pneumonia
- Identify the risk factors for mortality to improve site-of-care decisions
- Improve antibiotic selection in the empiric therapy of community-acquired pneumonia
- Recognize the risk of avian influenza and community-acquired methicillin-resistant *Staphylococcus aureus*

Key words: community-acquired methicillin-resistant *Staphylococcus aureus;* CURB-65; Patient Outcomes Research Team (PORT) score; *Streptococcus pneumoniae*

Community-acquired pneumonia (CAP) affects 5.6 million adults annually in the United States and causes 1.7 million hospitalizations per year.[1] Combined mortality rates for pneumonia and influenza indicate that this is the sixth-leading cause of death in the United States, accounting for 83,000 deaths annually. It is the cause of 46% of all deaths from infectious disease.[2] Although causative pathogens are identified in <50% of cases,[3] the specific organisms that require coverage include typical organisms such as *Streptococcus pneumoniae, Haemophilus influenzae,* and *Moraxella catarrhalis.* Atypical organisms, including *Mycoplasma pneumoniae, Chlamydia pneumoniae,* and *Legionella pneumophila* may have a presentation that is more subacute, with nonproductive cough and a chest radiograph that appears characteristically worse than the patient's clinical appearance, but this presentation is not uniform by any means and does not allow clinical identification from patients with infection from usual organisms.[4]

When the latest Infectious Diseases Society of America/American Thoracic Society (ATS) CAP guideline is used as a framework, patients with CAP are classified into one of two groups, each with a list of likely pathogens.[5] Stratification is based on an assessment of the need for a specific site of therapy (outpatient, inpatient ward, or ICU), the presence of comorbidities, and the likelihood for drug-resistant *S pneumoniae* (DRSP), enteric Gram-negative organisms, and *Pseudomonas aeruginosa.* Not every patient should be considered at risk for infection with DRSP. Specific risk factors have been identified, and there are regional differences in resistance rates. The role of enteric Gram-negative organisms in CAP is controversial, but these organisms do not need to be considered unless specific risk factors are present; one of these risk factors includes residence in a nursing home.

S pneumoniae is the most common pathogen, and it may even account for pneumonia in patients who have no pathogen identified by routine diagnostic testing (Table 1). Although the incidence of DRSP is increasing, available data show that the rate of mortality in patients with CAP is adversely affected by drug-resistant pneumococci only when minimum inhibitory concentration values to penicillin are ≥4 mg/L.[6] The impact of organisms at lower levels of resistance remains uncertain. Some studies[7] have been unable to detect treatment

Table 1. *Organisms Associated with Community-Acquired Pneumonia**

Patient Type	Etiology
Outpatient	*S pneumoniae* *M pneumoniae* *H influenzae* *C pneumoniae* Respiratory viruses
Inpatient (non-ICU)	*S pneumoniae* *M pneumoniae* *C pneumoniae* *H influenzae* Legionella spp Aspiration Respiratory viruses
Inpatient (ICU)	*S pneumoniae* *S aureus* Legionella spp Gram-negative bacilli *H influenzae*

*Adapted from Mandell et al.[5]

failures when patients with drug-resistant strains of *S pneumoniae* are treated with antibiotics that do not have *in vitro* activity against the pathogen. Treatment failures have been described among patients with infection treated with macrolides when pneumococci exhibit macrolide resistance and fluoroquinolones when pneumococci exhibit fluoroquinolone resistance.[8,9] The mechanism of macrolide resistance does not appear to influence the risk of macrolide failures.[10]

All patients with CAP could potentially be infected with *C pneumoniae*, *M pneumoniae*, and Legionella sp (the "atypical" pathogens), either alone or as part of a mixed infection; thus, all patients should receive therapy to account for this possibility.[11] A meta-analysis[12] has suggested that clinical outcomes are satisfactory when outpatients are treated with β-lactams alone without atypical coverage. However, most of the trials selected for this meta-analysis were for antibiotic registration purposes, and the patients were highly selected. These trials examined late clinical outcomes, and differences in rates of recovery could easily be missed by this analysis. This meta-analysis applied only to outpatients and does not speak to the appropriate management of hospitalized patients with CAP. There are considerable data to suggest that atypical coverage (either with macrolides or fluoroquinolones) is associated with better clinical outcomes, including reduced lengths of hospital stay and rates of mortality.[13,14]

When patients with CAP are admitted to the ICU, the organisms responsible include *S pneumoniae*, *Staphylococcus aureus*, Legionella sp, and enteric Gram-negative organisms.[15] *P aeruginosa* has been recovered from some patients with severe CAP, but this organism should only be considered when patients have well-identified risk factors present. In a prospective study, Arancibia and coworkers[16] identified that probable aspiration, previous hospital admission, previous antimicrobial treatment, and the presence of pulmonary comorbidity were independent predictors of Gram-negative pneumonia. Similarly, pulmonary comorbidity and previous hospital admission were independent predictors of pneumonia caused by *P aeruginosa*.

Patients should be investigated for the presence of microorganisms when the usual empiric regimen would not be sufficient, especially when the patient has clinical or epidemiologic considerations suggesting the presence of unusual organisms.[5] All patients with CAP should undergo chest radiography to establish the diagnosis and the presence of complications (pleural effusion, multilobar disease).[5] All outpatients should have a careful assessment of disease severity, but sputum culture and Gram stain are not required. All admitted patients with CAP should have an assessment of gas exchange (oximetry or arterial blood gas), routine blood chemistry and blood counts, and a collection of two sets of blood cultures. The standard recommendation for blood cultures has recently been challenged.[17]

The risk of bacteremia is increased among patients with underlying liver disease, demonstrating hypotension (systolic BP <90 mm Hg), tachycardia (pulse rate ≥125 beats/min), extremes of temperature (<35°C or ≥40°C), and exhibiting certain abnormal laboratory features (BUN ≥30 mg/dL, sodium <130 mmol/L, WBC count <5,000 μL or >20,000 μL). The risk of bacteremia is significantly decreased among patients who have received antibiotics previously. When researchers used a decision support tool whereby no samples for blood cultures would be drawn if the risk of bacteremia was low, one blood culture if the risk of bacteremia was moderate, and two blood cultures if the risk of bacteremia was high, 88% of bacteremias would be detected and 38% fewer blood cultures would be drawn.[17]

If a drug-resistant pathogen or an organism not covered by usual empiric therapy is suspected, sputum culture should be obtained, and a Gram stain should be used to guide interpretation of culture results. Routine serologic testing is not recommended for any population with CAP. For patients with severe CAP, Legionella and pneumococcal urinary antigen should be measured, and aggressive efforts at establishing an etiologic diagnosis should be made, including the collection of bronchoscopic samples of lower respiratory secretions in selected patients, although the benefit of such efforts has not been proven.[5]

The admission decision can be difficult, and prognostic scoring rules (the Patient Outcomes Research Team [PORT] and British Thoracic Society [BTS] rules) are adjunctive tools to support, but not replace, this process.[18–20] In general, hospitalization is needed if patients have multiple risk factors for a complicated course. Patients may also need to be hospitalized for a variety of nonmedical reasons, and such social factors should also be incorporated into the admission decision process.

Admission to the ICU is needed for patients with severe CAP, defined as the presence of either one of two major criteria or the presence of two or three minor criteria (modified ATS). The major criteria include need for mechanical ventilation or septic shock. The minor criteria include systolic BP ≤90 mm Hg, multilobar disease, and Pa_{O_2}/fraction of inspired oxygen ratio <250.[5] Patients who have two of four criteria from the modified BTS rule also have more severe illness and should be considered for admission to the ICU. These criteria include respiratory rate ≥30 breaths/min, diastolic BP ≤60 mm Hg, BUN >7.0 mmol/L (>19.1 mg/dL), and confusion (*ie*, CURB [confusion, elevated urea, increased respiratory rate, decreased BP]). The modified ATS rule achieved a sensitivity of 69% and specificity of 97% in predicting admission to the ICU and a sensitivity of 94% and specificity of 93% for predicting mortality.[21] When two variables were used to predict outcome, the BTS-CURB criteria did not perform nearly as well as the modified ATS rules.[21]

Patients should initially be treated empirically based on the likely pathogens for each of the sites of care, although when culture results become available, organism-specific therapy may be possible for some patients. All populations should be treated for the possibility of atypical pathogen infection (Table 2). For outpatients or non-ICU inpatients with risk factors for these other organisms, therapy should be with either a β-lactam/macrolide combination or an antipneumococcal fluoroquinolone alone (Table 2). Although both regimens appear therapeutically equivalent, particularly among inpatients, in the outpatient treatment of the more complicated patient, an antipneumococcal fluoroquinolone may be more convenient than a β-lactam/macrolide combination.

All admitted patients should receive their first dose of antibiotic therapy as soon as possible after arrival to the hospital.[22] Although 4 h has been the recommended standard, it is not clear that every patient must be treated that quickly because the diagnosis of pneumonia often takes >4 h to establish and treatment should not be started until other diagnostic possibilities have been excluded. In the ICU-admitted patient, current data do not support the use of an antipneumococcal fluoroquinolone alone, and therapy should be with a β-lactam plus either a macrolide or fluoroquinolone, using a regimen with two antipseudomonal agents in appropriate, at-risk patients (Table 3). The more recent Infectious Diseases Society of America guidelines use a similar format to the ATS guidelines and have similar antibiotic recommendations.[16] The additional twist is the recognition that the use of antibiotics in the previous 3 months is a significant predictor of antibiotic resistance to that class.

Accordingly, the guidelines recommend use of an alternative class of therapy if an agent has been used within the past 3 months. Retrospective studies[23] have suggested that combination antibiotic therapy (usually a β-lactam plus a macrolide) is superior to single-agent therapy (usually a β-lactam alone) among severely ill patients with bacteremic pneumococcal pneumonia. In a prospective, international, observational study,[24]

Table 2. *Outpatient Treatment**

1. Previously healthy and no use of antimicrobials within the previous 3 mo
   - A macrolide
   - Doxycyline
2. Presence of comorbidities such as chronic heart, lung, liver, or renal disease; diabetes mellitus; alcoholism; malignancies; asplenia; immunosuppressing conditions or use of immunosuppressing drugs; or use of antimicrobials within the previous 3 mo (in which case an alternative from a different class should be selected)
   - A respiratory fluoroquinolone (moxifloxacin, gemifloxacin, or levofloxacin [750 mg])
   - A β-lactam plus a macrolide
3. In regions with a high rate (>25%) of infection with high-level (minimum inhibitory concentration, 16 g/mL) macrolide-resistant *S pneumoniae*, consider use of alternative agents listed above in (2) for patients without comorbidities (moderate recommendation; level III evidence)

*Adapted from Mandell et al.[5]

Table 3. *Inpatient Treatment**

Inpatient, non-ICU
A respiratory fluoroquinolone
A β-lactam plus a macrolide
Inpatient, ICU
A β-lactam (cefotaxime, ceftriaxone, or ampicillin-sulbactam) plus either azithromycin (level II evidence) or a respiratory fluoroquinolone (for penicillin-allergic patients, a respiratory fluoroquinolone and aztreonam are recommended)
Special concerns
If Pseudomonas is a consideration:
An anti-pneumococcal, anti-pseudomonal β-lactam (piperacillin-tazobactam, cefepime, imipenem, or meropenem) plus either ciprofloxacin or levofloxacin (750 mg); or
The above β-lactam plus an aminoglycoside and azithromycin; or
The above β-lactam plus an aminoglycoside and an anti-pneumococcal fluoroquinolone (for penicillin-allergic patients, substitute aztreonam for above β-lactam)

*Adapted from Mandell et al.[5]

combination antibiotic therapy was superior to monotherapy but only for severely ill patients. Whether a respiratory fluoroquinolone is equivalent to two agents cannot be ascertained from the available data.

Most patients with CAP will have an adequate clinical response within 3 days; when the patient has met appropriate criteria, a switch to oral therapy should be made.[25] Criteria for switch include improvement in cough and dyspnea, afebrile (<37.8°C) on two occasions 8 h apart, decreasing WBC count, and functioning GI tract with adequate oral intake. Even if the patient is febrile, a switch in therapy can occur if other clinical features are favorable. If the patient has met criteria for a switch, oral therapy can be started and the patient discharged on the same day if other medical and social factors permit. Switch therapy is simpler and quicker if a respiratory fluoroquinolone is used rather than a β-lactam/macrolide combination. Outcomes are identical to patients staying in hospital longer to complete their course of therapy.[26]

Length of stay has been shown to be related to three quality-of-care measures: initial administration of antibiotics in the emergency department, appropriate antibiotic selection, and shortened door to needle time.[27–30] Initiation of antibiotic therapy in the emergency department led to shorter hospital stays for CAP by approximately 2 days in one report.[28]

The following have been listed as quality indicators in the assessment of care of the CAP patient:

- Antibiotics administered in a timely way, within either 4 h or 8 h of hospital admission;
- Oxygen assessment or therapy within 8 to 24 h of hospital arrival;
- Blood specimen for culture drawn before the administration of antibiotics in the hospitalized patient;
- Administration of antibiotics with activity against all likely causative pathogens, preferably the least-expensive efficacious regimen;
- Counseling patients regarding smoking cessation;
- Switching from IV to oral antibiotics if the patient is clinically improving and hemodynamically stable, with discharge within 24 h of switching to oral therapy;
- Chest radiography within 24 h of hospital admission; and
- Use of methods to increase vaccination rates against influenza and pneumococcus; and No discharge home for patients who are unstable on the day of discharge.[30]

In a metaanalysis,[3] the overall mortality rate among 33,148 patients reported in 127 studies was 13.7%, ranging from 5.1% in a population that included both hospitalized and ambulatory patients, to 13.6% for hospitalized patients. In the elderly, the mortality rate was 17.6%, whereas among nursing home patients, it was 30.8%, and among those admitted to the ICU was 36.5%. When *S pneumoniae* was responsible, the mortality rate was 12.3%, a rate similar to that found when no pathogen could be identified (12.8%). Certain pathogens such as *P aeruginosa*, other Gram-negative organisms (such as *Klebsiella pneumoniae*), and *S aureus* had greater associated mortality rates. An episode of CAP in young adults without significant comorbidity is not a predictor of poor medium-term survival.[31] Increasing age, comorbid cerebrovascular and cardiovascular disease, an altered mental status, and increasing blood glucose are independent predictors of decreased medium-term (*ie*, up to 3 years) survival.[31]

Treatment failure rates with guideline-driven empiric therapy have been reported as high as 15%.[32] Risk factors for treatment failure that have been identified include liver disease, pneumonia risk class, leukopenia, multilobar CAP, pleural effusion, and radiographic signs of cavitation. Independent factors associated with a lower risk of treatment failure include influenza vaccination, initial treatment with fluoroquinolones, and a concurrent diagnosis of COPD. Failure of empiric therapy increases the rate of mortality in patients with CAP 11-fold after adjustment for risk class. Modification of these risk factors is possible and should encourage prospective randomized trials.

Emerging Threats

Community-Acquired Methicillin-Resistant S aureus

Community-acquired methicillin-resistant *S aureus* (MRSA) has emerged as a cause of CAP over the past several years.[33] It is quite distinct from hospital-acquired MRSA from an epidemiologic, genetic, and clinical perspective. Community-acquired MRSA tends to be less resistant to antimicrobial agents than hospital-acquired MRSA strains, and it almost always contains a type IV Staphylococcus cassette chromosome *mec* type IV gene (SCC *mec* IV) in addition to the genes for Panton-Valentine leukocidin, an extracellular cytotoxin that is a virulence factor for primary skin infections and pneumonia. Although community-acquired MRSA is not common, it may cause pneumonia that is typically characterized by a short duration of illness and focal necrotizing infiltrates. The disease may be rapidly progressive, so consideration of this entity is important in the management of severely ill patients with CAP.

In general, these strains are usually susceptible *in vitro* to vancomycin, linezolid, trimethoprim-sulfamethoxazole, doxycycline, and fluoroquinolones. In addition, they are often susceptible to clindamycin, but the presence of *in vitro* inducible resistance should be determined before the drug is administered. The initial choice in most published series has been IV vancomycin, although linezolid appears to be at least equivalent to vancomycin in the treatment of nosocomial MRSA pneumonia. The efficacy of treatment with trimethoprim-sulfamethoxazole in systemic infections caused by MRSA was comparable with vancomycin, and it has been effective alone and in combination with rifampin in patients with soft-tissue infections caused by community-acquired MRSA.

Avian Influenza

Avian influenza is an infectious disease of birds caused by type A strains of the influenza virus. Migratory waterfowl, most notably wild ducks, are the natural reservoir of avian influenza viruses, and these birds are also the most resistant to infection. Domestic poultry, including chickens and turkeys, are particularly susceptible to epidemics of rapidly fatal influenza. H5N1 variants demonstrated a capacity to directly infect humans in 1997 and have done so again in Vietnam in January 2004. The spread of infection in birds increases the opportunities for direct infection of humans. If more humans acquire infection over time, the likelihood also increases that humans with concurrent infection with human and avian influenza strains could serve as a "mixing vessel" for the emergence of a novel subtype with sufficient human genes to be easily transmitted from person to person. Such an event would mark the start of an influenza pandemic. In published series, symptoms of fever, sore throat, cough and, in several of the fatal cases, severe respiratory distress secondary to viral pneumonia developed.[34] Previously healthy adults and children and some with chronic medical conditions were affected. Antiviral drugs, some of which can be used for both treatment and prevention, are clinically effective against influenza A virus strains in otherwise-healthy adults and children but have some limitations.

Newer Studies

A metaanalysis was performed on randomized controlled trials of antibacterials for CAP in outpatients aged ≥ 18 years.[35] Clinical success and rate of mortality were compared between different oral antibiotic classes, and antibacterials with atypical coverage (macrolides and fluoroquinolones) were specifically compared with other antibacterials. In total, 13 eligible studies involving a total of 4,314 patients were included. No significant difference was detected regarding clinical success or mortality, regardless of atypical coverage or between antibacterial classes with similar atypical coverage. It was not possible to demonstrate any advantage of specific antibacterials for mild CAP in relatively healthy outpatients.

In contrast, a retrospective cohort study[36] was conducted in patients with pneumonia and clinical criteria of severe sepsis. Severe sepsis was present in 30.1% of subjects, of whom 43.9% received macrolides. The rate of mortality was 20.3% at 30 days and 24.5% at 90 days. In the multivariable analysis, the use of macrolide was associated with a decreased rate of mortality at 30 days and at 90 days in patients with severe sepsis and in patients with macrolide-resistant pathogens.

A prospective multinational observational study[37] was conducted to develop a propensity score for combination therapy vs monotherapy based on baseline patient and infection characteristics. Patients were matched by the propensity score and the 30-day mortality and hospital stay were examined. Patients treated with monotherapy (β-lactam alone) were older, had a greater chronic diseases score, and had a different clinical presentation compared with patients treated with combination therapy (β-lactam, macrolide). The unadjusted rate of mortality was significantly greater when monotherapy was used (22% vs 7%). Among patients in the monotherapy group matched to patients in the combination group, the mortality in these groups was identical when the propensity score was used. The benefit of combination therapy vs monotherapy cannot be reliably assessed in observational studies because the propensity to prescribe these regimens differs markedly.

In a retrospective analysis, 2,209 Medicare patients with bacteremic pneumonia, admitted to hospitals from either home or a nursing facility, were stratified according to the type of antibiotic treatment.[38] Multivariate modeling was performed to assess the relationship between the class of antibiotic used and several outcome variables. The initial use of any antibiotic active against atypical organisms was independently associated with a decreased risk of 30-day mortality and hospital admission within 30 days of discharge. Further analysis revealed that the benefits of atypical coverage were associated with the use of macrolides but not the use of fluoroquinolones or tetracyclines. Initial antibiotic treatment including a macrolide agent is associated with improved outcomes in Medicare patients hospitalized with bacteremic pneumonia. However, this study did not address the possibility that a fluoroquinolone as monotherapy is equally as effective as combination therapy with a macrolide/β-lactam.

To compare clinical outcomes of patients with CAP treated with and without atypical coverage, a secondary analysis was performed with the use of two comprehensive international databases.[39] Patients treated with atypical coverage had decreased time to clinical stability, decreased length of stay, decreased rate of total mortality, and decreased CAP-related mortality. These findings would support empiric therapy for all hospitalized patients with CAP with a regimen that covers atypical pathogens.

In a prospective observational study of 2,457 patients, 57 patients (2.3%) died ≤ 48 h after admission.[40] The overall rate of mortality was 7.7%. Independent factors associated with early death were increased age, altered mental status at presentation, multilobar pneumonia, shock at admission, pneumococcal bacteremia, and discordant empiric antibiotic therapy. Currently, early mortality is relatively low and is caused by pneumonia-related factors. Because pneumococcal bacteriemia and discordant antibiotic therapy, mainly attributable to a lack of coverage against *P aeruginosa*, are significant risk factors, appropriate early intervention may improve clinical outcome.

In a prospective multicenter trial, CRP levels were measured on admission and on days 3 and 7.[41] Etiology could be determined in 47.4%; in 38.8%, initial antibiotic therapy was appropriate. A decrease of <60% in CRP levels in 3 days and a decrease of <90% in CRP levels in 7 days were both associated with an increased risk of having received inappropriate empiric antibiotic treatment. Consecutive CRP measurements may be useful in the first week in follow-up of antibiotic treatment for severe CAP, and delayed normalization of CRP levels is associated with a greater risk of having received inappropriate antibiotic treatment.

A retrospective national cohort study in which the authors used the Department of Veterans Affairs administrative data involving mainly elderly men (n = 8,652) examined the role of statins and angiotensin-converting enzyme (ACE) inhibitors on the rate of mortality among patients admitted to hospital with pneumonia.[42] A total of 9.9% of subjects died within 30 days of presentation. In this cohort, 18.1% of subjects were receiving statins and 33.9% were receiving ACE inhibitors. After adjusting for potential confounders, current statin use and ACE inhibitor use were significantly associated with decreased 30-day mortality.

In a prospective observational study[43] of patients admitted to the hospital with CAP, the use of statins, ACE inhibitors, β-blockers, and aspirin was recorded. On multivariate logistic regression, statin use was associated with significantly lower 30-day mortality and development of complicated pneumonia. There was no effect on requirement of mechanical ventilation or inotropic support. On multivariate logistic regression, statin use was independently protective against a CRP that failed to decrease by ≥50% at day 4.

In a secondary analyses of the Community-Acquired Pneumonia Organization database of hospitalized patients with CAP and pneumococcal bacteremia and patients with CAP and negative blood culture findings, investigators modeled all-cause mortality and CAP-related mortality by the use of logistic regression analysis and time-to-clinical stability and length of hospital stay by the use of Cox proportional hazards models.[44] The multivariable regression analysis revealed a lack of association of pneumococcal bacteremic CAP and time to clinical stability, length of hospital stay, all-cause mortality, and CAP-related mortality. This finding suggests that factors related to severity of disease are confounders of the association between pneumococcal bacteremia and poor outcomes and the presence of pneumococcal bacteremia by itself should not be a contraindication for the de-escalation of therapy in clinically stable hospitalized patients with CAP.

In a prospective, observation study involving 193 patients, 39% had a pathogen identified. Of these pathogens, 15% were viruses, 20% were bacteria, 4% were mixed, and the rest were unknown.[45] Influenza, human metapneumovirus, and respiratory syncytial virus accounted for most viral infections. Compared with patients with bacterial infection, patients with viral infection were older, more likely to have cardiac disease, and were more frail. There were few clinically meaningful differences in presentation and no differences in outcomes according to the presence or absence of viral infection. This study suggests that viral infections are common in adults with pneumonia, raising issues of incidental nosocomial transmission.

In a secondary analysis[46] of a multicenter observational study conducted among 457 patients with ICU-admitted CAP, the presence of radiographic progression and bacteremia was determined. Logistic regression analysis indicated that the groups with radiographic progression plus bacteremia or radiographic progression alone had a greater risk for shock than patients without either finding, whereas bacteremic patients had no increased risk. In addition, patients with radiographic progression plus bacteremia or radiographic progression alone had an increased risk of ICU death compared with patients without either finding, whereas bacteremic patients had no increased risk. This finding suggests that in patients with severe CAP, radiologic progression of pulmonary infiltrates in the first 48 h is a poor prognostic feature, whereas bacteremia does not affect outcomes.

In an observational retrospective study[47] of 500 consecutive CAP patients, those who experienced clinical failure were identified. Clinical failure occurred in 13%. The most common etiologies for clinical failure related to CAP were severe sepsis (33%), acute myocardial infarction (28%), and progressive pneumonia (19%). All cases of severe sepsis occurred in the first 72 h of hospitalization. The most common etiology for clinical failure unrelated to CAP was the development of hospital-acquired pneumonia (45%). The development of severe sepsis early during hospitalization is the primary etiology for clinical failure related to CAP.

Clinical, laboratory, and functional data were prospectively collected on 1,813 adults with CAP admitted to hospital outside of influenza season.[48] The cohort consisted of 352 vaccine recipients and 352 matched control subjects. Influenza vaccination was associated with a 51% reduction of mortality outside influenza season. Adjustment for age, sex, and comorbidities did not alter these findings. More complete adjustment for confounding (*eg*, functional and socioeconomic status) markedly attenuated these benefits. This result would suggest that previous observational studies may have overestimated the mortality benefits of influenza vaccination.

A prognostic index was derived in 1,117 adult CAP patients and was validated among 646 consecutive patients discharged from hospitals at a later time.[49] In the derivation cohort, preillness functional status, Charlson index, and the severity on admission were independently associated with 90-day mortality, and a scoring system was developed. The 90-day mortality was 0.7% in the low-risk group, 3.5% in the intermediate-risk group, and 17.3% in the high-risk group. The results in the validation cohort were very similar. The prognostic index accurately stratified patients hospitalized for CAP into low-, intermediate-, and high-risk groups for 90-day mortality on discharge.

In a randomized controlled trial[50] in 596 patients with COPD, the role of pneumococcal vaccination in preventing pneumonia was determined. There were 58 first episodes of CAP caused by pneumococcus or of unknown etiology. There was no significant difference between the intervention and nonintervention arms among all patients. However, the efficacy of pneumococcal vaccination in younger patients with severe airflow obstruction was 91%. Pneumococcal vaccination was effective in preventing CAP in patients with COPD <65 years of age and in those with severe airflow obstruction but was ineffective among the other groups of patients with COPD.

In a database analysis[51] of 62,918 adults hospitalized with CAP, 12% had a record of previous pneumococcal vaccination. Vaccine recipients were less likely to die of any cause during hospitalization than were individuals with no record of vaccination, even after adjustment for the presence of comorbid illnesses, age, smoking, and influenza vaccination and under varying assumptions about missing vaccination data. Vaccination also lowered the risk of respiratory failure and other complications and reduced median length of stay by 2 days compared with no vaccination.

In a systematic review[52] of 15 randomized controlled trials comprising 2,796 total subjects, the role of short-course therapy was examined. Short-course regimens primarily studied the use of azithromycin (n = 1) also were analyzed. Of the extended-course regimens, three studies used the same antibiotic, whereas nine involved an antibiotic of the same class. Overall, there was no difference in the risk of clinical failure, mortality, or bacterial eradication between the short-course and extended-course regimens. This finding would suggest that adults with mild-to-moderate CAP can be safely and effectively treated with an antibiotic regimen ≤7 days.

Conclusion

Significant progress has been made in the management of patients with CAP. With the widespread development of clinical practice guidelines and the identification of processes of care that lead to well-documented improvement in outcomes, the prognosis of this disease should improve. Physicians need to be cognizant of the threats posed by community-acquired MRSA and possible pandemic influenza.

References

1. Niederman MS, McCombs JS, Unger AN, et al. The cost of treating community acquired pneumonia. Clin Ther 1998; 20:820–837
2. Merchant S, Mullins CD, Shih YT. Factors associated with hospitalization costs for community-acquired pneumonia. Clin Ther 2003; 25:593–610
3. Fine MD, Smith MA, Carson CA, et al. Prognosis and outcomes of patients with community acquired pneumonia: a meta-analysis. JAMA 1996; 275:134–141
4. Fang GD, Fine M, Orloff J, et al. New and emerging etiologies for community-acquired pneumonia with implications for therapy: a prospective multicenter study of 359 cases. Medicine 1990; 69:307–316
5. Mandell LA, Wunderink RG, Anzueto A, et al. Infectious Diseases Society of America/American

Thoracic Society consensus guidelines on the management of community-acquired pneumonia in adults. Clin Infect Dis 2007; 44:S27–S72

6. Feikin D, Schuchat A, Kolczak M, et al. Mortality from invasive pneumococcal pneumonia in the era of antibiotic resistance, 1995–1997. Am J Public Health 2000; 90:223–229
7. Yu VL, Chiou CC, Feldman C, et al. An international prospective study of pneumococcal bacteremia: correlation with *in vitro* resistance, antibiotics administered, and clinical outcome. Clin Infect Dis 2003; 37:230–237
8. Vanderkooi OG, Low DE, Green K, et al. Predicting antimicrobial resistance in invasive pneumococcal infections. Clin Infect Dis 2005; 40:1288–1297
9. Davidson R, Cavalcanti R, Brunton JL, et al. Resistance to levofloxacin and failure of treatment of pneumococcal pneumonia. N Engl J Med 2002; 346:747–750
10. Daneman N, McGeerA, Green K, et al. Macrolide resistance in bacteremic pneumococcal disease: implications for patient management. Clin Infect Dis 2006; 43:432–438
11. Marston BJ, Plouffe JF, File TF Jr., et al. Incidence of community-acquired pneumonia requiring hospitalization: results of a population-based active surveillance study in Ohio. The Community-Based Pneumonia Incidence Study Group. Arch Intern Med 1997; 157:1709–1718
12. Mills GD, Oehley MR, Arrol B. Effectiveness of β-lactam antibiotics compared with antibiotics active against atypical pathogens in non-severe community acquired pneumonia: meta-analysis. BMJ 2005; 330:456–460
13. Martinez JA, Horcajada JP, Almeld M, et al. Addition of a macrolide to a [beta]-lactam-based empirical antibiotic regimen is associated with lower in-hospital mortality for patients with bacteremic pneumococcal pneumonia. Clin Infect Dis 2003; 36:396–398
14. Gleason PP, Meehan TP, Fine JM, et al. Associations between initial antimicrobial therapy and medical outcomes for hospitalized elderly patients with pneumonia. Arch Intern Med 1999; 159:562–572
15. Ruiz M, Ewig S, Marcos M, et al. Etiology of community-acquired pneumonia: impact of age, comorbidity, and severity. Am J Respir Crit Care Med 1999; 160:397–405
16. Arancibia F, Bauer TT, Ewig S, et al. Community-acquired pneumonia due to Gram-negative bacteria and *Pseudomonas aeruginosa:* incidence, risk and prognosis. Arch Intern Med 2002; 162:1849–1858
17. Metersky ML, Ma A, Bratzler DW, et al. Predicting bacteremia in patients with community-acquired pneumonia. Am J Respir Crit Care Med 2004; 169:342–347
18. Fine MJ, Auble TE, Yealy DM, et al. A prediction rule to identify low-risk patients with community-acquired pneumonia. N Engl J Med 1997; 336:243–250
19. Lim WS, van der Eerden MM, Laing R, et al. Defining community acquired pneumonia severity on presentation to hospital: an international derivation and validation study. Thorax 2003; 58:377–382
20. Ewig S, Ruiz M, Mensa J, et al. Severe community-acquired pneumonia: assessment of severity criteria. Am J Respir Crit Care Med 1998; 158:1102–1108
21. Ewig S, de Roux A, Bauer T, et al. Validation of predictive rules and indices of severity for community acquired pneumonia. Thorax 2004; 59:421–427
22. Houck PM, Bratzler DW, Nsa W, et al. Timing of antibiotic administration and outcomes for Medicare patients hospitalized with community-acquired pneumonia. Arch Intern Med 2004; 164:637–644
23. Waterer GW, Somes GW, Wonderink RG. Monotherapy may be suboptimal for severe bacteremic pneumococcal pneumonia. Arch Intern Med 2001; 161:1837–1842
24. Baddour LM, Yu VL, Klugman KP, et al. Combination antibiotic therapy lowers mortality among severely ill patients with pneumococcal pneumonia. Am J Respir Crit Care Med 2004; 170:440–444
25. Rhew DC, Tu GS, Ofman J, et al. Early switch and early discharge strategies in patients with community-acquired pneumonia: a meta-analysis. Arch Intern Med 2001; 161:722–727
26. Fine MJ, Stone RA, Lave JR, et al. Implementation of an evidence-based guideline to reduce duration of intravenous antibiotic therapy and length of stay for patients hospitalized with community-acquired pneumonia: a randomized controlled trial. Am J Med 2003; 115:343–351
27. Meehan TP, Fine MJ, Krumholz HM, et al. Quality of care, process, and outcomes in elderly patients with pneumonia. JAMA 1997; 278:2080–2084
28. Battleman DS, Callahan M, Thaler HT. Rapid antibiotic delivery and appropriate antibiotic selection reduce length of hospital stay of patients with community-acquired pneumonia. Arch Intern Med 2002; 162:682–688

29. Marrie TJ, Lau CY, Wheeler SL, et al. A controlled trial of a critical pathway for treatment of community-acquired pneumonia. JAMA 2000; 283:749–755
30. Rhew DC, Goetz MB, Shekelle PG. Evaluating quality indicators for patients with community-acquired pneumonia. Jt Comm J Qual Improv 2001; 27:575–590
31. Waterer GW, Kessler LA, Wunderink RG. Medium term survival after hospitalization with community-acquired pneumonia. Am J Respir Crit Care Med 2004; 169:910–914
32. Menendez R, Torres A, Zalacain R, et al. Risk factors of treatment failure in community acquired pneumonia: implications for disease outcome. Thorax 2004; 59:960–965
33. Vandenesch F, Naimi T, Enright MC, et al. Community-acquired methicillin-resistant *Staphylococcus aureus* carrying Panton-Valentine leukocidin genes: worldwide emergence. Emerg Infect Dis 2003; 9:978–984
34. The Writing Committee of the World Health Organization (WHO). Consultation on human influenza A/H5: avian influenza A (H5N1) infection in humans. N Engl J Med 2005; 353:1374–1385
35. Maimon N, Nopmaneejumruslers C, Marras TK. Antibacterial class is not obviously important in outpatient pneumonia: a meta-analysis. Eur Respir J 2008; 31:1068–1076
36. Restrepo MI, Mortensen EM, Waterer GW, et al. Impact of macrolide therapy on mortality for patients with severe sepsis due to pneumonia. Eur Respir J 2009; 33:153–159
37. Paul M, Nielsen AD, Gafter-Gvili A, et al. The need for macrolides in hospitalised community-acquired pneumonia: propensity analysis. Eur Respir J 2007; 30:525–531
38. Metersky ML, Ma A, Houck PM, Bratzler DW. Antibiotics for bacteremic pneumonia. Chest 2007; 131:466–473
39. Arnold FW, Summersgill JT, LaJoie AS, et al. A worldwide perspective of atypical pathogens in community-acquired pneumonia. Am J Respir Crit Care Med 2007; 175:1086–1093
40. Garcia-Vidal C, Fernández-Sabé N, Carratalà J, et al. Early mortality in patients with community-acquired pneumonia: causes and risk factors. Eur Respir J 2008; 32:733–739
41. Bruns AHW, Oosterheert JJ, Hak E, et al. Usefulness of consecutive C-reactive protein measurements in follow-up of severe community-acquired pneumonia. Eur Respir J 2008; 32:726–732
42. Mortensen EM, Pugh PJ, Copeland LA, et al. Impact of statins and angiotensin-converting enzyme inhibitors on mortality of subjects hospitalised with pneumonia. Eur Respir J 2008; 31:611–617
43. Chalmers JD, Singanayagam A, Murray MP, et al. Prior statin use is associated with improved outcomes in community-acquired pneumonia. Am J Med 2008; 121:1002–1007
44. Bordón J, Peyrani P, Brock GN, et al. The presence of pneumococcal bacteremia does not influence clinical outcomes in patients with community-acquired pneumonia. Chest 2008; 133:618–624
45. Johnstone J, Majumdar SR, Fox JD, et al. Viral infection in adults hospitalized with community-acquired pneumonia. Chest 2008; 134:1141–1148
46. Lisboa T, Blot S, Waterer GW, et al. Radiologic progression of pulmonary infiltrates predicts a worse prognosis in severe community-acquired pneumonia than bacteremia. Chest 2009; 135:165–172
47. Aliberti S, Amir A, Peyrani P, et al. Incidence, etiology, timing, and risk factors for clinical failure in hospitalized patients with community-acquired pneumonia. Chest 2008; 134:955–962
48. Eurich DT, Marrie TJ, Johnstone J, et al. Mortality reduction with influenza vaccine in patients with pneumonia outside "flu" season: pleiotropic benefits or residual confounding? Am J Respir Crit Care Med 2008; 178:527–533
49. Capelastegui A, España PP, Quintana JM, et al. Development of a prognostic index for 90-day mortality among patients discharged after hospitalization for community-acquired pneumonia. Thorax 2009; 64:496–501
50. Alfageme I, Vazquez R, Reyes N, et al. Clinical efficacy of anti-pneumococcal vaccination in patients with COPD. Thorax 2006; 61:189–195
51. Fisman DN, Abrutyn E, Spaude KA, et al. Prior pneumococcal vaccination is associated with reduced death, complications, and length of stay among hospitalized adults with community-acquired pneumonia. Clin Infect Dis 2006; 42:1093–1101
52. Li JZ, Winston LG, Moore DH, Bent S. Efficacy of short-course antibiotic regimens for community-acquired pneumonia: a meta-analysis. Am J Med 2007; 120:783–790

Pneumoconiosis

David W. Kamp, MD, FCCP

Objectives:

- Review the epidemiology, pathophysiology, and clinical manifestations of silicosis and coal worker's pneumoconiosis
- Understand the pulmonary manifestations of asbestos-induced diseases of the lung (asbestosis and rounded atelectasis) and of the pleura (effusions and plaques)
- Discuss the malignancies associated with asbestos exposure (bronchogenic carcinoma and mesothelioma)
- Briefly review a variety of other pneumoconioses (talcosis, berylliosis, and hard metal lung disease)

Key words: asbestos; coal; lung cancer; mesothelioma; pulmonary fibrosis; silica

---

Pneumoconiosis is a 19th century Greek term (*pneumo*, meaning "breath"; *konis*, meaning "dust") that describes lung diseases associated with mineral dust exposure. The term has evolved to imply the putative dust (*eg*, silicosis/silica, asbestosis/asbestos, berylliosis/beryllium, stannosis/tin) or workers who are at risk (coal workers' pneumoconiosis [CWP], hard metal lung disease). The International Labor Organization (ILO) defines pneumoconiosis as the accumulation of mineral dusts inciting tissue reactions that range from minimal stromal reactions that are reversible to interstitial fibrosis that results in permanent scarring.[1] The term is often further restricted to non-neoplastic pathology excluding asthma, chronic bronchitis, and emphysema, all of which can occur with occupational dust exposure. The patient with pneumoconiosis typically presents with nonspecific respiratory symptoms (*eg*, cough and dyspnea) and an abnormal chest radiograph finding. A careful occupational history to ascertain the cause of a particular patient's complaints (*ie*, whether acute or chronic, malignant or nonmalignant) is absolutely essential. This history is especially important, given the large number of workers exposed and the significant rate of morbidity and mortality associated with mineral dust exposure.

Silicosis

Definition

Silicosis is a chronic lung disease that is caused by the inhalation of crystalline silica (usually quartz and, less commonly, cristobalite, tridymite, coesite, and stishovite) and is characterized by progressive parenchymal nodules and pulmonary fibrosis. Silica or silicon dioxide is the most abundant mineral in the crust of the earth and is used in a wide range of industrial products. Amorphous or noncrystalline silica particulates (*eg*, diatomite and vitreous silica) are relatively less fibrogenic, but when they are combined with metal complexes to form silicates, as occurs with asbestos, mica, or talc, they induce unique forms of pulmonary toxicity, each of which will be reviewed separately.

Silica-associated lung disease is among the earliest lung diseases described and has been the most intensively studied occupational lung disease. In 1556, Agricola described the pulmonary effects of inhaled dusts from mining and the production of metals; van Dumerbroek in 1672 noted similar problems in stone cutters.[2]

Epidemiology

Silicosis is the most prevalent chronic occupational disease worldwide. The risk of silicosis is directly proportional to the particle concentration, the duration of exposure, and the silica content of different rock types, which ranges from nearly 100% (sandstone and flint) to $<10\%$ (shale). In 2006, the National Institute for Occupational Safety and Health (NIOSH) estimated that each year >1 million US workers are at risk for the development of silicosis and that >200 workers die from silicosis, with hundreds more becoming disabled.[3] The dust control measures and workplace permissible exposure limits (PELs) that have been established by most industrial countries have significantly decreased the number of deaths caused by silicosis. However, the number of silicosis-associated deaths among persons 15 to 44 years of age has not decreased significantly in the United States.[4,5] Further, 30 to 50% of the workplaces inspected between 1979 and 1982 had at least one air sample containing a concentration of >100 μg/m³, which is greater than the Occupational Safety and Health Administration (OSHA) PEL for an 8-h work exposure.

Industries/Occupations at Risk

Some of the major industries in which workers are at high risk for silica exposure are listed in Table 1, along with some examples of hazardous occupations. These examples include industries that involve work in mines, in quarries, with stone work, and in foundries; in the use of abrasives; and in ceramic production. Another high-risk group includes persons working in road maintenance that involves "cut and repair," where potentially increased levels of silica exposure occur during the cutting, breaking up, and removal of concrete. A careful occupational history for silica exposure is essential for any patient presenting with pulmonary nodules, masses, or interstitial lung disease. This history is particularly important given the long latency between toxic exposure and appearance of the disease, the large number of workers exposed in past years before stringent work safety measures were invoked in the 1970s, and the fact that silicosis, like most pneumoconioses, can progress in the absence of additional exposure.

Pathology

There are three distinct forms of silicosis, as follows: chronic (the most common), acute, and accelerated. The chronic form is characterized by silicotic nodules that typically are located in the peribronchial regions with interstitial extension, <1 cm in diameter, well-formed, spherical, hard, and light gray (Fig 1, *A*). This is in contrast to the heavily black-pigmented, stellate nodules that are associated with coal exposure (Fig. 1, *B*). The silicotic nodule has three components, as follows: (1) a central area of dense, acellular, hyalinized collagen-containing silica particles that are visible with polarized light; (2) a mid-zone of concentrically layered collagen; and (3) a peripheral thick capsule consisting of dust-laden macrophages and lymphocytes mixed with collagen. Silicotic nodules, which can develop decades after exposure,

Table 1. *Some High-Risk Industries and Occupations Associated With Silica Exposure**

Industries (Examples)	Occupations
Mining, tunneling, and excavating	
Underground: gold, copper, iron, tin	Miner, driller, tunneler
Surface: coal, iron, foundation excavation	Drill operator
Quarrying	
Granite, slate, sandstone	Digger, driller, hammerer
Stonework	
Granite sheds, monument masonry	Cutter, dresser, polisher, grinder
Foundries	
Iron and noniron metals	Molder, caster, knockout man
Abrasives	
Production: metal polish, paint fillers	Crusher, mixer, abrasive work
Sandblasting, oil rigs, tombstones	
Ceramics	
Pottery, stoneware, oven bricks	Oven-brick maker
Others (glass making, boiler scaling, gemstone worker, dental technician)	

*Modified from Becklake and Cowie .[1]

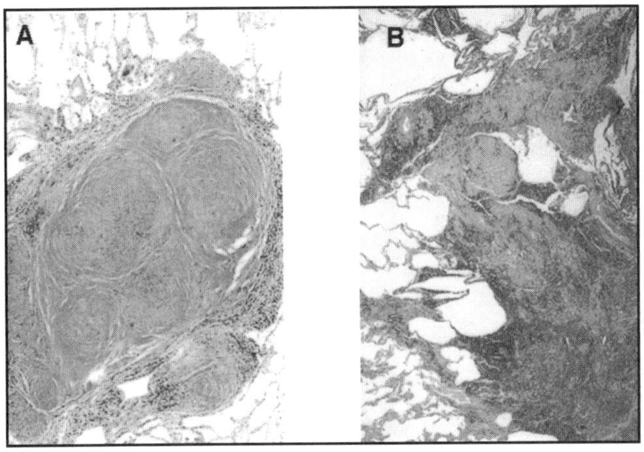

Figure 1. *A*, silicotic nodule. *B*, coal macule.

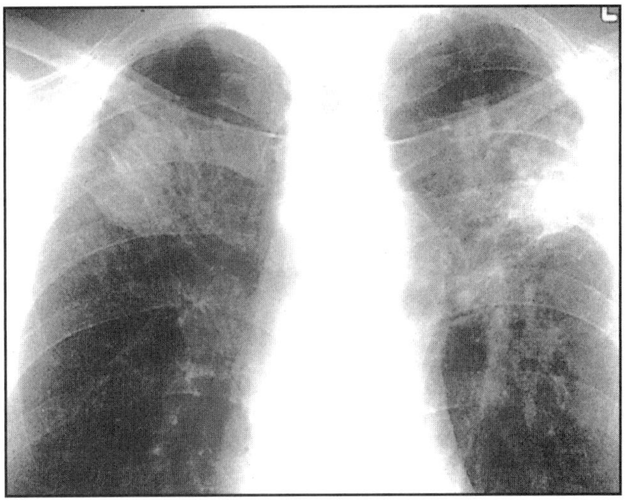

Figure 3. Progressive massive pulmonary fibrosis due to silica exposure.

typically are scattered throughout the upper lung zones, sparing the majority of the lung parenchyma and thereby causing minimal symptoms (Fig 2).

Simple silicosis, which is the earliest stage of chronic silicosis, can become complex silicosis as the nodules expand, affecting the bronchioles and vasculature and eventually coalescing into large masses (progressive pulmonary fibrosis [PMF]) that can undergo necrosis (Fig 3). However, the presence of central cavitation should raise concern about tuberculosis (TB). The adjacent lung may show signs of retraction and emphysema. If silica is mixed with other dusts (*eg*, coal, mica, and kaolin), then the nodules become less distinct and more stellate in appearance. Silicotic nodules may also form in the hilar and mediastinal lymph nodes, which can become calcified (so-called *egg-shell calcification*, as shown in Fig 4) and may impinge on the airways (broncholith). Silicotic nodules can form outside the lungs (*eg*, liver, spleen, bone marrow, and kidney). In the kidney, silicon nephropathy can have a variable presentation from mild renal insufficiency to rapidly progressive renal failure associated with necrotizing vasculitis.

Acute silicosis is characterized by diffuse fluid-filled alveolar spaces that consist of eosinophilic, proteinaceous, and surfactant-containing material. The interstitial space typically shows extensive alveolar epithelial cell damage with hypertrophic alveolar type II cells as well as small focal nodules and fibrosis.

Pathogenic Mechanisms

The risk for silicosis depends on the level of particle exposure (dose and duration) as well as the content and type of silica inhaled.[6] The precise relationship between specific silica subtypes and the development of pulmonary fibrosis is unclear, but quartz, cristobalite, and tridymite are more fibrogenic than amorphous silica. Silica particles

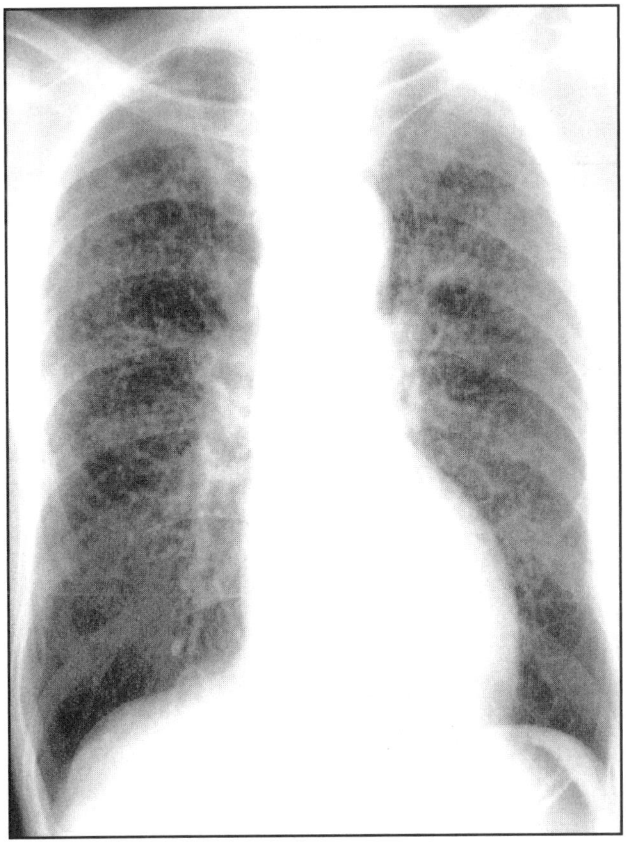

Figure 2. Simple silicosis.

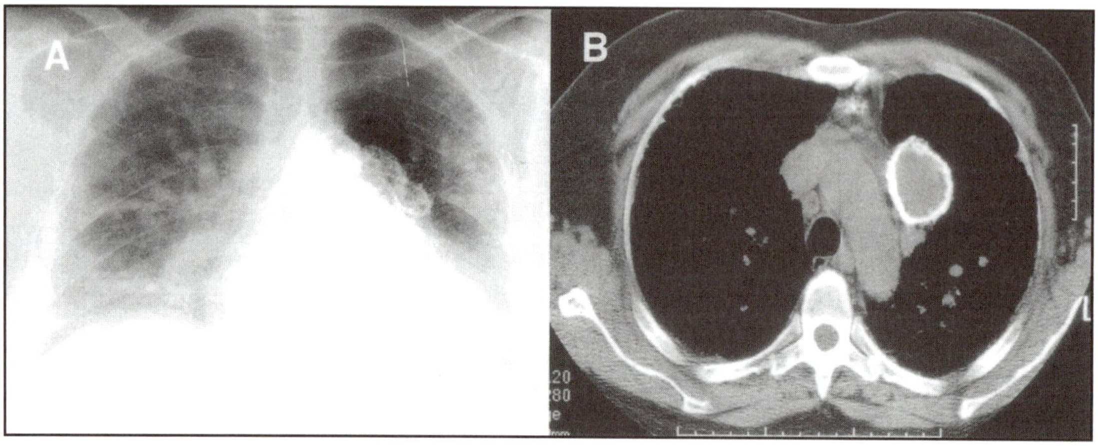

Figure 4. *A*, chest radiograph from a patient with silicosis showing left hilar adenopathy with egg-shell calcification. *B*, chest CT scan demonstrating egg-shell calcification.

that are <5 μm in size can make their way to the distal alveoli, where they are ingested by alveolar macrophages (AMs), which are the first line of alveolar defense. Silica-activated AMs subsequently release reactive oxygen species (ROS), reactive nitrogen species, fibronectin, and various cytokines and growth factors. In particular, silica and other particulates activate the expression of transforming growth factor-β, resulting in excess extracellular matrix deposition. Silica also can directly injure alveolar type I cells, which leads to the formation of hyperplastic type II cells. If extensive alveolar damage occurs, as seen with intense exposure to high levels of silica, surfactant production and processing are altered, resulting in acute silicosis. PMF, which can occur with both silica and coal exposure, may ensue over time but may also occur in association with a mycobacterial infection.

Figure 5 depicts some of the key pathogenic events leading to silicosis and highlights the overlapping molecular pathways that are activated by

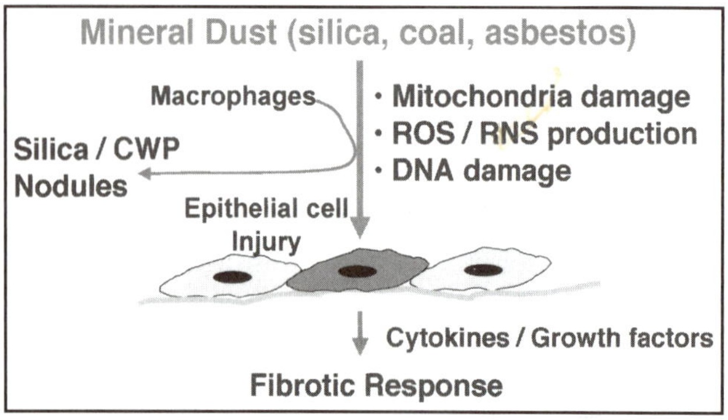

Figure 5. A simplified hypothetical model underlying mineral dust-induced pulmonary toxicity.

other mineral dusts such as coal and asbestos. The precise mechanisms underlying the distinct clinical manifestations of each mineral dust are unknown but likely relate in part to the differences in the deposition patterns of the various dusts into the distal airways, the chemical composition of each particulate, and the genetic background of the worker in whom the host response is regulated. A recent case–control study involving 183 silicosis patients and 111 silica-exposed miners in China identified several interesting genetic polymorphisms that will need to be verified by a larger cohort.[7]

Clinical Features

Patients with silica-induced lung disease can present with chronic, accelerated, or acute onset of disease, depending on the intensity and duration of the silica exposure. Chronic silicosis, the most common form, typically occurs after low-dose silica exposure for >20 years. The prevalence estimates of silicosis in exposed workers varies from 0.4 to 11% after 20 years of exposure to the OSHA PEL of 100 $\mu g/m^3$ to 1.2 to 53% after a cumulative exposure of 4 mg/m^3.[8] A study of US foundry workers[9] showed a 12% prevalence of chest radiograph changes after 30 years and that black patients were twice as likely to have abnormalities as white patients. Most patients with chronic simple silicosis are relatively asymptomatic, and the diagnosis of disease is established based on the occupational exposure history and characteristic chest radiograph findings. A lung biopsy generally is reserved for patients with atypical occupational exposure or chest radiograph findings. Silicotic nodules are generally small (1 to 3 mm), symmetrical, upper lobe—predominant lesions that favor the posterior aspects of the lungs but can involve other lung zones. Calcification is evident in 10 to 20% of the pulmonary nodules.

Complicated silicosis consists of conglomerated nodules that can eventually form mass-like PMF lesions. The PMF lesions, unlike those in bronchogenic carcinoma, typically are symmetrical in location and may have an "angel wing" appearance. Eggshell calcification (Fig 4) is infrequent; if present, it strongly suggests a silicosis diagnosis but is not pathognomonic. Over time, the mass lesions tend to contract, especially in the upper lobes, resulting in a rim of emphysema surrounding the mass. Although central necrosis similar to TB may develop in the mass, active TB should be suspected whenever a lesion changes in size or cavitates. As the disease progresses, patients may note exertional dyspnea, cough, and sputum production. Inspiratory crackles and digital clubbing are unusual and suggest an alternative cause such as another interstitial lung disease, bronchogenic carcinoma, or infection. In a study[10] of 243 patients with silicosis/mixed-dust pneumoconiosis and 62 patients with idiopathic pulmonary fibrosis (IPF), the prevalence of chronic interstitial fibrosis, as defined by chest CT scan, was 12% in the silicosis/mixed-dust exposure group, of which 75% of the lesions were IPF-like. Cor pulmonale and cyanosis can occur in the advanced phase of silicosis.

Patients with accelerated and acute forms of silicosis typically present within months to a few years after intense silica exposure rather than decades. Dyspnea occurs after 5 to 15 years of high levels of occupational exposure to material with moderate levels of quartz-containing silica. These patients often progress to respiratory failure and death. Patients with acute silicosis generally present within several months to years after intense exposure to high levels of silica (*eg*, from sandblasting, surface drilling, tunneling, silica flour milling, and ceramic production), often with little or no respiratory protection. The chest radiograph is characterized by a diffuse alveolar pattern similar to that found in patients with alveolar proteinosis. In these patients, dyspnea, cough, and weight loss appear, which rapidly progress to respiratory failure and death.

Pulmonary function tests (PFTs) correlate poorly with the presence of nodules as assessed by chest CT scan. Patients with early silicosis may show normal volumes, air flows, and diffusing capacity of the lung for carbon monoxide (DLCO). As the disease progresses or the level of silica exposure increases, a progressive restrictive pattern with a reduced DLCO typically is found in these patients.[11,12] Occasionally, an obstructive or mixed pattern may be evident. In patients with simple silicosis, the chest radiographic abnormalities are typically more impressive than the PFT changes. However, when compared with patients with simple silicosis, patients with conglomerate, accelerated, or acute silicosis invariably demonstrate significant and progressive restrictive physiology and reduced DLCO.

Complications

TB can occur at any stage of silicosis, but generally the rate increases as silicosis progresses. Pulmonary TB must always be considered in patients with PMF, a group with a significantly increased risk of morbidity and mortality. There is a threefold greater risk of pulmonary TB in patients with chronic silicosis than in healthy individuals.[13] Silica exposure alone in the absence of silicosis is also a risk factor for pulmonary TB, and the increased risk persists after exposure to silica has stopped.[14] Current smokers have a dose-dependent increased risk of developing TB compared with other silicotic patients after correcting for confounders.[15] Because silica impairs AM function, the risk for various mycobacterial infections such as *Mycobacterium tuberculosis, Mycobacterium kansasii,* and *Mycobacterium avium-intracellulare* is increased.

A clinical suspicion of pulmonary TB may be thwarted by relatively nonspecific complaints such as fever, weight loss, hemoptysis, malaise, or increased dyspnea, all of which can be found in patients with PMF or a variety of other infections. Because of impaired host defense mechanisms and decreased drug penetration into silicotic nodules, antituberculous therapy should be extended for at least 2 months beyond the typical 6-month course for patients who demonstrate no cavities on the chest radiograph and who have a smear result that is negative for acid-fast bacilli.[13] For patients with silicosis who present with active pulmonary TB with cavities and have smears positive for acid-fast bacilli, the recommended treatment duration is for 11 months rather than 9 months. TB prophylaxis should be continued for 12 months with isoniazid alone or for 4 months if a four-drug regimen consisting of isoniazid, rifampin, ethambutol, and pyrazinamide is used. Close posttreatment follow-up of patients with silica-mycobacterial infections is necessary because of the high rate of relapse.[13]

The risk for lung cancer in workers who have been exposed to silica but do not have disease is controversial. In 1997, the International Agency for Research on Cancer reviewed the available experimental and human epidemiologic data and concluded that there was sufficient evidence implicating silica in the form of quartz or cristobalite as a group I carcinogen (*ie*, carcinogenic in humans).[8,16] At least 20 studies have suggested that men with silicosis have a twofold to fourfold increased risk of dying of lung cancer. However, the risk from confounding variables (*eg*, smoking and exposures to other dust, such as asbestos) in some of these studies[12,17] is unclear. It is also uncertain whether the lung cancer risk is restricted to workers with silicosis because pulmonary fibrosis *per se* is a well-known risk factor for lung cancer. Some studies[18,19] have noted a dose–response relationship between lung cancer mortality rate and cumulative silica exposure among workers without silicosis. In contrast, a 2006 analysis[20] of 28 cohort, 15 case–control, and 2 proportionate mortality ratio studies concluded that the carcinogenic role of silica alone in the absence of silicosis remains unclear.

Crystalline silica exposure has also been causally attributed to a variety of other diseases, such as various collagen vascular diseases (*eg*, rheumatoid arthritis, scleroderma, vasculitis, and systemic lupus erythematosus); sarcoidosis; glomerulonephritis; and hepatosplenic silicosis.[12,16] However, these associations are relatively rare and have not been well established.

Management

There is no established treatment that can prevent or reduce the pulmonary toxicity associated with silica exposure. Because pulmonary fibrosis is irreversible in workers with chronic silicosis and is directly related to the level of silica exposure, any additional silica exposure must be avoided. NIOSH recommends an exposure limit of 50 μg/m³, whereas OSHA recommends a PEL of 100 μg/m³ despite the fact that these levels have been associated with the development of silicosis.[8,9,12] There are several NIOSH-approved air-purifying respirators with replaceable N95 filters that have been recommended for silica-exposed workers. For the workers who have the greatest risk and who are involved with abrasive blasting, the only approved respirator is the type CE abrasive blasting respirator that completely covers the head and operates in a positive-pressure mode. Table 2 lists the recommended chest radiograph surveillance guidelines from various groups for silica-exposed workers.[21] Treatment may be indicated to prevent silica-associated complications, as described previously, as well as assistance with pulmonary disability that may ensue in the advanced phases of silicosis. Lung transplantation has been performed in a small number of patients with advanced silicosis, but it has a limited role in the management of silicosis, given the late age of onset of severe pulmonary disability.

Coal Workers' Pneumoconiosis

Definition

CWP, also known as *black lung*, is a distinct pathologic entity that results from chronic exposure to coal dust, graphite, and other forms of carbon. Some of the mineral and elemental contaminants commonly found within coal include pyrite; kaolinite; ankerite; quartz; titanium dioxide; calcite; and trace metals, such as cadmium, copper, nickel, iron, lead, and zinc. CWP is distinguished from silicosis partly by the unique pathologic changes and the fact that carbon tends to be less fibrogenic than quartz. However, mixed-dust exposures are well documented. The Mine Safety and Health Administration respirable coal dust PEL is 2 mg/m³, whereas NIOSH has set a standard of 1 mg/m³.[16] Coal is ranked into four types based on the carbon content, geologic age, and presence of contaminating minerals and oxygen. The four types of coal are lignite, subbituminous,

Table 2. *Pneumoconiosis Chest Radiograph Surveillance Guidelines**

Particulate	Frequency[†]
Silica	
• OSHA	Preplacement; every 5 years if <20 years of exposure; every 2 years if >20 years of exposure; at employment termination
• WHO	Preplacement; then after 2–3 years of silica exposure; then every 2–5 years of silica exposure and thereafter
• ACOEM	Preplacement; every 3 years if <10 years of exposure; every 2 years if >10 years of exposure; at employment termination
Asbestos	
• OSHA	Preplacement; every 5 years if <10 years of exposure; every 5 years if >10 years of exposure up to age 35 then every 2 years up to age 45; then annually thereafter or at employment termination if ≥0.1 fiber/cm³ exposure
• WHO	Preplacement; every 3–5 years if <10 years of exposure; every 1–2 years if >10 years of exposure; annually if >20 years of exposure

[*]Adapted from Schwerha JJ. Occupational Medicine Forum. J Occup Environ Med 2008; 50:101–104.
[†]Frequency of recommended chest radiographs by either the Occupational Safety and Health Administration (OSHA), World Health Organization (WHO) or American College of Occupational and Environmental Medicine (ACOEM); may be increased at the discretion of the managing physician.

bituminous, and anthracite. Bituminous coal accounts for nearly 43% of the US coal reserves; it is contaminated with low levels of silica and, in the Pittsburgh area, surface-active iron (0.119 mg/100 mg), which may account for its greater pathogenicity.[22]

Epidemiology

Underground miners, compared with surface or strip miners, have the greatest risk for the development of CWP. In the 1950s and 1960s, there was an increase in mortality rate among coal miners in part because of CWP.[1,2,16] The extensive dust-control measures invoked in the 1960s through the 1970s in the United States and in other industrialized countries resulted in a substantial reduction in the prevalence and mortality rate of CWP. It is estimated that >100,000 workers currently are employed in the coal-mining industry in the United States and that the estimated prevalence of CWP, defined as an ILO chest radiograph abnormality of 1/0 or greater, varies from 3 to 14%, depending on the mining region, with the highest prevalence occurring in workers with >30 years of mining work.[2,16] Fortunately, complicated CWP or PMF develops in <0.5% of workers with CWP.[2] The risk for PMF is directly proportional to the radiographic profusion score and the levels of quartz in the coal being mined.

Pathology

The initial lung tissue reaction to coal dust is the formation of a coal macule and, when combined with surrounding focal emphysema, defines simple CWP. Coal macules are typically up to 4 mm in size and tend to form at the junctions of respiratory bronchioles in the upper lungs (Fig 1, *B*). The macule, consisting of coal dust–laden macrophages and fibroblasts, enlarge, loosen the connections of the alveolar walls to the bronchioles, and thereby cause focal areas of emphysema. Unlike the concentric collagen arrangement in silicotic nodules, the nodules associated with CWP have haphazardly arranged collagen bundles filled with dark-staining anthracotic pigment and lack the birefringent particles found in silicosis tissue, which can be seen with polarized light. However, coal-induced macules are similar to silicosis in that they can enlarge and coalesce, resulting in masses that encroach on the alveolar ducts and alveoli. In patients with either CWP or silicosis, when these masses are >1 cm radiographically, the PMF label can be used.

Pathogenesis

CWP and silicosis are both closely related yet distinct. The severity of CWP is closely associated with the levels of coal dust rather than quartz.

The prevalence of CWP is greater in anthracite coal miners than in bituminous coal miners in part because of the greater levels of crystalline silica and in part because of the greater levels of carbon-centered free radicals. Coal mine dust fractured by grinding contains more free radicals than unfractured dust and is a better predictor of the toxic potential of the dust.[22] As outlined in Figure 5, many of the patho-physiologic events implicated in mediating CWP are similar to those involved with silica. Although coal and carbon are not toxic to AMs, the combination of coal and quartz is. Coal dust is generally less fibrogenic than silica and tends to blunt the effects of quartz.[23] In a study[24] of 253 coal miners, genetic polymorphisms for genes encoding for tumor necrosis factor-α and lymphotoxin-α were associated with an increased risk for CWP. A role for interleukin (IL)-18, a lymphokine that regulates neutrophil activation and the production of proinflammatory cytokines and ROS, in decreasing coal-induced fibrotic lung disease was suggested in a longitudinal study of 200 miners.[25] These findings suggest that interactions between environmental dusts and certain genes are critically involved in determining disease expression in patients with CWP, which is similar to the situation with other pneumoconioses.

Clinical Features

In 1831, the first case of CWP was described, in a British coal miner. Although coal was believed to be relatively inert and the pulmonary toxicity largely caused by silica, subsequent studies established CWP as a distinct entity.[16] The clinical manifestations of CWP that are similar to silicosis include simple CWP, complicated CWP, and PMF. However, unlike silica, chronic bronchitis is a more prominent feature, and an accelerated or acute-onset form of the disease does not occur. Simple CWP is the most common and typically occurs after low-dose coal exposure for ≥20 years. Most patients with simple CWP are relatively asymptomatic but can develop cough and sputum production. The diagnosis is based on the occupational exposure history and characteristic chest radiograph findings. Nodules associated with coal exposure are generally small (*ie*, 1 to 3 mm), haphazardly arranged lesions that favor the posterior aspects of the upper lobes but can involve other lung zones. A lung biopsy generally is reserved for patients with an atypical occupational exposure or chest radiograph findings.

The onset of dyspnea on exertion typically is seen in patients with complicated CWP or PMF. A rim of emphysema surrounding the large nodules is a prominent feature in patients with CWP and, at this stage of the disease, PFTs generally reveal a mixed obstructive and restrictive defect. There is a well-described association between CWP and rheumatoid arthritis (Caplan syndrome), so any clinical evidence of rheumatoid arthritis should also be carefully evaluated. Similar to silicotic masses, central necrosis may develop, raising the specter of a complicating mycobacterial infection. The presence of crackles or clubbing is unusual and suggests an alternative cause for the lesion, such as another interstitial lung disease, bronchogenic carcinoma, or infection. Cor pulmonale and cyanosis can occur in the advanced phase of CWP.

As reviewed in detail elsewhere,[26] the radiographic findings of CWP are better detected by high-resolution CT (HRCT) of the chest as compared with chest radiograph. The characteristic HRCT findings include: (1) focal emphysema, (2) punctate opacities, (3) subpleural nodules, (4) PMF, (5) cavitating masses, (6) diffuse interstitial pulmonary fibrosis, and (7) bronchiectasis.

As in silicosis, PFT abnormalities correlate poorly with the presence of nodules as assessed by chest imaging. Patients with early CWP may show normal volumes, flows, and DLCO. As the disease progresses or the levels of coal dust exposure increase, a progressive restrictive pattern with a reduced DLCO or a mixed obstructive/restrictive pattern is often evident resulting from the focal emphysematous changes around the coal macule.[11,12] Expiratory airflow limitation occurs independently of the stage of CWP. Coal dust levels have an inverse relationship with FEV_1. Patients with complicated CWP or PMF caused by coal exposure invariably demonstrate a severe and rapidly progressive combined obstructive and restrictive defect with a reduced DLCO.

Management

As with silicosis, there is no established treatment to prevent or reduce the fibrogenic effects of coal exposure and the complicating mycobacterial infections that occur in both diseases. An unexplained dichotomy is that the risk of lung cancer in coal miners is lower, but in patients with silicosis, the risk is greater than that in the general population when adjusted for age and smoking status.[12] Premature death is limited to patients with complicated CWP or PMF. A 23-year follow-up study[27] of 8,899 coal miners who were initially examined between 1969 and 1971 at 31 US coal mines showed an increase in mortality from nonmalignant respiratory diseases (*eg*, pneumoconiosis and COPD) but not from lung cancer. Management is also centered on the diagnosis and prevention of the coal-associated complications that were described previously as well as assistance with pulmonary disability that may ensue in the advanced phases of CWP.

Asbestos-Related Diseases

Definition

Asbestos is a generic term for a group of naturally occurring hydrated silicate fibers, the tensile strength and resilient structural and chemical properties of which are ideal for a variety of construction and insulation purposes. The word asbestos, which is derived from the Greek word for "inextinguishable" or "unquenchable," was first used in the late 1300s.[28] However, industrial production of asbestos did not occur until the 1850s. All forms of asbestos cause nonmalignant inflammatory pulmonary diseases (*ie*, pleural effusions, pleural plaques, rounded atelectasis, and asbestosis) and malignant pulmonary diseases (*ie*, mesothelioma and broncho-genic carcinoma).[29–31]

Epidemiology

The first cases of asbestos-associated fibrosis were described in the early 1900s, and the term *asbestosis* was coined by Cooke[32] in 1927. Asbestos-associated bronchogenic carcinoma in patients with asbestosis was well-recognized by the mid-1950s; the association with mesothelioma was established by the 1960s. Despite a dramatic decrease in its use since the 1970s, asbestos-induced pulmonary diseases continue to be a significant health concern for multiple reasons. First, >30 million tons of asbestos have been mined, processed, and used in the United States since the early 1900s.[29] Second, an estimated 27 million workers in the United States were exposed to aerosolized asbestos fibers between 1940 and 1979.[33] Third, there is a long interval (called the *latency period*) between fiber exposure and the development of asbestosis or mesothelioma (15 to 40 years), requiring long-term, careful follow up of occupationally exposed workers. Fourth, exposures from consumer products and from fibers released during structural renovation are a source of possible morbidity and mortality for both occupationally exposed workers and the general population.[30,34]

Although the prevalence of asbestosis in the United States has not been established, in 2000 there were an estimated 20,000 hospital discharges listing "asbestosis" and 2,000 deaths in which asbestosis was the primary or contributing cause.[34] Surveys[28] in Europe and the United States have shown a doubling of the prevalence of asbestos-associated pleural disease, including mesothelioma, from the early 1970s until 2000. It is estimated that the total number of asbestos-associated deaths in the United States may exceed 200,000 by the year 2030.[35] Given these facts, it is not surprising that asbestos-related diseases have inundated our legal system, resulting in recent very large class-action lawsuits (68,000 individual claims were made in the year 2000 alone) and the bankruptcy of many old-line industrial companies.[28]

Asbestos is a well-recognized human carcinogen, but whether a threshold level exists that does not increase the risk of malignancy is unknown.[28,30,36] OSHA established a PEL for fibers >5 mm long with a 3:1 aspect ratio assessed by phase-contrast light microscopy of 0.1 fibers per cubic centimeter over an 8-h period for all fiber types. Epidemiologic studies have convincingly shown that all types of fibers increase the malignant risk associated with occupational exposure greater than the OSHA PEL. There is considerable controversy regarding the malignant risks associated with nonoccupational exposure, especially to chrysotile, which accounts for >95% of global asbestos consumption.[28,30,36] Few well-designed epidemiologic studies have directly assessed the risk of malignancy from low-dose asbestos exposure. A large-scale, retrospective population study[37] of 405 hospital-based patients and control subjects concluded that 5 years of exposure to the current OSHA PEL would produce a fourfold excess of pleural mesotheliomas. As reviewed in detail elsewhere,[36] several recent studies have documented more precisely an increased risk from environmental asbestos exposure that appears to be approximately 10 times lower than that observed with occupational asbestos exposure.

Industries/Occupations at Risk

Asbestos exposure arises from the following three principal sources: (1) mining and milling of the fibers; (2) industrial applications of asbestos (*eg*, textiles, cement, friction materials, insulation, shipbuilding, repairing brake linings, lagging, or pipe cutting); and (3) nonoccupational exposure to airborne asbestos. The development of asbestosis is directly associated with both the magnitude and duration of the asbestos exposure.[6,29,33] Although a single well-documented case[38] of asbestosis caused by brief inhalational exposure has been described, the overwhelming majority of patients have had significant occupational asbestos exposure over a prolonged period. Airborne asbestos levels in public buildings are generally several orders of magnitude below the current OSHA standard, but greater levels occur during renovation and demolition. Although asbestos-induced lung cancer and mesothelioma were well-recognized in the United States by the early 1960s, industrial production continued until 1973 when it reached a peak of 803,000 metric tons.[28] By 1998, it had decreased to 16,000 metric tons.

Pathophysiology

The toxic effects of asbestos depend on the cumulative dose and the time since the initial exposure. Essentially, all adverse effects of asbestos arise from inhalation. There are two classes of asbestos fibers: serpentine and amphibole fibers. Serpentine fibers (*eg*, chrysotile) are curly-stranded, curved structures, whereas amphiboles (*eg*, crocidolite, amosite, and tremolite) are straight, rod-like fibers.

The physical properties of the different asbestos fibers have been implicated in the pathogenesis of asbestos-induced diseases for many years. Amphibole fibers may be more toxic than the serpentine chrysotile, but this area is one of considerable controversy because tremolite, which is an amphibole, is a frequent contaminant that has been implicated as a contributor to the toxicity of chrysotile. Compared with chrysotile, amphibole fibers accumulate more readily in the distal lung parenchyma, are not cleared as effectively, and are more durable (their estimated half-life in the lungs is on the order of months vs decades, respectively).[6,30] Chrysotile-induced asbestosis typically requires a threefold greater lung fiber concentration compared with amphiboles, but chrysotile injures lung parenchymal and pleural cells and can induce asbestosis, lung cancer, and mesothelioma in humans.[6,31]

Although fiber length has been shown to be important in the fibrogenic and malignant capacity of asbestos in animal and *in vitro* models, the results of human studies have been less impressive.[6,30] The discrepancies between animal and human data are in part attributed to the confounding effects of cigarette smoke, which reduces lung fiber clearance.[6] Asbestos-induced lung cancer has been attributed to the "amphibole hypothesis" that fiber structural characteristics (*ie*, length, diameter, and aspect ratio) are the basis for lung malignancies.[6,30] This concept has been questioned because fiber physical properties alone appear to be insufficient to account for asbestos pulmonary toxicity, but they may partly contribute to lung injury.

Extensive investigations conducted during the last 20 years have convincingly shown that ROS and reactive nitrogen species are important second messengers of toxicity caused by asbestos.[6,30,36,39] The mechanisms underlying free radical generation by asbestos are in part caused by reactions occurring at surface sites on the mineral dusts, by mitochondrial dysfunction, and by the activation of AMs or neutrophils attempting to take up the fibers. Once inside macrophages, asbestos fibers maybe coated with iron that is derived from hemosiderin and can be redox-activated. These coated fibers, called *ferruginous bodies*, can be seen with various types of fibers, including asbestos, and as such are also known as *asbestos bodies*. Asbestos fibers cause pulmonary toxicity in a manner similar to silica and coal via many of the same pathogenic pathways as shown in Figure 5. By mechanisms that remain uncertain, asbestos-induced mitochondrial ROS signaling in lung epithelial cells stabilizes p53 and promotes p53-dependent transcription of various proteins involved in tumor suppression, cell cycle arrest, apoptosis, and cell survival.[36]

Benign Asbestos Pleural Effusions

The latent period between asbestos exposure and the development of a benign asbestos pleural effusion varies from <1 year (shortest latency of all the asbestos-related diseases) to >40 years. The clinical presentation ranges from being asymptomatic with total resolution or a blunted costophrenic angle to pleuritic chest pain associated with fever, dyspnea, and bloody pleural fluid. The pleural fluid is usually unilateral, left-sided, and exudative yet rarely contains ferruginous bodies. The erythrocyte sedimentation rate often is elevated. A diagnosis can be made only after the appropriate exposure history, the exclusion of all other causes (especially malignancy), and close follow-up for 2 to 3 years. Although this has not been firmly established, benign asbestos pleural effusion has no clear prognostic implications for the development of pleural plaques or malignancy.[28]

Pleural Plaques

Pleural plaques occur in 20 to 60% of occupationally exposed workers [40,41] and in 2 to 6% of nonoccupationally exposed individuals.[42] The most common lesions are circumscribed or localized pleural plaques, which are discrete areas of fibrosis on the parietal pleura. Plaques serve as a marker of asbestos exposure and little else. They consist of dense collagenous material that develops in the mid-lower ribs and on the diaphragm (Fig 6). Electron microscopic studies may reveal noncoated fibers and, rarely, ferruginous bodies. Over time, typically >30 years, these lesions calcify. The frequency with which plaques occur varies widely based on the sex (male > female), age (up to 50% of shipyard workers older than the age of 70 years), and the number of years of occupational and nonoccupational exposure.[28] The clinical consequences of circumscribed plaques are minimal. In most patients, plaques are an incidental finding on a routine chest radiograph. PFT results are invariably normal unless they are confounded by another process. Conventional chest CT scans combined with selective high-resolution cuts are often useful

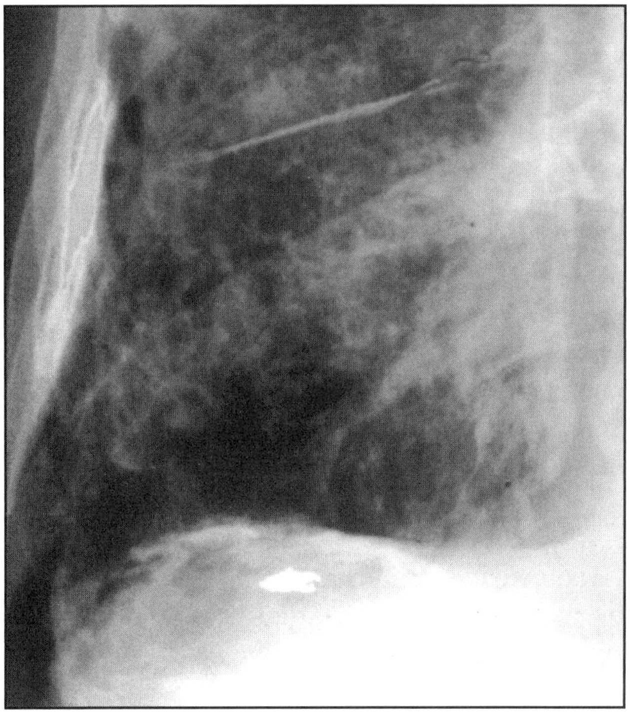

Figure 6. Asbestos-induced pleural plaques demonstrated on the diaphragm, parietal pleura, and interlobar fissure.

to better define the extent of the plaques and to clarify whether confounding processes (*eg*, asbestosis, lung mass, fat tissue, or serratus anterior and external oblique muscles) contribute to the chest radiographic abnormalities.[28,43]

There is no firm evidence that pleural plaques increase the risk of mesothelioma or lung cancer. In a review[44] of 13 studies of the relationship between pleural plaques and the risk for lung cancer, 10 of the studies were deemed appropriate to address this issue; in none of the 10 was there a direct relationship found. In 1997, an International Expert Meeting[45] concluded that the presence of parietal pleural plaques alone were insufficient for attributing lung cancer to asbestos. Only 6.5% of 234 patients with lung cancer and some asbestos exposure had pleural plaques without histologic asbestosis.[46] However, a review[47] of 38 asbestos cohort studies demonstrated a direct relationship between the cumulative asbestosis rate and the rate of excess lung cancers. Thus, patients with asbestos-induced pleural plaques without asbestosis have a minimally elevated risk for the development of bronchogenic carcinoma. A reasonable periodic monitoring program for such patients would include assessing current asbestos exposure risks, advising the patient of the importance of smoking cessation, and obtaining an intermittent chest radiograph (Table 1).

Diffuse pleural plaques are a more widespread form of pleural fibrosis involving the visceral and parietal pleural surfaces, resulting in blunting of the costophrenic angle. These lesions, which can be unilateral or bilateral, are relatively infrequent and, unlike circumscribed plaques, diffuse pleural plaques may result in restrictive pulmonary physiology and functional impairment.

Rounded Atelectasis

Rounded atelectasis is a distinct form of pleural/parenchymal thickening that is characterized by its major radiographic finding, the "comet tail" sign. As pleural fibrosis progresses, it can entrap the underlying healthy lung and bronchovascular tissue. These patients present with a pleural-based mass that appears similar to bronchogenic carcinoma but can be distinguished from it based on the characteristic asbestos exposure history, the relative stability of the lesion >2 to 3 years, other radiographic signs of asbestos exposure, and the comet tail sign pointing toward the hilum on the chest CT scan. The uncertain nature of the lesion may occasionally necessitate a biopsy by means of percutaneous needle aspiration or, rarely, video-assisted thoracoscopic surgery. The mechanisms by which rounded atelectasis occurs are unclear, but the pathways implicated include the local fusion of the visceral and parietal pleura by the fibrotic process, the regional shrinkage of connective tissue along the visceral pleura, and/or the absorption of pleural effusions.[28]

Malignant Mesothelioma

Malignant mesothelioma is a rare tumor that is caused by all forms of asbestos. It occurs in the following two sites: the parietal pleura and the peritoneum. It is much more frequent in the parietal pleura, possibly because inhalation is the typical route of pathogenicity. The incidence of malignant mesothelioma has increased for decades, largely as a result of the extensive use of asbestos from World War II until the 1970s; the incidence is expected to peak sometime between 2010 and 2020 because of the extraordinarily long interval from the time of exposure to the onset of disease.[48,49] Malignant mesothelioma occurred in nearly 2% of asbestos textile workers exposed to approximately one fiber per cubic centimeter >50 years and accounts for approximately 8% of the deaths among asbestos workers.[50] In industrial countries, the yearly incidence of mesothelioma is 2 cases per million person-years among women and 10 to 30 cases per million person-years among men but as much as 270 to 366 cases per million person-years in men who have been exposed to crocidolite asbestos.[49,51] Although occupational asbestos exposure can be documented in 50 to 85% of patients with malignant mesotheliomas, nonoccupational exposure, radiation, chemical carcinogens, viruses, and chronic pleural disease also have been implicated.[30,36] Unlike bronchogenic carcinoma, there is no synergistic interaction between asbestos and cigarette smoke affecting the incidence of mesothelioma.

The typical clinical presentation of a patient with malignant pleural mesothelioma is an elderly (age range, 50 to 70 years) man (male/female ratio, 5:1) with an insidious onset (median time from symptom onset to diagnosis, 3 months to 2 years) of nonspecific complaints such as fever, weight loss, night sweats, and fatigue.[49] Dyspnea (50 to 70%), nonpleuritic chest pain (approximately 60%), and cough (approximately 30%) also may be present. Physical examination and chest radiographic findings consistent with a pleural effusion are seen in 80 to 95% of patients.[28] A mediastinal shift toward the side of the pleural effusion is seen occasionally and indicates a potentially trapped lung. Chest CT scanning is more sensitive than a chest radiograph for detecting pleural plaques, differentiating a pleural effusion from a tumor, assessing the extent of diaphragmatic as well as hilar and mediastinal lymph node involvement, and identifying areas of asbestosis. MRI of the chest is a promising approach for distinguishing between benign pleural plaques and malignant mesothelioma.[52]

The chest radiographic findings of malignant pleural mesothelioma, although often very suggestive, are not specific enough to establish a definitive diagnosis. Differentiating malignant mesothelioma from metastatic adenocarcinoma, benign pleural mesothelioma, or reactive mesothelial cells is challenging. No single immunohistochemical marker or ultrastructural feature is pathognomonic.

A diagnosis of mesothelioma begins with a strong clinical suspicion based on the appropriate exposure history. Pleural fluid cytology is diagnostic in only 25 to 33% of patients, closed needle pleural biopsy is diagnostic in 21 to 77% of patients, and video-assisted thoracoscopic surgery is occasionally diagnostic.[28] A panel of immunohistochemical stains of pleural tissue is often helpful.

Adenocarcinomas, with which mesothelioma is often confused, show periodic acid-Schiff-positive vacuoles and stain positively with carcinoembryonic antigen and Leu-M1 (CD15 antigen). The findings of these stains typically are negative in mesotheliomas. However, mesothelioma cells generally stain positively for vimentin. Mesotheliomas may also elevate pleural fluid hyaluronic acid levels, but this test is not always readily available. Newer markers of mesothelioma include calretinin, a calcium-binding protein that strongly stains 88% of malignant mesotheliomas, as opposed to adenocarcinoma, where it binds weakly in approximately 50%.[48] Also, simian virus-40 DNA is detected in approximately 66% of malignant mesotheliomas but not in surrounding normal mesothelial cells.[48] Simian virus-40 is not necessary for inducing mesotheliomas but may contribute to its development, especially in the nearly 20% of patients with mesothelioma who have not knowingly been exposed to asbestos.

Reviews published during the past several years examining whether various biomarkers (*eg*, mesothelin, megakaryocyte potentiating factor, osteopontin, soluble mesothelin-related protein, and others) are useful for discriminating between asbestos-exposed individuals with malignant mesothelioma as compared with other benign (*eg*, asbestosis, pleural plaques, etc) and malignant conditions (*eg*, lung cancer) have been limited by a significant number of false-positive results and negative studies [53-55] Complementary DNA microarray technology has been used to identify nearly 300 genes of the > 6,500 genes surveyed that could serve as useful markers of human mesothelioma.[56] The translational significance of these recently described biomarkers awaits the outcome of ongoing large prospective studies investigating the diagnostic accuracy and the relationship between biomarker levels and mortality. A combination of these pathologic techniques and the traditional history, clinical presentation, and chest radiographic findings should establish a definitive diagnosis.

Unlike lung cancer, there is no widely accepted staging system for patients with diffuse malignant pleural mesothelioma. There are five different staging systems, but none of them has been adequately validated in comparative trials involving a sufficient number of patients.[28,57] Some of the favorable prognostic factors identified include the following: (1) absence of a 5% total body weight loss at the time of diagnosis; (2) tumor confined to the ipsilateral parietal pleura; (3) epithelioid cell type; (4) good performance status; (5) young age; and (6) platelet count < 400,000 cells/µL.

No standard therapeutic regimen has been clearly shown to substantially alter the median survival time, which remains a dismal 6 to 18 months, with a 5-year survival rate of < 5%.[28,48] Single-modality therapy, including various chemotherapeutic agents, radiation therapy, intrapleural chemotherapy, intrapleural immunotherapy (*eg*, interferon-γ or IL-2), or surgery (*eg*, pleurectomy or extrapleural pneumonectomy), for highly selected patients rarely prolongs survival beyond several months.[48,49,57] A large phase III study[58,59] showed that cisplatin, which is the single most efficacious chemotherapeutic agent (response rate, approximately 17 to 23%; median survival time, 9 months), is more effective when combined with pemetrexed (response rate, 41%; median survival time, 12 months). Multimodality therapy with various combinations of chest surgery, chemotherapy, and radiation has been adapted. In 183 patients who were treated with taxol, carboplatin, extrapleural pneumonectomy, and radiation therapy, the overall median survival time was 17 months, and the 5-year survival rate was 14%.[60] However, 2-year and 5-year survival rates of 68% and 46%, respectively, were observed for highly selected patients with stage I disease and epithelial-type histopathology. Although select patients may survive longer when managed with multimodality therapy, no randomized, multicenter, phase III studies have shown that this approach is superior to any other therapy.

Asbestosis

Asbestosis is a slowly progressive, diffuse pulmonary fibrotic process caused by the inhalation of asbestos fibers. There is a latency period of at least 20 to 40 years from the time of initial exposure to the development of respiratory symptoms. The earliest symptom of asbestosis is insidiously progressive exertional dyspnea that often progresses inexorably regardless of further asbestos exposure. Cough with sputum production is generally attributed to exposure to cigarette smoke rather than asbestos. Patients with asbestosis may have bibasilar fine end-inspiratory crackles (32 to 64%), clubbing (32 to 42%) and, in the advanced stages, signs of cor pulmonale.[29,33]

The chest radiograph usually reveals small parenchymal opacities in the lower lung zones with a nodular and/or reticular pattern that is similar to that seen in patients with IPF. Unlike IPF, pleural involvement is a hallmark of asbestos exposure. Pleural plaques are usually present but may be absent in 10 to 20% of patients.[43] In the early stages of asbestosis, the interstitial and pleural involvement begin in the mid to lower lung zones, resulting in a hazy, ground-glass appearance that blurs the heart border (called the shaggy heart sign) and the diaphragm on the chest radiograph.[40] Neither the mediastinal nor hilar lymph nodes are enlarged. Honeycombing and upper lobe involvement develop in the advanced stages of asbestosis.

Because the chest radiographic changes associated with asbestosis may be subtle, a HRCT scan is frequently obtained because of its greater sensitivity. The characteristic HRCT scan findings of asbestosis, although nonspecific, include the following: (1) subpleural linear densities parallel to the pleura; (2) parenchymal bands 2 to 5 cm in length, often contiguous with the pleura; (3) thickened interlobular septal lines; and (4) honeycombing.[43] In a study[61] of 169 asbestos-exposed workers with a normal chest radiograph findings, HRCT scan findings consistent with asbestosis were noted in 57 patients (33.7%). These workers also had reductions in both vital capacity and DLCO and an increased dyspnea score in comparison with workers who had normal HRCT scan findings.

Pulmonary function abnormalities in patients with asbestosis demonstrate restricted lung volumes and diminished DLCO, but otherwise, their spirometry results are normal.[29,33,62] Abnormal spirometry results (FEV_1, <75% predicted) generally reflect concomitant exposure to cigarette smoke. Although controversial, some groups have suggested[62] that asbestos alone may cause airways obstruction in part attributable to the large airways inflammation resulting from fiber deposition along the respiratory bronchioles and alveolar duct bifurcations.

A diagnosis of asbestosis is based on several characteristic features and does not require histopathologic evaluation for compensation purposes.[29,33] An American Thoracic Society (ATS) expert panel concluded originally in 1986[33] and again in 2004[29] that a clinical diagnosis of asbestosis is established, in the absence of lung tissue, by the following: (1) a reliable exposure history, (2) an appropriate latency period, (3) characteristic chest radiograph abnormalities of 1/1 or greater based on the ILO scale, (4) reduced lung volumes and/or DLCO, and (5) end-inspiratory crackles. The 2004 ATS statement[29] encompassed chest radiograph as well as HRCT scan abnormalities in the clinical definition and established the role of BAL fluid (*ie*, showing more than one asbestos body per milliliter, which is indicative of a high probability of substantial occupational asbestos exposure), whereas asbestos fiber analysis was deemphasized. For patients with an atypical presentation, the most definitive evidence supporting the diagnosis of asbestosis is lung tissue demonstrating asbestos bodies in the setting of diffuse interstitial pulmonary fibrosis. Asbestosis can have a patchy distribution that favors the lower lung zones, similar to that of IPF. The early phase of asbestosis is characterized by peribronchiolar fibrosis with normal distal alveoli. In the advanced stages of asbestosis, the fibrotic process, similar to that in IPF, extends into the distal airspaces and is associated with traction bronchiectasis and honeycombing. Conglomerate lesions are unusual unless the worker has been exposed to a mixed dust containing silica.

Asbestosis is generally a slowly progressive process that culminates in respiratory failure. In seven studies[63] involving >2,200 asbestos workers who were followed up from 1 to 17 years after their initial diagnosis of asbestosis, progression occurred in 5 to 31% of the patients, as assessed by changes in the chest radiograph or PFT results. Risk factors predicting the progression of asbestosis include the following: cumulative asbestos exposure (total amosite/crocidolite fiber burden, >100,000 fibers per gram of dry lung); duration of exposure; and crocidolite exposure.[63] A study[64] of the mortality of

655 male workers with asbestosis found that of the 233 workers who died, 20% died from asbestosis, 39% died from lung cancer, 9% died from mesothelioma, and 32% died from other causes. Given the long latency between exposure and disease as well as the direct relationship between asbestos consumption in > 33 countries and mortality from asbestos-related diseases (*eg*, asbestosis, mesothelioma, and lung cancer), the ILO has called for a total worldwide asbestos ban.[65]

Lung Cancer

By the mid-1950s, epidemiologic data firmly supported a relationship between asbestosis and lung cancer. In the mid-1980s, the Environmental Protection Agency and the World Health Organization's International Agency for Research declared asbestos a proven human carcinogen. From a 2001 review[66] of 23 studies of the associations among asbestos, cigarette smoke, and lung cancer, it was concluded that asbestos causes lung cancer in nonsmokers despite the small numbers of such workers available for study. Moreover, a multiplicative or synergistic interaction rather than an additive model better described the association between asbestos and cigarette smoke. This distinction implies that the combined attributable lung cancer risk exceeds the sum of the risk of each agent. The mechanisms underlying this synergistic effect are not fully known but are caused in part by impaired lung fiber clearance and enhanced DNA damage.[6,39] Early studies suggested that tumor location and histology differ in asbestos- and cigarette smoke-exposed individuals, but this has been refuted by others as reviewed elsewhere. Asbestos-induced lung cancers can occur in any lobe of the lung, and the distribution of the four major histopathologic lung cancer types is similar to the distribution pattern among patients with cigarette smoke-induced lung cancer.[67,68]

Considerable controversy surrounds the hypothesis that excess lung cancer risk in those persons with an occupational asbestos exposure is limited to workers with asbestosis. There is general agreement that histologically and radiographically defined asbestosis, in addition to other forms of pulmonary fibrosis, significantly increase the risk of lung cancer. Weiss[47] reviewed 34 cohort studies and reported a direct correlation between the rate of asbestosis and lung cancer, suggesting that asbestosis is a better predictor of excess lung cancer risk than measures of asbestos exposure. Others[69] have challenged this conclusion, arguing that asbestos exposure, and not asbestosis, causes lung cancer.

Because it is not necessary to have emphysema to implicate cigarette smoke as a cause of lung cancer, it might not be necessary to have asbestosis for implicating asbestos as the attributable cause of lung cancer. This controversy is not likely to be resolved soon because of the nonuniform definition of asbestosis used in the various studies (*eg*, clinical vs histopathologic) and the uncertain biological scenario whereby the molecular mechanisms underlying interstitial fibrosis are required to develop a malignancy. Oksa et al[70] showed that lung cancer developed in 11 of 24 patients with progressive asbestosis (46%), whereas lung cancer developed in only 5 of 54 patients with stable asbestosis (9%). They postulated that the progression of asbestosis, in addition to cigarette smoke and asbestos exposure, is an independent predictor of lung cancer risk in patients with asbestosis.

Asbestos can act at all the critical steps in the formation of a malignant clone of cells (*eg*, initiation, promotion, and progression) and, as such, is not dependent on the presence of fibrosis. Asbestos-exposed workers can have mutations in the *k-ras* gene at codon 12 in lung cancers without radiographic determination of asbestosis, suggesting that these two events are not necessarily linked.[30] Thus, it is unclear whether asbestosis is simply a marker of high-dose asbestos exposure or a necessary requirement for attributing an individual's lung cancer to asbestos. Until more definitive studies have clarified this controversy, lung cancer attribution should be based on the merits of each patient's carcinogen exposure history combined with the appropriate clinical history and laboratory findings.

Talc Pneumoconiosis

Definition/Occupations

Talc is a heterogeneous term that includes hydrated magnesium silicates, and it is used commercially to describe mixed materials that may contain minimal amounts of talc. Relatively pure talc, which is widely used in the cosmetic industry, is mined primarily in Vermont, the French Pyrenées, and Italy. Less pure talc (approximately 60%) that is contaminated with asbestos, carbonates, and silica is mined from other areas (*eg*, New York, Texas, and California) and is used extensively for a variety of industrial purposes. Talc is found near the surface of the earth and is mined in open pits. Rock containing talc is crushed into a fine powder, bagged, and shipped for numerous commercial uses in the manufacturing of ceramics, rubber products, chemicals, cosmetics, and pharmaceuticals and as a filler in paint, paper, soaps, and roofing material.

Epidemiology

Talc pneumoconiosis, also known as *talcosis*, typically develops in heavily exposed occupational workers.[2] The first case of talc pneumoconiosis was described in 1896. With modern dust control measures in mines and in industrial talc plants, the incidence of talcosis is a relatively rare one today. Because talc is frequently contaminated with other mineral dusts, other lung diseases occur in talc-exposed workers. Although widely used by consumers, talc rarely causes disease except in adults exposed to massive amounts of baby powder. Also, talcosis can develop in drug abusers who inject or inhale crushed tablets containing talc.

Pathophysiology

The toxic manifestations of talc depend on the purity of the material to which the workers are exposed. Nodular lesions in the respiratory bronchioles similar to those seen in silicosis are characteristic but, unlike silicosis, talc is rarely seen in the nodule, nor are birefringent silica crystals visible. Multinucleated giant cells can occur, but focal and diffuse fibrosis occurs in the later stages. A mixed nodular and diffuse fibrotic process may be evident pathologically as well as radiologically. In IV drug abusers, talc granulomas may be seen in the interstitium as well as in the pulmonary arteries, resulting in pulmonary hypertension and cor pulmonale. Drug abusers may also present with very severe emphysematous changes associated with areas of granulomatous inflammation and fibrosis surrounding the talc.[71]

Clinical Features/Management

The nodular form of talcosis is similar, both clinically and radiographically, to silicosis in that patients are typically asymptomatic despite substantial chest radiographic abnormalities. A nonproductive cough and dyspnea may develop many years after the initial exposure. The onset of diffuse fibrosis results in cough and dyspnea, bibasilar inspiratory crackles on examination, and chest radiographic abnormalities that are similar to those seen in silicosis and other forms of pulmonary fibrosis. PFT abnormalities are minimal in the nodular form of talcosis but can demonstrate a restrictive defect with a reduced DLCO once fibrosis occurs. There is no proven treatment for talc pneumoconiosis; therefore, the prevention of further exposure is the key to management. There have been anecdotal reports of a benefit from steroid therapy in symptomatic patients with talcosis whose disease is progressing.

Beryllium Lung Disease

Definition/Occupations

Beryllium is a rare light metal that is extracted from beryl ore that is mined in the United States, Brazil, and China, and is refined in the United States, Japan, and Russia. Beryllium has a very high melting point and a very low density, elasticity, and coefficient of thermal expansion. It also is permeable to radiation. These properties make it ideally suited for use in heat shields, rotor blades, radiograph tubes, and parts for microwave equipment and nuclear reactors.[2,72] Shortly after beryllium was first used commercially in phosphors for fluorescent lights in the United States in the 1930s, its toxic properties were recognized. Since then, an estimated 800,000 workers have had past or current beryllium exposure, resulting in chronic berylliosis in nearly 1 to 21% of the workers.[2,72] Beryllium can cause the following two types of pathologic conditions acute pneumonitis caused by short-term, high-level exposure and chronic disease caused by long-term, low-level exposure causing a granulomatous inflammation similar to sarcoidosis. Worker exposure to beryllium occurs primarily in the aerospace, nuclear, computer, and electronics industries.

Pathophysiology

Acute beryllium pneumonitis is caused by direct acute lung injury resulting from the inhalation of high levels of beryllium particles. Beryllium also incites an antigen-specific immune response that can cause a noncaseating granulomatous inflammatory reaction that is histopathologically similar to that seen in patients with sarcoidosis. Persistent low-level beryllium exposure results in chronic berylliosis, which is manifested by chronic interstitial fibrosis, often with bullous changes, as well as systemic involvement in the skin, liver, spleen, lymph nodes, myocardium, kidney, bones, and salivary glands. T lymphocytes from the lung and blood of patients with berylliosis proliferate when exposed *in vitro* to beryllium salts, which act as an antigen or hapten. This reaction serves as an important early marker for diagnosing berylliosis and also has been implicated in the pathogenesis of lung fibrosis.[2,73] Up to 16% of beryllium workers are sensitized to beryllium as assessed in the lymphocyte proliferation test.[2]

Clinical Features/Management

Acute beryllium disease is now relatively rare because of improved industrial hygiene methods, but when it does occur, beryllium acts as a direct irritant. The diagnosis should be suspected when there is high-level beryllium exposure in association with acute pneumonitis, conjunctivitis, periorbital edema, nasopharyngitis, and tracheobronchitis. These patients typically present with dyspnea, cough, sputum production, chest pain, tachycardia, crackles, and hypoxemia. Chest radiographs typically reveal diffuse alveolar infiltrates, whereas PFT results show a restrictive process with a reduced DLco. Patient management includes eliminating further beryllium exposure, providing supplemental oxygen if needed, supportive measures and, in more advanced forms, a therapeutic trial of steroids. Most patients fully recover, although chronic berylliosis may develop in up to 25% of patients.[2]

Chronic berylliosis develops after a latent period ranging from months to as long as 10 years after the onset of low-level beryllium exposure.[2,72] The diagnosis should be suspected in patients with an appropriate exposure history who present with dyspnea (the most common complaint), cough, chest pain, weight loss, fatigue, and arthralgias and who have an abnormal chest radiograph finding, with a reticular-nodular infiltrate seen predominately in the upper lung lobes (although all lobes can be involved). The chest radiographic pattern is similar to that found with sarcoidosis, including mediastinal and bilateral hilar adenopathy. A beryllium lymphocyte transformation test should be performed to document sensitization. Although an estimated 50% of beryllium-sensitized workers have evidence of chronic beryllium disease at the time of an initial presentation, a 2005 longitudinal study[74] showed that chronic berylliosis will develop in 31% of disease-free sensitized workers (especially machinists) within 3.8 years (range, 1.0 to 9.5 years), whereas the disease never develops in the remaining 69% $>$4.8 years of follow-up. However, there is insufficient evidence to recommend performing routine beryllium lymphocyte transformation tests for screening asymptomatic workers.[75]

Large calcified masses and pleural reactions can be seen, whereas nearly one-third of the patients have bilateral hilar adenopathy. PFT results show reduced volumes and DLco. Although the clinical course of chronic berylliosis is variable, most patients have a slow, inexorable decline that can result in cor pulmonale in nearly one-third of patients. Treatment options are sparse but of prime importance is the elimination of further beryllium exposure; often, a course of steroids is administered. Although there are no controlled studies demonstrating their efficacy, most reports have shown that removal from further beryllium exposure and the use of steroids result in a favorable response both clinically and radiographically; however, similar to the situation with sarcoidosis, many cases recur when steroid therapy is discontinued. Data from a large beryllium registry[2] involving 689 patients demonstrated excess mortality from lung cancer and nonmalignant beryllium disease. Notably, a recent study documented 16 cases of nonoccupational, environmental chronic beryllium disease in residents surrounding a beryllium manufacturing facility.[76]

Hard Metal Lung Disease

Definition/Occupations

As shown in Table 3, various hard metals can induce a wide range of lung diseases. Although the majority of the hard-metal lung diseases arise from occupational exposure, environmental exposures have been reported (*eg*, mercury-induced chemical pneumonitis). Metal-induced pulmonary toxicity can be caused by either antigen-specific immunologic reactions or nonspecific immune/inflammatory responses caused in part by oxidative stress similar to that depicted in Figure 5.[2,77]

Cobalt

The main components of commercially available hard metal include tungsten and titanium carbides (70 to 95%); cobalt (5 to 25%); and small amounts of various other metals (*eg*, nickel, chromium, tantalum, and vanadium). Because tungsten is inert, cobalt is the primary culprit that causes pulmonary toxicity associated with hard-metal exposure. Cobalt is used as a hardener and binder of metal alloys of, for example, tungsten, aluminum, chrome, molybdenum, and beryllium. Cobalt exposure may occur in occupations such as machinist, metal tool maker, polisher, grinder, saw sharpener, and dental driller.

Occupational exposure to cobalt is associated with the following three pulmonary manifestations: (1) airways obstruction that resembles occupational asthma; (2) acute interstitial pneumonitis with features of hypersensitivity pneumonitis; and (3) chronic diffuse interstitial fibrosis that can progress to end-stage fibrosis. Patients with cobalt-induced chronic interstitial fibrosis present with the insidious onset of exertional dyspnea, cough, weight loss, and restrictive pulmonary physiology. Pathologic findings include desquamative interstitial pneumonitis, giant cell interstitial pneumonitis, and varying degrees of bronchiolitis obliterans, interstitial fibrosis, and sarcoid-like granulomas. A characteristic diagnostic feature is the presence of odd-appearing giant multinucleated cells. An immune mechanism involving suppressor T lymphocytes is implicated in mediating cobalt pulmonary toxicity.[76] Also, genetic factors involving the allelic substantiation of a glutamic acid in position 69 of the human leukocyte antigen-DPβ chain has been identified in workers with cobalt-induced chronic interstitial lung disease.[78] Furthermore, the combination of cobalt and other metallic carbides can induce an oxidative stress on the lungs. Limiting exposure below the PEL of 50 mg/m^3 is mandatory. Once cobalt-related lung disease has occurred, the worker should be moved to other sites at which no cobalt exposure can occur. Progression can occur without further cobalt exposure; occasionally, cor pulmonale and death may occur many years after the initial exposure. In a 13-year follow-up[79] of lung function changes in 122 workers exposed to cobalt-containing compounds, pulmonary fibrosis did not develop in one person, whereas a significant decrease in FEV_1 occurred only in workers who were cigarette smokers. There were no

Table 3. *Some Representative Hard Metal-Induced Lung Diseases**

Agent	Histopathology	Occupational Exposure
Aluminum	Interstitial fibrosis; sarcoid-like granuloma	Aluminum miner/refineries
Beryllium	Sarcoid-like granulomas; ILD	Beryllium miner/aerospace, nuclear, and electronics work
Cadmium	Acute pneumonitis; ILD; emphysema	Lead or zinc smelter; batteries (Brazier disease)
Cobalt	Giant-cell ILD; sarcoid-like granuloma; obstructive airways	Metal hardener for tungsten carbide (tool grinders, metal polisher, dental drills)
Iron	Dust macule, ILD	Iron miner/welder
Mercury	Tracheobronchitis; pneumonitis; pulmonary edema	Electrical industry; scientific equipment; catalyst work

*ILD = interstitial lung disease.

associations with polymorphisms in glutamic acid in position.[69]

Siderosis

Occupations involving iron exposure (*eg*, mining, smelting, welding, and steel making) can lead to siderosis. It is often a relatively benign condition, usually noted as an incidental finding or as an abnormality on a chest radiograph with dense linear opacities in an asymptomatic iron worker. Occasionally, iron can induce respiratory symptoms, restrictive pulmonary physiology, and pulmonary fibrosis in heavily exposed workers.[80] Pathologic findings range from the characteristic iron dust macule to interstitial fibrosis. There is no specific treatment other than the prevention of further iron exposure.

Metal Fume Fever

Metal fume fever is a set of flu-like symptoms that occur within 4 to 12 h after the start of the work shift in metal workers after exposure to high levels of metal fumes, especially zinc oxide. Fumes of metal oxides of arsenic, boron, cadmium, chromium, copper, magnesium, manganese, nickel, and titanium can cause similar symptoms.[77] It was initially defined in brass foundry workers in the mid-1800s and in steel welders in the early 1900s.[76] These patients present with fever at temperatures from 102 to 104°F associated with a metallic taste in the mouth, throat irritation, cough, dyspnea, malaise, fatigue, myalgias, arthralgias, sweats, and shaking chills. The syndrome typically is associated with mild airflow obstruction and minimal chest radiographic findings and resolves in >24 to 48 h.[77] Metal fume fever is caused by dose-related toxicity rather than immunologic sensitization because there is no latency period. Studies have shown that workers with metal fume fever have increased levels of various cytokines (*eg*, tumor necrosis factor-α, IL-6, and IL-8) in their BAL fluid, presumably released from AMs, that likely mediate this syndrome.[77] An unexplained feature of this syndrome is the development of tolerance so that symptoms diminish on successive days of exposure but recur after a brief absence away from work.

Acknowledgment: This work was supported in part by a Merit Review grant from the Department of Veterans Affairs. The author is grateful for the comments of David Cugell.

Annotated References

1. Cowie RL, Murray J, Becklake MR. Pneumoconioses. In: Mason RJ, Broaddus C, Murray JF, et al, eds. Textbook of respiratory medicine. 4th ed. Philadelphia, PA: WB Saunders, 2005; 1748–1782
   An excellent overview of the topic. Includes references.
2. King TE, Kamp DW, Panos RJ. Pneumoconiosis, chronic interstitial fibrosis and bronchiolitis. In: Witorsch P, Spagolo SV, eds. Air pollution and lung disease in adults. Boca Raton, FL: CRC Press, 1994; 207–284
   A concise summary of the relevant diseases. Includes 273 references.
3. National Institute for Occupational Safety and Health. Silicosis. Publication No. 2006-110 Available at: http://www.cdc.gov/niosh/docs/2006-110/. Accessed April 9, 2008
4. National Institute for Occupational Safety and Health, Division of Respiratory Disease Studies. Silicosis deaths among young adults: United States, from 1968 to 1994. JAMA 1998; 280:13–14
5. National Institute for Occupational Safety and Health. Hazard review: health effects of occupational exposure to respirable crystalline silica. Washington, DC: Department of Health and Human Services, NIOSH, 2002; 1–127; Publication No. 2002-129
6. Mossman BT, Churg A. Mechanisms in the pathogenesis of asbestosis and silicosis. Am J Respir Crit Care Med 1998; 157:1666–1680
7. Wu F, Xia Z, Qu Y, et al. Genetic polymorphism of IL-1A, IL-1, IL-1RN, NFKB1, FAS, and FASL and risk of silicosis in a Chinese occupational population. Am J Indust Med 2008; 51:843–51
8. Finkelstein MM. Silica, silicosis, and lung cancer: a risk assessment. Am J Ind Med 2000; 38:8–18
9. Roseman KD, Reill MJ, Rice C, et al. Silicosis among foundry workers: implications for the need to revise the OSHA standard. Am J Epidemiol 1996; 144:890–900
10. Arakawa H, Johkoh T, Honma K, et al. Chronic interstitial pneumonia in silicosis and mix-dust pneumoconiosis. Chest 2007; 131:1870–1876

11. Wang X-R, Christiani DC. Respiratory symptoms and functional status in workers exposed to silica, asbestos, and coal mine dusts. J Occup Environ Med 2000; 42:1076–1084
12. Greenberg MI, Waksman J, Curtis J. Silicosis: a review. Dis Mon 2007; 53:394–416
A relatively current review of silicosis. Includes 79 references.
13. American Thoracic Society, Centers for Disease Control and Prevention, Infectious Diseases Society of America. Treatment of tuberculosis. Am J Respir Crit Care Med 2003; 167:603–662
14. Hnizdo E, Murray J. Risk of pulmonary tuberculosis relative to silicosis and exposure to silica dust in South American gold miners. Occup Environ Med 1998; 55:496–502
15. Leung CC, Yew WW, Law WS, et al. Smoking and tuberculosis among silicotic patients. Eur Respir J 2007; 29:745–750
16. Castranova V, Vallyathan V. Silicosis and coal workers' pneumoconiosis. Environ Health Perspect 2000; 108(suppl):675–684
An excellent review of silicosis and CWP emphasizing recent clinical developments and pathogenic mechanisms. Includes 130 references.
17. Weill H, McDonald JC. Exposure to crystalline silica and risk of lung cancer: the epidemiologic studies. Thorax 1996; 51:97–102
18. Checkoway H, Hughes JM, Weill H, et al. Crystalline silica exposure, radiologic silicosis, and lung cancer mortality in diatomaceous earth industry workers. Thorax 1999; 54:56–59
19. Cassidy A, Mannetje A, van Tongeren M, et al. Occupational exposure to crystalline silica and risk of lung cancer. Epidemiology 2007; 18: 36–43
20. Pelucchi C, Pira E, Piolatto G, et al. Occupational silica exposure and lung cancer risk: a review of epidemiologic studies from 1996 to 2005. Ann Oncol 2006; 17:1039–1050
21. Schwerha JJ. Occupational Medicine Forum. J Occup Environ Med 2008; 50:101–104.
An excellent reference documenting the recommended radiographic follow-up in patients with pneumoconiosis.
22. Kamp DW, Vallyathan V. Influence of mineral dust surface characteristics and generation of reactive species. In: Vallyathan V, Castranova V, Shi X, eds. Oxygen/nitrogen radicals: lung biology in health and disease series (vol 187). New York: Marcel Dekker, 2004; 139–160
23. Wallace WE, Harrison JC, Grayson RL, et al. Aluminosilicate surface contamination of respirable quartz particles from coal mine dusts and from clay works dusts. Ann Occup Hyg 1994; 38:439–45
24. Nadif R, Jedlicka A, Mintz M, et al. Effect of TNF and LTA polymorphisms on biological markers of response to oxidative stimuli in coal miners: a model of gene-environment interaction; tumour necrosis factor and lymphotoxin α. J Med Genet 2003; 40:96–103
25. Nadif R, Mintz M, Marzec J, et al. IL18 and IL18R1 polymorphisms, lung CT and fibrosis: a longitudinal study in coal miners. Eur Respir J 2006; 28:1100–1105
26. Blum T, Kollmeier J, Ott S, et al. CT for diagnosis and grading of dust-induced occupational lung disease. Curr Opin Pulm Med 2008; 14:135–140
27. Attfield MD, Kuempel ED. Mortality among United States underground coal miners: a 23-year follow up. Am J Ind Med 2008; 51:231–245
28. Cugell DW, Kamp DW. Asbestos and the pleura: a review. Chest 2004; 125:1103–1117
A summary of the various effects of asbestos on the pleura. Includes 120 references.
29. Guidotti TL, Miller A, Christiani D, et al. Diagnosis and initial management of nonmalignant diseases related to asbestos. Am J Respir Crit Care Med 2004; 170:691–715
The ATS 2004 consensus statement about the criteria for diagnosing and managing asbestos-induced nonmalignant diseases containing excellent representative histopathologic and radiographic examples as well as 160 references.
30. Kamp DW, Mossman BT. Asbestos-associated cancers: clinical spectrum and pathogenic mechanisms. Clin Occup Environ Med 2002; 2:753–778
31. Hein MJ, Staynor LT, Lehman E, et al. Follow up study of chrysotile textile workers: cohort mortality and exposure-response. Occup Environ Med 2007; 64:616–625
32. Cooke WE. Pulmonary asbestosis. BMJ 1927; 2:1024–1025
33. Murphy RL, Becklake MR, Brooks SM, et al. The diagnosis of nonmalignant diseases related to asbestos. Am Rev Respir Dis 1986; 134:363–368
The ATS consensus statement about the criteria for diagnosing asbestos-induced nonmalignant diseases.
34. O'Reilly KMA, McLaughlin AM, Beckett WS, et al. Asbestos-related lung disease. Am Fam Physician 2007; 75:683–688

35. Nicholson WJ, Perkel G, Selikoff IJ. Occupational exposure to asbestos: population at risk and projected mortality; from 1980 to 2030. Am J Ind Med 1982; 3:259–311
36. Kamp DW. Asbestos-induced lung diseases: an update. Transl Res 2009; 153:143–152.
A recent review emphasizing epidemiology and pathogenesis. Includes 106 references.
37. Iwatsubo Y, Pairon JC, Boutin C, et al. Pleural mesothelioma, dose-response relation at low levels of asbestos exposure in a French population-based case-control study. Am J Epidemiol 1998; 148:133–142
38. Barbers RG, Abraham JL. Asbestos occurring after a brief inhalational exposure: usefulness of BAL in diagnosis. Br J Ind Med 1989; 46:106–110
39. Shukla A, Gulumian M, Hei T, et al. Multiple roles of oxidants in the pathogenesis of asbestos-induced diseases. Free Radic Biol Med 2003; 34: 1117–1129
40. Merchant JA. Human epidemiology: a review of fiber type and characteristics in the development of malignant and nonmalignant disease. Environ Health Perspect 1990; 88:287–293
41. Miller A, Lilis R, Godbold J, et al. Relationship of pulmonary function to radiographic interstitial fibrosis in 2,611 long-term asbestos insulators. Am Rev Respir Dis 1992; 145:263–270
42. Rogan WJ, Ragan NB, Dinse GE. Radiograph evidence of increased asbestos exposure in the United States population from NHANESI and NHANESII, from 1973 to 1978. Cancer Causes Control 2000; 11:441–449
43. Kim JS, Lynch DA. Imaging of nonmalignant occupational lung disease. J Thorac Imaging 2002; 17:238–260
44. Weiss W. Asbestos-related pleural plaques and lung cancer. Chest 1993; 103:1854–1859
45. Henderson DW, Rantanen J, Barnhart S, et al. Asbestos, asbestosis, and cancer: the Helsinki criteria for diagnosis and attribution; a consensus report of an international expert group. Scand J Work Environ Health 1997; 28:311–316
46. Roggli VL, Sanders LL. Asbestos content of lung tissue and carcinoma of the lung: a clinicopathologic correlation and mineral fiber analysis of 234 cases. Ann Occup Hyg 2000; 44:109–117
47. Weiss W. Asbestosis: a marker for the increased risk of lung cancer among workers exposed to asbestos. Chest 1999; 115:536–549
48. Robinson BWS, Lake RA. Advances in malignant mesothelioma. N Engl J Med 2005; 353: 1591–1603
Excellent update on the clinical-pathologic features of mesothelioma as well as more recent treatment strategies. Includes 98 references.
49. Boutin C, Schlesser M, Frenay C, et al. Malignant pleural mesothelioma. Eur Respir J 1998; 12:972–981
50. Peto J, Doll R, Herman C, et al. Relationship of mortality to measures of environmental asbestos pollution in an asbestos textile factory. Ann Occup Hyg 1985; 29:305–355
51. McDonald JC, Sebastien P, McDonald AD, et al. Epidemiologic observations on mesothelioma and the implications for nonoccupational exposure. In: Bignon J, Peto J, Saracchi R, eds. Nonoccupational exposure to mineral fibers. Lyon, France: International Agency for Research on Cancer, 1989; 420–427; IARC Science publication No. 90
52. Boraschi P, Neri S, Braccini G, et al. Magnetic resonance appearance of asbestos-related benign and malignant pleural disease. Scand J Work Environ Health 1999; 25:18–23
53. Creaney J, Yeoman D, Demelker Y, et al. Comparison of osteopontin, megakaryocyte potentiating factor, and mesothelin proteins as markers in the serum of patients with malignant mesothelioma. J Thorac Oncol 2008; 3:851–857
54. Amati M, Tomasetti M, Mariotti L, et al. Assessment of biomarkers in asbestos-exposed workers as indicators of cancer risk. Mutat Res/Gene Toxicol and Environ Mutag 2008; 655:52–58
55. van Meerbeeck JP, Hillerdal G. Screening for mesothelioma: more harm than good. Am J Respir Crit Care Med 2008; 178:781–782.
56. Rihn BH, Mohr S, McDowell SA, et al. Differential gene expression in mesothelioma. FEBS Lett 2000; 480:95–100
57. Sterman DH, Kaiser LR, Albelda SM. Advances in the treatment of malignant mesothelioma. Chest 1999; 116:504–520
58. Vogelzang NJ, Rusthoven JJ, Symanowski J, et al. Phase III study of pemetrexed in combination with cisplatin vs cisplatin alone in patients with malignant pleural mesothelioma. J Clin Oncol 2003; 21:2636–2644
59. Janne PA. Comprehensive review: chemotherapy for malignant pleural mesothelioma. Clin Lung Cancer 2003; 5:98–106

60. Sugarbaker DJ, Flores RM, Jaklitsch MT, et al. Resection margins, extrapleural nodal status, and cell type determine postoperative long-term survival in trimodality therapy of malignant pleural mesothelioma. J Thorac Cardiovasc Surg 1999; 117:54–65
61. Staples CA, Gamsu G, Ray CS, et al. High resolution CT and lung function in asbestos-exposed workers with normal chest radiographs. Am Rev Respir Dis 1989; 139:1502–1508
62. Miller A, Lilis R, Godbold J, et al. Relationship of pulmonary function to radiographic interstitial fibrosis in 2,611 long-term asbestos insulators. Am Rev Respir Dis 1992; 145:263–270
63. Becklake MR. Asbestos and other fiber-related diseases of the lungs and pleura. Chest 1991; 100:248–254
64. Berry G. Mortality of workers certified by pneumoconiosis medical panel as having asbestosis. Br J Ind Med 1981; 38:130–137
65. Lin R-T, Takahashi K, Karjalainen A, et al. Ecological associations between asbestos-related diseases and historical asbestos consumption: an international analysis. Lancet 2007; 369:844–849
66. Lee PN. Relation between exposure to asbestos and smoking jointly and the risk of lung cancer. Occup Environ Med 2001; 58:145–153
67. Roggli VL, Sanders LL. Asbestos content of lung tissue and carcinoma of the lung: a clinicopathologic correlation and mineral fiber analysis of 234 cases. Ann Occup Hyg 2000; 44:109–117
68. Weiss W. Asbestosis and lobar site of lung cancer. Occup Environ Med 2000; 57:358–360
69. Henderson DW, Roggli VL, Shilkin KB, et al. Is asbestosis an obligate precursor for asbestos-related lung cancer? In: Peters GA, Peters BJ, eds. Asbestos health effects, treatment and control (vol 11). Charlottesville, VA: The Michie Co., 1995; 103–169
70. Oksa P, Klockars M, Karjalainen A, et al. Progression of asbestosis predicts lung cancer. Chest 1998; 113:1517–1521
71. Schmidt RA, Glenny RW, Godwin JD, et al. Panlobular emphysema in young IV ritalin abusers. Am Rev Respir Dis 1991; 143:649–656
72. Kreiss K, Day GA, Schuler CR. Beryllium: a modern industrial hazard. Annu Rev Public Health 2007; 28:259–277

A recent update of beryllium-induced pulmonary toxicity. Includes 75 references.

73. Newman LS. Significance of the blood beryllium lymphocyte proliferation test. Environ Health Perspect 1996; 104(suppl):953–956
74. Newman LS, Mroz MM, Balkissoon R, et al. Beryllium sensitization progresses to chronic beryllium disease. Am J Respir Crit Care Med 2005; 171:54–60
75. Borak J, Woolf SH, Fields CA. Use of the beryllium lymphocyte proliferation testing for screening of asymptomatic individuals: an evidence-based assessment. J Occup Environ Med 2006; 48:937–947
76. Maier LA, Martyny JW, Liang J, et al. Recent chronic beryllium disease in residents surrounding a beryllium facility. Am J Respir Crit Care Med 2008; 177:1012–1017
77. Kelleher P, Pacheco K, Newman LS. Inorganic dust pneumoconiosis: the metal-related parenchymal disorders. Environ Health Perspect 2000; 108 (suppl):685–696

An *excellent comprehensive review of the area. Includes 196 references.*

78. Potolicchio I, Mosconi G, Forni A, et al. Susceptibility to hard metal lung disease is strongly associated with the presence of glutamate 69 in HLA-DP β chain. Eur Respir J 1997; 27:2741–2743
79. Verougstraete V, Mallants A, Buchet J-P, et al. Lung function changes in workers exposed to cobalt compounds. Am J Respir Crit Care Med 2004; 170:162–166
80. Akbar-Khanzadeh F. Short term respiratory function changes in relation to work shift welding fume exposure. Int Arch Occup Environ Health 1993; 64:393–397

Hospital-Acquired and Ventilator-Associated Pneumonia

Ronald R. Grossman, MD, FCCP

Objectives:

- Identify the key respiratory pathogens causing hospital-acquired pneumonia/ventilator-associated pneumonia
- Develop a systematic approach to the diagnosis of hospital-acquired pneumonia/ventilator-associated pneumonia
- Improve the initial therapeutic choices for the management of hospital-acquired pneumonia/ventilator-associated pneumonia

Key words: clinical pulmonary infection score; hospital-acquired pneumonia; *Pseudomonas aeruginosa; Staphylococcus aureus;* ventilator-associated pneumonia

Definition

Pneumonia that develops ≥48 h after admission to the hospital and was not incubating at the time of admission is defined as *hospital-acquired pneumonia* (HAP).[1] *Ventilator-associated pneumonia* (VAP) refers to pneumonia that occurs >48 to 72 h after endotracheal intubation among patients treated in an ICU setting.[1,2] *Health-care-associated pneumonia* refers to patients admitted to the hospital with pneumonia that may have been received via IV therapy at home, wound care, or specialized nursing care through a health-care agency, family, or friends or via self-administered IV medical therapy in the 30 days before pneumonia.[3,4] They may have attended a hospital or hemodialysis clinic or received IV chemotherapy in the 30 days before pneumonia. They also may have been admitted to an acute care hospital for 2 or more days in the 90 days before pneumonia or resided in a nursing home or a long-term care facility.

Epidemiology

HAP is the second most common nosocomial infection in the United States and is associated with high rates of mortality and morbidity.[1] Hospital length of stay increases by an average of 7 to 9 days per affected patient and is associated with costs >$40,000 per patient.[3,5] HAP occurs at a rate of between 5 and 10 cases per 1,000 hospital admissions, with the incidence increasing by as much as 6- to 20-fold in patients receiving mechanical ventilation.[3,6,7]

HAP accounts for up to 25% of all ICU infections and for >50% of the antibiotics prescribed.[8] VAP occurs in 9 to 27% of all intubated patients.[3,5] The risk of VAP is greatest early in the course of hospital stay and then abates somewhat. The risk has been estimated to be 3% per day during the first 5 days of ventilation, 2% per day during days 5 to 10 of ventilation, and 1% per day after this.[9] Nosocomial pneumonia is less common when patients are managed with noninvasive ventilation.[10–12]

Previous guidelines[13] identified that early-onset pneumonia frequently was caused by community pathogens. Early-onset HAP and VAP, defined as occurring within the first 4 days of hospitalization, are more likely to be caused by antibiotic-sensitive bacteria. Late-onset HAP and VAP (≥5 days) are more likely to be caused by multidrug-resistant (MDR) pathogens and are associated with increased patient mortality and morbidity. However, patients with early-onset HAP who have received antibiotics or who have had hospitalization within the past 90 days have similar pathogens to those patients with late-onset HAP or VAP and should be treated similarly (Table 1).[14]

The crude mortality rate for HAP may be as high as 30 to 70%, but the mortality related to HAP or "attributable mortality" has been estimated to be between 33% and 50% in several case-matching studies of VAP.[15] Increased mortality rates are associated with bacteremia, especially with *Pseudomonas aeruginosa* or Acinetobacter species; medical rather than surgical illness; and treatment with ineffective antibiotic therapy.[15,16] Strangely, the authors of some studies[17–19] using similar methodology have not identified any attributable mortality caused by VAP.

Etiology

The most frequent isolated pathogens from respiratory secretions are aerobic Gram-negative

Table 1. *Risk Factors for MDR Pathogens Causing HAP, Health-Care-Associated Pneumonia, and VAP**

Antimicrobial therapy in preceding 90 d
Current hospitalization of ≥5 d
High frequency of antibiotic resistance in the community or in the specific hospital unit
Presence of risk factors for health-care-associated pneumonia
Hospitalization for ≥2 d in the preceding 90 d
Residence in a nursing home or extended-care facility
Home infusion therapy (including antibiotics)
Long-term dialysis within 30 d
Home wound care
Family member with MDR pathogen
Immunosuppressive disease and/or therapy

*Adapted from American Thoracic Society/Infectious Diseases Society of America.[34]

bacilli, such as *P aeruginosa, Escherichia coli, Klebsiella pneumoniae,* and Acinetobacter sp.[3–6,20–25] Infections caused by Gram-positive cocci, such as *Staphylococcus aureus,* particularly methicillin-resistant *S aureus* (MRSA), are increasing, particularly among patients with diabetes mellitus, head trauma, and those hospitalized in ICUs.[26,27] Rates of polymicrobial infection vary widely but appear to be increasing and are especially high in patients with ARDS.[28–30]

The etiology of HAP and the frequency of specific MDR pathogens vary by hospital, patient population, exposure to antibiotics, type of ICU patient, and changes over time.[31,32] Local surveillance data are crucial in monitoring the emergence of MDR pathogens and should drive the formulation of local guidelines. Anaerobic lung infection may follow aspiration in nonintubated patients but is very uncommon in patients with VAP.[21,33]

Elderly residents of long-term care facilities have been found to have a spectrum of pathogens that more closely resemble late-onset HAP and VAP.[23,24] This observation has led to the development of the term *health care-associated pneumonia.* This designation essentially identifies patients from health-care facilities who are at increased risk for infection with resistant pathogens.[34] Rates of *Legionella pneumophila* vary considerably between hospitals, and disease occurs more commonly with serogroup 1 when the water supply is colonized or there is ongoing construction.[35,36] Nosocomial virus and fungal infections are uncommon causes of HAP and VAP in immunocompetent patients. Outbreaks of influenza have occurred sporadically, and the risk of infection can be substantially reduced with widespread effective infection control, vaccination, and use of anti-influenza agents.[37–39]

Pathogenesis

The severity of the patient's underlying disease, previous surgery, exposure to antibiotics, other medications, and exposure to invasive respiratory devices and equipment may lead to airway colonization and contribute to the pathogenesis of HAP and VAP.[40,41] Aspiration of oropharyngeal pathogens or leakage of secretions containing bacteria around the endotracheal tube cuff are the primary routes of bacterial entry into the lower respiratory tract.[42–44] Inhalation or direct inoculation of pathogens into the lower airway, hematogenous spread from infected IV catheters, and bacterial translocation from the GI tract lumen are uncommon pathogenic mechanisms.[44] Infected biofilm in the endotracheal tube, with subsequent embolization to distal airways, is another source of entry of infected material into the lung.[45] The stomach and sinuses may be potential reservoirs of nosocomial pathogens that contribute to bacterial colonization of the oropharynx, but the importance of these routes is debated.[46,47]

Diagnosis

The standard diagnostic criteria in VAP include at least two of the following three findings: fever, leukocytosis, and purulent tracheal secretions, usually with abnormal findings on chest radiographic studies. When these conditions occur, the likelihood of VAP is high.[48] The presence of a radiographic infiltrate in a patient with fever, leukocytosis, or purulent tracheobronchial secretions has high diagnostic sensitivity but low specificity. When all four criteria are present, specificity improves but sensitivity decreases to <50%, which is clinically unacceptable.[49] The only study[48] examining interobserver diagnostic reliability found no major differences between individual physicians or those grouped by level or training.

Pugin and coworkers[50] developed the clinical pulmonary infection score (CPIS), which combines clinical, radiographic, physiologic (Pao_2/fraction of inspired oxygen), and microbiologic data into a single numerical result to improve the specificity of clinical diagnosis. When the CPIS exceeded 6, a good correlation with positive quantitative culture findings of bronchoscopic and nonbronchoscopic BAL fluid specimens was observed. These findings have not been reproduced by other investigators, but the accuracy of the CPIS score is improved if a Gram stain of a deep respiratory tract culture is added to the evaluation.[51,52]

These findings suggest that the presence of abnormal clinical manifestations, combined with abnormal radiographic findings, can be used for initial screening for VAP. However, the lack of specificity with this method suggests that additional procedures are needed, such as cultures of lower respiratory tract secretions.

All patients with suspected VAP should have blood cultures collected. The physician ordering the culture should recognize that a positive result can indicate the presence of either pneumonia or extrapulmonary infection.[53] A diagnostic thoracentesis to rule out a complicating empyema or parapneumonic effusion should be performed if the patient has a large pleural effusion or if the patient with a pleural effusion appears toxic. Samples of lower respiratory tract secretions should be obtained from all patients with suspected HAP and should be collected before changes of antibiotic. Samples can include an endotracheal aspirate, BAL fluid sample, or protected specimen brush sample.[54–56] A sterile culture of respiratory secretions in the absence of a new antibiotic in the past 72 h virtually rules out the presence of bacterial pneumonia, but viral or Legionella sp infection are still possible. If these patients have clinical signs of infection, an extrapulmonary site of infection should be investigated.[57]

A reliable tracheal aspirate Gram stain can be used to direct initial empiric antimicrobial therapy and may increase the diagnostic value of the CPIS.[58] The presence of a new or progressive radiographic infiltrate and at least two of three clinical features (fever >38°C, leukocytosis or leukopenia, and purulent secretions) represent the most accurate clinical criteria for starting empiric antibiotic therapy.[51] If a clinical strategy is used, reevaluation of the decision to use antibiotics based on the results of semiquantitative lower respiratory tract cultures and serial clinical evaluations, by day 3 or sooner, is appropriate.[59–61]

Singh and coworkers[60] demonstrated that a modified CPIS of ≤6 for 3 days is an objective criterion to select low-risk patients for early discontinuation of empiric treatment of HAP. Tests that identify pathogens on the basis of qualitative cultures will lead to treatment for more organisms than diagnostic techniques based on quantitative cultures.[57,62–64] Nonbronchoscopic sampling can reliably obtain lower respiratory tract secretions for quantitative cultures if bronchoscopic sampling is not immediately available.[65] The use of a bronchoscopic bacteriologic strategy has been shown to reduce 14-day mortality but not the 28-day mortality, compared with a clinical strategy, in one study[57] of suspected VAP.

Three other smaller studies demonstrated no advantage of an invasive diagnostic approach. A randomized controlled trial[66] comparing the utility of bronchoscopic lavage with quantitative culture of BAL fluid or endotracheal aspirate with nonquantitative culture of the aspirate identified no significant difference in the 28-day mortality rate (the primary outcome), the rate of targeted therapy, days alive without antibiotics, hospital or ICU length of stay, or maximum organ dysfunction scores. Delays in the initiation of appropriate antibiotic therapy can increase the rate of mortality of VA and, thus, therapy should not be delayed for the purpose of performing diagnostic studies in patients who are clinically unstable.[37,67,68]

Therapy

Initial empiric therapy should be selected based on the absence or presence of risk factors for MDR pathogens. These risk factors include prolonged duration of hospitalization (≥5 days), admission from a health-care-related facility, and recent prolonged antibiotic therapy (Table 1).[14] Choice of specific agents should be dictated by local microbiology, cost, availability, and formulary restrictions (Tables 2 and 3).[69,70] Patients with health-care-related pneumonia should be treated for potentially drug-resistant organisms regardless of when during the hospital stay the pneumonia begins. Inappropriate therapy (failure of the etiologic pathogen to be sensitive to the administered antibiotic) is a major risk factor for excess mortality

Table 2. *Initial Empiric Antibiotic Therapy for HAP or VAP in Patients With No Known Risk Factors for MDR Pathogens, Early Onset, and Any Disease Severity*

Potential Pathogens	Recommended Antibiotic
Streptococcus pneumoniae *Haemophilus influenzae* Methicillin-sensitive *S aureus* Antibiotic-sensitive enteric Gram-negative bacilli *E coli* *K pneumoniae* Enterobacter species Proteus species *Serratia marcescens*	Ceftriaxone; or levofloxacin, moxifloxacin, or ciprofloxacin or ampicillin/sulbactam or ertapenem

Table 3. *Initial Empiric Therapy for HAP, VAP, and Health-Care-Associated Pneumonia in Patients With Late-Onset Disease or Risk Factors for MDR Pathogens and All Disease Severity*

Potential Pathogens	Combination Antibiotic Therapy
Pathogens listed in Table 2 and MDR pathogens	Antipseudomonal cephalosporin (cefepime, ceftazidime); or
P aeruginosa	Antipseudomonal carbepenem (imipenem or meropenem); or
K pneumoniae (extended-spectrum β-lactamase positive)	β-lactam/β-lactamase inhibitor (piperacillintazobactam) plus
Acinetobacter species	Antipseudomonal fluoroquinolone (ciprofloxacin or levofloxacin; or
MRSA	Aminoglycoside (amikacin, gentamicin, or tobramycin)
L pneumophila	Plus linezolid or vancomycin

and length of stay for patients with HAP, and antibiotic-resistant organisms are the pathogens most commonly associated with inappropriate therapy.[67] In selecting empiric therapy for patients who have recently received an antibiotic, an effort should be made to use an agent from a different antibiotic class because recent therapy increases the probability of inappropriate therapy and can predispose to resistance to that same class of antibiotics.[70] Initial antibiotic therapy should be administered promptly because delays in administration may add to excess mortality resulting from VAP.[68,71,72]

Empiric therapy of patients with severe HAP or VAP requires the use of antibiotics at optimal doses to ensure maximum efficacy.[73] Initial therapy should be administered IV to all patients, with a switch to oral/enteral therapy in selected patients with a good clinical response and a functioning intestinal tract. Highly bioavailable agents, such as the quinolones and linezolid, may be easily switched to oral therapy in such patients. Combination therapy should be used if patients are likely to have infection with MDR pathogens.[68] No data have documented the superiority of this approach compared with monotherapy, except to enhance the likelihood of initially appropriate empiric therapy. If patients receive combination therapy with an aminoglycoside-containing regimen, the aminoglycoside can be stopped after 5 to 7 days in responding patients.[74] Monotherapy with selected agents can be used for patients with severe HAP and VAP in the absence of resistant pathogens.[73] Patients in this risk group should initially receive combination therapy until the results of lower respiratory tract cultures are known and confirm that a single agent can be used. If patients receive an initially appropriate antibiotic regimen, therapy can be shortened from the traditional 14 to 21 days to periods as little as 7 days, provided that the etiologic pathogen is not *P aeruginosa* and that the patient has a good clinical response.[75,76]

If *P aeruginosa* pneumonia is documented, combination therapy is recommended. The principal justification is the high frequency of development of resistance on monotherapy.[74] Although combination therapy will not necessarily prevent the development of resistance, combination therapy is more likely to avoid inappropriate and ineffective treatment of patients.[67] If Acinetobacter sp are documented to be present, the most active agents are the carbapenems, sulbactam, colistin, and polymyxin. There are no data documenting an improved outcome if these organisms are treated with a combination regimen.[77] If extended-spectrum β-lactamase—positive Enterobacteriaceae sp are isolated, the use of third-generation cephalosporins should be avoided and carbapenems considered.[78] Linezolid is an alternative to vancomycin for the treatment of MRSA VAP. A subset analysis of two prospective randomized trials[79,80] has indicated that the use of linezolid may be superior to vancomycin. This agent may also be preferred if patients have renal insufficiency or are receiving other nephrotoxic agents, but more data are needed. Antibiotic restriction can limit epidemics of infection with specific resistant pathogens. The heterogeneity of antibiotic prescriptions, including formal antibiotic cycling, may be able to reduce the overall frequency of antibiotic resistance. However, the long-term impact of this practice is unknown.[81,82]

A serial assessment of clinical parameters should be used to define the response to initial empiric therapy.[59,61] Modifications of empiric therapy should be made on the basis of this information in conjunction with microbiologic data. Clinical improvement usually takes 48 to 72 h, and thus, therapy should not be changed during this time unless there is rapid clinical decline. Nonresponse to therapy is usually evident by day 3 and can be ascertained by an assessment of clinical parameters.[59,61] Serum procalcitonin may act as a prognostic marker in VAP, with increased levels despite the use of therapy predicting a poor outcome.[83] The responding patient's antibiotics should be reduced and his or her therapy narrowed to the most focused regimen possible on the basis of culture data.[69] The nonresponding patient should be evaluated for noninfectious mimics of pneumonia, unsuspected or drug-resistant organisms, extrapulmonary sites of infection, and complications of pneumonia and its therapy. Diagnostic testing should be directed to whichever of these causes is likely.[84]

New Developments

Twice-weekly quantitative surveillance cultures of endotracheal aspirates may assist in the early prescription of appropriate antibiotic treatments for patients who acquire VAP.[85] This strategy may improve clinical outcomes, potentially may reduce antibiotic resistance in patients in critical care units and related complications, and may reduce hospitalization costs. Antibiotic selection based on the available results of pre-VAP endotracheal aspirate cultures was adequate in 38 of 40 patients (95%) in a recent small study.[86] In contrast, had the guidelines of the American Thoracic Society/Infectious Diseases Society of America guidelines[34] and Trouillet et al[14] been used, empiric antibiotic treatment would have been adequate in 68% and 83% of patients, respectively. The main reason for the inadequate coverage using the published guidelines was the failure of the guidelines to inform the empiric treatment selection in the coverage of highly resistant pathogens. Before this strategy can be widely adopted, prospective randomized trials are needed to confirm this observation. This approach to the diagnosis and management of nosocomial pneumonia has been summarized in the recently published American Thoracic Society guidelines for the management of adults with HAP, VAP, and health-care--associated pneumonia.[34]

In a prospective, observational, cohort study, variables independently associated with ICU rate of mortality were derived from 441 patients with VAP.[85] Results were converted into a four-variable score based on the PIRO (predisposition, insult, response, organ dysfunction) concept for ICU mortality risk stratification in VAP patients. The VAP PIRO score identified four independent variables associated with mortality (comorbidities [COPD, immunocompromise, heart failure, cirrhosis, or chronic renal failure], bacteremia, systolic BP <90 mm Hg, and ARDS), allowing assessment of severity. On the basis of observed mortality for each VAP PIRO score, patients were stratified into three levels of risk: (1) mild, 0 to 1 points; (2) high, 2 points; and (3) very high, 3 to 4 points. The VAP PIRO score was associated with greater risk of death in the high-risk group and the very-high-risk group. The use of this scoring may improve prediction of outcomes, allowing the more appropriate use of medical resources.

Sixty episodes of VAP treated with appropriate therapy (*H influenzae*, 15 episodes; methicillin-sensitive *S aureus*, 15 episodes; *P aeruginosa*, 15 episodes; and MRSA 15 episodes), and 30 episodes with initial inappropriate therapy, all caused by *P aeruginosa*, were compared in a prospective observational study.[87] A significant delay in the resolution of hypoxemia was observed in VAP episodes caused by MRSA and *P aeruginosa* with inappropriate antibiotic therapy when compared with the remaining pathogens. MRSA VAP was associated with longer respiratory support independent of the appropriateness of initial antibiotic therapy. More aggressive management may be required for these difficult to treat pathogens.

A prospective randomized trial compared conventional and continuous aspiration of subglottic secretions (CASS) procedures in ventilated patients after major heart surgery.[88] CASS was a safe procedure that reduced the use of antimicrobial agents in the overall population and the incidence of VAP in at-risk patients (ventilated for >48 h). The cost of the CASS tube was \$12.60 (€9) vs \$2.10 (€1.5) for the conventional tube. This is more evidence to support the use of these more expensive endotracheal tubes, at least in patients undergoing major heart surgery.

In a prospective observational study involving 105 consecutive patients receiving mechanical ventilation and undergoing BAL, BAL fluid soluble triggering receptor expressed on myeloid cells-1 concentration was measured to determine the diagnostic utility of this measurement.[89] Receiver operating curve analysis and multivariate logistic regression analysis demonstrated that measurement of soluble triggering receptor expressed on myeloid cells-1 was inferior to clinical parameters for the diagnosis of VAP. Previous studies had suggested this measurement may assist in the diagnosis of VAP, and therefore, these findings are disappointing.

In a prospective, randomized, controlled, unblinded, multicenter study, patients with nosocomial tracheobronchitis were randomly assigned to receive or not receive IV antibiotics for 8 days.[90] Antimicrobial treatment was associated with a greater number of days free of mechanical ventilation and lower rates of VAP and ICU rate of mortality. However, antibiotic treatment had no significant impact on total duration of mechanical ventilation. This study and previous ones demonstrate the importance of nosocomial tracheobronchitis as a precursor to VAP and suggest therapy at this early stage may improve outcomes.

References

1. Tablan OC, Anderson LJ, Besser R, et al. Guidelines for preventing health-care-associated pneumonia, 2003: recommendations of the CDC and the Healthcare Infection Control Practices Advisory Committee. MMWR Recomm Rep 2004; 53(RR-3):1–36
2. Craven DE, Kunches LM, Kilinsky V, et al. Risk factors for pneumonia and fatality in patients receiving continuous mechanical ventilation. Am Rev Respir Dis 1986; 133:792–796
3. Chastre J, Fagon JY. Ventilator-associated pneumonia. Am J Respir Crit Care Med 2002; 165: 867–903
4. Fagon JY, Chastre J, Hance AJ, et al. Nosocomial pneumonia in ventilated patients: a cohort study evaluating attributable mortality and hospital stay. Am J Med 1993; 94:281–288
5. Rello J, Ollendorf DA, Oster G, et al. Epidemiology and outcomes of ventilator-associated pneumonia in a large US database. Chest 2002; 122:2115–2121
6. Celis R, Torres A, Gatell JM, et al. Nosocomial pneumonia: a multivariate analysis of risk and prognosis. Chest 1988; 93:318–324
7. Torres A, Aznar R, Gatell JM, et al. Incidence, risk, and prognosis factors of nosocomial pneumonia in mechanically ventilated patients. Am Rev Respir Dis 1990; 142:523–528
8. Richards MJ, Edwards JR, Culver DH, et al. Nosocomial infections in medical ICUs in the United States: National Nosocomial Infections Surveillance System. Crit Care Med 1999; 27: 887–892
9. Cook DJ, Walter SD, Cook RJ, et al. Incidence of and risk factors for ventilator-associated pneumonia in critically ill patients. Ann Intern Med 1998; 129:433–440
10. Brochard L, Mancebo J, Wysocki M, et al. Noninvasive ventilation for acute exacerbations of chronic obstructive pulmonary disease. N Engl J Med 1995; 333:817–822
11. Antonelli M, Conti G, Rocco M, et al. A comparison of noninvasive positive-pressure ventilation and conventional mechanical ventilation in patients with acute respiratory failure. N Engl J Med 1998; 339:429–435
12. Hilbert G, Gruson D, Vargas F, et al. Noninvasive ventilation in immunosuppressed patients with pulmonary infiltrates, fever, and acute respiratory failure. N Engl J Med 2001; 344:817–822
13. American Thoracic Society. Hospital-acquired pneumonia in adults: diagnosis, assessment of severity, initial antimicrobial therapy, and preventive strategies. Am J Respir Crit Care Med 1996; 153:1711–1725
14. Trouillet JL, Chastre J, Vuagnat A, et al. Ventilator associated pneumonia caused by potentially drug-resistant bacteria. Am J Respir Crit Care Med 1998; 157:531–539
15. Heyland DK, Cook DJ, Griffith L, et al. The attributable morbidity and mortality of ventilator-associated

pneumonia in the critically ill patient. Am J Respir Crit Care Med 1999; 159:1249–1256

16. Rello J, Ausina V, Ricart M, et al. Impact of previous antimicrobial therapy on the etiology and outcome of ventilator-associated pneumonia. Chest 1993; 104:1230–1235
17. Chastre J, Trouillet JL, Vuagnat A, et al. Nosocomial pneumonia in patients with acute respiratory distress syndrome. Am J Respir Crit Care Med 1998; 157:1165–1172
18. Bregeon F, Ciais V, Carret V, et al. Is ventilator-associated pneumonia an independent risk factor for death? Anesthesiology 2001; 94:554–560
19. Papazian L, Bregeon F, Thirion X, et al. Effect of ventilator-associated pneumonia on mortality and morbidity. Am J Respir Crit Care Med 1996; 154:91–97
20. Craven DE, Steger KA. Epidemiology of nosocomial pneumonia: new perspectives on an old disease. Chest 1995; 108:1S–16S
21. Dore P, Robert R, Grollier G, et al. Incidence of anaerobes in ventilator-associated pneumonia with use of a protected specimen brush. Am J Respir Crit Care Med 1996; 153:1292–1298
22. Yu VL, Kroboth FJ, Shonnard J, et al. Legionnaires' disease: new clinical perspective from a prospective pneumonia study. Am J Med 1982; 73:357–361
23. El Solh AA, Sikka P, Ramadan F, et al. Etiology of severe pneumonia in the very elderly. Am J Respir Crit Care Med 2001; 163:645–651
24. El Solh AA, Aquilina AT, Dhillon RS, et al. Impact of invasive strategy on management of antimicrobial treatment failure in institutionalized older people with severe pneumonia. Am J Respir Crit Care Med 2002; 166:1038–1043
25. Lim WS, Macfarlane JT. A prospective comparison of nursing home acquired pneumonia with community acquired pneumonia. Eur Respir J 2001; 18:362–368
26. Fridkin SK. Increasing prevalence of antimicrobial resistance in intensive care units. Crit Care Med 2001; 29:N64–N68
27. Rello J, Torres A, Ricart M, et al. Ventilator associated pneumonia by Staphylococcus aureus: comparison of methicillin-resistant and methicillin-sensitive episodes. Am J Respir Crit Care Med 1994; 150:1545–1549
28. Torres A, Puig de la Bellacasa J, Xaubet A, et al. Diagnostic value of quantitative cultures of bronchoalveolar lavage and telescoping plugged catheters in mechanically ventilated patients with bacterial pneumonia. Am Rev Respir Dis 1989; 140:306–310
29. Luna CM, Vujacich P, Niederman MS, et al. Impact of B AL data on the therapy and outcome of ventilator-associated pneumonia. Chest 1997; 111:676–685
30. Markowicz P, Wolff M, Djedaini K, et al. ARDS Study Group: multicenter prospective study of ventilator-associated pneumonia during acute respiratory distress syndrome: incidence, prognosis, and risk factors. Am J Respir Crit Care Med 2000; 161:1942–1948
31. Johanson WG Jr., Pierce AK, Sanford JP, et al. Nosocomial respiratory infections with Gram-negative bacilli: the significance of colonization of the respiratory tract. Ann Intern Med 1972; 77:701–706
32. Rello J, Sa-Borges M, Correa H, et al. Variations in etiology of ventilator-associated pneumonia across four treatment sites: implications for antimicrobial prescribing practices. Am J Respir Crit Care Med 1999; 160:608–613
33. Marik PE, Careau P. The role of anaerobes in patients with ventilator-associated pneumonia and aspiration pneumonia: a prospective study. Chest 1999; 115:178–183
34. American Thoracic Society, Infectious Diseases Society of America. Guidelines for the management of adults with hospital-acquired, ventilator-associated and healthcare-associated pneumonia. Am J Respir Crit Care Med 2005; 171:388–416
35. Stout J, Yu VL, Vickers RM, et al. Potable water supply as the hospital reservoir for Pittsburgh pneumonia agent. Lancet 1982; 1:471–472
36. Yu VL, Kroboth FJ, Shonnard J, et al. Legionnaires' disease: new clinical perspective from a prospective pneumonia study. Am J Med 1982; 73:357–361
37. El-Ebiary M, Torres A, Fabregas N, et al. Significance of the isolation of Candida species from respiratory samples in critically ill, non-neutropenic patients. Am J Respir Crit Care Med 1997; 156:583–590
38. Krasinski K, Holzman RS, Hanna B, et al. Nosocomial fungal infection during hospital renovation. Infect Control 1985; 6:278–282
39. Pachucki CT, Pappas SA, Fuller GF, et al. Influenza among hospital personnel and patients: implications for recognition, prevention, and control. Arch Intern Med 1989; 149:77–80
40. Kollef MH. The prevention of ventilator-associated pneumonia. N Engl J Med 1999; 340:627–634

41. Craven DE, Steger KA. Nosocomial pneumonia in mechanically ventilated adult patients: epidemiology and prevention in 1996. Semin Respir Infect 1996; 11:32–53
42. Valles J, Artigas A, Rello J, et al. Continuous aspiration of subglottic secretions in preventing ventilator-associated pneumonia. Ann Intern Med 1995; 122:179–186
43. Cook D, De Jonghe B, Brochard L, et al. Influence of airway management on ventilator-associated pneumonia: evidence from randomized trials. JAMA 1998; 279:781–787
44. Bergmans DC, Bonten MJ, van Tiel FH, et al. Cross-colonisation with Pseudomonas aeruginosa of patients in an intensive care unit. Thorax 1998; 53:1053–1058
45. Inglis TJ, Millar MR, Jones JG, et al. Tracheal tube biofilm as a source of bacterial colonization of the lung. J Clin Microbiol 1989; 27:2014–2018
46. Bonten MJ. Controversies on diagnosis and prevention of ventilator-associated pneumonia. Diagn Microbiol Infect Dis 1999; 34:199–204
47. Rouby JJ, Laurent P, Gosnach M, et al. Risk factors and clinical relevance of nosocomial maxillary sinusitis in the critically ill. Am J Respir Crit Care Med 1994; 150:776–783
48. Fagon J, Chastre J, Hance A. Evaluation of clinical judgment in the identification and treatment of nosocomial pneumonia in ventilated patients. Chest 1993; 103:547–553
49. Sutherland K, Steinberg K, Maunder R, et al. Pulmonary infection during the acute respiratory distress syndrome. Am J Respir Crit Care Med 1995; 152:550–556
50. Pugin J, Auckenthaler R, Mili N, et al. Diagnosis of ventilator-associated pneumonia by bacteriologic analysis of bronchoscopic and nonbronchoscopic "blind" bronchoalveolar lavage fluid. Am Rev Respir Dis 1991; 143:1121–1129
51. Fabregas N, Ewig S, Torres A, et al. Clinical diagnosis of ventilator associated pneumonia revisited: comparative validation using immediate post-mortem lung biopsies. Thorax 1999; 54:867–873
52. Fartoukh M, Maitre B, Honore S, et al. Diagnosing pneumonia during mechanical ventilation: the clinical pulmonary infection score revisited. Am J Respir Crit Care Med 2003; 168:173–179
53. Luna CM, Videla A, Mattera J, et al. Blood cultures have limited value in predicting severity of illness and as a diagnostic tool in ventilator-associated pneumonia. Chest 1999; 116:1075–1084
54. Marquette CH, Herengt F, Mathieu D, et al. Diagnosis of pneumonia in mechanically ventilated patients: repeatability of the protected specimen brush. Am Rev Respir Dis 1993; 147:211–214
55. Michaud S, Suzuki S, Harbarth S. Effect of design-related bias in studies of diagnostic tests for ventilator-associated pneumonia. Am J Respir Crit Care Med 2002; 166:1320–1325
56. Souweine B, Veber B, Bedos JP, et al. Diagnostic accuracy of protected specimen brush and bronchoalveolar lavage in nosocomial pneumonia: impact of previous antimicrobial treatments. Crit Care Med 1998; 26:236–244
57. Fagon JY, Chastre J, Wolff M, et al. Invasive and noninvasive strategies for management of suspected ventilator-associated pneumonia: a randomized trial. Ann Intern Med 2000; 132:621–630
58. Cook D, Mandell L. Endotracheal aspiration in the diagnosis of ventilator-associated pneumonia. Chest 2000;117:195S–197S
59. Dennesen PJ, Van der Ven AJ, Kessels AG, et al. Resolution of infectious parameters after antimicrobial therapy in patients with ventilator-associated pneumonia. Am J Respir Crit Care Med 2001; 163:1371–1375
60. Singh N, Rogers P, Atwood CW, et al. Short-course empiric antibiotic therapy for patients with pulmonary infiltrates in the intensive care unit: a proposed solution for indiscriminate antibiotic prescription. Am J Respir Crit Care Med 2000; 162:505–511
61. Luna CM, Blanzaco D, Niederman MS, et al. Resolution of ventilator-associated pneumonia: prospective evaluation of the clinical pulmonary infection score as an early clinical predictor of outcome. Crit Care Med 2003; 31:676–682
62. Sanchez-Nieto JM, Torres A, Garcia-Cordoba F, et al. Impact of invasive and noninvasive quantitative culture sampling on outcome of ventilator-associated pneumonia: a pilot study. Am J Respir Crit Care Med 1998; 157:371–376
63. Ruiz M, Torres A, Ewig S, et al. Noninvasive versus invasive microbial investigation in ventilator-associated pneumonia: evaluation of outcome. Am J Respir Crit Care Med 2000; 162:119–125
64. Sole Violan J, Fernandez JA, Benitez AB, et al. Impact of quantitative invasive diagnostic techniques in the management and outcome of

mechanically ventilated patients with suspected pneumonia. Crit Care Med 2000; 28:2737–2741
65. Campbell GD. Blinded invasive diagnostic procedures in ventilator-associated pneumonia. Chest 2000;117:207S–211S
66. The Canadian Critical Care Trials Group. A randomized trial of diagnostic techniques for ventilator-associated pneumonia. N Engl J Med 2006; 355: 2619–2630
67. Kollef MH, Sherman G, Ward S, et al. Inadequate antimicrobial treatment of infections: a risk factor for hospital mortality among critically ill patients. Chest 1999; 115:462–474
68. Luna CM, Aruj P, Niederman MS, et al. Appropriateness and delay to initiate therapy in ventilator-associated pneumonia. Eur Respir J 2006; 27:158–164
69. Ibrahim EH, Ward S, Sherman G, et al. Experience with a clinical guideline for the treatment of ventilator-associated pneumonia. Crit Care Med 2001; 29:1109–1115
70. Namias N, Samiian L, Nino D, et al. Incidence and susceptibility of pathogenic bacteria vary between intensive care units within a single hospital: implications for empiric antibiotic strategies. J Trauma 2000; 49:638–645
71. Trouillet JL, Vuagnat A, Combes A, et al. Pseudomonas aeruginosa ventilator-associated pneumonia: comparison of episodes due to piperacillin-resistant versus piperacillin-susceptible organisms. Clin Infect Dis 2002; 34:1047–1054
72. Garnacho-Montero J, Garcia-Garmendia JL, Barrero-Almodovar A, et al. Impact of the outcome of adequate empirical antibiotherapy in patients admitted to the ICU for sepsis. Crit Care Med 2003; 31:2742–2751
73. Leone M, Bourgoin A, Cambon S, et al. Empirical antimicrobial therapy of septic shock patients: adequacy and impact on the outcome. Crit Care Med 2003; 31:462–467
74. Fink MP, Snydman DR, Niederman MS, et al. Treatment of severe pneumonia in hospitalized patients: results of a multicenter, randomized, double-blind trial comparing intravenous ciprofloxacin with imipenem-cilastatin. Antimicrob Agents Chemother 1994; 38:547–557
75. Gruson D, Hilbert G, Vargas F, et al. Rotation and restricted use of antibiotics in a medical intensive care unit: impact on the incidence of ventilator-associated pneumonia caused by antibiotic-resistant Gram-negative bacteria. Am J Respir Crit Care Med 2000; 162:837–843
76. Chastre J, Wolff M, Fagon JY, et al. Comparison of 8 vs 15 days of antibiotic therapy for ventilator-associated pneumonia in adults: a randomized trial. JAMA 2003; 290:2588–2598
77. Garnacho-Montero J, Ortiz-Leyba C, Jimenez Jimenez FJ, et al. Treatment of multidrug-resistant Acinetobacter baumannii ventilator-associated pneumonia (VAP) with intravenous colistin: a comparison with imipenem-susceptible VAP. Clin Infect Dis 2003; 36:1111–1118
78. Paterson DL, Ko WC, Von Gottberg A, et al. Outcome of cephalosporin treatment for serious infections due to apparently susceptible organisms producing extended-spectrum β-lactamases: implications for the clinical microbiology laboratory. J Clin Microbiol 2001; 39:2206–2212
79. Wunderink RG, Rello J, Cammarata SK, et al. Linezolid vs vancomycin: analysis of two double-blind studies of patients with methicillin-resistant Staphylococcus aureus nosocomial pneumonia. Chest 2003; 124:1789–1797
80. Rubinstein E, Cammarata S, Oliphant T, et al. Linezolid (PNU-100766) versus vancomycin in the treatment of hospitalized patients with nosocomial pneumonia: a randomized, double blind, multicenter study. Clin Infect Dis 2001; 32:402–412
81. Kollef MH, Vlasnik J, Sharpless L, et al. Scheduled change of antibiotic classes: a strategy to decrease the incidence of ventilator-associated pneumonia. Am J Respir Crit Care Med 1997; 156:1040–1048
82. Gruson D, Hilbert G, Vargas F, et al. Strategy of antibiotic rotation: long-term effect on incidence and susceptibilities of Gram-negative bacilli responsible for ventilator associated pneumonia. Crit Care Med 2003; 31:1908–1914
83. Luyt C-E, Guerin V, Combes A, et al. Procalcitonin kinetics as a prognostic marker of ventilator-associated pneumonia. Am J Respir Crit Care Med 2005; 171:48–53
84. Meduri GU, Mauldin GL, Wunderink RG, et al. Causes of fever and pulmonary densities in patients with clinical manifestations of ventilator-associated pneumonia. Chest 1994; 106:221–235
85. Lisboa T, Diaz E, Sa-Borges M, et al. The ventilator-associated pneumonia PIRO score. Chest 2008; 134:1208–1216

86. Michel F, Franceschini B, Berger P, et al. Early antibiotic treatment for BAL-confirmed ventilator-associated pneumonia: a role for routine endotracheal aspirate cultures. Chest 2005; 127:589–597
87. Vidaur L, Planas K, Sierra R, et al. Ventilator-associated pneumonia. Chest 2008; 133:625–632
88. Bouza E, Pérez MJ, Muñoz P, et al. Continuous aspiration of subglottic secretions in the prevention of ventilator-associated pneumonia in the postoperative period of major heart surgery. Chest 2008; 134:938–946
89. Anand NJ, Zuick S, Klesney-Tait J, et al. Diagnostic implications of soluble triggering receptor expressed on myeloid cells-1 in bal fluid of patients with pulmonary infiltrates in the ICU. Chest 2009; 135:641–647
90. Nseir S, Favory R Jozefowicz E, et al. Antimicrobial treatment for ventilator-associated tracheobronchitis: a randomized, controlled, multicenter study. Critical Care 2008; 12:R62

Hypoxemic Respiratory Failure

Curtis N. Sessler, MD, FCCP

Objectives:

- Examine the causes of hypoxemic respiratory failure
- Review the pathophysiology, diagnostic criteria, clinical features, and epidemiology for acute lung injury (ALI) and the ARDS
- Examine management strategies for ALI/ARDS, including mechanical ventilation, medical management, and rescue therapy for refractory hypoxemia

Key words: acute lung injury; ARDS; hypoxemia; mechanical ventilation

Hypoxemic Respiratory Failure

Pulmonary Gas Exchange

The disruption of gas exchange, as a result of one or more of numerous pathophysiologic mechanisms, can cause a significant elevation in $Paco_2$, *ie*, hypercapnia, and/or a reduction in Pao_2, *ie*, hypoxemia. The normal range of Pao_2 varies with age as a result of the loss of effective alveoli during advancing age and can be approximated from the following equation: $Pao_2 = 100.1 - 0.32 \times$ (age in years). This equation assumes the individual is breathing ambient air and is near sea level. Pao_2 will decline progressively with increasing altitude greater than sea level as a result of decreasing barometric pressure and, thus, lower Po_2 of inhaled gas.

Hypoxemia and Hypoxia: Mechanisms and Measurement

Hypoxemia usually arises as a result of disrupted alveolar ventilation and/or perfusion that causes relative impaired or absent ventilation of perfused alveoli. The range of ventilation–perfusion mismatching of the 300 million or so alveoli runs the spectrum from near absence of ventilation (shunt-like) to absence of perfusion (dead space). In fewer cases, hypoxemia is the result of true shunting of venous blood that admixes with oxygenated blood, producing hypoxemia. These conditions cause an increased gradient between calculated PAO_2 and measured Pao_2, as calculated in the equation:

$$P(A - a)O_2 = (\text{barometric pressure} - 47 \text{ mm Hg}) \times 0.21 - Paco_2/RQ - Pao_2,$$

where 47 mm Hg represents the partial pressure of water vapor, RQ is the respiratory quotient (generally regarded to be 0.8 to 1.0), and $P(A\text{-}a)O_2$ is alveolar-arterial oxygen pressure difference.

While one is breathing ambient air at sea level, $PAO_2 = 150 - (Paco_2/0.8)$, and $P(A\text{-}a)O_2$ should be <10 to 15 mm Hg. In contrast, generalized alveolar hypoventilation without ventilation/perfusion mismatch can result in hypercapnia plus hypoxemia with a normal $P(A\text{-}a)O_2$. Supplemental oxygen often is administered for hypoxemia, and in this setting, the relative degree of hypoxemia is more accurately estimated by use of the ratio of Pao_2 to the fraction of oxygen of inhaled gas (Fio_2), or Pao_2:Fio_2, than with $P(A\text{-}a)O_2$. In the presence of diffuse parenchymal lung disease, the ratios <300 mm Hg and <200 mm Hg are general thresholds for moderate and severe hypoxemia, respectively.

Although hypoxemia represents low oxygen tension in blood, tissue hypoxia can occur through various mechanisms that impair oxygen delivery or utilization from a cellular perspective. Reductions in oxygen delivery include hypoxemic hypoxia from reduced oxygen tension in arterial blood, anemic hypoxia (in which reductions in oxygen content of blood is caused by reduced oxygen-carrying capacity via loss of hemoglobin or hemoglobin dysfunction), and circulatory hypoxia (in which depressed cardiac output or vascular factors impair oxygen delivery to tissue). Finally, metabolic forms of hypoxia occur at the cellular level when oxygen utilization is disrupted.

Clinical Manifestations and Causative Conditions of Hypoxemia

A variety of symptoms and clinical signs may accompany hypoxemia, including dyspnea, tachypnea, tachycardia, hypertension, cardiac arrhythmias (including bradycardia progressive to asystole in extreme cases), tremor, anxiety, delirium, and agitation. Often additional clinical manifestations are present that reflect the underlying causative condition(s). The pace of onset of clinical manifestations can be more gradual, as with slow progression of long-standing illness, or may be abrupt from rapidly progressive cardiopulmonary disease. Common clinical conditions which are associated with hypoxemic respiratory failure are listed in Table 1. Among these associated clinical conditions, acute lung injury (ALI)/ARDS represents a continuum of a syndrome of parenchymal lung disease characterized by high-protein alveolar edema and diffuse inflammation that usually has a specific underlying cause(s).

Management Principles for Hypoxemic Respiratory Failure

Care of the patient who has hypoxemic respiratory failure includes initial evaluation and stabilization, assessment and management of the underlying conditions, support of oxygenation and ventilation, application of interventions identified as being associated with improved outcomes, consideration of use of rescue therapies for refractory hypoxemia, and supportive care. General considerations for initial evaluation and stabilization and support of oxygenation and ventilation in hypoxemic respiratory failure are discussed here, whereas issues more directly related to ALI / ARDS, such as evidence-based interventions and rescue therapy for refractory hypoxemia, are addressed below.

Table 1. *Common Clinical Conditions Associated With Hypoxemic Respiratory Failure*

Acute lung injury (ALI)/ARDS
Pulmonary edema
Diffuse alveolar hemorrhage
Pulmonary embolism
Interstitial lung disease
Infectious pneumonia
Pneumonitis
Neoplasm
Pulmonary contusion
Atelectasis
Emphysema
Asthma
Chronic bronchitis
Bronchiolitis

Initial Evaluation and Stabilization: Basic life-support measures, including management of the airway and breathing, should be rapidly initiated. Life-threatening respiratory distress will often require urgent endotracheal intubation and mechanical ventilation. Assessment of oxygenation and ventilation by arterial blood gas analysis is useful, and pulse oximetry may provide continuous display of oxygenation, including response to therapy. Initial evaluation should also include timely detection and management of urgent conditions, such as airway obstruction or tension pneumothorax.

Supplemental Oxygen and Artificial Ventilation: Supplemental oxygen can be administered by a variety of interfaces, including face mask, face tent, and nasal cannula, with greater effective FIO_2 being delivered with a tight-fitting nonrebreather mask. Mechanical ventilation, with delivery of positive pressure breaths for alveolar ventilation, as well as positive end-expiratory pressure (PEEP) for alveolar recruitment and distention, can be provided by the use of a ventilator and delivered via an endotracheal or tracheostomy tube or with a tightly fitting mask applied to the face or nose. The addition of PEEP is particularly effective for improving oxygenation in the setting of diffuse lung disease and poorly compliant lungs as seen in ALI/ARDS and similar conditions. Details regarding positive pressure ventilation, including noninvasive positive pressure ventilation are discussed more extensively in other chapters.

ALI and ARDS

Definitions

ARDS was first described in 1967 as the acute onset of hypoxemic respiratory failure accompanied by diffuse pulmonary infiltrates in the absence of a cardiac failure and after an inciting event. Although broadly debated, specific diagnostic criteria based on readily available information form the basis for the American European consensus conference definitions, the essential elements of which are displayed in Table 2. It is noteworthy that exclusion of left atrial hypertension as the cause for pulmonary edema is inexact. For example, measurement of pulmonary capillary wedge pressure (PCWP), or more properly *pulmonary artery occlusion pressure*, is performed infrequently in current practice, and elevations in PCWP may reflect volume expansion in the setting of ALI as the result of sepsis-induced capillary leak, rather than heart failure, per se. In the ARDS Network (ARDSNet) randomized controlled trial (RCT) that compared fluid management guided by measurements from a central venous catheter vs a pulmonary artery catheter (PAC), 29% of patients with ALI had PCWP >18 mm Hg, nearly all of whom had normal or elevated cardiac output. Although increased alveolar capillary leak for protein as well as pulmonary inflammation, factors that might more accurately reflect the pathophysiology of ALI than other criteria, have been demonstrated in research settings, such measurements are not availability for widespread clinical use.

Clinical Features

Clinical features of ALI/ARDS at the onset of illness include manifestations of hypoxemia as described previously as well as signs and symptoms related to the underlying cause(s). When data from large RCTs are used, it is shown that most patients have sepsis, pneumonia, gastric aspiration, and/or trauma as the cause. It is noteworthy that the manifestations that are directly related to ALI/ARDS can change over time. In the early phase of ARDS, progressive hypoxemia and increased work of breathing caused by the development of pulmonary edema typically results in hypoxemia that is partially responsive to supplemental oxygen but may also lead to frank respiratory distress and ventilatory failure. The pace of onset varies, but in general, is faster with aspiration lung injury (90% of cases of ARDS develop within 48 h of insult) than sepsis (75% within 48 h) or trauma (65% within 48 h). Some patients recover quickly with effective transport of sodium and water from alveoli and re-epithelialization with type II pneumocytes, whereas others lapse into a condition characterized by ongoing inflammation and disorganized fibrosis. This "fibroproliferative" phase of ARDS often is heralded by ongoing fever, leukocytosis, and acute alveolar inflammation, with a predominance of neutrophils found in BAL fluid.

The chest radiograph typically demonstrates bilateral infiltrates that are patchy or confluent and often are described as alveolar or ground glass. In contrast to cardiogenic pulmonary edema, features such as cardiomegaly, pleural effusions, and widening of the vascular pedicle are not prominent. Although these infiltrates usually appear diffuse on chest radiograph, cross-sectional imaging with the use of CT reveals heterogeneity of infiltrates. Often there is consolidation involving dependent lung units with areas of near-normal appearing lung and atelectatic lung units in mid and upper lung zones, as seen in Figure 1. Interestingly, quickly after moving the patient from supine to

Table 2. *American European Consensus Criteria for ALI and ARDS*

All features must be present:

1. Acute onset (<7 days)
2. Hypoxemia
   a. ALI: Pao_2:Fio_2 <300 mm Hg
   b. ARDS: Pao_2:Fio_2 <200 mm Hg
3. Diffuse bilateral pulmonary infiltrates on frontal chest radiograph consistent with pulmonary edema; infiltrates can be patchy and/or asymmetric
4. absence of left atrial hypertension based upon clinical assessment or PCWP <18 mm Hg if measured.

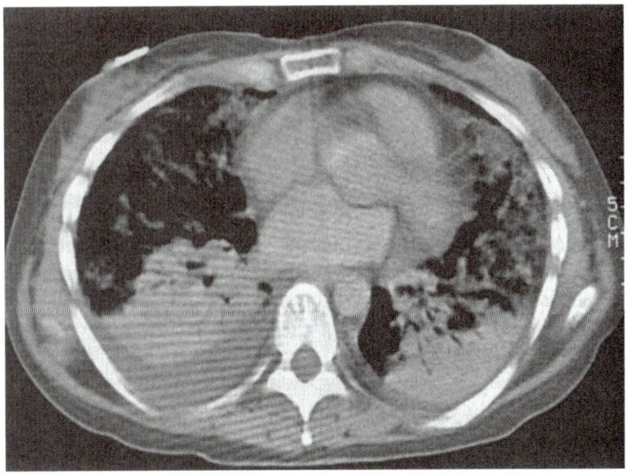

Figure 1. CT section of chest in a patient with ARDS that demonstrates dependent consolidation and areas of normal lung and atelectatic lung in the mid and anterior zones.

prone position, CT may demonstrate migration of consolidation and infiltrates to the ventral lung units which are now in a dependent position.

Causes of ALI/ARDS

The causes of ALI/ARDS often are categorized based on the mechanism of injury: direct (or epithelial) or indirect (or vascular). The more common causes are listed in Table 3 using this categorization. When one considers comprehensive epidemiology studies, sepsis, pneumonia, trauma, and gastric aspiration account for the majority of cases.

Pathophysiology of ALI / ARDS

The acute phase of ALI/ARDS is characterized by the accumulation of protein-rich edema fluid within the lung interstitium spaces and the alveoli as a result of increased permeability of the alveolar capillary endothelium and the alveolar epithelium, and a highly inflammatory lung injury. Net fluid accumulation is influenced by the influx of fluid and proteins as well as clearance which is normally primarily from lymphatic drainage of peribronchovascular edema fluid. Epithelial disruption is a primary cause of alveolar flooding, and injury to type I pneumocytes contributes to impaired transport of sodium, chloride, and water from alveoli. Further, surfactant is inactivated and diluted. As epithelium is sloughed, hyaline membranes are formed.

The injury to epithelium and endothelium is interwoven with an inflammatory injury. Neutrophils migrate from the vasculature into interstitium and alveoli, where they release inflammatory mediators, proteases, and oxidants. Neutrophils are recruited and activated in part because of release by alveolar macrophages of cytokines such as tumor necrosis factor-α, interleukin (IL)-1, IL-6, and IL-8. Other cellular sources of mediators also are important, because ALI/ARDS occurs in neutropenic patients. Additionally, fibroblasts are activated to produce extracellular matrix. Fibrin is abundant, as is collagen, particularly in a state of prolonged inflammation and fibrosis. Many patients quickly progress to a recovery phase characterized by phagocytosis of apoptotic neutrophils, clearance of sodium by the sodium pump of type II epithelial cells, and water efflux via aquaporins. The presence of alveolar and interstitial edema, fibrosis, and inflammation contributes to stiff poorly compliant lungs. Many alveoli are not functional gas exchange units because they are filled with fluid and/or inflammatory exudates, or are prone to collapse, and thus contribute to shunt-like gas exchange resulting in refractory hypoxemia. The reader is referred to excellent reviews by Ware and Matthay for further information.

Table 3. *Common Causes of ALI/ARDS*

Causes
Direct causes
Pulmonary infection
Aspiration injury (gastric contents, near drowning, blood, toxins)
Inhalation injury (smoke, toxins)
Trauma (contusion)
Embolism (amniotic fluid, fat, air)
Re-expansion injury
Reperfusion injury
Indirect causes
Severe sepsis
Shock
Nonpulmonary trauma
Transfusion-related lung injury
Cardiopulmonary bypass
Anaphylaxis
Medications (opioids, salicylates, amiodarone, tocolytics, chemotherapy)
Acute pancreatitis

Epidemiology of ALI/ARDS

Epidemiologic estimates of the incidence of ALI and ARDS vary widely from 1.5 to 75 per 100,000 annually but are highly dependent on the population studied, the definitions used, and other factors. Some of the best data regarding US cases comes from studies conducted in Seattle, in which Rubenfeld et al estimated crude incidence of 79.8 and 58.7 per 100,000 for ALI and ARDS, respectively. Extrapolated to the US population, 190,600 and 141,500 cases are estimated to occur annually.

The authors of these same studies reported in-hospital mortality rates of 38.5% and 41.1% for ALI and ARDS, respectively, by using data collected in 1999 and 2000. Of note, mortality rates tend to be lower for ALI/ARDS from trauma compared with cases arising after sepsis or gastric aspiration. An analysis of published reports suggests that mortality rates for ALI/ARDS have declined approximately 1% per year from 1994 to 2006. Mortality rates in recent large RCTs of patients with ALI, performed primarily in AMCs, reveal 30- to 60-day mortality rates of 25 to 30%.

Pulmonary function tends to return to near normal during the ensuing 12 months for survivors, with residual reduced diffusing capacity and exercise-induced hypoxemia seen in some patients. In contrast, quality of life is often impaired after ARDS and the causative event(s), with a high proportion of patients having neuropsychological problems and neuromuscular weakness as prominent components.

An Overview of Management of ALI/ARDS

Management of ALI/ARDS incorporates treatment of the underlying cause; support for gas exchange; supportive and preventative measures such as adequate nutrition and prophylaxis against deep venous thrombosis, stress gastric ulceration, and ventilator-associated pneumonia; application of evidence-based strategies for ventilation and medical care ALI/ARDS; and rescue therapies for refractory hypoxemia in selected cases. There is a long history of proposed therapies for ARDS, many subjected to large-scale RCTs. Yet very few interventions have been demonstrated to improve key outcomes, such as survival, or reduced duration of mechanical ventilation and length of stay (LOS) in ICU. There is general agreement that use of lung protective ventilation, including limiting tidal volumes (VTs) to ≤ 6 mL/kg of predicted body weight (PBW) is a key component of contemporary management. Some interventions improve physiologic parameters, like oxygenation, that have relevance for clinical management. Interestingly, there is not consistent concordance between physiologic improvement and enhanced outcome. Despite considerable investigation, some interventions such as systemic corticosteroids, prone positioning, and high levels of PEEP remain controversial despite extensive study. Management will be discussed as ventilatory management and medical management.

Ventilatory Management of ALI/ARDS

Ventilatory management goals for ALI/ARDS include enhancing the likelihood of survival, avoidance of ventilator- and airway-related complications, reducing the duration of mechanical ventilation and critical illness, supporting gas exchange, and relieving distress and excessive work of breathing. Key principles of ventilatory management are guided by observations from experimental results of clinical and animal-model investigations, and imaging studies that help to correlate structure and function. First, multiple lines of evidence demonstrate that effective alveolar volume is reduced substantially in ARDS, mimicking "baby" lungs in size, and that overdistention of functional alveoli impairs gas exchange and induces a state of inflammatory lung injury, so called ventilator-associated lung injury (VALI). Alveolar overdistention is typically produced by creation of excessive transpulmonary distending pressure during positive pressure breath delivery.

Second, many alveoli are prone to collapse either throughout the respiratory cycle or as lung volume and airway pressure decrease during exhalation. Recruiting these alveoli and maintaining them in an open state improves gas exchange and reduces VALI that is related to injury caused by repetitive alveolar collapse and recruitment. Third, high concentrations of oxygen are typically necessary to achieve sufficient cellular oxygenation, but if administered for prolonged periods are associated with pulmonary fibrosis in animal models. Thus, current ventilatory strategies for ARDS focus on using small VTs, sufficient PEEP to splint open alveoli, and supplemental oxygen. Also see the chapter on "Mechanical Ventilatory Support" for additional information about VALI and mechanical ventilation in ARDS.

Although earlier RCTs that compared low VTs positive pressure ventilation to conventional ventilation in patients with ALI/ARDS were not conclusive, the pivotal trial performed by the ARDSNet investigators in 861 patients with ALI/ARDS demonstrated a 10% absolute reduction in mortality. Patients randomized to receive VTs of 6 mL/kg PBW also had more ventilator-free and organ failure-free days compared with patients who received 12 mL/kg PBW VTs. Interestingly, there was no significant difference in barotrauma rates.

ARDSNet recommendations for mechanical ventilation in ARDS include the following: (1) use the volume-assist control mode, (2) set inspiratory flow greater than patient demand (usually >80 L/min), (3) start with VT = 8 mL/kg PBW and reduce VT by 1 mL/kg until 6 mL/kg PBW is reached, (4) aim for plateau inspiratory airway pressure (Pplat) < 30 cm H_2O, (5) increase respiratory rate, to a maximum of 35 breaths/min, to achieve pH = 7.3 to 7.45, (6) consider adding IV bicarbonate if necessary to achieve pH goals, (7) adjust FIO_2 and PEEP to achieve PaO_2 = 55 to 80 mm Hg or pulse oxygen saturation = 88 to 93% according to Table 4. Note that PBW (in kilograms) can be calculated as 50 + 2.3 × (height in inches – 60) for men and 45.5 + 2.3 × (height in inches – 60) for women.

Although the results are compelling for adoption of a low VT approach to mechanical ventilation, examination of actual clinical practice at ARDSNet hospitals and other academic medical centers (AMCs) years after publication of ARDSNet results indicates that clinicians often do not reduce lung volumes adequately. In fact, in one three-center study only 16% of patients with ALI/ARDS had VT < 8 mL/kg PBW. Barriers to adoption include clinician reluctance to relinquish control of the ventilator; lack of recognition of ARDS; and concerns for contraindications, discomfort, and impaired gas exchange. However, a recent report demonstrated that higher rates of compliance can be achieved by the use of a written protocol. The use of nomograms to easily identify hypoxemia that reaches the threshold for ALI or ARDS (Fig 2) and that quickly converts height in inches or cm to predicted body weight and to the target VT of 6 mL/kg (Fig 3) may help raise awareness and streamline the process of providing lung-protective ventilation.

It is noteworthy that the original ARDSNet 6 mL/kg VT approach (described previously) actually led to slightly worse oxygenation compared with 12 mL/kg VT. This finding contrasts with other smaller studies, such as those by Amato et al and Ranieri and coworkers, in which a more aggressive PEEP strategy was associated with better oxygenation. As a result of these observations and the considerable evidence from animal models of lung injury that greater PEEP may protect against injury from repetitive alveolar collapse and recruitment (the "atelectrauma" component of VALI), three large (>500 subjects) multicenter RCTs designed to compare a high PEEP strategy to

Table 4. *Adjustments to PEEP and FIO_2 During Mechanical Ventilation for ALI/ARDS According to the ARDS Network**

FIO_2	0.3	0.4	0.4	0.5	0.5	0.6	0.7	0.7	0.8	0.9	1.0	1.0
PEEP, cm H_2O	5	8	8	10	10	10	14	14	14	18	24	

*PEEP is increased in increments of 2 cm H_2O, FIO_2 by 0.1. From the ARDS Network N Engl J Med 2000, 342.1301–1308.

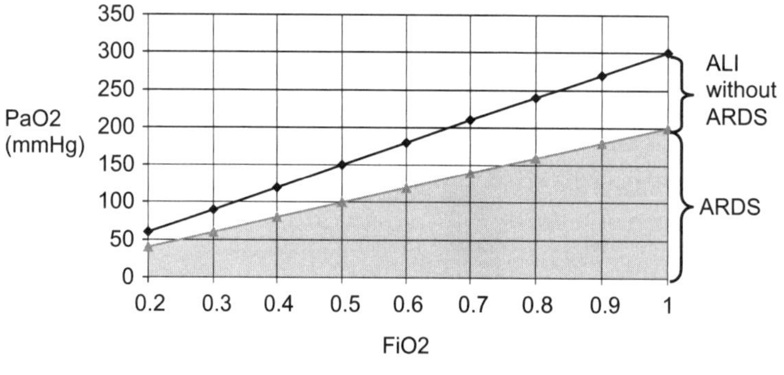

Figure 2. Graph of PaO_2 vs FiO_2 to easily identify if oxygenation criteria is present for ALI or ARDS. Find the point where the horizontal line for measured PaO_2 intersects the vertical line for FiO_2 and determine if this point is within the area that defines ARDS or ALI without ARDS.

Male		Female		Predicted body weight	6 ml/kg tidal volume
Height in inches	Height in cm	Height in inches	Height in cm	(in kg)	(in ml)
58	147	60	152	45.5	272
60	152	62	157	50	300
62	157	64	163	54.7	328
64	163	66	168	59	355
66	168	68	173	64	383
68	173	70	178	68.5	410
70	178	72	183	73	438
72	183	74	188	78	466
74	188	76	193	82	493

Figure 3. Table to identify VTs that corresponds to 6 mL/kg of PBW based on patient sex and height in inches or centimeters. Find the cell that most closely matches the height in inches or centimeters for a male (left) or female (right) and identify the corresponding VT listed in the same row. The PBW is also listed for the corresponding heights. Calculations are based on the following equations: man: PBW (in kg) $= 50 + 2.3 \times$ (height in inches -60); woman: PBW (in kg) $= 45.5 + 2.3 \times$ (height in inches -60).

traditional ARDSNet PEEP have been completed. All studies were similar in that PEEP averaged about 8 to 10 cm H_2O in the low PEEP arm and 10 to 16 cm H_2O in the high PEEP arm over the course of the first week of ARDS. Pao_2:Fio_2 ratios were uniformly greater and rescue therapy for hypoxemia used less frequently in patients randomized to the more aggressive PEEP strategy in these studies.

None of the studies demonstrated a difference in rates of mortality or barotrauma events; however, more organ failure-free and ventilator-free days were seen with greater PEEP in the study by Mercat and colleagues. In this study, the volume-assist control mode with VT = 6 mL/kg PBW was used and the PEEP was increased according to the Table 5 as long as the pressure plateau (Pplat) remained ≤ 30 cm H_2O. A word of caution regarding the more aggressive PEEP approach of Mercat et al; there was a trend for lower mortality for the three quartiles with more severe hypoxemia, but a trend for higher mortality in the quartile with Pao_2:Fio_2 was > 180 mm Hg. Accordingly, we would not support this approach if Pao_2:Fio_2 is > 180 mm Hg. In a recent study, esophageal pressure was used as a surrogate for pleural pressure to guide setting PEEP while avoiding excessive transpulmonary pressure. Better oxygenation and lung compliance was achieved, without increasing barotrauma in this pilot study.

Although the pivotal ARDSNet study prescribed using the volume-assist control mode, application of a pressure-targeted mode, as done by Amato et al, in his lung-protective strategy, is of interest to clinicians. A pressure-targeted mode may permit more fine-tuning of Pplat, PEEP, and inspiratory time to improve oxygenation while also adhering to VT $\leq$ 6 mL/kg PBW and acceptable Pplat. The "open ventilation" mode tested by Meade and colleagues incorporated pressure-targeted ventilation with I:E up to 1:1, greater Pplat to a maximum of 40 cm H_2O, higher PEEP (discussed previously), and recruitment maneuvers after disconnection from the ventilator. With this approach, they demonstrated superior oxygenation, fewer deaths caused by refractory hypoxemia, and no difference in mortality, barotrauma, or LOS in the ICU compared with traditional ARDSNet ventilation. A significant limitation of using pressure-targeted ventilator modes in ALI/ARDS is the loss of "control" over the VT and, thus, violation of the important goal of using low VT ventilation. For the same inspiratory pressure and inspiratory time settings, a more vigorous inspiratory effort or

Table 5. *Adjustments to PEEP and Fio_2 During Mechanical Ventilation for ALI/ARDS According to the "Increased Recruitment" Arm of the EXPRESS Trial**

Fio_2	0.3	0.4	0.5	0.6	0.7	0.8	0.9	1.0
PEEP, cm H_2O	5–10	10–18	18–20	20	20	20–22	22	22–24

*PEEP is adjusted upwards according to the table, unless Pplat > 30 cm H_2O while the patient is receiving volume-assist control ventilation with VT = 6 mL/kg PBW. PEEP is increased in increments of 2 cm H_2O, Fio_2 by 0.1. Note that a trend for greater mortality was noted for patients with Pao_2: $Fio_2 > 180$ mm Hg; thus, this strategy is *not* recommended for ALI without ARDS (*ie*, Pao_2: $Fio_2 > 200$ mm Hg. From Mercat et al. JAMA 2008; 299:646–655.

improvement in lung compliance will result in larger, and potentially excessive, VTs.

A modification of pressure-targeted controlled ventilation that permits inspiratory efforts to occur regardless of the phase of ventilation (*ie*, the so-called *bilevel ventilation*), may permit the use of less sedation. Additionally, there is evidence that unrestricted spontaneous breathing, particularly if the breaths are *not* pressure supported, promotes better aeration of dependent juxtadiaphragmatic lung zones. Investigators have demonstrated better gas exchange with measured decreases in shunt fraction and dead space, as well as increased cardiac index with the addition of unsupported spontaneous breaths throughout ventilation using a pressure-targeted mode. Some clinicians employ a form of bilevel ventilation with a very long inspiratory plateau and a very brief (<0.8 s) exhalation (the so-called *airway pressure release ventilation [APRV]*).

Although oxygenation may be improved with APRV, there are few data and no adequately powered RCTs that address important outcomes with this technique. Further, the very short exhalation time may be inadequate to fully empty the lungs, particularly if bronchospasm or secretions impede exhalation, potentially leading to life-threatening auto-PEEP. If a longer inspiratory time is used, we prefer using an expiratory time of ≥1 s to reduce the likelihood of this dangerous situation from occurring. Recruitment maneuvers are used by some clinicians to open alveoli that are then splinted open with PEEP. However, large-scale studies suggested the benefit is generally short-lived. Application of a recruitment maneuver, such as applying an inspiratory pressure at 40 cm H_2O for 40 s, may be reasonable after ventilator disconnection with the accompanying loss of alveolar distention.

High frequency oscillatory ventilation (HFOV) is perhaps the ultimate form of lung protective ventilation for ARDS since tidal volumes of <150 mL are delivered at rates of 180 to 300 breaths/min. Although HFOV has been demonstrated in RCTs to be equivalent to conventional ventilation, such studies were performed with the use of larger (10 to 12 mL/kg PBW) VTs and an RCT comparing HFOV to conventional ventilation with VT = 6 mL/kg PBW is needed. Use of HFOV adds significant complexity to patient management and use should be limited to centers with experience and immediately available on-site expertise to troubleshoot problems.

Nonventilatory Management of ALI/ARDS

Many pharmacologic interventions, as well as other nonventilatory treatment strategies, have been used in uncontrolled settings or tested in RCTs, most with negative results. Some experimental therapies, such as surfactant replacement, continue to undergo active investigation and are not readily available; thus, they are not discussed. Rather, we will focus on readily available interventions that have either compelling or controversial evidence from RCTs, including conservative fluid management with or without albumin administration, specialized nutritional formulations, and corticosteroids. Additional interventions, such as inhaled nitric oxide (INO) and prone positioning, will be considered within the context of rescue therapy for refractory hypoxemia.

Conservative Fluid Management: Typical management of a patient with ALI results in a net positive fluid balance of about 1 L/d. There is evidence from a large multicenter RCT from the ARDSNet investigators that a protocol-directed conservative approach to fluid management for patients with ALI leads to shorter duration of mechanical ventilation (more ventilator-free and ICU-free days) without negatively impacting renal function, when compared with a "liberal fluid management" conventional approach. There was no difference in mortality between groups but more electrolyte disorders (hypernatremia, hypokalemia, alkalosis) were noted.

The research protocol for conservative fluid management is complex, however. Each of 20 separate management cells is defined by the central venous pressure (CVP) using a central venous catheter (CVC) or PCWP using a PAC range and one or more of the following clinical characteristics: (1) the presence vs absence of shock (i.e., mean arterial pressure <60 mm Hg or any need for vasopressor), (2) urinary output (<0.5 mL/kg/h vs >0.5 mL/kg/h), or (3) ineffective circulation (cardiac output <2.5 L/min/m^2 or cold, mottled skin with delayed capillary refill time) or effective circulation. A simplified version (by collapsing several CVP ranges into one CVP range, and elimination of the "ineffective circulation" parameter because

Table 6. *Conservative Fluid Management Strategy for ALI**

CVP range, mm Hg	Shock Present	Shock Absent	
		Oliguric	Nonoliguric
≥9	Vasopressors	Diuretic†	Diuretic†
4–8	Fluid bolus	Fluid bolus	Diuretic†
<4	Fluid bolus	Fluid bolus	KVO fluids

*Shock indicates mean arterial pressure <60 mm Hg or use of any vasopressor. CVP = central venous pressure. Oliguria indicates urine output <0.5 mL/kg/h. KVO = "keep vein open" IV fluid rate.
†Diuretics are not given if a vasopressor was used within 12 h.

this was rarely present) is presented in Table 6. Of note, 75% of interventions performed during the study were when the patient was "stable," *ie*, normotensive and nonoliguric; this is the opportune time to eliminate excessive fluid by diuresis. Work by other investigators suggest that the addition of albumin infusion to patients with ALI and low (<5 mg/dL) serum protein as they are receiving furosemide diuresis leads to improved oxygenation, fluid balance, and hemodynamics.

Nutritional Supplementation: ALI/ARDS is an inflammatory disorder in which oxidants also play a role in lung injury. Altering the fatty acids that are incorporated into tissue lipids can modify the nature of lipid inflammatory mediators that are subsequently released. The arachidonic acid metabolites, in particular, are proinflammatory and may contribute to worsening lung injury. Several smaller RCTs have demonstrated that enteral administration of a nutrition product that contains gamma-linoleic acid, and eicosapentaenoic acid, and antioxidants to patients with ARDS is associated with better oxygenation, along with more ventilator-free days, more organ dysfunction-free days, and more ICU-free days. Additionally, the earlier multicenter RCT by Gadek and colleagues also demonstrated reduced alveolar inflammation with the specialized nutritional formulation. Although addition study in a larger multicenter RCT is needed, the simplicity, low cost, and safety of this intervention is attractive and such a nutritional product is on the market.

Corticosteroids: The use of glucocorticoids in the treatment of ALI/ARDS as a condition characterized by intense inflammatory and disordered fibrotic repair spans decades and has never been free of controversy. In the 1980s, four RCTs demonstrated the lack of benefit of high-dose, short-duration corticosteroids in *preventing* the development of ARDS in high risk patients. During the past two decades, four studies addressing the administration of corticosteroids early in the course of ALI/ARDS suggest that corticosteroids may be beneficial in reducing mortality but did not reach statistical significance (odds ratio 0.48, 95% confidence interval, 0.40 to 1.09) when pooled. A low-dose (1 mg/kg/d methylprednisolone to start, then taper) long-course (28-day) regimen yielded positive results (higher PaO_2:FIO_2, shorter duration of mechanical ventilation, shorter ICU LOS) vs placebo in an RCT; however, the results may be clouded by methodologic concerns of the study.

Some clinicians have given corticosteroids in modest doses (such as methylprednisolone [MP] 40 mg q6h) to treat unresolving or "fibroproliferative" ARDS that has been present >7 days. The condition is typically recognized by fever and leukocytosis without evidence of infection and persistent pulmonary infiltrates and hypoxemia requiring ongoing mechanical ventilation. A multicenter RCT performed by the ARDSNet investigators yielded mixed results, interpreted by the authors as showing no benefit. These results, however, deserve further review, and the study design bears closer scrutiny. Proponents of corticosteroid administration have long emphasized a longer course of therapy slowly tapered over several weeks, since more rapid tapering has been linked to relapse. The ARDSNet trial prescribed tapering the MP over only 2 days under selected circumstances including septic shock or successful extubation for 2 days. Critics argue that this rapid taper may have led to relapse and reintubation or to worsening shock since the administration of corticosteroids shortens the duration of vasopressor use in septic shock. The results show significantly more ventilator-free days through day 28 with MP vs placebo (11.2 vs 6.8 days), but higher rates of reintubation. Patients randomized to MP were first extubated 10 days earlier on average (14 days vs 24 days)\compared with the use of placebo. Patients randomized to MP also had significantly lower rates of shock and pneumonia, but did have significantly more adverse effects attributed to myoneuropathy.

Interestingly, structured evaluation for myoneuropathy disclosed no difference in the rates between groups. Randomization to MP was also associated with better oxygenation, lower Pplat, and better lung compliance than placebo. Mortality was similar between groups at 28, 60, and 180 days. Subset analysis demonstrated that among patients enrolled ≥14 days after onset of ARDS, those randomized to placebo had a significantly lower 60-day mortality rate (8%) than MP (35%), accounting for the difference in survival for the late persistent ARDS group. Although this is a subset analysis on a small number of patients (n = 48), the authors conclude (and we concur), that corticosteroids should not be initiated to treat unresolving ARDS after day 13, until more data are available. When RCT data are limited to patients with unresolving ARDS who had onset 1 to 13 days earlier and who received treatment for at least 1 week, a meta-analysis by Meduri et al shows better survival with MP (p = 0.01), although the population is limited to 245 subjects and includes studies with methodologic concerns.

Further research in well-designed studies and re-analysis of existing data are needed. Of note, measurement of procollagen peptide III in BAL fluid may prove helpful as a screening test for treatment, since patients who received MP had a significant lower mortality rate compared with placebo when this peptide was found in high amounts before treatment in the ARDSNet study. If MP is administered for unresolving ARDS, the following caveats should be considered: (1) starting MP >13 days after onset of ARDS should be avoided, (2) the MP dosage should be modest (0.5 mg/kg every 6 h to start) and tapered slowly, (3) active infection surveillance should be performed during MP therapy, and (4) the use of neuromuscular blocking agents (NMBA) concomitantly should be avoided.

Rescue Therapy for Refractory Hypoxemia

The incidence of refractory and/or life-threatening hypoxemia in ALI/ARDS is not known, although "refractory hypoxemia" was found in about 10% and rescue therapies (INO, prone positioning, almitrine) were used in 10 to 35% of patients in several recent multicenter RCTs for mechanical ventilation in ALI/ARDS. Although most patients with fatal ALI/ARDS die from multiple organ failure, some deaths are the result of refractory hypoxemia. Typically, these patients have oxygen desaturation with minimal movement, suctioning, or other minor stimulation that is very slow to recover. A number of the interventions discussed earlier have been associated with significantly improved oxygenation acutely, such as increased PEEP and APRV. Additionally several nonventilatory interventions are commonly used as rescue therapy for refractory and life-threatening hypoxemia, including neuromuscular blockade (NMB), INO, and prone positioning.

NMB: The administration of a NMB agent (NMBA) in ALI/ARDS can result in improved oxygenation, primarily when there is persistent patient-ventilator dyssynchrony. The frequency with which NMBA are used in ARDS is highly variable, ranging from <10 to >50% of patients in large multicenter RCTs. The dosage of NMBA can be titrated to achieve a range of effects, from synchronous breathing with the ventilator, to apnea, or even cessation of all movement. When NMBAs are used, the lowest effective dose is recommended, and the duration of therapy should be as brief as possible. Further, concomitant administration of corticosteroids is to be avoided because of the increased likelihood of persistent weakness caused by acute quadriplegic myopathy under these circumstances.

INO: NO is a gas with vasodilator properties in minute quantities (*ie*, 5 to 20 parts per million [ppm]). Mechanistically, INO is an attractive intervention. NO is delivered by inhalation to alveoli, which are ventilated, and then diffuses into capillaries, feeding these alveoli and thus increasing their perfusion while not entering nonfunctional alveoli. Increasing perfusion to all alveoli, such as with an IV vasodilator, would indiscriminately increase perfusion, thus potentially increasing the proportion of blood flow to shunt-like alveoli and worsening oxygenation. Additionally, NO is inactivated quickly; thus, it does not produce vasodilatation of systemic vessels that might result in systemic hypotension. In clinical studies, INO increases Pao_2 and decreases pulmonary artery pressure. In dose ranging studies, these effects tend to peak at concentrations of 20 to 40 ppm. The authors of RCTs demonstrate improved oxygenation in most patients, sometimes dramatically, but the effects tend to decline >2 to 4 days. None of the multicenter RCTs have shown that the administration of INO to patients with ALI/ARDS improves chances of survival or reduces ventilator time. Thus, the role of INO is largely as rescue therapy for refractory and life-threatening hypoxemia. Potential adverse effects of INO include methemoglobinemia and increased levels of nitrogen dioxide, neither of which is common unless high doses of INO (80 ppm) are used. Because the acquisition cost is quite high, use of INO should be carefully considered, and unless a clinically important improvement in oxygenation demonstrated, it should be discontinued in a timely fashion. Other inhaled vasodilators are being investigated as alternatives.

Prone Positioning: Placing hypoxemic patients who have ALI/ARDS in the prone position improves oxygenation in most. Principle mechanisms by which this occurs include (1) creating a more uniform distribution of ventilation, with more ventilation of dependent lung units, thereby more effectively matching ventilation and perfusion; (2) lifting the weight of the heart off of the left lower lobe, as the heart is now in a dependent position; and (3) promoting more effective drainage of secretions from the airways. Moving the patient from supine to prone and maintaining the patient in the prone position for an extended time period creates new concerns and potential complications. For example, deeper sedation is needed, and NMB is required in more patients, the incidence of new or worsening pressure sores increases, the likelihood of airway obstruction increases, and the likelihood of accidental removal of critical tubes and lines during position change is present. RCTs demonstrate a clear increase in oxygenation that is partially lost when the patient is returned to the supine position. Several large multicenter RCTs failed to demonstrate improvement in survival or reduction in LOS, although Mancebo et al noted a trend for improved survival and in post-hoc analysis Gattinoni and coworkers observed improved mortality among the sickest quartile of patients, both by severity of illness and by severity of hypoxemia. Prone positioning can be useful for severely hypoxemic patients with ALI/ARDS, but a healthy respect for the challenging process and use of measures to safeguard against complications is necessary. Additional RCTs that may further inform clinical practice are underway.

Summary and Conclusions

Hypoxemic respiratory failure has many causes, but ALI/ARDS is chief among these. Supplemental oxygen, often combined with positive pressure ventilation, usually is necessary as the underlying cause(s) is treated. Management of ALI/ARDS focuses on ventilatory strategies that support oxygenation and ventilation while limiting the potential injurious effects of mechanical ventilation on the vulnerable lung. Specifically, low V_T ventilation (6 mL/kg PBW) and increased levels of PEEP are the cornerstones. Nonventilatory measures include avoidance of excessive lung water, and consideration for using specialized nutritional products and corticosteroids in selected circumstances. Ancillary interventions such as administration of NMBAs, INO, and prone positioning may be necessary to combat life-threatening hypoxemia in selected cases. Future research will help define the role for novel interventions and new treatment strategies.

Annotated Bibliography

Adhikari NK, Burns KE, Friedrich JO, et al. Effect of nitric oxide on oxygenation and mortality in acute lung injury: systematic review and meta-analysis. BMJ 2007; 334:779

Meta-analysis shows little benefit from INO for routine use in ARDS, although oxygenation usually improves.

Amato MB, Barbas CS, Medeiros DM, et al. Beneficial effects of the "open lung approach" with low distending pressures in acute respiratory distress syndrome. A prospective randomized study on mechanical ventilation: am J Respir Crit Care Med 1995; 152:1835–1846

First RCT that promoted an "open lung" or lung protective approach. Criticized for high mortality rates. Meade study replicates study design and demonstrates equivalency to ARDSNet study parameters now 13 years later.

Angus DC, Clermont G, Linde-Zwirble WT, et al. Healthcare costs and long-term outcomes after acute respiratory distress syndrome: a phase III trial of inhaled nitric oxide. Crit Care Med 2006; 34:2883–2890

Poor quality of life after ARDS described.

Arroliga AC, Thompson BT, Ancukiewicz M, et al. Use of sedatives, opioids, and neuromuscular blocking agents in patients with acute lung injury and acute respiratory distress syndrome. Crit Care Med 2008; 36:1083–1088

Use of sedatives, opioids, and NMBAs was similar in low and high PEEP, and sedatives and opioids were associated with delayed weaning.

Ashbaugh DG, Bigelow DB, Petty TL, et al. Acute respiratory distress in adults. Lancet 1967; 2:319–323

Original description of ARDS.

Bernard GR, Artigas A, Brigham KL, et al. The American-European Consensus Conference on ARDS. Definitions, mechanisms, relevant outcomes, and clinical trial coordination: am J Respir Crit Care Med 1994; 149:818–824

Consensus definitions for ALI/ARDS.

Brower RG, Lanken PN, MacIntyre N, et al. Higher versus lower positive end-expiratory pressures in patients with the acute respiratory distress syndrome. N Engl J Med 2004; 351:327–336

ARDSNet RCT found better oxygenation but no other significant differences with a more aggressive PEEP strategy compared to the original ARDSNet protocol.

Calfee CS, Matthay MA. Nonventilatory treatments for acute lung injury and ARDS. Chest 2007; 131:913–920

Review of medical management. Substantial focus on fluid management.

Classic ARDSNet RCT showing lower mortality with lower VTs.

Dellinger RP, Zimmerman JL, Taylor RW, et al. Effects of inhaled nitric oxide in patients with acute respiratory distress syndrome: results of a randomized phase II trial. Inhaled Nitric Oxide in ARDS Study Group. Crit Care Med 1998; 26:15–23

Multicenter RCT showing improved oxygenation but no effect on mortality or ventilation duration with INO.

Derdak S, Mehta S, Stewart TE, et al. High-frequency oscillatory ventilation for acute respiratory distress syndrome in adults: a randomized, controlled trial. Am J Respir Crit Care Med 2002; 166:801–808

HFOV had outcomes similar to conventional ventilation, but with larger VTs than currently used. Complexity much higher than conventional ventilation.

de Wit M, Sessler CN. Acute respiratory failure. In: Rakel RE, Bope ET, ed. Conn's current therapy 2005. Philadelphia, PA: Elsevier Saunders, 2005; 247–253

Review of respiratory failure.

Gadek JE, DeMichele SJ, Karlstad MD, et al. Effect of enteral feeding with eicosapentaenoic acid, gamma-linolenic acid, and antioxidants in patients with acute respiratory distress syndrome. Enteral Nutrition in ARDS Study Group. Crit Care Med 1999; 27:1409–1420

Modest sized multicenter RCT showing less inflammation, better oxygenation, and shorter ventilator time for patients who received feeding modified for reducing lipid mediators and supplemented with antioxidants.

Gainnier M, Roch A, Forel JM, et al. Effect of neuromuscular blocking agents on gas exchange in patients presenting with acute respiratory distress syndrome. Crit Care Med 2004; 32:113–119

NMBA improved gas exchange substantially.

Gattinoni L, Chiumello D, Cressoni M, et al. Pulmonary computed tomography and adult respiratory distress syndrome. Swiss Med Wkly 2005; 135:169–174

One of a number of papers by Gattinoni examining structure-function relationships for ARDS using CT.

Gattinoni L, Tognoni G, Pesenti A, et al. Effect of prone positioning on the survival of patients with acute respiratory failure. N Engl J Med 2001; 345:568–573

Early RCT showing better oxygenation and subset analyses suggesting possible mortality benefit for the most severely ill patients.

Girard TD, Bernard GR. Mechanical ventilation in ARDS: a state-of-the-art review. Chest 2007; 131:921–929

Review, focusing on low VT ventilation.

Guerin C, Gaillard S, Lemasson S, et al. Effects of systematic prone positioning in hypoxemic acute respiratory failure: a randomized controlled trial. JAMA 2004; 292:2379–2387

Multicenter RCT demonstrates improved oxygenation but no other benefit to 8 h/d prone positioning.

Mancebo J, Fernandez R, Blanch L, et al. A multicenter trial of prolonged prone ventilation in severe acute respiratory distress syndrome. Am J Respir Crit Care Med 2006; 173:1233–1239

Another multicenter RCT showing proning improves oxygenation and has a trend for lower mortality when applied for 17 h/day x 10 d. They recommend early and prolonged proning for severe ARDS.

Marik PE, Pastores SM, Annane D, et al. Recommendations for the diagnosis and management of corticosteroid insufficiency in critically ill adult patients: consensus statements from an international task force by the American College of Crit Care Med Crit Care Med 2008; 36:1937–1949

SCCM consensus statement concludes that moderate dose glucocorticoids should be considered for early severe ARDS and before day 14 with unresolving ARDS and that steroids should be tapered and not stopped abruptly – as 2B recommendations. Note that no ARDSNet investigators were task force members.

Martin GS, Moss M, Wheeler AP, et al. A randomized, controlled trial of furosemide with or without albumin

in hypoproteinemic patients with acute lung injury. Crit Care Med 2005; 33:1681–1687
Addition of albumin to furosemide led to better oxygenation and hemodynamic stability.
Meade MO, Cook DJ, Guyatt GH, et al. Ventilation strategy using low tidal volumes, recruitment maneuvers, and high positive end-expiratory pressure for acute lung injury and acute respiratory distress syndrome: a randomized controlled trial. JAMA 2008; 299:637–645
Large multicenter RCT of mostly Canadian centers, published in the same JAMA issue with the Mercat paper. Both compare higher PEEP strategies to the traditional ARDSNet approach. All patients received 6 mL/kg VTs. Additionally, higher Pplat, pressure-targeted ventilation, and recruitment maneuvers (Amato-like parameters). Similar outcomes but better oxygenation with this approach, compared to ARDSNet.
Meduri GU, Golden E, Freire AX, et al. Methylprednisolone infusion in early severe ARDS: results of a randomized controlled trial. Chest 2007; 131:954–963
Recent study of methylprednisolone for early ARDS—positive results, but significant methodologic concerns with the study.
Meduri GU, Marik PE, Chrousos GP, et al. Steroid treatment in ARDS: a critical appraisal of the ARDS network trial and the recent literature. Intensive Care Med 2008; 34:61–69
Essentially a rebuttal and meta-analysis to the Steinberg ARDSNet RCT for corticosteroids and unresolving ARDS. Raises important questions about interpretation of the ARDSNet data and looks at reasons for re-examining.
Mercat A, Richard JC, Vielle B, et al. Positive end-expiratory pressure setting in adults with acute lung injury and acute respiratory distress syndrome: a randomized controlled trial. JAMA 2008; 299:646–655
Multicenter French RCT showing higher PEEP strategy had better oxygenation and more ventilator-free days, but no more barotrauma compared to the ARDSNet PEEP strategy. Mortality was unchanged.
Milberg JA, Davis DR, Steinberg KP, et al. Improved survival of patients with acute respiratory distress syndrome (ARDS): 1983-1993. JAMA 1995; 273:306–309
Older paper that showed improving ARDS outcomes at one center over a decade.
Peter JV, John P, Graham PL, et al. Corticosteroids in the prevention and treatment of acute respiratory distress syndrome (ARDS) in adults: meta-analysis. BMJ 2008; 336:1006–1009
Meta-analysis concludes that a possibility of reduced mortality and increased ventilator days with steroids started after the onset of ARDS is suggested.
Pontes-Arruda A, Aragao AM, Albuquerque JD. Effects of enteral feeding with eicosapentaenoic acid, gamma-linolenic acid, and antioxidants in mechanically ventilated patients with severe sepsis and septic shock. Crit Care Med 2006; 34:2325–2333
Compared to isocaloric feeding, this enteral feed was associated with better oxygenation and other outcomes in patients with sepsis and hypoxemic respiratory failure (ie, ALI/ARDS).
Ranieri VM, Suter PM, Tortorella C, et al. Effect of mechanical ventilation on inflammatory mediators in patients with acute respiratory distress syndrome: a randomized controlled trial. JAMA 1999; 282:54–61
Small but fascinating study that demonstrates beneficial effects of lung protective ventilation – low VTs + high PEEP on course of BAL and blood cytokine levels and physiologic and outcomes effects as compared to conventional ventilation.
Rubenfeld GD, Caldwell E, Peabody E, et al. Barriers to providing lung-protective ventilation to patients with acute lung injury. Crit Care Med 2004; 32:1289–1293
Large epidemiology study of ALI in Seattle area.
Rubenfeld GD, Cooper C, Carter G, et al. Incidence and outcomes of acute lung injury. N Engl J Med 2005; 353:1685–1693
Identifies reasons why physicians do not do low VT ventilation for ALI.
Sessler CN. Mechanical ventilation of patients with acute lung injury. Crit Care Clin 1998; 14:707–729
Review of mechanical ventilation for ALI/ARDS, including mechanisms of VALI in the context of ARDS pathophysiology.
Sessler CN. Sedation, analgesia, and neuromuscular blockade for high-frequency oscillatory ventilation. Crit Care Med 2005; 33:S209–S216
Review of sedation and NMB during ARDS and HFOV.
Steinberg KP, Hudson LD, Goodman RB, et al. Efficacy and safety of corticosteroids for persistent acute respiratory distress syndrome. N Engl J Med 2006; 354:1671–1684
Controversial ARDSNet placebo-controlled RCT showing methylprednisolone possible benefit (physiology and markedly more ventilator-free days) when started 7 to 13 days after ARDS onset, but higher mortality when started >13 days into ARDS.
Talmor D, Sarge T, Malhotra A, et al. Mechanical ventilation guided by esophageal pressure in acute lung injury. N Engl J Med 2008; 359:2095–2104
In a pilot RCT, guidance of setting PEEP by measured esophageal pressure as a surrogate for pleural pressure to estimate transalveolar pressure led to better oxygenation and

lung compliance without increasing barotrauma. Although there are technical concerns regarding accuracy of esophageal pressure, the concept of individualized setting of PEEP (rather than by a table) is attractive.

Taylor RW, Zimmerman JL, Dellinger RP, et al. Low-dose inhaled nitric oxide in patients with acute lung injury: a randomized controlled trial. JAMA 2004; 291:1603–1609

Multicenter RCT demonstrating no outcomes benefits to routine use of INO in ALI.

Umoh NJ, Fan E, Mendez-Tellez PA, et al. Patient and intensive care unit organizational factors associated with low tidal volume ventilation in acute lung injury. Crit Care Med 2008; 36:1463–1468

Use of a written protocol was highly associated with improved compliance with low V_T ventilation.

Ware LB, Matthay MA. Clinical practice. Acute pulmonary edema: N Engl J Med 2005; 353:2788–2796

Mechanisms of edema formation and clearance, plus other information regarding pulmonary edema.

Ventilation with lower tidal volumes as compared with traditional tidal volumes for acute lung injury and the acute respiratory distress syndrome. The Acute Respiratory Distress Syndrome Network. N Engl J Med 2000; 342:1301–1308

Ware LB, Matthay MA. The acute respiratory distress syndrome. N Engl J Med 2000; 342:1334–1349

Excellent review, including detailed analysis of mechanisms.

Wheeler AP, Bernard GR, Thompson BT, et al. Pulmonary-artery versus central venous catheter to guide treatment of acute lung injury. N Engl J Med 2006; 354:2213–2224

Management no better with PAC than CVC, but more minor complications with PAC. About 30% of patients with ALI had PCWP > 18 mm Hg, but normal cardiac output.

Wheeler AP, Bernard GR. Acute lung injury and the acute respiratory distress syndrome: a clinical review. Lancet 2007; 369:1553–1564

Review of current concepts.

Wiedemann HP, Wheeler AP, Bernard GR, et al. Comparison of two fluid-management strategies in acute lung injury. N Engl J Med 2006; 354:2564–2575

ARDSNet trial with complex conservative fluid management protocol resulted in shorter duration of ventilation by 2 days without worsening renal function.

Young MP, Manning HL, Wilson DL, et al. Ventilation of patients with acute lung injury and acute respiratory distress syndrome: has new evidence changed clinical practice? Crit Care Med 2004; 32:1260–1265

No, only a small percentage of patients had V_Ts < 8 mL/kg PBW and [mL/kg] virtually none < 6 mL/kg.

Zambon M, Vincent JL. Mortality rates for patients with acute lung injury/ARDS have decreased over time. Chest 2008; 133:1120–1127

By pooling many different studies, the authors conclude that mortality has fallen about 1% per year from 1994 to 2006.

Symptoms of Respiratory Disease

Richard S. Irwin, MD, FCCP

Objectives:

- Address the symptoms of respiratory disease commonly encountered by the pulmonologist
- Review the physiology, pathophysiology, complications, differential diagnosis, pathogenesis, diagnosis, and treatment of cough
- Review the physiology, differential diagnosis, pathogenesis, and diagnosis of wheeze
- Review the pathogenesis, differential diagnosis, diagnosis, and treatment of hemoptysis
- Review the physiology, differential diagnosis and pathophysiology, diagnosis, and treatment of dyspnea

Key words: cough; dyspnea; hemoptysis; wheeze

Respiratory symptoms are among the most common reasons for which patients seek medical care. The National Ambulatory Medical Care Survey, published in 2006 by the US Department of Health and Human Services,[1] showed that respiratory system-related symptoms were the most common symptoms for which patients made office visits in 1998, accounting for approximately 12% of the total. Other common system-related symptoms are shown in Table 1. Of all symptoms reported, cough of undifferentiated duration was the single most common complaint for which patients sought medical care of primary care physicians. Of the estimated 1.1 billion visits to office-based physicians in the United States from 2001 to 2002, 3.1%, or 34.1 million visits, were for cough. Because the common cold is the most common affliction of men and women, and it is almost always accompanied by an acute (*ie*, < 3 weeks in duration) and usually self-limited cough, it is likely that the greatest majority of the coughs seen by primary care physicians are acute in duration. With respect to the pulmonologist, referrals of patients with persistently troublesome chronic cough of unknown etiology have been shown to account for 10 to 38% of the outpatient practice.[2,3]

Cough

Healthy people rarely cough during waking hours or especially during sleep, and when they do, it is essentially devoid of any clinical importance. The lesser frequency of cough during sleep compared with wakefulness in normal subjects as well as in patients with chronic bronchitis and emphysema is likely the result of greater thresholds to coughing stimuli during sleep.[4] However, when cough is present and persistent, it can assume great clinical importance. Cough can be an important defense mechanism that helps clear excessive secretions and foreign material from the airway, it can be an important factor in the spread of infection, and it is one of the most common symptoms for which patients seek medical attention and spend health-care dollars. Voluntary coughing can be used as a means of providing cardiopulmonary resuscitation.

Table 1. *Spectrum/Frequency of Symptoms by System for Which Patients Sought Medical Care in the Office Setting in the United States in 2001 to 2002**

Reason for Visit	% of Symptoms
Symptoms related to respiratory system	11.8
Symptoms related to nervous system and eyes and ears.	8.6
Symptoms related to circulatory system	8.0
Symptoms related to musculoskeletal and connective tissue	7.9
Symptoms of a general nature	7.5
Symptoms related to endocrine, nutritional/metabolic/immunity disorders	5.3
Symptoms related to mental disorders	4.8
Symptoms related to skin and subcutaneous tissues	4.8
Symptoms related to genitourinary system	4.7
Symptoms related to digestive system	3.7

*Adapted from Schappert and Burt.[1]

Physiology/Pathophysiology of Cough

There are usually three phases involved in the active cough mechanism. Cough is usually preceded by a deep inspiration (inspiratory phase). This initial inspiration is important in producing an effective cough by permitting both expiratory pressure and flow to be maximal during the ensuing expiration. This high lung volume allows maximal expiratory flow rates. During the second compressive phase, intrathoracic pressure is increased sufficiently to produce flow rates necessary for effective cough during the expiratory phase. It is during this latter phase that the defense mechanism function of cough is carried out, that is, the removal of undesired material from the lower respiratory tract.

Although dynamic changes are taking place in the glottis (*eg*, vocal cords separate and vibrate, and the width of the glottis narrows at the aryepiglottic folds that shake secretions loose from the larynx), the same thoracic and abdominal muscles that were active during the compressive phase of cough contract further. The continued shortening of these muscles after the opening of the vocal cords serves to maintain the rapid flow of air by ensuring a high-pressure gradient between intrathoracic airways and the mouth. Numerous studies have noted that maximal intrathoracic pressures during a cough occur after the opening of the glottis, attesting to the contribution of the expiratory muscles in maintaining high pressures and therefore high flow. Along with the larynx and expiratory musculature, the tracheobronchial tree also undergoes dynamic changes that ensure an effective cough.

The single most important parameter in the production of an effective cough is the linear velocity of the moving column of air. The determinants of linear velocity are described by the following formula: velocity = flow/cross-sectional area. Therefore, an effective cough depends primarily on a small cross-sectional area and high flow rates.[5] Most important in maintaining the small cross-sectional area is the dynamic compression that the tracheobronchial tree undergoes during the forced expiration. The most important factor necessary for achieving high flow rates is the initial deep breath of a cough.

All clinically important disorders that mitigate the effectiveness of a cough interfere with the inspiratory or expiratory phases of cough, with most conditions affecting both, and respiratory muscles of sufficient strength are key to both phases. Disorders or interventions that might predominantly affect the compressive phase in a negative way are probably not clinically important. For instance, although vocal cord closure is an important component of the compressive phase, it is not essential for the production of effective cough pressures. The muscles of expiration appear to be the most important determinant in producing elevated intrathoracic pressures, and they are capable of doing so even when an endotracheal tube is in place.[6]

Cough can be predicted to be ineffective at the bedside if patients are unable to or can barely cough on command. However, there are few data that allow one to predict when cough is approaching a threshold for ineffectiveness that will prohibitively predict the risk of substantial gas exchange abnormalities, atelectasis, and/or suppurative disease of the lower respiratory tract. Observations in patients with myasthenia gravis have suggested that when maximal expiratory pressures are <40 cm H_2O (31 mm Hg), patients seemed to have difficulty in raising secretions without endotracheal suctioning.[7]

Complications of Cough/Cough Cardiopulmonary Resuscitation

During the expiratory phase of vigorous coughing, intrathoracic pressures up to 300 mm Hg, expiratory velocities up to 28,000 cm/s or 500 miles/h (*ie*, 85% of the speed of sound), and from 1 to 25 J of energy can be generated.[8] Although pressures, velocities, and energy of these magnitudes allow coughing to be an effective means of providing cardiopulmonary resuscitation in the conscious patient, they also cause a variety of complications, as summarized in Table 2.

Cough cardiopulmonary resuscitation has assumed an established place in clinical practice and has been found to be beneficial in the ECG-monitored, conscious patient with the following: (1) asystole, (2) profound bradycardia with hypotension, and (3) ventricular tachycardia.[8] Although voluntary coughing is unlikely to convert ventricular fibrillation to a more viable rhythm, it can maintain BP and oxygenation while the defibrillator

Table 2. *Complications of Cough*

Category	Examples
Cardiovascular	Arterial hypotension; loss of consciousness; rupture of subconjunctival/nasal/anal veins; massive intraocular suprachoroidal hemorrhage during *pars plana* vitrectomy; dislodgement/malfunctioning IV catheters; bradytachyarrhythmias
Constitutional symptoms	Excessive sweating; anorexia; exhaustion
GI	Malfunction of gastrostomy button; splenic rupture; inguinal herniation; cough-induced gastroesophageal reflux events; gastric hemorrhage after percutaneous endoscopic gastrostomy; hepatic cyst rupture; herniations (*eg*, inguinal, through abdominal wall, small bowel through laparoscopic trocar site); Mallory-Weiss tear
Genitourinary	Urinary incontinence; inversion of bladder through urethra
Musculoskeletal	Ranges from asymptomatic elevations of serum creatine phosphokinase to rupture of *rectus abdominis* muscles; rib fractures; diaphragmatic rupture; sternal wound dehiscence
Neurologic	Cough syncope/headache/dizziness; cerebrospinal fluid rhinorrhea; acute cervical radiculopathy; cervical epidural hematoma associated with oral anticoagulation; malfunctioning ventriculoatrial shunts; seizures; stroke caused by vertebral artery dissection; cerebral air embolism
Ophthalmologic	Spontaneous compressive orbital emphysema of rhinogenic origin; others are listed under cardiovascular category
Psychosocial	Fear of serious disease; lifestyle changes; self-consciousness
Quality of life	Decreased
Respiratory	Exacerbation of asthma; herniations of the lung (*eg*, intercostals and supraclavicular); hydrothorax in peritoneal dialysis; laryngeal trauma (*eg*, edema and hoarseness); pulmonary interstitial emphysema, with potential risk of pneumatosis intestinalis; pneumomediastinum; pneumoperitoneum; pneumoretroperitoneum; pneumothorax; subcutaneous emphysema; tracheobronchial trauma (*eg*, bronchitis and bronchial rupture)
Skin	Petechiae and purpura; disruption of surgical wounds

is being readied. It has been shown that patients with ventricular fibrillation, asystole, or heart block can maintain consciousness in catheterization laboratories or coronary care units with forceful, abrupt coughing at 1- to 3-s intervals for 39 to 92 s. Coughing produces hemodynamic changes that compare favorably with chest compressions. During the expiratory phase of vigorous coughing, systolic pressures approach 140 mm Hg, compared with 75 mm Hg during chest compressions. Cough cardiopulmonary resuscitation cannot be continued indefinitely because the act of coughing expends more than a modest amount of energy.

Differential Diagnosis and Pathogenesis of Cough

Cough can be caused by a multiplicity of disorders in a variety of locations. Because virtually any condition that stimulates cough receptors or afferent nervous pathways is capable of producing cough, only the most common disorders will be discussed in detail. They will be categorized according to the duration of cough into acute, subacute, and chronic types. Acute cough is one that lasts <3 weeks and is most commonly transient and of minor consequence (*eg*, the common cold); however, it can occasionally be potentially life threatening (*eg*, pulmonary embolism, congestive heart failure, or pneumonia). Subacute cough lasts from 3 to 8 weeks. It is most commonly caused by postinfectious cough that encompasses whooping cough and exacerbations of underlying conditions such as asthma and COPD. Chronic cough lasts >8 weeks and is persistently troublesome. Because there are patients with respiratory infections (*eg*, pertussis) more severe than the common cold who complain of cough for >3 weeks and have it spontaneously disappear by 8 weeks, it is reasonable to withhold a diagnostic workup for cough that follows an obvious respiratory infection for 8 weeks. However, when cough lasts >3 weeks and does not follow an obvious respiratory infection, the workup for cough should not wait 8 weeks. Finally, because acute cough may become chronic, the categories are not mutually exclusive.

With respect to the pathogenicity of cough, there are limited data that do not appear at this time to support one common mechanism. For example, although excessive mucus production may lead to cough by mechanically stimulating the afferent limb of the cough reflex and extraluminal masses by compressing/distorting submucosal airway receptors, an increased sensitivity of the afferent limb of the cough reflex appears to be an important pathogenetic mechanism common to patients who have a nonproductive cough caused by a variety of diseases (*eg*, asthma, upper respiratory infection, gastroesophageal reflux disease [GERD], and angiotensin-converting enzyme inhibitors [ACEIs]).

Acute Cough

The limited published studies on the spectrum and frequency of acute cough suggest acute upper respiratory tract infections primarily caused by the common cold[9,10] are the most common causes of the acute, transient cough (Table 3). Less common causes include potential life-threatening conditions that must always be considered. These conditions include pneumonia, aspiration syndromes, congestive heart failure, and pulmonary embolism.

Subacute Cough

The most common causes of subacute cough in immunocompetent adults include postinfectious cough[11] that includes *Bordetella pertussis* infection, bacterial sinusitis, and exacerbations of underlying conditions such as asthma, COPD, and bronchiectasis. When patients complain only of chronic cough after a respiratory tract infection and have normal chest radiographic findings, some authors[12] have referred to these coughs as *postinfectious in causation*. An important part of the definition is that the cough eventually resolves, seemingly on it own; however, on occasion, the resolution of the cough may be hastened by a brief course of an oral corticosteroids, inhaled corticosteroids, or ipratropium. The diagnosis is one of exclusion.

In adults, during outbreaks of *B pertussis* infection, the frequency of postinfectious cough increases to 25 to 50% in selected series. Although up to 28% of the cases reported to the Centers for Disease Control and Prevention on an annual basis occur in adults, it is clear that this is an underestimation because the disease is underappreciated. Whooping cough should be considered in all subjects who present with a cough-vomit syndrome even if the typical whoop (*ie*, the stridorous noise heard during inspiration following a prolonged fit of coughing) may be absent. *B pertussis*-specific serum acute IgA antibody by enzyme-linked immunosorbent assay is a sensitive test (albeit not perfectly sensitive) for the diagnosis and can distinguish between a response to natural infection and that from previous immunization. Treatment with a macrolide (or trimethoprim/sulfamethoxazole when macrolide cannot be administered) for the sick individual and prophylaxis for exposed persons have been found to be effective in decreasing the severity and transmission of the disease to others if therapy is begun early, within the first 8 days of the infection. It is reasonable to consider adding corticosteroids.

Table 3. *Spectrum of the Most Common Causes of Acute Cough in Immunocompetent Adults*

Common cold
Acute bronchitis
B pertussis infection
Exacerbations of underlying conditions (*eg*, COPD, asthma, bronchiectasis)
Allergic rhinitis

Chronic Cough

The most common causes of chronic cough in immunocompetent adults include the following: upper airway cough syndrome (UACS), previously referred to as *postnasal drip syndrome* (PNDS), which is caused by variety of rhinosinus conditions; (2) asthma; (3) GERD; (4) chronic bronchitis from cigarette smoking or other inhaled environmental irritants; (5) nonasthmatic eosinophilic bronchitis; and (6) bronchiectasis. These conditions, singly or in combination, have accounted for up to 94% of the causes of chronic cough in prospective studies.[2,3,13–15] Other conditions have constituted no > 6% of the causes in prospective studies.[2,3,13-15] These have included bronchogenic carcinoma, chronic interstitial pneumonia, sarcoidosis, left ventricular failure, ACEI-induced cough, and aspiration from a condition associated with pharyngeal dysfunction.

UACS

Because it is unclear whether the mechanisms of cough are postnasal drip itself or the direct irritation or inflammation of the cough receptors located in the upper airway, the 2006 ACCP Cough Guideline Committee recommended that the term *UACS* be used in preference to PNDS when referring to cough associated with upper airway conditions. The diagnosis of UACS is determined by prescribing medications that eliminate the discharge or inflammation and the complaint, such as cough. Although the pathogenesis of chronic cough attributed to UACS is not known for certain, available data[16] suggest that it arises from stimuli irritating the afferent limb of the cough reflex located in the hypopharynx and/or larynx. It is not known why only some individuals in the population who have a postnasal drip sensation and/or clear their throats have chronic cough, whereas most others with these same complaints do not. Any condition with the potential for irritating the upper respiratory tract may cause the UACS. Although GERD can irritate the upper respiratory tract and mimic UACS, cough and throat irritation in this setting will only resolve with treatment for GERD, not with therapy directed at causes of UACS such as those shown in Table 4.

The treatment options are somewhat dependent on the subcategory of disease. For instance, in nonhistamine-mediated rhinitides such as the common cold and perennial nonallergic rhinitis, an older-generation antihistamine/decongestant combination medication has been shown to be efficacious in double-blind, randomized, double-blind, prospective studies, and in four prospective, descriptive studies.[2,3,19,13,15]

In contradistinction, newer-generation, relatively nonsedating antihistamines, such as terfenadine in two studies[17,18] and loratadine plus pseudoephedrine in one study,[19] were found to be ineffective in treating the nonhistamine-mediated acute cough associated with the common cold in randomized, placebo-controlled trials. The older antihistamines are probably effective because of their anticholinergic properties. Other treatment options include intranasal corticosteroids and ipratropium; however, data on their use are limited.

Table 4. *Spectrum of Conditions Causing Chronic Cough Due to UACS*

Rhinitis
Allergic rhinitis
Drug-induced rhinitis
Environmental irritant rhinitis
Perennial nonallergic rhinitis
Postinfectious rhinitis
Vasomotor rhinitis
Sinusitis

On the basis of numerous controlled clinical trials in allergic rhinitis, there is good reason to believe that avoidance of allergens, intranasal corticosteroids and cromolyn, and all antihistamines will be efficacious for the treatment of the cough caused by histamine-mediated UACS. Allergen immunotherapy may be of long-term value but is not for immediate help.

Acute bacterial sinusitis in adults is most commonly caused by *Streptococcus pneumoniae* and *Haemophilus influenzae*. Other organisms include anaerobes, Streptococcal species, *Moraxella catarrhalis* (especially in children), and *Staphylococcus aureus*. Therapy includes antibiotics, intranasal corticosteroids to decrease inflammation, and decongestants such as oxymetazoline hydrochloride. It should be noted, however, that no prospective, randomized, double-blind studies have proven either nasal or oral decongestants to be efficacious in patients with documented acute or chronic sinusitis.

The treatment of chronic sinusitis is even less clear cut. However, although the role of bacterial infection and the importance of antibiotic therapy are controversial, four descriptive studies[2,3,13,15] have shown the following treatment regimen to be effective in eliminating the cough caused by UACS secondary to sinusitis: a minimum of 3 weeks of an antibiotic effective against *H influenzae*, mouth anaerobes, and *S pneumoniae*; a minimum of 3 weeks of oral treatment with an older-generation antihistamine/decongestant twice daily and 5 days of intranasal decongestants twice daily. When cough disappears with this therapy, intranasal corticosteroids have been administered for 3 months.

Asthma

Cough is a symptom that occurs in all asthmatics; sometimes, however, persisting cough can be the most troublesome symptom. In prospective, descriptive studies of patients with chronic cough attributable to asthma, cough has been the only symptom from 6.5 to 57% of the time. This is called *cough-variant asthma. A* diagnosis of asthma should be considered in the differential diagnosis of all patients with chronic cough because it is a common cause. Usually, patients with isolated cough do not have variable airflow obstruction at the time of presentation. The diagnosis of cough-variant asthma is suggested by the presence of airway hyperresponsiveness in a patient with chronic cough and only confirmed when cough goes away with asthma medications. The treatment of cough-variant asthma should be the same as that of asthma presenting with other symptoms. The most benefit is likely to be obtained with corticosteroids, either orally initially followed by inhaled corticosteroids if the symptoms are very severe, or with inhaled corticosteroids together with inhaled β_2-agonists to relieve acute symptoms. The inhaled medications should be delivered from a dry powder device or a pressurized metered-dose inhaler together with a spacer. Inhalation from a pressurized metered-dose inhaler can exacerbate cough acutely in some patients with asthma. The maximum symptomatic benefit of the inhaled corticosteroids is often not seen for 6 to 8 weeks.[20]

A therapeutic trial with systemic corticosteroids has sometimes been the only method used by some investigators[21] to attempt to establish a diagnosis of cough-variant asthma. This method for diagnosis is not recommended because other types of chronic cough (*eg*, chronic nonasthmatic eosinophilic bronchitis[22]) that are not associated with the physiologic abnormalities of asthma (*eg*, airway hyperresponsiveness or variable airflow obstruction) can respond to the same antiinflammatory medication.

Nonasthmatic Eosinophilic Bronchitis

There are patients who present with chronic cough as an isolated symptom, normal spirometry results, normal airway responsiveness to inhaled methacholine, and eosinophilic airway inflammation (*ie*, >3% of nonsquamous epithelial cells in induced-sputum samples are eosinophils). This condition is called *nonasthmatic eosinophilic bronchitis.*[22] The differences in functional association appear to be related to the localization of mast cells within the airway wall, with airway smooth-muscle infiltration occurring in patients with asthma and only epithelial infiltration in patients with nonasthmatic eosinophilic bronchitis. A few cases have been associated with occupational exposures to acrylates. Although this condition is considered to be distinct from asthma, it appears to be sensitive to inhaled or oral corticosteroids. The dose and duration of treatment differ between patients. The condition can be transient, episodic, or persistent unless treated, and occasionally, patients may require long-term prednisone treatment.

GERD

GERD, along with asthma and UACS, is one of the three most common causes of chronic cough in adults. Although GERD can cause cough by aspiration, it most likely causes chronic cough in patients with normal chest radiographic findings by a vagally mediated distal esophageal-tracheobronchial reflex mechanism.[23] When GERD is the cause of chronic cough, there may be no GI symptoms up to 75% of the time. A cough reflux self-perpetuating cycle is likely to exist whereby cough from any cause may precipitate further reflux. Therefore, in the management of patients with chronic cough, consideration should be given to breaking this cycle by searching for and treating other simultaneously contributing conditions.

Although far from perfect, the most sensitive and specific test for GERD is 24-h esophageal pH monitoring. In interpreting this test, it is essential not only to evaluate the duration and frequency of the reflux episodes, but also to determine the temporal relationship between reflux and cough episodes. Patients with normal standard reflux parameters may still have reflux diagnosed as a cause of cough if the temporal relationship exists. Although 24-h esophageal pH monitoring is the most sensitive and specific test in linking GERD and cough in a cause-effect relationship, it has its limitations. For example, there is no general agreement on how to best interpret the test, and it cannot detect nonacid reflux events that have been shown to be important in the pathogenesis of the disease.

Therefore, in patients with chronic cough caused by GERD, the 2006 ACCP Cough Guideline Committee recommends that the term *acid reflux disease*, unless it can be definitively shown to apply, should be replaced by the more general term *reflux disease*, so as not to mislead the clinicians into thinking that all patients with cough caused by GERD should improve with acid-suppression therapy.[23] The Committee also recommends empiric therapy for GERD when patients fit the following clinical profile that has been prospectively validated to be 92% accurate in predicting that cough will improve or disappear with antireflux therapy:

- Cough >8 weeks in duration
- Not exposed to environmental irritants or a present smoker
- Not receiving an ACEI
- Chest radiographic findings are normal or show nothing more than stable, inconsequential scarring
- Symptomatic asthma has been ruled out:
  - Cough has not improved with asthma therapy or
  - Methacholine inhalation challenge is negative
- UACS caused by rhinosinus diseases has been ruled out:
  - First-generation histamine type 1 antagonist has been used and cough failed to improve, and
  - "Silent" sinusitis has been ruled out; and
- nonasthmatic eosinophilic bronchitis has been ruled out:
  - Properly performed sputum study results are negative or
  - Cough has not improved with inhaled/systemic corticosteroids

When using empiric therapy as a diagnostic test, it is important to be aware that if empiric therapy fails, it cannot be assumed that GERD has been ruled out as a cause of cough because the empiric therapy may not have been intensive enough or medical therapy may have failed. The objective of therapy is to decrease the frequency and duration of reflux events and decrease the irritative nature of gastric secretions. Conservative, dietary, and lifestyle measures should be tried in all patients. These measures, in addition to acid-suppressing agents with or without prokinetic agents, have resulted in the resolution of cough in 70 to 100% of adults.[23] In patients who failed to respond to this therapy, antireflux surgery may be successful.[23]

Because it is not known what constitutes the minimum effective medical therapy for treating chronic cough caused by GERD, the following caveats should be considered: (1) drug therapy should not be used to the exclusion of dietary and lifestyle changes; (2) acid-suppression therapy alone may fail; (3) patients may not start to improve until 2 to 3 months of intensive medical therapy has been administered, including diet, lifestyle changes, and acid-suppressing and prokinetic agents; and (4) antireflux surgery may be successful when intensive medical therapy has failed. Failure of medical therapy can be determined by performing 24-h esophageal pH/impedance monitoring while the patient is continuing the most intensive medical therapy. This relatively new test has the ability to detect all reflux events by changes in impedance and can determine the percentage that is acidic and nonacidic in nature.

Chronic Bronchitis

Cough is one of the main features of chronic bronchitis. It is caused by inhalation of irritants and associated with airway inflammation, mucus hypersecretion, and impaired mucociliary clearance. It is important not to overdiagnose this condition as the cause of a cough-phlegm syndrome in patients who are not smokers and who are not exposed to environmental irritants because UACS, asthma, and GERD are more common causes of this syndrome.[15] Although most smokers have a chronic cough, they are not the group of patients who most commonly seek medical attention complaining of cough. Treatment should mainly target a reduction of sputum production and airway inflammation by removing environmental irritants, particularly through smoking cessation. Cough has been shown to disappear or markedly decrease in 94 to 100% of patients with smoking cessation; 54% of the time, cough resolution occurred within 4 weeks.[24] Ipratropium can decrease sputum production, but mucolytics are of no apparent benefit.[25] Although the effectiveness of systemic corticosteroids and antibiotics on cough has not been specifically studied, they are likely to be helpful in decreasing cough during the most severe exacerbations of COPD.[25]

Bronchiectasis

As a cause of chronic cough, bronchiectasis has been diagnosed in prospective studies[3,15] with a frequency of approximately 4%. Its diagnosis is established by compatible clinical history, chest radiographs, high-resolution CT scans of the thorax, and cough disappearance with specific therapy. Cough associated with flares of the disease can be treated successfully with a combination of chest physiotherapy, drugs to stimulate mucociliary clearance, and systemic antibiotics. Aerosolized antibiotics have been shown to be effective in cystic fibrosis (CF) patients with bronchiectasis, but their use in non-CF patients has not been proven to be of benefit.

Bronchogenic Carcinoma

Bronchogenic carcinoma is not a common cause of chronic cough (0 to 2%). It is very unlikely in patients who have never smoked. Chest radiography, sputum cytology, and flexible bronchoscopy are the most important initial tests to consider in evaluating for this entity. The chest radiograph is the most important initial diagnostic test for predicting whether a bronchogenic carcinoma is not a potential cause of chronic cough. The chest radiograph has a positive predictive value of 36 to 38% and a negative predictive value of 100%.[26] When the radiograph suggests that bronchogenic carcinoma or an inflammatory pulmonary parenchymal process are present in the context of chronic cough, bronchoscopy has a positive predictive value of 50 to 89% and negative predictive value of 100%.[26] In nonsmokers with chest radiographic findings that are normal or show nothing more than a stable, inconsequential scar, bronchogenic carcinoma is so unlikely to be the cause of chronic cough that other causes should initially be preferentially pursued.[26]

ACEI-Induced Cough

Cough caused by ACEIs is typically nonproductive and is associated with an irritating, tickling, or scratchy sensation in the throat. Cough appears to be a class effect of these drugs and not dose related. Cough has been shown to be caused by ACEIs from 0 to 3% of the time.[27] Cough may appear within a few hours to weeks or months after taking the first dose of the ACEI. Because no laboratory test will predict who will have an ACEI-induced cough, the diagnosis should be considered in any patient who has a cough while receiving an ACEI. Although cough caused by ACEIs typically comes on after variable periods of time after initiation of therapy, patients can present with cough initially as the result of another condition before initiation of the ACEI therapy and have cough subsequently be attributed solely to an ACEI when the original cough goes away. Therefore, no matter when cough starts in association with an ACEI, consider the diagnosis of ACEI-induced cough. Cough caused by ACEIs will disappear or substantially improve within 4 weeks of discontinuing the drug.[27] Although sulindac, indomethacin, nifedipine, picotamide, and inhaled sodium cromoglycate will provide symptomatic relief in some patients, definitive treatment is discontinuation of the drug.[27]

The incidence of cough associated with therapy with angiotensin-receptor blockers has been shown to be similar to that of control drugs such as hydrochlorothiazide. Therefore, these agents in most instances can be used in place of ACEIs when the ACEIs have to be stopped because of cough.

Habit Cough, Tic Cough, and Psychogenic Cough in Adult and Pediatric Populations

In adults, these are very uncommon causes of chronic cough. The methodologies used and the rigor of the diagnostic and therapeutic interventions reported in the literature are inconsistent. The putative clinical characteristics of habit cough and psychogenic cough, for the most part, have not been prospectively or systematically studied. Therefore, on the basis of expert opinion, the diagnoses of habit cough or psychogenic cough can be made only after an extensive evaluation is performed that includes ruling out tic disorders and uncommon causes of chronic cough and after cough improves with behavior modification or psychiatric therapy.[28] Short of a therapeutic trial, it is hard to distinguish habit cough from cough caused by UACS. Although the pediatric literature[28] suggests that the patients with psychogenic cough will have a barking or honking character to their coughs, the presence or absence of these characteristics is not diagnostically helpful in adults.

Chronic Interstitial Pulmonary Disease

In series of patients, this is an uncommon cause of chronic cough. In patients with chronic cough, before diagnosing interstitial lung disease as the sole cause, common etiologies such as UACS, asthma, and GERD should be considered. The cause of cough may be caused by a diagnosis other than interstitial lung disease at least 50% of the time. Therefore, the diagnosis of interstitial lung disease as the cause of cough should be considered a diagnosis of exclusion.[29]

Guidelines for Evaluating Acute Cough

A clinical approach is recommended for evaluating acute cough.[30] The approach initially consists of obtaining history, physical examination, and considering the need for laboratory investigations. Figure 1 is the suggested algorithm for managing adult patients with an acute cough. The most important initial clinical decision is to decide whether the patient does or does not have a potential life-threatening condition.

Guidelines for Evaluating Subacute Cough

A clinical approach is recommended for evaluating subacute cough.[30] The approach initially consists of obtaining history, physical examination, and considering the need for laboratory investigations. Figure 2 is the suggested algorithm for managing adult patients with a subacute cough. The most important initial clinical decision is to decide whether the subacute cough did or did not follow an obvious respiratory infection.

Guidelines for Evaluating Chronic Cough

A great deal is now known about how to successfully diagnose and treat chronic cough. For instance, the relative frequency of the disorders, alone and in combination, that can cause cough, as well as the sensitivity and specificity of various findings on medical history, physical examination, and the pertinent diagnostic tests (Table 5), are known from a number of clinical studies.[31] On the basis of this composite body of information, the 2006 ACCP Cough Guidelines Committee[30] recommends an initial empiric integrative approach to the management of chronic cough. Figure 3 is the suggested algorithm for managing adult patients with a chronic cough. After obtaining a history and performing a physical examination and chest radiography, the most important initial clinical decisions are to decide whether the etiology of the chronic cough is associated with an abnormal chest radiographic finding, smoking, or an ACEI. If it is not associated with any of these, the most common causes (UACS, asthma, nonasthmatic eosinophilic bronchitis, and GERD) should then be systematically considered.

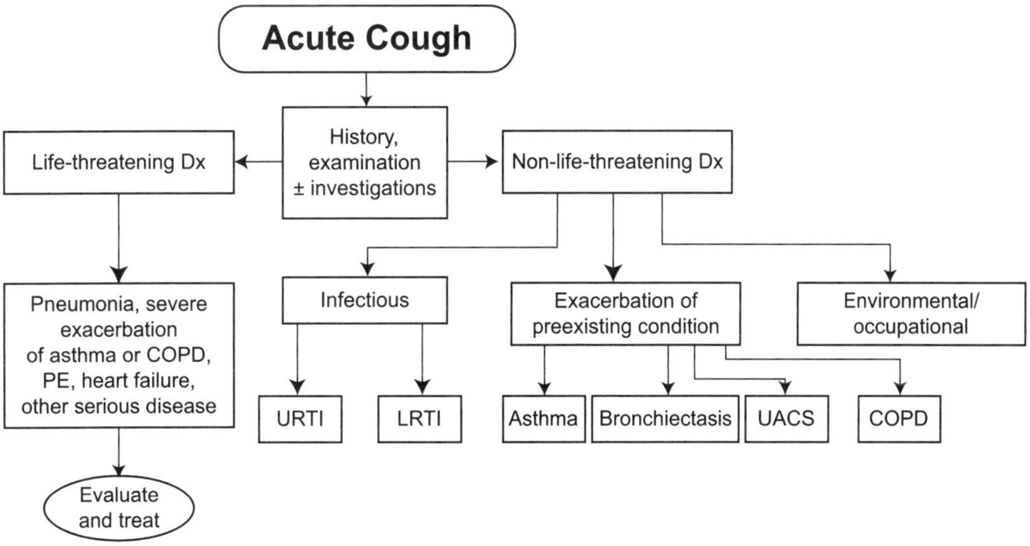

Figure 1. Acute cough algorithm for the management of patients ≥ 15 years of age with cough lasting < 3 weeks. Dx = diagnosis; LRTI = lower respiratory tract infection; PE = pulmonary embolism; UACS = upper airway cough syndrome; URTI = upper respiratory tract infection.

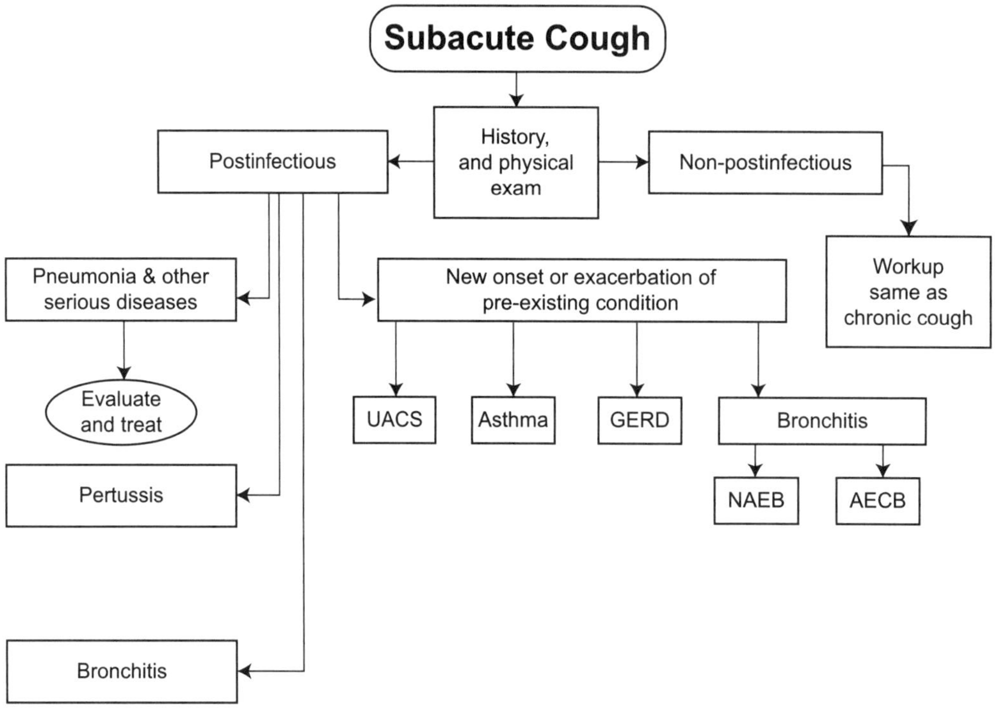

Figure 2. Subacute cough algorithm for the management of patients ≥15 years of age with cough lasting 3 to 8 weeks. AECB = acute exacerbation of chronic bronchitis; NAEB = nonasthmatic eosinophilic bronchitis; UACS = upper airway cough syndrome.

Table 5. *Testing Characteristics of Diagnostic Protocol**

Tests	Sensitivity, %	Specificity, %	PPV, %	NPV, %
Chest radiograph	100	54–76	36–38	100
Sinus radiograph	97–100	75–79	57–81	95–100
MIC	100	67–71	60–82	100
BaE	48–92	42–76	30–63	63–93
24-h esophageal pH	<100	66–100	89–100	<100
Bronchoscopy	100	50–92	50–89	100

*Data are from Irwin et al[3] and Smyrnios et al.[15] BaE = modified barium esophagography; MIC = methacholine inhalation challenge; NPV = negative predictive value; PPV = positive predictive value.

If the patient's cough persists after the empiric integrative evaluation, the following systematic, diagnostic approach that has been validated in immunocompetent patients with chronic cough is recommended: (1) Review the patient's history and perform a physical examination, concentrating on the anatomy of the cough reflex (Fig 4) and specifically the most common causes of chronic cough. The character of the cough (*eg*, paroxysmal, loose, and self propagating; productive or dry) and timing (*eg*, nocturnal, with meals) have not been shown in a prospective study[14] to be of diagnostic help. (2) Order a chest radiograph in nearly all patients. It is extremely useful for initially ranking differential diagnostic possibilities and directing laboratory testing. (3) Do not order additional laboratory tests in present smokers or patients receiving an ACEI until the response to cessation of smoking or discontinuation of the drug for 4 weeks can be assessed. (4) Depending on the results of the initial evaluation, smoking cessation, or discontinuation of the ACEI, the following may be obtained: sinus radiographs and allergy evaluation; spirometry prebronchodilator and postbronchodilator or methacholine inhalation challenge; modified barium esophagography and/or 24-h esophageal pH/impedance monitoring; sputum for microbiology and/or

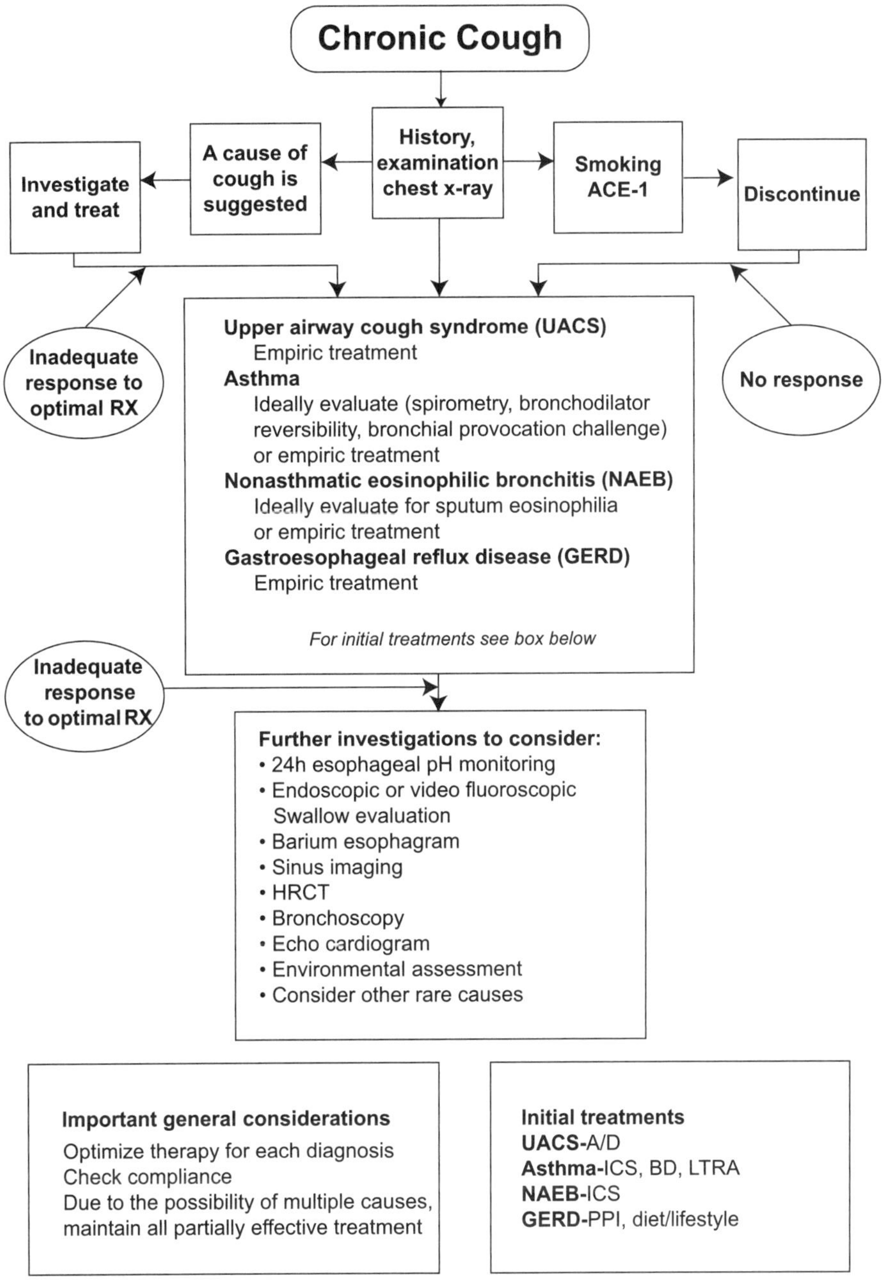

Figure 3. Chronic cough algorithm for the management of patients ≥15 years of age with cough lasting >8 weeks. A/D = antihistamine/decongestant; BD = bronchodilator; HRCT = high-resolution chest CT; ICS = inhaled corticosteroid; LTRA = leukotriene receptor antagonist; PPI = proton pump inhibitor.

cytology; flexible bronchoscopy; chest CT scan; and noninvasive cardiac studies. (5) Determine the cause(s) of cough by observing which specific therapy eliminates cough as a complaint. If the evaluation suggests more than one possible cause, therapies should be initiated in the same sequence in which the abnormalities were discovered. Because cough can be simultaneously caused by more than one condition, do not stop therapy that appears to be partially successful; rather, sequentially add to it.

Summary of Expected Results

The following is a summary of expected results when the aforementioned systematic, diagnostic approach is used[31]:

1. The cause can be determined from 88 to 100% of the time, leading to "specific therapy" with success rates between 84% and 98%.
2. Chronic cough is often simultaneously caused by more than one condition. A single cause has been found from 38 to 82% of the time,

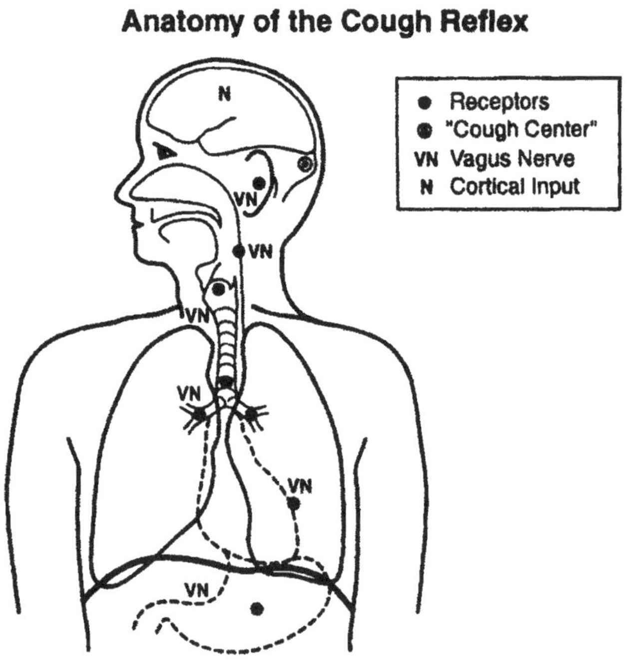

Figure 4. Schematic representation of the anatomy of the cough reflex. This representation comes from an amalgamation of clinical observations in man, and histologic and physiological results in experimental animal studies.

multiple causes from 18 to 62%. Multiply caused cough has been the result of three diseases up to 42% of the time.

3. Although most smokers have a cough, they have not been the group of patients who most commonly seek medical attention complaining of cough.
4. In adults of all ages and the elderly, UACS, asthma, and/or GERD are the three most common causes of chronic cough.
5. In prospective studies,[31] chronic cough in adults is most commonly (up to 94%) caused by six disorders: UACS, asthma, GERD, chronic bronchitis, noneosinophilic bronchitis, and bronchiectasis.
6. Cough has been shown in prospective studies[31] to be caused by four conditions (UACS, asthma, nonasthmatic eosinophilic bronchitis, and/or GERD) >99% of the time in nonsmoking adults who are not receiving an ACEI and who have a normal or nearly normal and stable chest radiographic findings.
7. Cough can be the sole clinical manifestation of asthma and GERD up to 57% and 75% of the time, respectively, and nonspecific bronchoprovocation challenge testing and 24-h esophageal pH monitoring have been shown to be extremely useful in making a diagnosis in these patients.
8. Unless the chest radiographic findings are abnormal, and this is an uncommon occurrence (no >7%), flexible bronchoscopy will have a very low diagnostic utility (approximately 4%).
9. The principal strength of the diagnostic protocol is in ruling out suspected possibilities. The principal limitation is that a positive test result cannot necessarily be relied on to establish the diagnosis because it has not always been shown to predict a favorable response to specific therapy (Table 5).
10. A carefully obtained history with detailed questioning of the character, timing, and complications of cough are not likely to be helpful in predicting the cause of chronic cough.

Treatment

We have learned a great deal about treatment of chronic cough. It can be divided into two main categories: (1) therapy that controls, prevents, or eliminates cough (antitussive therapy); and (2) therapy that makes cough more effective (protussive therapy). Antitussive therapy can be either specific or nonspecific. Specific therapy is directed at the etiology or operant pathophysiologic mechanism responsible for cough. Nonspecific therapy is directed at the symptom; it is indicated when specific therapy cannot be administered. There is a limited role for nonspecific therapy because of the high probability of one being able to determine the cause of chronic cough and prescribe specific therapy that can be successful 84 to 98% of the time,

Recommendations for specific therapy can be found in the section on specific diseases. When nonspecific antitussive therapy for chronic cough is indicated, dextromethorphan, codeine, and ipratropium bromide aerosol in patients with chronic bronchitis appear to be the agents of choice; they have been well studied and have been shown to be effective in double-blind, placebo-controlled studies.[32] To date, the clinical utility of protussive therapy remains to be determined in future studies that assess short-term and long-term effects of these agents on the patient's condition. The use of aerosolized hypertonic saline solution in patients with CF appears promising.

Wheeze

Wheeze is a continuous musical sound that lasts >80 to 100 ms.[33] The pathophysiologic mechanism(s) that generate wheezing are still not known. Although movement of airway secretions may play a role, flutter of airway walls narrowed almost to the point of closure is the most likely mechanism.[34] Wheeze can be high or low pitched, consist of single or multiple notes, occur during inspiration or expiration, and originate from airways of any size, from the large extrathoracic upper airway down to the intrathoracic small airways. Stridor refers to inspiratory wheezing loudest over the central airways.

Although the pitch of a wheeze is not determined by the site of its origin,[34] its timbre may theoretically provide a clue to its location. A polyphonic wheeze, consisting of multiple musical notes, is typically produced by dynamic compression of the large, more central airways.[34] Although monophonic wheezes, consisting of single musical notes, typically reflect disease in small airways and suggest asthma, especially when they are multiple, they have also been produced by diseases involving the extrathoracic large airways.[34] Although recognizing that the polyphonic or monophonic nature of expiratory wheezes may be helpful in suggesting the location of the wheeze, there are no studies that have evaluated their positive and negative predictive values in doing so.

Diagnostic Value of History and Physical Examination

Expiratory wheezing appreciated either by history or physical examination is lacking in sensitivity and specificity in diagnosing asthma.[35–38] Symptomatic asthma can present without wheeze, and wheezing associated with other conditions can mimic asthma. In a prospective study[35] of patients referred to a pulmonary clinic because of wheeze, a history of wheeze was predictive of asthma 35% of the time, and the physical finding of expiratory monophonic wheeze was predictive 43% of the time.

Inspiratory wheezing on physical examination is not specific for extrathoracic upper airway conditions, and it is not a sensitive sign of extrathoracic upper airway obstruction. Although inspiratory wheezing frequently accompanies expiratory wheezing during acute asthma, wheezing during asthma also may be heard only during inspiration.[36] Patients will have dyspnea on exertion when the site of upper airway obstruction is <8 mm in diameter, and stridor when the diameter is <5 mm.[39,40]

Because a wheeze can be caused by obstruction of any airway and because there is no characteristic of the wheeze of asthma that reliably distinguishes it from other conditions, it follows that wheezes should never be considered *a priori* caused by asthma. This finding has been confirmed by a study[35] that prospectively evaluated the acoustic spectrum and frequency of the causes of wheeze. This study also revealed that UACS, not asthma, was the most common cause of wheeze of unknown etiology in patients referred to a pulmonary outpatient clinic (Fig 5). Data from other studies[41,42] suggest that the expiratory wheeze associated with the UACS originated from the extrathoracic airway and most likely from the vocal cords.

An Approach to the Diagnosis of Wheeze

In evaluating patients with wheeze, it is important to be aware that "all that wheezes is not asthma; all that wheezes is obstruction." An approach to evaluating wheeze is to localize the site of the obstruction to either large or small intrathoracic airways or the extrathoracic airway using history, physical examination, lung function studies, and knowledge of the spectrum of differential diagnostic possibilities, especially those that have been shown to be the most common (Fig 5). Once diagnostic possibilities have been narrowed by history and physical examination, pulmonary function testing can be quite helpful in confirming a diagnosis.

Pulmonary Function Testing in the Evaluation of Wheeze

Pulmonary function testing can be helpful in localizing the site of obstruction causing the wheeze. Because the airway can be divided into three anatomic areas with different physiologic characteristics, obstructions in these three areas

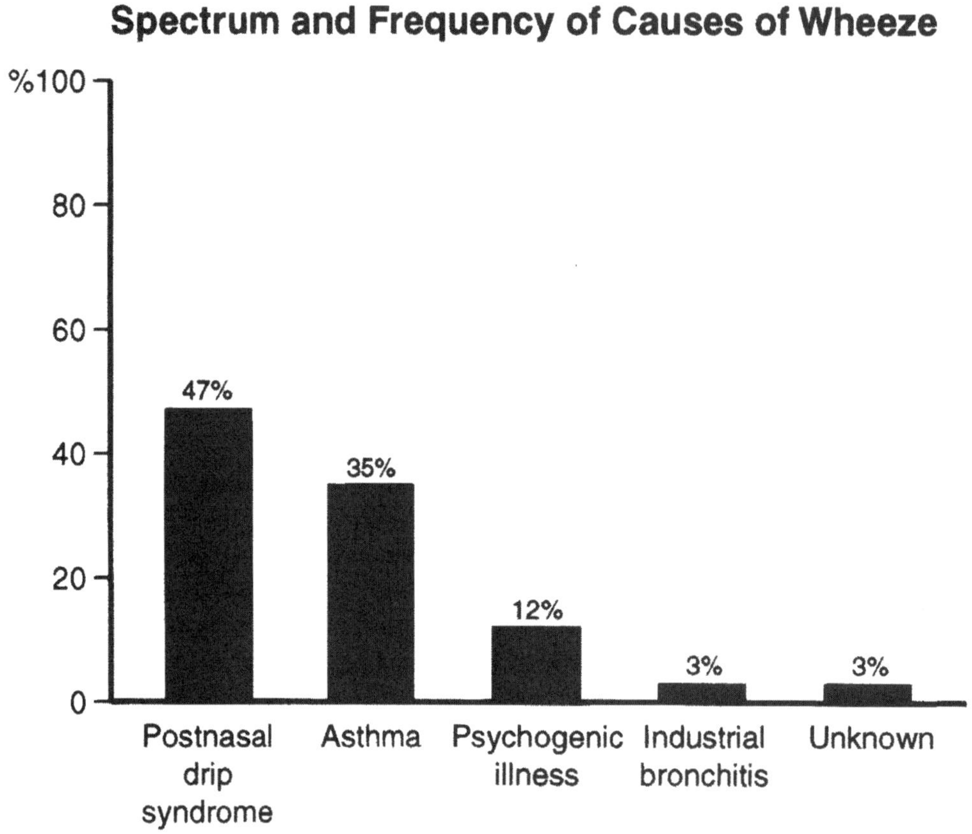

Figure 5. Spectrum and frequency of causes of wheeze in patients referred to a pulmonary clinic. PNDS is now referred to as UACS.

can be physiologically differentiated. The three areas include the following: (1) the extrathoracic upper airway that includes the nose, mouth, pharynx, larynx, and extrathoracic trachea; (2) the intrathoracic upper airways, including the intrathoracic trachea and bronchi down to the level of the 2-mm airways; and (3) the small airways that are < 2 mm in diameter (*ie*, airways that are beyond the eighth and ninth generations from the trachea).[43] From a physiologic standpoint, the distinguishing characteristics of these three anatomic areas are as follows: (1) the extrathoracic and intrathoracic large upper airways undergo different and opposite transmural pressure changes during the respiratory cycle (Fig 6); (2) airflow is predominantly turbulent through large airways and mostly laminar through small airways;[44] and (3) obstruction in the large airways impedes all the air in a uniform manner when there is one point of narrowing, whereas obstruction in small airways is almost always in multiple, scattered sites impeding airflow in a nonuniform manner.

Because spirometry and flow-volume loops during helium and air breathing are influenced by these phenomena, they can be routinely utilized to localize airway obstruction. Spirometry repeated after bronchodilator or systemic corticosteroid administration may demonstrate the presence of a substantial component of reversible airways disease consistent with asthma. In patients with normal or nearly normal baseline spirometry results, nonspecific bronchoprovocation challenge testing may show clinically significant bronchial hyperresponsiveness consistent with asthma.

Upper airway obstructing lesions are best identified by flow-volume loops (Fig 7). When there is only one site of obstruction, as usually occurs in the trachea, airflow is likely to remain constant during the middle portion of a maximum respiratory effort. If the obstruction is variable (*ie*, it allows the airway to respond to the normal transmural pressure change), it will be possible to distinguish an extrathoracic location from an intrathoracic location. A variable extrathoracic obstruction will typically only be seen

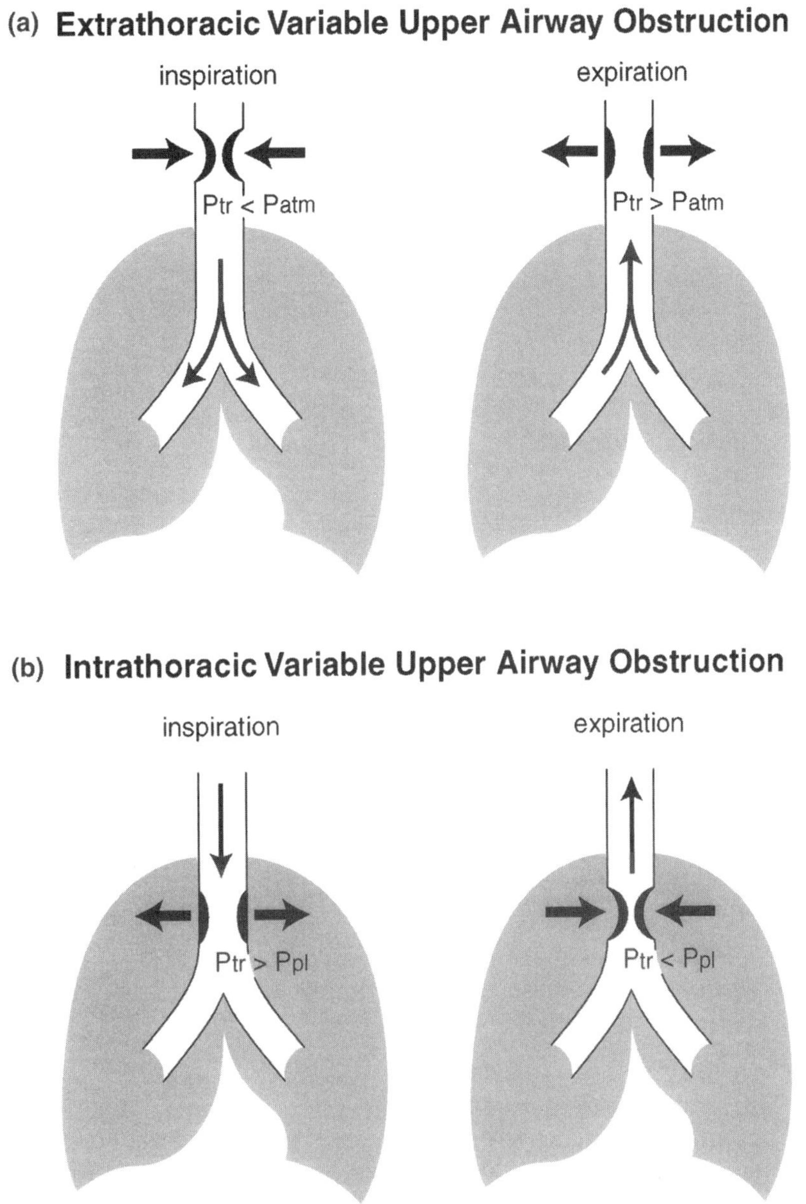

Figure 6. The effect of transmural pressure changes during inspiration and expiration on the severity of obstruction at different airway sites. *Top:* extrathoracic upper airway obstruction. During expiration, intrapleural pressure (Ppl) and subsequently intratracheal pressure (Ptr) are greater than atmospheric pressure (Patm). Therefore, the site of the obstruction widens. During inspiration, because Ppl and Ptr are less than Patm, the site narrows. *Bottom:* intrathoracic upper airway obstruction. During expiration, because Ppl is greater than Ptr, the site narrows. During inspiration, because Ptr is greater than Ppl, the site widens.

during maximal inspiratory effort (Fig 7). Because the extrathoracic airway will dilate during expiration, the maximal expiratory flow volume curve and spirometry will typically be normal. A variable intrathoracic obstruction will only be observed during a maximal expiratory effort (Fig 7), and spirometry will reveal values consistent with expiratory airflow obstruction. Spirometry alone cannot distinguish large from small intrathoracic airway diseases, because FEV_1, peak expiratory flow rate, and FEV_1/FVC percentage will be reduced in both situations. Because inspiratory flow rates are normally greater than expiratory flow rates when compared at lung volumes in the lower two thirds of the vital capacity (VC), the ratio of the two may distinguish variable extrathoracic from intrathoracic upper airway lesions.[45] When a variable extrathoracic lesion is present, inspiratory are less than expiratory flow rates (*eg*, forced inspiratory flow at 50% of VC / forced expiratory flow at 50% of VC is < 1).

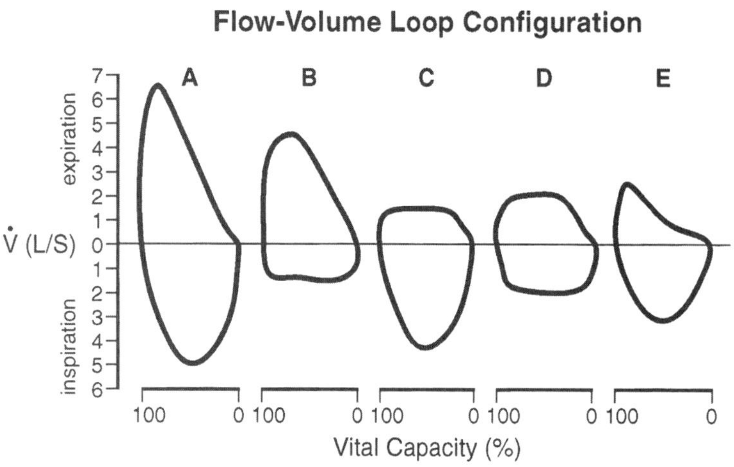

Figure 7. Schematic flow-volume loop configurations in a spectrum of airway lesions. *A*, normal; *B*, variable extrathoracic upper airway obstruction; *C*, variable intrathoracic upper airway lesion; *D*, fixed upper airway obstruction; and *E*, small airways obstruction.

If the upper airway obstruction is fixed (*ie*, it does not allow the airway to respond to normal transmural pressure changes), it cannot be localized physiologically to an extrathoracic or intrathoracic location. Nevertheless, the flow-volume loop will have a characteristic shape (Fig 7) that will suggest that the obstruction is in large rather than small airways (Fig 7). Airflow will be uniformly impeded during inspiration and expiration because there will be no difference between the amount of narrowing in inspiration and expiration. Because expiratory as well as inspiratory flow rates are decreased in a fixed upper airway obstruction, spirometry will reflect the expiratory flow limitation.

By comparing maximal expiratory flow-volume curves while patients first breathe room air and then a 20% oxygen to 80% helium mixture, it may also be possible to detect coexisting large and small airway intrathoracic obstructions.[44] Expiratory flow will substantially increase with the helium mixture when an obstruction occurs in large airways because the turbulent flow that occurs in this region increases when patients respire the less dense helium mixture.[46]

Differential Diagnosis of Wheeze

A large number of conditions located in a variety of anatomic airway locations (Table 6) can produce airway obstruction and present with expiratory or inspiratory wheezing. Asthma should be considered likely when patients present with episodic wheezing and other symptoms that respond favorably to conventional asthma medications (*eg*, inhaled bronchodilators). Although asthmatics with wheeze typically will present with reversible expiratory airflow obstruction demonstrated by spirometry, a restrictive ventilatory pattern also may be seen occasionally. A reversible restrictive lung disease has been described that is clinically indistinguishable from asthma.[47,48] The diagnosis of wheezing conditions other than asthma[49] should be considered when the initial evaluation suggests their presence or when wheeze does not respond to conventional asthma medications. Table 7 provides helpful hints[50,54] to aid in the differential diagnosis of the causes of wheezing.

Treatment

The treatment of wheezing depends on its cause (Tables 6, 7). Because the differential diagnosis of wheezing includes diseases that are potentially life threatening, it is important that the physician arrives at a specific diagnosis and institutes specific therapy. The failure of a therapy to correct wheezing should prompt the physician either to adjust the therapy or to search for an additional cause. The number of patients who have more than one simultaneous cause for wheezing is unknown.

Summary

Wheezes are not synonymous with asthma; they may occur with a variety of diseases. The protocol for the evaluation of wheeze places great emphasis on findings during history and physical examination. Unless the patients appear to be in imminent danger of respiratory failure, the

Table 6. *Differential Diagnosis of Wheeze*

Upper airway obstruction
Extrathoracic causes
UACS
Vocal cord dysfunction syndrome
Hypertrophied tonsils
Epiglottitis
Laryngeal edema
Laryngostenosis
Postextubation granuloma
Retropharyngeal abscess
Neoplasms
Anaphylaxis
Obesity
Klebsiella rhinoscleroma
Mobile supraglottic soft tissue
Relapsing polychondritis
Laryngocele
Abnormal arytenoid movement
Vocal cord hematoma
Bilateral vocal cord paralysis
Cricoarytenoid arthritis
Wegener granulomatosis
Intrathoracic causes
Tracheal stenosis due to intubation
Foreign body aspiration
Benign tracheal/bronchial tumors
Malignancies
Intrathoracic goiter
Tracheobronchomegaly
Acquired tracheomalacia
Herpetic tracheobronchitis
Right-sided aortic arch
Lower airway obstruction
Asthma
COPD
Pulmonary edema
Aspiration
Pulmonary embolism
Bronchiolitis
CF
Carcinoid syndrome
Bronchiectasis
Lymphangitic carcinomatosis
Parasitic infections

physician should, in stepwise fashion, address the following: (1) whatever is found in the history and physical examination, (2) the common causes of wheezing, and (3) less common causes evaluated in a physiologically oriented manner when common causes do not explain the patient's symptoms.

Hemoptysis

Hemoptysis is the spitting of blood derived from the lungs or bronchial tubes. Hemoptysis may be scant, producing the appearance of streaks of bright red blood in the sputum; or profuse, with expectoration of a large volume of blood. Massive hemoptysis is defined as the expectoration of 600 mL of blood within 24 to 48 h and may occur in 3 to 10% of all patients with hemoptysis.[55] Gross or frank hemoptysis produces a quantity smaller than massive hemoptysis and greater than blood streaking. Dark red clots may also be expectorated when blood has been present in the lungs for days.

Pseudohemoptysis is the expectoration of blood from a source other than the lower respiratory tract. It may cause diagnostic confusion when patients cannot clearly describe the source of their bleeding. Pseudohemoptysis[56] may occur when blood from the oral cavity, nares, pharynx, or tongue drains to the back of the throat and initiates the cough reflex; when blood is aspirated into the lower respiratory tract in patients who have hematemesis; and when the oropharynx is colonized with the red, pigment-producing, aerobic, Gram-negative rod, *Serratia marcescens.* This colonization may occur in hospitalized patients who have received broad-spectrum antimicrobial agents and mechanical ventilation. Other rare causes of pseudohemoptysis are self-inflicted injuries or other bizarre tactics in the malingering patient seeking hospitalization, and rifampin overdose (red man syndrome).

Etiology

Hemoptysis can be caused by a wide variety of disorders (Table 8).[56] The etiologies are considered here in three general categories: nonmassive, massive, and idiopathic.

Nonmassive Hemoptysis: Although bronchitis, bronchiectasis, lung carcinoma, and tuberculosis have always been among the most common causes of hemoptysis, their incidence varies depending on the study population. The more recent studies[55,57] have shown that bronchiectasis and tuberculosis have become less common and bronchitis more common. In 148 urban, adult, mostly indigent patients studied in Kansas City between 1977 and 1985, the causes of hemoptysis were bronchitis in

Table 7. *Diagnosis of Selected Wheezing Illnesses Other Than Asthma*

Illnesses	Distinguishing Features
Upper airway diseases	
UACS	History of postnasal drip, throat clearing, nasal discharge; physical examination shows oropharyngeal secretions or cobblestone appearance to the mucosa
Epiglottitis	History of sore throat out of proportion to pharyngitis; evidence of supraglottitis on endoscopy or lateral neck radiographs
Vocal cord dysfunction syndrome	Lack of symptomatic response to bronchodilators; presence of stridor plus expiratory wheeze in absence of increased alveolar-arterial pressure gradient; extrathoracic variable obstruction on flow-volume loops; paradoxical inspiratory and/or early expiratory adduction of vocal cords on laryngoscopy during wheezing; this syndrome can masquerade as asthma, be provoked by exercise, and often coexists with asthma
Retropharyngeal abscess	History of stiff neck, sore throat, fever, trauma to posterior pharynx; swelling noted by lateral neck or CT radiographs
Laryngotracheal injury caused by tracheal cannulation	History of cannulation of trachea by endotracheal or tracheostomy tube; evidence of intrathoracic or extrathoracic, variable obstruction on flow-volume loops, neck/chest radiographs, laryngoscopy or bronchoscopy, or all of these. Flow-volume loops with helium and air may reveal large airway obstruction superimposed on underlying small airway disease (*eg*, COPD).
Neoplasms	Carcinoid tumor is suspected when there is hemoptysis, unilateral wheeze, or evidence of lobar collapse on chest radiography or combinations of these; bronchogenic carcinoma in the same setting in a cigarette smoker; diagnosis is confirmed by bronchoscopy
Anaphylaxis	Abrupt onset of wheezing with urticaria, angioedema, nausea, diarrhea, and hypotension, especially after insect bites or administration of drug or IV contrast, or family history
Small airway diseases	
COPD	History of dyspnea on exertion and productive cough in cigarette smoker; because productive cough is nonspecific, it should only be ascribed to COPD when other cough phlegm syndromes have been excluded[47]; forced expiratory time >4 s, and there is decreased breath sound intensity; unforced wheezing during auscultation and irreversible, expiratory airflow obstruction on spirometry[47,48]
Pulmonary edema	History and physical examinations consistent with passive congestion of the lungs, ARDS, impaired lung lymphatics; abnormal chest radiograph, echocardiogram, radionuclide ventriculography, cardiac catheterization, or combinations of these
Aspiration	History of risk for pharyngeal dysfunction or GERD; abnormal modified barium swallow and/or 24-h esophageal pH monitoring
Pulmonary embolism	History of risk for thromboembolic disease; positive confirmatory test results
Bronchiolitis	History of respiratory infection, connective tissue disease, transplantation, ulcerative colitis, development of chronic airflow obstruction over months to few years rather than over many years in a nonsmoker; mixed obstructive and restrictive pattern on pulmonary function tests, and hyperinflation and fine nodular infiltrates on chest radiography
CF	Combination of productive cough, digital clubbing, bronchiectasis with Pseudomonas colonization/infection obstructive azoospermia; family history; pancreatic insufficiency and two sweat chloride determinations >60 mEq/L; some diagnoses are not made until adulthood; in one instance as late as age 69 yr[51]; when sweat test result is occasionally normal, definitive diagnosis may require nasal transepithelial voltage measurements and genotyping[52]
Carcinoid syndrome	History of episodes of flushing and watery diarrhea; elevated 5-hydroxyindoleaceticacid level in a 24-h urine specimen
Bronchiectasis	History of episodes of productive cough, fever, or recurrent pneumonias; suggestive chest radiographs or typical chest CT findings; allergic pulmonary aspergillosis should be considered when bronchiectasis is central
Lymphangitis carcinomatosis	History of dyspnea or previous malignancy; reticulonodular infiltrates with or without pleural effusions; suggestive high-resolution chest CT scan; bronchoscopy with biopsies
Parasitic infections	Consider in a nonasthmatic who has traveled to an endemic area and complains of fatigue, weight loss, fever; peripheral blood eosinophilia; infiltrates on chest radiograph; stools for ova and parasites for nonfilarial causes; blood serologic studies for filarial causes

Table 8. *Causes of Hemoptysis According to Category of Disease**

Tracheobronchial disorders
Acute tracheobronchitis
Amyloidosis
Aspiration of gastric contents
Bronchial adenoma
Bronchial endometriosis
Bronchial telangiectasia
Bronchiectasis
Bronchogenic carcinoma
Broncholithiasis
Chronic bronchitis
CF
Endobronchial hamartoma
Endobronchial metastases
Endobronchial tuberculosis
Foreign body aspiration
Mucoid impaction of bronchus
Tracheobronchial trauma
Tracheoesophageal fistula
Tracheoartery fistula
Localized parenchymal diseases
Acute and chronic nontuberculous pneumonia
Actinomycosis
Amebiasis
Ascariasis
Bronchopulmonary sequestration
Coccidioidomycosis
Congenital and acquired cyst
Cryptococcosis
Exogenous lipoid pneumonia
Histoplasmosis
Hydatid mole
Lung abscess
Lung contusion
Metastatic cancer
Mucormycosis
Nocardiosis
Paragonimiasis
Pulmonary endometriosis
Pulmonary tuberculosis
Sporotrichosis
Hematologic disorders
Anticoagulant therapy
Disseminated intravascular coagulation
Leukemia
Thrombocytopenia
Cardiovascular disorders
Aortic aneurysm
Bronchial artery rupture
Congenital heart disease
Congestive heart failure
Coronary artery bypass graft
Fat embolization
Hughes-Stovin syndrome
Mitral stenosis
Postmyocardial infarction syndrome
Pulmonary arteriovenous fistula
Pulmonary artery aneurysm
Pulmonary embolism
Pulmonary venous varix
Schistosomiasis
Subclavian artery aneurysm
Superior vena cava syndrome
Tumor embolization
Diffuse parenchymal diseases
Capillaritis (with or without systemic vasculitis)
Disseminated angiosarcoma
Farmer lung
Goodpasture syndrome
Idiopathic pulmonary hemosiderosis
IgA nephropathy
Inhaled isocyanates
Legionnaires disease
Mixed connective tissue disease
Mixed cryoglobulinemia
Polyarteritis nodosa
Scleroderma
Systemic lupus erythematosus
Systemic vasculitis
TMA toxicity
Viral pneumonitis
Wegener granulomatosis
Miscellaneous disorders
Idiopathic
Iatrogenic
Bronchoscopy
Cardiac catheterization
Needle lung biopsy

* This listing is not meant to be all-inclusive.

37%, bronchogenic carcinoma in 19%, tuberculosis in 7%, pneumonia in 5%, and bronchiectasis in 1%.[57] In 59 patients with hemoptysis >200 mL/d studied at Duke University between the years 1972 and 1981, the causes included bronchitis or bronchiectasis in 28%, cancer in 36%, CF in 7%, anticoagulation in 7%, and tuberculosis in 5%.[55] In a retrospective study[58] of hemoptysis in patients with HIV infection, the cause was identified for 78% of episodes. Of these, it was thought to be the result of pneumonia in 70%, Kaposi sarcoma in 12%, bronchiectasis in 5%, pulmonary embolism in 5%, bronchitis in 3%, endocarditis in 3%, and lung cancer in 3%. Of the 28 presumed pneumonias, disease was caused by bacterial etiology in 16 cases, *Mycobacterium tuberculosis* in 3 cases, *Pneumocystis jiroveci* in 3 cases, *Mycobacterium avium-intracellulare* in 3 cases, and fungal causes in 3 cases. Hemoptysis in this series when described was blood streaking in 77%, frank in 19%, and massive in 4% (as the result of Aspergillus sp and Pseudomonas sp infections). Although bleeding from tracheoartery fistula complicating tracheostomy, rupture of pulmonary artery from a balloon flotation catheter, and diffuse intrapulmonary hemorrhage may be submassive, they are discussed in the section on massive hemoptysis.

Massive Hemoptysis: The more frequent causes of massive hemoptysis are listed in Table 9. Virtually all causes of hemoptysis may result in massive hemoptysis, but it is most frequently caused by infection and cancer. Several series[56] report that >60% of cases are caused by tuberculosis, bronchiectasis, and lung abscess. Infection is also the cause of bleeding from aspergilloma and CF. In one series[57] of 22 patients, 27% of cases were caused by bronchitis, 18% were caused by tuberculosis, 9% were caused by aspergilloma, 4% were caused by bronchiectasis, and 4% were caused by sporotrichosis. In a series[55] from Duke University, 17 of 42 patients (40%) with massive hemoptysis had cancer and only 8 patients (19%) had bronchitis, bronchiectasis, or tuberculosis as a cause. Idiopathic hemoptysis is less frequent in patients with massive hemoptysis and usually constitutes <5% of cases.[57]

Rupture of a pulmonary artery complicates balloon flotation catheterizations in <0.2% of cases.[59] It is fortunate that this is rare because it carries a mortality approximating 40%.[59] Tracheoartery fistula is also an unusual but devastating condition, complicating approximately 0.7% of tracheostomies.[60] These two complications of procedures and diffuse intrapulmonary hemorrhage, usually attributable to an immunologically mediated disease, are most likely to be considered in the differential diagnosis of massive rather than submassive hemoptysis in ICU patients.

Idiopathic Hemoptysis: When one uses the systematic diagnostic approach outlined in Tables 10 and 11, the cause of hemoptysis can be found in most instances. In 2 to 32% of patients (average, 12%),[61,62] the cause cannot be determined. This condition, called *idiopathic* or *essential hemoptysis*, is seen most commonly in men between the ages of 30 and 50 years. Prolonged follow-up studies almost always fail to reveal the source of bleeding, although 10% continue to have occasional episodes of hemoptysis.[63] Consider Dieulafoy disease of bronchus (superficial bronchial artery) in the context of idiopathic hemoptysis; it can be involved in a subset of patients yet to be determined.[64]

Table 9. *Common Causes of Massive Hemoptysis*

Cardiovascular
Arteriobronchial fistula
Congestive heart failure
Pulmonary arteriovenous fistula
Diffuse intrapulmonary hemorrhage
Diffuse parenchymal disease
Iatrogenic
Malposition of chest tube
Pulmonary artery rupture
Tracheoartery fistula
Infections
Aspergilloma
Bronchiectasis
Bronchitis
CF
Lung abscess
Sporotrichosis
Tuberculosis
Malignancies
Bronchogenic carcinoma
Leukemia
Metastatic cancer
Trauma

Table 10. *Routine Evaluations for Hemoptysis*

History
Physical examination
CBC
Urinalysis
Coagulation studies
ECG
Chest radiography
± Bronchoscopy*

*Although bronchoscopy is not indicated in some conditions (*eg*, pulmonary embolism, aortopulmonary fistula, congestive heart failure), it should routinely be considered.

Table 11. *Examples of Special Evaluations for Hemoptysis According to Category of Disease**

Tracheobronchial disorders
Expectorated sputa for tuberculosis, parasites, fungi, and Cytology
Bronchoscopy (if not done)
Bronchography
High-resolution chest CT scan
Localized parenchymal diseases
Expectorated sputa for tuberculosis, parasites, fungi, and Cytology
Chest CT scan
Lung biopsy with special stains
Diffuse parenchymal diseases
Expectorated sputa for cytology
Blood for BUN, creatinine, anti-nuclear antibody,
Rheumatoid factor, complement, cryoglobulins,
Antineutrophil cytoplasmic antibody
Antiglomerular basement membrane antibody
Lung and/or kidney biopsy with special stains
Cardiovascular disorders
Echocardiogram
Arterial blood gas on 21% and 100% oxygen
Ventilation/perfusion scans
Pulmonary arteriogram
Aortogram, contrast CT scans
Hematologic disorders
Coagulation studies
Bone marrow

*This list is not meant to be all-inclusive.

Pathogenesis

The bronchial arteries are the chief source of blood for the airways (from mainstem bronchi to terminal bronchioles), for the supporting framework of the lung that includes the pleura, intrapulmonary lymphoid tissue, and the large branches of the pulmonary vessels, and for the nerves in the hilar regions. The pulmonary arteries supply the pulmonary parenchymal tissue, including the respiratory bronchioles. Communications between these two blood supplies, bronchopulmonary arterial and venous anastomoses, occur in the proximity of the junction of the terminal and respiratory bronchioles. These anastomoses allow the two blood supplies to complement each other.[65] For instance, if flow through one system is increased or decreased, a reciprocal change occurs in the amount of blood supplied by the other system. Arteriographic studies in patients with active hemoptysis have shown that the systemic circulation is primarily responsible for the bleeding in approximately 92% of cases.

The pathogenesis of hemoptysis depends on the type and location of the disease.[56] In general, if the lesion is endobronchial, the bleeding is from the bronchial circulation; if the lesion is parenchymal, the bleeding is from the pulmonary circulation. Moreover, in chronic diseases, repetitive episodes are most likely the result of increased vascularity in the involved area.

In bronchogenic carcinoma, hemoptysis results from necrosis of the tumor with its increased blood supply from bronchial arteries or from local invasion of a large blood vessel. In bronchial adenomas, bleeding is usually from rupture of the prominent surface vessels. In bronchiectasis, hemoptysis is usually the result of irritation by infection of the granulation tissue that has replaced the normal bronchial wall. In acute bronchitis, bleeding results from irritation of the unusually friable vascular mucosa.

The mechanism of hemoptysis in mitral stenosis is controversial, but the most likely explanation is rupture of the dilated varices of the bronchial veins in the submucosa of large bronchi caused by pulmonary venous hypertension. Pulmonary venous hypertension may also be responsible for the bleeding in congestive heart failure because it is associated with widening of the capillary anastomoses between the bronchial and pulmonary arteries.

Hemoptysis in pulmonary embolism may be caused by infarction, with necrosis of parenchymal tissue or hemorrhagic consolidation as the result of an excessive influx of bronchial arterial blood at systemic pressures through the bronchopulmonary anastomoses into the pulmonary circulation distal to the obstructing clot.

In tuberculosis, bleeding can occur for a variety of reasons. In the acute parenchymal exudative lesion, scant hemoptysis may result from necrosis of a small branch of a pulmonary artery or vein. In the chronic, parenchymal fibroulcerative lesion, massive hemoptysis may result from rupture of a pulmonary artery aneurysm bulging into the lumen of a cavity. The aneurysm occurs from tuberculous involvement of the adventitia and media of the vessel. When a healed and calcified tuberculous lymph node erodes the wall of a bronchus because of pressure necrosis, the patient may cough up blood as well as the calcified node (broncholith). In endobronchial tuberculosis, hemoptysis may result from acute tuberculous ulceration of the bronchial mucosa. In healed and fibrotic parenchymal areas of tuberculosis, bleeding may arise from irritation of granulation tissue in the walls of bronchiectatic airways in the same areas.

In traumatic rupture of the pulmonary artery by a balloon flotation catheter, risk factors include pulmonary hypertension, distal location of the catheter tip, excessive catheter manipulation in an attempt to obtain a pulmonary artery occluded pressure measurement, a large catheter loop in the right ventricle, and advanced age.[59] In tracheo-artery fistula complicating tracheostomy, bleeding is caused by trauma from the tracheostomy cannula and/or balloon.[60] Bleeding is usually caused by rupture of the innominate artery. The fistula can form at three tracheal locations: the stoma, the intratracheal cannula tip, and the balloon. Trauma at the stoma is caused by pressure necrosis, usually because the tracheostomy was created too low (below the fourth tracheal ring). It may also occur at the cannula tip because of excessive angulation of the cannula and at the balloon site caused by pressure necrosis because of excessive inflation pressures. Diffuse intrapulmonary hemorrhage attributable to immunologic diseases is caused by an inflammatory lesion, usually of capillaries.[66]

Diagnosis

General Considerations: The success rate in determining the cause of hemoptysis is excellent but variable. If one accepts the diagnosis of idiopathic (essential) hemoptysis as a distinct entity, the cause of hemoptysis can be determined in close to 100% of cases. If one does not accept this diagnosis, the cause can be determined in 68 to 98% of cases (average, approximately 88%).

The diagnostic workup of hemoptysis involves routine (Table 10) as well as special evaluations (Table 11). Routine evaluations are initially performed in every patient, whereas special studies are ordered only when the clinical setting suggests they are indicated. In general, each category of disease (Table 8) has its special studies.

Routine Evaluation: As in any diagnostic problem, a detailed history and physical examination must be performed. These should be performed in systematic fashion, not only to rule in the common causes of hemoptysis, but also to rule in the category of the cause (Table 8).

Although the amount of bleeding is generally not indicative of the seriousness of the underlying disease process, a history of the frequency, timing, and duration of hemoptysis may be helpful. For example, repeated episodes of hemoptysis occurring over months to years suggest bronchial adenoma and bronchiectasis, whereas small amounts of hemoptysis occurring every day for weeks are more likely to be caused by bronchogenic carcinoma. Bleeding attributable to bronchogenic carcinoma usually is of short duration because it is generally a late finding in these patients. In addition to having abnormal chest radiographic findings, these patients are usually >40 years of age and are almost invariably cigarette smokers.

Hemoptysis that coincides with the menses (catamenial) suggests the rare diagnostic possibility of pulmonary endometriosis, whereas bleeding associated with sexual intercourse or other forms of exertion suggests passive congestion of the lungs. Although hemoptysis may be a symptom at any age, it is distinctly uncommon in the young. When hemoptysis is present before the third decade of life, it suggests an acute tracheobronchitis, a congenital cardiac or lung defect, an unusual tumor, CF, a blood dyscrasia, or infectious pneumonia. No matter what the age, if a patient with pneumonia who is undergoing appropriate therapy has hemoptysis that persists for longer than the usual 24 h, an endobronchial lesion or coagulopathy should be suspected.[67]

A travel history can often be helpful in bringing certain endemic diseases to mind. This is true of coccidioidomycosis and histoplasmosis in the United States, of paragonimiasis and ascariasis in the Far East, and of schistosomiasis in South America, Africa, and the Far East. Chronic sputum production before hemoptysis suggest the diagnoses of chronic bronchitis, bronchiectasis, and CF. The presence of orthopnea and paroxysmal nocturnal dyspnea suggest the diagnoses of passive congestion of the lungs from mitral stenosis and left ventricular failure. A history of anticoagulant therapy suggests an intrapulmonary bleed from too large a dose or recurrent pulmonary embolism from too small a dose. The possibility of pulmonary embolism should always be considered when a patient who presents with hemoptysis has been at increased risk for deep venous thrombosis. The possibility of traumatic rupture of a pulmonary artery caused by to balloon flotation catheterization should always be considered when these catheters are used.

Although tracheoartery fistula must be considered in the differential diagnosis of hemoptysis in every patient with a tracheostomy,[60] it is fortunately an infrequent cause in this setting. When it occurs, the onset is almost always at least 48 h after the procedure. While the peak incidence is between the first and second week, and 72% of fistulas will bleed during the first 21 days after tracheostomy, hemorrhage from this complication can also occur as late as 18 months after the procedure. There is a sentinel bleed in 34 to 50% of cases. Before 48 h, bleeding from the stoma is usually the result of capillary bleeding from inadequate hemostasis. Whenever hemoptysis occurs in a patient who has an endotracheal tube or tracheostomy in place, trauma from suctioning, especially when coagulation is abnormal, should be considered a likely cause.

Although patients with diffuse intrapulmonary hemorrhage typically have hemoptysis, they may occasionally not expectorate at all but just complain of dyspnea[68] or the abrupt onset of fever, dyspnea, cough, and malaise. Therefore, lack of hemoptysis does not rule out a substantial intrapulmonary hemorrhage.[68] The diagnosis of trimellitic anhydride (TMA)-induced pulmonary hemorrhage should be suspected in workers exposed to high-dose TMA fumes. Exposure occurs when heated metal surfaces are sprayed with corrosion-resistant epoxy resin coatings. The syndrome requires a latent period of exposure and appears to be antibody mediated.[69] Respiratory failure with pulmonary infiltrates and hemoptysis have also been reported in a patient with a documented exposure and antibodies to isocyanates.[70]

In a patient with the triad of known upper airway disease, lower airway disease, and renal disease, systemic Wegener granulomatosis should be suspected. Although the diagnosis of systemic lupus erythematosus is readily considered in a patient known to have this disease, pulmonary hemorrhage can be the presenting manifestation. Goodpasture syndrome (antibasement membrane antibody-mediated disease) typically occurs in young men, and it has been reported to be associated with influenza infection, inhalation of hydrocarbons, and penicillamine ingestion. Therefore, it should be considered in these historical contexts.[56]

Diffuse alveolar hemorrhage should be suspected in patients who have undergone recent bone marrow transplantation when they present with cough, dyspnea, hypoxemia, and diffuse pulmonary infiltrates. This finding typically occurs with marrow recovery. Diffuse alveolar hemorrhage has been reported to occur in approximately 20% of patients during autologous bone marrow transplantation, and it has been associated with an 80% mortality.[71] The pathogenesis is thought to be related to damage caused by chemotherapy or radiation therapy compounded by return of inflammatory cells with marrow recovery.

Physical examination may be helpful in several ways. Inspection of the skin and mucous membranes may show telangiectasias, suggesting hereditary hemorrhagic telangiectasia, or ecchymoses and petechiae, suggesting a hematologic abnormality. Pulsations transmitted to a tracheostomy cannula should heighten suspicion of a tracheoartery fistula or risk of one. Inspection of the thorax may show evidence of recent or old chest trauma, and unilateral wheeze or crackles may herald localized disease such as bronchial adenoma or carcinoma. Although pulmonary embolism is not definitively diagnosed on physical examination, tachypnea, phlebitis, and pleural friction rub suggest this disorder. If crackles are heard diffusely on chest examination, passive congestion as well as other diseases causing diffuse intrapulmonary hemorrhage should be considered. Careful cardiovascular examination may rule in mitral stenosis, pulmonary artery stenosis, or pulmonary hypertension.

The routine laboratory studies listed in Table 10 are useful for the following reasons. The CBC count may suggest presence of an infection, hematologic disorder, or chronic blood loss. Idiopathic hemosiderosis or other causes of diffuse intrapulmonary hemorrhage may present only with diffuse pulmonary infiltrates and iron deficiency anemia from chronic bleeding into the lungs. Urinalysis may reveal hematuria and suggest the presence of a systemic disease associated with diffuse parenchymal disease. While there is simultaneous evidence of clinical involvement of the lungs and kidneys in 33% of cases of Goodpasture syndrome, there can be clinical lung involvement without renal disease in 33% and clinical renal involvement without lung disease in 33%.[56]

Coagulation studies may uncover a hematologic disorder that is primarily responsible for the hemoptysis or that contributes to excessive bleeding from another disease. The ECG may help suggest the presence of a cardiovascular disorder. Although as many as 30% of patients with hemoptysis have normal chest radiographic findings,[72] routine posteroanterior and lateral radiographs may be diagnostically valuable.

When pulmonary tumor or infection is not readily apparent, other radiographic signs that may suggest the cause and source of bleeding include radio-opaque foreign bodies that may give rise to hemoptysis even years after entry into the lungs; the disappearance of a calcified mediastinal lymph node after it has eroded the bronchial wall and is expectorated as a broncholith; aortic or pulmonary aneurysms that by dissection may erode into the bronchial tree; single or multiple pulmonary cavities that suggest pulmonary tuberculosis, fungal disease, parasitic disease, acute or chronic lung abscess, primary or metastatic neoplasm, septic pulmonary emboli, or Wegener granulomatosis; an intracavitary mass lesion that is indicative of a fungus ball (aspergilloma) or blood clot; and localized honeycombing that is consistent with bronchiectasis. The presence of a new infiltrate localized to the area subtending a balloon flotation catheter suggests a rupture of the pulmonary artery. The appearance of a new air-fluid level in a preexisting cavity or cyst suggests the location of the source of bleeding, as does a nonsegmental alveolar pattern that clears within a few days. A solitary pulmonary nodule with vessels going toward it suggests an arteriovenous malformation. In patients with hemoptysis caused by pulmonary embolism, a parenchymal density abutting a pleural surface with evidence of pleural reaction and/or effusion is usually present. The cardiac silhouette, vascular or parenchymal patterns, and presence of Kerley B lines may be useful in documenting cardiovascular disease.

When the chest radiograph shows diffuse pulmonary infiltrates, hemorrhage from bleeding disorders (*eg*, thrombocytopenia in the compromised host), lung contusion from blunt chest trauma, and passive congestion of the lungs should be considered, in addition to the diseases listed under diffuse alveolar hemorrhage in Table 8. In the earliest stages of diffuse intrapulmonary hemorrhage, chest radiographs may appear normal, but usually hemorrhage appears in a diffuse alveolar pattern. This progresses to a mixed alveolar-interstitial pattern and, then, when bleeding ceases entirely, an interstitial pattern, as hemosiderin deposition accumulates.

Even when findings of the history, physical examination, and chest radiograph are normal or there is an obvious cause of hemoptysis on the chest radiograph, bronchoscopy is invaluable for not only accurate diagnosis but for precise localization of the pulmonary hemorrhage. It is not uncommon for bronchoscopy to establish sites of bleeding different from those suggested by the chest radiograph.[73,74] Bronchoscopy may not be needed in patients with stable chronic bronchitis with one episode of blood streaking, particularly if it is associated with an exacerbation of acute tracheobronchitis in which the site of bleeding was recently documented by bronchoscopic examination; with acute lower respiratory tract infections; and with obvious cardiovascular causes of hemoptysis, such as congestive heart failure and pulmonary embolism. In localizing the bleeding site, the best results are obtained when bronchoscopy is performed during or within 24 h of active bleeding. The bleeding site can be localized in up to 93% of patients[74,75] with a flexible bronchoscope, and in up to 86% with the rigid instrument.[76] When the procedure is done within 48 h, localization of bleeding can drop to 51%.[77] When bronchoscopy is done after bleeding has ceased, accurate localization is likely to be reduced even further. Although the flexible bronchoscope is usually the instrument of choice in diagnosing lower respiratory tract problems, rigid bronchoscopy is preferred in cases of massive uncontrolled hemorrhage because patency of the airway is maintained more effectively during this procedure. There are data that show that obtaining a high-resolution chest CT before bronchoscopy may enhance the yield of bronchoscopy. With the exception of tracheoartery fistula, the tracheobronchial disorders that can be diagnosed by a bronchoscopic examination are listed in Table 8.

Bedside bronchoscopy should not be performed to rule in the diagnosis of tracheoartery fistula.[60] In tracheostomized patients with hemoptysis, bronchoscopy should be performed to rule out other causes, such as bleeding from suction ulcers, tracheitis, or lower respiratory tract disorders. If no other cause for hemoptysis can be found and bleeding has stopped or anterior and downward pressure on the cannula on the stomal site or overinflation of the tracheostomy balloon slows down or stops the bleeding, a surgical consultation should be sought immediately and the patient brought to the operating room for examination in a more controlled environment. In this setting, balloon deflation and removal of the tracheostomy tube are not advised unless airway protection with an endotracheal tube can be performed nearly simultaneously, followed by a definitive vascular repair should the diagnosis be correct. As long as tracheoartery fistula remains a diagnostic possibility, the tracheostomy balloon should not be deflated and the tracheostomy tube should not be removed without protecting the airway below the tracheostomy tube.

When there is no active bleeding, bronchoscopy with BAL fluid can be helpful in suggesting diffuse intrapulmonary hemorrhage. Return of bright red or blood-tinged lavage fluid from multiple lobes from both lungs suggests an active, diffuse intrapulmonary hemorrhage; hemosiderin-laden macrophages (*ie*, siderophages) on cytologic analysis from these same specimens suggest bleeding that has been ongoing. Because normal subjects may have siderophages in their alveoli, the diagnosis of diffuse alveolar hemorrhage requires a substantial number of siderophages to be recovered by BAL fluid ($\geq$ 20% of total alveolar macrophages).[78] Because carbon monoxide diffusing capacity is increased as the result of intra-alveolar RBCs binding carbon monoxide for 24 to 48 h after bleeding stops, this test may be helpful in diagnosing intra-alveolar hemorrhage in the stable patient without hemoptysis.

Although the diagnosis of unquestionable bronchiectasis can be made only with the aid of the bronchogram or high-resolution chest CT scan, a presumptive diagnosis can be made without bronchography. Bronchiectasis is visible on routine chest radiographs in up to 90% of cases,[79] and bronchoscopy can localize the bleeding to the corresponding abnormal areas. Angiography may determine the site of bleeding in up to 90 to 93% of cases.[75] When performed routinely, diagnostic angiography establishes a diagnosis not identified by bronchoscopy in only 4% of patients.[75] ^{99m}Tc-labeled colloid and RBC studies have been shown to be accurate and may be positive in 6 to 10 min.[79] Although the use of angiography may not be initially helpful in confirming rupture of the pulmonary artery caused by balloon flotation catheterzation if the rent has sealed, it can be extremely helpful in detecting a pseudoaneurysm that has formed in the healing process.[59] Identification of an unstable lesion is important because it should be obliterated to prevent future rupture and death.[59] Angiography has not been useful in diagnosing tracheoartery fistula.[60]

Special Evaluations: Depending on the results of the initial evaluation and the possible categories of cause of hemoptysis (Table 8), additional diagnostic evaluations should be systematically performed (Table 11). The diagnosis of Goodpasture syndrome is made by demonstrating linear deposition of IgG along the basement membrane of the lung or kidney and the presence of high titers of circulating anti-basement membrane antibody in the blood. Antibodies from patients with traditional Goodpasture syndrome react with the α3(IV) chain of type IV collagen. A patient with pulmonary hemorrhage from adenocarcinoma was initially misdiagnosed and initially incorrectly treated because he had increased levels of serum anti-glomerular basement membrane antibodies.[80] Once the cancer was subsequently diagnosed, it was determined that the patient did not have Goodpasture syndrome because antibodies did not show anti-α3(IV) reactivity. They only reacted to the α1(IV) chain. The choice of lung or kidney biopsy depends on the clinical setting. However, anti-IgG immunofluorescent staining of the kidney may be positive even in the absence of clinical evidence of renal disease.[81] Although Goodpasture syndrome is typically associated with IgG, there are also reports of a pulmonary-renal hemorrhagic syndrome associated with IgA.[82] The importance of this observation is that the immunoserologic testing must be designed to include both Igs.

Definitive diagnosis of the pulmonary vasculitides depends on histologic examination, including special stains and cultures that rule out tuberculosis and fungal diseases. Pulmonary capillaritis with hemorrhage has been reported in an ever-increasing number of conditions. The diagnosis can sometimes be made on transbronchial biopsy, thus avoiding the need for open-lung biopsy, but care must be taken to exclude infectious etiologies by using special stains. While high levels of IgG, IgA, and IgM antibody to trimellitic-coupled protein and trimellitic-conjugated erythrocytes have been found in patients with TMA-induced pulmonary disease, the diagnosis can be made clinically by obtaining a history of the exposure and ruling out other diseases (Table 8).

It is important to be aware that diseases may be considered (and therefore evaluated) in more than one category. For instance, the case of a patient with hemoptysis caused by overzealous anticoagulation may be evaluated in three categories: (1) a hematologic disorder that may cause (2) localized and (3) diffuse parenchymal disease. A patient with chronic bleeding from the tracheobronchial disorder of diffuse bronchial telangiectasis could present with diffuse as well as localized parenchymal disease (aspiration hemosiderosis). A patient with long-standing passive congestion of the lungs or a cardiovascular disorder might present with diffuse pulmonary hemosiderosis, whereas a patient with acute pulmonary edema usually presents with diffuse pulmonary infiltrates.

Differential Diagnosis

In evaluating patients with hemoptysis, it is necessary to rule out the causes of pseudohemoptysis. Unless the cause of pseudohemoptysis is definitively determined, the spitting up of blood must be assumed to be true hemoptysis. An upper airway lesion must not be assumed to be the cause of the bleeding unless it is seen bleeding actively at the time of examination.

Treatment

The treatment of hemoptysis can be divided into supportive and definitive categories. In prescribing definitive therapy, it is important to consider the cause, the amount of bleeding, and the patient's underlying lung function.

Supportive Care: Supportive care usually includes bed rest and mild sedation. Drugs with antitussive effects (all narcotics) should not be used. An effective cough may be necessary to clear blood from the airways and to avoid asphyxiation. Drugs with antiplatelet effects also should not be used. Depending on the results of oximetry and/or arterial blood gas analysis, supplemental oxygen should be administered. If bleeding continues and gas exchange becomes further compromised, endotracheal intubation and mechanical ventilation may become necessary. To facilitate flexible bronchoscopy with a sufficiently large suction port, an endotracheal tube with an internal diameter of at least 8 mm should be used, if possible. Other respiratory adjunctive therapy, such as chest physiotherapy and postural drainage, should be avoided. Fluid and blood resuscitation should be administered when indicated. The amount of hemoptysis should be continuously quantitated until it stops. The amount helps determine the patient's subsequent care.

Definitive Care—Nonmassive Hemoptysis: In definitive care for patients with scant or frank (submassive) hemoptysis, treatment is directed at the specific cause. For instance, suppurative bronchiectasis is treated with antibiotics plus a mucociliary escalator drug (*eg*, theophylline, β-adrenergic agonists). An acute exacerbation of chronic bronchitis associated with cigarette smoking is treated with a mucociliary escalator and cessation of cigarette smoking. Although the role of antibiotics in the context of hemoptysis caused by COPD has not been specifically studied, antibiotics have been shown to be helpful in patients with the most severe exacerbations of COPD. CF is treated with broad-spectrum antibiotics plus a mucociliary escalator drug. Bronchial adenoma and bronchogenic carcinoma should be resected whenever possible. Congestive heart failure is treated with combinations of drugs for preload and afterload reductions and inotropic agents when appropriate, mitral stenosis with diuretics, and pulmonary embolism with heparin. There are no data to support that patients with hemoptysis caused by pulmonary embolism bleed more with heparin. Therefore, do not initially withhold or undertreat these patients with nonmassive hemoptysis. The effects of overzealous anticoagulation are treated with cessation of blood thinning and perhaps fresh frozen plasma and vitamin K. Tuberculosis is treated with antituberculous drugs; appropriate antibiotic therapy is administered for acute infectious pneumonias.

Definitive Care—Massive Hemoptysis: In patients with massive hemoptysis, treatment is directed not only at the specific cause but also at abrupt cessation of bleeding. Death from massive hemoptysis is predominantly caused by asphyxiation, and the likelihood of death appears directly related to the rate of bleeding. Urgent management in all cases of massive hemoptysis must emphasize protecting the uninvolved lung from aspiration of blood and tamponading of the bleeding site. When tracheo-artery fistula may be present, the following steps should be considered:[60] if bleeding is immediate and profuse, there may be time only to overinflate the balloon, tamponading the potential bleeding site at the balloon, and apply downward and forward pressure on the top of the tracheostomy tube, tamponading the potential bleeding site at the stoma. If the arterial rupture is at the cannula tip, these efforts will not be helpful. If bleeding stops or slows either by these efforts or spontaneously, an endotracheal tube should be placed distal to the tip of the tracheostomy tube and an immediate surgical consultation requested. Ideally, an experienced surgeon should be present when the tracheostomy tube is removed; should crisp bleeding start again, the surgeon can attempt to finger tamponade/compress the bleeding artery (*eg*, usually the innominate) by bluntly dissecting down the anterior tracheal wall and behind the sternum to the vessel. The vessel, once reached, can be compressed against the back of the sternum. When the situation has been stabilized, clots can be gently suctioned from the distal trachea and the patient taken to the operating room for definitive repair.

When bleeding originates from below the primary carina, the bleeding lung should be kept dependent to minimize aspiration of expectorated blood. Numerous techniques have been advocated to help minimize aspiration and have proved helpful. A bronchoscopically positioned endobronchial balloon may provide effective tamponade. Hemoptysis caused by bleeding from all but the right upper lobe has been managed with balloon occlusion. Placement of a Carlen tube that intubates each mainstem bronchus separately is helpful, but the tube can be difficult to place; once in position, its small diameter may prevent subsequent diagnostic flexible bronchoscopy. In cases of persistent massive hemoptysis, diagnostic considerations may need to be delayed because placement of a Carlen tube may be necessary to ensure patient survival.

Urgent treatment to stop massive hemoptysis may involve laser bronchoscopy, iced saline solution lavage, angiographic embolization, supportive treatment only, or surgical resection. Use of a laser to stop hemoptysis has been successful in $>90\%$ of patients with cancer,[83] but recurrence of bleeding within a few weeks is typical. No large studies of patients with massive hemoptysis have been reported. Because the laser is useful only in patients with proximal airway lesions and is difficult to use during massive hemoptysis, laser therapy will probably not evolve into a common therapeutic tool for these patients. Bronchoscopically directed iced saline solution lavage of the bronchi leading to the site of hemorrhage has been reported to be successful in stopping hemorrhage in an uncontrolled series.[84]

Angiography can identify the bleeding site in $>90\%$ of cases[75,85] and, when combined with an embolization procedure, has been successful in stopping bleeding in massive hemoptysis in $>90\%$ of cases.[85] Several angiographic sessions may be required, and both systemic and pulmonary vessels may need to be studied. Fourteen percent of patients bleed again within 1 to 4 days, and multiple procedures are frequently necessary.[85,86] Once active bleeding ceases, 20% of patients bleed again during the next 6 months[87] and 22% by 3 to 5 years.[85] Angiographic embolization may be achieved with the use of gel foam or polyurethane particles and is aided by temporary balloon occlusion of the involved vessel.[85,88,89] Sclerosing agents have led to subsequent massive lung necrosis and should be avoided.[85]

Although early studies included several cases complicated by embolization of spinal arteries with subsequent paresis or paralysis, this complication appears rare when the procedure is performed by experienced angiographers.[85] Other complications, such as pleurisy or hematoma formation, are infrequent and usually are minor.[85] In patients with hemoptysis caused by trauma, urgent thoracotomy has been advocated, with the recommendation that it be performed with the patient in the supine position to minimize aspiration and that the bronchovascular trunk of the involved lung be clamped while the patient is stabilized to minimize the chance of air embolism while receiving positive pressure ventilation.

Survival from iatrogenic rupture of the pulmonary artery has been reported.[59] Several urgent maneuvers may prove helpful, and balloon tamponade and selective intubation should always be attempted. Balloon tamponade of the ruptured vessel with the Swan-Ganz balloon has been helpful. With the balloon deflated, the catheter should be withdrawn 5 cm, the balloon inflated with 2 mL of air, and the balloon allowed to float back into the hemorrhaging vessel to occlude it. Ideally, patients should immediately be intubated in the mainstem bronchus opposite the involved lung to minimize aspiration. In most patients, death from pulmonary artery rupture occurs before the bleeding lung can be identified. Because the catheter usually floats to the right pulmonary artery, when it is not known which pulmonary artery has been ruptured, selective intubation of the left mainstem bronchus or placement of a Carlen tube should be attempted. Selective intubation of the left mainstem bronchus might be facilitated by using a bronchoscope or suction catheter designed specifically to enter the left lung. All patients who stop bleeding require angiographic evaluation to help localize the arterial tear and check for the formation of a pseudoaneurysm.[59] At the time of angiography, embolization of the affected vessel should be performed if a pseudoaneurysm or a tear is found. Hemoptysis from a pseudoaneurysm usually occurs in the first day after formation but may occur weeks later.

Aside from repairing lesions such as a tracheoartery fistula, the role of emergency surgery for hemoptysis remains controversial. Several studies[90] have advocated emergency surgery for all patients with massive hemoptysis when feasible, citing older statistics that patients who have had surgery have a 19% mortality compared with 54% in the nonoperative group. A more recent study[55] challenges this, citing the following findings in 84 patients with hemoptysis of >200 mL/d: (1) there were no deaths in patients with <1 L/d of hemoptysis, even they did not undergo surgery; (2) the rate of mortality varied more with whether the patient was operable than with whether the patient underwent surgery (mortality in operable patients with hemoptysis of >1 L/d was 30% vs 65% in inoperable patients); and (3) the rate of mortality was greatly affected by diagnosis, in that no patient died from hemoptysis attributable to bronchitis, tuberculosis, bronchiectasis, or anticoagulation, whereas 80% of patients with cancer and hemoptysis of >1 L/d died. Others have advocated conservative nonsurgical treatment when hemoptysis is caused by infectious causes. In patients with CF, even with normal lung function, resection should be avoided because repeated episodes in other areas are likely to occur.

With respect to surgery, it is clear that no treatment preference can be recommended for all patients on the basis of reported studies. The trials of therapy span different decades of practice, have widely differing causes of hemoptysis in their populations, and employ several different definitions for massive hemoptysis. A review of the literature suggests the following strategy: (1) patients who are not candidates for surgery because of their pulmonary function, general medical condition, or diffuse nature of their lesions should be treated with selective embolization; (2) resectional surgery should be performed in operable patients when surgery is the definitive treatment for the underlying disease; and (3) all potentially operable patients who continue to bleed at rates of >1 L/d despite supportive, conservative care should undergo either surgical resection or embolization. The correct therapy in a given patient depends on the cause of the bleeding, lung function, availability of resources, and local expertise.

In patients with diffuse intrapulmonary hemorrhage, selective arterial embolization and surgery are not options. For immunologically mediated diseases, corticosteroids, cytotoxic agents, and other interventions are available. With respect to corticosteroid and cytotoxic drug therapies, the following generally apply[56]: (1) corticosteroids are used alone if the syndrome is self-limited; (2) cytotoxic therapy should be added when the disease is known to respond to cytotoxic therapy (*eg*, Wegener granulomatosis or Goodpasture syndrome); (3) cytotoxic agents can be used as steroid-sparing agents in patients whose disease has responded to corticosteroids but who are having side effects caused by corticosteroids; and (4) cytotoxic agents may be considered in immunologic lung disease that has not responded as expected to corticosteroids and for which no intercurrent disease process can be identified.

When corticosteroid therapy is administered alone for critically ill patients with immunologic lung diseases, the dose is 1 mg/kg/d of methylprednisolone IV or the equivalent dose of another corticosteroid. Larger doses, on the order of 7 to 15 mg/kg/d for 1 to 3 days, have been recommended to control progressive pulmonary hemorrhage and hypoxemia of Goodpasture syndrome, systemic lupus erythematosus, and some of the vasculitides.[56] In general, corticosteroids should be administered initially in around-the-clock divided doses until substantial improvement has occurred. They can then be administered once per day and tapered as the patient's condition dictates.

In general, patients with Goodpasture syndrome are treated in the following manner: (1) if patients present with severe pulmonary hemorrhage, methylprednisolone is initially administered at the higher dose of 7 to 15 mg/kg/d for 1 to 3 days; (2) plasmapheresis may be useful for the immediate and long-term reduction of anti-glomerular basement membrane antibody levels; and (3) short-term and long-term cyclophosphamide and plasmapheresis therapy are guided by the results of serially obtained serum anti-glomerular basement membrane antibody levels. If pharmacologic doses of corticosteroids control severe pulmonary hemorrhage and the plasmapheresis and cyclophosphamide therapy makes circulating anti-glomerular basement membrane antibody disappear, bilateral nephrectomy is unnecessary. On the basis of favorable case reports in life-threatening situations, consider recombinant activated factor VII as a temporizing measure in unstable patients without coagulopathic bleeding.[91]

Dyspnea

Dyspnea is a distressing sensation of difficult, labored, or unpleasant breathing. The word *distressing* is very important to this definition because labored or difficult breathing may be encountered by healthy individuals while exercising, which does not qualify as dyspnea because it may not be perceived as distressing. The sensation is often poorly or vaguely described by patients.

Physiology

The physiology of dyspnea remains unclear despite >40 years of active investigation. What is clear, however, is that a simplistic single neural pathway theory has been superceded by a complex, multiple neural pathway paradigm.[92] Because the respiratory system is extremely complex and redundant in its control mechanisms, it is quite likely that there are multiple stimuli, receptors, nerves, and neural pathways that mediate the sensation of dyspnea. This multiple neural pathway model of dyspnea suggests that dyspnea may arise caused by abnormalities in the afferent pathways, the efferent pathways, or the central control centers of the respiratory system (Fig 8). Because afferent pathways feed back to the CNS from virtually all levels of the efferent pathway, afferent dyspneic information from virtually all thoracic and upper abdominal organs (including the pharynx, larynx, airways, lung parenchyma, esophagus, heart, and stomach) may potentially impact the sensation.

On the basis of the vagus nerve, muscle afferent, and chemoreceptor experiments, it appears that hypercapnia, hypoxemia, and muscle afferent data that relate to load, effort, and impedance are the major dyspnogenic stimuli. An important role for vagal afferents has not been ruled out. With respect to the central integration of the afferent and efferent systems, it appears that the intensity of dyspnea can be modulated by learning, experience, and emotional/behavioral states.

Differential Diagnosis of Dyspnea

As with cough, a multiplicity of causes located in a variety of anatomic locations where the dyspnea pathways travel have been reported to cause dyspnea. Although the individual causes are too numerous to list,[92] they can be grouped into categories of diseases (Table 12). The spectra and frequencies of causes will vary depending on whether dyspnea is acute or chronic, on the age group studied, and on whether the patient presents as an inpatient, in the emergency department, or in an outpatient clinic (Fig 9) or office. Nevertheless, if the data from all studies reported in these varied settings are combined, one can conclude that cardiopulmonary diseases will cause 75 to 92% of cases in emergency department and hospitalized patients and 46 to 85% of cases in outpatients.[93,94] Moreover, in all settings, dyspnea appears to be attributable to one of five major causes 94% of the time: (1) cardiac,

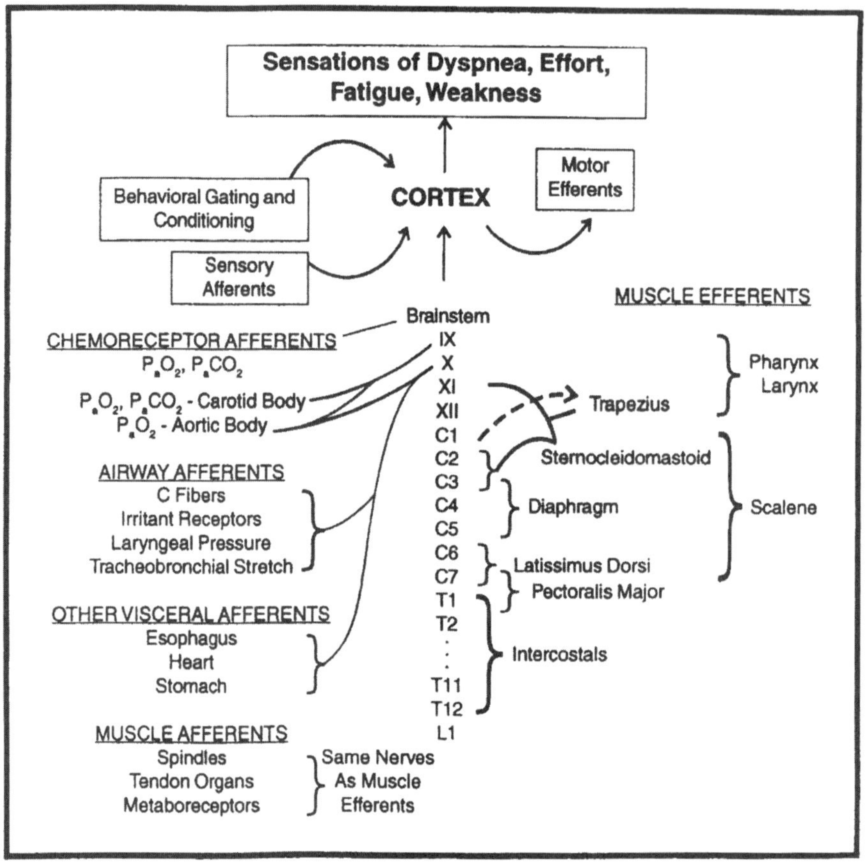

Figure 8. Schematic representation of the afferent and efferent motor nerves serving the respiratory system. The cortex integrates sensory afferent (*left side*) and efferent (*right side*) data with experience and produces sensations of dyspnea, effort, fatigue, and weakness. Reprinted with permission from Curley.[92]

Table 12. *Differential Diagnosis of Dyspnea According to Category of Disease*

Cardiac	Nutritional
Deconditioning/obesity	Oncologic
Dermatologic	Pharmacologic
Endocrine	Pregnancy
GI	Pulmonary
Hematologic	Psychiatric
Infectious	Renal
Larynx/upper airway	Rheumatologic
Neuromuscular	Vascular

(2) pulmonary, (3) psychogenic/hyperventilation, (4) GERD, and (5) deconditioning disorders. Approximately two thirds of cases, chronic dyspnea will be caused by four diseases: COPD, asthma, interstitial lung disease, and cardiomyopathy.[95]

Pathophysiology of Dyspnea

The mechanism by which diseases produce dyspnea varies with the disease. Some affect

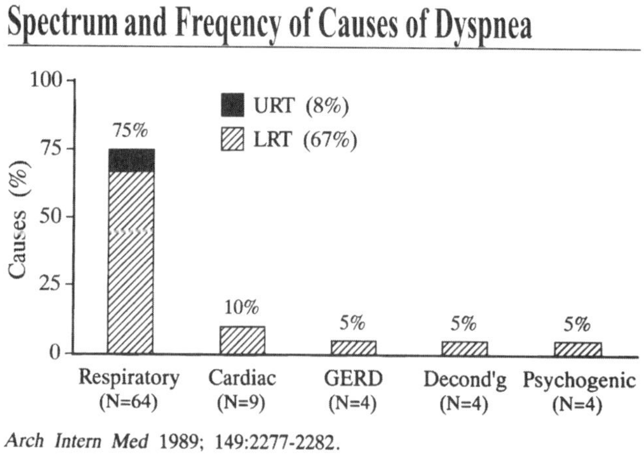

Figure 9. Representative spectrum and frequency of causes of chronic dyspnea evaluated in an outpatient pulmonary clinic. The 64 respiratory disorders included asthma in 25 cases, COPD in 12 cases, interstitial lung disease in 12 cases, UACS in 6 cases, bronchiectasis in 2 cases, tracheal stenosis in 1 case, kyphoscoliosis in 1 case, fibrothorax in 1 case, costochondritis in 1 case, lung cancer in 1 case, bronchiolitis obliterans in 1 case, and unilateral hyperlucent lung syndrome in 1 case. Upper respiratory tract disorders accounted for 8% of the causes of dyspnea. Decond'g = deconditioning; LRT = lower respiratory tract; URT = upper respiratory tract. Adapted from Pratter et al.[97]

afferent pathways, others affect efferent pathways, and others affect the central integrative sensory pathways. In most diseases, the precise mechanism by which dyspnea occurs is unknown or unstudied. Virtually all studies performed to elucidate the mechanism of dyspnea have been performed on patients with COPD or asthma.

The authors of studies[92] on the genesis of dyspnea in asthma reveal that mechanical, blood gas, and psychological factors probably all play a role. The intensity of dyspnea does not appear to correlate well with the degree of obstruction. It has most recently been shown[96] that asthmatic patients with a history of near-fatal attacks had a reduced response to hypoxia and a reduced sensation of dyspnea.

Compared with asthma, $Paco_2$ and Pao_2 appearto play a greater role in COPD, whereas the mechanical effects are similar.[92] Similar to COPD and asthma, dyspnea in interstitial lung disease is probably caused by abnormal gas exchange, impaired muscle function, or andactivation of intrapulmonary vagal afferents.[92] Compression of the tracheobronchial tree and laryngeal dysfunction probably cause dyspnea by creating airway obstruction similar to COPD and perhaps by triggering vagal afferent pathways.[92] Compression of lung tissue by pneumothorax, tumor, or pleural effusion likely leads to dyspnea by stimulating vagal afferents and altering gas exchange.[92] Distortion of the thoracic cage by kyphoscoliosis and similar chest wall deformities may alter gas exchange and muscle length-tension relationships.[92]

Cardiac diseases probably cause dyspnea by activating afferents, muscle efferents, and/or by causing gas exchange abnormalities.[92] The mechanism by which GERD causes dyspnea (it has been reported to do so 2 to 5% of the time[96,97,98]) is not known. Because patients may have normal lungs, exercise capacity, muscle strength, and gas exchange, dyspnea in patients who do not have laryngospasm and who do not aspirate may be attributable to the stimulation of vagal afferents. Hyperventilation syndrome, anxiety, panic, and other psychological diseases can cause dyspnea. Because these patients typically have normal cardiopulmonary function, normal efferent pathways, and no obvious afferent pathway defects, it is tempting to explain dyspnea as a perceptual central integrative problem. However, because dyspnea can be provoked during hyperventilation, disordered afferent pathways related to increased minute ventilation and metabolic disturbances associated with reducetion in $Paco_2$ may play a role.[92]

Deconditioning presumably increases the sensation of dyspnea by requiring an abnormally high minute ventilation to perform a task. This increased effort may be perceived as inappropriate to the level of difficulty of the task performed. Therefore, the cause is likely to be multifactorial involving afferent, efferent, and integrative pathways.[92] For speculative mechanisms of dyspnea associated with anemia, high levels of carbohydrate ingestion, and lung cancer, the reader is encouraged to read the chapter by Curley.[92]

Guidelines for Evaluating Acute Dyspnea

A clinical approach is recommended for evaluating acute dyspnea. It consists of obtaining a history and performing a physical examination and laboratory tests, considering potential life-threatening conditions first (*eg*, acute asthma, pulmonary embolism, pulmonary edema states, pneumonias).

Guidelines for Evaluating Chronic Dyspnea of Unknown Etiology

The following systematic, diagnostic approach has been validated in patients with chronic dyspnea who were evaluated in a university hospital, outpatient pulmonary clinic.[97] (1) Review the patient's history and perform a physical examination, concentrating on the anatomy of the potential origins of the dyspnea sensation (Fig 8) and, specifically, the most common causes of dyspnea: COPD, asthma, interstitial lung disease, cardiomyopathy, GERD, other respiratory diseases, and hyperventilation syndrome. Consider doing a provocative test for hyperventilation syndrome.[92] (2) Order a chest radiograph in nearly all patients. (3) Depending on the results of the initial evaluation and chest radio graphs, The following tests may be ordered:

- Pulmonary function testing to include spirometry before bronchodilator and after bronchodilator or methacholine, lung volumes, diffusing capacity, pulse oximetry at rest and during exercise, maximal inspiratory and expiratory mouth pressures, and flow-volume loops

- Noninvasive cardiac studies to include ECG, echocardiography, and stress testing
- Modified barium esophagography and/or 24-h esophageal pH monitoring
- Chest CT scan
- Comprehensive exercise tolerance test
- Other more invasive tests such as cardiac catheterization and lung biopsy

(4) Whenever possible, the final determination of the cause of dyspnea is made by observing which specific therapy eliminates dyspnea as a complaint. Because dyspnea may be simultaneously the result of more than one condition,[99] do not discontinue therapy that appears to be partially successful; rather, sequentially add to it.

Summary of Expected Results Using the Aforementioned Systematic Diagnostic Protocol

It should be possible to determine the cause of chronic dyspnea in nearly all cases that can lead to specific treatment that can be successful in 76% of cases.[97] COPD, asthma, interstitial lung disease, and cardiomyopathy are the most common causes of chronic dyspnea, accounting for 66% of cases; however, 13 other discrete disorders, including UACS, make up the remaining 33% of cases. A variety of respiratory disorders are the most common causes of chronic dyspnea, accounting for approximately 75% of the total.

When asthma is the cause of chronic dyspnea, dyspnea can be the sole presenting manifestation of this disease 20% of the time. The diagnosis of chronic dyspnea is more accurately determined by using objective test results combined with clinical impression, compared with clinical impression alone. Diagnoses of disease based only on history, physical examination, and chest radiographs are incorrect approximately 33% of the time.

The history and physical examination are most helpful in ruling out common diagnoses but are less useful in predicting the diagnosis. A previous diagnosis of asthma or a history of wheezing each have positive predictive values for asthma of $<50\%$. For COPD, a negative smoking history ruled out the diagnosis, but only 20% of smokers had COPD. A history of a previous diagnosis of COPD has a positive predictive value of only 45%. For interstitial lung disease, the presence of crackles on physical examination has a positive predictive value of 79%. However, the absence of crackles had a negative predictive value of 98%. For cardiovascular disease, crackles had a positive predictive value of only 21% but a negative predictive value of 92%.

The predictive values of positional or nocturnal dyspnea have not been studied. Nevertheless, they are likely to be nonspecific. Although trepopnea (*ie*, dyspnea that increases when one side is dependent) suggests asymmetric disease, it is more likely to be associated with common diseases such as COPD than a paralyzed hemidiaphragm.[92] Platypnea (*ie*, an increase in dyspnea in the upright posture) may result from pericarditis, ventilation-perfusion mismatch, ileus, or right-to-left shunt.[92] Orthopnea (*ie*, an increase in dyspnea on recumbency) has occurred in COPD, passive congestion of the lungs, and respiratory muscle weakness.[92] Nocturnal dyspnea has been associated with COPD, asthma, passive congestion of the lungs, and GERD.[92]

Several tests have been helpful in diagnosing the cause of dyspnea. Most are best at ruling out diagnoses (Table 13). Tests reported to have high negative predictive value include methacholine inhalation challenge that is 100% for ruling out asthma; spirometry that is 100% for ruling out COPD; diffusing capacity that is 95% for ruling out interstitial lung disease; and chest radiograph that is 91% for ruling out all diagnoses.[97] Few tests have a high positive predictive value, including methacholine inhalation challenge, which is 95% for ruling in asthma; diffusing capacity, which is 79% for ruling in interstitial lung disease; and chest radiography, which is 75% for ruling in all diagnoses. In addition to the known value of comprehensive exercise tolerance test to distinguish respiratory causes from cardiovascular causes of dyspnea, it is particularly helpful in diagnosing psychogenic dyspnea or deconditioning.

Treatment

Treatment for dyspnea can be either disease specific or disease nonspecific. Specific therapy treats the underlying disease. Nonspecific therapy treats the symptom. Whenever possible, the underlying cause of dyspnea should be identified and specific treatment prescribed. In a prospective

Table 13. *Predictive Values of Diagnostic Tests in the Evaluation of Chronic Dyspnea**

Test	Diagnosis	No.	PPV, %	NPV, %
Spirometry	COPD	84	32	100
Spirometry	Asthma	84	18	72
Spirometry	All diagnoses	84	80	56
Methacholine challenge	Asthma	62	95	100
Diffusing capacity	Interstitial lung disease	32	79	95
Echocardiogram	Cardiac	11	44	0
Radionuclide ventriculogram	Cardiac	9	66	0
Barium esophagram	GERD	15	33	83
Comprehensive endotracheal tube	All diagnoses	15	93	0
Chest radiograph	All diagnoses	84	75	91

*These data are adapted from Pratter et al.[97] See Table 5 for definition of abbreviations.

study,[97] the results of specific treatment yielded the following results: (1) chronic dyspnea improved in 76% of patients; (2) all patients with asthma, UACS, hyperventilation syndrome, deconditioning, and GERD improved; (3) 33% of patients with COPD, 58% with interstitial lung disease, and 78% with cardiomyopathy improved; (4) patients with interstitial lung disease and cardiomyopathy all continued to have some dyspnea despite treatment; and (5) when one of the less common diseases (*eg*, kyphoscoliosis, laryngeal edema) was the cause of dyspnea, therapy was helpful in only 12% of patients.

Specific treatment of asthma, COPD, and interstitial lung disease will be discussed by other authors in this volume; see the section on cough for recommendations for treatment of GERD. With respect to the hyperventilation syndrome, the authors of controlled studies[100] suggest that breathing retraining (*eg*, slow abdominal breathing) is very effective. Both obesity and deconditioning should respond to diet and exercise respectively.[101]

Nonspecific therapy for dyspnea has included conditioning regimens, nutrition, stress reduction and coping skills, oxygen, mechanical ventilation, respiratory muscle training, vagotomy, muscle vibration, acupuncture, and pharmacotherapy with narcotics, anxiolytics, and phenothiazines.[92] With respect to efficacy for dyspnea, the best case has been made for nutritional support. A randomized, controlled clinical trial[102] in patients with COPD showed that dyspnea decreased when protein malnutrition was improved. Although the use of anxiolytics may work in patients with panic disorders, the only two controlled clinical trials[103,104] of benzodiazepines showed that dyspnea was not improved in COPD patients. Although the results of studies with systemic narcotics are conflicting,[92] randomized controlled trials do not support use of nebulized morphine in COPD or interstitial lung disease[105,106] or acupuncture in nonmalignant breathlessness.[107] Finally, although a small double-blind randomized controlled clinical crossover pilot study[108] suggests that inhaled furosemide may alleviate the sensation of dyspnea in patients with COPD, the results must be confirmed in a larger, multicenter study before this can be routinely recommended.

Annotated References

Cough

1. Schappert SM, Burt CW. Ambulatory care visits to physicians' offices, hospital outpatient departments, and emergency department: United States, 2001–2002. National Center for Health statistics. Vital Health Stat 2006; 13:1–66

   This survey summarized data from an estimated 1.1 billion ambulatory visits during a 12-month period. Cough was the single most common complaint for which patients sought medical care.

2. Irwin RS, Corrao WM, Pratter MR. Chronic persistent cough in the adult: the spectrum and frequency of causes and successful outcome of specific therapy. Am Rev Respir Dis 1981; 123:413–417

   This prospective, descriptive study was the first to use and validate the anatomic, diagnostic protocol. It stud-

ied patients with chronic cough of unknown etiology, defined as cough that was at least 3 weeks in duration and persistently troublesome.

3. Irwin RS, Curley FJ, French CL. Chronic cough: the spectrum and frequency of causes, key components of the diagnostic evaluation and outcomes of specific therapy. Am Rev Respir Dis 1990; 141:640–647
This prospective, descriptive study revalidated the anatomic diagnostic protocol that had been modified to include 24-h esophageal pH monitoring to assess for "silent" GERD as a cause of chronic cough.
4. Power JT, Stewart IC, Connaughton JJ, et al. Nocturnal cough in patients with chronic bronchitis and emphysema. Am Rev Respir Dis 1984; 130:999–1001
This study showed that cough decreases during sleep, even in patients with a pathologic reason to cough. It is an important study to quote when others say that psychogenic cough should be considered because the patient does not cough at night.
5. Macklem PT. Physiology of cough. Ann Otol 1974; 83:761–768
Excellent review of the physiology of cough.
6. Gal TJ. Effects of endotracheal intubation on normal cough performance. Anesthesiology 1980; 52:324–329
This study clearly shows that an endotracheal tube passing through the vocal cords does not prevent cough from being an effective clearance mechanism.
7. Gracey DR, Divertie MB, Howard FM Jr. Mechanical ventilation for respiratory failure in myasthenia gravis: two-year experience with 22 patients. Mayo Clin Proc 1983; 58:597–602
One of very few studies that provides some objective data on how to assess when cough effectiveness is diminished. It suggests that maximal expiratory pressure may be useful in this regard.
8. Irwin RS. Complications of cough: ACCP evidence-based clinical practice guidelines. Chest 2006; 129(Suppl):54S–58S
This publication is the most comprehensive review of complications of cough.
9. French CT, Fletcher KE, Irwin RS. A comparison of gender differences in health-related quality of life in acute and chronic coughers. Chest 2005; 127:1991–1998
This prospective study suggests that >90% of the time acute cough is caused by an upper respiratory infection.
10. Curley FJ, Irwin RS, Pratter MR, et al. Cough and the common cold. Am Rev Respir Dis 1988; 138:305–311
This prospective, randomized, double-blind, placebo-controlled study demonstrated the prevalence of cough in the untreated common cold and also showed that a first-generation antihistamine-decongestant medication was effective in decreasing the severity and prevalence of cough caused by the common cold. It also provided evidence to support an upper airway mechanism in the pathogenesis of cough caused by PNDS.
11. Kwon N-H, Oh M-J, Min T-H, et al. Causes and clinical features of subacute cough. Chest 2006; 129:1142–1147
This prospective study reports the spectrum and frequency of causes of subacute cough. Postinfectious cough is the most common condition in this category of cough.
12. Braman SS. Postinfectious cough: ACCP evidence based clinical practice guidelines. Chest 2006; 129(Suppl):138S–146S
This publication is the most up-to-date and comprehensive discussion of postinfectious cough and includes a discussion regarding whooping cough.
13. Pratter MR, Bartter T, Akers S, et al. An algorithmic approach to chronic cough. Ann Intern Med 1993; 119:977–983
This prospective, descriptive study validates the anatomic diagnostic protocol. The protocol was modified by routinely and empirically treating for PNDS before ordering any tests. It introduces the concept of "silent" PNDS.
14. Mello CJ, Irwin RS, Curley FJ. Predictive values of the character, timing, and complications of chronic cough in diagnosing its cause. Arch Intern Med 1996; 156:997–1003
This prospective, descriptive study again revalidates the anatomic diagnostic protocol and showed that the character, timing, and complications of cough are not helpful in diagnosing the cause of chronic cough. It also showed that the spectrum and frequency of productive chronic cough were similar to those of dry cough.
15. Smyrnios NA, Irwin RS, Curley FJ. Chronic cough with a history of excessive sputum production: the spectrum and frequency of causes, key components of the diagnostic evaluation, and outcome of specific therapy. Chest 1995; 108:991–997
This prospective, descriptive study revalidated the anatomic diagnostic protocol in patients with productive cough (cough-phlegm syndrome) and showed that the spectrum and frequency of productive cough were similar to those of dry cough and that the most common causes of a cough-phlegm syndrome were PNDS,

asthma, and GERD and not chronic bronchitis.

16. Pratter MR. Chronic upper airway cough syndrome secondary to rhinosinus diseases (previously referred to as postnasal drip syndrome): ACCP evidence-based clinical practice guidelines. Chest 2006; 129(Suppl):63S–71S
This provides a comprehensive discussion of the upper airway cough syndrome and justification for changing the name from PNDS.
17. Gaffey MJ, Kaiser DL, Hayden FG. Ineffectiveness of terfenadine in natural colds: evidence against histamine as a mediator of common cold symptoms. Pediatr Infect Dis J 1988; 7:223–228
This randomized, controlled, clinical trial showed that a newer histamine type 1 antagonist was not effective in nonhistamine-mediated PNDS.
18. Berkowitz RB, Tinkleman DG. Evaluation of oral terfenadine for the treatment of the common cold. Ann Allergy 1991; 67:593–597
This randomized, controlled, clinical trial showed that a newer histamine type 1 antagonist was not effective in a nonhistamine-mediated PNDS.
19. Berkowitz RB, Connell JT, Dietz AJ, et al. The effectiveness of the nonsedating antihistamine loratadine plus pseudoephedrine in the symptomatic management of the common cold. Ann Allergy 1989; 63:336–339
This randomized, controlled, clinical trial showed that a newer histamine type 1 antagonist was not effective in a nonhistamine-mediated PNDS.
20. O'Byrne PM, Cuddy L, Taylor DW, et al. The clinical efficacy and cost benefit of inhaled corticosteroids as therapy in patients with mild asthma in primary care practice. Can Respir J 1996; 3: 169–175
This randomized, controlled, clinical trial showed that inhaled corticosteroids were effective in treating cough caused by asthma and how long it took before maximal benefit was achieved.
21. Dicpinigaitis PV. Chronic cough due to asthma: ACCP evidence-based clinical practice guidelines. Chest 2006; 129(Suppl):75S–79S
This is an evidence-based clinical practice guideline for managing cough caused by asthma that was endorsed by the American College of Chest Physicians, the American Thoracic Society, and the Canadian Thoracic Society.
22. Brightling CE. Chronic cough due to nonasthmatic eosinophilic bronchitis. Chest 2006; 129(Suppl):116S–121S
This publication discusses the latest information regarding nonasthmatic eosinophilic bronchitis.
23. Irwin RS. Chronic cough due to gastroesophageal reflux disease: ACCP evidence-based clinical practice guidelines. Chest 2006; 129(Suppl):80S–94S
A comprehensive state of the art discussion of cough caused by GERD.
24. Wynder EL, Kaufman PK, Lerrer RL. A short-term follow-up study on ex-cigarette smokers with special emphasis on persistent cough and weight gain. Am Rev Respir Dis 1967; 96:645–655
This prospective study showed how quickly cough caused by chronic bronchitis disappears when patients stop smoking cigarettes.
25. Braman SS. Chronic cough due to chronic bronchitis: ACCP evidence-based clinical practice guidelines. Chest 2006; 129(Suppl):104S–115S
Comprehensive discussion on managing cough caused by chronic bronchitis.
26. Kvale PA. Chronic cough due to lung tumors: ACCP evidence-based clinical practice guidelines. Chest 2006; 129(Suppl):147S–153S
Comprehensive discussion on managing cough caused by lung tumors.
27. Dicpinigaitis PV. Angiotensin-converting enzyme inhibitor-induced cough: ACCP evidence-based clinical practice guidelines. Chest 2006;129(Suppl):169S–173S
Comprehensive discussion on cough caused by ACEIs.
28. Irwin RS, Glomb WB, Chang AB. Habit cough, tic cough, and psychogenic cough in adult and pediatric populations: ACCP evidence-based clinical practice guidelines. Chest 2006; 129(Suppl):174S–179S
Comprehensive review of psychogenic, tic, and habit coughs in adults and children.
29. Brown KK. Chronic cough due to chronic interstitial pulmonary diseases: ACCP evidence-based clinical practice guidelines. Chest 2006; 129(Suppl):180S–185S
A comprehensive review of cough caused by interstitial lung diseases such as idiopathic interstitialfibrosis, sarcoidosis, and hypersensitivity pneumonitis.
30. Pratter MR, Brightling CE, Boulet L-P, et al. An empiric integrative approach to the management of cough: ACCP evidence-based clinical practice guidelines. Chest 2006; 129(Suppl):222S–231S
Algorithms that provide a "road map" that the clinician can follow are useful and are presented for acute, subacute, and chronic cough.
31. Diagnosis and management of cough: ACCP evidence-based clinical practice guidelines. Chest

2006; 129(Suppl):1S–292S
This document is the most comprehensive and up-to-date clinical practice guidelines on managing cough.
32. Bolser DC. Cough suppressant and pharmacologic protussive therapy: ACCP evidence-based clinical practice guidelines. Chest 2006; 129(Suppl):238S–249S
A comprehensive, evidence-based review of nonspecific cough agents; the few that have been shown to be effective are identified.

Wheeze

33. Pasterkamp H, Kraman SS, Wodicka GR. Respiratory sounds: advances beyond the stethoscope. Am J Respir Crit Care Med 1997; 156:974–987
This state-of-the-art review provides an update on all aspects of respiratory sound.
34. Forgacs P. The functional basis of pulmonary sounds. Chest 1978; 73:399–405
This review of the functional basis of lung sounds provides discussion of the topic by one of the "fathers" in the field and is easy to read and understand.
35. Pratter MR, Hingston DM, Irwin RS. Diagnosis of bronchial asthma by clinical evaluation: an unreliable method. Chest 1983; 84:42–47
This prospective, descriptive study was one of the first to show how unreliable clinical evaluation can be in the diagnsosis of asthma. It also reports the spectrum and frequency of causes of expiratory wheezing encountered in a pulmonary clinic practice.
36. Shim CS, Williams MH. Relationship of wheezing to the severity of obstruction in asthma. Arch Intern Med 1983; 143:890–892
This study shows that expiratory wheezing obtained by patient history or detected by physical examination is lacking in sensitivity and specificity in diagnosing asthma.
37. Marini JJ, Pierson DJ, Hudson LD, et al. The significance of wheezing in chronic airflow obstruction. Am Rev Respir Dis 1979; 120:1069–1072
Although unforced expiratory wheezing heard on physical examination has been shown to be significantly correlated with the severity of obstruction in patients with asthma and COPD, the correlations were not strong enough to permit consistent prediction for clinical purposes.
38. King DK, Thompson T, Johnson DC. Wheezing on maximal forced exhalation in the diagnosis of atypical asthma. Ann Intern Med 1989; 110: 451–455
Wheezing heard during forced expirations has not been shown to correlate with the severity of obstruction in COPD, nor has it been shown to be useful in diagnosing asthma.
39. Al-Bazzaz F, Grillo H, Kazemi H. Response to exercise in upper airway obstruction. Am Rev Respir Dis 1975; 111:631–640
This study provides experimental data associating degree of upper airway obstruction with dyspnea and stridor.
40. Geffin B, Grillo HC, Pontoppidan H. Stenosis following tracheostomy for respiratory failure. JAMA 1971; 216:1984–1988
This study provides additional data associating degree of upper airway obstruction with signs and symptoms.
41. Irwin RS, Pratter MR, Holland PS, et al. Postnasal drip causes cough and is associated with reversible upper airway obstruction. Chest 1984; 85:346–352
This study provides prospective data that expiratory wheezing indistinguishable from asthma can originate from the upper airway in the PNDS.
42. Curley FJ, Irwin RS, Pratter MR, et al. Cough and the common cold. Am Rev Respir Dis 1988; 138:305–311
This prospective, randomized, controlled clinical trial provides additional data that the expiratory wheezing in PNDS is associated with an extrathoracic, variable upper airway obstruction.
43. Macklem PT. Airway obstruction and collateral ventilation. Physiol Rev 1971; 51:368–436
This article reviews the anatomy and physiology of small airway diseases.
44. Gelb AF, Klein E. The volume of isoflow and increase in maximal flow at 50% of forced vital capacity during helium-oxygen breathing as tests of small air ways dysfunction. Chest 1977; 71:396–399
This study describes, demonstrates, and explains how helium-oxygen breathing during recording of flow-volume loops can be used to localize the site(s) of airflow obstruction.
45. Miller RD, Hyatt RE. Obstruction lesions of the larynx and trachea: clinical and physiologic characteristics. Mayo Clin Proc 1969; 44:145–161
This is a classic publication that reveals the usefulness of physiologic testing in distinguishing variable extrathoracic from variable intrathoracic upper airway lesions.
46. Kryger M, Bode F, Antic R. Diagnosis of obstruction of the upper and central airways. Am J Med 1976; 61:85–93
An excellent review article that covers the physiology, pathophysiology, and clinical aspects of diagnosing air-

way-obstructing lesions.

47. Kaminsky DA, Irvin CG. Anatomic correlates of reversible restrictive lung disease. Chest 1993; 103:928–931
This publication provides convincing data that diseases can present with reversible restrictive lung disease that is clinically indistinguishable from asthma.
48. Hudgel D, Cooper D, Souhrada J. Reversible restrictive lung disease simulating asthma. Ann Intern Med 1976; 85:328–332
This is another publication that reports that patients can have a reversible restrictive lung disease that is like asthma and responds to conventional asthma medications.
49. Smyrnios NA, Irwin RS. Wheeze. In: Irwin RS, Curley FJ, Grossman RF, eds. Diagnosis and treatment of symptoms of the respiratory tract. Armonk, NY: Futura Publishing Company, 1997; 117–153
This chapter is a comprehensive, extensively referenced review of all aspects of wheeze that discusses in detail the many diseases that comprise the differential diagnosis of wheeze.
50. Smyrnios NA, Irwin RS, Curley FJ. Chronic cough with a history of excessive mucus production: the spectrum and frequency of causes, key components of the diagnostic evaluation, and outcome of specific therapy. Chest 1995; 108:991–997
This prospective, descriptive study reports the spectrum and frequency of causes of cough-phlegm syndromes. Contrary to what had been believed, chronic bronchitis is not as common a cause of this syndrome as PNDS, asthma, or GERD. Consequently, if a patient has wheeze and a cough-phlegm syndrome, the diagnosis of COPD should not reflexively be made clinically.
51. Crapo RO. Pulmonary function testing. N Engl J Med 1994; 331:25–30
This review article provides guidelines for interpreting routine pulmonary function testing in determining whether or not the patient has reversible or irreversible airflow obstruction.
52. Webb J, Clark TJH, Chilvers C. Time course of response to prednisolone in chronic airflow obstruction. Thorax 1981; 36:18–21
This study reveals that significant reversibility in airflow obstruction may occur after weeks of systemic corticosteroids in patients who would have been thought to have irreversible disease based solely upon lack of bronchodilator response in the pulmonary function laboratory.
53. Brown RF, Dibenedetto R, Russell D, et al. Variant cystic fibrosis in an elderly man. South Med J 1986; 79:1430–1432
This report documents that CF should be considered a possibility in the proper context regardless of the patient's age.
54. Highsmith WE, Burch LH, Zhou Z, et al. A novel mutation in the cystic fibrosis gene in patients with pulmonary disease but normal sweat chloride concentrations. N Engl J Med 1994; 331:974–980
This article describes how to use new diagnostic methods in diagnosing CF when standard, traditional techniques have failed.

Hemoptysis

55. Corey R, Hla KM. Major and massive hemoptysis: reassessment of conservative management. Am J Med Sci 1987; 294:301–309
This article defines hemoptysis and reassesses the relative roles of surgery vs observation in patients with massive hemoptysis.
56. Irwin RS, Curley FJ, Robinson KA. Managing hemoptysis. In: Rippe JM, Irwin RS, Fink MP, et al, eds. Intensive care medicine. 6th ed. Boston, MA: Little, Brown and Company, 2008; 588–598
This chapter defines pseudohemoptysis and provides a differential diagnosis of the same. It also comprehensively reviews with extensive referencing the entire subject of hemoptysis.
57. Johnston H, Reiza G. Changing spectrum of hemoptysis: underlying causes in 148 patients undergoing diagnostic flexible fiberoptic bronchoscopy. Arch Intern Med 1989; 149:1666–1668
This is a representative article that deals with the spectra and frequencies of causes of hemoptysis from the late 1970s to the mid-1980s.
58. Nelson JE, Forman M. Hemoptysis in HIV-infected patients. Chest 1996; 110:737–743
This is a retrospective study that provides information on the spectra and frequency of causes of hemoptysis in HIV-positive patients.
59. Bartter T, Irwin RS, Phillips DA, et al. Pulmonary artery pseudoaneurysm: a potential complication of pulmonary artery catheterization. Arch Intern Med 1988; 148:471–473
This article summarizes what is known about rupture of a pulmonary artery by the balloon flotation catheter and reports the complication of pseudoaneurysm and how to recognize and treat it.
60. Schaefer OP, Irwin RS. Tracheo-artery fistula. J Intensive Care Med 1995; 10:64–75
This review article comprehensively discusses all

aspects of tracheoartery fistula as a complication of tracheostomy except for describing the surgical operations to correct the complication.

61. Lyons HA. Differential diagnosis of hemoptysis and its treatment. Basics of respiratory disease 1976; 5:26–30
This article reviews the spectra and frequencies of causes of hemoptysis and includes idiopathic or essential hemoptysis as a cause.
62. Rath GS, Schaff JT, Snider GL. Flexible fiberoptic bronchoscopy: techniques and review of 100 bronchoscopies. Chest 1973; 63:689–693
This study also includes idiopathic hemoptysis as a specific cause of hemoptysis.
63. Barrett RJ, Tuttle WM. A study of essential hemoptysis. J Thorac Cardiovasc Surg 1960; 40:468–474
The entity of essential (or idiopathic) hemoptysis is discussed in detail.
64. Savale L, Parrot A, Khalil A, et al. Cryptogenic hemoptysis: from a benign to a life-threatening pathologic vascular condition. Am J Respir Crit Care Med 2007; 175:1181–1185
From a cohort of 81 patients referred for crytogenic hemoptysis, an abnormal superficial vessel contiguous to the epithelium of the bronchial mucosa was found as the cause of hemoptysis (Dieulafoy disease) in 5 of 9 who underwent surgery. This diagnosis must be kept in mind.
65. Murray JF. Postnatal growth and development of the lung. In: Murray JF, ed. The normal lung: the basis for diagnosis and treatment of pulmonary disease. Philadelphia, PA: WB Saunders, 1976; 21
Provides a discussion of the anatomy of the bronchial and pulmonary circulations that is useful to review to better understand the pathogenesis of hemoptysis.
66. Schwarz MI, Sutarik JM, Nick JA, et al. Pulmonary capillaritis and diffuse alveolar hemorrhage: a primary manifestation of polymyositis. Am J Respir Crit Care Med 1995; 151:2037–2040
In addition to reporting pulmonary capillaritis and diffuse alveolar hemorrhage as a primary manifestation of polymyositis, this article briefly reviews the topic of pulmonary capillaritis.
67. Pratt LW. Hemoptysis. Ann Otol Rhinol Laryngol 63:296–309, 1954
Although patients with lung infections often have blood in their sputum, this article makes the point that hemoptysis that lasts for more than the usual 24 h suggests that an endobronchial lesion or coagulopathy are present.
68. Thomas HM III, Irwin RS. Classification of diffuse intrapulmonary hemorrhage [editorial]. Chest 1975; 68:483–484
In addition to providing a differential diagnosis of causes of diffuse intrapulmonary hemorrhage, this editorial makes the point that the lack of hemoptysis does not rule out a substantial intrapulmonary hemorrhage.
69. Zeiss CR, Leach CL, Smith LJ, et al. A serial immunologic and histopathologic study of lung injury induced by trimellitic anhydride. Am Rev Respir Dis 1988; 137:191–196
This publication demonstrates that intrapulmonary hemorrhage can be caused by inhaled TMA.
70. Patterson R, Nugent KM, Harris KE, et al. Immunologic hemorrhagic pneumonia caused by isocyanates. Am Rev Respir Dis 1990; 141:226–230
This study shows that inhaled isocyantes can also cause intrapulmonary bleeding.
71. Sisson JH, Thompson AB, Anderson JR, et al. Airway inflammation predicts diffuse alveolar hemorrhage during bone marrow transplantation in patients with Hodgkin's disease. Am Rev Respir Dis 1992; 146:439–443
Diffuse intrapulmonary hemorrhage is a complication of bone marrow transplantation.
72. Jackson CL, Diamond S. Hemorrhage from the trachea, bronchi, and lungs of nontuberculous origin. Am Rev Tuberc 1942; 46:126–137
This study demonstrates that chest radiographicfindings can be normal up to 30% of the time when hemoptysis is caused by a lower respiratory tract disease.
73. Kim JH, Follett JV, Rice JR, et al. Endobronchial telangiectasias and hemoptysis in scleroderma. Am J Med 1988; 84:173–174
This article documents that bronchoscopy can establish a site of hemoptysis different from that suggested by the chest radiograph.
74. Smiddy JF, Elliott RC. The evaluation of hemoptysis with fiberoptic bronchoscopy. Chest 1973; 64:158–162
This is another study showing that bronchoscopy can find a site of hemoptysis different than that suggested by the chest radiograph.
75. Saumench J, Escarrabill J, Padro L, et al. Value of fiberoptic bronchoscopy and angiography for diagnosis of the bleeding site in hemoptysis. Ann Thorac Surg 1989; 48:272–274
If flexible bronchoscopy is performed within 24 h of active bleeding, there is a high yield of being able to localize the specific site.
76. Pursel SE, Lindskog GE. Hemoptysis. Am Rev

Respir Dis 84:329–336, 1961
Even rigid bronchoscopy has an excellent chance of localizing the specific site of bleeding in hemoptysis if the procedure is performed early.

77. McGuinness G, Beacher JR, Harkin TJ, et al. Hemoptysis: prospective high-resolution CT/ bronchoscopic correlation. Chest 1994; 105:1155–1162
If there is a delay of 48 h in doing bronchoscopy, the frequency of being able to identify the site of bleeding decreases substantially.
78. De Lassence A, Fleury-Feith J, Escudier E, et al. Alveolar hemorrhage: diagnostic criteria and results in immunocompromised hosts. Am J Respir Crit Care Med 1995; 151:157–163
Provides guidelines for interpreting the results of BAL fluid (percentage of siderphages) in determining whether or not the patient has recently had diffuse alveolar hemorrhage.
79. Fraser RG, Pare JAP, Pare PD, et al. Diseases of the airways. In: Fraser RG, Pare JAP, Pare PD, et al, eds. Diagnosis of diseases of the chest (vol 3) 3rd ed. Toronto, Canada: WB Saunders, 1990; 2186–2206
Discusses the performance of routine chest radiography when the patient is suspected to have bronchiectasis.
80. Kalluri R, Petrides S, Wilson CB, et al. Anti-al(IV) collagen autoantibodies associated with lung adenocarcinoma presenting as the Goodpasture syndrome. Ann Intern Med 1996; 124:651–653
Discusses the different components of collagen and specifically the collagen in basement membranes as they relate to the diagnosis of Goodpasture syndrome.
81. Zimmerman SW, Varanasi UR, Hoff B. Goodpasture's with normal renal function. Am J Med 1979; 66:163–171
Immunofluorescent staining can be diagnostic of Goodpasture syndrome even when the patient has no evidence of renal disease.
82. Border WA, Baehler RW, Bhathena D, et al. IgA anti-basement membrane nephritis with pulmonary hemorrhage. Ann Intern Med 1979; 191:21–25
Pulmonary-renal syndrome mimicking Goodpasture syndrome can be caused by IgA ephropathy.
83. Clarke CP, Jackson KA, Moreland M, et al. Bronchoscopic use of the neodymium-yttrium-aluminum-garnet laser for lesions of the trachea and bronchus. Med J Aust 1989; 150:260–262
When hemoptysis is the result of bronchogenic carcinoma, the use of laser therapy can successfully stop the bleeding.
84. Conlan AA. Massive hemoptysis: review of 123 cases. J Thorac Cardiovasc Surg 1983; 85:120–124
Bronchoscopically directed iced saline solution lavge of the site of hemoptysis is reported to stop hemorrhage.
85. Rabkin JE, Astafjev VI, Gothman LN, et al. Transcatheter embolization in the management of pulmonary hemorrhage. Radiology 1987; 163:361–365
Reviews the role of interventional radiology in controlling intrapulmonary bleeding.
86. Hickey NM, Peterson RA, Leech JA, et al. Percutaneous embolotherapy in life-threatening hemoptysis. Cardiovasc Intervent Radiol 1988; 11:270–273
Reviews the role ofinterventional radiology in controlling intrapulmonary bleeding and emphasizes the point that multiple procedures may be necessary.
87. Stoll JF, Bettmann MA. Bronchial artery embolization to control hemoptysis: a review. Cardiovasc Intervent Radiol 1988; 11:263–269
Reviews the role of interventional radiology in controlling intrapulmonary bleeding and gives rates of rebleeding.
88. Uflacker R. Bronchial artery embolization in the management of hemoptysis: technical aspects and long-term results. Radiology 1985; 157:637–644
Reviews the role of interventional radiology and temporary balloon occlusion in controlling intrapulmonary bleeding.
89. Jardin M, Remy J. Control of hemoptysis: systemic angiography and anastomoses of the internal mammary artery. Radiology 1988; 168:377–383
Reviews the role of interventional radiology and temporary balloon occlusion in controlling bleeding.
90. Crocco JA, Rooney JJ, Fankushen DS, et al. Massive hemoptysis. Arch Intern Med 1968; 121:495–498
This older study recommends emergency surgery for massive hemoptysis over conservative therapy; more recent studies do not support this recommendation.
91. MacDonald JA, Fraser JF, Foot CL, et al. Successful use of recombinant Factor VII in massive hemoptysis due to community-acquired pneumonia. Chest 2006; 130:577–579
Recombinant Factor VII may be a useful temporizing measure in unstable patients with life-threatening pulmonary hemorrhage even when there is no coagulopathy.

Dyspnea

92. Curley FJ. Dyspnea. In: Irwin RS, Curley FJ, Grossman RF, eds. Diagnosis and treatment of symptoms of the respiratory tract. Armonk, NY: Futura Publishing Company, 1997; 55–111
This extensively referenced chapter comprehensively

and critically reviews all aspects of dyspnea.

93. Fedullo AL, Swineburne AJ, McGuire-Dunn C. Complaints of breathlessness in the emergency department: the experience at a community hospital. NY State J Med 1986; 86:4–6
This study provides data on spectrum and frequency of causes of dyspnea evaluated in an emergency department.
94. Pearson SB, Pearson EM, Mitchel JRA. The diagnosis and management of patients admitted to hospital with acute breathlessness. Postgrad Med 1981; 57:419–424
This study provides data on spectrum and frequency of causes of dyspnea evaluated in hospitalized patients.
95. Mustchin CP, Tiwari I. Diagnosing the breathless patient. Lancet 1982; 2:907–908
This study provides data on spectrum and frequency of causes of dyspnea evaluated in hospitalized patients.
96. DePaso WJ, Winterbauer RH, Lusk JA, et al. Chronic dyspnea unexplained by history, physical examination, chest roentgenogram, and spirometry: analysis of a seven-year experience. Chest 1991; 100:1293–1299
This study reports the spectrum and frequency of causes of dyspnea evaluated in the outpatient setting.
97. Pratter MR, Curley FJ, Dubois J, et al. Cause and evaluation of chronic dyspnea in a pulmonary disease clinic. Arch Intern Med 1989; 149:2277–2282
This study reports the spectrum and frequency of causes of dyspnea evaluated in the outpatient setting
98. Kikuchi Y, Okabe S, Tamura G, et al. Chemosensitivity and perception of dyspnea in patients with a history of near-fatal asthma. N Engl J Med 1994; 330:1329 1334
This study shows that asthmatics with a history of near-fatal attacks have a reduced response to hypoxia and reduced sensation of dyspnea.
99. Martinez FJ, Stanopoulos I, Acero R, et al. Graded comprehensive cardiopulmonary exercise testing in the evaluation of dyspnea unexplained by routine evaluation. Chest 1994; 105:168–174
This study reports the spectrum and frequency of causes of dyspnea evaluated in the outpatient setting. The frequency of GERD as the cause was 2%.
100. Lum LC. The syndrome of chronic habitual hyperventilation. In: Hill OW, ed. Modern trends in psychosomatic medicine. London, UK: Buttersworth, 1976; 196
Of 640 patients treated with slow abdominal breathing, Lum reported that 70% were rendered asymptomatic, 20 to 25% were improved, and 5 to 10% failed to respond.
101. Reardon J, Awad E, Normandin E, et al. The effect of comprehensive outpatient pulmonary rehabilitation on dyspnea. Chest 1994; 105:1046–1052
Deconditioned COPD patients were randomized to a noninterventional group or a group that underwent 12 3-h sessions over 6 weeks of an education and exercise program. Dyspnea in the interventional group significantly improved.
102. Rogers RM, Donahoe M, Costantino J. Physiologic effects of oral supplemental feeding in malnourished patients with chronic obstructive pulmonary disease: a randomized control study. Am Rev Respir Dis 1992; 146:1511–1517
This study demonstrates that malnourished COPD patients had a reduction in dyspnea after a 3-month refeeding intervention.
103. Woodcock AA, Gross ER, Geddes DM. Drug treatment of breathlessness: contrasting effects of diazepam and promethazine in pink puffers. BMJ 1981; 283:343–346
This controlled clinical trial failed to show a reduction in dyspnea in patients with COPD when a benzodiazepine was used.
104. Eimer M, Cable T, Gal P. Effects of clorazepate on breathlessness and exercise tolerance in patients with chronic airflow obstruction. J Fam Pract 1985; 21:359–362
This controlled clinical trial failed to show a reduction in dyspnea in patients with COPD when a benzodiazepine was used.
105. Foral PA, Malesker MA, Huerta G, et al. Nebulized opioids use in COPD. Chest 2004; 125:691–694
106. Baydur A. Nebulized morphine: a convenient and safe alternative to dyspnea relief? Chest 2004; 125 363–365
These two studies review the lack of efficacy of inhaled opioids for relief of dyspnea in COPD and interstitial lung disease.
107. Lewith GT, Prescott P, Davis CL. Can a standardized acupuncture technique palliate disabling

breathlessness? A single-blind, placebo-controlled crossover study. Chest 2004; 125:1783–1790
Although there have been very few studies assessing the efficacy of acupuncture for dyspnea relief, this study failed to demonstrate that acupuncture is efficacious.

108. Ong K-C, Kor A-C, Chong W-F, et al. Effects of inhaled furosemide on exertional dyspnea in chronic obstructive pulmonary disease. Am J Respir Crit Care Med 2004; 169:1028–1033
This pilot study suggests that inhaled furosemide may help alleviate dyspnea in patients with COPD. These results

Notes

Mechanical Ventilatory Support

Curtis N. Sessler, MD, FCCP

Objectives:

- Review the determinants of oxygenation and ventilation
- Compare the different modes of mechanical ventilatory support
- Examine the role and methods for noninvasive positive-pressure ventilation
- Examine the value of monitoring and ventilator graphics in understanding patient-ventilator dyssynchrony
- Describe the complications associated with mechanical ventilatory support, including auto-positive end-expiratory pressure (PEEP) and ventilator-associated lung injury
- Review the importance of patient-focused ventilation, particularly differentiating ventilation strategies for obstructive lung disease and for ARDS
- Review the rationale and results of studies supporting a lung-protective ventilation strategy for acute lung injury/ ARDS
- Examine structured protocols on liberation from mechanical ventilation and the endotracheal tube

Key words: intrinsic positive end-expiratory pressure; mechanical ventilation; noninvasive ventilation; respiratory failure; weaning

---

Mechanical ventilatory support is used as a key component in the management of both hypoxemic respiratory failure and hypercapnic respiratory failure, topics that are discussed in more detail in other chapters. The principle techniques for providing artificial ventilation have changed during the past century. Negative pressure support (PS) achieved widespread use in the polio epidemic in the 1920s with the Drinker iron lung, followed by introduction of other negative-pressure devices. However, positive-pressure ventilation, which typically is delivered through an artificial tracheal airway, has achieved broad acceptance, whereas negative-pressure ventilation is rarely used in current practice. Although the patient-ventilator interface for positive-pressure ventilation is most often an endotracheal (ET) tube or tracheostomy tube, the less-invasive approach of using a tightly fitting full-face (oronasal) or nasal mask has achieved widespread use in the treatment of selected forms of respiratory failure. Advances in mechanical ventilator technology during the past 50 years have included efficient demand valves for triggered ventilation delivery, computerized integration of physiologic measurements and gas-delivery parameters, accurate gas-blending systems, and advanced monitoring and safety systems that have resulted in more options for the clinician to match mechanical ventilation (MV) to patient needs, better patient-ventilator interactions, and greater patient safety. Experience with MV in the treatment of patients with ARDS illustrates that proper MV influences not just gas exchange but also survival and other important outcomes.

Physiology of Ventilation and MV

Delivery of a breath occurs when there is a change in transpulmonary pressure, which is the pressure differential between the mouth and the pleural space. During a spontaneous breath, respiratory muscle contraction causes chest wall expansion and diaphragmatic descent that creates negative pressure within the pleural space. Entering through the trachea, inspired gas moves via bulk flow down the pressure gradient through the conducting bronchi and bronchioles to the respiratory units, where gases move by diffusion within alveoli and respiratory bronchioles, and then by diffusion through the alveolar-capillary membrane to the pulmonary capillaries. Negative-pressure ventilators simulate the action of the respiratory muscles by creating subatmospheric pressure surrounding the chest, thus expanding the thoracic cavity in a manner that is physiologically similar to spontaneous breathing. The loss of effective diaphragm movement in the negative-pressure ventilation system, however, yields less-efficient alveolar ventilation and gas distribution.

Similar to spontaneous breathing and negative pressure ventilation, positive-pressure ventilators generate transpulmonary pressure, favoring bulk flow of gases down the trachea and the conducting airways. However, this is created by positive pressure within the airway, forcing air down the trachea, sufficient to overcome pleural pressure to achieve gas delivery to respiratory lung units. It is noteworthy that pleural pressure is often actually a positive pressure at rest as a result of the resistive forces associated with chest wall, abdominal, or pleural factors. Common examples of increased pleural pressure include large pleural effusions or pneumothoraces, increased chest wall thickness and/or rigidity from obesity or burn eschar, and diaphragmatic elevation from pregnancy, ascites, obesity, or intraabdominal hypertension. For example, plateau airway pressures of 30 cm H_2O may be associated with a transpulmonary pressure of only 20 cm H_2O in a patient who is obese and who has a pleural pressure of + 10 cm H_2O.

Distribution of inspired gases within the thorax differs between spontaneous breathing and controlled positive-pressure ventilation, particularly when the patient is in the supine position. With positive-pressure ventilation, gases are delivered preferentially to zones of least resistance, generally the more anterior lung units. In contrast, diaphragmatic descent in spontaneous ventilation more effectively inflates the inferiorly and dependently positioned juxta-diaphragmatic lung units, improving ventilation/perfusion matching of these units. Techniques to enhance ventilation of these lung units via spontaneous breathing and by prone positioning often yield improved oxygenation.

Positive-Pressure Ventilation

Although the notion of forcing gas down the trachea to inflate the gas exchange lung units with oxygen-enriched gas is a seemingly straightforward concept, there are many variables to be considered for safe and effective MV. The principles of MV will be discussed in the context of the primary derangements of respiratory failure, key parameters of positive-pressure ventilation, conventional modes of ventilation in widespread use, additional commercially available modes of ventilation, and specialized modes and techniques.

Oxygenation and Ventilation

A conceptual framework for understanding the key determinants of oxygenation and ventilation during MV is displayed in Figure 1. Although achieving acceptable oxygenation and ventilation is certainly inter-related, approaching the issues separately can be useful to emphasize key elements. Hypoxemia is a common component of respiratory failure, and the most straightforward solution is to increase the fraction of inspired oxygen (FIO_2). Adjustments in airway pressure can have an important impact on oxygenation as well, particularly for patients who have extensive parenchymal lung disease. Considerable ventilation/perfusion mismatching with a large component of underventilated or shunt-like alveoli contributes greatly to hypoxemia and is often responsive to increases in airway pressure through alveolar recruitment and retention. PEEP is typically added at low levels (*ie*, 5 cm H_2O) to help splint open alveoli even in the absence of diffuse lung disease; however, PEEP is generally increased to recruit and retain alveoli that are prone to cyclic collapse as airway pressures decrease during exhalation.

Although alveolar distention throughout the respiratory cycle is best accomplished by applying greater levels of PEEP, other adjustments that increase mean airway pressure (MAP)—particularly by increasing the duration of inspiratory distending pressure, *ie*, inspiratory time (TI)—can improve alveolar ventilation and oxygenation. Excessive alveolar pressure can be detrimental, however, by the following actions: (1) overdistending functional alveoli, thus increasing dead space; (2) increasing intrathoracic pressure thereby reducing venous return, cardiac output, and oxygen delivery; (3) overstretching alveoli, thereby producing ventilator-associated lung injury (VALI); and (4) causing alveolar rupture, thereby producing air-leak barotraumas. Ventilation can be conceptualized by understanding the parameters related to delivery of individual breaths, the frequency of breath delivery, and how conventional modes of ventilation differ regarding breath delivery.

Breath Delivery and Principal Modes of MV

Volume and Pressure-Targeted Breaths: As displayed in Figure 1, each breath the patient receives can be defined by the 3 "Ts": (1) the "target" for delivery, *ie*, volume or pressure; (2) the "trigger" or signal to initiate the breath; and (3) the "termination" criteria that signals the end of the inspiratory phase and beginning of the expiratory phase. Breath characteristics can

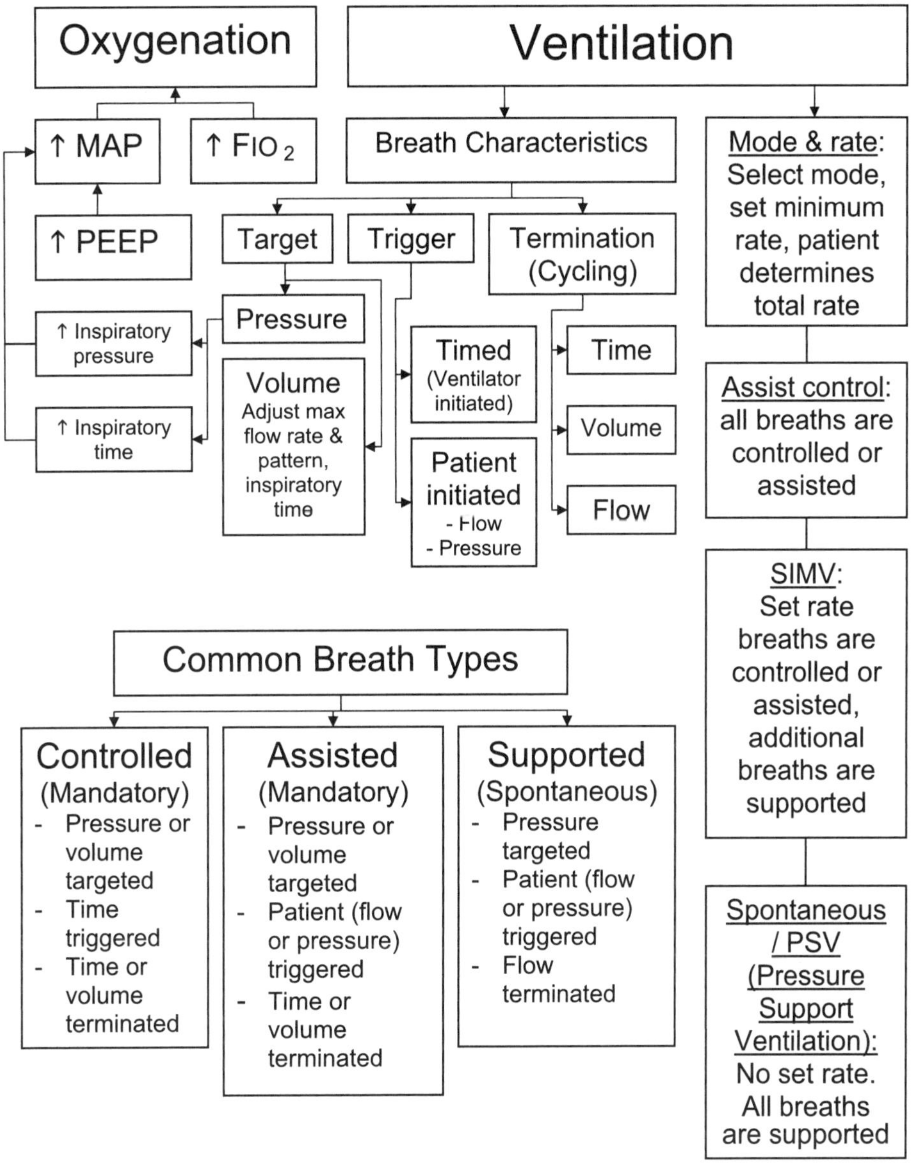

Figure 1. Mechanical ventilation parameters that influence oxygenation and ventilation. Oxygenation is controlled by adjusting FIO_2 and parameters that change MAP. Ventilation is determined by breath characteristics, ventilator mode, and respiratory rate, including minimum mandatory breaths and additional patient breaths. Each breath can be defined by the delivery target (pressure or volume) and the signals to initiate and to terminate the breath. There are three types of breaths as defined by initiation and termination signals: ventilator-initiated mandatory breath, patient-initiated mandatory breath, and patient-initiated spontaneous breath. The mode determines the type of breaths that can be mandatory and those that are in addition to the minimum set rate.

be determined by the clinician (ie, mandatory controlled or assisted breath) or influenced by clinician settings and patient effort (ie, pressure-supported spontaneous breath). These parameters differ in the common modes of ventilation (Table 1). An important concept is that mandatory breaths are "guaranteed," both in terms of a minimum number of breaths each minute, as well as delivery of a predetermined volume or a predetermined pressure and Ti. In contrast, spontaneous breaths are dependent on patient effort for both breath initiation as well as breath duration.

Mandatory breaths can be volume or pressure-targeted, whereas spontaneous breaths are only pressure-targeted in conventional modes. The patient interacts with the ventilator via sensors that are in-line pressure or flow transducers that respond to the patient's spontaneous efforts. Data suggest that flow-triggered sensors are more sensitive to the patient's efforts than are the demand sensors triggered by changes in pressure, unless the pressure transducer is positioned at the distal end of the ET tube. However, clinically available

Table 1. *Comparison of Principal Modes of Ventilation*

Mode of ventilation	AC Mode	SIMV	Spontaneous/PSV
Mandatory breaths	Yes	Yes	No
Spontaneous breaths*	No	Yes	Yes
Volume or pressure	Either	Mandatory: either spontaneous: pressure only	Pressure
Advantages	Stabilization mode		Comfortable mode
Disadvantages	Respiratory alkalosis, air trapping with tachypnea	Less comfortable	Unreliable ventilation if there is apnea, weakness, deterioration in lung mechanics

*Spontaneous breaths are all initiated by the patient, and the termination of inspiration (and thus inspiratory time) is determined by the patient.

sensors are positioned inside the ventilators and, thus, the pressure or flow signal is dampened by the dead space of the ventilator tubing that connects the ET tube to the ventilator. Depending on the sensitivity and responsiveness of the ventilator, respiratory muscular efforts may not be sensed by the ventilator, causing poor ventilator/patient interaction. This asynchrony increases the imposed work of breathing (WOB) that the patient has to generate to initiate a breath.

Volume-Targeted Breaths—In volume-targeted breaths, a tidal volume (VT) is chosen, and the breath is delivered by applying an inspiratory flow rate (flow limitation) and pattern of delivery (square wave, sine wave, or decelerating or ramp pattern). Typical flow rates vary from 30 to 80 L/min, with greater flows resulting in shorter TI and shorter inspiratory/expiratory (I:E) ratios but greater peak inspiratory pressure (PIP). Similarly, square wave flow results in shorter TI and greater PIP, whereas the decelerating pattern has the opposite effects. Collaboration with a skilled respiratory therapist is important to fine-tuning these parameters. The breath is terminated and exhalation permitted after the set VT has been delivered. In some volume-targeted modes, the TI is also set, and exhalation begins after TI is concluded. The airway pressure that is generated to deliver the breath varies, increasing to a peak pressure as the lung is inflated. Airway pressures are dependent on the ventilator settings as well as lung and chest wall mechanics. For example, greater PIP can be result of faster flow rates or larger VT but also bronchospasm, ET obstruction, or tension pneumothorax, with no change in set flow or VT.

Pressure-Targeted Breaths—In contrast to volume-targeted breaths, pressure-targeted (or pressure-limited) breaths do not guarantee the delivery of specific VT. The inspiratory pressure (Pi) and the TI will determine the VT. The Pi is set by the clinician in all conventional pressure-targeted modes, but TI can be determined by the clinician (as in a mandatory breath) or by the patient (as with a spontaneous breath). If the Pi and TI are held constant but lung mechanics change, the VT may be larger or smaller. For example, the resolution of pulmonary edema would improve lung compliance, which would result in a larger VT for the same Pi and TI, whereas new onset of bronchospasm would be associated with a smaller VT from increased airway resistance.

Breath Initiation (Trigger), Breath Termination, Breath Frequency, and Principle Modes of Ventilation—The frequency of breath delivery is dependent on the signal(s) to initiate the breath, the mode of ventilation, the minimum set rate for mandatory breaths, and patient effort. The influence of ventilator mode on respiratory frequency and type of breaths is compared in Table 1 and illustrated in hypothetical cases in Table 2. For ventilator-initiated (or -controlled) mandatory breaths, the breath is initiated when a clinician-determined time interval has been reached. For example, if a frequency of 10 breaths/min is set, a new breath will be initiated every 6 s. Among the conventional modes of ventilation (Table 1), the frequency of mandatory breaths can be set with the assist control (AC) mode or synchronized intermittent mandatory ventilation (SIMV) mode. Mandatory breaths can also be initiated by the patient (*ie*, patient-initiated [or -assisted] mandatory breath; see Fig 1). This feature promotes patient comfort by recognizing a patient's inspiratory effort and delivering a mandatory breath that has the same clinician-determined characteristics as if ventilator-initiated.

Table 2. *Hypothetical Examples of Varying the Drive to Breath, the Number of Patient Inspiratory Efforts, and Clinician-Selected Parameters on Breath Types and Characteristics in Principal Modes of Ventilation**

Scenarios	Parameters					
	Mode set Frequency	Assist Control 10/min	Assist Control 10/min	SIMV 10/min	SIMV 10/min	Spontaneous
	Pressure or volume	Pressure	Volume	Mandatory: pressure, Supported: pressure	Mandatory: volume, Supported: pressure	Supported: pressure
A. Baseline (12 inspiratory efforts/min)	Mandatory breaths	12 total, mix of controlled and assisted	12 total, mix of controlled and assisted	10 total, mix of controlled and assisted	10 total, mix of controlled and assisted	0
	Spontaneous breaths	0	0	2	2	12
B. Apnea	Mandatory breaths	10 controlled 0 assisted	10 controlled 0 assisted	10 controlled 0 assisted	10 controlled 0 assisted	0
	Spontaneous breaths	0	0	0	0	0
C. 30 patient inspiratory efforts/min	Mandatory breaths	30 total, most assisted since tachypneic	30 total, most assisted since tachypneic	10 total, 0-10 controlled, the rest assisted	10 total, 0-10 controlled, the rest assisted	0
	Spontaneous breaths	0	0	20	20	30
D. ↓set f to 2/min; there are 12 patient inspiratory efforts/min	Mandatory breaths	12 total, 2 controlled; 10 assisted	12 total, 2 controlled; 10 assisted	2 total probably all controlled	2 total probably all controlled	0
	Spontaneous breaths	0	0	10	10	12
E. Pulmonary edema develops	Tidal volume Peak airway pressure	Decreases No change	No change Increases	Decreases No change	No change Increases	Decreases No change

*Five examples of ventilator modes are presented. The rate is set at 10 breaths/min for all except the spontaneous mode. Five scenarios are presented in which different numbers of patient inspiratory efforts are made (A, B, and C), there is a reduction in the set rate to 2 breaths/min (D), or pulmonary edema develops (E). For the first four scenarios, the expected effect on mandatory and spontaneous breaths is depicted. In scenario E, the effect on V_T and peak airway pressure is illustrated.

The AC and SIMV modes differ in the number of mandatory breaths permitted. With the AC mode, a minimum frequency (for example, 10 breaths/min) is set; however, all additional breaths that the patient triggers are also mandatory breaths. In contrast, with SIMV, the number of breaths that are mandatory is always determined by the clinician-set minimum frequency. Any addition breaths are treated as "spontaneous" breaths that may be pressure "supported" (see scenarios C and D in Table 2 for examples). For SIMV, ventilator manufacturers apply different algorithms that determine whether an inspiratory effort triggers an assisted mandatory breath or a spontaneous pressure-supported breath. For example, with some ventilator models, the delivery of a mandatory breath is followed by a "refractory period," during which time a patient's inspiratory effort will trigger a spontaneous breath but not a mandatory breath. Finally, in the spontaneous mode, the patient determines both the onset and termination of each breath, thus controlling both the frequency of breathing and the T_I (which generally varies from breath to breath). These spontaneous breaths are usually pressure supported. The spontaneous mode with all breaths receiving PS is widely referred to as pressure support ventilation (PSV). In the spontaneous mode, V_T typically varies from breath to breath and will also change with alterations in lung mechanics.

Summary and Comparison of Principle Modes of Ventilation: AC, SIMV, and Spontaneous Modes: The three principle modes of ventilation are compared in Table 1. Among these modes, an international prospective surveillance study performed in 1998 of > 5,000 mechanically ventilated adults showed that AC was the most commonly applied mode, with nearly two thirds of patients with acute exacerbation of COPD and 60% of patients with ARDS receiving AC ventilation. Only 10 to 15% of patients with COPD or ARDS received SIMV with or without PS, whereas nearly 10% of patients with COPD had PSV, and 10 to 15% of patients with ARDS received pressure-controlled ventilation (PCV). The effect of hypothetical changes in respiratory frequency or respiratory drive and changes in lung mechanics on ventilatory parameters for the three principle modes are displayed in Table 2.

AC Ventilation—AC ventilation may be volume or pressure targeted, and all breaths have the same settings (V_T for volume targeted, Pi and T_I for pressure targeted). The clinician sets the minimal number of breaths per minute. In addition, inspiratory efforts trigger the ventilator to supply additional mandatory breaths. Usually, AC ventilation is used when the operator desires to minimize the amount of WOB that the patient has to perform. AC ventilation cannot be used as a weaning mode because all breaths the patient takes are mandatory breaths that are associated with minimal WOB regardless of the minimum frequency setting (see scenario C in Table 2). Because all breaths are mandatory breaths, hyperventilation in this setting can be detrimental because of the resulting high minute ventilation and associated respiratory alkalosis but also in the potential for "stacking" of breaths that could result in an increase in airway pressure caused by auto-PEEP and dynamic hyperinflation (scenario D in Table 2).

SIMV—Intermittent mandatory ventilation (IMV) was originally developed as a bridge between controlled mandatory ventilation and spontaneous breathing. With controlled mandatory ventilation, all breaths are ventilator-initiated mandatory breaths, and patient inspiratory efforts do not result in any airflow or ventilation, an uncomfortable sensation. With IMV, the patient's inspiratory effort promotes delivery of a spontaneous breath from a reservoir bag that contains gas with the same F_{IO_2} as for mandatory breaths. The size of the breath is determined by patient effort and lung mechanics. Most modern ventilators use "synchronized" IMV, which permits the patient to initiate a mandatory breath (*ie*, an "assisted" mandatory breath), or initiate a spontaneous breath. Current ventilators allow support of the spontaneous breaths with a predetermined pressure (*ie*, a PS breath). Thus with SIMV, there is a combination of controlled mandatory, assisted mandatory, and pressure-supported spontaneous breaths. Whether an assisted or supported breath is produced is dependent on the timing of the inspiratory effort. Over the course of a minute, the total number of mandatory breaths, including both controlled and assisted breaths, cannot exceed the preset frequency. Although the original intention of SIMV was to speed the transition from full ventilatory support to spontaneous breathing by gradually decreasing the number of mandatory breaths, clinical trials actually demonstrate SIMV to be inferior to PSV for weaning patients off ventilator support. Patient comfort can be impaired in this mode as well, with the patient receiving three different breath types.

Spontaneous Ventilation/PSV—Spontaneous ventilation requires patient effort for the initiation of all breaths. Additionally, the termination of all breaths is determined by a reduction in inspiratory effort that is reflected in a decrease in flow below a preset percentage of peak flow. This has been called *flow-cycled termination*. If PEEP is applied, then continuous positive airway pressure (CPAP) is present because the patient's airway pressure is positive during inspiration and expiration. Virtually all clinicians now augment spontaneous breaths with PS, usually in the 5 to 25 cm H_2O range, often referred to as PSV. With PSV, flow commences when a pressure or a flow sensor is triggered. The duration of the added PS is determined by the spontaneous inspiratory flow, related to patient inspiratory effort. PSV cycles off when the spontaneous inspiratory flow decreases to a preset level (usually approximately 25% of the peak flow). The amount of pressure can be adjusted to achieve comfortable breathing, with acceptable VT and respiratory rate (frequency, or *f*). Research suggests the PSV is the most comfortable mode of ventilation for the alert patient. Additionally, the amount of PS can be reduced, thus placing a greater requirement on the patient for WOB during transition from ventilatory support to spontaneous breathing.

In the past, PSV was a popular approach to weaning. The patient was placed on spontaneous mode and the PS level sequentially lowered, increasing the amount of patient WOB. The patient with adequate respiratory muscle strength and reserve experiences minimal change in the breathing pattern (*f*, VT, and thoracoabdominal synchrony) as the PS level is reduced. However, if the patient is not ready to assume all the required WOB, *f* will increase, and VT will decrease as the PS level is sequentially diminished. In current approaches to liberation of the ventilator, PSV (5 to 8 cm H_2O) is often used to overcome the added WOB that accompanies the resistance of breathing through the ET tube during a spontaneous breathing trial. Because mandatory breaths are not provided in this mode, reliance on the patient for initiating each breath as well as having sufficient respiratory drive and respiratory muscle strength to achieve adequate minute ventilation is an important limitation to consider if the patient is likely to become apneic or weak. Further, as with any pressure-targeted mode, deterioration in lung mechanics can result in hypoventilation despite previously effective PS settings.

Some Additional Commercially Available Modes of Ventilation

PCV: PCV is a controlled mode of ventilation (no spontaneous breaths) that previously was popular for the ventilatory management of ARDS, particularly with extended duration of the inspiratory phase in excess of inspiratory phase, so-called *pressure controlled inverse ratio ventilation* or *PC-IRV*. Recall that the I/E ratio is normally 1:2 to 1:4. PC-IRV uses I/E ratios of ≥1:1, with ratios of 3:1 occasionally used. PCV is similar to pressure-targeted AC or SIMV but without assisted or spontaneous breaths. With PCV, the ventilator rapidly achieves the clinician-set Pi, which is usually delivered in a decelerating waveform. The operator sets the duration of inspiration (and thus the VT varies) by varying the TI (time cycled) or by setting the I/E ratio. Inspiratory flow from the ventilator to the patient will continue until the preset TI or the I/E ratio has occurred. In the time-cycled mode, if the preset pressure is achieved early in the inspiratory cycle, an inspiratory hold will occur. The increase in MAP seen with PC-IRV can be effective for alveolar recruitment and retention and has been associated with better oxygenation. Outcome studies have not demonstrated greater survival or short duration of MV with PC-IRV. The major disadvantages of PCV are the need for heavy patient sedation and the variability of delivered VT and minute ventilation with changes in respiratory mechanics.

Bilevel Ventilation and Airway Pressure Release Ventilation (APRV): Bilevel ventilation is, in essence, a modification of SIMV in which mandatory breaths are pressure-targeted and PS is used to augment spontaneous breaths. The unique feature of bilevel ventilation is that spontaneous breaths can be performed throughout the respiratory cycle. Thus, in contrast to other pressure-targeted modes, including SIMV, AC, and PCV, the patient can take spontaneous breaths even during a prolonged lung inflation. Mandatory breaths are delivered by increasing airway pressure to a new greater level of pressure for a set time, and exhalation occurs when airway pressure is decreased to the PEEP level.

The frequency is set as with any mandatory breaths and like SIMV or AC can be initiated by the ventilator (*ie*, controlled) or initiated by the patient (*ie*, assisted).

PS can be applied to augment spontaneous breaths, but as a safety feature, the amount of PS is added relative to the PEEP level. For example, if PEEP is 10 cm H_2O and the Pi is 15 cm H_2O, then the plateau airway pressure will be 25 cm H_2O. An increase to 20 cm H_2O PS would increase the peak pressure of spontaneous breaths taken during the expiratory phase to 30 cm H_2O (*ie*, 10 cm H_2O PEEP + 20 cm H_2O PS)—this sets the upper limit for PS. Spontaneous breaths taken while at an inspiratory plateau pressure of 25 cm H_2O would only be augmented to the 30 cm H_2O limit; thus, an effective PS pressure of only 5 cm H_2O is provided. Bilevel ventilation is a potentially attractive mode for ARDS, combining the advantages of ventilation with pressure-targeted prolonged inspiratory breaths, yet by permitting spontaneous ventilations at any time in the respiratory cycle, reducing the requirement for sedation and neuromuscular blockade.

The term *APRV* has different connotations depending on locale. Bilevel ventilation with I/E ratio of 1:1 has been called APRV in some European studies; however, in the United States, the term APRV is generally applied to pressure-targeted ventilation with a very long Ti and a very brief (*ie*, < 0.8 s) expiratory time. Typically, exhalation to a set PEEP of zero is often performed; however, the actual PEEP is probably considerably greater as a result of intrinsic or auto-PEEP that develops from incomplete exhalation. In European clinical studies, bilevel ventilation with 1:1 I/E ratio and no PS for spontaneous breaths was associated with improved gas exchange and patient comfort. There is a paucity of outcomes studies that demonstrate improved outcomes for APRV with short expiratory time. An important concern for the very brief expiratory time is the abrupt development of life-threatening auto-PEEP caused by increased expiratory resistance from retained secretions or bronchospasm.

Proportional-Assist Ventilation (PAV): PAV was designed to deliver positive-pressure ventilation in proportion to respiratory resistance and elastance. PAV attempts to incorporate a feedback loop from the spontaneous breathing pattern to better proportion subsequent positive-pressure breaths. This requires real-time, ongoing measurement of these parameters with rapid adjustments of PAV to keep pace with changes in patient effort and resistance, which can be significant even when there are no clinical changes in the patient's status. Conceptually, this form of ventilation should optimize patient-ventilator interaction. However, a recently published study examining WOB with PAV vs PSV failed to show superiority of PAV over PSV during quiet breathing or when dead space was added to the circuit.

Noninvasive Positive-Pressure Ventilation (NPPV)

NPPV is widely used in a variety of settings of respiratory failure. NPPV is delivered through a tight-fitting full-face (oronasal) or nasal mask. It can be delivered via a pressure-targeted or volume-targeted mode delivered with a conventional ICU ventilator or a portable ventilator specifically designed for bilevel positive airway PS. The mask is connected to the ventilator via a single inspiratory and expiratory line fitted with a special exhalation valve or by dual lines such as used with conventional MV. The operator sets the inspiratory positive airway pressure as well as the expiratory positive airway pressure. These setting are analogous to PS and PEEP, respectively. This bilevel ventilator can be used in a spontaneous mode or in a spontaneous/timed mode that is the equivalent of SIMV plus PSV. Being a pressure-targeted mode of ventilation, bilevel NPPV does not guarantee delivery of a constant VT or minute ventilation. A limitation to NPPV is that the monitoring systems in conventional ventilators may be too sensitive to air leaks that occur around the mask. Recently, bilevel pressure devices have incorporated more sophisticated alarm systems to circumvent this problem.

NPPV has been used in many forms of respiratory failure. Among the many proposed indications, acute hypercapnic respiratory failure in the patient with COPD has the strongest evidence base for recommendation. Several multicenter randomized controlled trials (RCTs) have demonstrated lower intubation rates, shorter duration of MV, and improved survival. Additional indications with demonstration of improved outcomes include treatment of cardiogenic pulmonary edema, fever and pulmonary infiltrates in immunocompromised hosts, postextubation respiratory distress caused by upper-airway obstruction, and persistent weaning failure with extubation to NPPV. It is important to recognize that patients who require emergent ET intubation are poor candidates for NPPV, such as those with overt respiratory distress or cardiopulmonary arrest. Additionally, suitable candidates for NPPV are those who are hemodynamically stable, have sufficiently alert mental status (Glasgow coma scale score >10), lack of facial trauma or deformity, and adequate clearance of respiratory secretions.

Correction of profound hypoxemia is often not possible with NPPV, even with additional sources of supplemental oxygen. During NPPV, one must avoid air leaks, eye irritation, and nasal abrasions. Careful attention by respiratory therapists and bedside nurses, including the establishment of a good mask fit and careful titration of airway pressures to tolerance, will help with the success of NPPV. It is particularly important to continuously re-evaluate tolerance of NPPV and to identify in a timely fashion impending failure of NPPV. Experts recommend that if NPPV has not resulted in clear improvement within 2 h of onset, ET intubation and conventional ventilation should be strongly considered. Signs of improvement include reduced respiratory distress (*ie*, less tachypnea and use of accessory muscles, better thoracoabdominal coordination), or physiologic improvement as determined by arterial blood gas analysis or breathing pattern analysis. It is worth considering that many studies are modest in size, patients enrolled represent a small percentage of patients with acute respiratory failure at those centers, and blinding subjects and investigators to the intervention is impossible. Finally, the sobering results of a multicenter RCT that demonstrated a *greater* mortality rate for non-COPD patients who experienced extubation failure and were randomized to NPPV (vs usual care) emphasize the importance of close observation and rapid reintubation for a patient who is not responding to NPPV.

Monitoring During MV

Airway pressures, volumes, flow, and other variables can be monitored during ventilation. Monitoring incorporates continuous measurement of key parameters, display of numerical and graphic data to enhance visual inspection, establishment of thresholds that define acceptable limits for key parameters, and use of visual and audible alarms that alert clinicians of breaches in established thresholds. Key safety measurements include low ventilation or low pressure alarms that might indicate ventilator disconnection or loss of airway, apnea alarms, and high airway pressure alarms. Elevation of PIP is important to detect and should prompt investigation of potential causes. The following equation provides clues as to reasons for elevated PIP:

PIP = flow × resistance + plateau pressure (Pplat)

where Pplat = VT/compliance + PEEP. Thus, PIP elevation might be caused by increased airway resistance, in which case the Pplat would be unchanged. Common causes of increased airway resistance include bronchospasm and ET tube narrowing by secretions or a patient's biting of the tube. Elevation of both PIP and Pplat is typically produced by parenchymal lung disease (pulmonary edema, pneumonia, auto-PEEP); pleural disease (pneumothorax); chest wall abnormality (obesity); or increased abdominal pressure (ascites, pregnancy).

Close examination of graphic display of airway pressure, flow, and volume vs time can provide important clues as to patient-ventilator asynchrony, the likelihood that auto-PEEP is present, and the mode and settings of positive-pressure ventilation. Some of the recognized forms of patient—ventilator asynchrony include ineffective triggering, double triggering, auto triggering, and flow asynchrony. Ineffective triggering is considerably more common than the others, with double triggering second in frequency in prospective studies. An example of ineffective triggering is displayed in Figure 2, with the arrow corresponding to the event. Ineffective triggering occurs when an inspiratory effort by the patient does not create change in airway pressure or flow of sufficient magnitude to initiate a positive pressure breath. The characteristic findings seen on the graphic display include a transient peak in flow and concomitant dip in airway pressure (that is the result of the patient's inspiratory effort) that does not result in a triggered positive pressure breath. The most common cause of ineffective triggering is auto-PEEP, often in the

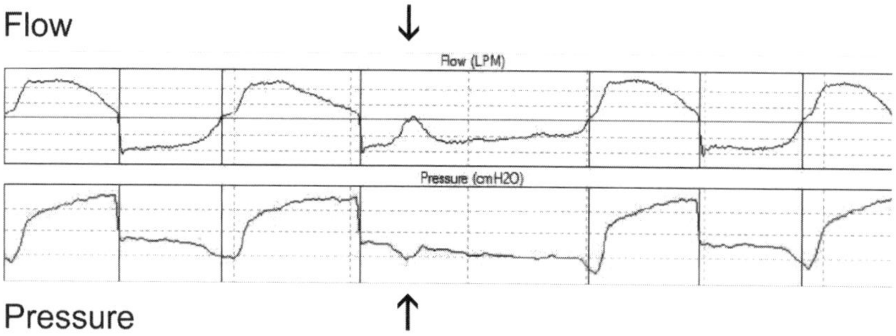

Figure 2. Ineffective triggering patient-ventilator dyssynchrony. Graphic display of flow and pressure over time demonstrates two conventional breaths followed by an ineffective trigger in which patient inspiratory effort (arrows) does not trigger a breath.

setting of COPD. Worsening airflow obstruction, tachypnea, high trigger sensitivity, and excessive PS can exacerbate auto-PEEP. Double-triggering is identified by the presence of two positive pressure breaths separated by a very brief expiratory phase (less than one half of the preceding T_I; Fig 3). Often the patient's ventilatory demand is high, and the set ventilator time is too brief, leading to a decrease in airway pressure early in exhalation that triggers an immediate second positive pressure breath.

Complications of Positive-Pressure Ventilation

Complications of MV and artificial airways are important issues to address proactively to prevent, recognize in a timely fashion, and manage appropriately. Some of the more common complications are listed in Table 3. Several complications require additional discussion.

Pulmonary Barotrauma

Air leaks typically develop from rupture of alveoli, particularly alveoli that abut fixed structures such as bronchi and vessels. With continued leaking, such as with positive-pressure ventilation, air then tracks in a path of least resistance, often along the bronchovascular bundles toward the hila of the lung, rupturing into mediastinum, and then through the thoracic inlet to produce subcutaneous emphysema. Eventually, air ruptures into the pleural space, producing a pneumothorax. It is important to recognize lesser forms of barotrauma, such as subcutaneous emphysema or pneumomediastinum, so that adjustments can be made to reduce ventilatory pressures and halt the progression.

Dynamic Hyperinflation and Auto-PEEP

Avoidance of overinflation of the lung relies on delivery of appropriately sized tidal breaths delivered with appropriate transpulmonary pressure plus allowance of full exhalation before initiating the next breath. Failure to adhere to these concepts increases the likelihood of developing dynamic hyperinflation from overinflation and presence of auto-PEEP (also called intrinsic PEEP or occult PEEP) from failure to fully deflate (*ie*, "stacking" breaths). Both are potentially dangerous conditions that might contribute to respiratory compromise

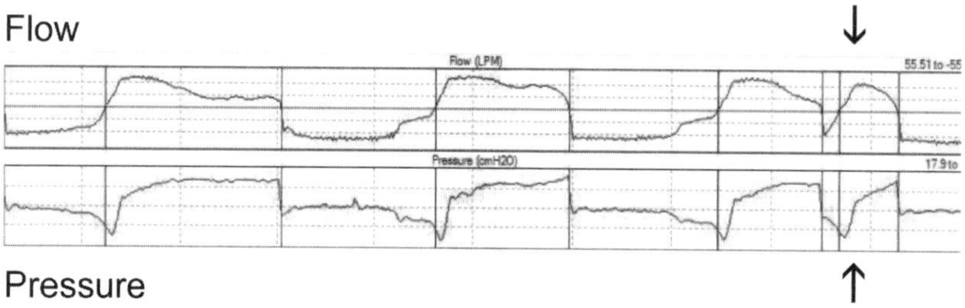

Figure 3. Double-triggering patient-ventilator dyssynchrony. Graphic display of flow and pressure over time demonstrates three conventional breaths followed by a double-triggered breath (arrows). See text for definition.

Table 3. *Complications of MV and Artificial Airways*

Oxygen toxicity
Pulmonary barotrauma: air leak
Pneumothorax
Pneumomediastinum/pneumopericardium/subcutaneous emphysema
Pulmonary interstitial emphysema and air cysts
Systemic air embolism
Dynamic hyperinflation and auto-PEEP or intrinsic PEEP
Hemodynamic compromise
Alveolar overdistention
Altered diaphragm/chest wall position and function, impairing ventilation
VALI
Volutrauma
Atelectrauma
Biotrauma
Multiple organ dysfunction
Ventilator-associated pneumonia
Tracheomalacia
Trauma and dysfunction of vocal cords
Trauma to lip, teeth, oral cavity, nose, pharynx
Unplanned extubation
Endotracheal tube malposition
Bronchial intubation
Esophageal intubation
Tracheostomy bleeding, stoma problems, decannulation
GI bleeding from stress ulceration/gastritis

and hemodynamic compromise. Hyperinflation can overdistend alveoli, increasing the likelihood of rupture as well as compressing the alveolar capillaries, thus converting functional alveoli to dead space. Additionally, hyperinflation can place the diaphragm in a flattened, mechanically disadvantaged position that contributes to smaller VT, which in turn promotes tachypnea, thus exacerbating air trapping by further reducing exhalation time. Auto-PEEP is also a common cause of ineffective triggering patient-ventilator asynchrony because the patient must overcome the auto-PEEP with decrease in intrathoracic pressure of sufficient magnitude to be sensed by the ventilator. When extreme, hypotension can progress to frank shock and even to cardiopulmonary arrest, typically with pulseless electrical activity. Mechanisms include reduced venous return, plus a component of altered right and left heart chamber filling, and increased right ventricular afterload from the increased intrathoracic pressure.

A common scenario is the patient with airflow obstruction who is tachypneic in the setting of positive-pressure ventilation, thus causing insufficient exhalation time and progressive hyperinflation and auto-PEEP. Another situation is the use of very short exhalation time (*ie*, < 1s), such as with APRV, in which even mild bronchospasm or respiratory secretion retention can impair exhalation, producing incomplete emptying. Unexpected auto-PEEP can occur in patients without obvious risk factors. Finally, manual ventilation with an Ambu bag is often performed too rapidly and with uncontrolled VTs, thus causing transient hyperinflation. A manual rate of 12 breaths/min is generally recommended.

The development of serious hyperinflation can be subtle and can be recognized by wheezing exhalation persisting up to the next positive pressure breath, respiratory efforts (chest movement) without ventilator triggering, characteristic findings of ineffective trigger on ventilator graphics, hyperinflation on chest radiograph, or a decrease in the VT if the patient is receiving positive-pressure ventilation in a pressure-targeted mode. Auto-PEEP is not directly measured during conventional ventilation, thus the designation *occult PEEP*. One can temporarily occlude the exhalation port by pressing a button on most modern ventilators, creating a no-flow state that allows equilibration of the pressure in the ventilator tubing (where the pressure is sensed) with the pressure deep within the lung. Total PEEP is measured, and one subtracts the extrinsic (or set) PEEP, yielding an estimation of auto-PEEP.

Often the presentation is more dramatic with hypotension and decreasing oxygen saturation. Life-threatening hyperinflation can be immediately treated by disconnecting the ET or tracheostomy tube from the ventilator, thus allowing passive exhalation—that may take ≥ 15 s—and prevent delivery of additional breaths. This exhalation is often followed by rapid and dramatic improvements in BP and oxygenation. More definitive treatment includes bronchodilators, sedation to reduce spontaneous respirations, and ventilator adjustment to increase expiratory time (reduce respiratory rate, lower VT, and perhaps increase inspiratory flow rate). If the patient is breathing spontaneously and has auto-PEEP-induced ineffective trigger breaths, extrinsic PEEP can be increased to a level several cm H_2O less than measured auto-PEEP to reduce the magnitude of pressure decrease the patient must generate to trigger a breath. The magnitude of inspiratory effort by the patient can be measured by the use of an esophageal balloon that displays changes in pleural pressure during these efforts.

Ventilator-Associated Lung Injury

There is considerable experimental evidence from animal models and accumulating evidence from patients that MV can be injurious, producing alveolar trauma and a systemic inflammatory response. It is hypothesized that excessive alveolar volume coupled with increased transalveolar pressure results in shearing forces that disrupt the fragile alveolar architecture. These deleterious effects are thought to be the worst when there is local inhomogeneity of ventilation. This has been called *volutrauma* because experiments in animal models identify alveolar distention, rather than the distending pressure per se, as the most important parameter. Additionally, the cyclical inflation and deflation of alveoli produces damage and inflammation, or so-called *atelectrauma*. The subsequent mechanical damage to lung tissue activates inflammatory mediators that act as a pulmonary source for multiple-organ failure in patients with acute lung injury (ALI) or ARDS and, to a lesser extent, in patients who do not satisfy criteria for ALI/ARDS. Figure 4 is an illustrated depiction of the major pathophysiologic and altered gas exchange events documented in ALI, with superimposed similar effects of MV on the lung that are derived from animal model research and human studies. The similarities are striking. Initially shown in animal models, but more recently in patients with ALI, the application of low VTs, *ie*, 6 mL/kg of predicted body weight in humans, is associated with reduced inflammation, less lung injury, shorter duration of MV, and improved survival. Further, many studies demonstrate that the application of PEEP at a level above the LIP prevents the cyclic alveolar collapse and reduced lung injury and inflammation.

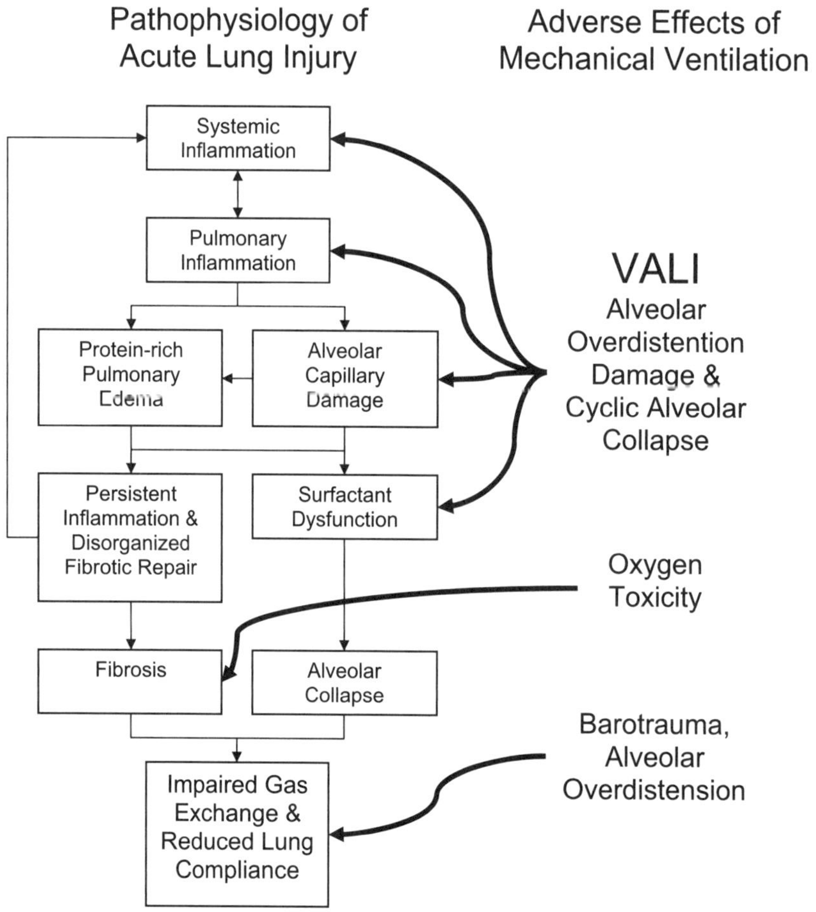

Figure 4. Hypothetical depiction of the pathophysiology of ALI and adverse effects of MV as related to components of lung injury.

Patient-Focused MV

The goals of MV include improving hypoxemia and hypercapnia, relief of suffering and distress such as dyspnea, providing respiratory support during circumstances in which the patient experiences an impaired drive to breathe (*ie*, general anesthesia), and applying evidence-based strategies to promote survival and timely recovery. Lung-protective strategies and permissive hypercapnia supersede goals of normalization of gas exchange. One can conceptualize stages of respiratory failure and MV support as stabilization, maintenance, and recovery.

Initiating MV

MV may be required when there is a failure of oxygenation or ventilation. Life-threatening respiratory distress or cardiopulmonary arrest requires immediate attention and emergent ET intubation, followed by initiation of MV. NPPV should be considered for many patients with progressive respiratory insufficiency, particularly those with respiratory failure as the result of COPD exacerbation or cardiogenic pulmonary edema who have suitably alert mental status and hemodynamic stability. Caveats regarding patient selection and early monitoring and management for the response to NPPV are discussed.

A strategy for providing full ventilatory support that will provide adequate ventilation and oxygenation is usually sufficient. However, some patients with respiratory failure have ARDS or have significant airflow obstruction from an exacerbation of asthma or COPD, conditions that require specific ventilatory strategies that differ substantially based on difference in pulmonary physiology. Ventilatory strategies for severe airflow obstruction and for ALI/ARDS are compared in Table 4.

MV During Airflow Obstruction

Status asthmaticus as well as acute exacerbation of COPD is associated with marked limitation of expiratory airflow. Such a state increases the likelihood of developing dynamic hyperinflation (increased end-inspiratory pressure and volume) and auto-PEEP (increased lung volume and intrathoracic pressure at the end of exhalation) as discussed previously. Additionally, such hyperinflation increases the likelihood of developing barotrauma. Ventilatory management includes adjusting the ventilator to prevent development of dynamic hyperinflation and auto-PEEP in addition to the early recognition and timely management of worsening of airflow obstruction. Key tenets of management include providing sufficient sedation (and possibly neuromuscular blockade) to control tachypnea, reducing the set respiratory rate (*ie*, *f*) to provide an expiratory phase of sufficient duration to allow near-complete emptying, and using small V_T. Of note, reducing the respiratory rate from 20 breaths/min to 10 breaths/min will more than double the expiratory time. Examination of the flow vs time graphics and examining the patient's chest for continued wheezing as one progressively increases the expiratory time can help identify when flow is near completion. Minute ventilation decreases significantly with these measures and development of hypercapnia is commonplace. Interestingly, because reductions in V_T and f can reduce the severity of alveolar hyperinflation and dead space ventilation, the increase in P_{CO_2} can be blunted as the number of perfused alveoli increases. Many clinicians have become comfortable with permissive hypercapnia with a pH in the 7.2 to 7.1 range, although a safe lower limit is not well defined. Follow-up of patients who were allowed to remain hypercapnic showed no long-term deleterious effects. Permissive hypercapnia is contraindicated in patients with intracranial hypertension (in whom hypercapnia could induce cerebral vasodilation and worsen the intracranial pressure) and in patients with an irritable myocardium (in whom hypercapnia may induce cardiac arrhythmias). Some clinicians administer IV bicarbonate in an attempt to maintain a pH >7.2 or so, but others do not. If a pressure-targeted mode is used, care must be taken to monitor V_T, for as the airflow obstruction improves, V_T is likely to increase significantly.

MV for ALI/ARDs

Considerable experimental evidence from various animal models has demonstrated that larger V_Ts and higher plateau or transpulmonary pressures are associated with ALI. CT examination of

Table 4. *Comparison of Ventilatory Strategies for Severe Airflow Obstruction and for ALI/ARDS Using ARDSNet Guidelines or Alternative Strategies Supported by Results of RCTs*

Variables	Severe Airflow Obstruction	ALI/ARDS: ARDSNet Strategy	ALI/ARDS: Alternative Strategy
F_{IO_2}	To achieve Sp_{O_2} of 88–93% or Pa_{O_2} of 55–80 mm Hg	To achieve Sp_{O_2} of 88–93% or Pa_{O_2} of 55–80 mm Hg*	To achieve Sp_{O_2} of 88–93% or Pa_{O_2} of 55–80 mm Hg
Mode of ventilation	Varies	AC mode	AC mode
Pressure or volume	Either	Volume	Pressure
Target VT	< 8 mL/kg PBW†	6 mL/kg PBW	6 mL/kg PBW
Total rate, breaths/min	Low (10–12)	25 (to 35 if needed)	25 (to 35 if needed)
I/E target	1:5	1:2–1:1	1:3–1:1
PEEP	Minimal‡	Modest; use PEEP-F_{IO_2}*	More aggressive; use PEEP-F_{IO_2}*
Target Pplat	< 30 cm H_2O	< 30 cm H_2O	< 40 cm H_2O
Recruitment maneuvers	No	No	Yes, after ventilator disconnection
Sedation/NMB	Yes, sufficient to prevent tachypnea; avoid NMB if possible	Yes	Yes (less sedation if bilevel mode is used)
Permissive hypercapnia	Ok; P_{CO_2} may be very high	Ok; pH ≥ 7.3	Ok; pH ≥ 7.3

*See Table 5.
†Male PBW (in kilograms) = 50 + 2.3 × (height in inches − 60); Female PBW (in kilograms) = 45.5 + 2.3 × (height in inches − 60).
‡Consider adding PEEP if significant auto-PEEP is present or there is WOB from ineffective triggering dyssynchrony. PEEP should be set to about 2 cm H_2O less than auto-PEEP.

the lungs of patients with ARDS reveals a small volume of normal or atelectatic lung, supporting the notion of "baby"-sized lungs in ARDS. Some earlier RCTs demonstrated improved outcomes in ARDS when patients were ventilated with lower VTs (and other ventilatory adjustments) compared with conventional volumes, but in some trials, no difference was found.

In 2000, publication of the result of the ARDS Network pivotal RCT that documented significantly lower rates of mortality among patients who received VT of 6 mL/kg predicted body weight compared with those who received 12 mL/kg has set the standard for MV for ALI/ARDS. There were also more ventilator-free and organ failure-free days but no difference in the frequency of barotrauma nor in oxygenation. The key components of the National Heart, Lung and Blood Institute ARDS Clinical Network (ARDSNet) approach to ventilating patients with ALI/ARDS are summarized in Table 4. The ARDSNet approach to MV for ARDS has been widely endorsed as an evidence-based cornerstone of management of critically ill patients. However, several groups of investigators, including ARDSNet investigators, have demonstrated in subsequent real-life studies years after publication of ARDSNet results that clinicians are not using low VTs. In one study in which three centers were examined, only 16% of patients had VT < 8 mL/kg predicted body weight (PBW), and virtually none were ≤ 6 mL/kg. Barriers to adoption include lack of willingness to relinquish ventilator control, recognition of ARDS, and concerns for contraindications, discomfort, and impaired gas exchange. Improved compliance with low VT ventilation was strongly associated with use of a written protocol in a one study.

On the basis of an earlier study by Amato and coworkers, more recent smaller studies by Ranieri et al and Villar et al, as well as other evidence, investigators have addressed some of the finer points of MV for ARDS/ALI, including the use of greater PEEP, use of a pressure-targeted rather than a volume-targeted mode, and the addition of recruitment maneuvers. There are now three large-scale (> 500 subjects in each) RCTs that address using a greater PEEP level—stratified by oxygenation—compared directly with the original ARDSNet study parameters and PEEP levels. In all studies, PEEP average approximately 8 to 10 cm H_2O in traditional ARDSNet ventilation and 10 to 16 cm H_2O with the greater PEEP strategy. All groups received VTs of 6 mL/kg PBW. In the Assessment of Low Tidal Volume and Increased End-Expiratory Volume to

Obviate Lung Injury trial, Brower and the ARDSNet investigators demonstrated better oxygenation but no difference in rate of mortality, ventilator-free days, or barotrauma.

In 2008, Meade and colleagues compared pressure-targeted ventilation with allowable Pplat up to 40 cm H_2O, greater PEEP, and recruitment maneuvers to ARDSNet ventilation. The experimental approach resulted in better oxygenation, including less mortality caused by refractory hypoxemia, and less frequent use of rescue therapy but no difference in rate of mortality, duration of MV, or incidence of barotrauma. Also, in 2008, Mercat and coworkers compared an "increased recruitment" strategy with sufficient PEEP applied to increase Pplat to 28 to 30 cm H_2O vs ARDSNet ventilation. The increased recruitment group had better oxygenation, fewer cases of refractory hypoxemia, less need for rescue therapy, and more organ failure-free and ventilator-free days. No difference in barotrauma or rate of mortality was noted, although there was a trend ($p=0.06$) for lower mortality with more severe hypoxemia. The approach used by Mercat et al probably caused alveolar overdistention in patients with milder lung injury and lower levels of PEEP and should probably be avoided in this subgroup.

We conclude that greater PEEP levels, such as guided by PEEP-FIO_2 in Table 5, should be considered, particularly if more severe hypoxemia is present. Recent work suggests that esophageal pressure monitoring can help individualize setting PEEP that improves gas exchange. Evidence for use of recruitment maneuvers is less compelling, with only transient improvement in oxygenation and potential for transient hemodynamic compromise in one large RCT. Use of a recruitment maneuver (typically 40 cm H_2O inflation held for 40 s) seems most likely to help when performed after ventilator disconnection and loss of alveolar distention.

Adjunctive and Alternative Therapy for Refractory Hypoxemia and ARDS

As many as one third of patients with ARDS receive adjunctive therapy, such as inhaled nitric oxide and prone positioning for refractory hypoxemia. Additionally, novel ventilatory approaches, including high-frequency oscillatory ventilation (HFOV), may be considered. Inhaled nitric oxide (INO) is a vasodilator that, when administered in very small doses (1 to 20 ppm) by inhalation, can increase perfusion to aerated alveoli without causing systemic vasodilatation. As a result about three fourths of ARDS patients will experience a >10% increase in PaO_2. Although INO can occasionally have dramatic effects in selected cases, its effects are often relative short-lived (48 h), and large RCTs have failed to show benefits in rates of mortality or duration of MV.

Prone positioning is accomplished by transferring the mechanically ventilated patient for supine to prone position where they remain for 8 to12 h or longer. Prone positioning promotes a more-even distribution of ventilation relative to perfusion, removes the weight of the heart from compressing lung tissue, and aids in respiratory secretion clearance. Oxygenation is improved in approximately three fourths of ARDS patients, but PaO_2 reverts to near-baseline values when patients resume the supine position. Outcomes studies demonstrate no benefit in rate of mortality or duration of MV, and the use of greater doses of sedation and neuromuscular blockade, risk for tube or catheter dislodgment, and potential for pressure sores must be considered. HFOV has been investigated as the ultimate form of lung-protective ventilation because very small VTs are delivered 180 to 300 times/min. In contrast to high-frequency jet ventilation, HFOV ventilation is delivered with active inspiration and active exhalation. Its management can be complex and subjective. Troubleshooting of patient deterioration is more complex than with conventional ventilation, as is ventilator adjustment. HFOV can lead to impressive improvement in gas exchange in selected cases, but although HFOV has been demonstrated in a multicenter RCT to be equivalent to convention ventilation for ARDS, it has not been compared with low VT ventilation. More research is needed to confirm its role.

Weaning and Liberation From Ventilation

Weaning and Liberation: Evolving Concepts

Traditionally, separation of the patient from MV has primarily been a process of progressively reducing the proportion of ventilation that is supported artificially, *ie*, *weaning* from the

Table 5. *PEEP-F_{IO_2} Values for Table 4**

	F_{IO_2}											
Variables	0.3	0.4	0.4	0.5	0.5	0.6	0.7	0.7	0.8	0.9	1.0	1.0
ARDSNet protocol												
PEEP, cm H_2O	5	5	8	8	10	10	10	14	14	14	18	24
Alternative approach†												
PEEP, cm H_2O	5–10		10–18		18–20	20		20	20–22	22		

*PEEP is increased in increments of 2 cm H_2O; F_{IO_2} increased by 0.1.
†From Meade et al. JAMA 2008; 299:637–645.

ventilation, while increasing the WOB that the patient undertakes until it is judged that the patient is capable of breathing independently, at which time the ET tube is removed. Different approaches were used, most commonly progressive reducing in PS in the PSV mode, decreasing the mandatory breath rate in SIMV mode, or increasing the duration of spontaneous breathing trials in AC.

As a result of clinical trial results, clinicians now focus on identifying the patient who, as judged by successfully passing a number of conditions, has a high likelihood of breathing independently off the ventilator and tolerating removal of the ET tube, without the process of progressively reducing support. Historically, measures of respiratory muscle strength, endurance, and gas exchange such as negative inspiratory force, vital capacity, minute ventilation, maximum voluntary ventilation, respiratory rate, or f/V_T, were relied on. Effective programs to liberate the patient from MV incorporate evidence-based structured techniques, thus improving frequency and consistency of measurements and actions, are multidisciplinary and team based, incorporate criteria to proceed to the next step (thus eliminating unnecessary delays), integrate clinical judgment, and have been demonstrated to improve outcomes. The concepts and criteria are based on the pathophysiology of respiratory failure and also recognize the importance of nonpulmonary organ dysfunction in readiness to proceed.

Protocol Based Liberation from MV

In 1996, Ely and colleagues developed a multistep protocol to identify resolution of respiratory failure and in a RCT demonstrated faster weaning, shorter duration of ventilation, and fewer complications (unplanned extubation, prolonged ventilation, reintubation, and tracheostomy). This protocol incorporated daily screening of all mechanically ventilated patients by respiratory therapists for hemodynamic stability, cessation of sedative infusions, adequate oxygenation, low PEEP level, adequate cough, and adequate respiratory muscle strength as judged by $f/V_T \leq 105$ while breathing without support. Patients who successfully passed this screening protocol underwent a 2-h spontaneous breathing trial (SBT) with 5 cm H_2O CPAP or T tube. Those who passed were deemed likely (85% likelihood) to be successfully extubated. This protocol has served as a basic template for many weaning protocols (specific criteria) and structured approaches (daily performance by respiratory therapists and nurses). Most, but not all, published reports of such protocols have demonstrated shorter duration of ventilation, shorter ICU length of stay (LOS), cost savings, and/or other benefits. It is worth noting, however, that strict adherence to overly conservative criteria can actually delay weaning and/or extubation.

Evidence-Based Consensus Recommendations: In December 2001, a collective task force composed of representatives from the American College of Chest Physicians, American Association for Respiratory Care, and Society of Critical Care Medicine published evidence-based guidelines for weaning and discontinuation of MVS. Table 6 summarizes key recommendations regarding all aspects of the process. They offer specific recommendations for assessment of discontinuation potential (*ie*, screening) as follows: (1) evidence for some reversal of the underlying cause for respiratory failure; (2) adequate oxygenation ($Pa_{O_2}/F_{IO_2} \geq 150$ to 200, PEEP ≤ 5 to 8 cm H_2O, $F_{IO_2} \leq 0.4$ to 0.5), and pH ≥ 7.25;

Table 6. *Components of Protocols for Discontinuation of Ventilation*

Parameters	Measures
Medical stability	Presence of shock, use of vasopressors, pH
Mental status	Use of continuous sedative infusion, sedation scale criteria
Oxygenation	F_{IO_2}, PEEP, Pa_{O_2}/F_{IO_2} ratio
Lung mechanics	f/V_T, pH
Ventilatory endurance	SBT
Secretion clearance	Cough strength, sputum volume/ suction frequency
Airway patency	Cuff-leak test
Miscellaneous factors	Condition improving?

(3) hemodynamic stability (no active myocardial ischemia or clinically significant hypotension); and (4) capability to initiate an inspiratory effort. These recommendations serve as a solid basis for current recommendations; however, newer data allow us to readdress these and other parameters.

Components of Protocols to Assess Discontinuation of Ventilation

There are many factors that can influence the success a patient has for tolerating withdrawal of ventilatory support and removal of the ET tube. Some of the parameters and criteria that can affect this process are listed in Table 6, and several deserve additional comment. There is considerable evidence that mental status is an important determinant of timely recovery from MV because overly sedated patients may have an impaired drive to breathe and an inability to protect the airway once the ET tube is removed. Level of conscious is assessed in protocols indirectly by the use of continuous infusion of sedatives or directly with the use of a sedation scale.

Shorter duration of MV has been demonstrated in numerous prospective studies that use strategies to reduce oversedation, including daily interruption of sedation, intermittent (rather than continuous) sedative and opioid administration, and matching patient characteristics to drugs. In one study, the combination of a daily awakening trial plus a SBT was superior to SBT alone. The combination of poor cough, high sputum volume, and poor mental status is a particularly worrisome combination, even if the patient is capable of passing an SBT. In one study, 80% of patients who met this combination of findings were reintubated. Adequacy of oxygenation after extubation is important to predict. However, some protocol criteria may inadvertently delay extubation if the criteria are too restrictive. For example, some protocols require $F_{IO_2} \leq 0.4$, PEEP ≤ 5 cm H_2O, and/or $Pa_{O_2}/F_{IO_2} \geq 200$, yet many patients who have P_{O_2} = 95 mm Hg on F_{IO_2} of 0.5 will have adequate oxygenation postextubation. In fact, oxygenation criteria ($Pa_{O_2}/F_{IO_2} > 180$ mm Hg) was the most common weaning criterion never passed in a large cohort of patients who were successfully extubated. In 1991, Yang and Tobin found f/V_T to be a reliable measure of lung mechanics and good predictor of successful discontinuation. However, some patients, particularly smaller individuals and those with parenchymal lung disease, may have a more rapid, shallow pattern of breathing. As noted previously, investigators have demonstrated that incorporating $f/V_T < 105$ as a screening criterion delayed weaning. Some protocols use greater thresholds (*ie*, <125) or omit f/V_T from their protocol.

SBT: The SBT is widely considered to be the pivotal test, incorporating the assessment of lung mechanics and endurance. The patient is placed on low-level ventilatory support intended to overcome the added WOB of breathing through the ET tube, or without any support for a period of 30 to 120 min and observed for deterioration in vital signs or ventilatory failure. This is however, considerable variability in several parameters with different criteria for the mode and settings of ventilatory support, duration of SBT, and termination (failure) criteria. Although T tube, "flow-by," CPAP, or PSV is often used as low-level ventilatory support, automatic tube compensation (ATC) is emerging as a form of "smart" PSV. ATC is designed to provide enough PS to overcome the resistance of breathing through an artificial airway. This pressure is recalculated every 5 ms and is based on the tube size and type (ET vs tracheostomy) plus instantaneous flow measurement. Thus, greater pressure is provided if the tube has a smaller diameter or if flow is faster. In one study, ATC was superior to CPAP for overall success (SBT completed and extubation for >48 h).

Airway Patency and Postextubation Stridor: Although clinicians have long recognized the importance of postextubation stridor in extubation failure, recent research has helped clarify the importance and validated tools for assessment. Postextubation stridor is observed in 5 to 30% of patients, depending on the patient population. Those who develop stridor tend to be sicker, have longer duration intubation, and are more likely to have had a difficult intubation and/or self-extubation. By deflating the ET tube cuff and detecting airflow around the tube (either by measurement using comparison of volume exhaled through the tube before and after cuff deflation, or simply hearing a leak), one increases the ability to predict postextubation stridor. "Cuff leak" > 18% was identified as being a good predictor (85% sensitive, 72% specific) of postextubation stridor in one study, although thresholds of > 15 to 25% have been identified by others. Administration of methylprednisolone (MP) (40 mg q6h × 4 doses) to patients with poor cuff-leak (< 24%) was effective in reducing likelihood of postextubation stridor (6% vs 30% with no MP) in one study. In another study, giving MP at a dose of 20 mg q4h × 4 doses before extubation was effective in reducing postextubation stridor for unselected patients.

Recommendations for Weaning and Liberation

All endotracheally intubated mechanically ventilated patients should undergo daily evaluation to determine their potential for discontinuation of ventilation. This should be a structured, evidence-based protocol that incorporates key components in a multidisciplinary team-based approach that promotes efficiency. Interestingly, computerized weaning that is integrated within mechanical ventilators is being explored as a means of standardizing and streamlining the process, with shorter duration of MV and shorter ICU LOS demonstrated in one study. The author's recommendations for specific components and caveats related to these parameters are listed in Table 7. It is worth acknowledging that knowledge regarding weaning and extubation continuous to evolve, that some recommendations are based on opinion and lower-level evidence, and that clinical skills play an important and complementary role. An important component of the weaning process is to recognize that the patient who fails this evaluation repeatedly and/or who fails extubation should undergo evaluation for possible causes of failure, such as those listed in Table 8. Finally it is worth considering extubation followed by immediate institution of NPPV for the patient with COPD who has failed SBT. In a small RCT, NPPV was superior to conventional management for patients who failed three SBTs, in regards to duration of MV, ICU LOS, and hospital LOS. However, one must carefully consider reasons for SBT failure and troubleshoot potential causes before using this approach.

Tracheostomy

Tracheostomy has been available for many years as a surgically placed artificial airway that permits longer-term placement compared with an ET tube. Tracheostomy is considered to be more stable, more comfortable, and is associated with lower doses of sedative and opioid medications. Bedside percutaneous dilatational tracheostomy (PDT) is achieving widespread acceptance as an alternative to traditional approaches in which an open surgical technique is performed in the operating room. Meta-analyses of prospective studies indicate that PDT is associated with less infection, scarring, and expense, with a trend for fewer complications but greater rates of obstruction/decannulation. The optimal timing of tracheostomy remains unsettled, although a small meta-analysis indicated shorter duration of MV and shorter ICU LOS with "early" tracheostomy. Some experts favor early tracheostomy for patients with Acute Physiology and Chronic Health Evaluation *II* > 25 or combination of impaired mental status and poor oxygenation because these groups tend to have long courses of respiratory failure. Discontinuation of MV in the patient with a tracheostomy is generally by traditional weaning. This is typically accomplished by progressively increasing the duration of periods without ventilatory support, often using oxygen delivered directly via the tracheostomy tube, and omitting the ventilator circuit.

Summary and Conclusions

MV is a life-saving modality for treating respiratory failure and to providing gas exchange support. There are many subtleties in effective management that include adopting a patient-focused approach, using evidence-based strategies for MV as well as for discontinuation of ventilation, and avoiding complications related to MV and the artificial airway.

Table 7. *Recommendations for Evaluation of the Ability To Tolerate Discontinuation of Ventilation and Extubation**

Screening Criteria
1. Is patient hemodynamically stable (not in shock, no more than minimal vasopressor requirement)?
2. Is underlying cause of respiratory failure improving?
3. Is the patient alert or have easy arousal (opens eyes to voice) and cognition (follows simple commands)? Perform daily interruption of sedation in patients in whom this is feasible.
4. Is cough strength moderate or better and suctioning frequency no more than every 2 h?
5. Is Pa_{O_2}/F_{IO_2} ratio > 150 and PEEP < 8 cm H_2O?
6. Is f/V_T ratio < 125? Consider eliminating f/V_T ratio

Cuff-leak test
1. Is air movement around ET tube with cuff deflated > 15%? If cuff leak is < 25%, consider administering MP (see text)

SBT
1. Does patient tolerate breathing on minimal support for 60 min? Consider using ATC as mode of ventilatory support during SBT, if available

*All intubated patients receiving MV should undergo screening. Those who satisfy the criteria but fail mental status testing (screening criterion 3) should have sedation interrupted (*ie*, discontinue all IV sedative and opioid drugs) and repeat testing for screening criteria. Patients who satisfy the screening criteria should undergo a cuff-leak test. If the cuff leak is < 15%, MP should be administered (four doses of 40 mg IV every 6 h or 20 mg IV every 4 h). Patients who satisfy the screening criteria and who pass the cuff leak test should undergo SBT testing; if patients pass the SBT, they should be extubated.

Table 8. *Modifiable Factors Related to Failure of Weaning From MV*

Unresolved precipitating process
Reversible airflow obstruction
Increased endotracheal tube resistance
Excessive respiratory secretions
Impaired mental status
Respiratory depressant medications
Excessive sedative and opioid medications
Metabolic alkalosis
Electrolyte imbalance
Hemodynamic instability
Ischemic heart disease
Infection and sepsis
Malnutrition
Overfeeding
Neuromuscular disorders
Psychological factors

Annotated Bibliography

Acute Respiratory Distress Syndrome Network. Ventilation with lower tidal volumes as compared with traditional tidal volumes for acute lung injury and the acute respiratory distress syndrome. N Engl J Med 2000; 342:1301–1308

Large, multicenter, randomized sentinel trial with 861 patients showed that patients receiving MV with low V_T (6.2 mL/kg ideal weight, Pplat ≤ 30 cm H_2O) had significantly lower rates of mortality ($p = 0.007$) than patients receiving MV with conventional V_T (12 mL/kg, Pplat ≤ 30cm H_2O) as well as fewer days receiving MV.

Acute Respiratory Distress Syndrome Network. Higher versus lower positive end-expiratory pressures in patients with the ARDS. N Engl J Med 2004; 351:327–336

Greater PEEP levels improved oxygenation but did not improve survival in this controlled, multi-institutional, randomized trial.

Adhikari NK, Burns KE, Friedrich JO, et al. Effect of nitric oxide on oxygenation and mortality in acute lung injury: systematic review and meta-analysis. BMJ 2007; 334:779

Meta-analysis: no mortality benefit, better oxygenation, but more renal failure with INO.

Amato MBP, Barbas CSV, Medeiros DM, et al. Beneficial effects of the "open lung approach" with low distending pressures in ARDS. Am J Respir Crit Care Med 1995; 152:1835–1844

A controlled trial that suggests that maintaining alveolar patency while avoiding alveolar overdistention results in improved outcome for patients with ARDS. This was an impetus to the ARDS Network trial of low V_T ventilation.

Brochard L, Rauss A, Benito S, et al. Comparison of three methods of gradual withdrawal from ventilatory support during weaning from mechanical ventilation. Am J Respir Crit Care Med 1994; 150:896–903

This study concludes that SIMV is not a preferred weaning mode.
Brower RG, Morris A, MacIntyre N, et al. Effects of recruitment maneuvers in patients with acute lung injury and acute respiratory distress syndrome ventilated with high positive end-expiratory pressure. Crit Care Med 2003; 31:2592–2597
As studied, recruitment maneuvers did not accomplish much in this ARDSNet substudy.
Cheng KC, Hou CC, Huang HC, et al. Intravenous injection of methylprednisolone reduces the incidence of postextubation stridor in intensive care unit patients. Crit Care Med 2006; 34:1345–1350
Four doses of MP, 40 mg q6h, significantly reduced postextubation stridor.
Cohen JD, Shapiro M, Grozovski E, et al. Extubation outcome following a spontaneous breathing trial with automatic tube compensation versus continuous positive airway pressure. Crit Care Med 2006; 34:682–686
Automatic tube compensation ("smart" PSV) during SBT was better than CPAP for overall weaning success.
Dellinger RP, Zimmerman JL, Taylor RW, et al. Effects of inhaled nitric oxide in patients with acute respiratory distress syndrome: results of a randomized phase II trial. Inhaled Nitric Oxide in ARDS Study Group. Crit Care Med 1998; 26:15–23
Multicenter RCT: better oxygenation, not much else, with INO.
Derdak S, Mehta S, Stewart TE, et al. High-frequency oscillatory ventilation for acute respiratory distress syndrome in adults: a randomized, controlled trial. Am J Respir Crit Care Med 2002; 166:801–808
HFOV was equivalent to conventional but greater VT ventilation for ARDS. This study needs repeating with a low VT strategy.
Ely EW, Baker AM, Dunagan DP, et al. Effect on the duration of mechanical ventilation of identifying patients capable of breathing spontaneously. N Engl J Med 1996; 335:1864–1869
Classic RCT demonstrating benefit of identifying when patients are ready to be liberated from the ventilator.
Esteban A, Frutos F, Tobin MJ, et al. A comparison of four methods of weaning patients from mechanical ventilation: Spanish Lung Failure Collaborative Group. N Engl J Med 1995; 332:345–350
SIMV is not a preferred weaning mode.
Esteban A, Frutos-Vivar F, Ferguson ND, et al. Noninvasive positive-pressure ventilation for respiratory failure after extubation. N Engl J Med 2004; 350:2452–246
RCT demonstrated a greater rate of mortality with NPPV after extubation failure. Patients with COPD were excluded.
Ferrer M, Esquinas A, Leon M, et al. Noninvasive ventilation in severe hypoxemic respiratory failure: a randomized clinical trial. Am Rev Respir Crit Care Med 2003; 168:1438–1444
NPPV can reduce the rate of mortality in some hypoxemic respiratory failure groups.
Gattinoni L, Tognoni G, Pesenti A, et al. Effect of prone position on the survival of patients with acute respiratory failure. N Engl J Med 2001; 345:568–573
Randomized, unblinded, controlled trial of 304 patients failed to show improvement in 10-day or 6-month mortality. The study was criticized for using only 6 h/d of prone positioning in many patients.
Girard TD, Kress JP, Fuchs BD, et al. Efficacy and safety of a paired sedation and ventilator weaning protocol for mechanically ventilated patients in intensive care (Awakening and Breathing Controlled trial): a randomised controlled trial. Lancet 2008; 371:126–134
Combination of daily interruption of sedation and SBT better than SBT alone.
Griffiths J, Barber VS, Morgan L, et al. Systematic review and meta-analysis of studies of the timing of tracheostomy in adult patients undergoing artificial ventilation. BMJ 2005; 330:1243
Meta-analysis of timing of tracheostomy.
Huang C-J, Lin H-C. Association between adrenal insufficiency and ventilator weaning. Am J Respir Crit Care Med 2006; 173:276–280
Treatment of patients who were found to have adrenal insufficiency with hydrocortisone resulted in significantly shorter duration of weaning and improved weaning success.
International consensus conferences in intensive care medicine: ventilator-associated lung injury in ARDS: this official conference report was cosponsored by the American Thoracic Society, The European Society of Intensive Care Medicine, and The Societé de Réanimation de Langue Française, and was approved by the ATS Board of Directors, July 1999. Am J Respir Crit Care Med 1999; 160:2118–2124
Detailed review of experimental evidence, risk factors, monitoring, and prevention of VALI.
Kress JP, Pohlman AS, O'Connor MF, et al. Daily interruption of sedative infusions in critically ill patients undergoing mechanical ventilation. N Engl J Med 2000; 342:1471–1477
Daily interruption of continuous IV sedation significantly shortened length of MV and days in the ICU.
Lightowler J, Wedzicka J, Elliot M, et al. Non-invasive positive pressure ventilation to treat respiratory failure resulting from exacerbations of chronic obstructive

pulmonary disease: Cochrane systematic reviews and meta-analysis. BMJ 2003; 326:184–189
This Cochrane analysis solidifies the role of NPPV in COPD.
MacIntyre NR, Cook DJ, Ely EW, et al. Evidence-based guidelines for weaning and discontinuing ventilator support. Chest 2001; 120:375S–395S
Provides basis for approaches to weaning.
Meade MO, Cook DJ, Guyatt GH, et al. Ventilation strategy using low tidal volumes, recruitment maneuvers, and high positive end-expiratory pressure for acute lung injury and acute respiratory distress syndrome: a randomized controlled trial. JAMA 2008; 299:637–645
Recent large Canadian RCT that showed that pressure-targeted, liberal PEEP, recruitment, and more liberal Pplat while keeping V_T *at 6 mL/kg PBW was as good as traditional ARDSNet ventilation for mortality and duration of MV but had better oxygenation.*
Mercat A, Richard JC, Vielle B, et al. Positive end-expiratory pressure setting in adults with acute lung injury and acute respiratory distress syndrome: a randomized controlled trial. JAMA 2008; 299:646–655
Recent large RCT demonstrating more ventilator-free days in addition to better oxygenation and less requirement for "rescue therapy" for hypoxemia; no clear mortality benefit was demonstrated.
Nava S, Ambrosino N, Clini E, et al. Noninvasive mechanical ventilation in the weaning of patients with respiratory failure due to chronic obstructive pulmonary disease: a randomized, controlled trial. Ann Intern Med 1998; 128:721–728
This sentinel study demonstrated the superiority of NPPV over MV through an ET tube in COPD patients with hypercapnic respiratory failure.
Nava S, Carbone G, DiBattista N, et al. Noninvasive ventilation in cardiogenic pulmonary edema: a multicenter randomized trial. Am Rev Respir Crit Care Med 2003; 168:1432–1437
This study established that NPPV could improve oxygenation and reduce the need for intubation in patients with cardiogenic pulmonary edema. However, the rate of mortality was not affected nor was it worse with bilevel positive airway pressure vs CPAP.
Putensen C, Mutz NJ, Putensen-Himmer G, et al. Spontaneous breathing during ventilatory support improves ventilation-perfusion distributions in patients with acute respiratory distress syndrome. Am J Respir Crit Care Med 1999; 159:1241–1248
Improved gas exchange and hemodynamics with bilevel ventilation (called APRV using 1:1 I:E ratio).
Ranieri VM, Suter PM, Tortorella C, et al. Effect of mechanical ventilation on inflammatory mediators in patients with acute respiratory distress syndrome: a randomized controlled trial. JAMA 1999; 282:54–61
Combination of low V_T *and high PEEP was associated with decreases in inflammatory mediators in BAL fluid and blood, compared with conventional ventilation in ARDS*
Rubenfeld GD, Cooper C, Carter G, et al. Barriers to providing lung-protective ventilation to patients with acute lung injury. Crit Care Med 2004; 32:1289–1293
We do not follow low V_T *ventilation recommendations and here's why.*
Sessler CN. Mechanical ventilation of patients with acute lung injury. Crit Care Clin 1998; 14:707–729
Review of the topic is presented.
Sessler CN, Varney K. Patient-focused sedation and analgesia in the ICU. Chest 2008; 133:552–565
Comprehensive recent review of sedation and analgesia in patients on MV.
Talmor D, Sarge T, Malhotra A, et al. Mechanical ventilation guided by esophageal pressure in acute lung injury. N Engl J Med 2008; 359:2095–2104
In a pilot RCT, guidance of setting PEEP by measured esophageal pressure as a surrogate for pleural pressure to estimate transalveolar pressure led to better oxygenation and lung compliance without increasing barotrauma. Although there are technical concerns regarding accuracy of esophageal pressure, the concept of individualized setting of PEEP (rather than by a table) is attractive.
Tanios MA, Nevins ML, Hendra KP, et al. A randomized, controlled trial of the role of weaning: Predictors in clinical decision making. Crit Care Med 2006; 34:2530–2535
Addition of f/V_T *(rapid shallow breathing index) to weaning protocol slowed weaning by 1 day, although duration of MV was identical as extubation failure.*
Taylor RW, Zimmerman JL, Dellinger RP, et al. Low-dose inhaled nitric oxide in patients with acute lung injury: a randomized controlled trial. JAMA 2004; 291:1603–1609
Five ppm of INO improved oxygenation for 24 h, but no outcomes benefits were seen.
Umoh NJ, Fan E, Mendez-Tellez PA, et al. Patient and intensive care unit organizational factors associated with low tidal volume ventilation in acute lung injury. Crit Care Med 2008; 36:1463–1468
Use of a written protocol was highly associated with improved compliance with low V_T *ventilation.*
Varelmann D, Wrigge H, Zinserling I, et al. Proportional assist vs pressure support ventilation in patients with

acute respiratory failure: cardiorespiratory responses to artificially increased ventilatory demand. Crit Care Med 2005; 33:1968–1975

PAV, even when combined with an automatic tube compensation program, did not reduce WOB significantly better than PSV.

Villar J, Kacmarek RM, Perez-Mendez L, et al. A high positive end-expiratory pressure, low tidal volume ventilatory strategy improves outcome in persistent acute respiratory distress syndrome: a randomized, controlled trial. Crit Care Med 2006; 34:1311–1318

RCT of 108 patients showing better outcomes with low VT *and high PEEP.*

Vitacca M, Ambrosino N, Clini E, et al. Physiologic response to pressure support ventilation delivered before and after extubation in patients not capable of totally spontaneous autonomous breathing. Am J Respir Crit Care Med 2001; 164:638–641

This study demonstrates that NPPV decreased diaphragm energy expenditure to the same degree as applying PS in intubated patients.

Walsh TS, Dodds S, McArdle F. Evaluation of simple criteria to predict successful weaning from mechanical ventilation in intensive care patients. Br J Anaesth 2004; 92:793–799

Patients who are successfully weaning often do not have PaO_2*:*FIO_2 *> 180 mm Hg. Other parameters addressed as well.*

Ware LB, Matthay MA. The acute respiratory distress syndrome. N Engl J Med 2000; 342:1334–1349

This article reviews ARDS.

Wheeler AP, Bernard GR. Acute lung injury and the acute respiratory distress syndrome: a clinical review. Lancet 2007; 369:1553–1564

This article reviews ARDS.

Yang KL, Tobin MJ. A prospective study of indexes predicting the outcome of trials of weaning from mechanical ventilation. N Engl J Med 1991; 324:1445–1450

This classic article defines the rapid shallow breathing index.

Young M. Tidal volumes used in acute lung injury: why the persistent gap between intended and actual clinical behavior? Crit Care Med 2006; 34:543–544

Clinicians do not follow low VT *recommendations reliably.*

Unusual and Uncommon Pulmonary Disorders

Jay H. Ryu, MD, FCCP

Objectives:

- Discuss several unusual and uncommon pulmonary disorders
- Describe clinical manifestations and facilitate recognition of these disorders
- Discuss management options for these disorders

Key words: Birt–Hogg–Dubé syndrome; constrictive bronchiolitis; IgG4 sclerosing disease; pulmonary alveolar proteinosis; pulmonary amyloidosis; spontaneous pneumomediastinum

Rare (orphan) disease is defined as a disease or condition affecting < 200,000 persons in the United States.[1a] An estimated 25 million people in the United States have 1 of the > 6,000 rare diseases. The failure to diagnose a rare or unusual disease is generally attributable to the failure to consider the diagnosis in the first place.

The diagnosis of unusual pulmonary disorders is facilitated by considering a broad differential diagnosis at the outset and recognizing characteristic clinical context and imaging features associated with these disorders. Histopathology can be helpful but needs to be correlated with the clinical and radiologic features in formulating the final clinicopathologic diagnosis. Rational treatment and accurate assessment of prognosis depend on an accurate diagnosis.

IgG4-Related Sclerosing Disease

In 2001, Hamano et al[1a] reported the findings of high serum IgG4 concentrations and dense lymphoplasmacytic infiltrates containing IgG4-positive plasma cells in the pancreas in 20 patients with sclerosing pancreatitis (also called *autoimmune pancreatitis*). Subsequently, similar IgG4-related lesions were identified in other organs such as the bile duct, salivary gland, lacrimal gland, liver, kidney, retroperitoneum (retroperitoneal fibrosis), aorta (inflammatory aneurysm), as well as the lung. It is now known that IgG4-related sclerosing disease can be localized to one or two organs or present with systemic multisystem disease.[2,3]

IgG4-related sclerosing disease manifests similar histopathologic findings in different organs and is characterized by diffuse lymphoplasmacytic infiltrate consisting of extensive IgG4-positive plasma cells and T lymphocytes along with fibrotic changes.[2] Other histopathologic features may include eosinophilic infiltration and obliterative angiitis.

Quantitatively, IgG4 is the smallest subclass of IgG and accounts for only 3 to 6% of total IgG in normal serum. The IgG subclasses exhibit differences in their effector functions. Involvement of immunologic mechanisms appears likely in IgG4-related sclerosing disease, but exactly what role IgG4 plays in the pathogenesis and pathophysiology of this disorder remains unclear.[2] The target antigens in this inflammatory disorder and the trigger for the serum IgG4 elevation also are not known.

IgG4 sclerosing disease occurs in adults, more commonly men than women, with a median age of 60 years (range, 17 to 80 years).[2,3] Manifestations of IgG4-related sclerosing disease commonly include pancreatic involvement, but extrapancreatic lesions without pancreatic involvement can occur.[2,3] Systemic symptoms including fever also may be seen.

Intrathoracic manifestations of IgG4-related sclerosing disease may include focal parenchymal lesions (*eg*, inflammatory pseudotumor, plasma-cell granuloma); interstitial infiltrates (organizing pneumonia, nonspecific interstitial pneumonia patterns); mediastinal/hilar lymphadenopathy; and mediastinal fibrosis.[2,4] Malignancy, *eg*, lung cancer, may be suspected on initial presentation. Radiologically, the manifestations include solitary nodule or mass, round-shaped ground-glass opacities, bilateral interstitial infiltrates consisting of reticular and ground-glass opacities, and thickening of bronchovascular bundles and interlobular septa. On ^{18}F-fluorodeoxyglucose PET scanning, abnormal

[18]F-fluorodeoxyglucose uptake is observed in pancreatic and extrapancreatic lesions.

Serum IgG4 levels and immunostaining of the biopsy specimen with anti-IgG4 antibody are useful in making the diagnosis.[2] Although the serum IgG4 level was initially reported to be increased in nearly all patients with autoimmune pancreatitis,[1a] the prevalence of increased IgG4 levels appears to be lower in patients presenting with various extrapancreatic lesions of IgG4-related sclerosing disease.

In patients with intrathoracic abnormalities associated with extrathoracic inflammatory or fibrotic lesions, particularly pancreatitis, the diagnosis of IgG4-related sclerosing disease should be considered. Even in the absence of extrathoracic manifestations, some unusual cases of intrathoracic lesions such as mediastinal fibrosis and focal inflammatory lesions may be IgG4 related in origin.

IgG4-related sclerosing disease responds well to corticosteroid therapy.[2–4] The starting dose of prednisone is typically 30 to 60 mg/d for 1 to 2 weeks followed by gradual tapering of the dose over the subsequent several weeks to a low maintenance dose, *eg*, 10 mg/d. In the absence of recurrent disease, corticosteroid therapy is eventually discontinued.

Pulmonary Alveolar Proteinosis

Pulmonary alveolar proteinosis (PAP), also known as *pulmonary alveolar phopholipoproteinosis*, is a rare parenchymal lung disease that is characterized by accumulation of lipoproteinaceous material in the alveoli. Most cases (90%) are idiopathic; the remaining cases consist of congenital and secondary forms of PAP.[5–7] The congenital form is caused by mutations in the genes encoding surfactant proteins or the receptor for granulocyte-macrophage colony-stimulating factor (GM-CSF). Secondary PAP occurs in association with hematologic or immunodeficiency disorders, inhalation of chemicals or inorganic dusts (*eg*, silica), or certain pulmonary infections. PAP results from impaired surfactant metabolism by macrophages caused by alterations in GM-CSF signaling. In most cases of idiopathic PAP, anti-GM-CSF antibodies are detectable in the serum and BAL fluid.

The median age at the time of diagnosis of idiopathic PAP is 39 years; most patients are 20 to 60 years of age.[5] Clinical features are nonspecific. Although most patients present with insidious onset of exertional dyspnea and cough, some patients may be asymptomatic.[5,6] Less common symptoms include fever, fatigue, weight loss, chest pain, and hemoptysis. Inspiratory crackles are heard in 20 to 50% of patients; digital clubbing is uncommon.[5,6]

Mildly increased levels of serum lactate dehydrogenase are common. Increased levels of lung surfactant protein A and D and mucin-like glycoprotein (KL-6) in the serum have also been found in patients with PAP; however, these findings are nonspecific and not limited to this disease.[5,6] Patients affected by PAP may have periodic acid-Schiff (PAS)-positive material or increased levels of surfactant protein A in their sputum, but these also are nonspecific findings. Serologic testing for anti-GM-CSF autoantibodies is not a routinely available assay.

Chest radiography usually reveals bilateral, patchy airspace infiltrates.[8] Less commonly, an interstitial pattern may be seen. Infiltrates often are more prominent in the perihilar regions, and this "bat-wing" pattern may be mistaken for pulmonary edema. High-resolution CT (HRCT) of the chest demonstrates ground-glass and/or consolidative infiltrates in patchy or diffuse distributions. Sharp demarcation of the infiltrates from surrounding normal lung tissue is commonly observed. Reticular opacities or interlobular septal thickening are present within the airspace infiltrates, creating a "crazy-paving" pattern.[8,9] This pattern is characteristic, but not specific, for PAP, and it can be seen in diffuse alveolar damage superimposed on usual interstitial pneumonia ("exacerbation" of idiopathic pulmonary fibrosis), acute interstitial pneumonia, ARDS, cardiogenic pulmonary edema, and drug-induced lung disease.[8,9] Pulmonary function testing demonstrates a restrictive defect with a reduced diffusing capacity.[6,10]

In an appropriate clinical setting, the diagnosis of PAP may be made by BAL fluid, which typically yields a milky effluent.[5,10] Under light microscopy, this fluid shows large amounts of PAS-positive lipoproteinaceous material. Transbronchial biopsy also provides the diagnosis in most cases and demonstrates accumulation of granular, PAS-positive, lipoproteinaceous material within the alveolar spaces with preserved alveolar architecture, although thickening of the alveolar septa and interstitial fibrosis may occur in some cases.[10] In the absence of a superimposed infection, very few inflammatory cells are seen in the lung tissue. Surgical biopsy is now less frequently required to confirm a PAP diagnosis.

The treatment standard for PAP is whole-lung lavage, during which repeated instillation and drainage of the lung with aliquots of isotonic saline solution (up to a total volume of 20 to 30 L) is performed until the run off is clear.[5,6,10] This procedure is performed via a bronchoscope passed through a double-lumen endotracheal tube with the patient under general anesthesia. Chest percussion is performed during the lavage procedure to facilitate removal of the lipoproteinaceous material. The main indication for treatment is limiting exertional dyspnea associated with hypoxemia. Approximately 85% of patients show improvement after lung lavage. The median duration of clinical benefit is approximately 15 months. Eventually, 60 to 70% of patients require repeat lavage. Lung lavage is associated with improved survival.[5,6] Consistent with its proposed importance in surfactant clearance, preliminary experience with GM-CSF administration in PAP has shown favorable responses in 40 to 50% of patients, with some patients experiencing a complete response.[10,11] GM-CSF has been administered subcutaneously (dose range, 5 to 20 µg/kg/d) or via aerosolization (dose range, 250 to 500 µg bid every other week).[6,12]

The clinical course of patients with PAP is variable; spontaneous resolution can occur as well as progression to respiratory failure.[5,6] Five- and 10-year survival rates in PAP are 75% and 68%, respectively. [5,6] Death caused by PAP is uncommon and usually related to respiratory failure or uncontrolled infection. Superimposed infection, especially with opportunistic pathogens such as Nocardia, may occur and disseminate. Lung transplantation is an option in those individuals with progressive disease that is not adequately responding to medical therapy. Recurrent PAP after double-lung transplantation has been reported.[13]

Pulmonary Amyloidosis

Amyloidosis is a heterogeneous group of acquired or inherited diseases characterized by deposition of amyloid in the extracellular tissue space. Amyloid, a fibrillar, insoluble, proteinaceous material, can deposit in the tracheobronchial tree or pulmonary parenchyma in either localized or diffuse pattern.[14] This pulmonary involvement can occur as part of a systemic process or be isolated to the lung.[14,15]

The most frequent types of amyloidosis are the AL (primary) and AA (secondary) types. AL amyloidosis can occur alone or in association with multiple myeloma or another plasma-cell dyscrasia. AA amyloidosis occurs with chronic inflammatory or infectious disorders. The frequency of pulmonary involvement is low with secondary and familial amyloidosis, whereas pulmonary involvement by AL (primary) systemic amyloidosis is relatively common.

Patients with pulmonary amyloidosis with or without previous amyloidosis may present to pulmonologists for an evaluation of respiratory symptoms or abnormal findings on chest imaging. Laryngeal and tracheobronchial forms of pulmonary amyloidosis may be seen as focal nodules/plaques or diffuse submucosal infiltration and usually occur as localized amyloidosis. Diffuse endobronchial involvement is recognizable bronchoscopically as shiny, pale plaques with scattered focal stenoses. Symptoms associated with airway involvement depend on the extent of luminal compromise and include dyspnea, cough, hemoptysis, wheeze, atelectasis, and recurrent pneumonias.

Pulmonary parenchymal involvement manifests as single or multiple nodules or diffuse parenchymal infiltrates. The nodular form is often detected incidentally on chest radiography. These nodules may grow slowly, cavitate, or calcify. A diffuse interstitial pattern is usually seen with systemic AL amyloidosis. HRCT reveals bilateral nodular and/or reticular pattern with septal thickening.[16] Pleural effusions may occur as the result of pleural involvement or from heart failure caused by cardiac amyloidosis. Other pulmonary manifestations are mediastinal and/or hilar adenopathy, mediastinal masses, and obstructive sleep apnea resulting from macroglossia.

The diagnosis of pulmonary amyloidosis is achieved by obtaining biopsy material that reveals the characteristic apple-green birefringence with polarized microscopy after staining with Congo red.[14,15] Tracheobronchial and diffuse parenchymal forms of pulmonary amyloidosis can be diagnosed by bronchoscopy, although the endoscopist must be prepared for potential patient bleeding. Lung nodules are diagnosed by needle aspiration biopsy or surgical resection. Diagnosis of pulmonary amyloidosis should lead to an evaluation to identify the underlying cause or condition leading to amyloid deposition, if it is not already known, as well as the extent of involvement.

The treatment of amyloidosis varies with different types of pulmonary involvement and the underlying cause of amyloidosis. Treatment of diffuse parenchymal amyloidosis associated with AL (primary) amyloidosis is directed against the underlying plasma cell dyscrasia. This is also true for hilar/mediastinal adenopathy. The prognosis is poor for patients with primary systemic amyloidosis who have pulmonary involvement. Symptomatic tracheobronchial involvement with localized stenosis can be treated with bronchoscopic laser or surgery. Recently, external beam therapy has been reported to be effective in the treatment of tracheobronchial amyloidosis.[17] The use of bevacizumab, an antivascular endothelial growth factor antibody, has been reported to be effective in managing refractory pleural effusions patients with primary (AL) systemic amyloidosis.[18] Treatment of AL systemic amyloidosis involves systemic chemotherapy and peripheral stem-cell transplantation.

Birt-Hogg-Dubé Syndrome

Birt-Hogg-Dubé (BHD) syndrome is a rare, inheritable disorder (autosomal dominant) that is associated with cystic lung disease and pneumothoraces.[19] Recent reports suggest that BHD may be an underdiagnosed cause of pneumothorax. BHD was first described in 1977 and is characterized by the cutaneous triad of fibrofolliculomas (hamartoma of the hair follicle), trichodiscomas, and skin tags, along with a propensity for renal tumors. It is caused by germline mutations in the BHD (*FLCN*) gene that lies on chromosome 17 and encodes a tumor-suppressor protein, folliculin.[20,21] Folliculin is highly expressed in a variety of tissues, including the skin, kidney, and lung.

Characteristic skin lesions of BHD typically appear as firm, dome-shaped papules in adulthood during the third or fourth decades of life and occur predominantly on the face, scalp, neck, and upper chest.[19] Renal tumors associated with BHD syndrome include oncocytic hybrid tumor, chromophobe renal-cell carcinoma, clear-cell carcinoma, and papillary renal-cell carcinoma.[19]

Patients with BHD syndrome who present with cystic lung disease or a history of pneumothoraces tend to be middle aged without a previous diagnosis of the underling genetic syndrome.[21,22] Approximately 90% of adult patients with BHD will have lung cysts of varying degrees on CT.[21] Approximately 25% of patients with BHD will experience pneumothorax, which will typically occur during third to sixth decades of life.[21,22] Some germline mutations of the BHD gene can cause pulmonary manifestations (cystic lung disease and pneumothorax) in the absence of skin or kidney lesions.[20] Histopathologic features in the lung are nonspecific and include intraparenchymal air-filled spaces surrounded by normal parenchyma or a thin fibrous wall.[22]

Cystic lung disease seen in BHD syndrome needs to be distinguished from other lung diseases characterized by multifocal or diffuse cystic changes, including lymphangioleiomyomatosis, pulmonary Langerhans-cell histiocytosis, lymphocytic interstitial pneumonitis, and Pneumocystis pneumonia.[23] Pulmonary lymphangioleiomyomatosis, whether occurring in a sporadic form or associated with tuberous sclerosis complex, affects women of childbearing age almost exclusively. It can be associated with renal tumors (angiomyolipomas) and may at times be difficult to distinguish from BHD.[24] Lymphocytic interstitial pneumonia and Pneumocystis pneumonia both cause parenchymal changes aside from cysts, such as ground-glass opacities, consolidation, nodules, and reticular opacities.[23] In addition, both of these disorders usually are symptomatic and are associated with specific clinical contexts. Pulmonary Langerhans-cell histiocytosis encountered in adults is usually a smoking-related interstitial lung disease and is characterized by irregular cystic lesions and nodules that predominantly affect the upper and mid lung zones with relative sparing of the bases.[25] Rarely, metastatic neoplasms, such as adenocarcinomas and low-grade sarcomas, can present with cystic lung lesions.[23]

The diagnosis of BHD has obvious implications on family members and the need for their evaluation. Patients with BHD who experience pneumothorax are at high risk of recurrence and should be managed accordingly, *ie*, consider pleurodesis. These patients also need to be screened for renal neoplasms.[21]

Constrictive Bronchiolitis

Constrictive bronchiolitis (also called obliterative bronchiolitis or bronchiolitis obliterans) is a form of obstructive lung disease that results from bronchiolar scarring and narrowing.[26,27] Bronchioles are small airways (internal diameter ≤ 2 mm that do not contain cartilage in their walls. Membranous and terminal bronchioles are purely air-conducting, and respiratory bronchioles (≤ 0.5 mm in diameter) contain alveoli in their walls. Constrictive bronchiolitis can be seen in a variety of clinical settings, most recognizably in organ transplant recipients, *ie*, obliterative bronchiolitis syndrome.[26,27] Outside of organ transplant recipients, constrictive bronchiolitis may present as obstructive lung disease of obscure etiology (*eg*, no smoking history) or abnormal CT findings suggestive of small airways disease with air trapping.

The types of constrictive bronchiolitis can be classified by etiology into following groups[26]:

- Allograft recipients;
- Postinfectious (viruses, mycoplasma, bacteria, fungi);
- Connective tissue diseases (rheumatoid arthritis, systemic lupus erythematosus, etc);
- Inhalational injury (*eg*, "popcorn lung" caused by diacetyl[28]);
- Ingested toxins (*eg*, *Sauropus androgynus*);
- Chronic hypersensitivity pneumonitis;
- Drugs (such as penicillamine, lomustine, cocaine);
- Other associations, including inflammatory bowel diseases, microcarcinoid tumorlets, paraneoplastic pemphigus, menstrual associations; and
- Cryptogenic constrictive bronchiolitis.

Patients with constrictive bronchiolitis typically present with slowly worsening exertional dyspnea, sometimes accompanied by a chronic cough.[26,29] On auscultation, the lungs usually sound clear without adventitious sounds. Wheezing may be heard in some patients. Evidence of expiratory slowing and hyperinflation will be observed in more severe cases. Pulmonary function testing will demonstrate airflow obstruction, usually without significant reversibility.

Chest radiography typically shows hyperinflation in the absence of any parenchymal infiltrates. HRCT reveals a mosaic pattern with patchy areas of air trapping.[26,29–31] Scattered changes of bronchiectasis may be seen in some patients.

The treatment of constrictive bronchiolitis varies with the underling cause.[26,29] Causative exposure or underlying disease needs to be controlled. In general, corticosteroids administered systemically or by inhaled route are relatively ineffective in reversing the airflow obstruction.[26,29] In organ transplant recipients, administration of macrolides, *eg*, azithromycin, 250 mg three times per week, has demonstrated some beneficial effects.[32,33]

Spontaneous Pneumomediastinum

Pneumomediastinum is defined as the presence of free air in the mediastinum. Pneumomediastinum can be spontaneous, traumatic, or iatrogenic (surgical and endoscopic procedures). Spontaneous pneumomediastinum (SP) is defined as the presence of air in the mediastinum without preceding traumatic or procedural injury and is subdivided into primary (no apparent lung disease) and secondary (known lung disease) categories.

Potential sources of air into the mediastinum in cases of SP include airways, lung, or esophagus. The proposed pathophysiology involves the development alveolar rupture with dissection of air along the interstitium and bronchovascular tissue sheath following a centripetal pattern toward the hilum and the mediastinum. Rarely, pneumomediastinum may be caused by a mediastinal infection with a gas-producing organism.

Preexisting lung diseases are identified in approximately one half of patients with SP and include asthma, chronic obstructive lung disease, and interstitial lung diseases.[34,35] Precipitating events preceding SP may include coughing, sneezing, vomiting, exercise or athletic activities, inhalational drug use, Valsalva maneuver during childbirth, and the playing of wind instruments.[34] These activities are associated with increase alveolar pressure. In some patients, no precipitating event can be identified.[35,36]

SP is typically encountered in young men and women in their third and fourth decades of life but can be encountered in subjects over a wide range of ages.[34–36] Presenting clinical manifestations usually consist of chest pain and/or dyspnea. Other common symptoms may include dysphagia, odynophagia, neck pain and swelling, and dysphonia. In some patients, SP may be detected radiologically in the absence of any relevant symptoms.

Crepitations from subcutaneous emphysema may be present in the neck or chest wall.[34–36] The Hamman sign (a mediastinal crunching or clicking sound that is synchronous with the heart beat) is uncommon. The use of plain chest radiography (posteroanterior and lateral views) is usually sufficient to reveal the presence of mediastinal air.[35] However, chest radiographic findings may be normal up to 30% of the time.[34,35,37] Thus, CT is the diagnostic standard for pneumomediastinum.

The presence of pneumomediastinum is commonly viewed as an ominous finding, with potentially catastrophic complications. However, SP is generally not associated with identifiable pathologic cause such as esophageal or tracheobronchial rupture.[34–38] In the absence of worrisome symptoms such as severe dysphagia, fever, leukocytosis, or hemodynamic instability, extensive diagnostic evaluation is unnecessary and conservative management suffices. Resolution of pneumomediastinum and symptoms occurs over the following 1 to 2 weeks. Associated pneumothorax may develop in 10 to 30% of patients, but these patients do not require drainage in most cases. Recurrence of pneumomediastinum is unusual.[34–38]

References

1. Office of Rare Diseases, National Institutes of Health. Disease information from NORD. Available at http://www.rarediseases.org/info/about.html. Accessed June 15, 2009

1a. Hamano H, Kawa S, Horiuchi A, et al. High serum IgG4 concentrations in patients with sclerosing pancreatitis. N Engl J Med 2001; 344:732–738

2. Kamisawa T, Okamoto A. IgG4-related sclerosing disease. World J Gastroenterol 2008; 14:3948–3955
3. Pickartz T, Mayerle J, Lerch MM. Autoimmune pancreatitis. Nat Clin Pract Gastroenterol Hepatol 2007; 4:314–323
4. Neild GH, Rodriguez-Justo M, Wall C, et al. Hyper-IgG4 disease: report and characterisation of a new disease. BMC Med 2006; 4:23
5. Seymour JF, Presneill JJ. Pulmonary alveolar proteinosis: progress in the first 44 years. Am J Respir Crit Care Med 2002; 166:215–235
6. Trapnell BC, Whitsett JA, Nakata K. Pulmonary alveolar proteinosis. N Engl J Med 2003; 349: 2527–2539
7. Inoue Y, Trapnell BC, Tazawa R, et al. Characteristics of a large cohort of patients with autoimmune pulmonary alveolar proteinosis in Japan. Am J Respir Crit Care Med 2008; 177:752–762
8. Frazier AA, Franks TJ, Cooke EO, et al. From the archives of the AFIP: pulmonary alveolar proteinosis. Radiographics 2008; 28:883–899; quiz 915
9. Johkoh T, Itoh H, Muller NL, et al. Crazy-paving appearance at thin-section CT: spectrum of disease and pathologic findings. Radiology 1999; 211:155–160
10. Ioachimescu OC, Kavuru MS. Pulmonary alveolar proteinosis. Chron Respir Dis 2006; 3:149–159
11. Venkateshiah SB, Yan TD, Bonfield TL, et al. An open-label trial of granulocyte macrophage colony stimulating factor therapy for moderate symptomatic pulmonary alveolar proteinosis. Chest 2006; 130:227–237
12. Wylam ME, Ten R, Prakash UBS, et al. Aerosol granulocyte-macrophage colony-stimulating factor for pulmonary alveolar proteinosis. Eur Respir J 2006; 27:585–593
13. Parker LA, Novotny DB. Recurrent alveolar proteinosis following double lung transplantation. Chest 1997; 111:1457–1458
14. Lachmann HJ, Hawkins PN. Amyloidosis and the lung. Chron Respir Dis 2006; 3:203–214
15. Utz JP, Swensen SJ, Gertz MA. Pulmonary amyloidosis: the Mayo Clinic experience from 1980 to 1993. Ann Intern Med 1996; 124:407–413
16. Pickford HA, Swensen SJ, Utz JP. Thoracic cross-sectional imaging of amyloidosis. AJR Am J Roentgenol 1997; 168:351–355
17. Neben-Wittich MA, Foote RL, Kalra S. External beam radiation therapy for tracheobronchial amyloidosis. Chest 2007; 132:262–267
18. Hoyer RJ, Leung N, Witzig TE, et al. Treatment of diuretic refractory pleural effusions with bevacizumab in four patients with primary systemic amyloidosis. Am J Hematol 2007; 82:409–413
19. Schmidt LS, Nickerson ML, Warren MB, et al. Germline BHD-mutation spectrum and phenotype analysis of a large cohort of families with Birt–Hogg–Dubé syndrome. Am J Hum Genet 2005; 76:1023–1033

20. Gunji Y, Akiyoshi T, Sato T, et al. Mutations of the Birt–Hogg–Dubé gene in patients with multiple lung cysts and recurrent pneumothorax. J Med Genet 2007; 44:588–593
21. Toro JR, Pautler SE, Stewart L, et al. Lung cysts, spontaneous pneumothorax, and genetic associations in 89 families with Birt–Hogg–Dubé syndrome. Am J Respir Crit Care Med 2007; 175:1044–1053
22. Ayo DS, Aughenbaugh GL, Yi ES, et al. Cystic lung disease in Birt–Hogg–Dubé syndrome. Chest 2007; 132:679–684
23. Ryu JH, Swensen SJ. Cystic and cavitary lung diseases: focal and diffuse. Mayo Clin Proc 2003; 78:744–752
24. Ryu JH, Moss J, Beck GJ, et al. The NHLBI lymphangioleiomyomatosis registry: characteristics of 230 patients at enrollment. Am J Respir Crit Care Med 2006; 173:105–111
25. Vassallo R, Ryu JH. Pulmonary Langerhans' cell histiocytosis. Clin Chest Med 2004; 25:561–571
26. Ryu JH, Myers JL, Swensen SJ. Bronchiolar disorders. Am J Respir Crit Care Med 2003; 168: 1277–1292
27. Visscher DW, Myers JL. Bronchiolitis: the pathologist's perspective. Proc Am Thorac Soc 2006; 3: 41–47
28. van Rooy FGBGJ, Rooyackers JM, Prokop M, et al. Bronchiolitis obliterans syndrome in chemical workers producing diacetyl for food flavorings. Am J Respir Crit Care Med 2007; 176:498–504
29. Cordier JF. Challenges in pulmonary fibrosis: 2. Bronchiolocentric fibrosis. Thorax 2007; 62:638–649
30. de Jong PA, Dodd JD, Coxson HO, et al. Bronchiolitis obliterans following lung transplantation: early detection using computed tomographic scanning. Thorax 2006; 61:799–804
31. Kang E-Y, Woo OH, Shin BK, et al. Bronchiolitis: classification, computed tomographic and histopathologic features, and radiologic approach. J Comp Assist Tomogr 2009; 33:32–41
32. Gottlieb J, Szangolies J, Koehnlein T, et al. Long-term azithromycin for bronchiolitis obliterans syndrome after lung transplantation. Transplantation 2008; 85:36–41
33. Verleden GM, Vanaudenaerde BM, Dupont LJ, et al. Azithromycin reduces airway neutrophilia and interleukin-8 in patients with bronchiolitis obliterans syndrome. Am J Respir Crit Care Med 2006; 174:566–570
34. Caceres M, Ali SZ, Braud R, et al. Spontaneous pneumomediastinum: a comparative study and review of the literature. Ann Thorac Surg 2008; 86:962–966
35. Macia I, Moya J, Ramos R, et al. Spontaneous pneumomediastinum: 41 cases. Eur J Cardiothorac Surg 2007; 31:1110–1114
36. Newcomb AE, Clarke CP. Spontaneous pneumomediastinum: a benign curiosity or a significant problem? Chest 2005; 128:3298–3302
37. Takada K, Matsumoto S, Hiramatsu T, et al. Management of spontaneous pneumomediastinum based on clinical experience of 25 cases. Respir Med 2008; 102:1329–1334
38. Jougon JB, Ballester M, Delcambre F, et al. Assessment of spontaneous pneumomediastinum: experience with 12 patients. Ann Thorac Surg 2003; 75:1711–1714

Notes

Mediastinal and Other Neoplasms

Jay H. Ryu, MD, FCCP

Objectives:

- Discuss the anatomic compartments of the mediastinum
- Discuss the diagnostic approach to mediastinal lesions and management options
- Discuss uncommon intrathoracic neoplasms

Key words: carcinoid; germ-cell tumors; hamartoma; lymphadenopathy; lymphomas; mediastinal tumors; mediastinum; neurogenic tumors; salivary gland type carcinoma

Mediastinum

The mediastinum is the intrathoracic compartment located between the two pleural cavities. It includes those structures bounded by the thoracic inlet, diaphragm, sternum, vertebral bodies, and pleura. Several different schemes exist in subdividing the mediastinum into compartments.[1] For this discussion, we will use the three-compartment model: anterior, middle, and posterior. The anterior compartment refers to the retrosternal space that is anterior to the heart and the great vessels; it includes the thymus and lymph nodes as well as adipose and connective tissue. The posterior compartment extends from the posterior heart border and trachea to the posterior aspect of the vertebral bodies. It includes the descending aorta, azygous veins, esophagus, autonomic ganglia and nerves, thoracic duct, and lymph nodes. In between is the middle compartment, which contains the heart, ascending aorta and aortic arch, brachiocephalic vessels, main pulmonary arteries and veins, vena cavae, lymph nodes, trachea, and main bronchi.

Mediastinal Tumors

The differential diagnosis of a mediastinal mass is facilitated by identifying its location within the mediastinal compartments (Table 1). Thus, CT scanning is the most important imaging procedure in the diagnosis of mediastinal lesions. CT also can be used to define the density of the mass (fat, fluid,

Table 1. *Mediastinal Masses According to Compartments*

Location	Disorder
Anterior	Thymoma and other thymic tumors Lymphomas Germ cell tumors Thyroid goiter and other thyroid tumors Metastases Miscellaneous: parathyroid tumors, mesenchymal neoplasms (*eg*, lipoma, leiomyoma, lymphangioma), and Morgagni hernia
Middle	Lymphomas Metastases Nonmalignant lymphadenopathy (*eg*, infections, sarcoidosis, silicosis, and Castleman disease) Mediastinal cysts Vascular lesions Miscellaneous (*eg*, lymphangiomas and hernias)
Posterior	Neurogenic neoplasms Esophageal lesions Miscellaneous (*eg*, lateral meningocele, extramedullary hematopoiesis, descending aortic aneurysm, and Bochdalek hernia)

air, calcification, heterogeneous attenuation) and effect on adjacent structures (compression, infiltration). Sometimes, a confident diagnosis can be established based on CT features, *eg*, teratoma, mediastinal goiter, and pericardial cyst. MRI typically adds little additional information beyond that provided by CT scanning, but it may be useful in patients with contraindication to the use of iodinated IV contrast or when additional characterization of musculoskeletal or neurovascular anatomy is needed, *eg*, neurogenic tumor with intraspinal extension.[2]

In general, the diagnostic approach to mediastinal masses includes consideration of the following parameters: location; radiologic characteristics; clinical context (*ie*, age, symptoms, concurrent and previous illnesses); and tempo (*ie*, assess from evolution of clinical manifestations and comparison to previous imaging studies). Approximately 25 to 30% of mediastinal masses occurring in adults are malignant, with a higher risk in those masses appearing in the anterior mediastinum and in children.[3] Symptomatic patients are also more likely to have a malignancy (50%) compared with those without symptoms (10 to 20%).[3] Patients with mediastinal masses may experience localized symptoms (related to compression or invasion of adjacent mediastinal structures, metastatic sites), constitutional symptoms, or symptoms related to paraneoplastic syndromes. Overall, the most frequent mediastinal lesions are thymoma, neurogenic neoplasms, lymphomas, and foregut cysts.

Anterior Mediastinal Lesions

Thymoma

Thymoma is defined as a low-grade epithelial neoplasm of the thymus, and it is typically located in the superior aspect of the anterior mediastinum. It is the most common mediastinal neoplasm in most published case series.[3] Grossly, most thymomas are encapsulated firm masses but may have necrotic, hemorrhagic, or cystic components. Invasive thymomas tend to infiltrate the surrounding mediastinal structures. Microscopically, thymomas are composed of a mixture of neoplastic thymic epithelial cells and nonneoplastic T lymphocytes.[4,5] Accordingly, thymomas are subclassified as predominantly epithelial, predominantly lymphocytic, or mixed lymphoepithelial types.[4,5] The predominantly epithelial cell type category displays a greater rate of recurrence and tumor-related deaths than other subtypes. Thymomas are also subclassified based on the type of neoplastic cells present; polygonal-cell type, spindle-cell type, and mixed-cell type. Precise histologic subclassification can be difficult because histologic heterogeneity is common within thymomas. Several schemes exist for classification of thymomas.

Thymoma usually occurs in adults, particularly during the fourth and fifth decades of life.[3,5,6] One half to two thirds of patients present with symptoms such as cough, chest pain, dyspnea, dysphagia, constitutional symptoms, or symptoms related to one or more of the parathymic syndromes. These parathymic syndromes occur in 30 to 50% of patients with thymoma and include myasthenia gravis (most common), pure red cell aplasia, hypogammaglobulinemia Good syndrome, and connective tissue diseases.[7] The remaining cases are discovered as asymptomatic mediastinal mass on routine chest radiography.[3,5] Thymoma appears on chest radiography as a rounded, well-circumscribed, anterior mediastinal mass.[3] On CT, thymoma is typically homogeneous, discrete soft-tissue mass, but at times, it may exhibit heterogeneous attenuation related to hemorrhage, necrosis, or cystic changes.

The diagnosis of thymoma may be obtained by ultrasound or CT-guided core needle biopsy or surgical excision.[3,6] Local invasive disease may be observed in approximately one third of cases, but lymph node and hematogenous spread are relatively rare. Anatomic staging of thymoma is based on assessment of capsular invasion at the time of surgery and on microscopic examination. Thymomas can be classified into three categories for staging: encapsulated, invasive, or metastatic.

Optimal treatment for thymoma is complete surgical excision.[5,6,8] Adjunctive chemotherapy and radiation therapy are used for locally invasive or metastatic disease.[6] In patients with thymoma associated with myasthenia gravis who are <55 to 60 years of age, thymectomy yields improvement in the neurologic disease, although the benefit of thymectomy is not immediate, with remission rate gradually increasing during the following 5 to 10 years.[7] Thymectomy in patients with pure red cell aplasia results in 40 to 50% remission rate, whereas those with hypogammaglobulinemia do not benefit from thymic resection. The overall 5-year survival rate associated with encapsulated thymomas is 75%, whereas patients with invasive thymomas have a 5-year survival rate of 50%.[5,8]

Other Thymic Tumors

Thymic carcinoma is a rare epithelial malignancy with malignant histologic features (high or low grade) and typically presents as a large, poorly defined, infiltrative anterior mediastinal mass.[9,10] Thymic carcinoma typically occurs in the fifth and sixth decades of life and has predominance in male patients.[9,10] Most patients present with respiratory and/or systemic symptoms. Regional lymph node and pulmonary metastases as well as pleural and/or pericardial effusions frequently are noted at presentation. Surgical resection is the preferred treatment, when feasible.[10] Response to adjuvant cisplatin-based chemotherapy and radiotherapy are generally poor, with 5-year survival rates of approximately 30%.[10]

Thymic carcinoid is a rare, malignant neuroendocrine neoplasm that is associated with similar clinical and radiologic presentation as for thymic carcinoma.[11,12] Approximately one third of patients experience ectopic hormone production, including Cushing syndrome (most common), multiple endocrine neoplasia syndrome type I, syndrome of inappropriate antidiuretic hormone secretion, and carcinoid syndrome. Surgical resection, when feasible, is the treatment of choice.[11,12]

Thymolipoma is a rare benign neoplasm that is composed of mature thymic and adipose tissue as demonstrated on a CT scan. It usually affects young adults. Treatment is surgical resection, and the prognosis is excellent.[8,12] Thymic cyst is another rare mediastinal lesion and appears as a unilocular or multilocular lesion, often with calcification, on CT. It may be acquired or congenital.[12] Surgical resection is the recommended treatment.

Lymphomas

Lymphomas represent 4 to 5% of the estimated new cases of cancer overall and 3% of cancer deaths in the United States.[13] Lymphoma involves the mediastinum usually as part of widespread disease; in < 10% of patients, lymphoma is limited to the mediastinum.[14] Primary mediastinal lymphomas occur typically in the anterior mediastinum and more commonly presents as Hodgkin disease (HD) than non-Hodgkin lymphoma (NHL).[14,15] Patients with primary mediastinal lymphoma are usually young adults who may or may not be symptomatic (local or constitutional symptoms) at the time of diagnosis.

Radiologic studies[14,15] generally demonstrate a lobulated mass or bulky adenopathy in the anterior mediastinum. The diagnosis of lymphoma requires an adequate biopsy specimen obtained by surgical excision of an enlarged lymph node or extranodal mass. Core needle biopsy may also yield adequate tissue. Treatment of mediastinal HD consists of radiotherapy and/or chemotherapy; both treatment modalities usually are instituted in the treatment of NHL. Prognosis is better for those with mediastinal HD compared with NHL.[3,14]

Germ-Cell Tumors

Mediastinal germ-cell tumors consist of a diverse group of benign and malignant neoplasms that are usually located in the anterior mediastinum. Germ-cell tumors are uncommon neoplasms that most frequently present as testicular tumors, but approximately 5% of these tumors can primarily arise in extragonadal locations such as the mediastinum.[16] Germ-cell tumors account for 15% of anterior mediastinal tumors in adults.[3,16–18] Like primary gonadal germ-cell tumors, they are most common in young men (usually in the third decade of life). Germ-cell tumors are generally classified into the following three groups: teratomas, seminomas, and nonseminomatous tumors.[3,16–18]

Teratomas (benign or mature) account for 60 to 70% of mediastinal germ-cell tumors and contain varying amounts of tissues derived from at least two of the three primitive germ layers: ectoderm, endoderm, and mesoderm. Teratoma typically affects children and young adults. The majority of patients with benign teratomas are asymptomatic, and the tumor is discovered incidentally.[3,16] Characteristic but uncommon symptoms include expectoration of hair (trichoptysis) or sebaceous debris attributable to a communication between the tumor and the airways. Radiologically, mediastinal teratomas are well-circumscribed round or lobular masses that may contain fat (75%), calcification (20 to 50%), or cystic changes (80%).[3,16] Occasionally, teeth or bone may be recognized and are very suggestive of the diagnosis. Malignant degeneration of this tumor can occasionally occur. Treatment of mediastinal teratoma is surgical excision performed through a median sternotomy or posterolateral thoracotomy.[16,18] Thoracoscopic resection has also been reported.[18]

Primary mediastinal seminoma is the second most common form of mediastinal germ-cell tumor but is the most common malignant germ-cell tumor in this location.[3,16] Mediastinal seminomas typically are found in men in the third and fourth decades of life who are usually symptomatic, most commonly with chest pain. Increased serum level of β-human chorionic gonadotrophin (β-hCG) is noted in a minority of patients, and serum α fetoprotein (AFP) level is usually within normal range. Radiologically, mediastinal seminoma manifests as a large, lobular, well-circumscribed, homogeneous mass. Fine-needle aspiration biopsy is often adequate to make the diagnosis. Pure seminomas are very radiosensitive, but if nonseminomatous components, *eg*, embryonal carcinoma, are present, these tumors tend be more aggressive and do not readily respond to radiation therapy. Patients with locally advanced disease may be treated with chemotherapy, followed by resection of residual tumor. At the time of diagnosis, 60 to 70% of patients have metastatic disease that requires cisplatin-based combination chemotherapy with or without radiation.[3,16]

Nonseminomatous germ-cell tumors include choriocarcinoma, embryonal carcinoma, endodermal sinus tumor, teratocarcinoma, and mixed germ-cell neoplasms. These rare tumors are commonly grouped together because of therapeutic and prognostic similarities, including rapid growth and poor outlook. These tumors typically occur in young men (usually in the third and fourth decades of life), and they are commonly associated with symptoms that include chest pain, hemoptysis, cough, fever, weight loss, gynecomastia, or superior vena caval syndrome.[3,18] Serum tumor markers, AFP and β-hCG, are increased in approximately 80% and 30% of patients, respectively.[16] Radiologically, these tumors present as large, irregularly shaped heterogeneous masses with areas of necrosis, hemorrhage, or cystic changes, along with evidence invasion into adjacent structures and metastases.[3] Treatment usually involves cisplatin-based combination chemotherapy, followed by surgical resection of residual neoplasm.[3,18] Serial monitoring of serum AFP and β-hCG is helpful in assessing the response to therapy and detecting early recurrence.

Thyroid

Intrathoracic goiter can present as an anterior mediastinal mass and usually results from extension of a cervical thyroid goiter into the mediastinum. An intrathoracic goiter can cause symptoms by compressing the trachea or esophagus but, more commonly, symptoms are absent. Although most intrathoracic goiters are benign, 10 to 15% may contain thyroid cancer or lymphoma.[3,19] On chest radiography, intrathoracic goiter is seen as a mass associated with tracheal narrowing or deviation or as superior mediastinal widening. CT demonstrates a lobular, discrete mass with heterogeneous attenuation. Caution needs to be exercised in the administration of iodinated radiocontrast dye because iodine may induce hyperthyroidism. Symptomatic goiters are surgically excised, usually through a cervical incision.[20,21]

Other Anterior Mediastinal Masses

Although rare in occurrence, lesions arising from parathyroid tissue can produce an anterior mediastinal mass, including parathyroid cysts, carcinomas, and adenomas. These tumors tend to be small and are usually detected by CT. Other rare causes of anterior mediastinal masses include mesenchymal tumors (such as lipoma, leiomyoma, and lymphangioma) and Morgagni hernia. Occasionally, metastatic disease may present as an anterior mediastinal mass without a preceding cancer diagnosis.

Middle Mediastinal Masses

The differential diagnosis of middle mediastinal masses is broad and includes lesions of many causes.

Mediastinal Lymphadenopathy

There are many neoplastic and nonneoplastic diseases that can cause mediastinal and/or hilar lymphadenopathy.[3] Metastatic mediastinal/hilar lymphadenopathy may be seen with lung cancer, lymphomas, and cancers of extrapulmonary origin.[15] Infections, particularly fungi and mycobacteria, are also commonly associated with mediastinal and/or hilar lymphadenopathy. There are many other disorders that cause mediastinal lymphadenopathy and include sarcoidosis, drugs (*eg*, phenytoin), silicosis, amyloidosis, and Castleman disease. The diagnostic approach to mediastinal lymphadenopathy requires integration of the radiologic findings, clinical context, and tempo of the disease process.

Mediastinal Cysts

Primary mediastinal cysts are benign lesions usually found in the middle mediastinum and include bronchogenic cyst, enteric cyst, and pericardial cyst.[3,22,23] Bronchogenic cyst is the most common. Bronchogenic cysts are lined with ciliated respiratory epithelium and contain serous fluid, mucus, blood, or purulent material. Bronchogenic cysts typically are found in adults.[24,25] Patients are commonly asymptomatic at presentation, although symptoms can be produced from airway compression or communication of the cyst with the airway. These cysts are most commonly located in the subcarinal or paratracheal regions but are occasionally in the lung. Radiologically, bronchogenic cysts appear as homogeneous, nonenhancing masses of variable attenuation depending on the composition of the fluid.[23] When water attenuation is seen, it can be highly suggestive of the diagnosis. Definitive diagnosis can be obtained by CT-guided, bronchoscopic, or endoscopic aspiration of the cyst fluid.[24,25] Most bronchogenic cysts are surgically excised, but fluid aspiration and observation are other management options.[24,25]

Enteric cysts are lined by enteric or stratified squamous epithelium and are usually seen in the middle or posterior mediastinum.[24] The majority of enteric cysts are encountered in children. They may cause symptoms by compression of the trachea or esophagus, as well as mucosal ulceration, hemorrhage, or cyst rupture if the cyst contains gastric or pancreatic mucosa.[3] Surgical excision is the treatment of choice.[24] Prognosis after complete excision is excellent.[24]

Pericardial cysts are lined by mesothelial cells and appear as well-circumscribed lesions abutting the heart (most commonly in the area of the right cardiophrenic angle), the diaphragm, and the anterior chest wall.[23] CT demonstrates a unilocular lesion with characteristic water attenuation and a thin cystic wall. Most pericardial cysts are congenital but they can be acquired lesions. These cysts are usually asymptomatic but can occasionally cause cardiac compromise.[26] These lesions do not require intervention unless symptoms or diagnostic uncertainty exists.[22]

Vascular Lesions

Vascular lesions, such as aneurysms and fistulas, constitute approximately 5 to 10% of all mediastinal masses and may radiologically resemble neoplasms. The diagnosis is usually established by contrast-enhanced CT, MRI, and/or angiography.

Other Middle Mediastinal Masses

Lymphangiomas are rare congenital or acquired disorders involving the lymphatic vessels.[27] Although most commonly found in the neck, they can also occur in the mediastinum and appear as solitary or multilobulated cystic masses. These lesions are considered benign in nature but can slowly enlarge and infiltrate adjacent structures.[27,28] Total resection is optimal, if feasible. Mediastinal lipomatosis is a benign condition characterized by abnormal adipose tissue accumulation in the mediastinum. It is associated with endogenous and exogenous steroid excess, as well as obesity. CT reveals diagnostic features.[29]

Posterior Mediastinum

Neurogenic Tumors

The most common cause of posterior mediastinal masses is neurogenic neoplasm, which accounts for 75% of primary posterior mediastinal neoplasms.[30] Neurogenic tumors may arise from the peripheral, autonomic, or paraganglionic nervous systems. Ninety percent of neurogenic neoplasms occur in the paravertebral gutters. The majority (70 to 80%) of neurogenic neoplasms are benign; the occurrence of multiple lesions suggests the diagnosis of neurofibromatosis and the associated risk of malignant transformation.[3]

Approximately one half of neurogenic tumors are first detected on chest radiography in asymptomatic patients.[3] CT helps to define the location, characteristics, and margins of the mediastinal mass. Approximately 10% of mediastinal neurogenic tumors extend through the neural foramen into the spinal canal, creating a dumbbell shape (*ie*, "dumbbell tumor"). In this setting, MRI is more sensitive than CT in delineating the extension through neural foramen and spinal canal involvement.[2]

Peripheral nerve sheath tumors are the most common type (40 to 65%) of mediastinal neurogenic tumors and include schwannoma (also called neurilemmoma), neurofibroma, and malignant peripheral nerve sheath neoplasm.[3,30] They are most commonly found in asymptomatic adults in the third and fourth decades of life. The vast majority of schwannoma and neurofibromas are benign and slow growing. They usually arise from a posterior spinal nerve root. Radiologically, schwannomas and neurofibromas are well-circumscribed, round, or lobular posterior mediastinal masses.[3] Associated abnormalities may be seen in the ribs, vertebral bodies, and neural foramina as the result of pressure and erosion caused by the enlarging mass. The treatment of choice is surgical resection. Combined thoracic and neurosurgical approach may be needed for dumbbell tumors.[31]

Malignant peripheral nerve sheath neoplasms are rare spindle-cell sarcomas (<5% of nerve sheath tumors) and include malignant neurofibrosarcomas, malignant schwannomas, and neurogenic fibrosarcomas. Approximately one half of these are associated with neurofibromatosis.[30] Pain and enlarging mass are common presenting manifestations of this tumor, which appears radiologically as a sharply marginated, round, heterogeneous mass on CT. Evidence of local invasion and/or metastases may also be revealed. Complete surgical resection is the optimal treatment; in patients with unresectable tumors, adjuvant chemotherapy and radiation are options.[3,30,32]

Neoplasms of the sympathetic ganglia arise from nerve cells and include ganglioneuroma, ganglioneuroblastoma, and neuroblastoma. These tumors are more common in the pediatric population, and most are malignant.[3,30] Ganglioneuroblastoma and neuroblastoma are aggressive malignancies that usually affect children in the first decade of life. Treatment for limited disease is surgical resection. Management of advanced disease includes chemotherapy and radiation. Ganglioneuromas are benign neoplasms and occur in older children and young adults. One half of patients are symptomatic from local effects of the tumor or intraspinal extension. CT demonstrates a well-circumscribed paraspinal mass that may be associated with skeletal displacement or erosion. MRI may be needed to exclude intraspinal extension.[3] Complete surgical resection is the treatment of choice and may necessitate a combined thoracic and neurosurgical approach.

Mediastinal paraganglionic tumors are very rare and may arise from either sympathetic or parasympathetic cells.[33] They can occur in all three compartments of the mediastinum. Paravertebral paragangliomas occur in young adults and may be functional, *ie*, secrete catecholamines. Catecholamine-secreting paragangliomas may be associated with neurofibromatosis 1, von Hippel-Lindau disease, Carney triad, and multiple endocrine neoplasia type 2.[34] Mediastinal paragangliomas generally behave as low-grade, indolent neoplasms.[30,33] The treatment of choice is surgical excision.

Other Posterior Mediastinal Masses

Hiatal hernias are common and may manifest radiologically as a retrocardiac mass. Lateral thoracic meningoceles are rare and consist of redundant meninges that protrude through the neural foramen.[35] CT scans demonstrate a well-circumscribed, paraspinous cystic lesion (homogeneous water attenuation) that is continuous with the thecal sac. Symptomatic lesions are treated with surgical excision.

Extramedullary hematopoiesis refers to the proliferation of hematopoietic cells outside of the bone marrow in conditions of compromised tissue oxygenation. Most cases are associated with hemoglobinopathies manifesting severe, chronic anemia such as thalassemia major, hereditary spherocytosis, hemolytic anemia, or sickle-cell anemia.[36,37] Myeloproliferative disorders and other chronic illnesses associated with persistent anemia may also lead to extramedullary hematopoiesis. Extramedullary hematopoiesis can be seen in the posterior mediastinum as one or multiple, inhomogeneously contrast-enhancing paravertebral masses.[36,37] The diagnosis can be confirmed with percutaneous fine-needle aspiration or thoracoscopic biopsy, if needed. Extramedullary hematopoiesis usually regresses with treatment of anemia and the underlying condition or with radiation therapy.

Thoracic duct cyst is a rare lesion that can present in the posterior mediastinum and occasionally in the neck (left supraclavicular fossa). It may arise as a congenital anomaly or related to inflammatory or traumatic injuries. Symptomatic worsening or increase in size of the lesion after meals is a diagnostic clue.[38] The diagnosis can be established by needle aspiration of the chylous fluid within the cyst or lymphangiography.

Uncommon Thoracic Tumors

There are many types of uncommon to rare tumors that may be encountered in the thorax.[39–41]

Among these, more frequently encountered tumors include the carcinoid tumor, salivary gland-type carcinomas (mucoepidermoid carcinoma and adenoid cystic carcinoma), and hamartoma.

Carcinoid

Bronchial carcinoid tumors are malignant neoplasms with neuroendocrine differentiation and account for 1 to 2% of all thoracic tumors.[42,43] There is no clear association with smoking. Carcinoid tumors have been histologically subclassified into typical (more common) and atypical types.[39,42] Atypical tumors have greater mitotic activity and necrosis.

Patients with typical bronchial carcinoids usually present in the fifth decade of life, whereas those with atypical carcinoids present later.[39,42] The majority of carcinoid tumors are central or perihilar in location. Patient often present with symptoms related to bronchial obstruction (*eg*, recurrent pneumonias or wheezing) or vascularity of the tumor (*eg*, hemoptysis).[43] Bronchial carcinoids are occasionally associated carcinoid syndrome caused by release of serotonin and other vasoactive substances into the systemic circulation.[43] Rarely, biopsy or manipulation of a bronchial carcinoid results in acute carcinoid syndrome. Bronchial carcinoids can also cause Cushing syndrome and acromegaly as a result of the ectopic production of adrenocorticotrophic hormone and growth hormone-releasing factor, respectively.[42,43]

Radiologically, bronchial carcinoids may manifest obstructive pneumonia, discrete ovoid hilar mass or, occasionally, a peripheral nodule. CT helps identify the location and extent of the tumor as well as the presence or absence of mediastinal lymphadenopathy. MRI appears to be more sensitive than CT in detecting hepatic metastases (the most common metastatic site). Somatostatin receptor scintigraphy using a radiolabeled somatostatin analog such as ^{111}In-octreotide can sometimes be helpful in localizing the primary tumor and in staging.[43]

Carcinoids are generally attached to the bronchus by a broad base but can be polypoid and create a ball-valve effect. Caution should be used in biopsy of these vascular tumors (typically pink to red mass). Typical carcinoid tumors are usually indolent in behavior, and hilar/mediastinal nodal metastases are uncommon.[42,43] However, atypical carcinoids have an aggressive course, and metastasis to mediastinal lymph nodes are seen in 20 to 60% of cases. Atypical carcinoids are associated with a greater recurrence rate compared with the typical type. The 5-year survival rate associated with atypical carcinoid is 40 to 60%, compared with 85 to 100% for the typical carcioid.[42,44]

Surgical resection of the tumor with complete mediastinal lymphadenectomy is the treatment of choice for localized bronchial carcinoid tumors.[42,43] Surgical resection of liver metastases may be of benefit in patients with limited hepatic disease.[43] Hepatic artery occlusion or embolization is an option for patients who are not candidates for hepatic resection.[43]

Octreotide, a somatostatin analog, and interferon are used in the treatment of metastatic carcinoid tumors.[42] Cytotoxic chemotherapy has had a limited therapeutic effect.[43] Radiolabeled somatostatin analogs and biological agents targeting the vascular endothelial growth factor pathway are being investigated.[42]

Salivary Gland-Type Carcinomas

Mucoepidermoid carcinoma and adenoid cystic carcinoma are the most common forms of salivary gland-type carcinomas that can occur in the thorax, accounting for 0.1 to 0.2% of all thoracic tumors.[45] Both are considered low-grade malignancies, and lymph node spread is rare to uncommon. Neither tumor has a clear association with smoking.

Mucoepidermoid carcinoma is derived from minor salivary gland tissue in the proximal tracheobronchial tree.[46] This tumor usually appears as an endobronchial mass in the trachea or major bronchi.[45,46] Histologically, mucoepidermoid carcinoma consists of three components: mucus-secreting, squamous, and intermediate cells.[46] Pulmonary mucoepidermoid carcinoma occurs in a wide range of patients, from children to elderly. Patients usually present with cough, hemoptysis, wheezing, or obstructive pneumonia. CT may identify an endobronchial lesion or findings of obstructive pneumonia. Surgical resection is the treatment of choice and complete resection portends an excellent prognosis.

Adenoid cystic carcinomas (previously called cylindroma) also arise in the trachea or a major bronchus in most cases. It occurs in adults, most commonly in the fifth decade of life.[45,47] Dyspnea, cough wheeze, and hemoptysis are the most common presenting symptoms. Surgical resection is the treatment of choice; however, this tumor has a propensity to recur locally and metastasize.[45,47] Late recurrence as long as 15 to 20 years after initial resection has been reported. Median survival after resection is approximately 6 years.[45,47] Radiation and palliative laser therapy are used for unresectable tumors.

Hamartoma

Hamartoma is defined as a benign tumor-like malformation that is composed of abnormal and disorganized mixture of tissue elements. Pulmonary hamartoma typically consists of a combination of cartilage, connective tissue, smooth muscle, fat, and respiratory epithelium.[48] Hamartoma is the most common benign neoplasm to occur in the lung, accounting for approximately 75% of all benign lung tumors and 4% of solitary pulmonary nodules.[48]

Pulmonary hamartomas occur in all patient age groups; the greatest incidence is in the fourth to seventh decades of life.[48,49] The majority of pulmonary hamartomas are located in the periphery of the lung and are not associated with symptoms.[48,49] Radiologically, hamartoma appears as a solitary, round, or lobulated opacity with smooth margins, generally measuring 1 to 3 cm in size. Calcification is detected in approximately 25% of hamartomas, appearing as small flecks throughout the lesion; the classic appearance of "popcorn" calcification is infrequent. Areas of fat density are seen by CT in up to one half of cases. Hamartomas grow slowly, if at all. Diagnostic confirmation, if needed, requires tissue diagnosis that can be obtained by transthoracic needle aspiration biopsy, bronchoscopy, or thoracoscopy.

References

1. Aquino SL, Duncan G, Taber KH, et al. Reconciliation of the anatomic, surgical, and radiographic classifications of the mediastinum. J Computr Assist Tomogr 2001; 25:489–492
2. Thompson BH, Stanford W. MR imaging of pulmonary and mediastinal malignancies. Magn Reson Imaging Clin N Am 2000; 8:729–739
3. Duwe BV, Sterman DH, Musani AI. Tumors of the mediastinum. Chest 2005; 128:2893–2909
4. Suster S. Diagnosis of thymoma. J Clin Pathol 2006; 59:1238–1244
5. Thomas CR, Wright CD, Loehrer PJ. Thymoma: state of the art. J Clin Oncol 1999; 17:2280–2289
6. Casey EM, Kiel PJ, Loehrer PJ Sr. Clinical management of thymoma patients. Hematol-Oncol Clin N Am 2008; 22:457–473
7. Tormoehlen LM, Pascuzzi RM. Thymoma, myasthenia gravis, and other paraneoplastic syndromes. Hematol-Oncol Clin N Am 2008; 22:509–526
8. Wright CD, Kessler KA. Surgical treatment of thymic tumors. Semin Thorac Cardiovasc Surg 2005; 17:20–26
9. Moran CA, Suster S. Thymic carcinoma: current concepts and histologic features. Hematol-Oncol Clin N Am 2008; 22:393–407
10. Eng TY, Fuller CD, Jagirdar J, et al. Thymic carcinoma: state of the art review. Int J Radiat Oncol Biol Phys 2004; 59:654–664
11. Detterbeck FC, Parsons AM. Thymic tumors. Ann Thorac Surg 2004; 77:1860–1869
12. Strollo DC, Rosado-de-Christenson ML. Tumors of the thymus. J Thorac Imaging 1999; 14:152–171
13. Jemal A, Siegel R, Ward E, et al. Cancer statistics, 2008. CA Cancer J Clin 2008; 58:71–96
14. Ryu J, Habermann T. Pulmonary lymphoma: primary and systemic disease. Semin Respir Crit Care Med 1997; 18:341–352
15. Sharma A, Fidias P, Hayman LA, et al. Patterns of lymphadenopathy in thoracic malignancies. Radiographics 2004; 24:419–434
16. Wood DE. Mediastinal germ cell tumors. Semin Thorac Cardiovasc Surg 2000; 12:278–289
17. Strollo DC, Rosado-de-Christenson ML. Primary mediastinal malignant germ cell neoplasms: imaging features. Chest Surg Clin N Am 2002; 12:645–658
18. Takeda S, Miyoshi S, Ohta M, et al. Primary germ cell tumors in the mediastinum: a 50-year experience at a single Japanese institution. Cancer 2003; 97:367–376
19. Strollo DC, Rosado de Christenson ML, Jett JR. Primary mediastinal tumors. Part 1: tumors of the anterior mediastinum. Chest 1997; 112:511–522
20. de Perrot M, Fadel E, Mercier O, et al. Surgical management of mediastinal goiters: when is a

sternotomy required? Thorac Cardiovasc Surg 2007; 55:39–43
21. Netterville JL, Coleman SC, Smith JC, et al. Management of substernal goiter. Laryngoscope 1998; 108:1611–1617
22. Zambudio AR, Lanzas JT, Calvo MJR, et al. Nonneoplastic mediastinal cysts. Eur J Cardiothorac Surg 2002; 22:712–716
23. Jeung M-Y, Gasser B, Gangi A, et al. Imaging of cystic masses of the mediastinum. Radiographics 2002; 22:S79–S93
24. Cioffi U, Bonavina L, De Simone M, et al. Presentation and surgical management of bronchogenic and esophageal duplication cysts in adults. Chest 1998; 113:1492–1496
25. Patel SR, Meeker DP, Biscotti CV, et al. Presentation and management of bronchogenic cysts in the adult. Chest 1994; 106:79–85
26. Patel J, Park C, Michaels J, et al. Pericardial cyst: case reports and a literature review. Echocardiography 2004; 21:269–272
27. Faul JL, Berry GJ, Colby TV, et al. Thoracic lymphangiomas, lymphangiectasis, lymphangiomatosis, and lymphatic dysplasia syndrome. Am J Respir Crit Care Med 2000; 161:1037–1046
28. Park JG, Aubry M-C, Godfrey JA, et al. Mediastinal lymphangioma: Mayo Clinic experience of 25 cases. Mayo Clin Proc 2006; 81:1197–1203
29. Nguyen KQ, Hoeffel C, Le LH, et al. Mediastinal lipomatosis. South Med J 1998; 91:1169–1172
30. Reeder LB. Neurogenic tumors of the mediastinum. Semin Thorac Cardiovasc Surg 2000; 12:261–267
31. Shadmehr MB, Gaissert HA, Wain JC, et al. The surgical approach to "dumbbell tumors" of the mediastinum. Ann Thorac Surg 2003; 76:1650–1654
32. Wright CD, Mathisen DJ. Mediastinal tumors: diagnosis and treatment. World J Surg 2001; 25:204–209
33. Suster S, Moran CA. Neuroendocrine neoplasms of the mediastinum. Am J Clin Pathol 2001; 115(suppl):S17–27
34. Young WF Jr. Paragangliomas: clinical overview. Ann New York Acad Sci 2006; 1073:21–29
35. Chen KM, Bird L, Barnes P, et al. Lateral meningocele syndrome: vertical transmission and expansion of the phenotype. Am J Med Genet 2005; 133A:115–121
36. Koch CA, Li C-Y, Mesa RA, et al. Nonhepatosplenic extramedullary hematopoiesis: associated diseases, pathology, clinical course, and treatment. Mayo Clin Proc 2003; 78:1223–1233
37. Berkmen YM, Zalta BA. Case 126: extramedullary hematopoiesis. Radiology 2007; 245:905–908
38. Dool JJ, de Bree R, van den Berg R, et al. Thoracic duct cyst: sclerotherapy as alternative for surgical treatment. Head Neck 2007; 29:292–295
39. Brambilla E, Travis WD, Colby TV, et al. The new World Health Organization classification of lung tumours. Eur Respir J 2001; 18:1059–1068
40. Chan AL, Shelton DK, Yoneda KY. Unusual primary lung neoplasms. Curr Opin Pulm Med 2001; 7:234–241
41. Gimenez A, Franquet T, Prats R, et al. Unusual primary lung tumors: a radiologic-pathologic overview. Radiographics 2002; 22:601–619
42. Kulke MH. Clinical presentation and management of carcinoid tumors. Hematol-Oncol Clin N Am 2007; 21:433–455; vii-viii
43. Gustafsson BI, Kidd M, Chan A, et al. Bronchopulmonary neuroendocrine tumors. Cancer 2008; 113:5–21
44. Thomas CF Jr., Tazelaar HD, Jett JR. Typical and atypical pulmonary carcinoids: outcome in patients presenting with regional lymph node involvement. Chest 2001; 119:1143–1150
45. Molina JR, Aubry MC, Lewis JE, et al. Primary salivary gland-type lung cancer: spectrum of clinical presentation, histopathologic and prognostic factors. Cancer 2007; 110:2253–2259
46. Liu X, Adams AL. Mucoepidermoid carcinoma of the bronchus: a review. Arch Pathol Lab Med 2007; 131:1400–1404
47. Gaissert HA, Grillo HC, Shadmehr MB, et al. Long-term survival after resection of primary adenoid cystic and squamous cell carcinoma of the trachea and carina. Ann Thorac Surg 2004; 78:1889–1896; discussion 1896–1887
48. Whyte RI, Donington JS. Hamartomas of the lung. Semin Thorac Cardiovasc Surg 2003; 15:301–304
49. Gjevre JA, Myers JL, Prakash UB. Pulmonary hamartomas. Mayo Clin Proc 1996; 71:14–20

Notes

Pathology of Airway Disease and Organizing Pneumonia

Henry D. Tazelaar, MD, FCCP

Objectives:

- Review the morphologic characteristics of COPD
- Summarize the pathology of disease affecting small and large airways
- Review the histopathologic features of asthma
- Review the complex constellation of histologic abnormalities in patients with allergic bronchopulmonary fungal disease, including bronchocentric granulomatosis, and mucoid impaction of bronchi
- Review and contrast the histologic characteristics of organizing pneumonia and constrictive (obliterative) bronchiolitis

Key words: allergic bronchopulmonary fungal disease; obstructive airway disease; obliterative bronchiolitis; organizing pneumonia; pathology

Obstructive Pulmonary Disease

Emphysema

Emphysema is defined as "a condition of the lung characterized by abnormal, permanent enlargement of airspaces distal to the terminal bronchiole, accompanied by destruction of their walls, and without obvious fibrosis." [1] Four major types of emphysema are found in four different clinical settings[2]:

Centriacinar:

- Most common form of emphysema.
- Most common correlate of severe airflow obstruction in smokers.[3]
- Also seen in coal workers, *ie*, simple coal worker's pneumonoconiosis.
- Upper lobes most often are affected.
- Destruction of alveoli affects the alveoli immediately adjacent to second- and third-order respiratory bronchioles. Lung at the periphery of the lobule appears normal.
- In severe cases, there is overlap with panacinar.

Panacinar:

- α_1-Protease inhibitor deficiency (ZZ), IV drug abuse, Ritalin, Swyer-James syndrome, aging lung.
- Involves destruction of entire acinus.
- Lower lobes most affected initially.

Distal Acinar:

- Least common form of emphysema.
- Not usually associated with airflow obstruction.
- Acini adjacent to pleura and interlobular septa most destroyed.
- Upper lobes most often involved.
- May contribute to spontaneous pneumothoraces and bullae formation in tall, asthenic male adolescents.

Paracicatricial Airspace Enlargement (So-Called Irregular or "Scar" Emphysema):

- Airspace enlargement next to foci of fibrosis.
- May not have clinical correlate depending on underlying disease, *eg*, Langerhans' cell histiocytosis.

Blebs and Bullae

- *Bleb*: Air within the visceral pleural layers, so a form of interstitial "emphysema." (The term *emphysema* really being a misnomer here by the aforementioned definition.)[4]
- *Bullae:* Emphysematous space >1 cm in diameter in the distended state.[4]

Chronic Bronchitis

The clinical definition of chronic bronchitis is productive cough of unknown cause occurring on most days for ≥3 or more months for at least 2 successive years. The pathologic definition usually refers to a nonspecific combination of goblet-cell metaplasia of bronchial luminal lining cells, thick ened basement membrane, submucosal gland hyperplasia, smooth muscle hypertrophy, and chronic inflammation.

Obviously, pathology is not the way to make the diagnosis! The Reid index is used to measure the thickness of mucous gland layer/thickness of bronchial wall (normal <0.4). The submucosal gland hyperplasia appears to contribute the most to mucus hypersecretion, but goblet cell metaplasia likely also contributes. The pathogenesis of chronic bronchitis appears related to inflammatory mechanisms in which neutrophils appear to play a key role.[5]

Significance of Small Airways and Obstructive Lung Disease

Small airways *disease* probably is a term that should be abandoned, as it has meant many different things since it was first introduced and does not refer to a specific disease.[4] The thickness of small airways in patients who smoke (caused by fibrosis, inflammation, and mucus), however, does appear to correlate with emphysema.[6]

Asthma

As with chronic bronchitis, pathology is not diagnostic in patients with asthma.[4] However, there are characteristic macroscopic and microscopic findings. Macroscopic findings in patients dying of status asthmaticus are mucous plugging of airways, air trapping; in late/longstanding disease: saccular bronchiectasis, especially in the upper lobe.

Microscopic findings include thickened basement membranes; intraluminal mucous plugs with Charcot–Leyden crystals; Curschmann spirals (*ie*, coiled mucus plugs); creola bodies (*ie*, small groups of shed epithelial cells); goblet-cell metaplasia; submucosal gland hyperplasia; inflammation, including eosinophils, mast cells, and mononuclear cells; and smooth-muscle hypertrophy.

Miscellaneous Diseases Affecting Large and Small Airways

Allergic Bronchopulmonary Fungal Disease

Allergic bronchopulmonary fungal disease syndrome affects asthmatic patients and patients with cystic fibrosis and results from an allergic reaction to fungi. Although Aspergillus sp are the most notorious fungi to cause this allergic phenomenon (allergic bronchopulmonary aspergillosis), multiple other fungi can cause the disease. Diagnostic criteria include the presence of six, including the first five, of the following[7,8]:

- History of asthma or cystic fibrosis (10 to 15% of cases);
- Immediate skin reactivity to fungal (usually Aspergillus sp) extract;
- Precipitating antibodies to fungi (usually Aspergillus sp);
- Elevated total serum IgE (>1,000 ng/mL);
- Elevated IgE and/or IgG to fungi, usually *Aspergillus fumigatus* antigens;
- Central bronchiectasis;
- Recurrent pulmonary infiltrates;
- Peripheral eosinophilia (>500 μL).

Pathology includes a complex constellation of findings in various combinations: bronchiectasis, mucoid impaction of bronchi, bronchocentric granulomatosis (BCG), eosinophilic bronchiolitis, chronic eosinophilic pneumonia, bronchiectasis, and mucoid impaction of bronchi.[4,9] Macroscopic findings include dilated large airways filled with tenacious mucous plugs and casts of variable color from green–grey to yellow–white. Microscopic findings include lamellated mucus as seen in other allergic syndromes such as allergic fungal sinusitis rich in eosinophils in various stages of degeneration and Charcot–Leyden crystals, rare degenerating fungal hyphae (*ie*, not as many as one would see in an infection), and bronchocentric granulomatosis, which are extremely rare (most cases of possible BCG are not BCG but true infection).

In BCG, bronchioles appear replaced by necrotizing granulomas centrally located within the airway. Fungal hyphae may be identified in the necrotizing granuloma, but they should be rare and noninvasive. Airways adjacent to those with BCG may contain an exudate not unlike that described previously in the context of mucoid impaction of bronchi.

Acute Bronchiolitis

There are many causes of acute bronchitis,[9] most significantly infection and aspiration (may be associated with foreign material, *eg*, food). The pathology includes ulceration of mucosa, inflammation, usually including neutrophils, and intraluminal exudate.

Chronic Bronchiolitis

Chronic bronchiolitis[10] is a nonspecific pathologic term used to describe the presence of chronic inflammation and/or fibrosis around and in wall of bronchiole and the presence of peribronchiolar metaplasia. Usually, it is part of the spectrum of pathology found in a variety of primary airway diseases and as a component of many classically "interstitial" diseases, *eg*, extrinsic allergic alveolitis.

Respiratory (Smokers') Bronchiolitis

Respiratory bronchiolitis is an incidental finding in smokers.[11] It may be responsible for asymptomatic small nodules on imaging in smokers and is defined as the presence of pigmented macrophages within respiratory bronchioles and surrounding alveoli. Mild chronic inflammation and fibrosis of bronchiole may be found. Histology is the same as in respiratory bronchiolitis-interstitial lung disease.

Follicular Bronchiolitis

Follicular bronchiolitis[12] is a form of lymphoid hyperplasia associated with connective tissues diseases (especially Sjögren syndrome and rheumatoid arthritis) and immunodeficiencies. It is described as chronic inflammation with germinal centers around bronchioles.

Diffuse Panbronchiolitis

Diffuse panbronchiolitis is a form of bronchiolitis associated with sinusitis. Predominantly seen in Japanese adults, it is associated with human leukocyte antigen BW54. Macroscopic findings include bronchiectasis and hyperinflation. Microscopic findings are not entirely specific but include acute and chronic inflammation of respiratory bronchioles, follicular bronchiolitis, interstitial foamy macrophages, and intraluminal exudate containing neutrophils.

Constrictive (Obliterative) Bronchiolitis

This entity can be found in multiple clinical settings, including lung transplantation (chronic rejection), bone marrow transplantation (graft vs host disease), drug toxicity, connective tissue disease, and idiopathic disease. Common exposures include diacetyl (popcorn worker's lung), sulfur mustard gas, and infection (*eg*, postadenoviral). Pathology includes bronchiolar and peribronchiolar fibrosis with narrowing and eventual obliteration of the lumen. Constrictive bronchiolitis may be preceded by acute and chronic bronchiolitis, but histology is similar regardless of etiology.

Organizing Pneumonia (Bronchiolitis Obliterans Organizing Pneumonia)

Organizing pneumonia (OP)[13,14] is a myxoid-appearing intraluminal (alveolar, alveolar duct, and terminal and respiratory bronchioles) fibroblastic proliferation ("fibrosis") associated with mild chronic interstitial inflammation. The term *OP* is now preferred over *bronchiolitis obliterans organizing pneumonia* (BOOP) because the bronchiolitis obliterans component (which could be called *proliferative* obliterative bronchiolitis) is often difficult to appreciate pathologically[47] and because it is rare for patients to present with "bronchiolitis."

OP may appear in clinical settings or as a histologic component of the following: idiopathic (cryptogenic OP); connective tissue disease; drug reaction (*eg*, bleomycin, amiodarone); resolving bacterial and viral infection; extrinsic allergic alveolitis; nonspecific interstitial pneumonia (may be seen focally in 50% of cases); radiation; reaction to tumor; infarct; Wegener granulomatosis; and chronic eosinophilic pneumonia.

Pathology is the same regardless of clinical category: polypoid plugs of proliferating fibroblasts in alveoli and alveolar ducts (strictly speaking, this would have constituted the OP of BOOP) and terminal respiratory bronchioles (the BO of BOOP), mild interstitial pneumonia confined to areas of organization, intra-alveolar foamy macrophages (from a failure to clear secretions as the result of small airway obstruction), and no collagen (dense) fibrosis.

Relationship Between Proliferative Obliterative Bronchiolitis in OP and Constrictive Obliterative Bronchiolitis

The exact relationship between the two diseases is uncertain. In most cases, they appear to be separate and distinct entities with different clinical, radiographic, and morphologic features.

In certain circumstances, such as lung transplant recipients, silo filler's disease and, occasionally, rheumatoid arthritis, there is evidence to suggest that intraluminal organization localized to membranous and respiratory bronchioles can cause obstructive airways disease and can "progress" to a lesion that is indistinguishable from the late stage of constrictive bronchiolitis.

[Note to participants regarding references: There are some primary sources quoted, but the textbooks have additional photographs worth studying.]

References

1. Snider G, Keinerman J, Thurlbeck W. The definition of emphysema. Report of a National Heart, Lung, and Blood Institute, Division of Lung Diseases workshop. Am Rev Respir Dis 1985; 132:182–185
2. Travis W, Colby TV, Koss MN, et al. Non-neoplastic disorders of the lower respiratory tract. In: Atlas of nontumor pathology. Washington, DC: American Registry of Pathology and the Armed Forces Institute of Pathology, 2002
3. West W, Nagai A, Hodgkin JE, et al. The National Institutes of Health Intermittent Positive Pressure Breathing trial—pathology studies. III. The diagnosis of emphysema. Am Rev Respir Dis 1987; 135:123–129
4. Churg A, Myers J, Tazelaar H, et al. Thurlbeck's pathology of the lung. 3rd ed. New York, NY: Thieme Medical Publishers, 2005
5. Barnes P. Chronic obstructive pulmonary disease. N Engl J Med 2000; 343:269–280
6. Hogg J, Chu F, Utokaparch S, et al. The nature of small-airway obstruction in chronic obstructive pulmonary disease. N Engl J Med 2004; 350:2645–2653
7. Greenberger PA, Patterson R. Diagnosis and management of allergic bronchopulmonary aspergillosis. Ann Allergy 1986; 56:444–448
8. Cockrill BA, Hales CA. Allergic bronchopulmonary aspergillosis. Annu Rev Med 1999; 50:303–316
9. Leslie KO, Wick MR. Practical pulmonary pathology: a diagnostic approach. Philadelphia, PA: Churchill Livingstone, 2005; 813
10. Visscher D, Myers J. Bronchiolitis: the pathologist's perspective. Proc Am Thorac Soc 2006; 3:41–47
11. Fraig M, Shreesha U, Savici D, et al. Respiratory bronchiolitis: a clinicopathologic study in current smokers, ex-smokers, and never-smokers. Am J Surg Pathol 2002; 26:647–653
12. Aerni MR, Vassallo R, Myers JL, et al. Follicular bronchiolitis in surgical lung biopsies: clinical implications in 12 patients. Respir Med 2008; 102:307–312
13. Katzenstein A, Askin F. Surgical pathology of nonneoplastic lung disease. 4th ed. Philadelphia, PA: W.B. Saunders, 2006; 503
14. Elicker B, Pereira CA, Webb R, et al. High-resolution computed tomography patterns of diffuse interstitial lung disease with clinical and pathological correlation. J Bras Pneumol 2008; 34: 715–744

Pathology of Diffuse and Neoplastic Disease

Henry D. Tazelaar, MD, FCCP

Objectives:

- Review morphologic characteristics and potential etiologies of diffuse alveolar damage
- Review and contrast morphologic characteristics of the "idiopathic" interstitial pneumonias
- Review histopathologic features of diffuse lung disease with specific histologic features, including Langerhans cell histiocytosis, hypersensitivity pneumonia, sarcoidosis, lymphangioleiomyomatosis, pulmonary alveolar proteinosis, Wegener granulomatosis, hot tub lung, and pulmonary rejection
- Review certain infectious pathogens that can be identified on the basis of their morphologic characteristics in tissue sections
- Discuss the morphology of neuroendocrine tumors and other lung cancers

Key words: granulomatous disease; infection; interstitial lung disease; neoplasia; transplant

Diffuse Lung Disease

Diffuse Alveolar Damage/Acute Interstitial Pneumonia

Diffuse alveolar damage (DAD) is the most common pathologic correlate of ARDS.[1,2] Causes include pulmonary edema; septic shock; oxygen toxicity; drugs; radiation; infection (influenza; *Pneumocystis carinii* pneumonia); and trauma. DAD is associated with connective tissue disease *eg*, acute lupus pneumonitis, and its idiopathic variant is represented by acute interstitial pneumonia and Hamman-Rich syndrome.[3,4]

Microscopic Pathology:

- The disease is temporally uniform (homogenous); microscopically, the lungs look the same from field to field. There are two phases: acute and organizing (often overlapping caused by attempted repair at the same time there is ongoing injury). Acute (exudative) includes interstitial edema, type I pneumocyte sloughing, and the formation of hyaline membranes; organizing includes proliferating/reactive type II pneumocytes and interstitial fibroblasts with focal airspace organization. (These areas may look like typical organizing pneumonia.) Acute and organizing thrombi within vessels are common. Metaplastic bronchiolar epithelium may be *very* atypical and mimic carcinoma.

Differential Diagnosis:

- Cryptogenic organizing pneumonia;
  More subacute course;
  Process is patchy around bronchioles;
  Hyaline membranes are not seen; and
  Organization is only intraalveolar and intraluminal, not interstitial.

"Idiopathic" Interstitial Pneumonias

Idiopathic interstitial pneumonias comprise a heterogeneous group of pneumonias with acute, *eg*, acute interstitial pneumonia, and more chronic presentations. The American Thoracic Society/European Respiratory Society endorses the classification scheme shown in Table 1.[4] Although causes for other interstitial pneumonias are not always known, *eg*, sarcoidosis, the idiopathic interstitial pneumonias are characterized histologically by varying combinations of interstitial fibrosis, organization, and chronic inflammation in both or either the interstitium and alveolar spaces *without* the presence of granulomas or specific cell types, *eg*, Langerhans cells.

Usual Interstitial Pneumonia

Clinical findings of usual interstitial pneumonia (UIP)[5–7]: idiopathic disease = clinical diagnosis of idiopathic pulmonary fibrosis (IPF).

- Common in connective tissue disease, as a manifestation of drug reaction and rarely as manifestation of chronic hypersensitivity pneumonitis.[8] Gross findings include lower lobe and peripheral predominant fibrosis and a

Table 1. *Clinical and Pathologic Classification of Idiopathic Interstitial Pneumonias**†

Clinical Diagnosis	Pathologic Pattern
AIP, Hamman-rich disease idiopathic diffuse alveolar damage	DAD
IPF, cryptogenic fibrosing alveolitis	UIP
DIP	Desquamative interstitial pneumonia
RB-ILD	Respiratory bronchiolitis
Nonspecific interstitial pneumonia	Nonspecific interstitial pneumonia: cellular and fibrotic variants
Cryptogenic organizing pneumonia (formerly idiopathic bronchiolitis obliterans organizing pneumonia)	Organizing pneumonia
Lymphocytic interstitial pneumonia	Lymphocytic interstitial pneumonia

*The American Thoracic Society/European Respiratory Society endorses some separate terms to describe the disease clinically and pathologically because some pathologic patterns may be associated with known disease, *ie*, they are not idiopathic, *eg*, usual interstitial pneumonia occurring in the setting of rheumatoid arthritis is still UIP, but it is not IPF.
†From ATS/ERS.[4]

honeycomb appearance. Microscopic findings include the following:

Geographic heterogeneity: looks different from field to field, *eg*, variegated fibrosis worse in subpleural and paraseptal regions. Areas of normal lung (usually centrilobular) are found between areas of fibrosis.

Temporal heterogeneity (refers to type of "fibrosis"): dense collagen and fibromyxoid fibroblastic foci (look similar to small flat areas of organizing pneumonia) are observed.

Inflammatory infiltrate usually consists of chronic inflammatory cells. Germinal centers and dense lymphoid infiltrates are associated with UIP in connective tissue diseases, *eg*, rheumatoid arthritis.[9] A total of 70% of patients are smokers; therefore, pigmented alveolar macrophages, as seen in *respiratory bronchiolitis* (RB) and *desquamative interstitial pneumonia* (DIP), are common.

Honeycomb changes are most advanced at the bases and periphery.

Work by some investigators[10,11] but not all[12] has shown a correlation between survival and the number of "fibroblast foci," a finding that suggests the critical pathway to end-stage fibrosis is not "alveolitis" (as has been supposed for many years) but ongoing epithelial damage and repair.

Differential Diagnosis: (1) DIP (also see Table 2) diffuse macrophage accumulation and temporally uniform; (2) cryptogenic organizing pneumonia; injury is temporally uniform, areas of recent organization are more pronounced and intraalveolar, and areas of dense collagen deposition are absent;

Table 2. *Idiopathic Interstitial Pneumonias: Contrasting Pathologic Features*

Variables	NSIP	UIP	DIP/RB-ILD	AIP
Temporal appearance	Uniform	Variegated	Uniform	Uniform
Inflammation	Prominent	Patchy	Scant	Scant
Collagen	Patchy fibrosis	Prominent	Patchy (none to minimal in RB-ILD)	Minimal
Fibroblast proliferation	No	Typical	Rare	Late
Organizing pneumonia-like foci, %	50	No	No	Focal
Honeycomb change	No	Yes	No	Rare
Intraalveolar macrophages	Focal	Focal	Diffuse (DIP), patchy (RB-ILD)	No
Hyaline membranes	No; in "accelerated" form	No	No	Focal

(3) nonspecific interstitial pneumonia; fibrosis is geographically and temporally more uniform; (4) accelerated idiopathic pulmonary fibrosis; foci of diffuse alveolar damage are present.[13–15]

Accelerated Idiopathic Pulmonary Fibrosis[13–15]

Underlying UIP can be recognized clinically (previous history of slowly progressive interstitial fibrosis with characteristic features of IPF), radiographically, and/or on the basis of findings at the time of surgical lung biopsy. Wedge lung biopsy will show underlying UIP with DAD or, likely as the result of sampling, either just DAD or just UIP. In some cases, only organizing pneumonia is seen.

Nonspecific Interstitial Pneumonia/Fibrosis

Findings for nonspecific interstitial pneumonia/fibrosis[16,17] include geographic homogeneity (looks same from field to field), fibrosis and interstitial thickening with inflammation, and is NOT variegated. Some cases lack fibrosis altogether. Fibrosis, when present, is not worse in subpleural and paraseptal regions, but uniform. Honeycomb appearance is absent, with rare exceptions. There is also temporal homogeneity: refers to type of fibrosis. Dense collagen may be present but, when present, is the only type present, and fibromyxoid fibroblastic foci are absent, with rare exceptions.

DIP

DIP[18,19] is closely related to respiratory bronchiolitis-interstitial lung disease (RB-ILD; see next section). A total of ~90% of patients are cigarette smokers. DIP is much more uniform at low magnification and lacks the variegated appearance of UIP. Alveolar septa are thickened by an inflammatory infiltrate that often includes mononuclear cells and occasional germinal centers. The most striking (and definitional) feature is the presence of numerous lightly pigmented macrophages within most of the distal air spaces. Collagen fibrosis occurs and may be associated with a honeycomb appearance.

RB-ILD

RB-ILD[20–23] is a diagnosis of exclusion, as the histology of RB may be seen in any active or past smoker. Microscopic findings include RB (pigmented alveolar macrophages in and around respiratory bronchioles) and a lacks of significant fibrosis, interstitial inflammation, or germinal centers.

Differential Diagnosis: RB-ILD and DIP represent points along a spectrum, and some cases fall somewhere in between; therefore, their separation may not always be possible. Such cases may be diagnosed as smoking-related interstitial lung disease.

Lymphoid Interstitial Pneumonia

Lymphoid interstitial pneumonia (LIP)[24–26] is a distinct clinicopathologic syndrome that can occur in a variety of settings (Table 3). Microscopic findings include exquisitely interstitial and bronchovascular infiltrate of small lymphocytes and plasma cells. Immunophenotypic studies have demonstrated that T cells predominate in the alveolar septal infiltrates, whereas B lymphocytes predominate in the peribronchiolar zones with polyclonal plasma cells. Poorly formed non-necrotizing granulomas with multinucleated giant cells are present in a minority of cases. There is polyclonal light-chain expression in the plasma cell component in HIV and non-HIV–associated cases.

Table 3. *Clinical Features of Lymphocytic Interstitial Pneumonia*

Variables	HIV-Negative	HIV-Positive
Female/male ratio	2.2:1	
Mean age, yr	51	13 to 77
Symptoms, %		
Dyspnea	69	80
Cough	62	60
Fever	22	60
Weight loss	22	100
Adenopathy	>95	
Autoimmune diseases, %	Common	Uncommon
Sjögren syndrome	20	Yes
Mortality, %	>30	>75
Mean survival, mo	20	10.4

Langerhans Cell Histiocytosis

Microscopic findings of Langerhans cell histiocytosis[1,3,5] include (1) bronchiolocentric nodular to stellate lesions; (2) variable fibrosis; and (3) a diagnostic cell, *ie*, Langerhans cell with convoluted nuclei (kidney-bean shaped, grooved, resemble buttocks). They usually are admixed with some eosinophils and smoker's macrophages. Immunohistochemical findings include S100 protein+, CDla+, Langerin+, HLR-DR+. On electron microscopy, Birbeck granules (pentilaminar structure with a "tennis racket" morphology) appear. "Cystic" change is seen radiographically: Langerhans cell histiocytosis results from dilated bronchioles, paracicatricial airspace enlargement (so-called scar emphysema), and necrosis in the center of the lesions. As lesions age, they become less cellular and more fibrotic and may be confused with the chronic interstitial pneumonias. The process appears to start as a polyclonal one, but clonality may develop.[27]

Hypersensitivity Pneumonitis/Extrinsic Allergic Alveolitis

Microscopic findings of hypersensitivity pneumonitis/extrinsic allergic alveolitis[1,3,5] include a classic triad (seen in ~80% of patients who undergo biopsy with a clinical diagnosis): (1) Cellular interstitial pneumonia composed mainly of lymphocytes, plasma cells, and macrophages occasionally admixed with eosinophils (only 10% of cases) and neutrophils; (2) chronic bronchiolitis with organizing pneumonia; and (3) vague poorly formed nonnecrotizing granulomas or giant cells. Fibrosis may develop and be indistinguishable from UIP.[28] well-proven cases clinically have been reported to resemble nonspecific interstitial pneumonia, cryptogenic organizing pneumonia, and UIP.[8,29]

Hot Tub Lung

Hot tub lung[30–32] may represent an infection or a hypersensitivity reaction to *Mycobacterium avium-intracellulare* organisms. Microscopic findings include non-necrotizing granulomatous inflammation (although the granulomas often are larger and more exuberant than those seen in classic hypersensitivity pneumonitis) and patchy, chronic interstitial pneumonia that resembles that found in hypersensitivity pneumonitis.

Sarcoidosis

The diagnosis of sarcoidosis[1,3,5] usually requires the pathologic presence of granulomatous inflammation. Transbronchial biopsy has become the method of choice and can be expected to yield a diagnosis in nearly 80% of patients, including 70% with stage 1 disease. The likelihood of obtaining a diagnostic biopsy is related to the number of specimens obtained, and the best results require a minimum of 4 specimens in patients with stage 2 or 3 disease and as many as 10 in patients with stage 1 disease.

Microscopic findings (berylliosis looks identical):

- Granulomatous inflammation without bronchiolitis or cellular interstitial pneumonia;
- Granulomas;
  - Compact, well-circumscribed collections of epithelioid histiocytes and multinucleated giant cells surrounded by a rim of lymphocytes and collagen fibrosis;
  - Central necrosis (~20% of cases);
  - Distribution along lymphatic routes (bronchovascular bundles, interlobular septa, and visceral pleura);
- Multinucleated giant cells may contain a variety of cytoplasmic inclusions which should not be confused with foreign material (however, these are not specific for sarcoid);
  - Schaumann (conchoidal) bodies (blue, calcified);
  - Asteroid bodies: star-shaped protein;
  - Sheet-like and needle-shaped birefringent crystalline inclusions (often endogenous calcium oxalate);
- Granulomatous vasculitis (~70% of cases);
- Nodular sarcoidosis (coalescence of the granulomas combined with dense collagen fibrosis);
- Necrotizing sarcoidosis-sarcoid background of lymphangitic nonnecrotizing granulomatous inflammation associated with broad foci of parenchymal necrosis and vasculitis.

Table 4. *Differential Diagnosis of Diffuse Lung Disease With Small Granulomas**

	Hypersensitivity Pneumonitis	Sarcoidosis	Hot Tub Lung
Interstitial pneumonia	+–+++	–	+
Chronic bronchiolitis	++–+++	–	++–+++
Granulomas			
Well formed	+–+++	+++	+++
Single giant cells	+–++	–	–
Necrosis	–	+	+
Organizing pneumonia	+–++	–	+–++
Cultures	–	–	*Mycobacterium avium intracellulare*

*+ = rare; ++ = occasional; +++ = prominent feature.

Differential diagnosis of disease with small granulomas is discussed in Table 4.

Pulmonary Alveolar Proteinosis

Pulmonary alveolar proteinosis (PAP)[1,3,5,33,34] is due to a defect in alveolar macrophage function caused by granulocyte/macrophage colony-stimulating factor antibodies. The etiologies of pulmonary alveolar proteinosis are listed in Table 5. Microscopic findings include the accumulation of granular eosinophilic material in alveoli (positive with stains for periodic acid Schiff), minimal (if any) interstitial pneumonia, and late fibrosis. Electron microscopy shows lamellar bodies of surfactant.

Lymphangioleiomyomatosis

The gross findings of lymphangioleiomyomatosis[1,3,5] include randomly distributed cystic airspaces with thin walls involving upper and lower lobes. The main pathology includes a disorderly proliferation of smooth muscle cells, cystic "emphysematous" spaces (common) that usually contain smooth-muscle bundles within at least a portion of their walls, and hemosiderin laden macrophages that may be present within air spaces as the result of pulmonary hemorrhage. Immunohistochemistry of smooth muscle cells is positive for HMB45, actin, desmin, melan A, and estrogen and progesterone receptor protein

Other pathology includes micronodular pneumocyte hyperplasia, or circumscribed proliferations of cytologically bland type 2 pneumocytes in a pattern resembling bronchioloalveolar adenocarcinoma.[35] Evidence suggests that lymphangioleiomyomatosis cells may either metastasize or develop from progenitor cells capable of migrating to the lung.[36]

Table 5. *Classification of PAP*

- Primary PAP
- Secondary PAP
  - Immunocompromised patients, hematologic disorders (polycythemia vera, leukemias, idiopathic thrombocytopenic purpura, multiple myeloma),
- AIDS
  - Infections, Nocardia, *Pneumocystis mycobacteria*
  - Environmental inhalants, dusts (silica, aluminum), toxins (solvents, insecticides, cleansers)
  - Neoplasms

Eosinophilic Pneumonia

There are two types of eosinophilic pneumonia, chronic and acute. Histologic feature of chronic eosinophilic pneumonia[1,3,5] are constant regardless of clinical context (Table 6). The major abnormality is filling of distal air spaces by a cellular exudate of eosinophils and histiocytes, including multinucleated giant cells. Relative proportions of the two cell types are variable, alveolar septa are thickened and contain a similar inflammatory infiltrate, and OP is a frequent associated finding.

Table 6. *Associations and Causes of Chronic Eosinophilic Pneumonia Pathology*

Allergic bronchopulmonary fungal disease
Simple pulmonary eosinophilia
Systemic infection (parasites, fungi)
Connective tissue disease, especially rheumatoid arthritis
Radiation (ipsilateral or contralateral)
Cigarette smoking, especially at initiation or with change of brands*
Drugs esp. salicylates, antibiotics†
Churg Strauss syndrome
Hodgkin lymphoma
Inflammatory bowel disease
Lung cancer

*From Uchiyama H, Suda T, Nakamura Y, et al. Alterations in smoking habits are associated with acute eosinophilic pneumonia. Chest 2008; 133:1174–1180.
†From Allen JN. Drug-induced eosinophilic lung disease. Clin Chest Med 2004; 25:77–88.

In acute eosinophilic pneumonia, there is diffuse alveolar damage with prominent tissue eosinophilia.[1,3,5]

Wegener Granulomatosis

Classic pathology includes the following:

- Necrotizing granulomatous inflammation with geographic borders (appears more like parenchymal necrosis than a true granuloma since the foci usually lack significant numbers of epithelioid histiocytes);
  - Centrally in foci of necrosis there is amorphous eosinophilic to basophilic debris with remnants of necrotic neutrophils and other inflammatory cells (so-called *dirty necrosis*);
  - Early lesions described as "palisading granulomas" and microabscesses;
    - Palisading granulomas are tiny granulomas composed of a single layer of palisading epithelioid histiocytes that either radiate around a central point or surround a central eosinophilic structure resembling a collagen bundle. As the palisaded granulomas enlarge, they become more microabscess-like;
- Necrotizing segmental (involving portion of the wall) vasculitis of arteries and veins; and
- Randomly dispersed, darkly staining multinucleated giant cells common variants.
- Common variants include: (1) presentation as a solitary pulmonary nodule limited to the lung; (2) hemorrhage with or without capillaritis (vasculitis involving capillaries recognized by presence of neutrophils in alveolar walls); (3) bronchocentric; (4) organizing pneumonia-like; and (5) eosinophilic pneumonia-like.
- c-ANCA titers are positive in approximately 90% of patients with active generalized disease, 60 to 85% of patients with active limited disease, and 30 to 35% of patients with quiescent disease. Positive p-antineutrophil cytoplasmic antibody titers generally representing autoantibodies directed against myeloperoxidase are less specific but have been reported to be positive in some patients with Wegener granulomatosis.

Pneumoconioses

Asbestos-related reactions (Table 7): the pneumoconioses[5,37] is "asbestosis." Macroscopically, firm, fibrotic lungs with areas of honeycomb change can be found, whereas microscopically, marked interstitial fibrosis with minimal inflammatory infiltrate are found, as well as UIP-like reactions. The presence of asbestos bodies, fibrosis, and exposure history are needed for a definitive diagnosis.

Asbestos bodies are iron-encrusted fibers (one type of ferruginous body, which is a more generic term) that typically are beaded and dumbbell shaped with a thin translucent core. There are no generally accepted criteria defining how many asbestos bodies must be identified in any given case for a diagnosis of asbestosis, but the presence of even a single asbestos body in a routine tissue section usually signifies "above-background" asbestos exposure.

Table 7. *Pulmonary Complications of Asbestos Exposure**

Pleural disease
Effusion
Fibrosis
Plaques
Pseudoneoplasms (rounded atelectasis)
Parenchymal lung disease
Asbestosis
Asbestos airways disease
Neoplasms
Malignant mesothelioma
Bronchogenic carcinoma (especially in cigarette smokers)

*From Churg and Green.[37]

Table 8. *Morphologic Classification of Silicosis*

Simple (nodular) silicosis
Silicotic nodules ≤1 cm
Upper lung zones
Complicated silicosis
Conglomerate nodules >1 cm
Upper and middle lung zones
Acute silicosis (silicoproteinosis)
Alveolar proteinosis
Silicotuberculosis

Silicosis

Gross findings of silicosis (Table 8) include firm, discrete, rounded lesions with variable amounts of black pigment and nodules in a lymphatic distribution (*ie*, around bronchovascular bundles, in subpleural and paraseptal areas).

Microscopic findings include:

- Discrete foci of concentric layers of hyalinized collagen;
  Abundant dust-filled histiocytes; and
  Birefringent particles (usually); often a mix of silica and silicates);

When necrosis is present, complication by tuberculosis should be considered. Nodules may expand and eventually coalesce to form larger masses; when these masses measure >1 cm in diameter, they are referred to as conglomerate nodules (complicated silicosis).

Pulmonary Infections

See Tables 9–12 for a listing of pulmonary infections.[1,5]

Pathology of Lung Transplantation[38, 39]

Primary graft failure in lung transplantation is described as the immediate deterioration of pulmonary function after successful revascularization of the graft. Diffuse alveolar damage is found microscopically in the most severe cases.

Rejection

The grading scheme is strictly pathologic and does not rely on clinical parameters (*eg*, for the diagnosis of obliterative bronchiolitis syndrome):

- Grade 0, negative for rejection: normal pulmonary parenchyma without evidence of mononuclear infiltration or alveolar hemorrhage;
- Grade 1, minimal acute rejection: infrequent perivascular mononuclear infiltrates venules are usually involved before arterioles. The mononuclear cell cuff is usually more than two to

Table 9. *Comparison of Pulmonary Fungal Pathogens**

Variables	Histo	Cocci	Blasto	Crypto	Asper	Mucor	Candida
Tissue reaction							
Necrotizing granulomas	Yes	Yes	Yes	Yes/no	No	No	No
Vascular invasion/infarct	No	No	No	No	Yes	Yes	No
AC inflammation/abscess	No	No	Yes	No	No	No	Yes
Morphology							
Budding yeast	Yes	No	Yes	Yes	No	No	Yes
Lavage size, microns	3	3	30–60	8–15	4–7		3–6
Shape	Oval	No	Round	Irregular	Hyphae	Hyphae	Dimorphic
Spherules/endospores	No	Yes	No	No	No	No	No
Thick cell wall	No	Yes	Yes	No	No	No	No
Mucin-positive capsule	No	No	No	Yes	No	No	No
Hyphae	No	Rare	No	No	Yes	Yes	Rare
Size, microns					3–5	10–15	
Septate					Yes	No	
Branching					45°	90°	
Pseudohyphae	No	No	No	No	No	No	Yes

*Data are from Katzenstein and Askin.[1] AC = acute; Histo = Histoplasma; Cocci = Coccidioides; Blasto = Blastomyces; Crypto = Cryptococcosis; Asper = Aspergillus; Mucor = Zygomycetes.

Table 10. *Comparison Between Actinomyces and Nocardia*

Variables	Actinomyces	Nocardia
Sulfur granules	Yes	No
Special stains		
Gram	Yes	Yes
GMS	Yes	Yes
Acid fast*	No	Yes

*Modified acid fast (Fite stain) substituting weak acid for decolorization.

Table 11. *Staining Characteristics of Pneumocystis*

Stains	Frothy Exudate	Cysts	Sporozoites
HE	Yes	No	No
Papanicolaou	Yes	No	No
Ultraviolet fluorescence		Yes	Yes
GMS		Yes	No
Gram-Weigert		Yes	No
Cresyl-Echt violet		Yes	No
PAS-Gridley		Yes	No
Toluidine blue		Yes	Yes
Wright stain		No	Yes
Giemsa		No	Yes
Methylene blue		No	Yes
Monoclonal antibodies (immunofluorescence/ immunoperoxidase)		Yes	Yes

Table 12. *Morphology of Selected Viral Pathogens*

Variables	CMV	Herpes	Adenovirus	Respiratory Syncytial Virus
Tissue response				
Interstitial pneumonia	Yes	No	No	No
Necrotizing bronchopneumonia	Yes/no	Yes	Yes	Yes
Bronchiolitis	Rare	Yes	Yes	Yes
Tracheobronchitis	No	Yes	Yes	Yes
DAD	Yes/no	Uncommon	Yes	Uncommon
Giant-cell pneumonitis	No	No	No	Yes
Inclusions				
Intranuclear	Yes	Yes	Yes	No
Cowdry A	No	Yes	Yes	No
Ground glass	No	Yes	No	No
Cytoplasmic	Yes	No	No	No
"Smudge" cells	No	No	Yes	No

three cells thick and is composed of small round, plasmacytoid, and transformed lymphocytes;

- Grade 2, mild acute rejection: frequent perivascular inflammatory cell infiltrates surrounding venules and arterioles. Infiltrates are readily recognizable and are usually five to six cells in thickness in the vascular adventitia nd no obvious infiltration is found by inflammatory cells into the adjacent alveolar septae or airspaces;

- Grade 3, moderate acute rejection: all of the histologic features of mild acute rejection. Inflammatory cell infiltrate extends into perivascular and peribronchiolar alveolar septae and airspaces;
- Grade 4, Severe acute rejection: diffuse perivascular, interstitial, and airspace infiltrates of inflammatory cells, including neutrophils. Alveolar pneumocyte damage usually is associated with necrosis, airspace hemorrhage, and sometimes a necrotizing vasculitis. Antibody-mediated rejection and pulmonary hemorrhage, capillaritis, and complement deposition are present.

Neoplasia[5,40]

Squamous Cell Carcinoma

Gross findings vary from small to large, obstructive lesions that commonly are cavitated. Microscopic findings include keratinization and intercellular bridges. Variants include papillary, clear cell, small cell, and basaloid. Immunohistochemistry is thyroid transcription factor 1–, cytokeratin 5/6, and p63+.

Adenocarcinoma

Adenocarcinomas are more commonly peripheral. Microscopically, they are gland forming (majority) or contain mucin by special stains (solid variant). They can be acinar, papillary, solid, and bronchioloalveolar. Immunohistochemistry is chromogranin/synaptophysin: 10 to 20%+, cytokeratin 7+ and cytokeratin 20±, and thyroid transcription factor 1+. k-ras mutations can be present.

Bronchioloalveolar Carcinoma

In bronchioloalveolar carcinoma there are nodules or areas of consolidation, more commonly peripheral. Mucinous subtypes usually replace entire lobe and show preservation of underlying architecture with large pools of mucus within airspaces. Microscopic findings include nonmucinous, mucinous, and mixed variants. The epithelium is well differentiated, uniform, and grows along intact alveolar walls, and there is no invasion into underlying stroma. Multifocality with microsatellite lesions is common. The differential diagnosis: atypical adenomatous hyperplasia, (1) cytologic atypia is less marked, and (2) typically <0.5 cm.

Small Cell Carcinoma

A total of 70% of cases present as perihilar mass. Extensive lymph node metastases are common. Small cell carcinoma typically is peribronchial; endobronchial lesions are uncommon. Microscopically, small cell carcinomas are round-to-fusiform nuclei, nuclear molding, faint or absent nucleoli, and have scant cytoplasm. Extensive necrosis may be found, and 5% of small cell carcinoma may be combined with a nonsmall cell component. Immunohistochemically, 20% of cases may be negative classic for neuroendocrine markers.

Large Cell Carcinoma

Large cell carcinomas are central or peripheral and are typically large. They appear microscopically as having a "sheets and nests" growth pattern with extensive necrosis, large nuclei with prominent nucleoli, and no evidence of squamous or glandular differentiation by light microscope. Variants include large cell neuroendocrine carcinoma, basaloid, lymphoepithelioma-like, and clear cell carcinoma. On electron microscopy, 80% show

Table 13. *Working Formulation for Classification and Grading of Pulmonary Allograft Rejection**

A. Acute rejection (perivascular, interstitial and alveolar inflammation)
Grade 0 – None
Grade 1 – Minimal
Grade 2 – Mild
Grade 3 – Moderate
Grade 4 – Severe
B. Airway inflammation
Grade 0 – None
Grade 1R – Low grade
Grade 2R – High grade
Grade X – Not gradable
C. Chronic airway rejection – bronchiolitis obliterans
0 – Absent
1 – Present
D. Chronic vascular rejection – accelerated graft vascular sclerosis
Antibody-mediated rejection

*From Stewart et al.[39]

glandular differentiation; 10% show squamous differentiation.

Carcinoid Tumorlet

A carcinoid tumorlet is usually an incidental microscopic finding. Multiple tumorlets may mimic metastatic tumor, *eg*, breast cancer.[41,42] They rarely are associated with syndrome of airflow obstruction.[41] Microscopically, nests of neuroendocrine cells (≤0.5 cm) are found embedded in fibrotic stroma. They are usually adjacent to the bronchiole.

Neuroendocrine Cell Hyperplasia

Neuroendocrine cell hyperplasia[43] is defined as increased neuroendocrine cells within bronchiolar epithelium.

Typical and Atypical Carcinoids

Microscopic, neuroendocrine cells with organoid, trabecular, insular, palisading ribbon, and rosette-like architecture are found. They have round-to-oval nuclei with finely granular chromatin and inconspicuous nucleoli. Sromal changes include bone, cartilage, dense fibrosis, and amyloid. Atypical carcinoids have 2–10 mitoses per 10 high powered fields and/or focal necrosis.

Large Cell Neuroendocrine Carcinoma

Microscopic findings include organoid, palisading, trabecular patterns; large, polygonal nuclei and low nuclear/cytoplasmic ratio with frequent nucleoli; and high mitotic rate (>10 mitoses /10 high powered fields). Necrosis can be prominent. Immunohistochemistry: chromogranin 80%+, synaptophysin 40%+, and bombesin 40%+. By definition, one of the aforementioned neuroendocrine markers must be positive.

Lymphomatoid Granulomatosis-Lymphoma

Lymphomatoid granulomatosis-lymphoma was described at a time when the existence of extranodal lymphomas was not accepted, but this disease is a malignant lymphoma.[44,45] It appears with a nodular consolidation; nodules may have central necrosis. Microscopically, nodules or diffuse infiltrates of lymphoid cells appear; central necrosis and cavitation can be seen in larger nodules; prominent vascular invasion is usually seen. The cell population is heterogeneous, but large atypical cells are malignant. Most cells are positive for T-cell markers (CD4, CD8), but the majority of the malignant cells are B cells. They show either immunoglobulin gene rearrangements (B-cell) or T-cell receptor rearrangements (in the few that represent T-cell lymphomas). Epstein–Barr virus DNA often is detected by in situ hybridization.

References

[Note to participants regarding references: there are some primary sources quoted, but the textbooks have additional photographs worth studying.]

1. Katzenstein A, Askin F. Surgical pathology of non-neoplastic lung disease. 4th ed. Philadelphia, PA: Saunders Elsevier, 2006
2. Parambil JG, Myers JL, Aubry MC, et al. Causes and prognosis of diffuse alveolar damage diagnosed on surgical lung biopsy. Chest 2007; 132:50–57
3. Travis W, Colby T, Koss M, et al. Non-neoplastic disorders of the lower respiratory tract. In: Atlas of nontumor pathology. Washington, DC: American Registry of Pathology and the Armed Forces Institute of Pathology, 2002
4. American Thoracic Society/European Respiratory Society International Multidisciplinary Consensus Classification of the Idiopathic Interstitial Pneumonias. This joint statement of the American Thoracic Society (ATS), and the European Respiratory Society (ERS) was adopted by the ATS board of directors, June 2001 and by the ERS Executive Committee, June 2001. Am J Respir Crit Care Med 2002; 165:277–304
5. Churg A, Myers J, Tazelaar H, et al. Thurlbeck's pathology of the lung. 3d ed. New York, NY: Thieme Medical Publishers, 2005
6. Katzenstein A, Askin F. Surgical pathology of non-neoplastic lung disease. 4th ed. Philadelphia, PA: W.B. Saunders, 2006; 503
7. Katzenstein AL, Mukhopadhyay S, Myers JL. Diagnosis of usual interstitial pneumonia and distinction from other fibrosing interstitial lung diseases. Hum Pathol 2008; 39:1275–1294

8. Trahan S, Hanak V, Ryu JH, et al. Role of surgical lung biopsy in separating chronic hypersensitivity pneumonia from usual interstitial pneumonia/idiopathic pulmonary fibrosis: analysis of 31 biopsies from 15 patients. Chest 2008; 134:126–132
9. Atkins SR, Turesson C, Myers J, et al. Morphologic and quantitative assessment of CD20+ B cell infiltrates in rheumatoid arthritis-associated nonspecific interstitial pneumonia and usual interstitial pneumonia. Arthritis Rheum 2006; 54:635–641
10. King T, Jr., Schwarz M, Brown K, et al. Idiopathic pulmonary fibrosis: relationship between histopathologic features and mortality. Am J Respir Crit Care Med 2001; 164:1025–1032
11. King T, Jr., Tooze J, Schwarz M, et al. Predicting survival in idiopathic pulmonary fibrosis: scoring system and survival model. Am J Respir Crit Care Med 2001; 164:1171–1181
12. Hanak V, Ryu JH, de Carvalho E, et al. Profusion of fibroblast foci in patients with idiopathic pulmonary fibrosis does not predict outcome. Respir Med 2008; 102:852–856
13. Churg A, Müller NL, Silva CIS, et al. Acute exacerbation (acute lung injury of unknown cause) in UIP and other forms of fibrotic interstitial pneumonias. Am J Surg Pathol 2007; 31:277–284
14. Parambil J, Myers J, Ryu J. Histopathologic features and outcome of patients with acute exacerbation of idiopathic pulmonary fibrosis undergoing surgical lung biopsy. Chest 2005; 128:3310–3315
15. Kim D, Park JH, Park BK, et al. Acute exacerbation of idiopathic pulmonary fibrosis: frequency and clinical features. Eur Respir J 2006; 27:143–150
16. Katzenstein A, Fiorelli R. Nonspecific interstitial pneumonia/fibrosis. Histologic features and clinical significance. Am J Surg Pathol 1994; 18:136–147
17. Travis WD, Hunninghake G, King TE Jr., et al. Idiopathic nonspecific interstitial pneumonia: report of an American Thoracic Society project. Am J Respir Crit Care Med 2008; 177:1338–1347
18. Aubry M, Wright J, Myers J. The pathology of smoking-related lung diseases. Clin Chest Med 2000; 21:11–35, vii
19. Ryu J, Colby T, Hartman T, et al. Smoking-related interstitial lung diseases: a concise review. Eur Respir J 2001; 17:122–132
20. Fraig M, Shreesha U, Savici D, et al. Respiratory bronchiolitis: a clinicopathologic study in current smokers, ex-smokers, and never-smokers. Am J Surg Pathol 2002; 26:647–653
21. Vassallo R, Jensen EA, Colby TV, et al. The overlap between respiratory bronchiolitis and desquamative interstitial pneumonia in pulmonary Langerhans cell histiocytosis: high-resolution CT, histologic, and functional correlations. Chest 2003; 124:1199–1205
22. Myers J, Veal CF Jr., Shin MS, et al. Respiratory bronchiolitis causing interstitial lung disease. A clinicopathologic study of six cases. Am Rev Respir Dis 1987; 135:880–884
23. Yousem S, Colby T, Gaensler E. Respiratory bronchiolitis-associated interstitial lung disease and its relationship to desquamative interstitial pneumonia. Mayo Clin Proc 1989; 64:1373–1380
24. Saldana M, Mones J. Lymphoid interstitial pneumonia in HIV infected individuals. Prog Surg Pathol 1991; 12:181–215
25. Koss M, Hockhholzer L, Langloss JM, et al. Lymphoid interstitial pneumonia: clinicopathological and immunopathological findings in 18 cases. Pathology 1987; 19:178–185
26. Cha S, Fessler MB, Cool CD, et al. Lymphoid interstitial pneumonia: clinical features, associations and prognosis. Eur Respir J 2006; 28:364–369
27. Yousem S, Colby TV, Chen YY, et al. Pulmonary Langerhans' cell histiocytosis: molecular analysis of clonality. Am J Surg Pathol 2001; 25:630–636
28. Churg A, Muller NL, Flint J, et al. Chronic hypersensitivity pneumonitis. Am J Surg Pathol 2006; 30:201–208
29. Ohtani Y, Saiki S, Kitaichi M, et al. Chronic bird fancier's lung: histopathological and clinical correlation. An application of the 2002 ATS/ERS consensus classification of the idiopathic interstitial pneumonias. Thorax 2005; 60:665–671
30. Khoor A, Leslie KO, Tazelaar HD, et al. Diffuse pulmonary disease caused by nonturberculous mycobacteria in immunocompetent people (hot tub lung). Am J Clin Pathol 2001; 115:755–762
31. Hanak V, Kalraa S. Hot tub lung: presenting features and clinical course of 21 patients. Respir Med 2006; 100:610–615
32. Aksamit T. Hot tub lung: infection, inflammation, or both? Semin Respir Infect 2003; 18:33–39
33. Seymour J, Presneill J. Pulmonary alveolar proteinosis: progress in the first 44 years. Am J Respir Crit Care Med 2002; 166:215–235
34. Trapnell B, Whitsett J, Nakata K. Pulmonary alveolar proteinosis. N Engl J Med 2003; 349:2527–2539

35. Muir T, Leslie KO, Popper H, et al. Micronodular pneumocyte hyperplasia. Am J Surg Pathol 1998; 22:465–472
36. Karbowniczek M, Astrinidis A, Balsara B, et al. Recurrent lymphangiomyomatosis after transplantation: genetic analyses reveal a metastatic mechanism. Am J Respir Crit Care Med 2003; 167:976–982
37. Churg A, Green F. Pathology of occupational lung disease. 2nd ed. Baltimore, MD: Williams & Wilkins, 1998
38. Stewart S. Pathology of lung transplantation. Semin Diagn Pathol 1992; 9:210–219
39. Stewart S, Fishbein MC, Snell GI, et al. Revision of the 1996 working formulation for the standardization of nomenclature in the diagnosis of lung rejection. J Heart Lung Transplant 2007; 26:1229–1242
40. World Health Organization classification of tumours. In: Travis WD, et al., eds. Pathology and genetics of tumours of the lung, pleura, thymus and heart. Lyon: IARC Press, 2004
41. Aubry MC, Thomas CF, Jett JR, et al. Significance of multiple carcinoid tumors and tumorlets in surgical lung specimens: analysis of 28 patients. Chest 2007; 131:1635–1643
42. Darvishian F, Ginsberg MS, Klimstra DS, et al. Carcinoid tumorlets simulate pulmonary metastases in women with breast cancer. Hum Pathol 2006; 37:839–844
43. Armas OA, White DA, Erlandson RA, et al. Diffuse idiopathic pulmonary neuroendocrine cell proliferation presenting as interstitial lung disease. Am J Surg Pathol 1995; 19:963–970
44. Liebow A, Carrington C, Friedman P. Lymphomatoid granulomatosis. Hum Pathol 1972; 3:457–558
45. Myers J, Kurtin PJ, Katzenstein AL, et al. Lymphomatoid granulomatosis. Evidence of immunophenotypic diversity and relationship to Epstein-Barr virus infection. Am J Surg Pathol 1995; 19:1300–1312

Pleural Disease

Steven A. Sahn, MD, FCCP

Objectives:

- Understand the pathogenesis of pleural fluid (PF) formation in health and disease
- Appreciate the clinical presentation, radiographic features, and the most common causes of pleural effusions
- Appreciate the diagnostic value of PF analysis
- Understand the management of patients with pleural effusions, especially malignant and parapneumonic effusions
- Understand the pathogenesis, causes, clinical features, and management of patients with spontaneous pneumothorax

Key words: effusions; empyema; exudates; malignant pleural pleural disease; pneumothorax; transudates

Table 1. *Mechanisms of PF Formation in Disease**

Mechanism	Clinical Example	Classification
Increased PMV	Congestive heart failure	Transudate
Decreased peri-PMV	Atelectasis	Transudate
Decreased Pπ	Hypoalbuminemia	Transudate
Increased capillary permeability	Pneumonia	Exudate
Impaired lymphatic drainage	Yellow nail syndrome	Exudate
Peritoneal-pleural communication	Hepatic hydrothorax	Transudate
Thoracic duct rupture	Chylothorax	Exudate
PEEVO	Duropleural fistula	Transudate

*PEEVO = pleural effusion of extravascular origin; PMV = microvascular pressure; Pπ = oncotic pressure.

Pathogenesis of Pleural Effusions

Normal Pleural Fluid

In the normal pleural space, there is approximately 0.1 to 0.2 mL/kg body weight of pleural fluid (PF). Normal PF is clear, with <500 nucleated cells/μL; the differential is approximately 2% neutrophils, 0% basophils, 7 to 11% lymphocytes, 61 to 77% macrophages, and 9 to 30% mesothelial. PF pH has been reported in the range of 7.60 to 7.64, and there is a biocarbonate gradient (PF minus serum equals 8 mEq/L).[1,2]

Anatomy

The parietal pleura is supplied by systemic capillaries (intercostal vessels) that are situated close to mesothelial surface. The visceral pleura is supplied by the bronchial circulation that is situated a greater distance from mesothelial surface.[3] The formation of PF is a function of parietal pleura. An ultrafiltrate of parietal pleural capillaries increases interstitial pressure and promotes movement of fluid into pleural space between the mesothelial cell junctions. PF is resorbed from the pleural space with movement through the stomata of parietal pleura. The PF then moves into lymphatic lacunae and subsequently lymphatic ducts and well-formed lymphatic channels and ultimately into mediastinal lymph nodes. A clinically-relevant pleural effusion develops when PF formation exceeds resorption.[1] The mechanisms for PF formation and clinical examples are shown in Table 1.

Assessment of the Patient with a Pleural Effusion

Symptoms of Pleural Effusions

The patient may present with symptoms such as pleuritic chest pain (lupus pleuritis) or without symptoms, *eg*, most patients with a benign asbestos pleural effusion (BAPE). When patients with a pleural effusion are symptomatic, dyspnea and chest pain are the most common findings. Dyspnea may be caused by a large or massive pleural effusion in a patient with normal lungs, a moderate effusion in patients with some underlying lung disease, and a small-moderate effusion in patients with severe lung disease. A large effusion causes ipsilateral mediastinal shift, depression of the ipsilateral diaphragm, outward movement of the ipsilateral chest wall, and lung compression when there is no endobronchial lesion or fixed mediastinum. Dyspnea is perceived by the patient with a large-to-massive pleural effusion because of its effect on the previously mentioned structures with input from neurogenic receptors in the lung and chest wall.

Patients with a pleural effusion may present with pleuritic chest pain, which is associated with pleural inflammation. Pleuritic chest pain has been described as having a "stitch in the side" or a "stabbing" or "shooting" pain that may be exacerbated by deep inspiration, cough, or sneezing. Any maneuver resulting in chest wall splinting, such as manual pressure over the chest wall, will minimize the pain. However, a splinting maneuver will not differentiate between other causes of pleuritic-like chest pain, such as rib fractures or from inflammation of the pleura per se.

Value of PF Analysis

The clinician should recognize that PF analysis (PFA) in isolation will establish a definitive diagnosis, such as malignancy or empyema, in only a minority of patients. However, the number and specific definitive diagnoses will vary with the population being studied. In a prospective study of 129 patients with pleural effusion, thoracentesis provided a definitive diagnosis in only 18% of patients and a presumptive diagnosis in 55% of patients. In the remaining 27% of patients, the PF findings were unhelpful diagnostically because the values were compatible with two or more clinical possibilities.[4] However, in a number of these patients, the findings were useful in excluding other possible diagnoses, such as infection. Therefore, history and physical examination, radiologic evaluation, and ancillary blood tests are crucial in formulating a pretest diagnostic probability. PFA is a valuable test that may not provide a definitive diagnosis but can offer a confident clinical diagnosis if there is a thoughtful prethoracentesis evaluation. However, the more knowledgeable the clinician is concerning PFA, the more likely undiagnosed pleural effusions will decrease. The clinician who is more informed about PFA should be able to "make a confident clinical diagnosis" in virtually all patients with a pleural effusion.[5] Diagnoses that can be established "definitively" by PF analysis are shown in Table 2.[5,6]

Virtually all patients with a newly discovered pleural effusion should have a thoracentesis performed to obtain a diagnosis to guide management. Exceptions would be a secure clinical diagnosis, such as typical congestive heart failure (CHF) and a very small volume of fluid as with viral pleurisy. Observation is warranted in the aforementioned examples; however, if the clinical

Table 2. *Diagnoses That Can Be Established "Definitively" by PFA**

Disease	Diagnostic PF Tests
Empyema	Observation (pus, putrid odor)
Malignancy	Positive cytology; high salivary amylase level in absence of esophageal rupture
Lupus pleuritis	Presence of LE cells; ANA $\geq$ 1:320; and pleural fluid/serum > 1.0
Tuberculous effusion	Positive acid-fast bacilli stain or culture
Esophageal rupture	High amylase (salivary), low PF pH; presence of food particles or squamous epithelial cells on cytology
Fungal effusion	Positive potassium hydroxide stain or culture
Chylothorax	Triglyceride > 110 mg/dL (high likelihood); presence of chylomicrons definitive
Hemothorax	Hematocrit (pleural fluid/blood $\geq$ 0.5)
Urinothorax	Creatinine (pleural fluid/serum > 1.0)
Peritoneal dialysis	Protein (< 0.5 g/dL) and pleural fluid/serum glucose ratio > 2.0
Rheumatoid pleurisy	pH, 7.00, glucose < 30 mg/dL and LDH > 1,000 IU/L (highly likely if empyema excluded); characteristic cytology definitive
Duropleural fistula	Presence of β_2-transferrin
Glycinothorax	Glycine in PF (complication of transurethral surgery with glycine bladder infusion)
EVM of a CVC	Glucose PF/S > 1.0 with glucose infusion; PF protein < 0.5 g/dL with saline infusion; white fluid with high triglycerides with lipid infusion
Biliopleural fistula	Green fluid; bilirubin PF/S > 1.0

*LDH = lactate dehydrogenase; EVM of CVC = extravascular migration of central venous catheter.

situation changes or deteriorates, a thoracentesis should be performed promptly. Approximately 30 mL of PF is all that is necessary for a complete PFA. In 2009, most clinicians use ultrasound guidance for thoracentesis for safety purposes; the use of ultrasonography virtually excludes the possibility of a pneumothorax caused by needle puncture.

Observation of PF

Some diagnoses can be established at the bedside by visual inspection of the fluid (Table 3). For example, if pus is aspirated from the pleural space, the diagnosis of empyema is established and, if the pus has a putrid odor, anaerobic organisms are causative. A chylothorax can be suspected if there is milky fluid; however, this appearance could also be caused by empyema or a cholesterol effusion.

Table 3. *Observations of Pleural Effusions Helpful in Diagnosis**

Observations	Suggested Diagnosis
Color of fluid	
Pale yellow (straw)	Transudate, some exudates
Red (bloody)	Malignancy, BAPE, PCIS, or pulmonary infarction if trauma excluded
White (milky)	Chylothorax or cholesterol effusion; EVM of CVC with lipid infusion
Brown	Long-standing bloody effusion; rupture of amoebic liver abscess
Black	*Aspergillus niger* infection
Yellow-green	Rheumatoid pleurisy
Color of enteral tube	Feeding tube has entered pleural
Feeding or central Venous line infusate	EVM of CVC
Greenish tint	Biliopleural fistula
Character of fluid	
Pus	Empyema
Viscous	Mesothelioma
Debris	Rheumatoid pleurisy
Turbid	Inflammatory exudates
Anchovy paste	Rupture of amebic liver abscess
Satin-like sheen	Cholesterol effusion
Looks like water	Duropleural fistula
Looks like urine	Urinothorax
Odor of fluid	
Putrid	Anaerobic empyema
Ammonia	Urinothorax

*See Table 2 for abbreviations not used in the text.

The finding of ≥80% lymphocytes limits the possibilities of the exudative pleural effusion (Table 4). The most common of these diagnoses worldwide is a tuberculous pleural effusion. Although these diagnoses do not always have ≥80% lymphocytes, when this degree of lymphocytosis is present, one of these diagnoses is virtually always present.[6]

PF eosinophilia is defined as a PF eosinophil count of ≥10% of the total nucleated cells (Table 5). Interleukin-5 appears to be an important chemotactic factor attracting bone marrow-produced eosinophils into the pleural space. In patients who require thoracotomy for spontaneous pneumothorax, eosinophilic pleuritis is commonly encountered within hours of the pneumothorax. Although eosinophils appear to move rapidly into the pleural space after a pneumothorax, after a hemothorax, eosinophils do not appear in PF for 7 to 14 days.[7] Interestingly, PF eosinophilia is associated with delayed peripheral blood eosinophilia after a traumatic hemothorax that does not resolve until all eosinophils have left the pleural space.

Table 4. *Lymphocyte-Predominant (>80%) Exudative Pleural Effusions**

Disease	Comment
Tuberculous effusion	usually 90 to 95% lymphocytes; acutely, may be neutrophil-predominant
Chylothorax	2,000 to 20,000 lymphocytes/μL; most common cause is NHL
Lymphoma	Often 100% of nucleated cells are lymphocytes; diagnostic yield on cytology or pleural biopsy higher with NHL
Yellow nail syndrome	A cause of benign persistent effusion; protein discordant exudate
Chronic rheumatoid pleurisy	Often associated with an unexpandable lung
Sarcoidosis	Usually >90% lymphocytes; effusion in <2% of sarcoid patients; discordant exudate (by protein only)
Post-CABG effusions (>2 mo) including PCIS	82 to 99% lymphocytes; unilateral on left or bilaterally
Acute lung rejection	PF may be first manifestation of rejection

*Consistently but not always >80%; other exudates rarely have 80% lymphocytes. NHL = non-Hodgkin lymphoma.

Table 5. *PFE**

Disease	Comment
Pneumothorax	Lung and pleural tissue eosinophilia within a few hours after pneumothorax
Hemothorax	May take 1–2 wk to develop after blood enters pleural space
Benign asbestos pleural effusion	30% incidence of PFE; up to 50% eosinophils in PF
Pulmonary embolism	Associated with infarction and hemorrhagic effusion
Parasitic disease	Paragonimiasis, hydatid disease, amebiasis, ascariasis
Fungal disease	Histoplasmosis, coccidioidomycosis
Drug-induced	Dantrolene, bromocriptine, nitrofurantoin, valproic acid, and others
Carcinoma	5 to 8% with PFE
Churg-Strauss syndrome	Pleural effusions in 30% with marked PFE and peripheral eosinophilia
Lymphoma	Hodgkin disease (rare)
Tuberculous pleurisy	Rare

*PF eosinophils/total nucleated PF cells of >10%.

PF Glucose and pH

PF glucose and pH should be measured on all exudative effusions because: (1) they can narrow the differential diagnosis; (2) in a parapneumonic effusion, they provide information helpful in management strategies; and (3) in malignant effusions, it provides information relating to extent of pleural involvement with tumor, ease of diagnosis, prognosis, and management.[8] The finding of a pleural effusion with a pH <7.30 signifies substantial accumulation of hydrogen ions in the pleural space. There is a direct relationship between the pH of PF and glucose; if the pH is low, the glucose is low, and when the pH is normal, the glucose is normal. This correlation suggests that the pathophysiologic processes responsible for this biochemical phenomenon are interrelated (Table 6).

The mechanism responsible for a low pH and glucose in complicated parapneumonic effusions and empyema and esophageal rupture (an aerobic empyema) is an increased rate of glucose utilization by neutrophil phagocytosis and bacterial metabolism with the accumulation of the end-products of glycolysis, CO_2, and lactic acid, causing the pH to decrease.[9] In contrast, in malignant pleural effusions and chronic rheumatoid pleural effusions, the mechanism of low pH and glucose is related to an abnormal pleural membrane that inhibits the efflux of CO_2 and lactate from the pleural space rather than increased PF metabolism.[10]

Transudates vs Exudates

Chemical analysis helps to determine whether the fluid is an exudate, which results from infection, inflammation, malignancy, or impaired zlymphatic drainage from the pleural space. A transudate, which is caused by imbalances in hydrostatic and oncotic pressures, is associated with a normal pleura. Light and colleagues[11] have proposed a diagnostic rule for categorizing pleural effusion as an exudate. The rule defines an exudative effusion if any one of the following criteria are fulfilled: (1) a PF lactate dehydrogenase (LDH) level >0.67, *ie*, the upper limit of normal for the laboratory serum LDH value; (2) a PF/serum protein ratio >0.5; and (3) a PF/serum LDH ratio >0.6. The use of a three-test combination with "and/or" rule maximizes diagnostic sensitivity for detecting exudative pleural effusions but lowers specificity.

A high diagnostic sensitivity is desirable when screening for conditions, such as exudative effusions, that have important clinical implications. A metaanalysis of 1,444 patients[11] determined that all of the following tests have statistically similar

Table 6. *Diagnoses Associated With Pleural Fluid Acidosis (pH <7.30) and Low Glucose Concentration (PF/Serum <0.5)**

Diagnosis	pH Incidence (%)	Glucose (mg/dL)
CPPE and empyema	4.50–7.29 (~100)	0–40
Esophageal rupture	5.50–7.00 (~100)	0–59
Chronic tuberculous empyema	6.90–7.05 (100)	0–30
Chronic rheumatoid pleurisy	7.00 (~100)	0–30
Malignancy	6.95–7.29 (30)	30–59
Tuberculous effusion	7.00–7.29 (20)	30–59
Lupus pleuritis	7.00–7.29 (20)	30–59

*CPPE = complicated parapneumonic effusion.

diagnostic accuracy compared with the Light criteria: PF protein concentration >3.0 g/dL; PF/serum protein ratio >0.5; PF LDH greater than two-thirds the upper limits of normal of serum LDH; PF/serum LDH ratio >0.6; PF cholesterol >45, 54, 55, or 60 mg/dL; PF/serum cholesterol ratio >0.3; and albumin gradient <1.2 g/dL.[12]

In a receiver operating characteristic analysis of 200 consecutive patients with pleural effusions, a PF LDH of 163 IU/L (serum upper limits of normal, 200; ratio ≥0.82) was the best cutoff point for an exudate (area under the curve, 0.89), followed by PF/serum total protein ratio of 0.5 (area under the curve, 0.86).[13] If serum tests are not available, single tests or test combinations that rely only on PF results can be used with an excellent diagnostic accuracy. A Bayesian approach with application of likelihood ratios to pretest estimates of the probability of an exudative effusion improves diagnostic accuracy. For example, a PF/serum protein ratio of 0.70 has a much greater likelihood of being an exudate than a ratio of 0.51 (Tables 7, 8).[14]

Transudates

CHF

CHF is the most common transudate and most common cause of pleural effusions in the elderly. CHF PF is a consequence of pulmonary venous hypertension; a pulmonary capillary wedge pressure ≥24 mm Hg in the acute setting is strongly associated with bilateral pleural effusions.[15] These patients have the classic signs and symptoms of CHF; fine crackles usually are present, most prominently in the bases.

The chest radiograph most commonly shows bilateral effusions (R > L) with cardiomegaly and evidence of interstitial and alveolar edema. Kerley B lines may be observed. An isolated right effusion, 8%, and isolated left effusion, 4%, may occur. The severity of pulmonary edema correlates directly with the volume of PF.[16] Unless CHF develops after an acute myocardial infarction, the absence of cardiomegaly in a patient with bilateral effusions should raise the possibility of another cause of the bilateral effusions.

PFA reveals a serous fluid with <500 mononuclear cells/μL. Serum and PF glucose are equivalent and range from pH 7.45 to 7.55. Both

Table 7. *Causes of Transudative Pleural Effusions**

Disease	Comment
CHF	Diuresis can result in exudate by protein and LDH
Hepatic hydrothorax	Occurs frequently without clinical ascites
Nephrotic syndrome	Small, subpulmonic, and bilateral effusions
Peritoneal dialysis (CAPD)	Small, right-sided effusion most common; acute, massive, right hydrothorax can occur shortly after initiating dialysis
Hypoalbuminemia	Anasarca virtually always present; serum albumin level, <1.5 g/dL
Urinothorax	Caused by ipsilateral obstructive uropathy
Atelectasis	Small effusion caused by decreased peri-PMV
Constrictive pericarditis	Bilateral effusions due to pulmonary and systemic hypertension
Trapped lung	A result of remote pleural inflammation
Superior vena caval obstruction	Probably caused by acute systemic venous hypertension
Duro-pleural fistula	CSF leak into pleural space after disk surgery or trauma
Ventriculopleural shunt	30% incidence of symptomatic effusions
Ventriculoperitoneal shunt	Effusion can form with intrathoracic migration of catheter
EVM of CVC	Most common with left subclavian lines; transudate with saline solution or glucose infusion

*CAPD = continuous ambulatory peritoneal dialysis; CSF = cerebrospinal fluid. See Table 2 for other abbreviations not used in the text.

the PF protein and LDH may reach "exudative" levels after diuresis, which can be confirmed[16] with use of the serum- PF albumin gradient (≥1.2 supports a transudate).[17]

The diagnosis of pleural effusions from CHF is presumptive with the compatible clinical presentation. However, an elevated brain natriuretic peptide and compatible echocardiogram demonstrating a low left ventricular ejection fraction or diastolic dysfunction supports the diagnosis.[18]

Treatment includes reducing microvascular pressure with diuretics, angiotensin-converting enzyme inhibitors, spironolactone, and digitalis.

Table 8. Causes of Exudative Pleural Effusions

Infection	
	Bacterial pneumonia
	Tuberculous
	Parasites
	Fungal disease
	Atypical pneumonias
	Nocardia, Actinomyces
	Subphrenic abscess
	Rupture of amebic liver abscess
	Hepatic abscess
	Splenic abscess
	Viral hepatitis
	Spontaneous esophageal rupture
Malignancy	
	Carcinoma
	Lymphoma
	Leukemia
	Mesothelioma
	Sarcoma (angio, Kaposi)
Inflammatory and others	
	Pancreatic disease (acute; pancreaticopleural fistula)
	BAPE
	Pulmonary embolism
	Radiation therapy
	Uremic pleuritis
	Sarcoidosis
	PCIS
	Hemothorax
	ARDS
Connective tissue disease/vasculitis	
	Lupus pleuritis
	Rheumatoid pleurisy
	Mixed connective tissue disease
	Churg-Strauss syndrome
	Wegener granulomatosis
	Familial Mediterranean fever
Lymphatic abnormalities	
	Chylothorax
	Yellow nail syndrome
	LAM
	Noonan syndrome
	Lymphangiectasia
Movement of fluid from abdomen to pleural space	
	Acute pancreatitis
	Pancreaticopleural fistula
	Meigs syndrome
	Carcinoma
	Lymphoma
	Chylous ascites
Lung entrapment	
	Cholesterol effusion (TB; rheumatoid pleurisy)
	CPE/empyema
	CABG Surgery
Endocrine dysfunction	
	Hypothyroidism
	Ovarian hyperstimulation syndrome
Iatrogenic	
	Esophageal instrumentation
	Esophageal sclerotherapy
	Central venous catheter misplacement/migration
	Drug induced
	Enteral feeding tube misplacement into pleural space
	Leakage of percutaneous biliary drainage tube
	CABG surgery

If medical management is not completely effective, a unilateral pleurodesis for these medically refractive effusions is a reasonable option; however, bilateral pleurodesis is probably contraindicated because of the risk of the patient not being able to clear the heart failure fluid into the pleural spaces.

Hepatic Hydrothorax

Hepatic hydrothorax is defined as a pleural effusion in the setting of cirrhosis of the liver with portal hypertension and typically hypoalbuminemia; other causes of a transudative effusion must be excluded.[19] Although clinical ascites is usually present, up to 16% of patients develop an hepatic hydrothorax in the absence of clinical ascites.[20] The pathogenesis of these effusions is attributable to transdiaphragmatic movement of the ascitic fluid into the pleural space through congenital diaphragmatic defects that are rendered patent by the increased peritoneal pleural pressure.

The patients typically have stigmata of cirrhosis and present with the insidious onset of dyspnea with exertion. The chest radiograph usually demonstrates a small-to-moderate right effusion 70% of the time; an isolated left pleural effusion and bilateral effusions have each been reported in approximately 15% of patients.[21] The heart is typically normal in size and massive effusions, occupying the entire hemithorax, occur in only 5% of patients. PFA demonstrates a serous or sanguinous fluid with <500 mononuclear cells/μL. PF serum and glucose are equivalent and the pH ranges from 7.45 to 7.55.

The diagnosis is presumptive in the proper clinical setting with evidence of a low PF total protein (commonly < 1.0 g/dL) and an LDH clearly in the transudative range. The clinical diagnosis can be confirmed by demonstrating radionuclide passage from the ascitic fluid to the pleural space.

Medical treatment entails sodium restriction, a loop diuretic, and spironolactone. Approximately 25% of patients have a refractory hepatic hydrothorax.[22] If medical treatment fails, transjugular intrahepatic portosystemic shunt should be considered to manage the refractory ascites.[23] Video-assisted thoracoscopic surgery to patch diaphragmatic defects and perform talc poudrage has been used but is associated with a high rate of morbidity and mortality in these very ill patients. Chemical pleurodesis via chest tube has a low success rate. Furthermore, chest tube drainage in these individuals is contraindicated because it promotes infection, depletes protein and lymphocytes, and increases the risk of renal failure and often creates a prolonged fluid leak after removal of the chest tube. Liver transplantation is the best treatment for decompensated hepatic cirrhosis and, therefore, for patients with hepatic hydrothorax.

Clinical manifestations that should suggest that the patient may have spontaneous bacterial pleuritis are increased temperature, new-onset dyspnea, abdominal pain, and encephalopathy.[24] In this situation, an immediate thoracentesis with bedside inoculation of blood culture bottles should be performed.

Atelectasis

Atelectasis is a common cause of pleural effusions in the ICU (40% of patients on admission and 60% during medical ICU stay)[25]; pleural effusions are also observed postoperatively, especially after upper-abdominal surgery, thoracotomy, and coronary artery bypass grafting (CABG) surgery. Atelectasis may also be observed after pulmonary embolism without an infarction, an endobronchial obstruction from lung cancer, acute pancreatitis, splenic infarction, and subphrenic or hepatic abscess and the absence of a sympathetic effusion. The pleural effusion from atelectasis develops from decreased perimicrovascular pressure that favors fluid movement from the parietal pleural interstitium into the pleural space until the pressure gradient returns to normal.

Clinically, patients with an atelectatic pleural effusion may be asymptomatic or complain of dyspnea or chest pain. These patients may have an increased alveolar-arterial (A-a) oxygen (O_2) gradient. The chest radiograph typically shows small unilateral or bilateral effusions with minimal evidence of volume loss with a normal heart size and classic plate-like densities.

PF analysis shows a serous fluid with < 500 mononuclear cells/μL with a pH > 7.45 and a glucose level similar to serum glucose. The diagnosis is presumptive based on the patient's presentation. Treatment depends on the underlying disease and chest physiotherapy typically results in rapid resolution in the post-surgical patients.

Nephrotic Syndrome

Effusions develop in 20 to 25% of patients with nephrotic syndrome. The development of these effusions is associated with the degree of hypoalbuminemia. The effusions form because of decreased oncotic pressure, which at times may be associated with an increase in perimicrovascular pressure.

Individuals with nephrotic syndrome and pleural effusions are typically asymptomatic because the effusions are typically small. Patients become dyspneic when they develop volume overload. These effusions tend to occur when the albumin concentration is reduced to ≤ 1.8 g/dL.[26] The chest radiograph typically shows small bilateral effusions that are frequently subpulmonic and a normal heart size. On PFA, the fluid is serous with < 500 mononuclear cells/μL, a pH > 7.45, and a PF and serum glucose that are equivalent. The diagnosis is presumptive in the appropriate clinical setting with a low serum albumin. These patients, who are in a hypercoagulable state because of a loss of clotting inhibitors in the urine, may develop renal vein thrombosis and subsequent pulmonary embolism. Pulmonary embolism should always be considered in patients with nephrotic syndrome who develop pleuritic chest pain when the pleural effusion is significantly larger on one side orthe PF is hemorrhagic, exudative, or neutrophil predominant.[27] Management entails treating the underlying disease and preventing volume overload.

Trapped Lung

Trapped lung, the end stage of an infectious or inflammatory pleural effusion, presents as a persistent transudative effusion months to years after the acute pleural process. It is a relatively uncommon cause of a pleural effusion, representing < 5% of effusions in the Medical University of South Carolina database of > 1,000 patients. Trapped lung is one of the three forms of an unexpandable lung; the other two causes of an unexpandable lung are an endobronchial lesion, usually secondary to carcinoma of the lung, and chronic atelectasis, which may eventually resolve over time without intervention. Trapped lung is caused by visceral pleural restriction when a fibrous membrane covers a portion of the visceral pleura, preventing lung expansion to the chest wall. The increased negative intrapleural pressure favors PF formation until a new steady state is established.[28]

Patients with trapped lung may present with an asymptomatic pleural effusion seen on a routine chest radiograph or with dyspnea on exertion months to years after the acute pleural injury. Common causes of trapped lung include a complicated parapneumonic effusion or empyema, hemothorax, tuberculous pleural effusion, uremic pleuritis, rheumatoid pleurisy, and after CABG surgery. During a therapeutic thoracentesis, patients often develop severe, anterior, substernal chest pain as a result of the decrease in pleural pressure, which is quickly resolved by allowing air to enter through the pleural catheter.[29] The pleural effusion in trapped lung after thoracentesis reaccumulates relatively rapidly during a period of 72 h and does not result in relief of dyspnea.

The chest radiograph typically shows a small-to-moderate unilateral effusion without significant mediastinal shift.[29] PFA shows a serous fluid with a low nucleated cell count, typically < 500/μL, and a mononuclear predominance characterized by a lymphocytosis > 50% of the total nucleated cells. On a number of occasions, the protein is in the range expected for an exudate. We still believe that the fluid should be considered a transudate and that the pleural protein concentration depends on the plasma protein concentration, the protein reflection coefficient, solvent filtration into the pleural space (wash-down effect), and bulk flow of fluid via the pleural lymphatics. Finding a transudate by these criteria in effusions of vascular origin almost always indicates a normal protein reflection coefficient but also increased filtration and increased lymphatic bulk flow conditions, narrowing the differential diagnosis considerably.

Although the PF of trapped is by definition of vascular origin and the absence of inflammation and malignancy implies a normal protein reflection coefficient, solvent filtration may not be increased, and lymphatic bulk flow may be impaired. On the basis of these considerations, we do not interpret an isolated increase in PF protein concentration as unequivocal evidence of an abnormal protein reflection coefficient that would imply active inflammation.[29] The diagnosis of a trapped lung is established by finding an initial negative pleural liquid pressure on manometry that decreased precipitously after removal of PF. These patients typically have a pleural elastance of > 15 cm of H_2O per liter of fluid removed. Failure of the lung to expand on chest radiograph after removal of all fluid, in the absence of bronchial obstruction, also substantiates the diagnosis.

Treatment of trapped lung is reassurance if the patient is asymptomatic and decortication if the patient is symptomatic and the underlying lung is normal. Decortication for a trapped lung may be successful years after the diagnosis.

Hypoalbuminemia

The precise incidence of hypoalbuminemia is unknown. However, it is commonly seen in hospitalized patients with AIDS, patients with other chronic illnesses, and those in medical ICUs. The pathogenesis of these effusions is decreased oncotic pressure that generally requires a serum albumin of < 1.8 g/dL. It is highly unlikely a patient with hypoalbuminemia presents with an isolated pleural effusion without concomitant anasarca.

The patient typically has small bilateral pleural effusions and is generally not dyspneic at rest or with minimal activity; however, those patients with significant underlying pulmonary disease or heart disease may be breathless on exertion. The chest radiograph typically shows small-to-moderate bilateral effusions with a normal heart size. On PFA, the clinician will find paucicellular levels (ie, <500 total nucleated cells/μL) that are predominantly mononuclear. PF pH is 7.45 to 7.55, and the PF glucose is equivalent to the serum glucose. LDH and protein are clearly in the transudative range. Hypoalbuminemia-induced pleural effusions are a clinical diagnosis in a patient with a very low serum albumin and when other possible causes of the effusions have been excluded. The treatment is to maximize nutrition and prevent protein loss either through the GI track or kidneys.

Continuous Ambulatory Peritoneal Dialysis

Small right-sided, or less commonly, bilateral pleural effusions develop in approximately 2% of patients on continuous ambulatory peritoneal dialysis (CAPD). Acute, massive, right-sided pleural effusions may occur, usually in women in 1 month (range 1 day to 2 years) after starting peritoneal dialysis.[30] The pathogenesis of these effusions is peritoneal to pleural movement of fluid through diaphragmatic defects that become enlarged from acute increases in peritoneal pressure during dialysis. Multiparity and peritonitis are risk factors for the development of pleural effusions with CAPD.

The majority of these patients are asymptomatic, but some with enlarging effusions have insidious onset of dyspnea with exertion. Patients with acute massive effusions may present with acute respiratory failure and are often diagnosed as uncontrolled congestive heart failure.[31]

The chest radiograph typically shows a small right-sided or bilateral effusions or a massive effusion with an acute hydrothorax. PFA shows a serous fluid with a very low total protein (usually <0.5 g/dL) and glucose in the range of 200 to 2,000 mg/dL. The LDH ranges from 6 to 15 IU/L and the fluid contains <100 mononuclear cells/μL. Diagnosis is established with a high degree of clinical confidence in the patient on CAPD who has a PF total protein value of <0.5 g/dL and a PF/serum glucose ratio >2. Treatment is observation for patients who are asymptomatic with small pleural effusions. Patients with a large refractory symptomatic effusion or with an acute massive right effusion should be changed to hemodialysis. There have been reports of video-assisted thoracoscopic surgery pleurodesis used to successfully manage patients on CAPD.[32]

Urinothorax

The precise incidence of urinothorax is unknown; however, approximately 40 cases have been reported in the literature. It is highly likely that many cases are underdiagnosed and underreported. The most common cause of urinothorax is obstructive uropathy, where urine exudes from the capsule of the kidney and moves into the mediastinum or directly into the pleural space via the diaphragm due to a pressure gradient. Reported causes of urinothorax include bladder and prostate cancer, posterior urethral valves, renal cysts, nephrolithiasis, surgical ureteral manipulation, blunt trauma to the kidney, renal transplantation, ileal conduit with ureteral obstruction, bladder laceration, and pregnancy.[33,34]

The most common presenting symptom of a urinothorax is dyspnea after surgery or trauma. Occasionally a small asymptomatic urinothorax is found on a routine postoperative chest radiograph. The interval between the precipitating event and urinothorax has been reported to be from 8 h to 2 months, with most patients diagnosed within 48 h of the event.[33]

The chest radiograph typically shows a small-to-moderate pleural effusion ipsilateral to the obstructed kidney; however, there are reports of bilateral and contralateral effusions.[33,34] In most instances, there is no other abnormality on the chest radiograph.

On PFA, the fluid looks like and smells like urine. It has between 23 and 1,500 mononuclear cells/μL and typically has a protein <1.0 g/dL; the pH ranges from 7.00 to 8.00 and PF and serum glucose concentrations are equivalent.[35] The diagnosis is established by finding a PF/serum creatinine difference of >1.0; the range reported in the literature is 1.1 to 15.7. The PF/serum creatinine difference needs to be measured before relief of the obstruction because the latter will cause a rapid reversal in the PF/serum creatinine difference. Urinothorax is the only cause of a low pH (<7.30) transudate with a normal arterial pH.[35] Treatment is relief of the urinary obstruction, which results in a rapid reversal of the PF/serum creatinine difference, an increase in PF pH, and rapid resolution of the pleural effusion.

Exudates

Parapneumonic Effusions

A parapneumonic effusion is defined as a pleural effusion associated with pneumonia or lung abscess. An uncomplicated parapneumonic effusion is a small-to-moderate effusion that resolves with antibiotics only without pleural space sequelae. A complicated parapneumonic effusion requires pleural space drainage for resolution of pleural sepsis. An empyema, or pus in the pleural space, represents the end stage of a complicated parapneumonic effusion and always requires pleural space drainage. A parapneumonic effusion is the most common cause of an exudative effusion. A total of 40 to 57% of patients with bacterial pneumonia will develop parapneumonic effusions. However, only a small percentage (10 to 15%) have complicated effusions, and empyema develops in only 5 to 10%.[36]

The stages of a parapneumonic effusion are as follows: (1) exudative (capillary leak) with an estimated time period of 5 to 7 days; (2) fibrinopurulent or bacterial invasion and fibrin formation stage, which tends to occur after 7 days up to 2 weeks; and (3) the organizational or empyema stage, which generally occurs within 2 to 4 weeks of onset of the pleural effusion.[36,37] The most common organisms causing empyema are anaerobic bacteria, staphylococcus, Gram-negative aerobes, and the pneumococcus. At some time during the fibrinopurulent stage, the clinician loses the ability to treat the patient with antibiotics alone, and drainage is required.

The patient initially presents with symptoms typical of pneumonia: fever, pleuritic chest pain, cough with purulent sputum, and increasing dyspnea with exertion. The presence of these symptoms cannot determine whether the patient has a complicated or uncomplicated parapneumonic effusion, and therefore chest imaging, clinical factors, and PFA are often helpful in this determination.[36,37] An effusion $>40\%$ of the hemithorax on chest radiograph, the presence of an intrapleural air-fluid level, the presence of loculation or multiloculations, marked pleural thickening >5 mm, or enhancement of the pleural membranes on chest CT scan increase the likelihood that the patient has a complicated parapneumonic effusion or empyema. An anaerobic infection, prolonged pneumonia history, failure to respond to antibiotic therapy, virulence of the underlying bacterial pathogen, and hypoalbuminemia also suggest the presence of a complicated parapneumonic effusion.[36,37]

On PFA, the finding of purulent fluid establishes the presence of an empyema and always requires pleural space drainage. A positive bacterial culture, low PF pH of 7.20 to 7.30, a low glucose concentration <60 mg/dL, or a PF to serum ratio <0.5, or a high LDH >1000 IU/L are strong indicators for the need for pleural space drainage. It appears that the pH is the most sensitive of these parameters.[36,38]

The diagnosis of a parapneumonic effusion is relatively straightforward. In the clinical setting of pneumonia, PFA shows a neutrophil-predominant, concordant exudate (by both LDH and protein criterion) supporting the diagnosis of a parapneumonic effusion. Uncomplicated parapneumonic effusions require antibiotics only without dose escalation. Complicated parapneumonic effusions require appropriate antibiotics and pleural space drainage, which may be performed with a small-bore chest tube inserted under ultrasound guidance.[36,37,39,40] The use of fibrinolytic agents is controversial and clearly depends on the stage of the parapneumonic effusions. In the early fibrinolytic stage, fibrinolytics may shorten the clinical course. In established empyemas, the Multicenter Intrapleural Streptokinase trial showed that streptokinase was of no benefit in decreasing the rate of mortality or need for surgery in a large number of patients.[41] Empyemectomy and decortication by thoracoscopy or thoracotomy is necessary in patients with established empyemas to resolve pleural sepsis and to prevent severe pleural fibrosis or development of an unexpandable lung. In patients who are too debilitated to undergo surgery, open drainage is an option.[36,40]

Viral and Mycoplasma Pneumonia

Pleural effusions caused by viral infections tend to be small and self-limited and may develop in up to 20% of patients. However, because of the small volume of PF and spontaneous resolution in most patients; PF is usually not sampled. The majority of institutions are not equipped to perform viral cultures and, therefore, these effusions are typically not recognized. However, a pleural effusion develops in approximately 40% of patients with adenovirus 3 and 7. Adenovirus infection is endemic throughout the year and occurs in all age groups, although it is more common in school-aged children.[42]

The PF is a paucicellular exudate with a predominance of mononuclear cells. In the acute phase, there may be an increased number of neutrophils. The diagnosis is established by documenting increasing complement fixation titers or culturing the virus from the fluid.

Hantavirus, which has been reported predominantly from the Four Corners area of the United States (*ie*, New Mexico, Arizona, Utah, and Colorado) is the virus transmitted to humans via contact with deer mice. Pleural effusions are caused by either cardiac dysfunction or increased vascular permeability. The fluid can be either transudate in the initial phase with cardiac dysfunction or an exudate with vascular leak. Chest radiograph shows a normal-sized heart and bilateral infiltrates with blood tests documenting thrombocytopenia, a left shift in the myeloid series, and enlarged immunoblastoid lymphocytes.[43]

Patients with *Mycoplasma pneumoniae* infection can develop bronchopneumonia involving one or multiple lobes. A small pleural effusion occurs in 5 to 20% of patients.[44] The diagnosis is established by finding specific antibody titers or by isolating *M pneumoniae* from the PF. Positive polymerase chain reaction results from PF samples are associated with the abnormality observed on chest radiographs.[45] Macrolides are the drug of choice, and no specific treatment is necessary for the pleural effusion.

Malignant Pleural Effusions (Carcinoma, Lymphoma)

Malignant pleural effusions are the second most common cause of exudates. Lung and breast carcinoma represent approximately 60% of all malignant pleural effusions, with lymphoma representing approximately 10%.[46,47] Malignant pleural effusions in lung cancer result from ipsilateral tumor invasion into the pulmonary artery with embolization to the visceral pleural surface. Malignant cells migrate into the pleural space and adhere to the parietal pleural surface. Bilateral malignant pleural effusions in lung cancer develop from liver metastasis and the same pathologic process in the contralateral side.[47] With breast cancer, an ipsilateral malignant effusion occurs when there is metastasis through the chest wall lymphatics or hematogenous spread via the liver. In Hodgkin lymphoma, the effusion is predominantly caused by a lymphatic obstruction, whereas in non-Hodgkin lymphoma there is more commonly direct pleural invasion.[47] Non-Hodgkin lymphoma is one of the most common causes of a chylothorax.

Bilateral pleural effusions in the setting of malignancy are associated with mediastinal node involvement or bilateral parenchymal metastasis. Bilateral effusions also may occur years after mediastinal radiation secondary to either constrictive pericarditis or mediastinal lymphatic fibrosis. Lymphangitic carcinomatosis is seen with adenocarcinoma of the lung, breast, stomach, pancreas, prostate, and thyroid. A paramalignant effusion is defined as PF developing in the setting of a known malignancy but malignant cells are not found in the PF. Lymphatic obstruction appears to be the most important mechanism of a paramalignant effusion and is also associated with larger effusions.[47] In most series of patients with malignant effusions, <5% are transudates. Transudates may be caused by early lymphatic obstruction or endobronchial obstruction resulting in atelectasis or concomitant congestive heart failure. The course of a paramalignant effusion and a malignant effusion has not been compared.

Patients with a malignant effusion generally present with the insidious onset of exertional dyspnea and cough, typically with a known malignancy.[47] Chest radiographs may show a large-to-massive pleural effusion with contralateral mediastinal shift or bilateral effusions with a normal heart size or an apparent large effusion with ipsilateral shift. Any unilateral effusion in an elderly patient should suggest a possible malignancy. A massive pleural effusion (occupying the entire hemithorax) is most commonly to the cause of malignancy. Bilateral malignant effusions are most common with a nonlung primary. With an apparent large effusion without contralateral shift, the most likely diagnosis is lung cancer with obstruction of the ipsilateral mainstem bronchus. The classic triad of lymphangitic carcinoma is ipsilateral mediastinal adenopathy, Kerley B-lines, and a pleural effusion.

PFA is variable in a malignant pleural effusion. The fluid may be serous or grossly hemorrhagic and is typically a concordant exudate. Approximately 10 to 14% of patients with a malignant pleural effusion will have an elevated PF amylase (salivary) concentration that is virtually diagnostic of adenocarcinoma of the lung in an individual who clearly does not have esophageal perforation. A low PF pH and glucose in a malignant pleural effusion is associated with poorer survival, a greater yield on initial PF cytology, and poorer response to chemical pleurodesis than those with normal pH malignant pleural effusions.[7,46–48]

A malignant pleural effusion is diagnosed by finding malignant cells either in PF or on pleural biopsy. The yield of cytology and pleural biopsy depends on the stage of the disease, with the more advanced disease being associated with greater sensitivities; therefore, the sensitivity of cytology ranges from 45 to 90% and percutaneous pleural biopsy from 30 to 50% with thoracoscopy being the most sensitive diagnostic test with yields of 95 to 100% depending on the expertise of the operator.[46]

Treatment of patients with malignant pleural effusion is palliative; outpatient therapeutic thoracentesis for patients with far-advanced disease and contralateral mediastinal shift is appropriate. Chemical pleurodesis with talc poudrage or slurry for refractory effusions with dyspnea relieved by thoracentesis is an additional option. An indwelling catheter for failed pleurodesis or lung entrapment is an outpatient procedure, and the patient can manage his or her effusion at home.[49] Pleurectomy is rarely performed for failed pleurodesis unless there is an expected survival >6 months. All patients with a suspected malignant effusion should undergo pleural manometry to determine whether the lung is completely expandable, making the patient a candidate for pleurodesis. If the lung is not fully expandable, pleurodesis is futile. In these patients, an indwelling catheter should be placed for palliation.[49]

Malignant Mesothelioma

Malignant mesothelioma is the most common primary malignant tumor of the pleura that arises from the mesothelial surfaces of the pleura. Mesothelioma may also occur in the peritoneal cavity and pericardium. The estimated incidence of mesothelioma in the United States is 2,200 cases/year, and it appears to be on the rise. The predominant cause of a malignant mesothelioma is exposure to asbestos, with approximately 40% of malignant mesothelioma patients having a documented asbestos exposure. The lifetime risk of mesothelioma is estimated to be as high as 18 to 30% of asbestos workers.[50] However, there is no direct correlation to the amount and duration of asbestos exposure. The latency period from asbestos exposure to the development of mesothelioma varies from 20 to 50 years.

The World Health Organization classification of pleural tumors recognizes four major histologic subtypes: epithelioid, sarcomatoid, desmoplastic, and biphasic.[50] The epithelioid variant is most common. Immunohistochemistry has essentially replaced electron microscopy as the gold standard for diagnosis. Pathologists typically use a panel of markers to confirm the diagnosis. Calretinin, CK5-6, Wilms' tumor-1 antigen, and D2-40 positivity support the diagnosis of malignant mesothelioma.[51]

The majority of patients with malignant mesothelioma present in the fifth to seventh decades of life. The most frequent presenting symptom is nonpleuritic chest pain (60%) followed by dyspnea (25%) and cough (20%). Some patients are asymptomatic at diagnosis with a unilateral pleural effusion found on a routine chest radiograph. The disease is usually unilateral.

The initial radiographic manifestation is frequently a large unilateral pleural effusion with contralateral shift; the majority of the lesions are right-sided. Mesothelioma also may present as a pleural mass or with diffuse pleural thickening. A small percentage of patients will show evidence of asbestosis. In the later stages of disease, the patient develops ipsilateral mediastinal shift as the lung is encompassed by the tumor. CT will detect invasion of the chest wall, ribs, and mediastinal structures and can be used for staging.

There are no specific biomarkers in PF for the diagnosis of malignant mesothelioma. The effusions are typically exudative with protein concentration > 4 g/dL and are lymphocyte predominant. PF LDH levels often are > 600 IU/L. Patients with advanced disease present with extensive pleural involvement and a low PF pH and glucose, portending a poor prognosis as well as a poor response to pleurodesis. Other poor prognostic factors at the time of diagnosis include thrombocytosis, leukocytosis, anemia, fever, sarcomatoid or mixed histology, > 65 years of age, poor performance status, and male gender.[50,52]

Recent chemotherapy trials have demonstrated some evidence of antitumor activity with anthracyclines, platinum derivatives, and antimetabolites. Pleurodesis may be effective early in the course if lung entrapment is not present. Pleurectomy has been shown to be more successful than talc pleurodesis in reducing the recurrence of the pleural effusion. There are some long-term survivors after extrapleural pneumonectomy, when there is a component of a multimodality treatment suggesting that this procedure may alter the natural history of the disease in appropriately selected patients who are in early stages.[53] Other approaches to treatment are still in clinical trials including immunotherapy, targeted therapy, and gene therapy.[50]

Pulmonary Embolism

Pleural effusions occur in 40 to 50% of patients with angiogram-documented pulmonary embolism. A pleural effusion results from ischemia, leading to increased capillary permeability and the leak of protein-rich fluid into the pleural space. The effusion can also be the result of atelectasis secondary to chest pain. A large, hemorrhagic pulmonary infarction can rarely result in a hemothorax in a patient who is treated with heparin.

The presence of a pleural effusion does not alter the symptoms and signs of pulmonary embolism. Ipsilateral pleuritic chest pain, acute onset of dyspnea, tachypnea, and tachycardia are the typical findings. The patient may be afebrile or have a low-grade fever, but rarely exceeding 101.5°F (38.6°C). Hemoptysis may occur with a pulmonary infarction. Virtually all patients with a pleural effusion from pulmonary embolism have ipsilateral chest pain.

The chest radiograph typically shows a small unilateral pleural effusion virtually always less than one third of the hemithorax.[53] The effusion is present on the initial presentation in approximately 90% of cases. A radiographic infarction is seen in approximately one half of the patients and is usually in the lower lobe. A pleural effusion in association with a radiographic infarction tends to be larger than if no radiographic infarct is present but its volume is still less than onethird of the hemithorax.[55,56]

PFA in pulmonary embolism is highly variable.[54,57] One small study[55] showed that approximately 20% of patients with a pulmonary embolism had a transudative effusion. An exudative effusion may be hemorrhagic with neutrophil or mononuclear cell predominance depending on the timing of the thoracentesis in relationship to the acute pulmonary embolus. The PF and serum glucoses are equivalent, and the pH is typically > 7.30. The classic bloody, neutrophil-predominant exudate is present in only approximately one third of patients. The diagnosis of pulmonary embolism is best established by CT angiography; a ventilation/perfusion scan may be useful in situations in which the patient cannot receive IV contrast or the chest radiograph shows significant airspace disease or severe emphysema. A positive lower-extremity Doppler study and elevated d-dimer with a small ipsilateral neutrophil-predominant exudate makes the diagnosis highly likely.

Immediate anticoagulation with heparin should be instituted when the diagnosis is highly likely or definitively established. A hemorrhagic effusion or minimal hemoptysis is not a contraindication to anticoagulation. There are rare reports of hemothorax developing during heparin therapy in the setting of a large hemorrhagic infarction. No specific treatment is required for the pleural effusion of pulmonary embolism. A small effusion without radiographic infarction tends to peak in volume by 72 h and resolves in 7 to 10 days. Patients with a radiographic infarction and a larger pleural effusion usually require 14 to 21 days for resolution.[54–57]

Tuberculous Pleural Effusion

A tuberculous pleural effusion is the most common form of extrapulmonary tuberculosis, occurring in up to 10% of untreated purified protein derivative (PPD) converters. These effusions develop when a subpleural focus of tuberculosis ruptures into the pleural space followed by a cell-mediated immune response to the tuberculous antigens. A tuberculous pleural effusion can occur in the following two settings: (1) postprimary phase (3 to 6 months after the initial exposure) and (2) r-activation any time thereafter.[58–60]

These patients are typically symptomatic at presentation, exhibiting nonproductive cough (80%), chest pain (75%), which is usually pleuritic, and fever. Symptoms tend to be more acute in postprimary disease than with reactivation. The age of patients presenting with a tuberculous effusion tends to be increasing because more reactivation disease has been observed.[58]

The PPD skin test is positive in 69 to 100% of patients. A false-negative PPD results from the following: (1) circulating mononuclear cells that suppress sensitized T lymphocytes in the peripheral blood and skin but not in the pleural space; or (2) sequestration of PPD-reactive lymphocytes in the pleural space. Chest radiograph typically shows a unilateral small-to-moderate pleural effusion, which is more commonly on the right. A tuberculous pleural effusion is rarely massive. Bilateral pleural effusions are associated with hematogenous disease in 10% of HIV-positive patients and 5% in non-HIV–positive patients. Parenchymal infiltrates are noted in 33% on standard chest radiograph, whereas parenchymal lesions are seen more commonly (75%) on chest CT scan. Infiltrates are less commonly seen with postprimary disease. The effusion is ipsilateral to the infiltrate and is loculated in 30% of patients.[58,59]

PFA reveals serous fluid that may be serosanguineous in 10% but is never frankly bloody. The effusion is always an exudate with total protein >5.0 g/dL in 77% of patients. The total nucleated cell count ranges from 2,000 to 8,000 μL and is classically 90 to 95% lymphocytes; 90% of patients have >60% lymphocytes. Neutrophils are predominant with an acute presentation. PF eosinophilia or >5% mesothelial cells make the diagnosis of tuberculous pleural effusion unlikely.[61] The PF glucose is <60 mg/dL and the pH <7.30 in approximately 20% of patients. The PF pH is virtually never >7.40.[58]

Table 9. *Diagnosis of Tuberculous Pleural Effusion**

Tests	Sensitivity, %
Percutaneous pleural biopsy	
Histology	63–85
Culture	55–80
Pleural fluid culture	13–70
Sputum	4–50 (4% with isolated effusion on CXR)
Pleural biopsy acid-fast bacilli smear	5–18
Pleural fluid acid-fast bacilli smear	<5
N-PCR	51
VATS pleural biopsy	~100

*CXR = chest radiograph; N-PCR = nested polymerase chain reaction; VATS = video-assisted thoracoscopic surgery.

A combination of histology and culture of the pleural biopsy tissue, culture of PF, and sputum culture establishes the diagnosis in up to 86% of cases (Table 9).[58] A high PF adenosine deaminase (ADA) level of >40 to 60 U/L supports the diagnosis if rheumatoid arthritis and empyema are unlikely. An ADA level <40 U/L has a high negative predictive value for tuberculous pleural effusions. An ADA >50 IU/L with a lymphocyte/neutrophil ratio >75% makes a tuberculous effusion highly likely.[62]

Treatment is the same as for pulmonary tuberculosis[63]; however, because the organism load is low with a tuberculous pleural effusion, 6 months of isoniazid and rifampin appears to be effective therapy.[64] A tuberculous effusion usually resolves in 4 to 6 weeks with treatment or spontaneously but can persist for up to 16 weeks. Untreated, the recurrence rate is 65% within 5 years, mostly pulmonary without a pleural effusion.[65] Therefore, a patient with an undiagnosed lymphocyte-predominant exudate and positive PPD skin test needs to be treated with isoniazid prophylaxis if active disease has been excluded.[65] Corticosteroids are effective in resolving severe symptoms and in causing more rapid resolution of the pleural effusion but has no effect on residual pleural thickening.[66]

Pancreatic Disease (Acute Pancreatitis, Chronic Pancreatic Effusion [Pancreatopleural Fistula])

Approximately 3 to 17% of patients with acute pancreatitis will develop a left pleural effusion.[67]

Pleural effusions are much less common in patients with chronic pancreatitis. Those with acute pancreatitis develop a pleural effusion from transdiaphragmatic passage of amylase-rich PF into the pleural space with resultant increased capillary permeability from inflammatory mediators. The PF to serum amylase ratio is >1 and is explained by the rapid renal clearance of amylase and poor amylase clearance from the pleural space. A chronic, large recurrent pleural effusion is associated with chronic pancreatitis and pseudocyst formation. Pseudocysts develop in approximately 10% of patients with acute pancreatitis, and 50% of those patients with a pseudocyst will develop a pleural effusion.[68] The pleural effusion occurs when a fistulous track develops from the pseudocyst to the mediastinum, either pleural space, or the pericardial sac.[69] Patients with acute pancreatitis virtually always have abdominal symptoms and occasionally pleuritic pain and dyspnea. The major symptom with a chronic pancreatic effusion is dyspnea attributable to the large pleural effusion; chest discomfort and cough are typical in these patients who do not have abdominal symptoms but have a long history of alcohol abuse.[68,69]

The chest radiograph in acute pancreatitis is a small left-sided pleural effusion in 60% of cases but is right-sided in 30% and bilateral in 10%.[67] In addition, there is usually an elevated left diaphragm and evidence of left basilar atelectasis. In the setting of a chronic pancreatic effusion, the effusion is large or massive in size and typically unilateral on the left but can be right-sided or bilateral.[68,69] Pancreatic calcifications are typically observed on an abdominal film. The large pleural effusion usually recurs rapidly after thoracentesis because the fluid is rapidly generated from the pseudocyst along the pressure gradient.

PFA in acute pancreatitis reveals a turbid or hemorrhagic effusion that is neutrophil predominant and may have a total nucleated cell count of up to 50,000/μL. The PF and serum glucose concentrations are equivalent, and the pH ranges from 7.30 to 7.35. The PF/ serum amylase ratio is >1 and above the upper limits of normal of serum. The initial PF amylase may be normal but will be found to be elevated on a subsequent thoracentesis.[67] PF from a chronic pancreatic effusion is serous or hemorrhagic in appearance and is also a neutrophil-predominant exudate. However, these effusions have very high PF amylase levels, often >100,000 IU/L. The reported pH range is 7.28 to 7.50, with the vast majority being >7.30. The serum and PF glucose are equivalent.[68,69]

The diagnosis of an acute pancreatitis pleural effusion is established by finding a PF/ serum amylase ratio >1 or above the upper limits of normal of serum in the appropriate clinical setting. A very high PF amylase, > 50,000 to 100,000 IU/L, establishes the diagnosis of a chronic pancreatic effusion with pseudocyst formation and fistulous track in an alcoholic patient. Ultrasonography and CT can demonstrate the pseudocyst and the fistulous track.

There is no specific treatment for the pleural effusion of acute pancreatitis, which tends to resolve in 2 to 3 weeks as pancreatic inflammation subsides without pleural space sequelae. Patients with a chronic pancreatic effusion may respond to conservative therapy, which includes pleural space drainage, bowel rest, and hyperalimentation; however, conservative therapy is only successful in 50% of patients. In those with refractory chronic pancreatic effusions, percutaneous catheter drainage of somatostatin, the pseudocyst, or surgery are effective (Tables 10–12).[68,69]

Rheumatoid Pleurisy

Pleural effusions occur in rheumatoid arthritis in approximately 5% of patients; however, at autopsy, 50% of patients will have pleural fibrosis or an effusion (Table 13).[70] The pathogenesis for these effusions is local immune complex-mediated pleural inflammation. A chronic effusion may be seen with lung entrapment. Small fibrous plaques, rheumatoid nodules, or extensive fibrosis can involve the visceral pleura. There is an exfoliation of cells from the visceral pleural rheumatoid nodules that may produce an appearance of "debris" in the PF.[71] The low glucose and pH in rheumatoid effusions occur predominantly from an abnormal pleural membrane that inhibits glucose influx and hydrogen ion efflux from the pleural space.[72] Rheumatoid pleural effusions tend to occur in men (4:1 male/female ratio) who have rheumatoid nodules and moderate-to-severe active arthritis 5 to 10 years after the onset of articular disease.[70] However, effusions can occur up to 3 years before or after 20 years of the onset of rheumatoid arthritis.[70] At presentation, patients complain of pleuritic

Table 10. *Differentiating Features of Pleural Effusions From Acute and Chronic Pancreatitis*

Clinical Features	Acute Pancreatitis	Chronic Pancreatitis (Pancreaticoplueral Fistula)
Incidence	3–17%	Uncommon
Presenting symptom	Abdominal pain	Dyspnea
Size of effusion	Small	Large to massive
Site	Usually left sided	Usually left sided, can be bilateral or right sided
PF amylase, IU/L	500–10,000	May be >200,000
Pathogenesis	Increased vascular permeability	Direct fistulous communication from pancreatic pseudocyst
Outcome	Specific treatment not required	50% require surgical intervention, percutaneous drainage or somatostatin

Table 11. *Tests Useful in the Differential Diagnosis of Amylase-Rich Pleural Effusions*

Tests	Acute Pancreatitis	Chronic Pancreatic Effusion	Esophageal Rupture	Malignancy
Pleural fluid amylase concentration	Moderate	Extremely elevated	Minimal	Minimal
Pleural fluid /serum amylase	10:1	>20:1 (mean 63,000)	5:1	3:1
Pleural fluid amylase isoenzyme	Pancreatic	Pancreatic	Salivary	Salivary
Pleural fluid pH	7.30–7.39	7.28–7.39	5.50–7.00	7.05–7.40
Serum lipase	Elevated	Normal to minimally increased	Normal	Normal

Table 12. *Causes of Amylase-Rich Pleural Effusions*

Diagnosis	Type of Amylase Isoenzyme
Pancreatitis, pancreaticopleural fistula	Pancreatic
Carcinoma of the lung (usually adenocarcinoma)	Salivary (most common cause of salivary amylase-rich effusion)
Adenocarcinoma of ovary	Salivary
Lymphoma	Macroamylase/salivary
Esophageal rupture	Salivary
Chronic lymphatic leukemia	Salivary
Pneumonia	Salivary
Ruptured ectopic pregnancy	Probably salivary

chest pain and dyspnea or may be asymptomatic, usually without fever. Patients with rheumatoid pleurisy typically have high serum rheumatoid factors and presumably high levels of CCP antibodies. The chest radiograph typically shows a small-to-moderate unilateral effusion with a normal cardiac silhouette. However, in one third of patients, another manifestation of rheumatoid lung disease, such as rheumatoid nodules or interstitial lung disease, may be present.[70]

On PFA, the fluid may have several different appearances, including a yellowish-green tint, turbidity, milky, or debris-like.[70–72] The milky appearance suggests that the patient has longstanding lung entrapment and a cholesterol pleural effusion. The fluid typically contains a few hundred mononuclear cells (mostly lymphocytes) if there is an unexpandable lung without active disease, up to 15,000 mostly neutrophils/μL in acute rheumatoid pleurisy or with a cholesterol effusion with chronic inflammation. When the classic triad of a glucose <30 mg/dL, a pH of 7.00, and LDH >1,000 IU/L, the clinical diagnosis is highly likely as long as infection is excluded. Approximately 65% of patients on presentation with rheumatoid pleurisy will have a PF glucose

Table 13. *Differentiating Rheumatoid Pleurisy and Lupus Pleuritis**

Characteristics	Rheumatoid Pleurisy	Lupus Pleuritis
Frequency over course of disease	5%	50–75%
Onset	<3–5 to 10 yr after onset of articular disease	Any time; 5% as initial manifestation of SLE
Clinical	Men; active RA; with or without pleuritic pain	Flare up of disease
Chest radiograph	Small unilateral effusion	Unilateral or bilateral; with or without pericardial effusion
Appearance	Turbid, yellow-green, debris, milky	Serous-serosanguinous
Pleural fluid analysis	Low pH and glucose; increased LDH	Neutrophilic exudate; pH <7.30 and glucose PF/serum ratio <0.5 in 15–20% of patients
Diagnosis	Characteristic cytology (see text)	SLE cells present; PF ANA >1:320 and PF/serum ANA ratio >1 is suggestive
Treatment	Acute disease: corticosteroids; chronic disease: unknown	Corticosteroids
Resolution	3–4 mo (up to 1 yr)	2–4 wk
Residual	Pleural fibrosis; lung entrapment; cholesterol effusion	No sequelae or minimal pleural thickening

*ANA = antinuclear antibody; RA = rheumatoid arthritis.

<30 mg/dL, and 80% will have a glucose <50 mg/dL. PF complement is decreased, immune complexes are present, and rheumatoid factor is usually ≥1:320. Cytology is diagnostic by finding large, elongated tadpole-shaped cells with multinucleated giant cells with a background of granular material.[71] The cytologist should be advised that rheumatoid pleurisy is a possibility. The diagnosis is presumptive with the characteristic PF triad in the appropriate clinical setting; however, the cytologic appearance of the fluid is diagnostic.[70–75]

There are no controlled studies evaluating the effectiveness of corticosteroids or nonsteroidal antiinflammatory drugs. There are anecdotal reports of responses to corticosteroids; however, the course is variable, and it is uncommon for the effusion to resolve in <3 to 4 weeks. In fact, it usually takes several months but less than a year for resolution. Pleural thickening may be a residual in some patients evolving into a trapped lung that may require decortication.[76] A cholesterol effusion may develop over the course of several years.

Lupus Pleuritis

Pleural effusion or pleuritic chest pain during the course of systemic lupus erythematosus (SLE) occurs in 50 to 75% of patients.[77] Lupus pleuritis is a presenting manifestation of SLE in 5% of patients. At autopsy, 67% of patients with SLE will have pleural adhesions, pleural thickening, and pleural effusions (Table 13).[77] Pleuritis and pleural effusions result from a local immune response with low levels of complement and complement components found in PF. In addition, PF anti-DNA complexes may be involved. A specific immunofluorescent pattern of nuclear staining of pleural lining cells with either anti-IgM, anti-IgG or anti-C3 has been documented.[77,78]

Lupus pleuritis is typically associated with a flare of SLE. Patients are virtually always symptomatic with pleuritic chest pain (86 to 100%), pleural rub (71%), cough (65%), dyspnea (50%), and fever. The symptoms are similar in both native and drug-induced lupus. The chest radiograph typically shows small-to-moderate bilateral effusions; however, unilateral massive pleural effusions have been reported. Alveolar infiltrates, atelectasis, and an increased cardiac silhouette attributable to a pericardial effusion may be noted.[79]

PF analysis typically shows yellow or serosanguineous fluid. The total nucleated cell count ranges from 100 to 20,000/μL with either neutrophils in the acute setting or mononuclear cells predominating later. The glucose is <60 mg/dL and the pH is <7.30 in approximately 20% of patients. The presence of lupus erythematosus (LE) cells is diagnostic. A PF/serum antinuclear antibody (ANA) ratio of >1 and decreased complement levels support the diagnosis.[78,79] However, LE cells are not found in the PF of all patients with lupus pleuritis and are usually associated with the presence of serum LE cells, which may diminish the value of pleural LE cell positivity. Moreover, the detection of LE cells is not straightforward technically and may be subject to significant observer variation.

Pleuritic chest pain may respond to nonsteroidal antiinflammatory drugs but virtually always respond dramatically to corticosteroid therapy, although high doses may be needed for severe pleuritis or large effusions. In refractory cases, immunosuppressive agents, such as azathioprine, added to corticosteroids are sometimes but not always efficacious. Recurrent pleural effusions usually respond to pleurodesis. Asymptomatic lupus effusions require no treatment, usually resolve spontaneously, and have no prognostic significance. However, persistent pleuritic pain appears to be an adverse prognostic marker with a mean survival of <4 years.[77–79]

Postcardiac Injury Syndrome

Postcardiac injury syndrome (PCIS) occurs in up to 30% of patients after cardiac surgery and 1 to 15% after a myocardial infarction. The pleural effusion is most likely an immunologic response to cardiac injury. Patients with PCIS have increased levels of serum antimyocardial antibodies (AMA) compared with those without PCIS. PCIS may be triggered by a viral illness.[80]

PCIS is heralded by pleuritic chest pain in >90% of patients with fever, pericardial rub, dyspnea, and crackles (all >50%) 3 weeks (range 2 days to 1 year) after myocardial injury. These patients have an elevated erythrocyte sedimentation rate with a mean of 62 mm/h. Fifty percent of the patients have a leukocytosis. The chest radiograph is abnormal in 95% of patients, with pleural effusion occurring in 83%, either left-sided or bilateral, and right-sided effusion only in 17%. There is accompanying left lower-lobe infiltrates and an increased cardiac silhouette, most likely from a pericardial effusion.[81]

PFA demonstrates a serosanguineous or hemorrhagic effusion in 70% of patients. The PF is a concordant exudate, with both the protein and LDH being in the exudative range. The nucleated cell count ranges from 500 to 39,000/μL, depending on the timing of thoracentesis in relationship to the initial pleural injury. Neutrophils are predominant early. PF and serum glucose levels are equivalent, and the pH is >7.30. Low PF total hemolytic complement and complement components may be found and the PF to serum AMA is typically >1.[81]

The diagnosis is presumptive and is a diagnosis of exclusion. In the proper clinical setting, a PF/serum AMA ratio >1 and low PF complement levels when adjusted for the serum and PF protein concentrations support the diagnosis.[82]

Patients usually require antiinflammatory therapy for relief of symptoms, including prednisone in some cases. Approximately 50% of patients relapse and need additional antiinflammatory therapy. Corticosteroids typically result in rapid resolution of symptoms; however, the natural history of PCIS does not appear to be influenced by corticosteroids because their withdrawal often results in recurrence. Given the deleterious effects of corticosteroids on wound healing and the propensity of PCIS effusions to recur after their withdrawal, it is prudent to reserve corticosteroids for patients with moderate-to-severe persistent symptoms. Most patients have resolution without clinically important sequelae.[83]

Pleural Effusions After CABG Surgery (Not PCIS)

Small left pleural effusions virtually always occur postoperatively as the result of atelectasis from left phrenic nerve trauma (Table 14). Less commonly, a larger, left hemorrhagic effusion develops after internal mammary harvesting. These effusions may be asymptomatic or cause dyspnea and tend to persist for several months after surgery.[83–85]

The chest radiograph shows a small left-sided effusion with left lower-lobe atelectasis and an elevated left hemidiaphragm in the early postoperative period associated with phrenic nerve injury. In patients with internal mammary harvesting, a larger effusion may develop and persist for several months. A trapped lung may develop after 6 months and typically is a small, unilateral effusion that recurs rapidly after thoracentesis.[83]

Table 14. *Pleural Effusion Following CABG Surgery**

Type of Pleural Effusion	Description
Perioperative	Atelectasis
	Bloody effusions after IMA harvesting
	Others (CHF, PE, parapneumonic, chylothorax)
Early (within 1 mo)	PCIS
Late (2–12 mo)	PCIS
	Lymphocytic effusion of uncertain origin
	Constrictive pericarditis
	Lung entrapment
Persistent (≥6 mo)	Trapped lung

*PE = pulmonary embolism. From Heidecker J, Sahn SA. Clin Chest Med 2006; 27:267–283.

PF after internal mammary artery harvesting is hemorrhagic with a low number of nucleated cells, which are predominantly lymphocytic. The majority of post-CABG effusions resolve over weeks to months; however, some patients may require 1 to 3 therapeutic thoracenteses; less commonly, some progress to trapped lung with severe restriction requiring decortication.[29,82–84]

Chylothorax

When the thoracic duct or one of its major tributaries ruptures, chyle flows into the surrounding tissues. If the mediastinal pleura remain intact, chyle fills the mediastinum and forms a "chyloma" over the next several days before rupturing into the pleural space, usually on the right at the base of the pulmonary ligament. The thoracic duct, which has its origin in the cisterna chyli, is situated in the midline anterior to the first and second lumbar vertebrae. The thoracic duct travels through the aortic hiatus of the diaphragm approximately at the level of the tenth to twelfth thoracic vertebrae to the right of the aorta. Approximately at the fifth to sixth thoracic vertebrae, the duct enters the left posterior mediastinum and eventually joins the venous circulation where the left subclavian and internal jugular veins merge.

Therefore, disruption of the thoracic duct below T5 to T6 causes a right-sided chylothorax, whereas injury to the duct above this level results in a left chylothorax. However, significant anatomic variation exists in the path of the thoracic duct in almost half of the population.[86] Chyle is normally transported from the intestine to the lymphatic system into the blood. Long-chain triglycerides (containing ≥14 carbon units) and ingested fats are transformed into chylomicrons and low-density lipoproteins in the intestines and form chyle that enters the intestinal lymphatic vessels. In contrast, medium-chain triglycerides (containing ≤12 carbon units) are directly absorbed into the portal vein without entering intestinal lymphatics. Approximately 60% of the dietary fat enters the lymphatics, and 1,500 to 2,500 mL of chyle travels daily through these vessels.[86]

The most common cause of chylothorax is malignancy, particularly non-Hodgkin lymphoma. Cardiothoracic surgery, especially esophagectomy and surgery for congenital heart disease, are the most common causes.[87] However, the incidence of postoperative chylothorax remains at <1%. Trauma, including innocuous hyperextension of the thoracic spine, has also been reported. Several miscellaneous causes of chylothorax include lymphangioleiomyomatosis (LAM), with approximately 25% of patients with LAM developing chylothorax during the course of their disease and 9% as an initial presenting manifestation; other causes include lymphangiectasis, tuberculous lymphadenopathy, left subclavian vein thrombosis, filariasis, CABG surgery, chronic lymphocytic leukemia, Castleman disease (angiocentric or giant lymph node hyperplasia), sarcoidosis, Kaposi sarcoma, yellow nail syndrome, Noonan syndrome, multiple myeloma, Waldenström macroglobulinemia after thoracic radiation, and goiter.[87]

Patients with chylothorax present with subacute or insidious onset of dyspnea. The history may be a clue to its cause. However, after investigation, a number of chylothoraces are termed idiopathic; these are most likely caused by innocuous hyperextension of the spine or an occult malignancy. Patients with chylothorax are usually not febrile and do not have chest pain because chyle does not tend to invoke an inflammatory response. Chyle is bacteriostatic and, therefore, empyema is rare. Frequently, patients cough up chyle (chyloptysis). Sputum triglyceride concentrations have been reported to range from 662 to 2,600 mg/dL, which is greater than concurrent serum values. Chylomicrons have also been detected in sputum.

Table 15. *Differentiating a Chylothorax and a Cholesterol Effusion*

Characteristics	Chylothorax	Cholesterol Effusion
Incidence	Uncommon	Rare
Causes	Lymphoma, trauma, surgery, LAM	Rheumatoid arthritis or empyema, TB (a form of lung entrapment)
Onset	Acute or subacute	Insidious and chronic
Symptoms	Dyspnea	None; dyspnea
PFA	Milky, serous, turbid or bloody; >80% lymphocytes, protein discordant exudate; triglycerides >110 mg/dL (highly likely); cholesterol >60 to <200 mg/dL	Milky, satin-like sheen; neutrophil-predominant exudate; cholesterol >200 mg/dL; cholesterol/triglyceride ratio >1; triglyceride level may be >110 mg/dL
Diagnosis	Presence of chylomicrons	Presence of cholesterol crystals; cholesterol/triglyceride ratio >1 and cholesterol >200 mg/dL
Treatment	Manage underlying disease; pleurodesis	Observation; decortication

PFA shows fluid that is typically white and opalescent if fat is present; however, the fluid can be clear and yellow in the adult who has not eaten for 12 h or hemorrhagic if there is concomitant trauma. The supernatant of a chylothorax fails to clear after centrifugation. The primary cells in chyle are T lymphocytes, which typically represent >80% of the cellular population. The total nucleated cell count ranges from 400 to 6,800/μL. PF protein has been reported from 2.2 to 5.9 g/dL (Table 15).

In contrast to a cholesterol pleural effusion, the cholesterol levels in chyle are substantially lower and range from 65 to 220 mg/dL.[88] If the PF triglyceride is >110 mg/dL, there is a high likelihood that the patient has chylothorax. Conversely, if the triglyceride level is <50 mg/dL, it is highly unlikely that a chylothorax is present.[89] However, if the patient has been fasting for at least 12 h, the triglyceride concentration may be falsely low. If chylomicrons are present, the diagnosis is established definitively. Chylous fluid has been reported to have a pH from 7.40 to 7.80 and a glucose concentration of 78 to 200 mg/dL.[88] Measurement of the PF/serum glucose ratio assists in differentiating a chylous effusion (ratio <1.0) and pleural attributed to extravascular migration of a central venous catheter with glucose containing parenteral nutrition with lipid into the pleural space (ratio >1.0) (Table 15).[90]

There are two major principles that should be followed in managing a patient with a chylothorax. First, there should be a step-wise plan of care that begins with pleural space drainage if the patient is symptomatic and nutritional support with progression of pleural synthesis if necessary, which can be accomplished by various techniques. Second, prolonged drainage of a chylothorax should be avoided to prevent immunosuppression and malnutrition. Patients with a traumatic chylothorax are typically managed with chest tube drainage, bowel rest, and parenteral nutrition to minimize the flow of chyle and maintenance of fluid and electrolyte balance. Because most traumatic chylothoraces resolved within 10 to 14 days, protein loss and immunosuppression are usually minimal. If drainage is persistent after 2 weeks, >1,500 mL for 5 days, or if the patient develops significant weight loss or progressive loss of protein despite nutritional therapy, surgical intervention is indicated. There are recent reports of percutaneous catheterization and embolization of the thoracic duct in patients with traumatic chylothorax occurring after surgical procedures. Somatostatin and octreotide have been reported to decrease chyle production in postoperative chylothorax in small case series.[91]

LAM

LAM, a rare lung disease of unknown cause, is characterized by the proliferation and infiltration of the pulmonary interstitium with atypical muscle cells. In patients with LAM, progressive respiratory insufficiency and pleural complications, specifically pneumothorax and chylothorax, are clinical hallmarks.[92] Because the majority of initial episodes of pneumothorax or chylothorax occur before the diagnosis of LAM, their occurrence is often a sentinel event that leads the clinician to consider the diagnosis of LAM.

The incidence of pneumothorax in LAM, with a reported range of 39 to 76%, is one of the highest among diseases associated with secondary spontaneous pneumothorax.[91] Pneumothorax is commonly the presenting event that leads to the diagnosis of LAM. In a large retrospective study of pneumothorax from the LAM Foundation database, the prevalence of pneumothorax in 395 LAM patients during the course of their disease was 66% (260 patients).[93] Approximately 80% of these patients developed at least one pneumothorax before the diagnosis of LAM, with patients averaging 2.6 pneumothoraces before diagnosis. The rate of pneumothorax recurrence is remarkable in patients with LAM. In the LAM Foundation study, recurrence occurred in 140 (73% of 193 patients) who developed at least one pneumothorax.[93] The recurrences were ipsilateral (71%) and contralateral (74%), occurring at an average of 21.7 and 30 months after the initial pneumothorax, respectively, defining LAM as the disease with the highest rate of recurrence.[93] In patients with LAM, most pneumothoraces (81%) occurred at rest or with minimal activity. Bilateral simultaneous pneumothoraces have been reported in LAM; the LAM Foundation study identified 8 (4%) of 193 patients who developed bilateral simultaneous pneumothorax during the course of their disease, with several patients experiencing recurrent bilateral simultaneous pneumothoraces.[93]

The cardinal pathologic feature of LAM is a proliferation if immature smooth muscle cells along the peribronchial, perivascular, and perilymphatic structures.[93] Compression and obstruction of these conduits result in the development of airflow obstruction and pneumothorax, hemoptysis and alveolar hemorrhage, and chyloptysis and chylothorax, respectively. It has been suggested that bronchial obstruction by overgrowth of LAM cells is responsible for the obstructive pattern in trapped air and that the pathologic process ultimately leads to formation of diffuse, bilateral, thin-walled pulmonary cysts ranging in size from a few millimeters to a few centimeters in diameter.[94] The classic CT features of LAM include reticulonodular shadows, cysts or bullae, and hyperinflation.[95] Incidental small pneumothoraces occasionally are discovered on CT scan performed for other purposes. Patients with LAM should be counseled on the symptoms associated with pneumothorax and given explicit instructions to seek medical attention when a pneumothorax is suspected.

One of the major conclusions of the LAM Foundation study was that current experience with pneumothorax in LAM supports an early interventional procedure, either chemical pleurodesis or surgery, following the first pneumothorax.[93] The recommendation was put forth because of the high incidence of pneumothorax recurrence and associated rate of morbidity, including a life-long average of 1 month in the hospital for pneumothorax management in LAM patients who develop an initial pneumothorax.

However, interventional approaches for pneumothorax in LAM may affect candidacy and outcomes of lung transplantations. There are studies that have evaluated the outcomes of lung transplantation in LAM patients who had a pleural pleurodesis. However, a retrospective survey[96] of 34 patients with LAM who underwent lung transplantation at 16 centers in the United States and Europe showed that 27 received single-lung transplant, 6 received bilateral transplants, and one received a heart-lung transplant. Thirteen (38%) of 34 patients had previous pleurectomy or pleurodesis. Also, 18 (53%) of 34 patients had extensive pleural adhesions that were judged to be of moderate severity and severe intent. Moderate-to-severe hemorrhage occurred in four patients, leading to intraoperative death in one patient and repeat thoracotomy in two patients. Overall, posttransplantation survival in this cohort of LAM patients was similar to other chronic lung disease populations. It was concluded that although preoperative complications do occur in LAM patients who had bilateral pleural procedures, lung transplantation remains an important option that improves long-term outcomes.[96]

Chylothorax is a less common pleural complication of LAM than pneumothorax, with a prevalence of approximately 20 to 30% among all reported cases (see the section "Chylothorax"). Most chylothoraces are unilateral with no predilection for either hemithorax. Most, however, are large enough to require intervention. Pneumothoraces and chylothoraces in patients with LAM do not appear to occur simultaneously. Some patients with LAM develop chylous ascites before their chylothoraces. Patients with chylothorax have a subacute onset of dyspnea, with the average age of presentation being approximately 41 years of age compared with the average age of diagnosis of LAM of 34.[97] The occurrence of chylothorax in these patients did not correlate with the extent of lung involvement. Chylothorax in LAM most likely results from the obstruction of the lymphatic vessel by the infiltration of smooth muscle cells. Management of chylothorax in LAM is no different than for other causes of chylothorax.

Esophageal Perforation

The three distinct types of esophageal perforation are (1) traumatic (iatrogenic and barogenic), (2) inflammatory, and (3) neoplastic.[98] Iatrogenic causes account for most esophageal perforations, with the most common causative procedure being esophageal dilation which occurs 3 to 10 times more frequently than with diagnostic flexible fiberoptic esophagoscopy. Spontaneous esophageal rupture, more appropriately termed *barogenic rupture* (Boerhaave syndrome), is a relatively rare occurrence. Rupture is associated with vigorous vomiting. Mediastinitis and sepsis are responsible for the rates of high morbidity and mortality in this syndrome.[99]

The pathogenesis of esophageal rupture includes the following: (1) the esophageal tear always occurs longitudinally, (2) the tear always occurs in the lower half of the esophagus, (3) the rupture pressure is approximately 5 PSI, and (4) the mucosa is the most resistant layer.[100] The lower esophagus is more susceptible to rupture because the upper esophagus is buttressed by striated smooth muscle fibers, whereas the lower esophagus contains only unsupported smooth muscle. The left pleural space is predominantly involved after barogenic esophageal rupture because the esophagus deviates to the left to enter the esophageal hiatus, and therefore, the left lateral wall is in direct contact with the mediastinal pleura. However, perforation of the cervical esophagus usually does not involve the pleural space.

The most dramatic presentation of esophageal rupture is associated with barogenic perforation.[98] This entity is seen most commonly in men in their fourth-sixth decades of life with a history of alcoholism, dietary indiscretion, and malnutrition who present with severe epigastric pain that is pleuritic and may be misdiagnosed as an acute myocardial infarction, acute pancreatitis, perforated peptic ulcer, or empyema of the gallbladder. Pain typically follows severe vomiting and retching and is persistent and severe in the upper epigastrium. Reflex spasm of the upper abdominal muscles may focus the clinician on a primary abdominal process. Fever is universally present and occurs later than the chest pain. Dysphagia is invariably present. Pneumomediastinum is a constant feature of esophageal rupture. After esophageal-mediastinal perforation, a "crunch" may be auscultated over the left heart synchronous with the cardiac cycle.

The presence or absence of radiographic findings depends on the time interval between the perforation and the initial radiographic examination, the site of the perforation, and the integrity of the mediastinal pleura.[101] Early chest radiographs, within minutes of an esophageal perforation, are typically normal. Mediastinal widening with air-fluid levels indicates mediastinal infection and may take several hours to appear radiographically. Mediastinal emphysema virtually never appears before 1 h after perforation and never occurs in approximately 40% of patients. With intrathoracic esophageal perforation, mediastinal changes are more likely to occur. The presence and timing of pleural changes are linked to the integrity of the mediastinal parietal pleura. Rupture of the mediastinal parietal pleura occurs in most patients, with the rapid development of a hydropneumothorax or pyopneumothorax occurring. Most left-sided pleural lesions occur because 70% of barogenic esophageal ruptures develop in the left posterior lateral wall near the diaphragm.[102] Without pleural rupture, mediastinal and subcutaneous emphysema appear rapidly, and a small sympathetic pleural effusion attributed to mediastinitis develops insidiously in approximately 75% of patients.

When esophageal rupture is suspected, a contrast study of the esophagus should be performed immediately. The choice of contrast is limited to a water-soluble iodinated compound and barium sulfate. Barium has the advantage of increased radiographic density and better mucosal adherence. A disadvantage of barium is its ability to incite a foreign-body reaction with development of pleural and mediastinal granulomas and possibly fibrosis. Water-soluble contrast agents are rapidly absorbed and do not cause an inflammatory reaction; however, the limitations are related to hypertonicity. Therefore, aspiration of these compounds into the tracheobronchial tree can create significant inflammation and precipitate pulmonary edema. On chest CT, if air is found in the mediastinum in the appropriate clinical setting, an esophageal perforation is highly likely. Thoracentesis can establish the diagnosis once the mediastinal pleura have ruptured.

PFA will depend on whether the mediastinum is still intact. If mediastinitis alone is present without rupture into the pleural space, the PF is predominantly a neutrophilic exudate with a pH >7.30, glucose concentration >60 mg/dL, and amylase levels less than the upper limits of normal serum amylase. After mediastinal parietal pleural rupture, the patient develops an anaerobic empyema. The low PF pH and glucose are the result of enhanced glycolysis from neutrophil phagocytosis and bacterial metabolism causing increased carbon dioxide and lactic acid.[103] Therefore, finding a low pH, typically between 5.00 and 7.00, in association with a high amylase level, which is salivary on isoenzyme analysis, establishes the diagnosis. The PF at this stage should show high total protein and LDH levels (>1000 IU/L), the glucose concentration should be <60 mg/dL and may reach 0 mg/dL. Furthermore, PF cytologic analysis of high-speed cytocentrufication concentrates may show undigested food particles that confirm the diagnosis, which may not be detected on Gram stain and wet preparations. Squamous epithelial cells observed on cytologic examination also establish the diagnosis.

The patient with a barogenic esophageal rupture represents an emergency. On review[104] of 127 patients with esophageal perforation, it was reported that if primary closure was achieved within 24 h of rupture the outcome was excellent, with a 92% survival rate. After 24 h, survival was substantially worse, no specific treatment was clearly superior, and complications were frequent. Immediate primary repair of barogenic esophageal rupture includes mediastinal and pleural space drainage and prompt treatment with antibiotics that include anaerobic coverage.

BAPE

BAPEs are defined by exposure to asbestos, confirmation of the effusion by chest imaging or thoracentesis, absence of another disease related to the pleural effusion, and no development of a malignant tumor within 3 years.[105] The prevalence of BAPE is related to dose, with 7%, 3.7%, and 0.2% effusions with severe, indirect, and peripheral exposure, respectively. The latency of these effusions was shorter than for other asbestos-related disorders. BAPE was the most common asbestos-related abnormality during the first 20 years after asbestos exposure. BAPE was most common among asbestos pipe coverers, less common in asbestos product or paper machine operators, and least common among ship fitters, maintenance personnel, and welders. BAPE was the only manifestation within 10 years, and it was the most common abnormality during the first 20 years after asbestos exposure.[105]

Two thirds of patients report no symptoms during their effusion.[105] When symptomatic, the most common symptom was pleuritic pain in approximately 17% of patients and dyspnea in 9% of patients. Most BAPE effusions are small, unilateral effusions with a small number presenting bilaterally. In patients with BAPE, pleural plaques were seen in 20% of patients and asbestosis observed in <10%.[105] Follow-up chest radiographs show a blunted costophrenic angle in approximately 90% of patients and diffuse pleural thickening in approximately 50% of patients. Recurrent effusions develop in approximately 30% of patients, sometimes ipsilateral, but more often contralaterally.

PFA in 35 patients with BAPE showed a volume of fluid up to 2,000 mL. The mean volume of these effusions was 460 mL. Approximately onehalf of the pleural effusions were hemorrhagic, and in 26% the exudate demonstrated PF eosinophilia. Other cells in the effusion were predominantly lymphocytes with varying numbers of neutrophils and mesothelial cells. The PF glucose concentrations were similar to blood glucose.[106,107]

An unusual variant of pleural fibrosis, called rounded atelectasis, can result directly from a pleural effusion and often can be confused with possible tumor. Differentiation from a tumor can be problematic, but CT is of value in showing that the lesion simply represents peripheral atelectasis contiguous to the most significant pleural fibrosis and merely represents a form of peripheral lobar collapse.[108]

Uremic Pleural Effusion

At autopsy, 20% of uremic patients have fibrinous pleuritis.[109,110] In patients undergoing decortication for restriction from uremic pleuritis, both the visceral and parietal pleural surfaces are involved with a fibrotic peel covering both pleural surfaces. Pleural effusions from uremic pleuritis appear to result from increased pleural and pulmonary capillary permeability, possibly related to an immune complex injury.

It is estimated that 3 to 15% of patients with uremia develop pleuritis.[111,112] The typical clinical presentation is a patient who has been on dialysis for 1 to 2 years who presents with fever, chest pain, cough, and a transient pleural rub. Dyspnea is uncommon, and patients may be asymptomatic.

The chest radiograph typically shows a unilateral small-to-moderate effusion, but at times, the effusions can be bilateral and massive.[111,112] PF analysis typically shows a serosanguineous to bloody effusion, although the PF can be serous. The nucleated cell count is usually $<1,500/\mu L$, with a lymphocyte predominance averaging approximately 70% of the total nucleated cells. The PF is a concordant exudate by both protein and LDH, and the PF and serum glucose concentrations are equivalent. The pH is typically >7.30 if there is not significant systemic acidemia.[111,112] The PF/serum creatinine ratio is <1 differentiating this effusion from a urinothorax. The diagnosis is presumptive based on the PFA in the appropriate clinical setting. This effusion needs to be differentiated from a tuberculous pleural effusion because of the high risk of tuberculosis in this patient population.

The treatment of a uremic pleural effusion is continued dialysis; the effusion resolves in 75% of patients during a 4- to 6-week period but may recur. Decortication has been successful for those patients who develop severe restriction from lung entrapment.[113,114]

Yellow Nail Syndrome

Yellow nail syndrome (YNS) was first described by Samman and White[115] in 1964, who summarized a series of 13 patients and referred to several other reports from the 1920s and the early 1960s. Their patients had ankle edema and slow rates of nail growth (<0.2 mm/week compared with the normal rate of 0.5 to 1.2 mm/week). The authors suggested that an abnormality of lymphatics may explain the pathogenesis of the syndrome. Two years later, Emerson[116] described the full triad of slow-growing yellow nails, lymphedema, and pleural effusions, whereas Hiller and colleagues[117] in 1972 reported that the presence of two of the three symptoms were sufficient to establish the diagnosis.

YNS is a rare disease, and its diagnosis is based solely on clinical criteria. YNS has been reported from all five continents and includes all races. The male/female ratio has been approximated at 1:1.6.[118] The theory of impaired lymphatic drainage is supported by lymphangiographic findings in which most patients show a paucity of hypoplastic or dilated deficient lymphatics.[118] Electron microscopy has shown, in a single patient, normal lymphatics suggesting obstruction of lymph flow either in the major lymph vessels or at the lymph nodes. The age of onset varies from birth to as late as 65 years of age with a median age of 40 years. Approximately 90% of the reported cases have had yellow nails with the abnormal nails being the initial symptom in 37%. Onycholysis was often present, and some patients have noted that the fingernails acted as a barometer of the syndrome becoming deeply yellow during exacerbation of symptoms and not as impressive during periods of recession. Lymphedema of various degrees was encountered in 80% of the reported cases and was the initial symptom in 34%. The edema was variably pitting and nonpitting. The edema could be confined to the fingertips alone but was often more widespread.[118]

Sixty-three percent of the published cases had pleuropulmonary symptoms. In 29%, the initial symptoms were related to the respiratory tract. Pleural effusions were found in 36% of all cases. Patients often had a history of 10 to 20 years of recurrent episodes of chronic bronchitis associated with bronchiectasis, chronic sinusitis, pneumonia or pleuritis.

Diseases associated with YNS have included erysipelas, cellulitis and lymphangitis, and thyroid abnormalities, including Hashimoto thyroiditis, thyroid enlargement, hypothyroidism, and goiter. Of 97 patients, 6 (6%) developed malignancies. Hypogammaglobulinemia and nephrotic syndrome have also been reported in the setting of YNS.[118]

The PF in YNS is a straw-colored clear exudate with the total protein content generally being >3.0 g/dL and often >4.0 g/dL. In most cases, the PF LDH is <0.67 of the upper limits of normal of serum LDH but at times has been reported in the exudative range. The PF pH approximates 7.40; and the glucose is typically equivalent to the serum glucose, although there is a single report of a PF glucose of 10 mg/dL. The total cell count is <1,000/μL with a predominance (>80%) of lymphocytes.[117,118]

With the full triad, the diagnosis of YNS is easily established. However, signs and symptoms seldom appear simultaneously, and the full triad of the syndrome is not always present, giving rise to some differential diagnostic problems, especially concerning the nail changes.[118]

Treatment can be symptomatic with no specific therapy for YNS. However, there are reports of local steroid injection to the posterior nail folds demonstrating complete recovery, with normal nail growth in some patients. Other treatments that have been tried with variable success include biotin and periodic nail debridement. Lymphedema and pleural effusions, once present, seem to be persistent. Pleurodesis has been successful in preventing the recurrence of pleural effusions and has been accomplished after pleurectomy, chemical pleurodesis, and pleural abrasion. There have also been reports of vitamin E 400 IU twice daily to restore the nails to normal growth and color and improve lymphedema. No deaths attributable to YNS have been reported.[118]

AIDS

A large study from a single US hospital reported a 27% incidence of pleural effusions in 222 hospitalized patients with AIDS. Infection was the cause of the effusions in two thirds of patients, with bacterial pneumonia being the most common (31%).[119] *Pneumocystis jiroveci* pneumonia resulted in pleural effusions in 15% of the patients, and *Mycobacterium tuberculosis* was present in 8% of the population. Noninfectious causes were found in 34%, with hypoalbuminemia the most common cause in 19% of patients.[119]

In most patients, no respiratory symptoms were noted; however, patients with pneumonia, tuberculous effusion, Kaposi sarcoma, and lymphoma had systemic symptoms and dyspnea. The chest radiographs in these patients most commonly revealed small unilateral or bilateral pleural effusions; the largest effusions were seen with tuberculosis, Kaposi sarcoma, and lymphoma.[119]

PFA varies depending on the cause of the pleural effusion. In patients with hypoalbuminemic effusions, the serum albumin was <1.5 g/dL. Pleural effusions in HIV patients with tuberculosis appeared not to be different compared with those without HIV. *P jiroveci* effusions had a low number of nucleated cells with an LDH discordant exudate, most likely reflecting the serum LDH. The effusions with Kaposi sarcoma were hemorrhagic exudates with negative cytology.[119]

Patients with AIDS and effusions had lower CD4 counts and lower albumin concentrations than those AIDS patients without effusions. All cases of pleural tuberculosis in patients with AIDS from 1988 to 1994 reported to the state of South Carolina were reviewed. Twenty-two (11%) of the 202 AIDS patients with tuberculosis had pleural involvement compared with 6% in the patients without AIDS.[120] Associated features of AIDS tuberculous pleurisy included a substantial weight loss and lower lobe infiltrates; there was no difference in PF characteristics between AIDS patients with CD4 counts >200/μL compared with patients with a CD4 count <200/μL.[120] Follow-up with chest radiography in 20 patients showed complete resolution in 7, improvement in 10, and no improvement in 3.

Hypothyroid Pleural Effusion

A hypothyroid pleural effusion is a rare cause of an effusion and is defined as an effusion occurring solely from hypothyroidism without concomitant congestive heart failure, ascites, or other cause of pleural effusion.[121,122] The pathogenesis of the effusion is presumably increased capillary permeability. On presentation, the patient usually has obvious findings of hypothyroidism and may have no respiratory symptoms because the effusions are small and respiratory drives may be blunted. There appears to be no correlation between the development of the effusion and the thyroid-stimulating hormone concentration.[122] The chest radiograph typically shows a small unilateral or small bilateral pleural effusions with a heart of normal size. PFA reveals a protein discordant exudate that is serous or serosanguineous in appearance. There are a small number of mononuclear cells, and the PF and serum glucose are equivalent. The pH has been recorded as >7.30.[122] The diagnosis is presumptive and is one of exclusion; most effusions in a hypothyroid patient are caused by another disease, such as pneumonia. Other effusions are related to hypothyroid-induced congestive heart failure, pericardial effusion or ascites. The classic hypothyroid effusion will resolve over weeks with thyroid replacement.[122]

Pleural Disease After Radiation Therapy

Fifty years ago, radiation pleuritis was reported in 6% of patients treated for breast cancer with supervoltage radiation.[123] Currently, radiation therapy has been shown to cause pleuritis 6 weeks to 3 months after radiation therapy and is associated with a loculated exudative effusion. Late (a year or longer) manifestations of radiation therapy include mediastinal fibrosis, superior venal caval obstruction, and constrictive pericarditis.[124] Radiation pleuritis causes direct injury to the pleural and subpleural capillaries causing increased capillary permeability. The effects of late radiation fibrosis are manifested by impaired lymphatic drainage from the pleural space or imbalances in hydrostatic pressures.[124,125]

Many patients with radiation pleuritis are asymptomatic, but some manifest pleuritic chest pain or dyspnea 2 to 6 months after completion of radiation therapy, which is usually associated with radiation pneumonitis. Patients with remote radiation therapy may have dyspnea or signs of superior vena caval obstruction or have effusions from constrictive pericarditis. The chest radiograph of acute radiation pleuritis shows a small-to-moderate unilateral effusion with a tendency toward loculation. With mediastinal fibrosis, there may be small to moderate unilateral or bilateral effusion with a normal cardiac silhouette.

The PF analysis in radiation pleuritis is a nonspecific, lymphocyte-predominant exudate with reactive mesothelial cells. With the mediastinum fibrosis, the effusions are transudates caused by constrictive pericarditis.[124]

The diagnosis should be considered in any patient who has had previous radiation therapy and presents with either a transudative or exudative effusion. Effusions from radiation pleuritis may persist for months to years. Early use of corticosteroids may relieve symptoms and hasten resolution. With mediastinal fibrosis, malignancy must be excluded. Treatment is usually symptomatic; pericardectomy may be successful for the patient with constrictive pericarditis.

Drug-Induced Pleural Disease

A large number of drugs have been documented to cause pleural involvement (Table 16); however, the incidence is less than drugs implicated in parenchymal lung disease.[126–129] In the patient with an undiagnosed exudative effusion, a careful review of the their drug list must be done. Pleural involvement develops after a variable period of treatment ranging from a few days (nitrofurantoin) to several years (ergolines). Rarely, pleural involvement is noted after termination of the drug. The clinical imaging and pathologic pattern of pleural involvement should conform to earlier observations with the drug. Other drugs should be excluded as causative. Improvement should follow discontinuation of the drug, and pleural involvement should recur after reexposure. Additional supporting information for the diagnosis includes involvement of other serosal surfaces, such as the pericardium. Eosinophilia in PF, blood, and BAL fluid suggest a hypersensitivity reaction, whereas an elevated ANA or antineutrophil cytoplasmic antibodies titer suggests a drug-induced autoimmune condition. High titers of ANA or LE cells in PF are associated with drug-induced lupus pleuritis. The drugs associated with PF eosinophilia include clozapine, dantrolene, glicazide, isotretinoin, mesalazine, nitrofurantoin, propylthiouracil, sulfasalazine, and valproic acid. Eosinophilia is typically present in the blood, BAL fluid or pleural tissue concomitant with PF eosinophilia; there may be concomitant pulmonary infiltrates as well.

Drugs that produce pleural thickening include amiodarone, the ergolines, cyclophosphamide, and practalol.[126] Drug-induced pneumothorax can occur in patients with rheumatoid nodules, primary or metastatic lung tumors (particularly germ cell tumor or sarcoma), or lymphoma as the result of treatment with cytotoxic chemotherapy.

Pleuritic chest pain may be the most common symptom in patients with drug-induced as well as native lupus, whereas more intense pain and friction rubs have been described in patients with drug-induced pneumonitis or organizing pneumonia from nitrofurantoin, carbamazepine, and methacycline. Pleural effusions in association with drug-induced pneumonitis include methotrexate, mitomycin, nitrofurantoin, angiotensin-converting enzyme inhibitors, fenfluramine, amiodarone, and bleomycin. Furthermore, pleural effusions can be associated with drug-induced increased capillary permeability. Drugs that have caused ARDS with concomitant pleural effusions include the following: granulocyte-macrophage colony-stimulating factor, cytosine arabinoside, gemcitabine, and ethchlorvynol. Increased pulmonary capillary permeability has been noted with all-*trans*-retinoic acid and the ovarian hyperstimulation syndrome.

Pneumothorax

Pneumothorax, or air in the pleural space, is classified as spontaneous, traumatic, or iatrogenic (Table 17).

Primary Spontaneous Pneumothorax

The incidence of pneumothorax occurs in 7 to 18 per 100,000 patients/year for men and 1 to 6 per 100,000 patients/year for women. Air can enter the pleural space from rupture of an apical pleural bleb, which can be acquired from bronchial inflammation or be congenital. A pneumothorax may be precipitated by changes in barometric pressure. Small, ipsilateral, hemorrhagic pleural effusions are noted in approximately 10% of patients with primary spontaenous pneumothorax (PSP). PSP most commonly occurs in tall, thin boys and men ages 10 to 30 years. Smoking increases the risk approximately 20-fold in men and less in women. Ninety percent of PSPs occur at rest. Pleuritic chest pain and acute dyspnea are the most common symptoms, which typically resolve spontaneously within 24 h.[130]

A pneumothorax can be diagnosed on a standard chest radiograph when there is visualization of the visceral pleural line removed from the chest wall on an upright radiograph. An end-expiratory chest radiograph on lateral decubitus view with the affected side superior may be helpful in problematic cases. The expiratory radiograph will make the pneumothorax more apparent as the lung is compressed and therefore increases its density and the relative amount of air in the pleural space. An arterial blood gas shows mild-to-moderate hypoxemia and a respiratory alkalosis. The risk of recurrence after an initial PSP is 32 to 52%.[130] The recurrence rate increases with each subsequent pneumothorax. The recurrence rate does not appear to be affected by chest tube drainage (Table 18).

Patients should be treated with supplemental oxygen, which results in a fourfold increase in pneumothorax gas resorption. Observation is warranted with an asymptomatic patient and absence of progression over the course of 6 h. Simple aspiration is successful in 70% of patients with a moderate PSP.[131–133] A small-bore catheter can be left in place if simple aspiration is not effective or placed in a patient with a continued air leak and continued symptoms. The management of PSP is shown in Table 18.

Secondary Spontaneous Pneumothorax

The causes of secondary spontaneous pneumothoras (SSP) include the following: (1) diseases of the airways, (2) interstitial lung disease, (3) infection, (4) malignancy, and (5) others (see Table 18).[130] The peak incidence of SSP occurs later than PSP. Hyperexpansion of the distal air spaces from obstruction or inflammation in the airways can lead to alveolar rupture and retrograde movement of air along the bronchovascular bundle to the mediastinum with rupture through the mediastinal parietal pleura or direct rupture through the visceral pleura from an inflammatory parenchymal process.

Patients with SSP have more severe dyspnea than those with PSP because of their decreased pulmonary reserve. Chest pain is less common and severe than in PSP. However, these patients may

Table 16. *Drug-Induced Pleural Disease**

Drug	Presentation	Chest Radiograph	PFA	Comment
Procainamide	1 yr (1 mo–8 yr) of treatment prior (1.5 g/d) to polyarthralgias, fever, pleurisy; pleuritic pain and effusion in 67%	Infiltrates and effusion	Nonspecific exudate	Also exudative effusion with hydralazine and quinidine; positive ANA and anti-histone antibody
Nitrofurantoin	Acute: previous drug exposure; hours to days after drug; acute onset of fever, dyspnea, and cough; blood eosinophilia	Acute: lung infiltrates and effusions	May have eosinophilia	Symptoms resolve rapidly after drug stopped
	Chronic: insidious cough and dyspnea	Interstitial infiltrates usually without effusion; effusions always associated with infiltrates	Not reported	Sequelae dependent on length of drug therapy
Dantrolene	After 2 mo–3 yr of treatment; pleuritic chest pain and fever; some asymptomatic; blood eosinophilia	Unilateral effusion	Serosanguineous; eosinophilia common	Symptoms improve within days of stopping drug but CXR takes months to resolve
Methysergide	After 2 mo–6 yr of treatment; recurrent chest pain, dyspnea, and fever with pleural rub and effusions	Unilateral or bilateral loculated effusions and pleural thickening	Serous or serosanguineous exudate with low cell count	Symptoms resolve quickly but CXR resolves over months after drug is stopped
Procarbazine	With combination chemotherapy and hours after procarbazine: fever, chills, cough, dyspnea, crackles and blood eosinophilia	Bilateral interstitial lower lobe infiltrates with unilateral or bilateral effusions	Not reported	Symptoms and CXR clear rapidly after drug is stopped
Methotrexate	Afterintermittent or maintenance methotrexate; chest pain, fever, cough, and dyspnea	Effusion without infiltrates (low dose); diffuse infiltrates with small effusions (maintenance); thickening of fissures without effusion (high dose)	Not reported	Symptoms resolve days to weeks after drug stopped
Bromocriptine	1 wk–3 yr after drug; pleurisy, dyspnea, and cough	Interstitial infiltrates, effusion, and pleural thickening	Nonspecific exudate with a low number of cells	Structurally similar to methysergide; withdrawal of drug results in improvement of symptoms
Amiodarone	Dyspnea, cough, constitutional symptoms, pleuritic chest pain, pleural rub after 100 g of drug; pleural disease uncommon	Alveolar or interstitial infiltrates, pleural thickening, and unilateral or bilateral effusions	Serous or serosanguineous with low cell count; foamy macrophages present	Dose-related toxicity; stopping drug and steroids improves symptoms and CXR
Mitomycin	Asymptomatic or dyspnea, cough, chest pain after 36–40 mg/m^2 total dose	Interstitial infiltrates, pleural thickening, and small unilateral and bilateral effusions	Not reported	Isolated pleural disease does not occur; always associated with interstitial lung disease

(continued)

Table 16. *(Continued)*

Drug	Presentation	Chest Radiograph	PFA	Comment
Bleomycin	Effusions have occurred after 150 U; symptoms due to interstitial lung disease	Small bilateral effusions associated with interstitial lung disease	Not reported	Effusions resolve when interstitial disease treated with steroids
Valproic acid	Fever, chest pain or asymptomatic; peripheral eosinophilia often present	Unilateral or bilateral effusions; no parenchymal infiltrates	Exudate with high LDH > 1,000; IU/L 40 to 84% eosinophilia	Lymphoplasmacytic infiltrate and eosinophils on pleural biopsy. Effusions resolve over several weeks after drug discontinued

*Abbreviations as in Table 9.

Table 17. *Classification of Pneumothorax*

Types of Pneumothorax	Causes
Spontaneous pneumothorax	Primary: absence of clinical lung disease
	Secondary: a manifestation of clinical lung disease
Traumatic	Penetrating or blunt thoracic injury
Iatrogenic	Barotrauma
	Invasive procedures
	Insertion of central venous catheter
	Thoracentesis
	Pleural biopsy
	Transbronchial lung biopsy
	Transthoracic needle biopsy

have life-threatening hypoxemia, and hypotension occurs in 15%. The symptoms of SSP do not resolve spontaneously. A suspicion of pneumothorax should remain heightened in the COPD patient with dyspnea and unilateral chest pain. The presence of underlying lung disease often makes identification of the visceral pleural line problematic. A supine radiograph can show pneumothorax gas juxtacardiac or in the costophrenic sulcus and may produce a deep sulcus sign. CT scan may be necessary to diagnose a SSP. The arterial blood gas in patients with a SSP shows significant hypoxemia and concomitant hypercapnia (Table 19). Virtually all patients with SSP require chest tube drainage because the hypoxemia, hypercapnia, and respiratory distress can lead to an untoward event.[133] The management of SSP is discussed in Table 19.

Table 18. *Causes of SSP*

Types of SSP	Causes
Diseases of the airways	COPD
	Cystic fibrosis
	Status asthmaticus
Interstitial lung disease	LAM
	Langerhans cell histiocytosis
	Sarcoidosis
	Rheumatoid arthritis (usual interstitial pneumonia)
	Radiation fibrosis
	Idiopathic pulmonary fibrosis
Infectious disease	Pneumocystis pneumonia in AIDS
	Necrotizing Gram-negative pneumonia
	Anaerobic pneumonia
	Staphylococcal pneumonia
	M tuberculosis
Malignancy	Sarcoma
	Lung cancer
Others	Catamenial
	Pulmonary infarction
	Wegener granulomatosis
	Marfan syndrome
	Ehler-Danlos syndrome
	Birt-Hogge-Dubé syndrome

Tension Pneumothorax

The incidence of tension pneumothorax is 1 to 2% in patients who develop spontaneous pneumothoraces. Tension pneumothorax is most common with traumatic pneumothorax and pneumothorax occurring in patients on positive pressure ventilation. A tension pneumothorax develops when

Table 19. *Management of Spontaneous Pneumothorax*

Immediate Options	Comments
Supplemental oxygen	Results in fourfold increase in pneumothorax gas absorption
Observation	Small PSP, asymptomatic, no progression in 6 h
Simple aspiration	Successful in 70% of patients with moderate PSPs
Chest tube drainage	For virtually all patients with SSPs

Table 20. *Prevention of Recurrence of Spontaneous Pneumothorax*

Therapeutic Options	Comments
Chemical pleurodesis via chest tube	Reduces recurrence rate; talc slurry (most effective) and doxycycline used
Video-assisted thoracoscopic surgery	Stapling of large bleb with talc poudrage, pleural abrasion, or partial pleurectomy

pleural pressure exceeds atmospheric pressure during the entire respiratory cycle. It develops when there is unidirectional flow of air from the lung into the pleural space, and air accumulates in the pleural space because of a check-valve mechanism. Experimental data suggest that circulatory collapse in tension pneumothorax is related to decreased tissue oxygen delivery from hypoxemia rather than impaired venous return. The patient presents with severe respiratory distress, cyanosis, marked tachycardia, and hypotension. The ipsilateral hemithorax may be larger; however, at times it may be problematic to differentiate between the involved and noninvolved hemithorax. The predominant symptoms may be related to hemodynamic instability rather than respiratory distress. The chest radiograph shows the characteristic findings of contralateral mediastinal shift, depression of the ipsilateral diaphragm, lung collapse, and widening of the ipsilateral ribs.

With a high index of suspicion, immediate decompression of the involved hemithorax with insertion of a large-bore needle into the secondary intercostal space should be done without delay. With decompression, there is an immediate decrease in heart rate and respiratory rate, restoration of the BP, and improvement in oxygenation. As soon as the patient is stabilized, a standard chest tube should be inserted.

Iatrogenic Pneumothorax

Causes of iatrogenic pneumothorax include subclavian vein catheter insertion, thoracentesis, percutaneous pleural biopsy, transbronchial lung biopsy, and mechanical ventilation.[130]

References

1. Staub ND, Wiener-Kronish JP, Albertine KH. Transport through the pleura: physiology of normal liquid and solute exchange in the pleural space. In: Chretien J, Bignon J, Hirsch A, eds. The pleura in health and disease. New York: Marcel Dekker, 1985; 169–193
2. Stauffer JL, Potts DE, Sahn SA. Cellular content of the normal rabbit pleural space. Acta Cytol 1978; 22:570–574
3. Albertine KH, Wiener-Kronish JP, Roos PJ, et al. Structure, blood supply, and lymphatic vessels of the sheep's visceral pleura. Am J Anat 1982; 165:277–294
4. Collins TR, Sahn SA. Thoracentesis: clinical value, complications, technical problems and patient experience. Chest 1987; 91:817–822
5. Sahn SA. Approach to patients with pleural diseases. In: Light RW, Lee YCG, eds. Textbook of pleural diseases. 2nd ed. London: Hodder Arnold; 2008, 201–207
6. Heidecker JT, Kaplan AP, Sahn SA. Pleural fluid and peripheral eosinophilia from hemothorax: hypothesis for the pathogenesis of EPE in hemothorax and pneumothorax. Am J Med Sci 2006; 332:148–152
7. Sahn SA, Good JT Jr. Pleural fluid pH and malignant effusions: diagnostic, prognostic, and therapeutic implications. Ann Intern Med 1988; 108:345–349
8. Sahn SA, Reller LB, Taryle DA, et al. The contribution of leukocytes and bacteria to the low pH of empyema fluid. Am Rev Respir Dis 1983; 128:811–815
9. Good JT Jr., Taryle DA, Sahn SA. The pathogenesis of low glucose-low pH malignant effusions. Am Rev Respir Dis 1985; 131:737–741
10. Light RW, MacGregor I, Luchinger PC, et al. Pleural effusion, the diagnostic separation of transudates and exudates. Ann Intern Med 1972; 77:507–513

11. Heffner JE, Brown LK, Barbieri C. Diagnostic value of tests that discriminate between exudative and transudative effusions. Chest 1997; 111:970–979
12. Joseph J, Badrinath P, Basran G, et al. Is the pleural fluid transudate or exudate? A re-visit of the diagnostic criteria. Thorax 2001; 56:867–870
13. Heffner JE, Sahn SA. Multilevel likelihood ratios for identifying exudative pleural effusions. Chest 2002; 121:1916–1920
14. Wiener-Kronish JP, Matthay MA, Callen PW, et al. Relationship of pleural effusions to pulmonary hemodynamics in patients with congestive heart failure. Am Rev Respir Dis 1985; 132:1253–1256
15. Rabin CB, Blackman NS. Bilateral pleural effusion: its significance in association with a heart of normal size. J Mt Sinai Hosp 1957; 24:45–63
16. Romero-Candeira S, Fernandez C, Martin C. Influence of diuretics on concentration of proteins and other components of pleural transudates in patients with heart failure. Am J Med 2001; 110:681–686
17. Broaddus VC. Diuresis and transudative effusions-changing the rules of the game. Am J Med 2001; 110:732–735
18. Gegenhuber A, Mueller T, Dieplinger B, et al. Plasma B-type natriuretic peptide in patients with pleural effusions: preliminary observations. Chest 2005; 128:1003–1009
19. Lazaridis KN, Frank JW, Krowka MJ, et al. Hepatic hydrothorax: pathogenesis, diagnosis and management. Am J Med 1999; 107:262–267
20. Xiol X, Castellote J, Cortes-Beut R, et al. Usefulness and complications of thoracentesis in cirrhotic patients. Am J Med 2001; 111:67–69
21. Lieberman FL, Peters RL. Cirrhotic hydrothorax. Arch Intern Med 1970; 125:114–117
22. Sese E, Xiol X, Castellote J, et al. Low complement level and opsonic activity in hepatic hydrothorax: its relationship with spontaneous bacterial empyema. J Clin Gastroenterol 2000; 36:75–77
23. Chalasani N, Clark WS, Martin LG, et al. Determinates of mortality in patients with advanced cirrhosis after transjugular intrahepatic portosystemic shunting. Gastroenterology 2000; 118:138–144
24. Chen TA, Lo GH, Lai KH. Risk factors for spontaneous bacterial empyema in cirrhotic patients with hydrothorax. J Chinese Med Assoc 2003; 66:579–585
25. Mattison L, Coppage L, Alderman D, et al. Pleural effusions in the medical intensive care unit: prevalence, causes, and clinical implications. Chest 1997; 111:1018–1023
26. Abrass CK. Clinical spectrum and complications of nephrotic syndrome. J Invest Med 1997; 45:143–153
27. Llach F, Arieff AI, Massry SG. Renal vein thrombosis in nephrotic syndrome: a prospective study of 36 adult patients. Ann Intern Med 1975; 83: 8–14
28. Doelken P, Sahn SA. Trapped lung. Semin Respir Crit Care Med 2001; 22:632–636
29. Huggins JT, Sahn SA, Heidecker J, et al. Characteristics of trapped lung: pleural fluid analysis, manometry, air-contrast chest computed tomography. Chest 2007; 131:206–213
30. Rudnick MR, Coyle JF, Beck LH, et al. Acute massive hydrothorax complicating peritoneal dialysis: report of 2 cases and a review of the literature. Clin Nephrol 1979; 12:38–44
31. Lepage S, Bisson G, Verreault J, et al. Massive hydrothorax complicating peritoneal dialysis: isotopic investigation (peritoneopleural scintigraphy). Clin Nucl Med 1993; 18:498–501
32. Jagasia M, Cole F, Stegman M, et al. Video-assisted talc pleurodesis in the management of pleural effusions secondary to continuous ambulatory peritoneal dialysis: a report of three cases. Am J Kidney Dis 1996; 28:772–774
33. Salcedo J. Urinothorax: report of 4 cases and review of the literature. J Urol 1986; 135:805–808
34. Stark DD, Shanes JG, Baron RL, et al. Biochemical features of urinothorax. Arch Intern Med 1982; 142:1509–1511
35. Miller K, Wooten S, Sahn SA. Urinothorax: a cause of a low pH transudative pleural effusion. Am J Med 1988; 85:448–449
36. Sahn SA. Diagnosis and management of parapneumonic effusions and empyema. Clin Infect Dis 2007; 45:1480–1486
37. Sahn SA. Clinical commentary: management of complicated parapneumonic effusions. Am Rev Respir Dis 1993; 148:813–817
38. Heffner JE, Brown LK, Barbieri C, et al. Pleural fluid chemical analysis in parapneumonic effusions. Am J Respir Crit Care Med 1995; 151:1700–1708
39. Colice GL, Curtis A, Deslauriers J, et al. Medical and surgical treatment of parapneumonic effusions: an evidence-based guideline. Chest 2000; 118:1158–1171
40. Rahman NM, Chapman SJ, Davies RJO. The approach to the patient with a parapneumonic effusion. Clin Chest Med 2006; 27:253–266

41. Maskell NA, Davies CWH, Nunn AJ, et al (MIST 1 Trial). U.K. controlled trial of intrapleural streptokinase for pleural infection. N Engl J Med 2005; 352:865–874
42. Hong JY, Lee HJ, Piedra PA, et al. Lower respiratory tract infections due to adenovirus in hospitalized Korean children: epidemiology, clinical features, and prognosis. Clin Infect Dis 2001; 32:1423–1429
43. Bustamante EA, Levy H, Simpson SQ. Pleural fluid characteristics in Hantavirus pulmonary syndrome. Chest 1997; 112:1133–1136
44. Waites KB, Talkington DF. Mycoplasma pneumoniae and its role as a human pathogen. Clin Microbiol Rev 2004; 17:697–728
45. Narita M, Matsuzono Y, Itakura O, et al. Analysis of mycoplasmal pleural effusion by the polymerase chain reaction. Arch Dis Child 1988; 78:67–69
46. Antony VB, Loddenkemper R, Astoul P, et al. Management of malignant pleural effusions. Am J Respir Crit Care Med 2000; 162:1987–2001
47. Tremblay A, Michaud G. Single-center experience with 250 tunneled pleural catheter insertions for malignant pleural effusions. Chest 2006; 129:362–368
48. Heffner JE, Neitert PJ, Barbieri C. Pleural fluid pH as a predictor of survival for patients with malignant effusions. Chest 2000; 117:79–86
49. Sahn SA. Malignant pleural effusions. In: Fishman AP, Elias JA, Fishman JA, eds. Pulmonary diseases and disorders. 4th ed. New York: McGraw-Hill; 2008, 1505–1515
50. Sterman DH, Litzky LA, Albelda SM. Malignant mesothelioma and other primary pleural tumors. In: Fishman AP, Elias JA, Fishman JA, eds. Pulmonary diseases and disorders. 4th ed. New York: McGraw-Hill; 2008, 1536–1552
51. Curran D, Shamoud T, Therasse P, et al. Prognostic factors in patients with pleural mesothelioma: the European Organization for Research and Treatment of Cancer Experience. J Clin Oncol 1998; 16:145–152
52. Ordonez NG. What are the current best immunohistochemical markers for the diagnosis of epithelioid mesothelioma? A review and update. Human Path 2007; 38:1–16
53. Sugarbaker DJ, Flores RM, Jaklitsch MT, et al. Resection margins, extrapleural nodal status, and cell type determine postoperative long-term survival in trimodality therapy of malignant pleural mesothelioma: results of 183 patients. J Thorac Cardivasc Surg 1999; 117:54–65
54. Bynum LF, Wilson JE III. Radiographic features of pleural effusions in pulmonary embolism. Am Rev Respir Dis 1978; 117:829–834
55. Bynum LF, Wilson JE III. Characteristics of pleural effusions associated with pulmonary embolism. Arch Intern Med 1976; 136:159–162
56. Yap E, Anderson G, Donald J, et al. Pleural effusion in patients with pulmonary embolism. Respirology 2008; 13:832–836
57. Porcel JM, Madronero AB, Pardina M, et al. Analysis of pleural effusion in acute pulmonary embolism: radiological and pleural fluid data from 230 patients. Respirology 2007; 12:234–239
58. Gopi A, Madhvan S, Sharma S, et al. Diagnosis and treatment of tuberculous pleural effusion in 2006. Chest 2007; 131:880–889
59. Seibert AF, Haynes J Jr., Middleton R, et al. Tuberculous pleural effusion: twenty-year experience. Chest 1991; 99:883–886
60. Valdes L, Alvarez D, San Jose E, et al. Tuberculous pleurisy: a study of 254 patients. Arch Intern Med 1998; 158:2017–2071
61. Spriggs AI, Boddington MM. Absence of mesothelial cells from tuberculous pleural effusions. Thorax 1960; 15:169–171
62. Valdes L, Alvarez D, San Jose E, et al. Value of adenosine deaminase in the diagnosis of tuberculous pleural effusions in young patients in the region of high prevalence of tuberculosis. Thorax 1995; 50:600–603
63. Joint Tuberculosis Committee of the British Thoracic Society. Chemotherapy and management of tuberculosis in the United Kingdom: recommendations 1998. Thorax 1998; 53:536–548
64. Butt AK, Moers D, Stead WW. Tuberculous pleural effusion: six-month therapy with isoniadize and rifampin. Am Rev Respir Dis 1992; 145:1429–1432
65. Roper W, Waring JJ. Primary serofibrinous pleural effusion in military personnel. Am Rev Tuberculosis 1955; 71:616–634
66. Wyser C, Walzl G, Smedema J, et al. Corticosteroids in the treatment of tuberculous pleurisy: a double-blind, placebo-controlled, randomized study. Chest 1996; 110:333–338
67. Kaye MD. Pleuropulmonary complications of pancreatitis. Thorax 1968; 23:297–306
68. Uchiyama T, Suziki T, Adachi A, et al. Pancreatic pleural effusion: case report and review of 113 cases in Japan. Am J Gastroenterol 1992; 87:378–391

69. Tauseef A, Nandakumar S, Le V, et al. Pancreatico-pleural fistula. Pancreas 2009; 38:e26–e31
70. Walker WC, Wright V. Pulmonary lesions in rheumatoid arthritis. Medicine 1968; 47:501–520
71. Nosanchuk JS, Naylor B. A unique cytologic picture in pleural fluid from patients with rheumatoid arthritis. Am J Clin Pathol 1968; 50:330–335
72. Dodson WH, Hollingsworth JW. Pleural effusion in rheumatoid arthritis: impaired transport of glucose. N Engl J Med 1966; 275:1337–1342
73. Joseph J, Sahn SA. Connective tissue diseases and the pleura. Chest 1993; 104:262–270
74. Faurschou P, Francis D, Faarup P. Thoracoscopic, histological, and clinical findings in 9 cases of rheumatoid pleural effusion. Thorax 1985; 40:371–375
75. Sahn SA. Immunologic diseases of the pleura. Clin Chest Med 1986; 6:103–112
76. Brunk JR, Drash EC, Swineford O. Rheumatoid pleuritis successfully treated with decortication. Am J Med 1966; 251:545–555
77. Harvery AM, Shulman LE, Tumulty PA, et al. Systemic lupus erythematosus: a review of the literature and clinical analysis of 138 cases. Medicine 1954; 33:291–437
78. Pines A, Kaplinsky N, Olchovsky D, et al. Pleural-pulmonary manifestations of systemic lupus erythematosus: clinical features of its subgroups—prognostic and therapeutic implications. chest 1985; 88:129–135
79. Good JT Jr., Antony VB, King TE Jr., et al. Lupus pleuritis: clinical features and pleural fluid characteristics with special reference to antinuclear antibody titers. Chest 1983; 84:714–718
80. Engle MA, McCabe JC, Ebert PA, et al. The postpericardiotomy syndrome and antiheart antibodies. Circulation 1974; 49:401–406
81. Stelzner TJ, King TE Jr., Antony VB, et al. The pleuropulmonary manifestations of the postcardiac injury syndrome. Chest 1983; 84:383–387
82. Kim S, Sahn SA. Postcardiac injury syndrome: an immunologic pleural fluid analysis. Chest 1996; 109.570–572
83. Heidecker J, Sahn SA. The spectrum of pleural effusions following CABG surgery. Clin Chest Med; 2006; 27:267–284
84. Lee YC, Vaz MA, Ely KA. Symptomatic persistent post-coronary artery bypass graft pleural effusions requiring operative treatment: clinical and histologic features. Chest 2001; 119:795–800
85. Light RW. Pleural effusions after coronary artery bypass graft surgery. Curr Opin Pulm Med 2002; 8:308–311
86. Miller JJ. Anatomy of the thoracic duct and chylothorax. In: Shields T, Locicero J, Ponn R, et al, eds. General thoracic surgery. 6th ed. Philadelphia, PA: Lippincott, Williams & Wilkins; 2005, 879–888
87. Doerr C, Allan M, Nichols FR, et al. Etiology of chylothorax in 203 patients. Mayo Clin Proc 2005; 80:867–870
88. Agrawal V, Sahn SA. Lipid pleural effusions. Am J Med Sci 2008; 335:16–20
89. Staats BA, Ellefson RD, Budahn LL, et al. A lipoprotein profile of chylous and nonchylous pleural effusions. Mayo Clin Proc 1980; 55:700–704
90. Duntley P, Siever J, Korwes M, et al. Vascular invasion by central venous catheters: clinical features and outcomes. Chest 1992; 101:1633–1638
91. Browse NL, Allan D, Wilson N. Management of chylothorax. Br J Surg 1997; 84:1711–1716
92. Almoosa KF, McCormack FX, Sahn SA. Pleural disease in lymphangioleiomyomatosis. Clin Chest Med 2006; 27:355–368
93. Almoosa KF, Ryu J, Mendez J, et al. Management of pneumothorax in the lymphangioleiomyomatosis: effects on recurrence and lung transplantation complications. Chest 2006; 129:1274–1281
94. Sobonya RE, Quan SF, Fleishman JS. Pulmonary lymphangioleiomyomatosis: quantitative analysis of lesions producing air-flow limitation. Hum Pathol 1985; 16:1122–1128
95. Chu SC, Horiba K, Usuki J, et al. Comprehensive evaluation of 35 patients with lymphangioleiomyomatosis. Chest 1999; 115:1041–1052
96. Boehler A, Speich R, Russi EW, et al. Lung transplantation for lymphangioleiomyomatosis. N Engl J Med 1996; 335:1275–1280
97. Ryu J, Doerr CH, Fisher SD, et al. Chylothorax in lymphangioleiomyomatosis. Chest 2003; 123:623–627
98. Ferguson T. Esophageal perforations and mediastinal sepsis. In: Hardy J, ed. Critical surgical illness. 2nd ed. Philadelphia, PA: WB Saunders; 1980, 279–289
99. Campbell T, Andrews J, Neptune W. Spontaneous rupture of the esophagus (Boerhaave syndrome): necessity of early diagnosis and treatment. JAMA 1976; 235:526–528
100. MacKenzie M. A manual of diseases of the throat and neck including the pharynx, larynx, trachea,

oesophagus, nasal cavities and neck. London: Churchill Limitis; 1884
101. Parkin G. The radiology of perforated esophagus. Clin Radiol 1973; 24:324–332
102. Anderson R. Rupture of the esophagus. J Thorac Surg 1952; 24:369–388
103. Good JT, Antony V, Reller L, et al. The pathogenesis of the low pleural fluid pH in esophageal rupture. Am Rev Respir Dis 1983; 127:702–704
104. Bladergroen M, Lowe J, Postlethwait R. Diagnosis and recommended management of esophageal perforation and rupture. Ann Thorac Surg 1986; 42:235–239
105. Epler GR, McLoud TC, Gaensler EA. Prevalence and incidence of benign asbestos pleural effusion in a working population. JAMA 1982; 247: 617–622
106. Hillerdal G, Ozesmi M. Benign asbestos pleural effusion: 73 exudates in 60 patients. Eur J Respir Dis 1987; 71:113–121
107. Mattson SB. Monosymptomatic exudative pleurisy in persons exposed to asbestos dust. Scand J Respir Dis 1975; 56:263–272
108. Mintzer RA, Cugell DW. The association of asbestos-induced pleural disease and rounded atelectasis. Chest 1982; 81:457–460
109. Nidus BN, Matalon R, Cantaczino D, et al. Uremic pleuritis-a clinicopathological entity. N Engl J Med 1969; 281:255–256
110. Hopps HC, Wisler RW. Uremic pneumonitis. Am J Pathol 1955; 31:261–273
111. Berger HW, Ramnohan G, Neff MS, et al. Uremic pleural effusion: a study of 14 patients on chronic dialysis. Ann Intern Med 1975; 82:362–364
112. Jarratt M, Sahn SA. Pleural effusions in patients on chronic hemodialysis. Chest 1995; 108:470–474
113. Galen MA, Steinberg SM, Lowrie EG, et al. Hemorrhagic pleural effusion in patients undergoing chronic hemodialysis. Ann Intern Med 1975; 82:359–361
114. Rodelas R, Rakoswki TA, Argy WP, et al. Fibrosing uremic pleuritis during hemodialysis. JAMA 1980; 243:2424–2425
115. Samman PD, White WF. The yellow nail syndrome. Br J Dermatol 1964; 76:153–157
116. Emerson PA. Yellow nails, lymphedema and pleural effusion. Thorax 1966; 21:247–253
117. Hiller E, Rosenow EC III, Olsen AM. Pulmonary manifestations of yellow nail syndrome. Chest 1972; 61:452–458
118. Nordkild P, Kromann-Andersen H, Struve-Christensen E. Yellow nail syndrome: the triad of yellow nails, lymphedema, and pleural effusions. Acta Med Scand 1986; 219:221–227
119. Joseph J, Strange C, Sahn SA. Pleural effusions in hospitalized patients with AIDS. Ann Intern Med 1993; 118:856–859
120. Frye MD, Pozsik CJ, Sahn SA. Tuberculous pleurisy is more common in AIDS than in non-AIDS patients with tuberculosis. Chest 1997; 112:393–397
121. Schneierson SJ, Katz M. Solitary pleural effusion due to myxedema. JAMA 1958; 168:1003–1005
122. Goettehrer A, Roa J, Stanford GG, et al. Hypothyroidism and pleural effusions. Chest 1990; 98:1130–1132
123. Bachman AL, Macken K. Pleural effusions following supervoltage radiation for breast carcinoma. Radiology 1959; 72:699–709
124. Whitcomb ME, Schwarz MI. Pleural effusion complicating intensive mediastinal radiation therapy. Am Rev Respir Dis 1971; 103:100–107
125. Morrone N, Silva-Volpe VL, et al. Bilateral pleural effusion due to mediastinal fibrosis induced by radiotherapy. Chest 1993; 104:1276–1278
126. Rosenow E. Drug-induced bronchopulmonary pleural disease. J Allergy Clin Immunol 1987; 87:778–787
127. Huggins JT, Sahn SA. Drug-induced pleural disease. In: Camus P, Rosenow E, eds. Clin Chest Med 2004; 25:141–153
128. Camus P. Drug-induced pleural diseases. In: Bourous D, ed. Pleural disease. New York: Marcel Dekker; 2004, 317–352
129. Sahn SA. Drug-induced pleural disease. In: Camus P, Rosenow E, eds. Drug-induced iatrogenic lung disease. London: Hodder Arnold; 2009
130. Sahn SA, Heffner JE. Spontaneous pneumothorax. N Engl J Med 2000; 342:868–874
131. Harvey J, Prescott RJ. Simple aspiration versus intercostal tube drainage for spontaneous pneumothorax in patients with normal lungs: British Thoracic Society Research Committee. BMJ 1994; 309:1338–1339
132. Waki A, O'Sullivan RG, McCabe G. Simple aspiration versus intercostal tube drainage for primary spontaneous pneumothorax in adults. Cochrane Database Syst Rev 2007; 1:CD004479
133. Baumann MH. Management of spontaneous pneumothorax. Clin Chest Med 2006; 27:369–381

Pleural Pearls

Steven A. Sahn, MD, FCCP

Objectives:

- Understand the causes, pathophysiology, clinical presentation, diagnosis, and management of patients with trapped lung
- Understand the clinical presentation, pathophysiology, diagnosis, and management of patients with yellow nail syndrome
- Understand the epidemiology, pathogenesis, clinical presentation, diagnosis, and management of patients with thoracic endometriosis
- Understand the pathogenesis, clinical presentation, diagnosis, and management of patients with chronic tuberculous empyema
- Understand the causes, pathogenesis, clinical presentation, diagnosis, and management of patients with urinothorax
- Understand the causes, pathogenesis, diagnosis, and management of patients with a duropleural fistula
- Understand the causes, pathogenesis, diagnosis, and management of patients with a cholesterol pleural effusion
- Understand the pathogenesis, diagnosis, and management of patients with spontaneous bacterial pleuritis

Key words: cholesterol effusion; chronic tuberculous empyema; duropleural fistula; lung entrapment; spontaneous bacterial pleuritis; thoracic endometriosis; trapped lung; urinothorax; yellow nail syndrome

Trapped Lung

Trapped lung is one of a small number of causes of a persistent benign pleural effusion. This condition develops when a portion of the lung is covered by fibrous tissue that prevents its expansion to the chest wall, leaving a persistent, fluid-filled space. Trapped lung is an uncommon consequence of fibrinous or granulomatous pleuritis, in which a fibrous membrane covers the visceral pleura while the lung is separated from the chest wall. Trapped lung should be considered a consequence of abnormal healing in the pleural space with formation of scar tissue on the visceral pleura while the lung is partially collapsed.[1]

Pathophysiology

The diagnosis of trapped lung implies a chronic, constant-volume pleural effusion and a mechanical cause for the persistent fluid-filled pleural space. The pleural fluid in trapped lung typically has low total protein and lactate dehydrogenase (LDH) concentrations consistent with a transudative fluid; however, depending on the timing of the thoracentesis and the integrity of the parietal pleura, the protein concentration may be in the exudative range.[2] Transudative effusions of vascular origin, such as those associated with heart failure, are invariably caused by increased fluid filtration across the capillary endothelium. This increased fluid filtration in combination with a normal protein reflection coefficient results in a low total protein concentration in the effusate. Fluid egress from the pleural space fluid in these conditions is presumably by bulk flow via the parietal pleural lymphatics, preventing a secondary rise of total protein concentration in the effusion. There is currently no evidence that increased capillary fluid filtration is a feature of trapped lung. Furthermore, bulk flow from the pleural space also may be impaired in trapped lung as a result of the involvement of the parietal pleural lymphatics by a pleural peel and impairment of the pump function of the lymphatics during ventilation. A paucity of information is known about the pathophysiology of fluid persistence in trapped lung, and the finding of an exudate by total protein criterion should therefore not be interpreted as unequivocal evidence of an active pleural process.[2]

It is important to define the difference between a trapped lung and lung entrapment, which is associated with an active inflammatory or malignant process. A trapped lung is the end-stage of an unexpandable lung that is not caused by an endobronchial lesion or chronic atelectasis. All patients with a trapped lung must begin with lung entrapment connoting an active process (infection, inflammation [rheumatoid pleurisy] or malignancy) that generates pleural fluid, in addition to the fluid induced by an unexpandable lung. The mechanism of pleural fluid accumulation from an active inflammatory or infectious process or malignant condition may be associated with lung entrapment and differs from the single mechanism operative in trapped lung.[3]

In patients with trapped lung, there is no other explanation for the mechanical visceral pleural restriction of lung expansion or for the persistence of the pleural effusion. In contrast, with intense inflammation, as with empyema, there are other pathophysiologic mechanisms that produce pleural fluid in addition to the fluid induced by the hydrostatic imbalance. Lung entrapment, as can be present with malignancy, causes a pleural effusion by two mechanisms: a hydrostatic mechanism caused by the inability of the lung to expand to the chest wall because of visceral pleural tumor involvement and a capillary leak or lymphatic obstruction as a consequence of malignant infiltration. In contrast, a pleural effusion from trapped lung is solely caused by failure of lung expansion that results in hydrostatic imbalance. It follows therefore that a trapped lung would be a transudate and lung entrapment an exudate. A trapped lung, in reality, is the end stage of lung entrapment when the inflammatory process has resolved (Fig 1).

Pathophysiology

The generation and removal of pleural fluid in a trapped lung are operative under conditions found in the normal pleural space with intact hydrostatic and oncotic pressure gradients. The pleural fluid from a trapped lung exists because the forces promoting generation and removal of pleural fluid are in equilibrium. The loss of lung volume decreases pleural pressure and leads to decreased thoracic volume on the affected side. Moderate decreases in lung volume, such as with lobar atelectasis, lobectomy, or interstitial lung disease, usually do not result in a pleural effusion; the fact that trapped lung, with similar or slightly more volume loss, results in a pleural effusion requires explanation.

After lobectomy, the remaining lung expands, the diaphragm may be displaced upward, and the pleural space assumes its usual width with the remaining lung assuming the shape of the thoracic cavity. However, in trapped lung, the fibroelastic membrane usually involves only the dependent lung, although the entire lung may be involved. The affected lung is not only prevented from expanding by the fibrous membrane but also is restricted to conforming to the shape of the thoracic cavity. The unaffected lung expands normally during breathing and therefore will expand into any void left by the portion of lung that is unexpandable. For the effusion caused by the trapped lung to persist when it is only partially unexpanded, the shape of the

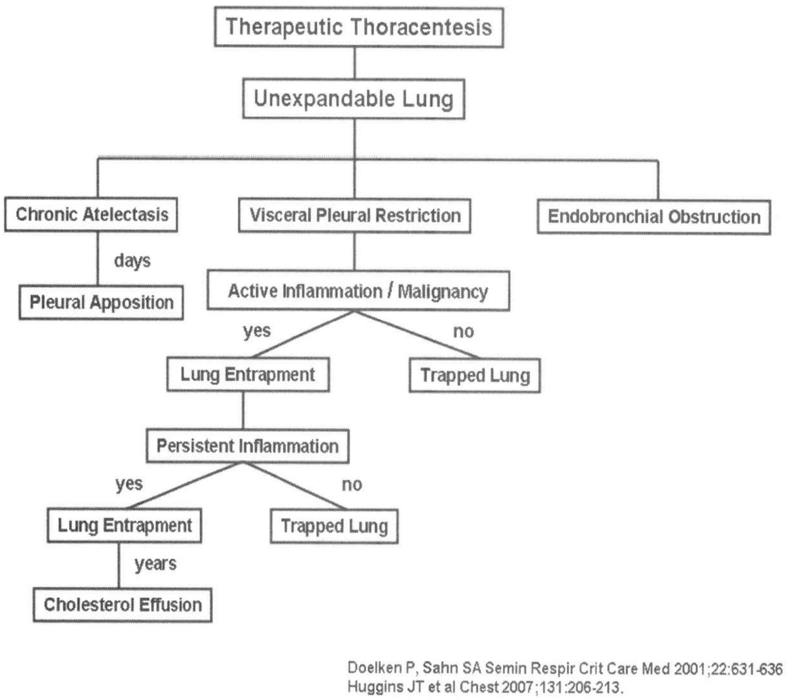

Figure 1. Flow chart of lung entrapment.

trapped lung must be sufficiently different from that of the opposing parietal pleural surface and the unaffected lung must be mechanically prevented from expanding into the space. Otherwise, the space would be obliterated during the reestablishment of negative pleural pressures after resolution of the inflammatory process. Conditions in the pleural effusion from a trapped lung are closer to the conditions along lobar margins, with wider separation of the pleural surfaces, a steeper pressure gradient, and more negative pressures.

The initial mean pleural liquid pressure in patients with trapped lung may be negative or minimally positive but rapidly and substantially decreases with fluid removal. A negative initial pleural pressure or minimally positive pleural pressure and an elastance (change in pleural pressure of >14.5 cm H_2O when 1 L of fluid is removed) in the absence of an active pleural process or endobronchial obstruction establishes the diagnosis of trapped lung.

Causes

A trapped lung can develop from an infection, a noninfectious inflammatory process, hemorrhage, or malignancy. A pleural effusion must have chronicity to allow for mature fibrous tissue to form on the visceral pleural surface while the pleural surfaces remain separated. Some conditions associated with the development of a trapped lung include coronary artery bypass grafting (internal mammary artery harvesting), infection (empyema), inflammation (rheumatoid pleurisy), and malignancy (lung cancer metastatic to the pleura). Because of the extensive number of cardiac surgeries performed currently, especially with use of internal mammary artery vascularization for coronary artery bypass grafting, cardiac surgery is one of the most common causes for trapped lung. Inadequate management of any of the previously mentioned conditions—whether therapy for the underlying condition, inadequate pleural space drainage, or both—can lead to the development of lung entrapment and eventually a trapped lung.

Clinical Presentation

Most patients with trapped lung present with an asymptomatic, chronic, unilateral pleural effusion discovered on a routine chest radiograph or suspected on physical examination. There is typically a remote history of pleurisy, pneumonia, an inflammatory pleural process, coronary artery bypass grafting surgery,[4] or chest trauma. The chest radiograph typically shows a small-to-moderate unilateral pleural effusion without significant mediastinal shift. In the asymptomatic patient, a trapped lung presents as a diagnostic dilemma rather than a condition requiring treatment. Some patients with trapped lung, however, have varying degrees of dyspnea and restrictive physiology on pulmonary function testing and therefore should be considered for decortication.

Diagnosis

The sole cause for the persistent pleural effusion in trapped lung is hydrostatic imbalance. The presence of malignancy, active infection, intense inflammation, a fibrinous exudate, or blood in the pleural space implies that other causes for fluid accumulation also are present, excluding the diagnosis of trapped lung. If trapped lung is suspected, a therapeutic thoracentesis with pleural manometry should be performed. A sterile, lymphocyte-predominant, low-protein, low-LDH effusion without malignant cells is compatible, but not diagnostic, of trapped lung. The diagnosis is established with a significant decrease (>14.5 cm H_2O/L of fluid removed) in pleural liquid pressure, in linear fashion, during fluid withdrawal.[5] The patient typically experiences significant, substernal chest pain from the increase in negative pleural pressure; relief via the allowance of air through the catheter into the pleural space confirms the diagnosis clinically. An air-contrast CT with the affected side superior confirms the diagnosis with visualization of a "thick visceral pleural peel." The patient does not obtain relief of dyspnea from the thoracentesis.

After thoracentesis, reaccumulation of fluid to the prethoracentesis volume generally occurs within 48 h to several days. Complete expansion of the lung after thoracentesis is inconsistent with the diagnosis of trapped lung. If the diagnosis is not established and the lung has not expanded after therapeutic thoracentesis, a chest CT scan should be obtained to exclude severe parenchymal disease; fiberoptic bronchoscopy should be considered to exclude endobronchial obstruction.

At thoracoscopy, a thin, resilient membrane is seen covering the lung surface and preventing reexpansion. On histologic examination, mature fibrosis is evident with few inflammatory cells. If chronicity and stability over time has been demonstrated, a diagnosis of trapped lung can be established with reasonable confidence. These patients often have a history of a persistent pleural effusion for months to years. The effusion resolves completely after decortication if the underlying lung is normal.

Management

A trapped lung can be prevented if there is appropriate management of the pleural space during the inflammatory process. For example, with a complicated parapneumonic effusion or empyema, appropriate antimicrobial therapy and timely drainage of the pleural space will typically prevent a fibrous peel from developing over the visceral pleural surface. Effusions after cardiac surgery and tuberculous pleuritis tend to resolve spontaneously or with the administration of drug therapy before the development of visceral pleural fibrosis. When an active pleural process has been excluded and there is no further explanation other than a mechanical cause for the persistent pleural effusion, a decision can be rendered regarding therapy. The asymptomatic patient with a small trapped lung does not appear to be at risk for a secondary infection or other complications and therefore will not benefit from decortication. In a symptomatic patient, the likelihood of improvement after decortication and the feasibility of surgery should be assessed. If the trapped lung is severely diseased reexpansion after decortication is problematic and therefore surgery would not be expected to result in symptomatic relief.

The underlying lung is best assessed with a chest CT scan. In contemplating surgery, the general health of the patient and the mechanics of surgery need to be carefully considered. Ideally, the elastic membrane that covers the visceral pleura can be easily separated from the pleura without creating significant air leaks. However, at times, a defined resection plane may not be present, increasing the likelihood of complications. Chest CT scan may be helpful by demonstrating extension of fibrous tissue from the pleura surface into the lung parenchyma. In the properly selected candidate, decortication can be achieved successfully years after the acute pleural injury.

Conclusion

Trapped lung should be included in the differential diagnosis of a stable, persistent pleural effusion. The diagnosis requires exclusion of an active pleural process. With trapped lung, there is failure of expansion of the lung after thoracostomy or thoracentesis with an initial negative or minimally positive pleural pressure and a high pleural space elastance. The fibrous membrane covering the visceral pleura can be demonstrated with an air-contrast CT scan after removal of pleural fluid. Asymptomatic patients with trapped lung do not require therapy. Patients with dyspnea on exertion and restrictive physiology should be considered for decortication if the underlying lung is normal.

Clinical Pearls

- Trapped lung, a result of visceral pleural restriction, is a cause of a persistent, benign, constant-volume effusion that is not associated with active pleural infection or inflammation or malignancy.
- Lung entrapment, a precursor of trapped lung, is associated with an active pleural process and an exudative effusion.
- There is no substantial relief of dyspnea with therapeutic thoracentesis in trapped lung, and substernal chest pain is a constant finding that is a consequence of a significant decrease in pleural pressure.
- A high pleural space elastance ($>$ 14.5 cm H_2O/L of fluid removed) confirms the diagnosis of trapped lung.
- A fibrous membrane covering the visceral pleura can be detected on an air-contrast CT scan.
- Asymptomatic patients with a trapped lung effusion do not require treatment.
- Decortication should be considered in patients with exertional dyspnea and restrictive physiology and normal underlying lung.

References

1. Doelken P, Sahn SA, Heidecker J. Trapped lung. Semin Respir Crit Care Med 2001; 22:631–635

2. Huggins JT, Sahn SA, Heidecker J, et al. Characteristics of trapped lung: pleural fluid analysis, manometry, and air-contrast chest CT. Chest 2007; 131:206–213
3. Lan R, Singh KL, Chuang M, et al. Elastance of the pleural space: a predictor for the outcome of pleurodesis in patients with malignant effusion. Ann Intern Med 1997; 126:768–774
4. Lee YCG, Vaz MAC, Ely KA, et al. Symptomatic persistent post-coronary artery bypass graft pleural effusions requiring operative treatment: clinical and histologic features. Chest 2001; 119: 795–800
5. Huggins JT, Doelken P. Pleural manometry. Clin Chest Med 2006; 27:229–240

Yellow Nail Syndrome

The differential diagnosis of a persistent, benign pleural effusion present for years includes lymphatic abnormalities, such as yellow nail syndrome (YNS), chylothorax, and lymphangiectasis and an unexpandable lung, such as trapped lung (postcoronary artery bypass grafting surgery) and lung entrapment (cholesterol effusion). Effusions that last several months, but not years, include benign asbestos pleural effusion, uremic pleurisy, rheumatoid pleurisy, postcardiac injury syndrome, and radiation pleuritis.

Definition and Diagnosis

YNS, first described more than 40 years ago, classically consists of the triad of yellow, slow-growing nails, lymphedema, and respiratory tract disease.[1,2] The latter includes pleural effusion, bronchiectasis, recurrent pneumonia, chronic bronchitis, and chronic sinusitis. However, the diagnosis can be established when two components of the triad are present.

Epidemiology and Pathophysiology

YNS is slightly more common in women and is a consequence of abnormal lymphatic vessels that result in impaired drainage and obstruction, leading to subungual edema, periorbital edema, lymphedema of the extremities, and pleural effusions. In addition, there is evidence that increased microvascular permeability contributes to the clinical findings. Lymphangiograms show a paucity of hypoplastic and dilated lymphatics.[3] The age of onset of symptoms ranges from birth to as late as 65 years of age, with a median of 40 years of age.[4]

Clinical Presentation

Yellow or unsightly nails are the initial finding in only one-third of patients. These patients' nails grow at approximately half the rate of the lower limits of normal nail growth. Other nail abnormalities seen in YNS include overcurvature, either transversely or longitudinally; thickening; onycholysis; cross-ridging; and loss of the lunulae and cuticles. Women frequently cover their unsightly nails with opaque nail polish that can obscure the finding from the unsuspecting observer. Lymphedema is seen in approximately 80% of patients during the course of the disease and is the initial symptom in approximately one-third of patients. Edema can be pitting or nonpitting and can be confined to the fingertips or eyelids only. Pleuropulmonary symptoms develop in approximately 60% of patients during the course of the disease, whereas a third present with a respiratory manifestation. Pleural effusions have been noted in 36% of recorded cases. Patients often provide a history of years of recurrent attacks of bronchitis (in a nonsmoker), bronchiectasis without a known cause, chronic sinusitis, or recurrent pneumonias. Chylothorax has also been reported. Symptoms seldom appear simultaneously, and the triad is not always present.

Pleural Fluid Analysis

The pleural fluid may be unilateral or bilateral, with the volume varying from small to massive. In most patients, the fluid is straw colored but can be sanguineous. The total protein concentration ranges between 3.5 and 4.5 g/dL, with an LDH concentration usually, but not exclusively, in the transudative range. The nucleated cell count is usually $<2{,}000/\mu L$ with a predominance ($>80\%$) of lymphocytes. The red blood cell count is usually $<10{,}000/\mu L$. The glucose level is equivalent to that in serum and the pH is approximately 7.40.

Management

Therapy is usually symptomatic. Local steroid injection and oral vitamin E have been reported to be successful in treating the yellow nails. After thoracentesis, fluid recurs over weeks to months. Chemical and surgical pleurodesis have been successful in those with symptomatic pleural effusions.[5,6] After pleurectomy in a single patient, there was remission of the yellow nails. Spontaneous partial or complete resolution of the nail abnormalities occurs in 30% of patients with occasional relapses. Lymphedema and pleural effusions appear to be persistent, and spontaneous recovery has not been reported. There is a single report of resolution of edema and chylothorax with octreotide.[7]

Clinical Pearls

- YNS should be considered in the differential diagnosis of a discordant exudative pleural effusion by protein criterion only with $\geq$80% lymphocytes that has been present for months or years.
- A history of bronchiectasis, chronic bronchitis (in a nonsmoker), chronic sinusitis, or recurrent pneumonias in association with a chronic pleural effusion or peripheral edema suggests the diagnosis.
- Slow nail growth is the most consistent nail finding and is more common than yellow discoloration of nails; women often cover their unsightly nails with opaque nail polish that may obscure the diagnosis from the unsuspecting observer.
- The triad of yellow, slow-growing nails, lymphedema, and respiratory tract disease is rarely present at the initial encounter; pleural effusion usually is a late manifestation that does not regress spontaneously.
- The diagnosis can be established when at least two components of the triad are present.
- Pleurodesis is successful for treating the symptomatic pleural effusion.

References

1. Samman PD, White WF. The "yellow nail syndrome." Br J Dermatol 1964; 76:153–157
2. Emmerson PA. Yellow nails, lymphedema and pleural effusion. Thorax 1966; 21:247–253
3. D'Alessandro A, Muzi G, Monaco A, et al. Yellow nail syndrome: does protein leakage play a role? Eur Respir J 2001; 17:149–152
4. Norkild P, Kromann-Andersen H, Struve-Christensen E. Yellow nail syndrome: the triad of yellow nails, lymphedema and pleural effusions. Acta Med Scand 1986; 219:221–227
5. David I, Crawford FA, Hendrix GH, et al. Thoracic surgical implications of the yellow nail syndrome. J Thorac Cardiovasc Surg 1986; 91:788–793
6. Sudduth D, Sahn SA. Pleurodesis for nonmalignant pleural effusions: recommendations. Chest 1992; 102:1805–1860
7. Makrilakis K, Pavlatos S, Giannikopoulos G, et al. Successful octreotide treatment of chylous, pleural effusion and lymphedema in the yellow nail syndrome. Ann Intern Med 2004; 141:246–247

Thoracic Endometriosis

Endometriosis is defined by the presence of endometrial glands in stroma outside the uterine cavitary and musculature. The growth and maintenance of these endometrial implants are dependent on the ovarian steroids; therefore, endometriosis occurs only in women of reproductive age or in those women who are receiving estrogen replacement therapy. Endometriosis typically involves the pelvic structures, particularly the ovaries, cul-de-sac, broad ligament, and uterosacral ligaments. However, on rare occasions, endometrial tissue can occur in the thorax, abdomen, brain, and skin.[1]

Epidemiology

Although the prevalence of pelvic endometriosis is approximately 1%, thoracic endometriosis is even less common. There were 110 cases of thoracic endometriosis reported in the English-language literature between 1966 and 1994.[2] These cases included catamenial pneumothorax, hemothorax, hemoptysis, chest pain, and pulmonary nodules. The term *catamenial* means "related to menses," which is an important historical feature that suggests the diagnosis. The most common form of thoracic endometriosis is catamenial pneumothorax. Catamenial pneumothorax occurred in 80

(73%) of 110 cases, catamenial hemothorax in 15 (14%), catamenial hemoptysis in 8 (7%), and lung nodules in 7 (6%).[2]

Pathogenesis

A number of hypotheses have been proposed to explain the pathogenesis of pelvic endometriosis. The most logical one is that retrograde menstruation results in endometrial tissue traversing the Fallopian tubes after failing to clear the peritoneal cavity. Movement of endometrial tissue from the peritoneal to pleural cavity can occur either through congenital diaphragmatic defects, which occur more commonly in the right diaphragm, or through the pelvic veins, with embolization to the pulmonary or the pleural capillaries.[3,4]

Clinical Presentation

At presentation, the mean age of women with thoracic endometriosis is 35 years (range, 19 to 54 years); the onset is typically several years after the peak age of onset of pelvic endometriosis. Of the 110 patients reported, 61 underwent laparoscopy or laparotomy; 51 (84%) had evidence of pelvic endometriosis. Pleural implants, however, were found in < 15% of patients who underwent thoracostomy or thoracotomy, whereas diaphragmatic defects and/or parenchymal cysts or blebs were observed in 25% of patients.

Patients with thoracic endometriosis typically have symptoms within 24 to 48 h of the onset of menstruation; however, catamenial symptoms may not occur with each menstrual cycle. Chest pain is the most common symptom, occurring in 90% of patients; dyspnea occurs in about 30%. Catamenial pneumothorax is almost exclusively (95%) a right-sided event, and the pneumothorax is typically small to moderate in size.[2,5]

Diagnosis

The diagnosis should be considered in a woman of reproductive age who presents with a pneumothorax (nonsmoker), hemothorax, hemoptysis, or chest pain associated with menses. The literature is replete with references to multiple episodes that are undiagnosed for years. Simply having knowledge about this disease should lead to earlier diagnosis and timely, specific therapy with decreased morbidity.

There have been isolated reports of the diagnosis being established by pleural fluid cytology, needle aspiration of lung lesions, cytology from bronchoscopic specimens, and visualization or biopsy of pleural lesions. Pulmonary and pleural nodules have been documented on chest CT within 48 to 72 h of the onset of menses.

Management

The goals of treatment are twofold: eradication or suppression of thoracic endometrial tissue and prevention of reseeding from the pelvis. Initial treatment usually consists of suppression of ectopic endometrium by inhibiting ovarian estrogen secretion. Therefore, oral contraceptives, progestins, danazol, or gonadotropin-releasing hormone analogs have all been used to suppress ovulation. Unfortunately, ovulation suppression appears to be effective in less than half of the patients.

The most effective form of therapy for patients with catamenial pneumothorax or hemothorax is pleurodesis. Pleurodesis is accomplished by thoracoscopic talc poudrage, thoracoscopic pleural abrasion, partial pleurectomy, and chemical pleurodesis through a chest tube. However, even with a successful pleurodesis, patients may still develop catamenial chest pain as long as endometrial tissue is present in the thorax. Recurrent symptoms are presumably the result of cyclical proliferation of the pleuropulmonary endometrial implants in response to ovarian estrogens. These symptoms can be relieved by hysterectomy with bilateral salpingo-oophorectomy but may recur if estrogen replacement therapy is initiated and dormant thoracic endometrial tissue is reactivated. Plication of the diaphragmatic defects has been successful in preventing pneumothorax in some patients.

Clinical Pearls

- Thoracic endometriosis is a clinical diagnosis in women who develop right-sided pneumothorax, hemothorax, chest pain, or hemoptysis in association with the onset of menses.
- Symptoms may be transient and may not occur with each menstrual cycle.

- Most patients have pelvic endometriosis diagnosed several years earlier.
- Suppression of ovulation prevents recurrence in <50% of patients.
- Pleurodesis is effective in preventing pneumothorax and hemothorax; however, catamenial chest pain may occur if endometrial tissue persists in the thorax.

References

1. Olive DL, Schwartz LB. Endometriosis. N Engl J Med 1993; 328:1759–1769
2. Joseph J, Sahn SA. Thoracic endometriosis syndrome: new observations from an analysis of 110 cases. Am J Med 1996; 100:164–170
3. Vinatier D, Roazi G, Cosson M, et al. Theories of endometriosis. Euro J Obstet Gynecol Reprod Biol 2001; 96:21–34
4. Cowl CT, Dunn WF, Deschamps C. Visualization of diaphragmatic fenestration associated with catamenial pneumothorax. Ann Thorac Surg 1999; 68:1413–1414
5. Johnson MM. Catamenial pneumothorax and other thoracic manifestations of endometriosis. Clin Chest Med 2004; 25:311–319

Chronic Tuberculous Empyema

Definition and Causes

Chronic tuberculous empyema, an entity distinct from and much less common than tuberculous pleural effusion, represents chronic, active infection of the pleural space. Chronic tuberculous empyema can occur in several settings: (1) progression of the primary tuberculous effusion (usually associated with a large to massive effusion) that has led to lung entrapment; (2) direct extension of infection into the pleural space from thoracic lymph nodes or a subdiaphragmatic focus; (3) hematogenous spread; (4) after oleothorax or after Lucite ball plombage; (5) postpneumonectomy; and (6) after therapeutic pneumothorax.[1]

Clinical Features

In patients with chronic tuberculous empyema, the inflammatory process may be present for years with a paucity of clinical symptoms. The prolonged asymptomatic course can be explained by the marked pleural thickening that virtually isolates the tubercle bacilli to the empyema cavity. These patients often come to clinical attention at the time of a routine chest radiograph or after the development of a bronchopleural fistula or empyema necessitatis.[1]

The onset of a bronchopleural fistula, which may be dramatic, with acute fever, dyspnea, and production of copious, mucopurulent sputum, not only heralds the disease but increases the risk of spread of the tubercle bacillus through infected sputum. Some patients may have insidious, constitutional symptoms, such as fatigue and weight loss, and also manifest low-grade fever and night sweats.[2]

Empyema necessitatis occurs when the encapsulated empyema erodes through the parietal pleura and discharges its contents. The most common site for empyema necessitatis is in the subcutaneous tissues of the chest wall; therefore, patients can present with a chest wall mass. Subsequent cutaneous rupture can occur, resulting in a pleurocutaneous fistula. Other sites of empyema necessitatis include the esophagus, vertebral column, retroperitoneum, pericardium, flank, and groin. Before the development of antituberculous medications, *Mycobacterium tuberculosis* was the most common cause of empyema necessitatis.

Radiographic Findings

The typical chest radiographic finding of chronic tuberculous empyema is a moderate-to-large, loculated pleural effusion with pleural calcification and enlargement of the overlying ribs due to the chronic infectious process. The diagnosis of chronic tuberculous empyema is confirmed clinically by finding a thick, calcific, pleural rind and rib thickening surrounding loculated pleural fluid on CT imaging. Chest CT findings of a thick-walled, well-encapsulated, calcific pleural mass associated with an extrapleural mass are virtually diagnostic of tuberculous empyema necessitatis.[3] Direct communication between the pleura and chest wall collections is rarely demonstrated because of the thin nature of the tract, which is below the resolution of the images obtained, or because the tract is tangential to the imaging plane and is missed by volume averaging. In addition to tuberculous empyema, the differential diagnosis of empyema necessitatis includes bacterial empyema, lung abscess, blastomycosis, and actinomycosis.

Pleural Fluid Analysis

The definitive diagnosis of tuberculous empyema is established at thoracentesis by finding purulent fluid that is smear positive for acid-fact *bacilli* and subsequently cultures *M tuberculosis.* Tuberculous empyemas typically have nucleated cell counts > 100,000/μL, with virtually all the cells being neutrophils. The pleural fluid is acidic, with pH usually < 7.20, and has a low glucose concentration, usually < 20 mg/dL. Pleural fluid protein concentration is typically > 5 g/dL, and the LDH is > 1,000 IU/L. Anaerobic and aerobic cultures should be performed because, on occasion, there is concomitant bacterial and mycobacterial infection.[1]

Complications

Complications that have been associated with chronic tuberculous empyema include pleural malignancy (most commonly non-Hodgkin lymphoma), superior vena cava syndrome, and pleural aspergillosis.[4]

Treatment

The principles of treatment, pleural space drainage and antimicrobial chemotherapy, are the same for both bacterial and tuberculous empyema. However, problems specific to chronic tuberculous empyema include the inability to reexpand the lung (lung entrapment) spontaneously with drainage and to achieve therapeutic drug levels in pleural fluid, which can lead to drug resistance.[2,5] Several patients have been described in whom chemotherapy for tuberculous empyema was complicated by progressive, acquired drug resistance. It is believed the mycobacteria are exposed to subtherapeutic concentrations of some or all the antituberculous drugs as the result of poor penetration of the agents into the empyema cavity because of a severely fibrotic and calcific pleura; it is possible that the subtherapeutic drug concentrations result in the emergence of resistant strains.

There is a single report of successful nonsurgical treatment of tuberculous empyema with serial, space-emptying thoracenteses and 24 months of isoniazid, rifampin, and ethambutol. Thoracentesis was repeated bimonthly for the first 2 months, monthly for 3 months, and less frequently as the fluid reaccumulated more slowly. Twenty-four months of therapy was chosen based on the rate of improvement of the pleural fluid by laboratory parameters.[6] Surgical options for chronic tuberculous empyema include standard decortication, decortication limited to the parietal side of the peel's sac, thoracoplasty, parietal wall collapse, open drainage, myoplasty, and omentopexy.[7–9]

Clinical Pearls

- Much less common than tuberculous pleural effusion, tuberculous empyema represents chronic, active infection in the pleural space.
- Tuberculous empyema may be present for years (up to 62 years) with a paucity of clinical symptoms.
- Tuberculous empyema may be discovered on routine chest radiograph or after the development of a bronchopleural fistula or empyema necessitatis.
- Chest CT is virtually diagnostic by finding a thick, calcific pleural rind and rib thickening surrounding loculated pleural fluid.
- Pleural fluid analysis shows purulent fluid that is smear positive for acid-fast bacilli.
- Anaerobic and aerobic cultures of the fluid should be performed because, on occasion, there is concomitant bacterial and mycobacterial infection.
- Problems associated with treatment include the inability to reexpand the lung and to achieve therapeutic drug levels in pleural fluid.

References

1. Sahn SA, Iseman MD. Tuberculous empyema. Semin Respir Infect 1999; 14:82–87
2. Iseman MD, Madsen LA. Chronic tuberculous empyema with bronchopleural fistula resulting in treatment failure and progressive drug resistance. Chest 1991; 100:124–127
3. Hulnick DH, Naidich DP, McCauley DI. Pleural tuberculosis evaluated by computed tomography. Radiology 1983; 149:759–765

4. Luchi K, Aozasa K, Yamamoto S, et al. Non-Hodgkin's lymphoma of the pleural cavity developing from long-standing pyothorax: summary of clinical and pathologic findings in thirty-seven cases. Jpn J Clin Oncol 1989; 19:249–257
5. Elliott AM, Berning SEN, Iseman MD, et al. The failure of drug penetration and acquisition of drug resistance in chronic tuberculous empyema. Tuberc Lung Dis 1995; 76:463–467
6. Neihart RE, Hof DF. Successful non-surgical treatment of tuberculous empyema in irreducible pleural space. Chest 1985; 88:792–794
7. Massard G, Rouge C, Wihlm JM, et al. Decortication is a valuable option for late empyema after collapse therapy. Ann Thorac Surg 1995; 68:888–895
8. Al-Kattan KM. Management of tuberculous empyema. Eur J Cardiothorac Surg 2000; 17:251–254
9. Tatsumura T, Koyama S, Yamamoto K, et al. A new technique for one-stage radical eradication of long-standing chronic thoracic empyema. J Thorac Cardiovasc Surg 1990; 99:410–415

Urinothorax

Pleural effusions associated with renal disease occur with nephrotic syndrome, salt and water excess leading to congestive heart failure, uremic pleurisy, peritoneal dialysis, perinephric abscess, and urinary tract obstruction.

Causes

An effusion secondary to obstructive uropathy has a unique pathogenesis and is termed *urinothorax*. With rare exception, hydronephrosis with extravasation of fluid into the perirenal space appears to be a prerequisite for the development of a urinothorax. Causes of urinothorax reported in the literature include bladder and prostate cancer, posterior urethral valves, renal cysts, nephrolithiasis, surgical ureteral manipulation, blunt kidney trauma, renal transplant, ileal conduit with ureteral obstruction, and bladder laceration.[1,2]

Pathogenesis

Obstructive uropathy leads to perirenal fluid accumulation and movement of urine transdiaphragmatically into the ipsilateral pleural space.[2] Removal of the obstructing lesion generally results in rapid resolution (within days) of the effusion. The pathogenesis of the low-pH transudate is not clearly established, although it is most likely related to the low pH of the extravasated urine with back-diffusion of hydrogen ions as the fluid passes from the retroperitoneal into the pleural space.[3] An alkaline urine at the time of extravasation could result in a pleural fluid pH up to 8.0.

Clinical Presentation

Depending on the size of the pleural effusion and the underlying pulmonary status, the patient may present with dyspnea or be asymptomatic. Other symptoms would depend on the cause of the urinary tract obstruction.[2,3]

Chest Radiograph

The chest radiograph should demonstrate a small-to-moderate effusion ipsilateral to the obstructed kidney; however, there are reports of bilateral and contralateral effusions.

Pleural Fluid Analysis

The pleural fluid looks and smells like urine. The fluid is a transudate that frequently has a pH <7.30. The total protein may be <1 g/dL if there is no significant proteinuria. The pleural fluid/serum creatinine ratio is >1.0 as long as urinary tract obstruction persists.[1,3]

Diagnosis

The effusion is often discovered on a routine postoperative chest radiograph. The diagnosis should be suspected in the setting of obstructive uropathy and can be confirmed by thoracentesis demonstrating a pleural fluid/serum creatinine ratio >1.0. The ratio of pleural fluid to serum creatinine appears to be specific for the diagnosis, especially if measured within the first few days of pleural fluid formation; an additional clue to the diagnosis is the finding of a low-pH transudate. The latter is a unique combination as all other low-pH effusions (pH <7.30) have been associated with exudates (empyema, complicated parapneumonic effusion, esophageal rupture, carcinoma, rheumatoid pleurisy, tuberculosis, and lupus pleuritis).

Treatment

Relief of obstruction results in rapid reversal of the pleural fluid/serum creatinine ratio and resolution of the effusion over several days without pleural space sequelae.

Clinical Pearls

- A urinothorax is typically an ipsilateral urine collection in the pleural space due to obstructive uropathy.
- Urinothorax is the only single cause of a low-pH transudate.
- A pleural fluid/serum creatinine ratio >1.0 is diagnostic of a urinothorax.
- The pleural fluid/serum creatinine ratio >1.0 and low pH will not be maintained once the urinary tract obstruction is relieved.
- The effusion resolves rapidly over a few days after the relief of obstruction, and there are no pleural sequelae.

References

1. Stark BD, Schanes JG, Baron RL, et al. Biochemical features of urinothorax. Arch Intern Med 1982; 142:1509–1511
2. Salcedo JR. Urinothorax: report of 4 cases and review of the literature. J Urol 1986; 135:805–808
3. Miller KS, Wooten S, Sahn SA. Urinothorax: a cause of low pH transudative pleural effusions. Am J Med 1988; 85:448–449

Duropleural Fistula

Definition

A duropleural fistula (DPF) or subarachnoid pleural fistula represents communication between the subarachnoid and pleural spaces.

Pathophysiology and Causes

The mechanism of a DPF involves disruption of the dural membrane and parietal pleura, allowing a tract to develop between the subarachnoid and pleural spaces. Once the fistula develops, a pressure gradient is established, which allows cerebrospinal fluid (CSF) to flow from the positive-pressure subarachnoid space to the negative-pressure pleural space.

Most cases of DPF are secondary to blunt and penetrating trauma, with a total of 23 cases reported since 1959.[1] The mechanism that results in a traumatic fistula can involve either a missile traversing both the pleural and subarachnoid spaces or a vertebral fracture that tears the dura and parietal pleura. A fistulous tract usually occurs between the upper thoracic subarachnoid space and the pleural space. With blunt trauma, the disruption occurs from extreme extension of the spine, resulting in the tearing of the relatively immobile nerve roots and dura. Significant chest wall compression may perforate the pleura against the bony prominence of the spine. Regardless of the cause, the DPF remains open because of the pressure gradient between the positive pressure of the subarachnoid space and the negative pressure in the pleural space.

Although laminectomy is a common neurosurgical procedure to treat spinal injuries, there have been only two reports of DPF as a complication.[2,3] Neurosurgery may be a more common cause than trauma; however, these DPFs may be recognized early by neurosurgeons and repaired without generating reports in the literature and requesting pulmonary consultation. DPF has been documented as a complication of thoracotomy in six cases and rupture of intrathoracic meningocele in one case.

Clinical Presentation

A high degree of suspicion is necessary to establish the diagnosis of a DPF. A DPF should be considered as a cause of a persistent transudative effusion. Symptoms that suggest a CSF leak include postural headaches, nausea, and vomiting. Often symptoms related to the effusion, such as chest pain, dyspnea, or fever, may be minimal or overshadowed by concomitant injuries, often delaying the diagnosis. In addition to the almost universal findings of severe spinal cord injury, other clues to the diagnosis may include pneumocephalus or meningitis.

Chest Radiograph

Shortly after the development of a DPV, the chest radiograph may be normal. Effusions range from small to massive depending on the size and duration of the fistula. Mediastinal widening may be an early manifestation, and once aortic injury has been excluded, a diagnosis of subarachnoid-mediastinal or subarachnoid-pleural fistula should be considered.

Pleural Fluid Analysis

Pleural fluid in nontraumatic DPF is clear and looks like water. The nucleated cell count is low and the pleural fluid glucose value is approximately 0.6 of the serum glucose. An important feature of the transudative effusion is that the total protein is consistently <1.0 g/dL (if precisely measured should be <0.05.); the LDH is also clearly in the transudative range.[1,4] Other causes of transudates with total protein consistently <1.0 g/dL include urinothorax, peritoneal dialysis, and extravascular migration of a central venous catheter with saline or glucose infusion. Previous authors have described both transudates and exudates in traumatic DPF. Because concomitant pleural processes secondary to trauma can be present, the diagnosis of DPF by pleural fluid analysis can be confounded by other pleural processes, such as hemothorax.[1] β_2-Transferrin is produced by neuraminidase activity in the brain and is found uniquely in the CSF and inner ear perilymph this protein is accepted as a sensitive and specific marker to identify CSF leaks into the pleural space following head or spine trauma or spinal surgery; testing for β_2-transferrin is available to practicing clinicians.[1,4,5]

Diagnosis

Although the presence of β_2-transferrin in pleural fluid diagnostic of DPF, definitive identification of the fistula requires radiographic visualization. Conventional myelography and radionuclide myelography are most commonly used. Several authors have concluded that isotope myelography is more sensitive than conventional myelography.[6] However, there are reports of false-negative results when myelography is used alone, with slow or intermittent leaks. CT scanning performed concomitantly with myelography will add to the delineation of the anatomic defect. In addition, the presence of contrast in the pleural space after myelography confirms the diagnosis in patients with slow CSF leaks.

Treatment

Because of the limited number of cases, there is no strong consensus regarding management of DPF. However, spontaneous resolution is rare, and most patients require either surgical ligation or closed-tube drainage for management. Of the 19 posttraumatic DPFs reported in one series, 13 (68%) patients were treated definitively with laminectomy or thoracotomy, while 3 (16%) patients responded to chest tube drainage. Two (11%) of 19 patients were treated with thoracentesis, although one was treated with "conservative" measures. In 9 (82%) of the 11 patients in whom laminectomy was performed, closure of the fistula was successful. The appropriate timing of surgical intervention is unknown. Some surgeons advocate chest tube drainage for up to 2 weeks before surgical intervention, whereas others recommend early intervention, noting the low rate of spontaneous closure.[7]

Clinical Pearls

- The most common reported cause of DPF is blunt or penetrating trauma; other causes include transthoracic diskectomy and thoracotomy.
- Symptoms that suggest CSF leak include postural headaches, nausea, and vomiting.
- DPF is a cause of a persistent, transudative pleural effusion.
- In nontraumatic cases, the pleural fluid looks like water, is paucicellular with a mononuclear predominance, has an alkaline pH, has a glucose level of approximately 0.6 of the serum glucose, and has a protein concentration <1 g/dL (typically <0.05).
- The presence of β_2-transferrin in the pleural fluid confirms the diagnosis.
- Definitive identification of the fistula requires radiographic visualization, either by radionuclide or conventional myelography.

- Spontaneous resolution is rare, and most patients require surgical closure for definitive treatment.

References

1. Lloyd C, Sahn SA. Subarachnoid pleural fistula due to penetrating trauma. Chest 2002; 122: 2252–2256
2. Monla-Hassan J, Eichenhorn M, Spickler E, et al. Duropleural fistula manifested as a large pleural transudate: an unusual complication of transthoracic diskectomy. Chest 1998; 114:1786–1788
3. Assietti R, Kibble MB, Bakay R. Iatrogenic cerebrospinal fluid fistula to the pleural cavity: case report and literature review. Neurosurgery 1993; 33:1104–1108
4. Huggins JT, Sahn SA. Duro-pleural fistula diagnosed by β2-transferrin. Respiration 2003; 70: 423–425
5. Skedros DG, Cass SP, Hirsch BE, et al. Beta-2 transferrin assay in clinical management of cerebral spinal fluid and perilymphatic fluid leaks. J Otolaryngol 1993; 22:341–344
6. Rosen PR, Chaudhuri TK. Radioisotope myelography in the detection of pleural-dural communication as a source of recurrent meningitis. Clin Nucl Med 1983; 8:28–30
7. Pollack II, Pang D, Hall W. Subarachnoid-pleural and subarachnoid mediastinal fistulae. Neurosurgery 1990; 26:519–525

Cholesterol Pleural Effusion

A cholesterol pleural effusion, also referred to as a *pseudochylous* or *chyliform effusion*, is characterized by a high lipid content that is not a consequence of leakage from the thoracic duct. It is thought to be a rare condition but probably occurs more commonly than reported in the literature. Some refer to *pseudochylothoraces* as lipid effusions with cholesterol crystals and to *chyliform effusions* as those without cholesterol crystals.[1–3]

Pathogenesis

The pathogenesis of these effusions has not been clearly elucidated. However, these effusions are a consequence of chronic pleural inflammation in the setting of lung entrapment and severe parietal pleural fibrosis that evolve over several years.[2] The origin of the elevated pleural fluid cholesterol has been attributed to local degeneration of pleural nucleated cells and RBCs. The lipoprotein pattern of a cholesterol effusion shows a shift of cholesterol binding towards the high-density lipoproteins, most likely occurring as the cholesterol is sequestered in the pleural space and undergoes a change in lipoprotein binding characteristics. Cholesterol in these effusions may be complexed with triglycerides and proteins.[4]

These chronic, inflammatory effusions result in "permanent" lung entrapment that causes persistence of the effusion as a result of hydrostatic imbalance; a concomitant, low-grade inflammatory process continues, as evidenced by a pleural fluid total protein and LDH in the exudative range with concomitant neutrophilia.[2] Over time, pleural fibrosis progresses and large cholesterol deposits are often demonstrated on histologic examination.

The high triglyceride concentration noted in some cholesterol effusions cannot be explained by local cellular degeneration and supports the hypothesis that plasma lipoproteins move into the pleural space bound to triglycerides.[4]

Causes

A literature review published in 1999 revealed 175 cases of cholesterol pleural effusions, with 78% in men (age range, 17 to 81 years). The majority of the cases were attributable to tuberculosis; rheumatoid pleurisy was a distant second in frequency. Other causes include paragonimiasis, lung cancer, empyema, hemothorax, and trauma (Table 1).[5]

Table 1. *Causes of Cholesterol Effusions**

Chronic tuberculous pleural effusion (most common)
Rheumatoid pleurisy (2nd most common)
Paragonimiasis
Lung cancer
Echinococcosis
Hemothorax
Collapse therapy for TB
Trauma
Hemothorax

*From Garcia-Zamalloa et al.[5]

Diagnosis

The cardinal feature of these effusions is a high cholesterol concentration, which is independent of the serum cholesterol. A cholesterol pleural effusion may be differentiated from a chylothorax by its etiology, chronicity, lack of symptoms, a cholesterol/triglyceride ratio > 1.0, and a total cholesterol level > 200 mg/dL (Table 2). The effusion can have a milky appearance or appear turbid with a satin-like sheen. These effusions also have been described as resembling "soft, white cheese" and "motor oil." Cholesterol crystals may be seen on microscopy. Cholesterol effusions typically have cholesterol concentrations from 300 to 1,500 mg/dL; however, lower levels may occur from a dilutional effect after repeated thoracenteses. Chylothoraces usually have cholesterol concentrations < 150 mg/dL. When the cholesterol concentration is > 200 mg/dL, the most likely diagnosis is a cholesterol effusion, regardless of the triglyceride levels. A chylous effusion is most likely when the triglyceride value is > 110 mg/dL and the cholesterol level is < 200 mg/dL.[2]

Management

These effusions represent the consequence of prolonged lung entrapment (hydrostatic imbalance) and chronic inflammation. The underlying disease should be treated if possible. If the effusion is small and the patient relatively asymptomatic, observation with reassurance is indicated. Decortication should be considered for the symptomatic patient with restrictive physiology as long as the underlying lung is relatively normal. However, the presence of an active inflammatory process would appear to make the prospect of successful decortication less likely.[6]

Clinical Pearls

- A cholesterol effusion is distinct from a chylothorax and is a consequence of chronic pleural inflammation and lung entrapment.
- Lung entrapment causes hydrostatic imbalance, whereas pleural inflammation leads to a capillary leak and with high total protein and LDH concentrations.
- The most common causes reported are chronic tuberculous empyema and rheumatoid pleurisy.
- The diagnosis can be suspected by observing fluid with a satin-like sheen and diagnosed if the cholesterol concentration is > 200 mg/dL and cholesterol crystals are seen microscopically.
- If the effusion does not resolve with treatment of the underlying disease, decortication should be considered for the symptomatic patient with restrictive physiology.

References

1. Coe JE, Aikawa JK. Cholesterol pleural effusion. Arch Intern Med 1961; 108:163–174

Table 2. *Differentiating a Cholesterol Effusion From Chylothorax**

Condition	Chylothorax	Cholesterol Effusion
Incidence	Uncommon	Rare
Causes	Lymphoma, trauma, surgery, lymphangioleiomyomatosis	Lung entrapment; tuberculosis, rheumatoid arthritis, empyema
Onset	Acute to subacute	Insidious; chronic course (years)
Symptoms	Dyspnea	None; dyspnea
Appearance	Serous, milky, turbid, bloody	Milky; satin-like sheen
Pleural fluid analysis	Protein-discordant exudate with ≥80% lymphocytes; triglycerides > 110 mg/dL	Neutrophil-predominant exudate; cholesterol, > 200 mg/dL; cholesterol/triglyceride ratio > 1.0
Diagnosis	Presence of chylomicrons; cholesterol > 60 and <200 mg/dL	Cholesterol >200 mg/dL; cholesterol crystals
Treatment	Manage underlying disease; pleurodesis	Observe; decortication

*From Agrawal V, Sahn SA.[2]

2. Agrawal V, Sahn SA. Lipid pleural effusions. Am J Med Sci 2008; 335:16–20
3. Hillerdal G. Chylothorax and pseudochylothorax. Eur Respir J 1997; 10:1157–1162
4. Hamm H, Pfalzer B, Fabel H. Lipoprotein analysis in a chyliform pleural effusion: implications for pathogenesis and diagnosis. Respiration 1991; 58:294–300
5. Garcia-Zamalloa A, Ruiz-Irastorza G, Aguayo FJ, et al. Pseudochylothorax: report of two cases and review of the literature. Medicine 1999; 78:1–13
6. Goldman A, Burford TH. Cholesterol pleural effusions: a report of three cases with cure by decortication. Dis Chest 1950; 18:586–594

Spontaneous Bacterial Empyema (Spontaneous Bacterial Pleuritis)

Definition

Spontaneous bacterial empyema is the term used in the literature when bacteria are cultured from pleural fluid of a cirrhotic patient with hepatic hydrothorax who has a neutrophil count >250/μL, similar to *spontaneous bacterial peritonitis* (SBP). It can also be diagnosed if pleural fluid culture is negative and the pleural fluid neutrophil count is >500 cells/μL, there is absence of an intra-abdominal source of infection, and the patient has not received antibiotics in the past 30 days. However, spontaneous bacterial empyema is a misnomer because, in the vast majority of cases, the pleural fluid is not purulent and, therefore, is not an empyema. The appropriate term should be *spontaneous bacterial pleuritis* (SBPL).

Pathogenesis

Conn reported the first case of SBP,[1] which has a prevalence of 10 to 20% in hospitalized patients with cirrhosis and clinical ascites. The organisms responsible for this infection are enteric bacteria, which may reach the ascitic fluid by migration across the bowel wall or through hematogenous spread. In normal individuals, enteric bacteria in portal blood are removed by the reticuloendothelial system. In patients with cirrhosis who have impaired reticuloendothelial system function, intrahepatic and portosystemic shunting of blood is likely to cause persistent bacteremia. Cirrhotic patients have a number of defects in host defenses, including defects in serum bactericidal function, chemoattraction, opsonization, and impaired cellular function of neutrophils and monocytes. In addition, ascitic fluid provides an excellent culture medium for bacteria.

Approximately 6% of patients with cirrhosis and clinical ascites have a pleural effusion (hepatic hydrothorax).[2] These effusions occur most commonly on the right side (70%) and less often on the left (15%) or bilaterally (15%). A hepatic hydrothorax develops as ascitic fluid moves into the pleural space through congenital diaphragmatic defects along a pressure gradient. This occurs more commonly on the right, as there are a greater number of diaphragmatic defects compared with the left hemidiaphragm.

Clinical Features

The exact incidence of SBPL is unknown. In addition to case reports, there have been only two retrospective series totaling 15 episodes and a prospective study of 24 episodes.[3,4] In the prospective trial, 120 patients with hepatic hydrothorax were hospitalized during a period of 4 years.[4] Ninety-five (79%) of the patients had detectable ascites in addition to their pleural effusion. Sixteen (13%) of the 120 patients had 24 episodes of SBPL. All patients had advanced cirrhosis, and most had been hospitalized on previous occasions with clinical signs of progressive liver dysfunction. Clinical ascites was not detectable during 6 (25%) of the 24 episodes of SBPL. In the 18 episodes with ascites, the ascitic fluid was infected in 14 (78%) patients and sterile in 4 (22%) patients. In 10 (43%) of the 24 episodes, SBPL was not associated with SBP (6 without ascites and 4 with noninfected ascites). Blood culture results were positive in 11 (46%) of 24 episodes, 4 of 10 patients without SBP, and 7 of 14 with SBP. Pleural fluid culture results were positive in 18 (75%) of the 24 episodes using a more sensitive method of culture (inoculation of pleural fluid into a tryptic soy broth blood culture bottle at the patient's bedside).[4–6]

The microorganisms identified in pleural fluid were *Escherichia coli* in eight patients, Streptococcus sp in four patients, Enterococcus sp in three patients, *Klebsiella pneumoniae* in two patients, and *Pseudomonas stutzeri* in one patient.[4] Six patients had culture-negative SBPL. The etiologic diagnosis was confirmed in four of the six culture-negative patients, two by ascitic fluid culture, one by blood culture, and one by both ascitic and blood cultures.

Only the pleural fluid LDH increased during infection; there was no significant change in total protein and glucose with SBPL. The absolute pleural fluid neutrophil count in the 24 episodes of SBPL was >1,000/μL in 21 (88%) episodes, with a range of 530 to 13,300/μL. In 8 (36%) of 22 episodes, the pleural fluid pH was <7.30 (range 7.04 to 7.50).[4]

Treatment

All patients were treated with antibiotics for 7 to 10 days. A chest tube was not inserted in any of the patients with SBPL.[4]

Outcome

Five (20%) of the 24 patients died. The causes of death were septic shock, esophageal variceal hemorrhage, and hepatic insufficiency. In the remainder of the patients, the infection was cured after 7 to 10 days of antibiotic treatment. Four of the 10 patients with SBPL who were discharged died between 1 and 19 months after their episode. In five patients, liver transplantation was performed 2 to 24 months after the episode of SBPL.[4]

Clinical Pearls

- SBPL is a frequent complication of hepatic hydrothorax; the 13% incidence is similar to that for patients with SBP with ascites.
- SBPL is rarely diagnosed because thoracentesis is not performed routinely in patients with hepatic hydrothorax, and hepatic hydrothorax in patients with clinical ascites is relatively uncommon.
- There are patients with culture-positive SBPL who have culture-negative SBP and *vice-versa*. Therefore, a thoracentesis should be performed, in addition to paracentesis and blood cultures, in cirrhotic patients with suspected infection.
- Ascites is not a prerequisite for SBPL, suggesting that enteric microorganisms reach the pleural space hematogenously.
- The inoculation of 10 mL of pleural fluid and ascitic fluid into a tryptic soy broth blood culture bottle at the patient's bedside increases the sensitivity for the diagnosis of both SBPL and SBP compared with traditional delayed inoculation techniques.
- If patients with SBPL do not have purulent fluid, they should be treated with antibiotics alone without the insertion of a chest tube, which can result in significant morbidity.

References

1. Conn HO. Spontaneous peritonitis and bacteremia in Laennec's cirrhosis caused by enteric organisms: a relatively common but rarely recognized syndrome. Ann Intern Med 1964; 60: 568–580
2. Lieberman FL, Hidemura R, Peters RL, et al. Pathogenesis and treatment of hydrothorax complicating cirrhosis with ascites. Ann Intern Med 1964; 61:385–401
3. Xiol X, Castellote J, Baliellis C, et al. Spontaneous bacterial empyema in cirrhotic patients: analysis of 11 cases. Hepatology 1990; 11:365–370
4. Xiol X, Castellvi JM, Guardiola J, et al. Spontaneous bacterial empyema in cirrhotic patients: a prospective study. Hepatology 1996; 23:719–723
5. Castellote J, Xiol X, Verdaguer R, et al. Comparison of 2 ascitic fluid culture methods in cirrhotic patients with spontaneous bacterial peritonitis. Am J Gastroenterol 1990; 85:1605–1608
6. Runyon BA, Antillon MR, Akriviadis EA, et al. Bedside inoculation of blood culture bottles with ascitic fluid is superior to delayed inoculation in the detection of spontaneous bacterial peritonitis. J Clin Microbiol 1990; 28:2811–2812

Lung Transplantation

Stephanie M. Levine, MD, FCCP

Objectives:

- Define the indications for lung transplantation
- Review the guidelines for recipient selection for lung transplantation
- Describe the relative and absolute contraindications to lung transplantation
- Describe outcomes after transplantation, including survival and physiologic results
- Review the complications after lung transplantation
- Give an overview of the immunosuppressive medications used in lung transplantation

Key words: acute rejection; cytomegalovirus; immunosuppression; lung transplantation; obliterative bronchiolitis

During the last 2.5 decades, lung transplantation (LT) has become a successful therapeutic option for patients with end-stage pulmonary parenchymal and vascular diseases. Dr. James Hardy at the University of Mississippi performed the first LT in 1963. However, the patient survived for only 18 days. Subsequent attempts at LT were complicated by bronchial anastomotic dehiscence and early graft failure, resulting in limited survival. Advances in donor and recipient selection, improved surgical techniques, new immunosuppressive drugs, and better management of infections have all contributed to improved survival. Despite these advancements, numerous complications still exist after LT.

According to the 2008 report from the International Society of Heart Lung Transplantation (ISHLT), 24,904 LT procedures have been performed worldwide; in 2006 alone, 2,168 procedures were performed. The 1-year, 3-year, 5-year, and 10-year survival rates are 78%, 63%, 51%, and 28%, respectively, as reported by the Registry of the ISHLT.[1] The major rate-limiting factors to the long-term survival of LT patients remain chronic rejection and infection.

Most LT referrals come from pulmonary physicians from outside of tertiary transplant centers. With the increase in the number of transplant recipients, much of the subsequent follow-up care is now conducted by the referring pulmonologist for logistical convenience and often is dictated by insurance company mandates. This section will attempt to concisely review the topic of LT for the pulmonary physician.

Indications for LT

Heart-Lung Transplantation

One of the original successful LT procedures, performed primarily in the late 1980s and early 1990s, was heart-lung transplantation (HLT). Currently, HLT is performed at only a few transplant centers and should be reserved for patients who cannot be treated by LT alone. The most frequent indications for HLT are Eisenmenger syndrome with a surgically uncorrectable cardiac anomaly or severe end-stage lung disease with concurrent severe heart disease.

Bilateral LT

Bilateral LT (BLT) is performed in patients with suppurative pulmonary lung disease (*ie*, cystic fibrosis [CF] and bronchiectasis). In fact, 28% of all BLTs are performed as treatment for CF. Initially, double-lung transplantation was the procedure of choice with the anastomosis performed at the level of the trachea; however, the rate of ischemic airway complications was prohibitive. Now, BLT (essentially, sequential single-lung transplantation [SLT]), in which the anastomoses are performed at the level of the mainstem bronchi, is the preferred surgical technique. Many centers also recommend BLT for younger patients with severe COPD (secondary to tobacco use [24% of BLTs] or α_1-antitrypsin deficiency [9% of BLTs]) because of a longer posttransplant life expectancy from the increased reserve provided during times of graft complications. In addition, most centers prefer to perform a BLT procedure in patients with primary pulmonary hypertension (PPH; 6% of BLTs). Although a single-lung allograft with normal pulmonary vasculature can accommodate the entire right ventricular output without elevation of pulmonary artery pressures, in times of graft compromise, such as rejection or infection, severe ventilation-perfusion abnormalities can develop. Overall, BLT procedures are now being performed more than SLT procedures.

SLT

SLT is performed for the treatment of obstructive nonsuppurative lung disease such as emphysema secondary to tobacco use or 1-antitrypsin deficiency (50% and 7%, respectively, of all SLTs are performed for these indications). SLT was initially thought to be a poor choice of procedure for the treatment of patients with COPD as the result of concerns of preferential ventilation to the compliant native lung, but these concerns have proven to be largely unfounded. Other indications for SLT include idiopathic pulmonary fibrosis (28% of all SLTs), familial pulmonary fibrosis, drug-induced or toxin-induced lung disease, occupational lung disease, sarcoidosis, limited scleroderma, lymphangioleiomyomatosis, eosinophilic granuloma, and other disorders resulting in end-stage fibrotic lung disease. SLT is rarely performed for pulmonary vascular disease (< 1% of SLTs); the immediate postoperative period can be difficult because of the large volume of blood flow going to the transplanted lung. The theoretical advantages of SLT include reduced rate of surgical morbidity, shortened hospitalization and, often, the avoidance of cardiopulmonary bypass. This procedure also results in the optimization of the use of donor organs, which are in critical shortage.

Guidelines for Recipient Selection

There has been a revision of the original consensus-based guidelines for the selection of LT candidates.[2] The new guidelines are also consensus based but have taken into consideration a greater body of evidence and transplant experience since the earlier version in 1998 and have several important modifications compared with the original guidelines (Table 1).

Table 1. *Guidelines for Recipient Selection for Lung Transplantation**

Criteria	Description
General selection criteria	Untreatable end-stage obstructive or restrictive pulmonary parenchymal or pulmonary vascular disease; No other significant medical diseases; Substantial limitation of daily activity; Limited life expectancy; Ambulatory with rehabilitation potential; and Satisfactory psychosocial profile and emotional support system
Age	≤ 65 yr
Relative contraindications	Critical or unstable medical condition; Systemic or untreated extrapulmonic disease; Colonization with resistant bacteria, fungus or atypical mycobacteria; Symptomatic osteoporosis; Severely limited functional status Mechanical ventilation; Ideal body weight < 70% or > 130% (body mass index > 30 kg/m^2);
Absolute contraindications	Extrapulmonic disease (*ie,* renal [creatinine clearance, < 50 mg/mL/min]); HIV infection; Malignancy within prior 2 yr; Hepatitis B antigen positivity; Hepatitis C biopsy-proven liver disease; Severe musculoskeletal disease; Substance addiction in prior 6 mo (including tobacco use); Absence of a reliable support system; Untreatable psychosocial problems; and medical noncompliance

*Modified from Orens et al.

Any patient with end-stage pulmonary or cardiopulmonary disease with the capacity for rehabilitation can be considered for transplantation. The patient should have untreatable end-stage pulmonary disease, no other significant medical illness, and a limited life expectancy. The candidate should be ambulatory with rehabilitation potential. The patient must be psychologically stable, committed to the idea of transplantation, and willing to comply with the rigorous medical protocols and regimens required for a successful LT outcome.

Age

The 2006 international guidelines for the selection of transplant candidates[2] now suggest an age limit of 65 years as, generally, but not firmly, the upper limit regardless of procedure type. Although this limit is somewhat arbitrary, numerous patients with end-stage pulmonary disease are young to middle aged, and there is a relative lack of available donors. In addition, older patients have a somewhat poorer outcome than younger patients.

Relative Contraindications

Systemic or Multisystem Disease: Transplantation is not contraindicated in patients with systemic diseases that are limited to the lungs such as scleroderma, systemic lupus erythematosus, polymyositis, and rheumatoid arthritis. These cases should be considered on an individual basis. Patients with diabetes mellitus, hypertension, or peptic ulcer disease should be evaluated carefully before being considered as candidates for LT, and they should only be accepted if their disease is well controlled and there is no resulting end-organ damage.

Patients with active sites of infection are not considered to be good transplant candidates. Treated tuberculosis and fungal disease pose a particular problem but are not contraindications for LT. Many centers will not consider performing a transplant in a patient with chronic colonization with a resistant organism (*eg*, *Burkholderia cepacia*, methicillin-resistant Staphylococcus species, atypical mycobacterium, or Aspergillus species). Centers should try to eradicate these organisms in the pretransplant period and consider each patient on an individual basis. However, if considered, these patients should be candidates only for BLT procedures because the remaining colonized lung could pose a serious threat to the new graft in the case of an SLT.

Osteoporosis: Osteoporosis has become a significant problem in the posttransplant period, and preexisting symptomatic osteoporosis has been identified as a relative contraindication to transplantation. Bone densitometry should be part of the pretransplant evaluation, and treatment should be initiated in those patients with evidence of osteoporosis that is symptomatic or in those who are asymptomatic.

Mechanical Ventilation: A requirement for invasive mechanical ventilation is a strong relative contraindication to transplantation, although LT has been performed successfully in small numbers of CF patients receiving mechanical ventilation. However, patients who are receiving noninvasive ventilatory support can be considered for transplantation.

Nutritional Status: To be considered for transplantation, patients should have a body weight of >70% or <130% of predicted ideal body weight. Those patients with poor nutritional status may be too weak to withstand the surgical procedure; those patients who are obese make more difficult surgical candidates and may have greater mortality rates than nonobese patients.[3]

Corticosteroids: Initial data implicated corticosteroids as a cause of tracheal bronchial dehiscence. At most centers, patients were required to have completely discontinued therapy with corticosteroids. This requirement certainly eliminated a large number of patients with chronic obstructive lung disease and pulmonary fibrosis. Subsequently, pretransplant low-dose therapy with corticosteroids has been proven to be acceptable for patients who cannot discontinue corticosteroid therapy completely. Currently, transplant programs will consider patients who can be maintained in the long term on a regimen of prednisone of ≤20 mg/d and may consider patients who are receiving greater doses.

Previous Thoracic Surgery: Previous thoracotomy or pleurodesis was once considered to be a relative contraindication to patients undergoing transplantation because of increased technical difficulties and increased bleeding. Despite these factors, transplantation can be successfully performed in these patients.

Absolute Contraindications

The 2006 international guidelines[2] identified several absolute contraindications to LT, including major organ dysfunction (*ie*, renal creatinine clearance of <50 mg/mL/min), HIV infection, hepatitis B-antigen positivity, and hepatitis C with biopsy-documented liver disease. Active malignancy within the previous 2 years is also a contraindication to transplantation. For patients with a history of breast cancer greater than stage 2, colon cancer greater than Duke A stage, renal carcinoma, or melanoma greater than or equal to level 2, the waiting period should be at least 5 years. Restaging is suggested before transplant listing.

Severe Musculoskeletal Disease: Severe nonosteoporotic skeletal disease, such as kyphoscoliosis, is often an absolute contraindication to transplantation, primarily because of the technical difficulties encountered during surgery.

Substance Abuse: Drug abuse and alcoholism are considered to be contraindications to transplantation because patients with these conditions are at high risk for noncompliance. Patients who continue to smoke despite having end-stage pulmonary disease are not candidates for LT. Transplant centers require patients to abstain from cigarette smoking, alcohol use, or narcotics use for 6 months to 2 years before being considered for LT evaluation.

Psychological Criteria: The patient must be well motivated and emotionally stable to withstand the extreme stress of the pretransplant and perioperative period. A history of noncompliance or significant psychiatric illness is an absolute contraindication, although many patients will present with reactive depression or anxiety in the terminal phase of their pulmonary illness.

Disease-Specific Guidelines for LT

One of the most difficult decisions when referring a patient for transplantation is defining the appropriate time for transplantation (also called the *transplant window*). The potential candidate should be sick enough to have a limited life expectancy but not so disabled that the individual will be unable to withstand the procedure. In 2006, revised guidelines were established to define the transplant window for specific diseases (Table 2).[2]

Table 2. *Disease-Specific Criteria for Lung Transplantation**

Disease	Criteria
COPD	BODE index ≥7 or at least one of the following: FEV_1 <20% predicted (nonreversible) and diffusing capacity <20% or homogenous emphysema on HRCT; Hospitalization with $Paco_2$ >50 mm Hg; Cor pulmonale or pulmonary hypertension; and O_2-dependent hypercapnic patients (refer early) BODE index >5 (refer to lung transplant center)
IPF	Diagnosis of usual interstitial pneumonitis with any of the following: Diffusing capacity <39% predicted; A decrease in FVC of ≥10% in 6 mo of follow-up; A decrease in pulse oximetry below 88% on a 6-min walk test; Honeycombing seen on HRCT; Histologic or radiographic evidence of UIP irrespective of vital capacity (refer to lung transplant center);
CF	FEV_1 of <30% predicted (refer); Clinical deterioration with FEV_1 of >30% predicted (exacerbation, hemoptysis, and pneumothorax) [refer]; $Paco_2$ of >50 mm Hg; Pao_2 on room air of <55 mm Hg; Pulmonary hypertension; and Young, female patients (refer early)
PPH	NYHA class III–IV despite vasodilator treatment; Cardiac index of <2 L/min/m^2; Right atrial pressure of >15 mm Hg; and Low (<350 m) or declining 6-min walk test distance

*IPF = idiopathic pulmonary fibrosis; UIP = usual interstitial pneumonitis. Adapted from Orens et al.

COPD

The variability in the natural course of COPD makes it especially difficult to predict when patients should be referred for LT. On the basis of the available data from several large studies in which authors determined the predictors of mortality in COPD, guidelines have been established. The 2006 revised guidelines recommend the inclusion of the BODE index (an index derived from measurements of body mass index, degree of airway obstruction, dyspnea score, and exercise capacity) when evaluating patients with COPD. The guidelines suggest that a BODE index score of ≥7 should be among the criteria for transplantation in patients with COPD, and a BODE index of 5 as appropriate for transplant referral. The guidelines also suggest that patients with COPD are in the transplant window if the FEV_1 is <20% of predicted without reversibility with bronchodilator administration, the diffusing capacity is <20% or there is homogenous distribution of emphysema on a high-resolution CT (HRCT) scan, the $Paco_2$ is 50 mm Hg, and/or cor pulmonale or pulmonary hypertension are present. Those patients who are hypercapnic and hypoxemic and require oxygen supplementation should be given preference.

A 1998 analysis[4] of transplant survival data has shown that patients with COPD may achieve a significant improvement in quality of life (QOL), but a clear survival benefit with transplantation has not been documented. Rehabilitation and long-term supplemental oxygen therapy, if the criteria are met, should be initiated while the patient is awaiting LT.

Idiopathic Pulmonary Fibrosis

On the basis of studies showing poor survival times in patients with idiopathic pulmonary fibrosis and the fact that most patients have a progressive downhill course despite receiving standard immunosuppressive therapy, patients with pulmonary fibrosis should be referred for transplantation early. In fact, this is the group of patients who have the greatest mortality rate while on the transplant list. The 2006 revised guidelines have suggested that these patients should be referred to a transplant center at the time of a diagnosis of usual interstitial pneumonitis and should undergo transplantation when diffusing capacity is $<39\%$ of predicted, when there is a decrease in FVC of $\geq 10\%$ in the 6 months of follow-up, when there is a decrease in pulse oximetric saturation to $<88\%$ on a 6-min walk test, or when honeycombing is seen on a HRCT scan.

CF

Although there has been an improvement in life expectancy for patients with CF, most patients still die from respiratory failure and cor pulmonale. The international guidelines have suggested that the following criteria be used to define the transplant window for patients with CF: $FEV_1 < 30\%$ of predicted or an FEV_1 30% of predicted with progressive deterioration, such as an increasing number of hospitalizations, a rapid deterioration in FEV_1, cachexia, and/or massive hemoptysis; $Pao_2 < 55$ mm Hg on room air; $Paco_2$ 50 mm Hg; or pulmonary hypertension. Female patients and patients <18 years old have a more progressive course and should be considered for LT earlier. In 2002, a predictive model[5] for selecting patients with CF was proposed to more accurately predict the survival effect of LT in these patients. The model includes the following: age, sex, percentage of predicted FEV_1, weight for age Z score, the presence of pancreatic sufficiency, diabetes mellitus, infection with *Staphylococcus aureus* or *B cepacia*, and the number of acute exacerbations requiring treatment. The use of the FEV_1 criteria and of a more complicated multivariate logistic model to define transplant referral for CF have been evaluated in a large group of CF patients.[6] The study found that these referral criteria had high negative predictive values (98% and 97%, respectively) but only modest positive predictive values (33% and 28%, respectively) and can result in premature transplant referral.

Recently, a controversial article on the impact of LT on survival in the pediatric CF population was published. The authors used data from the US Cystic Fibrosis Foundation registry and the Organ Procurement and Transplantation Network. The authors examined 514 children wait-listed for LT during a 10-year time period. A total of 248 patients underwent LT. Risk factors for survival on the waiting list and survival after LT were studied. The authors found that *B cepacia* was a risk factor for death both before and after LT, diabetes was a risk factor for death before LT but not after LT, older age affected post LT survival but not wait-list survival, and *S aureus* infection increased wait-list survival but decreased post LT survival. The authors concluded that of the 514 patients listed, 5 patients had a survival benefit, 76 had insignificant benefit, 118 patients had insignificant harm, and 315 had a significant risk of harm with LT.

This study included a large number of patients but was retrospective. In addition, QOL improvements were not addressed. Significant controversy has arisen over this article, including criticisms of the statistical methods used, resulting in subsequent published corrections by the authors, but without significant changes in the overall conclusions reached.[7]

Patients with CF often have multiple, resistant organisms that are defined as being resistant to all agents in two of the following classes: β-lactams, aminoglycosides, and/or quinolones. Panresistant colonization includes organisms, particularly *Pseudomonas aeruginosa* and *B cepacia*, that are resistant *in vitro* to all groups of antibiotics. As for the outcomes of CF patients with panresistant *P aeruginosa* and *B cepacia* vs those patients with organisms susceptible to therapy, including the number of postoperative ventilator days, the length of hospital stay, and the number of days receiving antibiotic therapy, the incidence of bronchitis and pneumonia, and 1-year survival rates appear to be similar between groups.

However, a subanalysis of those patients with *B cepacia* infection revealed that they had a lower 1-year survival rate (50%) compared with those with resistant *P aeruginosa* infection (90%). Another study[8] found a 1-year survival rate of 67% for *B cepacia*-positive CF patients, compared with 97% in *B cepacia*-negative CF patients. Some newer data have suggested that those patients with colonization with *B cepacia* of the genomovar III type have a particularly poor prognosis. Thus, colonization with *B cepacia* of the genomovar III type should be considered a strong relative contraindication for transplantation. A recent study examined the results of LT for CF in patients with panresistant organisms other than *B cepacia* (*eg*, *P aeruginosa*, *Stenotrophomonas maltophilia*, *Achromobacter xyloxoxidans*). The authors[9] found that there was decreased survival in patients with panresistant bacteria compared with patient with pansensitive bacteria (58.3% vs 85.6% at 5 years, respectively), but these survival rates were similar or better than those predicted by United Network for Organ Sharing.

PPH

On the basis of the extrapolation of data from the National Heart, Blood, and Lung Transplant Registry for PPH, selection guidelines have been established for patients with PPH. These guidelines suggest that patients who are in New York Heart Association (NYHA) functional class III or IV, despite receiving optimal therapy including vasodilators such as prostacyclin, and those with a depressed cardiac index (< 2 L/min/m^2), a right atrial pressure of 15 mm Hg, or low or declining 6-min walk test distances should be considered for transplantation. Other patients should be observed closely and reassessed for transplantation at 6-month intervals.

Pulmonary Hypertension Secondary to Congenital Heart Disease (Eisenmenger Syndrome)

Patients with this type of secondary pulmonary hypertension have been found to have a significantly better prognosis than those patients with primary disease. Therefore, because of the individuality of the progression of this disease, precise criteria for transplantation have not been established. In general, patients are usually referred to transplant centers when they are in NYHA functional class III or IV.

Pretransplant Evaluation

Once a patient is deemed to be a potential candidate for transplantation, several studies are usually performed for further assessment. Typically, these tests include pulmonary function tests, including lung volumes, spirometry, and diffusing capacity, and a measure of exercise performance such as a 6-min walk test. Cardiac evaluation includes an ECG and an echocardiogram, in addition to a functional cardiac study, such as dobutamine echocardiography and/or coronary angiography, in patients 40 years of age or those with significant risk factors for coronary artery disease. An HRCT scan is often obtained to look for bronchiectasis, which could indicate the necessity for a bilateral procedure, or to look for focal nodules that were not apparent on plain chest radiographs. Renal and liver functions are assessed by 24-h creatinine clearance and liver function tests, respectively. Serologies for hepatitis and HIV should also be obtained. The majority of these investigations can be performed at the referring center. In those patients being evaluated for SLT, a ventilation/perfusion scan with quantitation may suggest the preferred side to be transplanted if there is unequal distribution of perfusion.

While awaiting transplantation, patients should have close follow-up by the transplant center or their referring physician for both physiologic and emotional support. In those patients who are in the pretransplant phase for the treatment of suppurative lung disease, sputum cultures should be obtained at 3-month intervals to assist in the antibiotic regimen in the immediate postoperative period. Those patients who are able to should be involved in a rehabilitation program before undergoing transplantation.

Donor Allocation

Until the spring of 2005, as established by The United Network for Organ Sharing, lungs were allocated primarily by time on the waiting list and not by necessity. In the spring of 2005, the system for donor allocation for lungs was revised, and the assigned priority for lung offers became based on the lung allocation score (LAS), which is calculated using the following measures: (1) waiting list urgency measure (*ie*, the expected number of days lived without a transplant during an additional year on the waiting list); (2) posttransplant survival measure (*ie*, the expected number of days lived during the first year after transplant); and (3) the transplant benefit measure (*ie*, the posttransplant survival measure minus waiting list urgency measure).

It is too early to determine the effects that this new allocation system will have on LT, but preliminary data after the first year of the new allocation system suggest that patients with pulmonary fibrosis have moved significantly higher (*ie*, shorter wait time) on the waiting list in comparison with their ranking when the previous time accrual allocation system was used. The distribution of patients undergoing LT changed after the institution of the LAS, with more idiopathic pulmonary fibrosis and CF patients undergoing transplantation and fewer COPD patients. The mean LAS increased significantly after the institution of the LAS. Despite this, survival rates were comparable before and after the implementation of the LAS. Recent data suggest that the early results of the LAS appear to indicate that the LAS is achieving many of its goals. The long-term effects of the LAS remain to be determined, and further refinement of the system will be necessary.

Organs are first distributed locally, then regionally, and finally nationally. Currently, the average time spent on the waiting list is approximately 18 to 24 months; therefore, close management of the listed transplant patient is required. Despite this close attention, a significant percentage of patients die while awaiting transplantation. Non—heart-beating donors are now also being used in isolated cases for LT and may prove to partially alleviate the shortage of donor organs.

Living Donor Transplantation

Several institutions worldwide are now performing living donor transplantations. The primary indication for living donor transplantation is CF. Generally; two blood group-compatible living donors each provide a lower lobe to the recipient. Ideally, the donors should be larger than the recipient so that the donor lobes fill the hemithorax. This procedure is not performed at the majority of LT centers because of certain technical and ethical issues involved.

Donor Criteria

Donor organ shortage remains the greatest limiting factor in the numbers of LTs performed. The majority of potential lung donors are brain dead and, as stated previously, only a small number of living donor-related LT procedures have been performed. The usual donor selection criteria include age <60 to 65 years, no history of significant lung disease, and a limited smoking history. In addition, potential donors should have clear lung fields on chest radiographs and adequate gas exchange as assessed by a Pao_2 of 300 mm Hg on a fraction of inspired oxygen (Fio_2) equal to 1 and a positive end-expiratory pressure of 5 cm H_2O or a Pao_2/Fio_2 ratio of 250 to 300 mm Hg. A normal sputum Gram stain finding and/or endobronchial inspection are also part of the donor evaluation examination. Marginal or extended donors (*ie*, those not meeting all of the aforementioned criteria) are being used more frequently to expand the donor pool.[10,11] By instituting a protocol, including educational and donor management interventions, and changing donor classification and selection criteria, a single organ-procurement organization was able to increase the percentage of lungs procured per donor from 11.5 to 22.5% and the number of procedures performed without adverse recipient outcomes.[10]

Donors are excluded from potential lung donation if they have evidence of active infection, HIV infection, hepatitis infection, and/or malignancy. Donor and recipient compatibility are assessed by matching by A, B, and O blood types and chest wall size. Human leukocyte antigen (HLA) matching is not routinely performed in LT.

Surgical Procedure

For an SLT, the recipient surgery is performed via a posterolateral thoracotomy incision or sternotomy. The recipient left atrium and donor pulmonary vein undergo anastomosis first, followed by the bronchial anastomosis, and finally the arterial anastomosis. BLT is usually performed through a transverse thoracosternotomy (clam shell incision or median sternotomy). Cardiopulmonary bypass may be required in cases of pulmonary hypertension. Organ preservation remains a major area of research in LT. Currently, the lung can only be preserved for a period of approximately 4 to 6 h without experiencing significant ischemia/reperfusion injury. Newer preservative agents may increase this time period and permit a larger area for donor allocation.

Management After the Postoperative Period

Patients are typically discharged from the hospital within 7 to 14 days after surgery. Follow-up is in the outpatient clinic on a weekly, biweekly, and finally monthly basis. After this time, patients often return home for follow-up with the referring pulmonologist. Weekly monitoring includes measuring the levels of immunosuppressive medications such as cyclosporine or tacrolimus; a CBC count to monitor leukocyte concentrations, platelet counts because of therapy with azathioprine or mycophenolate mofetil; blood chemistry measurements to follow creatinine levels because of the use of therapy with cyclosporine or tacrolimus; a chest radiograph; routine spirometry and exercise oximetry; or a 6-min walk test. In addition, patients are given home spirometers and are instructed to bring in their home spirometry measurements at each visit.

Some institutions perform surveillance bronchoscopy on a routine schedule to detect asymptomatic rejection or infection, whereas other institutions reserve this procedure for clinical deterioration without compromised survival or rates of bronchiolitis obliterans syndrome (BOS).[12,13] The chest radiograph has not been shown to be specific for the early detection of rejection or infection.

Close monitoring of pulmonary function has also been studied as a way of detecting graft complications. Pulmonary function tests have been shown to have very low specificity and good sensitivity (85%) for the detection of graft complications but, again, are unable to distinguish rejection from infection. Therefore, pulmonary function tests remain the most sensitive test in the late postoperative period for detecting infection or rejection, although they cannot differentiate between these and other possible complications.

Outcome

Survival

Actuarial survival rates after transplantation are reported at 92%, 78%, 62%, and 50%, respectively, for 1 month, and 1, 3, and 5 years, as reported to the ISHLT Registry, [1] and are significantly lower than those reported for other types of solid-organ transplant recipients. Early mortality (*ie*, at <30 days) is most often to the result of primary graft failure, mortality between 30 days and 1 year is most often to the result of infection, and late mortality (*ie*, at 1 year) is most often related to rejection. Previously, there was no apparent survival difference between those patients undergoing SLT and BLT. However, it now appears that BLT recipients may have a survival advantage beginning at 3 years after LT. Patients undergoing HLT have lower survival rates. Survival rates are greater for patients undergoing LT for CF or COPD in comparison with those patients undergoing transplantation for idiopathic pulmonary fibrosis; older patients have a poorer long-term survival rate. Younger COPD patients (*ie*, <50 to 60 years of age) undergoing BLT appear to have a survival advantage over those undergoing SLT.

Physiologic Results

The degree of improvement in lung function postoperatively is the product of many factors. In the uncomplicated transplant recipients, one can expect a gradual improvement and ultimate plateau of lung function by 3 to 6 months after the procedure. In patients receiving a single lung, the FEV_1 can be expected to improve to 50 to 70% of predicted. SLT for the treatment of nonseptic obstructive lung disease results in moderate residual obstructive pulmonary dysfunction seen in spirometry findings. SLT in patients with underlying restrictive lung disease can be expected to have mild residual restrictive physiology. These results likely reflect the physiology of the remaining obstructed or restricted lung. After SLT procedures, the majority of the ventilation and perfusion goes to the transplanted lung. BLT procedures usually result in normal spirometry findings with an equal division of ventilation and perfusion. Those patients who undergo transplantation for PPH have no significant change in pulmonary function, marked improvement in gas exchange, and near-normal hemodynamics after transplantation, including a nearly complete recovery of right ventricular function.

The majority of those patients who undergo either LT procedure without complications are able to performed activities of daily living without compromise, although formal cardiopulmonary exercise testing generally reveals a reduction in maximum oxygen consumption to 40 to 60% of predicted in all transplant groups. The reasons for this remain unclear and do not appear to be cardiac or pulmonary in origin. The leading physiologic hypothesis is that the immunosuppressive agents may have an effect on peripheral skeletal muscles, resulting in impaired peripheral oxygen utilization.

QOL

QOL issues are a relatively recent area of research in LT. Several small studies have shown improvement in overall health-related QOL. The large majority of patients have expressed satisfaction with their transplant decision. Even if the survival benefit is in question, the improvement in QOL may be worth the sacrifice to many patients. Of interest, $\leq$40% of patients return to work on a part-time or full-time basis after transplantation.

Complications

Figure 1 shows some of the common post-transplant complications and the approximate time period in which they usually occur.

Primary Graft Dysfunction

The most significant early postoperative complication after LT is the development of primary graft dysfunction (PGD), pulmonary reimplantation response (PRR), or primary graft failure. It is estimated that up to 80% of patients will experience some degree of reimplantation injury, and in 15% of patients it can be severe. A 2005 consensus conference[14] attempted to standardize the grading of PGD based on gas exchange and the presence of radiographic infiltrates. When using the acute lung injury definition of ARDS as a PaO_2/FIO_2 ratio of < 200, the authors found that PGD has a reported incidence of 11 to 25%. PGD is characterized clinically by the presence of new radiographic infiltrates, a decrease in pulmonary compliance, an increase in pulmonary vascular resistance, and disrupted gas exchange.

Radiographic findings include patchy alveolar consolidation and/or dense perihilar haze and lower lobe alveolar consolidation. Pathology from biopsy specimens, autopsy specimens, or lung explants removed during retransplantation reveals diffuse alveolar damage. The typical course of PGD includes progressive worsening or stabilization over the subsequent hours up to 2 to 4 days, followed by resolution. However, PGD can persist for days after the surgery. It is thought that the likely mechanism for PGD is ischemia/reperfusion injury. Management includes the differentiation of other perioperative complications such as volume overload, rejection, infection, and venous anastomotic problems. The latter can be evaluated with a transesophageal echocardiogram. Treatment includes supportive care and therapy with diuretics. Reports[15,16] have documented the successful use of protective ventilatory strategies, nitric oxide, and/or extracorporeal membrane oxygenation in these patients. The prophylactic administration of inhaled nitric oxide was not found to be of benefit for hemodynamics, reperfusion injury, oxygenation, time to extubation, ICU or hospital stay, or 30-day mortality rate in one randomized, placebo-controlled trial[16] of 84 patients.

A large single center study[17] examined patients with primary graft failure. The investigators found an incidence of 15% for this complication, and it was associated with a prolonged hospital course, prolonged mechanical ventilation, a poor 1-year survival rate (40% vs 69%, respectively), and compromised function among survivors. The authors found no clear risk factors for primary graft failure, including age, sex, underlying disease, pulmonary artery pressure, type of transplant procedure performed, ischemic times, or use of cardiopulmonary bypass. The study did note that induction immunotherapy was used less frequently in those

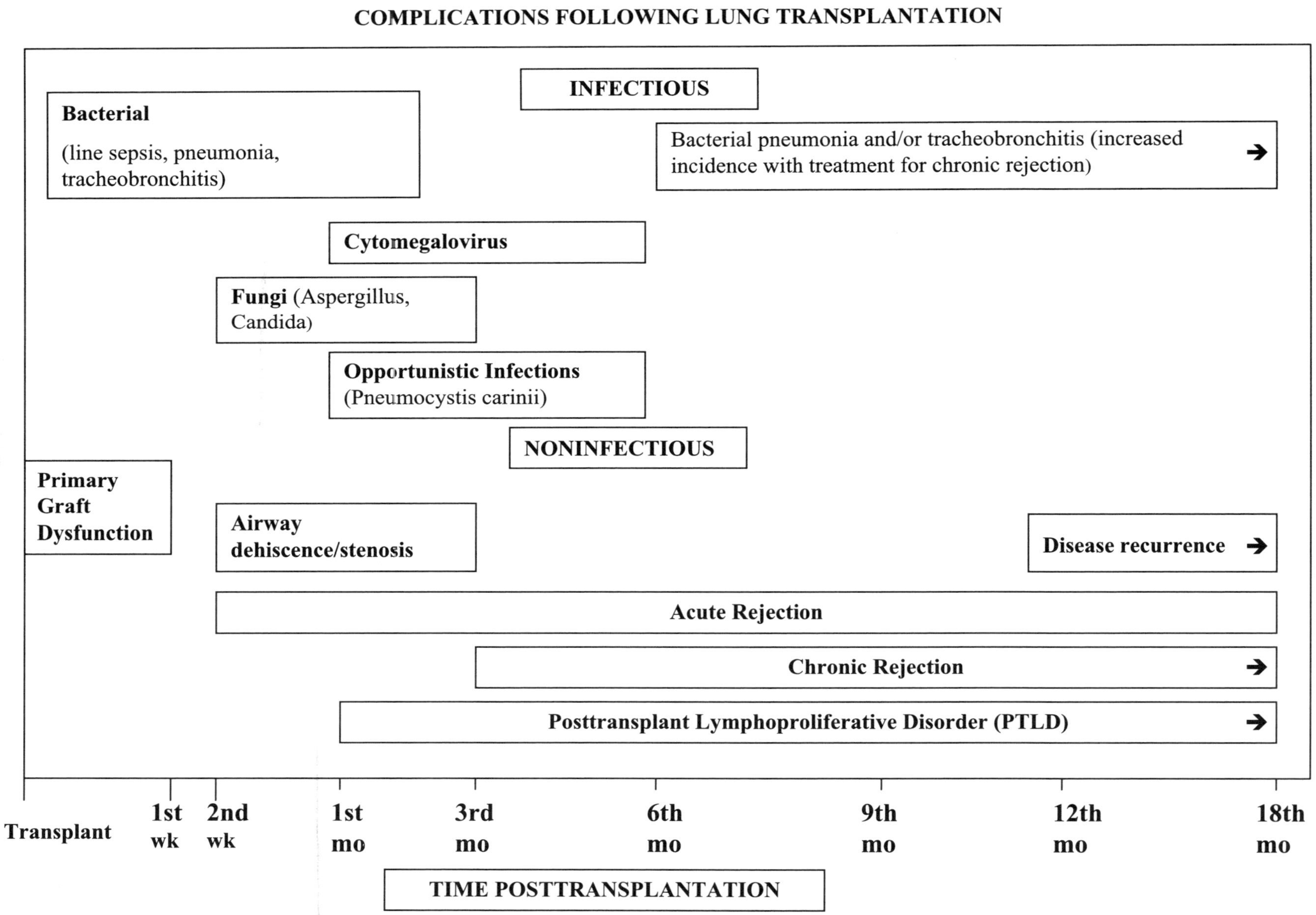

Figure 1. The common complications after LT and the typical time periods in which they develop. Reprinted with permission from Melo J, Levine SM. Lung transplantation for the referring pulmonologist. Pulm Crit Care Update 1999; 13:lesson 16.

patients in whom primary graft failure developed. A study[18] from a different large transplant center identified cardiopulmonary bypass as a risk factor for PRR and also observed prolonged mechanical ventilation and ICU stays in those patients with PRR. It did not observe a difference in survival rates between patients with and without PRR.

Another study[19] found the incidence of severe PGD to be 11.8% among 255 transplant recipients. Risk factors associated with the development of PGD when subjected to multivariate analysis included the following: a recipient diagnosis of PPH, donor of female sex, donor of African-American race, and donor age <21 and 45 years.[19] The technique used for preservation may also prove to be a risk factor for PGD. A French study[20] concluded that the development of PGD, even in the mildest form, is associated with a prolonged duration of mechanical ventilation in addition to increased ICU morbidity and mortality. The long-term outcomes in survivors, such as pulmonary function and incidence of bronchiolitis obliterans, vary among studies, with some reporting compromise and others reporting no long-term adverse effects.[21] Hemorrhage and phrenic nerve paralysis have also been reported in the early postoperative period.

Airway Complications

Airway problems were significant causes of morbidity and mortality after early attempts at LT and developed in 20 to 50% of transplant recipients. Airway complications can be classified into the early and late time periods. Early airway complications usually develop during the first 4 to 8 weeks. They present as a partial or complete anastomotic dehiscence and/or fungal anastomotic infection (usually Aspergillus or Candida species) or bacterial anastomotic infection (usually Staphylococcus or Pseudomonas species) anastomotic infection and can subsequently result in anastomotic strictures. Bronchomalacia can also develop.

The theoretical causes of airway complications include ischemia at the site of the anastomosis, infection, poor organ preservation, and/or rejection. Because revascularization of the bronchial circulation is generally not performed after LT, anastomotic techniques such as the omental wrap or pericardial fat have been developed, in which an intact portion of the omentum or pericardial fat is wrapped around the bronchial anastomosis; or the telescoping anastomotic technique, in which one bronchus overlaps one to two cartilaginous rings within the larger bronchus to improve blood flow. These techniques have resulted in a decrease in the incidence of anastomotic complications of 10 to 20%, with low rates of mortality and morbidity.

Clinically, patients with bronchial anastomotic complications, including stenosis and bronchomalacia, can present with cough, shortness of breath, wheezing, dyspnea on exertion, and worsening obstruction on pulmonary function testing. The characteristic flow-volume loop demonstrates a concave appearance in both the inspiratory and expiratory loops. Bronchial strictures or stenoses may also be visualized on chest radiographs, CT scans, and/or bronchoscopy. Partial or complete bronchial dehiscence can also present with mediastinal emphysema seen on chest radiographs or with air adjacent to the bronchial anastomosis seen on CT scans.

The therapeutic options for anastomotic complications include balloon dilation of a stricture, stent placement, laser therapy and, rarely, surgery. If anastomotic infection with fungal or bacterial organisms is suspected bronchoscopically or is diagnosed by endobronchial washing, brushing or biopsy culture, or histology, then therapy with appropriate antibiotics should be instituted.

Rejection

Graft rejection is categorized clinically according to the time of onset after transplantation and the histopathologic pattern. The three types of rejection are hyperacute, acute, or chronic. Hyperacute rejection is mediated by preexisting alloantibodies that immediately bind to the donor vascular epithelium, leading to vessel thrombosis via complement activation. Fortunately, this complication is a rare one in LT and will not be discussed further.

Acute Rejection: Acute rejection can develop in up to 50% of patients in the first postoperative month, and as many as 90% of patients will have at least one episode of acute rejection within the first year. The typical time period for acute rejection is 10 to 90 days after LT. It is not uncommon (20% of patients) for a single patient to experience two to three episodes within the first few months after transplantation that are either recurrent (*ie*, more than two episodes) or persistent (failure to resolve with standard therapy). Acute rejection is usually not seen as frequently after the first year after transplantation. Risk factors for acute rejection are poorly defined, but HLA mismatches and gastroesophageal reflux may have a correlation.

Clinically, patients with acute rejection present with cough, shortness of breath, malaise, and fever. Occasionally, the presentation is asymptomatic, and some centers advocate surveillance bronchoscopy to detect this, although outcome data are not available. A physical examination may reveal rales or wheezing. The utility of the chest radiograph depends on the time after transplantation. Typically, in the first month, the chest radiograph findings can be abnormal in up to 75% of rejection episodes; however, in those episodes of rejection occurring after 1 month after transplantation only 25% of patients have abnormal radiograph findings. The most common radiographic patterns noted with acute rejection include a perihilar flare, and alveolar, or interstitial, localized, or diffuse, infiltrates with or without associated pleural effusion.

Physiologic findings during periods of acute rejection include hypoxemia and deterioration in pulmonary function. Pulmonary function abnormalities are characterized by a decrease in FEV_1 of at least 10 to 15% from baseline as well as a decrease in the forced expiratory flow, midexpiratory phase of an expired vital capacity of 10 to 15%. Once again, these changes are nonspecific and can also be found in patients with infectious etiologies.

Because clinical criteria alone cannot differentiate among acute rejection, infection and, less common, graft complications, transbronchial biopsy with BAL fluid has emerged as the primary procedure for diagnosis. A diagnosis of acute rejection by transbronchial biopsy has ranged from 61 to 94%, and specificity has ranged from 90 to 100%. A histologic grading system for acute pulmonary rejection was initially proposed in 1990 and revised in 1996 and 2007.[22] Pathologically, acute rejection is characterized by perivascular, mononuclear, and lymphocytic infiltrates with or without airway inflammation and is graded histologically from A0 to A4, based on the degree of perivascular inflammation. In addition, airway involvement with lymphocytic bronchitis or bronchiolitis can develop and is graded from B0, B1R (low grade), B2R (high grade), and BX (ungradable). As rejection progresses, the perivascular lymphocytic infiltrates surrounding the venules and arterioles become dense and extend into the perivascular and peribronchiolar alveolar septa. In patients with severe rejection, the alveolar space may be involved, and parenchymal necrosis, hyaline membranes, and necrotizing vasculitis have been described.[22]

Once acute rejection has been diagnosed, treatment consists of the augmentation of immunosuppression. Methylprednisolone, 10 to 15 mg/kg/d IV for 3 days, followed by an increase in the maintenance prednisone regimen to 0.5 to 1 mg/kg/d with a taper over the next several weeks is a standard treatment regimen. Maintenance immunosuppression therapy should also be augmented. Typically, the resolution of symptoms occurs in days, and histologic follow-up in 3 to 4 weeks should show resolution. Recurrent or persistent acute rejection may initiate conversion in the baseline immunosuppression regimen. Lympholytic therapy, methotrexate, photopheresis, total lymphoid irradiation, and/or aerosolized cyclosporine therapy have been used with variable success. Therapy with mycophenolate mofetil initiated *de novo* has resulted in a decreased incidence of acute rejection in several small studies.

Obliterative Bronchiolitis: Chronic rejection has been equated with the histologic finding of obliterative bronchiolitis (OB) and remains a major cause of morbidity and mortality after LT and the leading single cause of death after the first posttransplant year. The current incidence of OB ranges from 35 to 50% among different centers. OB has been defined clinically by an obstructive functional defect and histologically by the obliteration of terminal bronchioles. The mean time to diagnose OB is 16 to 20 months after the LT procedure but has been reported as early as 3 months after transplantation. Some degree of OB will develop in 50% of transplant recipients by 5 years after transplant.

The etiology and risk factors for OB remain unclear. Several possible causes have been proposed, including uncontrolled acute rejection; lymphocytic bronchiolitis; cytomegalovirus (CMV) pneumonitis; CMV infection without pneumonitis; HLA-A mismatches; total HLA mismatches; the absence of donor antigen-specific hyporeactivity;

non-CMV infection; older donor age; and bronchiolitis obliterans with organizing pneumonia. The most consistently identified risk factor is acute rejection, particularly in those patients who experience recurrent, high-grade episodes of acute rejection. It is probable that lymphocytic bronchiolitis and CMV pneumonitis are also important risk factors for OB.[23,24] Other risk factors are being identified. In the past several years, gastric aspiration and gastroesophageal reflux disease (GERD) have been recognized as an important cause and/or contributing risk factor to the development of pulmonary dysfunction after LT, particularly BOS. Primary graft dysfunction may also be a risk factor for BOS. Clinically, OB can manifest as an upper respiratory tract infection and can be mistakenly treated as such. Other patients present without clinical symptoms but with gradual obstructive dysfunction seen on pulmonary function test results. FEV_1 has been the standard spirometric parameter used, but midexpiratory flow rates may be a more sensitive parameter for early detection.

Typically, chest radiographs are not helpful in the diagnosis of OB because most patients have radiographic findings that are unchanged from their baseline posttransplant radiographs. HRCT scans may reveal peripheral bronchiectasis, patchy consolidation, decreased peripheral vascular markings, trapped air, and bronchial dilation, which may aid in the diagnosis of OB. Trapped air on end-expiratory HRCT scans has been shown to be a sensitive (91%) and accurate (86%) radiologic indicator of OB but may not be able to provide an early diagnosis of this disorder.[25] BAL fluid neutrophilia, exhaled nitric oxide levels, bronchial hyperresponsiveness, and increased nitrogen washout may also be surrogate markers of BOS.

As with acute rejection, transbronchial biopsy is used to diagnose OB, although primarily to exclude other diagnoses. The classic pathologic finding is constrictive bronchiolitis. Unfortunately, the sensitivity for the diagnosis of OB by transbronchial biopsy is low (range, 15 to 87%), and the diagnosis of OB is often made by exclusion and is graded physiologically based on the degree of change in pulmonary function (*ie*, FEV_1) from baseline. Because of the variability in obtaining bronchioles by transbronchial biopsy, the ISHLT has established a BOS staging system.[26] This staging system is based on a reduction in FEV_1 in comparison with a posttransplant baseline FEV_1 with or without the pathologic documentation of OB. This staging system was revised by the ISHLT in 2002, and the new system includes an earlier BOS category of potential BOS using changes in FEV_1 and/or mid-flows compared with posttransplant baseline values (FEV_1, 81 to 90% of baseline values; and/or forced expiratory flow, midexpiratory phase, ≤75% of baseline values; Table 3).[24]

Once OB has been diagnosed histologically or clinically by the exclusion of alternate diagnoses, treatment is begun with high-dose methylprednisolone therapy followed by a tapering course of oral corticosteroids. Lympholytic agents such as antilymphocyte globulin, monoclonal antibody to the CD_3 lymphocyte receptor (OKT_3), or anti-interleukin (IL)-2 agents such as daclizumab can be considered for therapy if there is no clinical response to steroid treatment. Therapy may stabilize pulmonary function but uncommonly results in significant improvement. Other common physiologic scenarios may be relentless deterioration in pulmonary function despite therapy, gradual steady deterioration in pulmonary function, or a series of decreases in function with plateaus. A recent study found that the majority of patients had the steepest decrease in the percentage of predicted FEV_1 within the first 6 months after BOS diagnosis. The authors noted a steeper decrease in the first 6 months after the onset of BOS in patients with a diagnosis before LT of pulmonary fibrosis and in patients who were female. Patients with a rapid onset of BOS also had a steeper decrease in FEV_1 percentage of predicted. Recipients of an SLT had a worse percentage of predicted FEV_1 after diagnosis. After 24 months, the course of the percentage

Table 3. *Clinical Staging System for OB**

Stage†	FEV_1
0 (no OB)	>90% of baseline and $FEF_{25-75\%}$ of >75% of baseline
0-p (potential OB)	81–90% of baseline and/or $FEF_{25-75\%}$ of ≤75% of baseline
1 (mild OB)	66–80% of baseline
2 (moderate OB)	51–65% of baseline
3 (severe OB)	≤50% of baseline

*Adapted from Estenne et al. FEF = forced expiratory flow.
†Each stage is subdivided into a and b, where a is without histologic documentation of OB and b is with histologic documentation of OB. Adapted from the ISHLT staging system.

of predicted FEV_1 in BLT recipients was better than that in SLT recipients.[27]

Alternate immunosuppressive agents such as mycophenolate mofetil, tacrolimus, and sirolimus have also been associated with the stabilization of pulmonary function when used as rescue treatment for BOS. Methotrexate, total lympholytic radiation, aerosolized cyclosporine, photopheresis, and newer immunosuppressive agents have been used for treatment in refractory cases of OB. Inhaled corticosteroids may be added to therapy in cases of lymphocytic bronchiolitis. Small studies[28] have shown benefit from the use of low-dose azithromycin (via an antiinflammatory mechanism) for treating patients with BOS. Therapy directed toward GERD (both pharmacological and surgical) should also be considered.

Infection, including bronchiectasis, frequently complicates intensive immunosuppression therapy for OB and may result in death. Pseudomonas is a common offender, and aerosolized aminoglycoside antibiotics or suppressive quinolone treatment may be considered. Bronchomalacia can also develop. Survival rates after the diagnosis of OB have been reported at 74%, 50%, and 43%, respectively, at 1, 3, and 5 years in one small series.[29] Because most patients with OB can only be stabilized, strategies directed at prevention, early diagnosis, and treatment are necessary for the preservation of lung function. Retransplantation has been performed with variable results. Survival is somewhat less than that for patients receiving *de novo* transplants. In addition, the limited donor supply does not allow for the common practice of this procedure.

Humoral Rejection: Recently, humoral rejection has been described in LT recipients as a component of either acute or chronic rejection. Humoral rejection is suggested when high levels of donor-specific HLA antibodies are present in the serum of the recipient, and complement deposition is present in the tissue. Preliminary studies are examining the use of plasmapheresis, rituximab, and IV Ig in this setting.

Infectious Complications

Infections have been a major cause of early and late morbidity and mortality after transplantation, and they remain the leading single specific cause of death in the first posttransplant year. The incidence of infection is significantly greater than that reported in other solid-organ recipients and may be related to continuous environmental exposure of the allograft. Other predisposing factors include diminished cough reflex secondary to denervation, poor lymphatic drainage, decreased mucociliary clearance, recipient-harbored infection and, occasionally, the transfer of infection from the donor organ. Nosocomial infections at the site of the surgical wound, vascular access, and urinary tract or ventilator-associated pneumonias also occur in the early postoperative period. In most circumstances, the allograft or graft is the primary location of infection.

Bacterial Infections: Bacterial pneumonia is the most common life-threatening infection to develop in the early postoperative period and had once been reported to have an incidence as high as 35% in the first 2 postoperative weeks. Common organisms include *P aeruginosa* and Staphylococcus species. The incidence of perioperative bacterial pneumonia has been decreased to as low as 10% by broad-spectrum antibiotic prophylaxis, usually an antipseudomonal cephalosporin and clindamycin, and routine culture of the trachea of the donor and the recipient at the time of the surgery. Prophylactic therapy with antibiotics is usually discontinued at 3 days if the culture results are negative and are tailored to the cultured organisms if the results are positive. Patients with bronchiectasis who receive transplants usually receive postoperative bacterial prophylaxis for 7 to 10 days. The prevalence of bacterial pneumonia remains high during the first 6 months after transplantation and decreases subsequently, although a second late peak in incidence often occurs during the augmentation of immunosuppression for the treatment of chronic rejection. Bacterial infection caused by Staphylococcus or, less commonly, Pseudomonas species can develop at or distal to the site of the anastomosis in the early posttransplant period. Of interest, the incidence of lower respiratory tract infections does not appear to be increased in patients who receive transplants for CF in comparison with patients who receive transplants for other indications.

It is often difficult to distinguish pneumonia from other early graft complications such as reperfusion injury, pulmonary edema, rejection, and other infectious etiologies. In addition, differentiation between colonization and invasion may be difficult and often requires invasive procedures such as bronchoscopy with BAL fluid, quantitative sterile brush sample, and/or transbronchial biopsy.

Other Early Infections: Atypical pneumonias such as Legionella, Mycobacteria, and Nocardia species are uncommon in patients undergoing LT but have been reported to occur in 2 to 9% of recipients. The numbers of viral infections, such as those attributable to herpes simplex virus, have been significantly reduced with the common use of acyclovir or ganciclovir prophylaxis. Candidal infections may be seen in the early postoperative period but usually do not cause invasive disease. Trimethoprim sulfamethoxazole prophylaxis (usually on a three times per week schedule) has significantly reduced the incidence of Pneumocystis pneumonia to <1% in LT recipients.

Viral Infections (CMV): In the period 1 to 6 months after transplantation, CMV accounts for the majority of the viral infections in LT recipients. The typical time period for the development of CMV infection is 30 to 150 days postoperatively, with an incidence of illness (*ie*, infection and disease) of approximately 50%. Risk factors for CMV disease are dependent on the serology of the donor and recipient as well as the use of high-intensity immunosuppressive therapy, including cytolytic therapy. Approximately 25 to 35% of the time CMV disease develops in CMV-positive recipients from either positive or negative donors, whereas CMV-negative recipients have an 85% chance of the disease developing when implanted with a CMV-positive lung. There are data showing that CMV pneumonitis may contribute to the development of chronic rejection.[24]

CMV can cause a wide spectrum of disease from asymptomatic infection (*ie*, shedding of the virus in the urine or BAL fluid) to widespread dissemination. Various presentations of CMV in LT patients can include pneumonitis and, most commonly, gastroenteritis, hepatitis, and colitis. CMV pneumonitis can often be confused with acute rejection. Clinical findings of CMV pneumonitis include fever, cough, hypoxemia, the presence of an interstitial or alveolar infiltrate, and leukopenia. The diagnosis of invasive disease requires cytologic or histologic changes in cell preparation or tissue. Therefore, flexible bronchoscopy with transbronchial biopsy and BAL fluid is often necessary and can diagnose CMV pneumonia in 60 to 90% of patients.

The diagnosis of CMV infection may occasionally be made on the basis of positive cultures and the compatible clinical setting after other causes of pulmonary disease have been excluded bronchoscopically. The pathologic hallmark of CMV infection is a cytomegalic 250-nm cell containing a large central basophilic intranuclear inclusion. This inclusion is referred to as an *owl's eye* because it is separated from the nuclear membrane by a halo. These inclusions may be well seen with hematoxylin-eosin or Papanicolaou staining. The identification of CMV cytologically is very specific (98%) but lacks sensitivity (21%) for the presence of infection. Other pathologic findings in the lung parenchyma include a lymphocytic and mononuclear cell interstitial pneumonitis.

Ganciclovir is currently the mainstay of therapy for invasive CMV disease. Initial doses of 5 mg/kg bid for 3 to 4 weeks have been shown to reduce mortality from 60 to 80% to 15 to 20% in patients with symptomatic CMV pneumonitis. Some centers also use CMV-specific hyper-Ig in the treatment of CMV disease.

Prophylaxis against CMV infections has become a major strategy in most transplant centers. Initially, some centers attempted to match CMV-negative recipients with CMV-negative donors when possible; however, the limited donor supply did not allow the continuation of this practice. The use of CMV-negative blood products is advocated. Ganciclovir prophylaxis seems to be effective in delaying the onset of CMV infection. At some centers, prophylaxis is administered only to the CMV-mismatched patients (*ie*, a CMV-negative recipient receiving an organ from a CMV-positive donor). Other centers administer prophylaxis to all but the CMV-negative-to-CMV-negative patient group. Prophylactic treatment approaches usually include 2 to 4 weeks of therapy with ganciclovir (5 mg/kg qd), although some centers continue prophylaxis for up to 90 days, particularly in the donor-positive and recipient-negative subset of patients. In the groups with the greatest risk, CMV hyper-Ig may be added to the regimen. The oral form of ganciclovir may be of potential use in the LT population, but the data are inconclusive. Preemptive strategies such as the initiation of treatment when a high level of CMV blood antigenemia or polymerase chain reaction copies is detected may also delay and decrease the severity of CMV infection, and may become the standard of care.

Other viral infections that have been described in LT patients include herpes simplex virus (early after LT) respiratory syncytial virus, other paramyxoviruses (such as parainfluenza), influenza, metapneumovirus, and adenovirus. Acyclovir prophylaxis for herpes infection is initiated in most programs after the discontinuation of therapy with ganciclovir.

Fungal Infections: Fungal infections are more common in the LT recipient than in those who have received other solid-organ transplants. The overall incidence of invasive fungal infection in LT ranges from 10 to 22% and usually develops in the first few months after transplantation. Fungal infections account for the most significant morbidity and mortality of all infectious agents after transplantation, and the mortality rate can range from 40 to 70%.

Aspergillus species including *Aspergillus fumigatus*, *Aspergillus flavus*, *Aspergillus terreus*, and *Aspergillus niger* can be colonizing organisms or can result in infection presenting as indolent, progressive pneumonia or as an acute fulminant infection that rapidly disseminates. Aspergillus species exhibits the propensity to invade blood vessels and may present as an infarct or with hemoptysis. The radiographic findings of pulmonary aspergillosis include focal, lower-lobe infiltrates, patchy bronchopneumonic infiltrates, single or multiple nodules with or without cavitation, thin wall cavities, and opacification of the entire lung graft. A HRCT scan may reveal a halo sign thought to be pathognomonic for invasive aspergillosis. Other forms of presentation of Aspergillus infection can include pseudomembranous tracheobronchitis, often at and distal to the site of the anastomosis. The diagnosis of invasive aspergillosis requires the identification of organisms within tissues. These organisms can appear as septated hyphae that branch at acute angles, and can be detected with hematoxylin-eosin and methenamine silver staining.

Survival with Aspergillus infection has been improved with the early initiation of advanced generation azoles such as itraconazole and voriconazole and/or high-dose amphotericin therapy and a reduction in immunosuppressive therapy. Surgical resection may occasionally be required to maximize cure rates in patients with aspergillosis. Therapy with a lipid formulation of amphotericin B should also be considered in the management of invasive fungal infections in patients who are intolerant or in whom nephrotoxicity develops with conventional amphotericin B and in patients with progressive fungal infection despite therapy with conventional amphotericin. Prophylaxis with amphotericin B, azoles (particularly itraconazole for 3 to 6 months), or aerosolized amphotericin has shown promise in decreasing the incidence of Aspergillus infection after LT.

Candida species can cause a variety of syndromes in the patient undergoing LT, including mucocutaneous disease, line sepsis, wound infection and, rarely, pulmonary involvement. Fluconazole has emerged as an effective alternative for infections caused by *Candida albicans*, but amphotericin B is still the agent of choice for a widespread disease. Fluconazole appears to be less active against other Candida species such as *Candida glabrata* and *Candida krusei*.

Other rare causes of fungal infection in LT recipients have included *Cryptococcus neoformans*, as well as the dimorphic fungi such as coccidioides, histoplasma, and blastomyces. Azoles and amphotericin B remains the antifungal agents of choice for these infections, although azole agents can be used for maintenance therapy.

Mycobacteria: Mycobacterial diseases both typical and atypical have been successfully treated in the LT patient.

Vaccinations: Standard vaccination regimens should be used in patients in the LT population.

Posttransplant Lymphoproliferative Disorders

Posttransplant lymphoproliferative disorders (PTLDs) are reported more frequently after LT than after other types of solid-organ transplantation. Lymphomas comprise a majority (22%) of PTLDs. The PTLDs are composed of a heterogeneous group of lymphoid proliferations of variable clonality. The B-cell non-Hodgkin lymphomas are the most frequent form of PTLD and have been associated with Epstein-Barr virus (EBV) activity either serologically or by the identification of viral DNA in tissue. There is no clear correlation among episodes of rejection, specific immunosuppressive drugs, and the development of PTLD. The incidence of PTLD after LT has been reported to be

1.8% to 9.4%. Those patients who have negative EBV serology before transplantation and receive an organ from an EBV-positive donor resulting in seroconversion are at a significantly greater risk for the development of a PTLD. Children are at greater risk because of their frequent EBV-negative status.

The clinical features of PTLD in LT recipients include development in the first posttransplant year, involvement of the allograft, and radiographic findings of solitary or multiple pulmonary nodules. Disseminated disease has also been reported. Treatment includes the anti-CD20 monoclonal antibody rituximab, a reduction in immunosuppression, as well as consideration for adjunctive treatment with antiviral therapy, radiation, chemotherapy, surgery, and adoptive immunotherapies extrapolated from the bone marrow transplant population. Mortality may be significant with high-grade PTLD. An increased incidence of other nonlymphomatous malignancies has been reported in the LT population, and careful screening is recommended.

Miscellaneous Complications

The recurrence of primary disease has been described in patients who have received transplants for the treatment of sarcoidosis, lymphangiomyomatosis, giant-cell interstitial pneumonitis, desquamative interstitial pneumonia, idiopathic pulmonary hemosiderosis, bronchioalveolar carcinoma, eosinophilic granuloma, alveolar proteinosis, and diffuse panbronchiolitis. However, disease recurrence may be an incidental finding in some of these patients, particularly those with sarcoidosis.

Pleural effusions may develop because of the fact that the lymphatics are not reanastomosed after transplant and/or in the setting of rejection. Prolonged postoperative air leaks have been well described. Gastroparesis and an increased incidence of GI emergencies have also been described in LT recipients. GERD, both symptomatic and asymptomatic, is now known to be a significant problem after LT. This complication may be more common in those patient populations predisposed to the development of GERD, such as patients with CF. Osteoporosis remains a significant problem in the posttransplant period and is best managed with bisphosphonate agents such as alendronate or pamidronate.[30,31] Deep venous thrombosis and pulmonary embolism were reported to have an incidence of 8.6% in one series of LT recipients.[32] Hypogammaglobulinemia has also been described.

Immunosuppression

Because transplantation of a lung graft into a recipient invokes a specific immune response, the need to suppress the recipient's immune system exists immediately. Rejection results from the activation, differentiation, and proliferation of T lymphocytes acting against donor cells that are recognized as foreign, the major determinants of which are cell-surface markers known as HLAs. Current immunosuppressive regimens and strategies are based on the inhibition of this whole-cell response to foreign antigens.

Currently, most transplant centers use maintenance immunosuppression regimens including cyclosporine or tacrolimus, azathioprine or mycophenolate mofetil, and prednisone. In addition, in the first 2 weeks after LT, immunosuppression may be enhanced by the use of cytolytic agents such as OKT_3 (a monoclonal antibody to the OKT_3), antithymocyte globulin, or new human-derived IL-2 receptor antibodies such as daclizumab.

A typical maintenance immunosuppressive regimen consists of cyclosporine, 5 mg/kg bid (with dose adjusted to serum levels of 250 to 350 ng/mL); azathioprine, 1 to 2 mg/kg/d (adjusted to maintain a leukocyte count of 4,000 to 4,500 cells/µL); and prednisone, approximately 0.5 mg/kg/d for the first 3 months tapered over the next 3 months to 15 mg/d and to 5 mg/d by the 12th posttransplant month. Some programs have completely discontinued the use of prednisone after ≥1 year after transplantation. Tacrolimus may be used in lieu of cyclosporine at a dose of approximately 0.1 mg/kg bid (adjusted to a serum level of 8 to 15 ng/mL); and mycophenolate mofetil, 1 to 3 g/d, may be used in lieu of azathioprine.

All immunosuppressive drugs are wrought with complications, which can pose a significant problem after transplantation (Table 4). Cyclosporine and tacrolimus act by inhibiting IL-2 gene transcription, thus decreasing T-lymphocyte activation and subsequent proliferation. Chronic nephrotoxicity is a common complication of both agents and can develop in 25 to 75% of patients receiving

Table 4. *Immunosuppressive Drugs Used in Lung Transplantation*

Drug	Common Adverse Effects
Cyclosporine	Nephrotoxicity; hypertension; neurotoxicity (tremor, seizures, and headache); hyperlipidemia; hyperkalemia; hypomagnesemia; GI disturbance; hemolytic uremic syndrome; hirsutism; and gingival hyperplasia
Tacrolimus	Nephrotoxicity; hypertension; neurotoxicity (tremor, seizures, headache); hyperlipidemia; hyperkalemia; hypomagnesemia; GI disturbance; hemolytic uremic syndrome; hyperglycemia; and diabetes
Azathioprine	Leukopenia, macrocytic anemia, thrombocytopenia, hepatotoxicity, and pancreatitis
Mycophenolate mofetil	Diarrhea, abdominal pain, nausea, leukopenia, and anemia
Prednisone	Hyperglycemia, hypertension, hyperlipidemia, osteoporosis, myopathy, insomnia, cataracts, and weight gain
OKT_3	Cytokine release syndrome, hypotension, acute respiratory distress syndrome, and a septic meningitis
Antithymocyte globulin	Serum sickness, leukopenia, and thrombocytopenia
Sirolimus	Anemia, thrombocytopenia, leukopenia, anastomotic dehiscence (early postoperative period), hyperlipidemia, arthralgias, interstitial pneumonitis, and lower extremity edema

these drugs and, to some degree, in nearly 100% of patients with long-term use. Acute renal toxicity is usually related to dose and typically is reversible. In addition, other potentially nephrotoxic agents, including amphotericin B, trimethoprim-sulfamethoxazole, nonsteroidal antiinflammatory agents, and aminoglycoside antibiotics, which may compound the toxic effects of cyclosporine and tacrolimus, may be used in transplant patients. Both cyclosporine and tacrolimus are also associated with systemic hypertension, which can develop in up to 25 to 50% of LT recipients.

The occurrence of hypercholesterolemia has also been well described. The incidence of both posttransplant hypertension and hyperlipidemia may be lower with the use of tacrolimus than with cyclosporine. Other well-described side effects of tacrolimus and cyclosporine include neurologic toxicity such as tremors, paresthesias, headaches, confusion, depression, somnolence, seizures, white matter changes, coma, and death. Peripheral neurologic findings have also been described. Neurotoxicity appears to be significantly more common with tacrolimus therapy than with cyclosporine therapy. Cyclosporine use is also associated with hirsutism, gingival hyperplasia, and gastroparesis. Tacrolimus use is associated with hyperglycemia and diabetes. Both agents have been reported to cause a hemolytic uremic syndrome or thrombotic thrombocytopenic purpura.

It is important that physicians who are caring for transplant patients are aware of the numerous drug interactions with tacrolimus and cyclosporine. For example, use of the azoles results in a significant increase in cyclosporine and tacrolimus levels in the same dose. Likewise, the discontinuation of therapy with azole agents without increasing the dose of cyclosporine or tacrolimus can result in an acute and life-threatening drop in therapeutic levels of these drugs. Interactions with macrolide antibiotics, calcium-channel blockers, and gastric motility drugs have also been reported. Levels of both agents are decreased with the use of rifampin or anticonvulsant agents.

Azathioprine inhibits nucleic acid synthesis and suppresses the proliferation of lymphocytes. Toxicities of this drug include cytopenias such as leukopenia and thrombocytopenia. Macrocytic anemia can develop with long-term use. Pancreatitis and cholestatic hepatitis have been well described with azathioprine use.

Mycophenolate mofetil also inhibits purine synthesis and blocks lymphocyte proliferation. Typical side effects include GI symptoms such as diarrhea, nausea, and abdominal pain. In addition, leukopenia and anemia have been described.

Corticosteroids play a main role in posttransplant immunosuppression by binding to cytoplasmic glucocorticoid receptors, undergoing translocation into the nucleus, and then blocking cytokine transcription of genes and secretion from phagocytes. The side effects of corticosteroid use are well known and include hyperglycemia, hypertension, hyperlipidemia, osteoporosis, proximal myopathy, mood disturbance, cataract formation, and weight gain.

The lympholytic agents such as OKT_3 and antithymocyte globulin act by depleting CD_3 lymphocytes by lysis, opsonization, and phagocytosis. The administration of OKT_3 may be associated with the cytokine release syndrome manifested by hypotension, noncardiogenic pulmonary edema, renal insufficiency, and aseptic meningitis. Antithymocyte globulin is associated with leukopenia, thrombocytopenia, and serum sickness. It should not be administered to those patients who have manifested an allergic reaction to horse serum in the past.

Sirolimus is one of the newer available immunosuppressant agents. It is being used for cases of acute and chronic LT rejection and, in small studies, as *de novo* therapy after LT. Sirolimus is a macrocyclic triene antibiotic (structurally related to tacrolimus) with immunosuppressive, antitumor, and antifungal properties. Sirolimus has been demonstrated to block the proliferative response and the activation of T cells, B cells, and other cell lines by cytokines and growth factors, thus preventing cell-cycle progression and proliferation. In contrast, tacrolimus (FK-506) and cyclosporine inhibit the production of cytokines. The use of sirolimus in the immediate posttransplant period is discouraged because of the association with bronchial anastomotic dehiscence when used in combination with tacrolimus and corticosteroids. The major side effects of sirolimus include cytopenias (particularly thrombocytopenia and leukopenia), hyperlipidemia, arthralgias, and interstitial pneumonitis, which can become a serious problem in the LT recipient. Other side effects include those similar to the side effects described with cyclosporine and tacrolimus although, in general, the nephrotoxicity with this agent appears to be less that that of the other two agents. The role of sirolimus in the LT armamentarium remains to be established.

References

1. Christie JD, Edwards LB, Aurora P, et al. The Registry of the International Society for Heart and Lung Transplantation: twenty-fifth official adult lung and heart-lung annual report; 2008. J Heart Lung Transplant 2008; 27:957–969
2. Orens JB, Estenne M, Arcasoy S, et al. International guidelines for the selection of lung transplant candidates: 2006 update; a consensus report from the Pulmonary Scientific Council of the International Society for Heart and Lung Transplantation. J Heart Lung Transplant 2006; 25:745–755
3. Kanasky WF Jr., Anton SD, Rodrigue JR, et al. Impact of body weight on long-term survival after lung transplantation. Chest 2002; 121:401–406
4. Hosenpud JD, Bennett LE, Keck BM, et al. Effect of diagnosis on survival benefit of lung transplantation for end-stage disease. Lancet 1998; 351:24–27
5. Liou TG, Adler FR, Cahill BC, et al. Survival effect of lung transplantation among patients with cystic fibrosis. JAMA 2002; 286:2683–2689
6. Mayer-Hamblett N, Rosenfeld M, Emerson J, et al. Developing cystic fibrosis lung transplant referral criteria using predictors of 2-year mortality. Am J Respir Crit Care Med 2002; 166:1550–1555
7. Liou TG, Adler FR, Cox DR, Cahill BC. Lung transplantation and survival in children with cystic fibrosis. N Engl J Med 2007; 357:2143–2152
8. Chaparro C, Maurer J, Gutierrez C, et al. Infection with *Burkholderia cepacia* in cystic fibrosis: outcome following lung transplantation. Am J Respir Crit Care Med 2001; 163:43–48
9. Hadjiliadis D, Steele MP, Chaparro C, et al. Survival of lung transplant patients with cystic fibrosis harboring panresistant bacteria other than *Burkholderia cepacia*, compared with patients harboring sensitive bacteria. J Heart Lung Transplant 2007; 26:834–838
10. Angel LF, Levine DJ, Restrepo MI, et al. Impact of a lung transplantation donor-management protocol on lung donation and recipient outcomes. Am J Respir Crit Care Med 2006; 174:710–716
11. Bhorade SM, Vigneswaran W, McCabe MA, et al. Liberalization of donor criteria may expand the donor pool without adverse consequence in lung transplantation. J Heart Lung Transplant 2000; 12:1199–1204
12. Valentine VG, Taylor DE, Dhillon GS, et al. Success of lung transplantation without surveillance bronchoscopy. J Heart Lung Transplant 2002; 21:319–326
13. Levine SM. Transplant/Immunology Network of the American College of Chest Physicians. A survey of clinical practice of lung transplantation in North America. Chest 2004; 125:1224–1238
14. Christie JD, Carby M, Bag R, et al. Report of the ISHLT working group on primary lung graft dysfunction: part II. Definition: a consensus statement of the ISHLT. J Heart Lung Transplant; 2005; 24:1454–1459

15. Shargall Y, Guenther G, Ahya VN, et al. Report of the ISHLT working group on primary lung graft dysfunction: part VI. Treatment: a consensus statement of the ISHLT. J Heart Lung Transplant; 2005; 24:1489–1500
16. Meade MO, Granton JT, Matte-Martyn A, et al. A randomized trial of inhaled nitric oxide to prevent ischemia-reperfusion injury after lung transplantation. Am J Respir Crit Care Med 2003; 167:1483–1489
17. Christie JD, Bavaria JE, Pavlevsky HI, et al. Primary graft failure following lung transplantation. Chest 1998; 114:51–60
18. Khan S, Salloum J, O'Donovan PB, et al. Acute pulmonary edema after lung transplantation: the pulmonary reimplantation response. Chest 1999; 116:187–194
19. Christie JD, Kotloff RM, Pochettino A, et al. Clinical risk factors for primary graft failure following lung transplantation. Chest 2003; 124:1232–1241
20. Thabut G, Vinatier I, Stern JB, et al. Primary graft failure following lung transplantation: predictive factors of mortality. Chest 2002; 121:1876–1882
21. Arcasoy SM, Fisher A, Hachem RR, et al. Report of the ISHLT working group on primary lung graft dysfunction: part V. Predictors and outcomes: a consensus statement of the ISHLT. J Heart Lung Transplant; 2005; 24:1483–1488
22. Stewart S, Fishbein MC, Snell GI, et al. Revision of the 1996 working formulation for the standardization of nomenclature in the diagnosis of lung rejection. J Heart Lung Transplant 2007; 26:1229–1242
23. Sharples LD, McNeil K, Stewart S, et al. Risk factors for bronchiolitis obliterans: a systematic review of recent publications. J Heart Lung Transplant 2002; 21:271–281
24. Estenne M, Maurer JR, Boehler A, et al. Bronchiolitis obliterans syndrome 2001: an update of the diagnostic criteria. J Heart Lung Transplant 2002; 21:297–310
25. Leung AN, Fisher K, Valentine V, et al. Bronchiolitis obliterans after lung transplantation. Chest 1998; 113:365–370
26. Cooper JD, Billingham M, Egan T, et al. A working formulation for the standardization of nomenclature and for clinical staging of chronic dysfunction in lung allografts: International Society for Heart and Lung Transplantation. J Heart Lung Transplant 1993; 12:713–716
27. Lama VN, Murray S, Lonigro RJ, et al. Course of FEV_1 after onset of bronchiolitis obliterans syndrome in lung transplant recipients. Am J Respir Crit Care Med 2007; 175:1192–1198
28. Yates B, Murphy DM, Forrest IA, et al. Azithromycin reverses airflow obstruction in established bronchiolitis obliterans syndrome. Am J Respir Crit Care Med 2005; 172:772–775
29. Valentine VG, Robbins RC, Berry GJ. Actuarial survival of heart-lung and bilateral sequential lung transplant recipients with obliterative bronchiolitis. J Heart Lung Transplant 1996; 15:371–383
30. Spira A, Gutierrez C. Chaparro C, et al. osteoporosis and lung transplantation: a prospective study. Chest 2000; 117:476–481
31. Aris RM, Lester GE, Renner JB, et al. Efficacy of pamidronate for osteoporosis in patients with cystic fibrosis following lung transplantation. Am J Respir Crit Care Med 2000; 162:941–946
32. Izbicki G, Bairey O, Shitrit D, et al. Increased thromboembolic events after lung transplantation. Chest 2006; 129:412–416

Annotated Bibliography

Arcasoy SM, Fisher A, Hachem RR, et al. Report of the ISHLT working group on primary lung graft dysfunction: part V. Predictors and outcomes: a consensus statement of the ISHLT. J Heart Lung Transplant; 2005; 24:1483–1488
One article in a series of articles focusing on PGD.

Arcasoy SM, Kotloff RM. Lung transplantation. N Engl J Med 1999; 340:1081–1091
This is a concise review of the field of LT.

Belperio JA, Weigt SS, Fishbein MC, et al. Chronic lung allograft rejection: mechanisms and therapy. Proc Am Thorac Soc 2009; 6:108–121
This issue of this journal is devoted to LT.

Blondeau K, Mertens V, Vanaudenaerde BA, et al. Gastro-oesophageal reflux and gastric aspiration in lung transplant patients with or without chronic rejection. Eur Respir J 2008; 31:707–713
This study further examines the question of GERD and chronic rejection.

Boehler A, Estenne M. Post-transplant bronchiolitis obliterans. Eur Respir J 2003; 22:1007–1018
A review article discussing pathogenesis, risk factors, clinical presentation, diagnosis, and treatment of bronchiolitis obliterans.

Briffa N, Morris RE. New immunosuppressive regimens in lung transplantation. Eur Respir J 1997; 10:2630–2634

This article gives an excellent overview of the mechanisms of action of the immunosuppressive agents commonly used in LT.

Chaparro C, Maurer J, Gutierrez C, et al. Infection with *Burkholderia cepacia* in cystic fibrosis: outcome following lung transplantation. Am J Respir Crit Care Med 2001; 163:43–48

An article examining survival of LT patient with CF and resistant bacteria.

Christie JD, Carby M, Bag R, et al. Report of the ISHLT working group on primary lung graft dysfunction: part II. Definition: a consensus statement of the ISHLT. J Heart Lung Transplant 2005; 24:1454–1459

One article in a series of articles focusing on PGD.

Christie JD, Edwards LB, Aurora P, et al. The Registry of the International Society for Heart and Lung Transplantation: twenty-fifth official adult lung and heart-lung annual report; 2008. J Heart Lung Transplant 2008; 27:957–969

This is the annual report from the ISHLT. It presents data on indications, numbers, survival, rates of morbidity and mortality, and some complications after LT.

Cooper JD, Billingham M, Egan T, et al. A working formulation for the standardization of nomenclature and for clinical staging of chronic dysfunction in lung allografts: international Society for Heart and Lung Transplantation. J Heart Lung Transplant 1993; 12:713–716

This is the original article defining staging for the BOS.

Corris PA, Christie JD. Update in transplantation 2007. Am J Respir Crit Care Med 2008; 177:1062–1067

A succinct update on this subject.

de Antonio DG, Marcos R, Laporta R, et al. Results of clinical lung transplant from uncontrolled non-heart-beating donors. J Heart Lung Transplant 2007; 26:529–534

This article examines the use of non--heart-beating donors in LT.

DeSoyza A, McDowell A, Archer L, et al. Burkholderia cepacia complex genomovars and pulmonary transplantation outcomes in patients with cystic fibrosis. Lancet 2001; 358:1780–1781

This article examines transplant outcomes with different genomovars of B cepacia.

Estenne M, Maurer JR, Boehler A, et al. Bronchiolitis obliterans syndrome 2001: an update of the diagnostic criteria. J Heart Lung Transplant 2002; 21:297–310

This article includes the proposed new staging system for BOS, lists BOS risk factors, reviews the pathology of BOS, reviews surrogate markers of BOS, and discusses the response to treatment.

Gries CJ, Mulligan MS, Edelman JD, et al. Lung allocation score for lung transplantation: impact on disease severity and survival. Chest 2007; 132:1954–1961

This article examines the early impact of the LAS on waiting times, death on the waiting list, diseases transplanted, and early survival before and after the implementation of the LAS.

Hadjiliadis D, Steele MP, Chaparro C, et al. Survival of lung transplant patients with cystic fibrosis harboring panresistant bacteria other than *Burkholderia cepacia*, compared with patients harboring sensitive bacteria. J Heart Lung Transplant 2007; 26:834–838

An article examining survival of LT patient with CF and resistant bacteria.

Izbicki G, Bairey O, Shitrit D, et al. Increased thromboembolic events after lung transplantation. Chest 2006; 129:412–416

Another article on this subject.

Lama VN, Murray S, Lonigro RJ, et al. Course of FEV(1) after onset of bronchiolitis obliterans syndrome in lung transplant recipients. Am J Respir Crit Care Med 2007; 175:1192–1198

This study examined the progression in the percentage of predicted FEV_1 *after LT and attempted to identify risk factors for rapid decline.*

Levine SM, Angel L, Anzueto A, et al. A low incidence of post transplant lymphoproliferative disorder in 109 lung transplant recipients. Chest 1999; 116:1273–1277

This article presents data from a single center on PTLD. The article also reviews data from some of the other published series on this subject.

Levine SM, Peters JI. Fungal infection in the lung transplant recipient: update. Pulm Crit Care 1998; 12: Lesson 17

This is a review article describing the incidence, outcome, and varied clinical presentations of fungal infections in LT recipients.

Levine SM, Transplant/Immunology Network of the American College of Chest Physicians. A survey of clinical practice of lung transplantation in North America. Chest 2004; 125:1224–1238

This article presents the results of a large survey sent to all North American LT centers regarding the clinical practice of LT.

Levy RD, Ernst P, Levine SM, et al. Exercise performance after lung transplantation. J Heart Lung Transplant 1996; 15:1045–1058

This article examines exercise physiology in SLT and HLT groups.

Liou TG, Adler FR, Cahill BC, et al. Survival effect of lung transplantation among patients with cystic fibrosis. JAMA 2002; 286:2683–2689

This article proposes a detailed predictive model for a survival effect when referring CF patients for BLT.

Liou TG, Adler FR, Cox DR, et al. Lung transplantation and survival in children with cystic fibrosis. N Engl J Med 2007; 357:2143–2152

The purpose of this study was to determine the impact of LT on survival in children (< 18 years old) with CF.

Martinu T, Chen DF, Palmer SM. Acute rejection and humoral sensitization in lung transplant recipients. Proc Am Thorac Soc 2009; 6:54–65

A review of acute rejection including a discussion on humoral rejection.

Meade MO, Granton JT, Matte-Martyn A, et al. A randomized trial of inhaled nitric oxide to prevent ischemia-reperfusion injury after lung transplantation. Am J Respir Crit Care Med 2003; 167:1483–1489

A negative study of the use of nitric oxide to prevent reperfusion injury.

Mehrad B, Paciocco G, Martinez FJ, et al. Spectrum of aspergillus infection in lung transplant recipients: case series and review of the literature. Chest 2001; 119:169–175

This article reviews the various presentations of Aspergillus in the LT population.

Meyer DM, Bennett LE, Novick RJ, et al. Single vs bilateral, sequential lung transplantation for end-stage emphysema: influence of recipient age on survival and secondary end-points. J Heart Lung Transplant 2001; 20:935–941

This study supports the practice at some centers of performing BLT over SLT for younger patients with COPD as the result of a survival advantage.

Orens JB, Estenne M, Arcasoy S, et al. International guidelines for the selection of lung transplant candidates: 2006 update; a consensus report from the Pulmonary Scientific Council of the International Society for Heart and Lung Transplantation. J Heart Lung Transplant 2006; 25:745–755

These are updated consensus-determined guidelines regarding selection of LT candidates.

Pochettino A, Kotloff RM, Rosengard BR, et al. Bilateral versus single lung transplantation for chronic obstructive pulmonary disease: intermediate-term results. Ann Thorac Surg 2000; 70:1813–1818

This study also supports performing BLT in younger patients with COPD and SLT in older COPD patients.

Reams BD, McAdams HP, Howell DN, et al. Posttransplant lymphoproliferative disorder: incidence, presentation, and response to treatment in lung transplant recipients. Chest 2003; 124:1242–1249

Includes information on the treatment of PTLD with rituximab.

Shargall Y, Guenther G, Ahya VN, et al. Report of the ISHLT working group on primary lung graft dysfunction: part VI: treatment: a consensus statement of the ISHLT. J Heart Lung Transplant 2005; 24:1489–1500

One article in a series of articles focusing on PGD.

Sharples LD, McNeil K, Stewart S, et al. Risk factors for bronchiolitis obliterans: a systematic review of recent publications. J Heart Lung Transplant 2002; 21:271–281

A review of published human studies on the risk factors for OB.

Snyder LD, Palmer SM. Immune mechanisms of lung allograft rejection. Semin Respir Crit Care Med 2006; 27:534–543

A review of the immunology of graft rejection, including a discussion on humoral rejection.

Stewart S, Fishbein MC, Snell GI, et al. Revision of the 1996 working formulation for the standardization of nomenclature in the diagnosis of lung rejection. J Heart Lung Transplant 2007; 26:1229–1242

This is a revision of the pathology of acute and chronic rejection in LT recipients.

Trulock EP. Lung transplantation. Am J Respir Crit Care Med 1997; 155:789–818

This is the most comprehensive review of the field of LT. It is directed toward the pulmonary and critical care medicine audience.

United Network for Organ Sharing. Available at: http://www.unos.org. Accessed March 29, 2009

An important Web site for statistics regarding lung and other solid-organ transplants.

Young LR, Hadjiliadis D, Davis RD, et al. Lung transplantation exacerbates gastroesophageal reflux disease. Chest 2003; 124:1689–1693

This article describes the prevalence and possible etiologies of this complication.

Proc Am Thorac Soc 2009; 6:1–100

An entire issue devoted to many aspects of LT.

Rare Interstitial Lung Diseases: Pulmonary Langerhans Cell Histiocytosis, Lymphangioleiomyomatosis, and Cryptogenic Organizing Pneumonia

Joseph P. Lynch III, MD, FCCP

Objectives:

- Describe the salient epidemiologic, clinical, physiologic, and radiographic features of Langerhans cell histiocytosis (LCH), lymphangioleiomyomatosis (LAM), and cryptogenic organizing pneumonia (COP)
- Compare and contrast the salient features seen on high-resolution CT scans in these disorders
- Review the characteristic histopathologic features of each of these disorders and the role of immunohistochemical techniques or markers (for pulmonary LCH and LAM)
- Review the differing therapeutic strategies for these disorders

Key words: bronchiolitis obliterans organizing pneumonia; cryptogenic organizing pneumonia; cystic lung diseases; Langerhans cell granulomatosis; Langerhans cell histiocytosis; lymphangioleiomyomatosis; pulmonary eosinophilic granuloma;

Pulmonary Langerhans cell histiocytosis (LCH; also termed *Langerhans cell granulomatosis*) and lymphangioleiomyomatosis (LAM) are rare and poorly understood chronic lung disorders characterized by extensive cyst formation within the lung parenchyma. These disorders share certain features, but LAM affects exclusively women, whereas pulmonary LCH (PLCH) may affect either sex. Cryptogenic organizing pneumonia (COP), formerly termed *bronchiolitis obliterans organizing pneumonia* (BOOP), is a rare disease of unknown etiology characterized by dense alveolar infiltrates, subacute course, and excellent responsiveness to corticosteroid (CS) therapy. This chapter reviews the salient features of these disorders and presents approaches to diagnosis and therapy.

Pulmonary LCH

Pulmonary LCH is a rare disorder usually seen in smokers. It presents as chronic interstitial lung disease (ILD) or with pneumothoraces.[1,2] Histologically, the lesions of PLCH are identical to LCH (formerly termed *eosinophilic granuloma* or *histiocytosis X*), involving bone or extrapulmonary organs.[3] However, <20% of adults with PLCH manifest extrapulmonary involvement.[3-8] More importantly, LCH predominantly affects children, whereas isolated PLCH is a rare occurrence in children.[9] The clinical and radiographic features of PLCH overlap with those of myriad chronic ILDs. However, CT scans are highly characteristic and may distinguish PLCH from idiopathic pulmonary fibrosis and other chronic ILDs.

Epidemiology

The prevalence of PLCH is estimated at two to five cases per million persons.[1,3] PLCH accounts for <5% of cases of ILDs.[3] PCH typically occurs in adults 20 to 50 years of age; children are rarely affected.[3,4,8] PLCH is almost exclusively seen in Caucasian patients, suggesting a genetic predisposition.[3-5] However, no familial or inheritable trait has been identified. Multisystemic LCH in children or adults is monoclonal,[10] whereas PLCH is polyclonal, suggesting a reactive process.[11] The low proliferative rate of Langerhans cell (LCs) in PLCH suggests a nonmalignant process.[6,12] The authors of some studies suggest a distinct male predominance,[5,13] but others cite a slight female predominance.[4,6,7] These variations in incidence by sex may reflect differences in smoking habits of the populations studied.[1] More than 90% of cases of PLCH occur in smokers,[3-5,7,14] which suggests that constituents of cigarette smoke have a strong role in the pathogenesis.

Clinical Features

The clinical features and natural history of PLCH are variable. Symptoms of cough and dyspnea are present in twothirds of patients and often develop insidiously over the course of several months or years.[1] Pneumothoraces occurs in 6 to 20% of patients and may be the presenting feature.[1,4-6,15-17] Recurrent pneumothoraces may require surgical pleurodesis for control.[5,17] Rupture of subpleural cysts or blebs accounts for the predilection for recurrent pneumothoraces. Hemoptysis or wheezing occur in <5% of patients.[3] Constitutional symptoms of fever, malaise, weight loss, or anorexia are present in 15 to 30% of patients.[3-5] A total of 10 to 25% of patients are asymptomatic, with incidental findings on chest radiographs.[1,4-6]

Pulmonary arterial hypertension (PAH) is common in severe PLCH[18] and likely represents intrinsic pulmonary vascular disease. In a series of 21 patients with advanced PLCH who were awaiting lung transplantation, all had PAH (mean pulmonary arterial pressure, 59 mm Hg) that was disproportionate to the degree of pulmonary functional impairment or hypoxemia.[18] Histopathology demonstrated proliferative vasculopathy involving muscular arteries and veins with prominent venular involvement. A fatal case of veno-occlusive disease complicating PLCH was described.[19] Extrapulmonary involvement occurs in <20% of patients with PLCH.[3-7,13] Solitary punched-out lesions of bone and diabetes insipidus (from involvement of the pituitary) are the most common sites of extrapulmonary involvement.[1,3] Blood or serologic studies are not helpful. In contrast to chronic eosinophilic pneumonia, peripheral blood eosinophilia is not a feature of PLCH.[1]

The prognosis of PLCH is generally good, but disparate results have been reported in the literature. The disease stabilizes or improves spontaneously in approximately two thirds of patients, usually within 18 months of onset of symptoms.[4-7,15,16] However, the disease progresses in 15 to 30%, with destruction of lung parenchyma and respiratory impairment; fatality rates range from 2 to 27%.[4-7,13,16,20,21]

The risk of lung cancer appears to be increased in patients with PLCH.[22-24] In one study of 93 patients with PLCH, 5 developed bronchogenic carcinoma, for an annual risk of 1,040/100,000.[22] In contrast, none of 48 patients in a series from the National Institutes of Health had lung cancer.[7] Because virtually all patients are smokers, cigarette smoke likely contributes to the cancer risk. An association between lymphoma and PLCH has also been noted.[23,25]

Radiographic Features of the Chest

Conventional chest radiographs usually demonstrate diffuse reticular, reticulonodular, or cystic lesions with a predilection for the mid- and upper lung zones (Fig 1).[3-5] The costophrenic angles are usually spared.[4,5,15] Both nodular and cystic components are usually present concomitantly. The cystic radiolucencies correspond to walls of cysts or dilated bronchi or bronchioles. Reticular or reticulonodular lesions, typically ranging in size from 1 to 5 mm, represent the walls of cysts (from destroyed lung parenchyma) or peribronchiolar cellular lesions.[1] With advanced disease, volume loss and fibrosis may be extensive. Pneumothoraces occur in 6 to 20% of patients and may be the presenting feature (Fig 2).[4-6] Pleural thickening or effusions are uncommon.[15] Cavitation of nodules is occasionally observed on CT scans[1,15] but is not seen on plain radiographs. Hilar or mediastinal lymphadenopathy is rare.[1,4,26]

Chest CT Characteristics

Certain findings on thin-section high-resolution CT (HRCT) scans are highly suggestive of PLCH, and HRCT is far superior to conventional chest

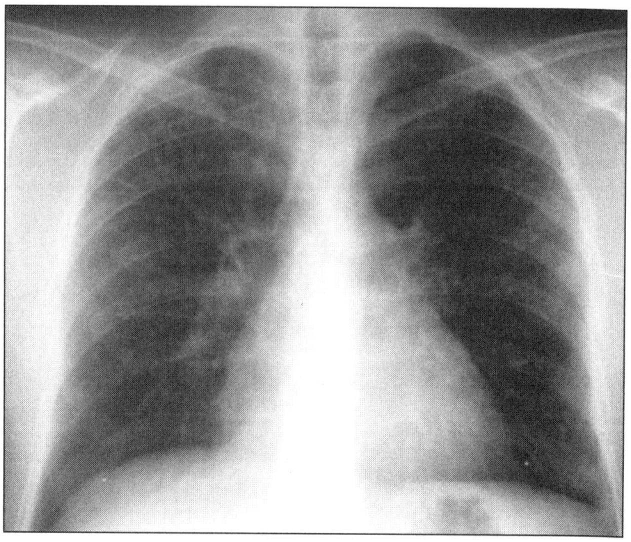

Figure 1. LCH. Posteroanterior chest radiograph demonstrating finely nodular densities throughout the lung parenchyma, with a predominance in the middle and upper lung fields, in a 44-year-old man with pulmonary LCH.

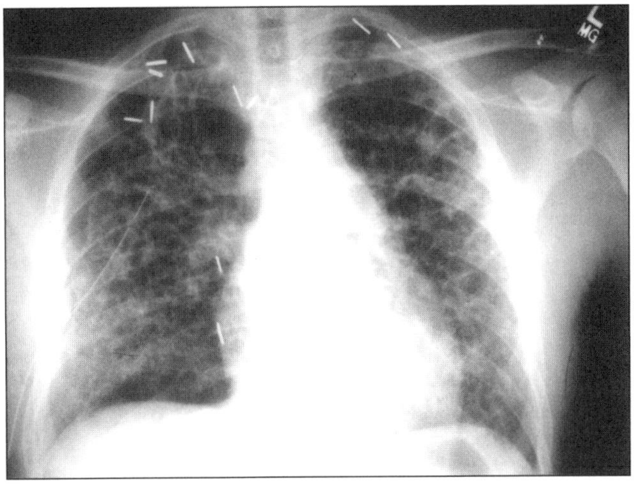

Figure 2. LCH. Posteroanterior chest radiograph demonstrating far advanced cystic and nodular changes throughout the lung parenchyma. A persistent right pneumothorax is evident, despite the presence of a right thoracoscopy tube. Surgical clips are from prior thoracotomies for attempted pleurodesis.

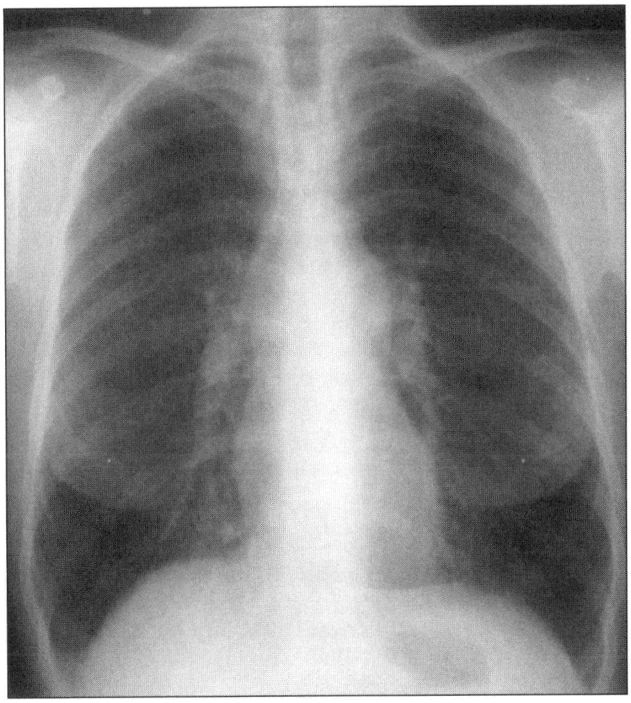

Figure 3. LCH. Posteroanterior chest radiograph demonstrating finely nodular densities throughout the lung parenchyma and hyperinflation in a 38-year-old woman with pulmonary LCH.

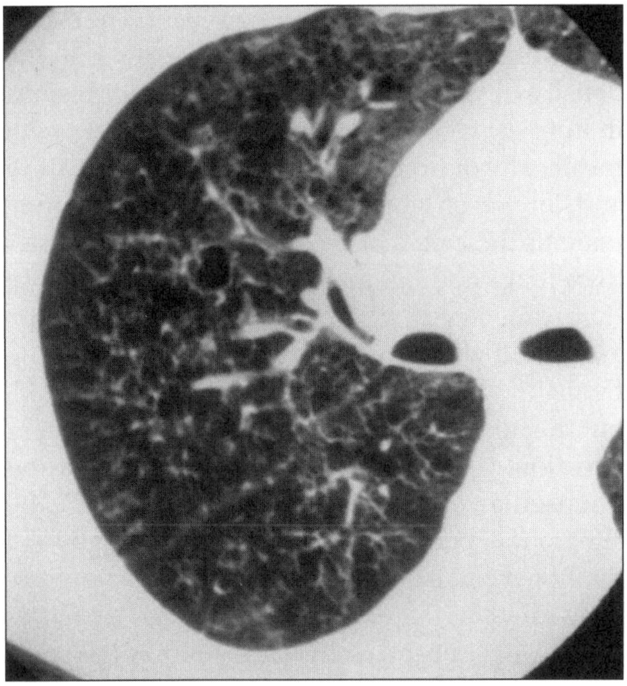

Figure 4. LCH. HRCT scan from the patient in Fig 3 reveals numerous cysts of various sizes throughout the lung parenchyma. Multiple small nodules can also be seen dispersed throughout the peribronchial regions and alveolar interstitium.

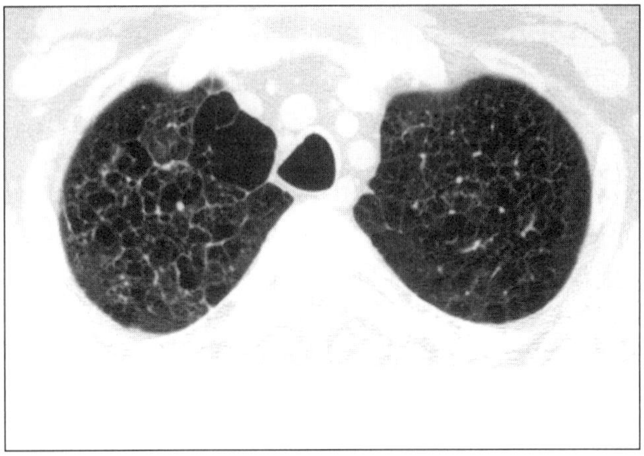

Figure 5. LCH. HRCT scan of the upper lobes from a 56-year-old man with progressive cough and dyspnea. Note the multiple well-defined cystic spaces and coalescence of blebs in the medial aspect of the right apex. A few tiny, scattered peribronchiolar nodules are also present. Transbronchial lung biopsy specimens demonstrated typical histologic features of LCH. S100 stains were also positive.

radiographs in discerning the cystic nature of the disease (Figs 3–5).[3,27,28] The combination of cystic and nodular lesions, with a proclivity to involve the upper lobes, strongly suggests PLCH.[1,29] There is no central or peripheral predominance. Multiple thin-walled cysts are observed in >85% of patients.[15,27,30] These cysts are usually round and <10 mm but may coalesce, occasionally exceeding 3 cm in size.[15,27] Nodules ranging in size from 1 to 15 mm are a prominent component of PLCH; they are found in approximately two thirds of patients.[15,27] The nodules surround small bronchioles and represent peribronchiolar granulomas. As the disease progresses, the nodules are replaced by cysts, some of which become confluent. The extent of nodular opacities on HRCT correlates with the density of granulomatous inflammatory lesions in lung tissue; cystic lesions on CT correlate with the density of cavitary lesions (both inflammatory and fibrotic) on biopsy.[8] Serial studies of individual patients indicate that lesions evolve from nodules to cavitary nodules and then to thick-walled and thin-walled cysts.[1,15,27] These cysts or nodules are associated with areas of intervening normal lung tissue.[15,27] The cystic radiolucencies resemble LAM, but the nodular component is lacking in LAM. In addition, LAM affects all lung zones, including the basilar regions. The cysts of PLCH lack the subpleural, peripheral, and basilar distribution of the honeycomb cysts noted in idiopathic pulmonary fibrosis (Fig 6, 7).[29] Ground-glass opacities (GGOs) have been described in 3 to 20% of patients with PLCH[3,14,15] but are rarely dominant. When GGOs are prominent, concomitant respiratory bronchiolitis-ILD often is present.[14] Pleural effusions and hilar adenopathy are rare.[1,15,29] However, mediastinal or paratracheal lymphadenopathy may be detected on CT scans in up to one third of patients.[3]

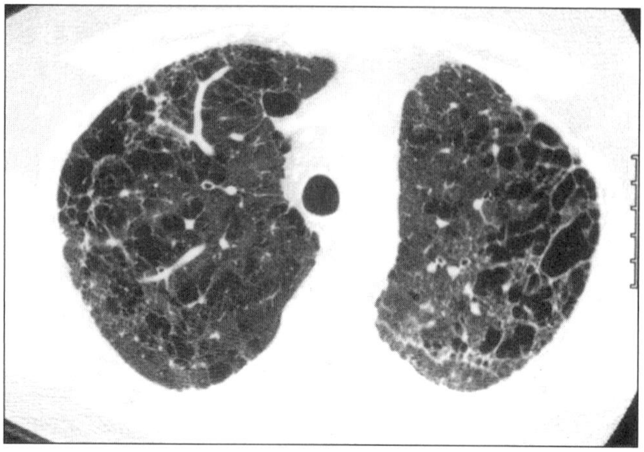

Figure 6. Idiopathic pulmonary fibrosis. HRCT scan from a 55-year-old woman with usual interstitial pneumonia (UIP) (documented by thoracoscopic lung biopsy) demonstrates extensive honeycombing throughout both lungs (upper lobes). Note that the cysts are distributed preferentially in the peripheral (subpleural) regions of the lung, with relative sparing of the central regions. This pattern differs from the more uniform distribution of cysts seen in patients with pulmonary LCH.

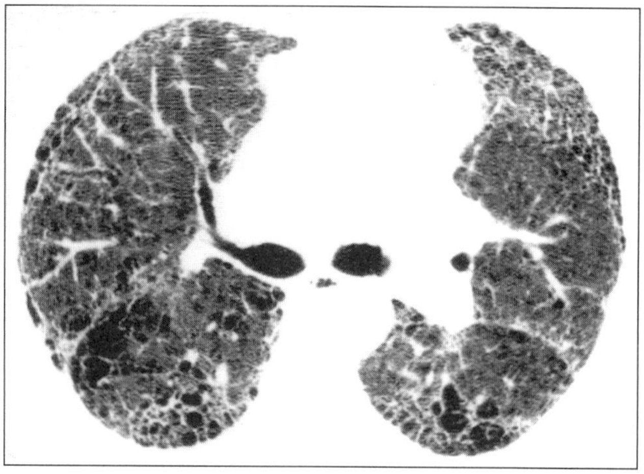

Figure 7. Idiopathic pulmonary fibrosis. HRCT scan from the patient in Fig 6 (lower lobes). Foci of honeycombing are noted throughout both lungs. Note the peripheral (subpleural) distribution of honeycomb cysts, with relative sparing of the central regions. In addition, prominent septal lines, bands, or fibrosis are apparent. This pattern differs from the more uniform distribution of cysts seen in patients with pulmonary LCH.

Pulmonary Function Tests

Pulmonary function tests (PFTs) are abnormal in >80% of patients with PLCH.[1,4-6,13,31] The diffusing capacity of the lung for carbon monoxide (DLCO) is reduced in >75% of patients.[3-6,13,15,31] Severe reductions in DLCO are associated with a worse prognosis and correlate with radiologic cyst formation. Reductions in vital capacity or total lung capacity (TLC) are present in 50 to 80% of patients.[4-7,13,31] Pure obstructive or mixed obstructive-restrictive patterns are present in one third of patients.[4-6,31] Air trapping (increased residual volume) occurs in nearly half of patients with PLCH, but hyperinflation (TLC >110% of predicted) is rare. Exercise tests typically demonstrate worsening gas exchange and increased dead space.[31] Aberrations in PFTs do not consistently correlate with radiographic findings. However, in a study of 26 cases of PLCH, correlations between PFTs and CT (semiquantitative) were noted.[32] The extent of cystic lesions on CT correlated inversely with FEV_1/FVC, Pao_2, DLCO, whereas nodular opacities did not. In most patients, PFTs improve or stabilize over time, but this finding is variable. Serial PFTs should be performed to monitor the course of the disease.

Histopathology

Histologically, PLCH is characterized by inflammatory, cystic, nodular, and fibrotic lesions distributed in a bronchocentric fashion.[4,6,31,33] Vasculitis is not a feature. The diagnosis of PLCH usually requires thoracoscopic lung biopsy, but transbronchial biopsies may be adequate provided the salient features are present.[7,13] Early in the course of the disease, the proliferation of atypical histiocytes (histiocytosis X cells or LCs) dominates.[4,6,34] Later, granulomatous inflammation ensues. Fibrosis is the end result of the chronic inflammatory cellular lesions. In individual patients, several histologic features may be present concomitantly (*eg*, histiocytic proliferation, granulomatous inflammation, fibrosis, healing, and repair).

The diagnosis of PLCH is suggested on low-power microscopy by numerous peribronchiolar nodules, numerous cysts, and a distinctive stellate or star-shaped pattern of fibrosis.[4,6] The stellate pattern of fibrosis was observed in 84 of 100 cases of PLCH reported by Friedman and colleagues.[4] The stellate border reflects extension of the cellular infiltrate into adjacent alveolar interstitium. Numerous discrete nodular infiltrates distributed throughout the lung, interspersed with large areas of normal lung parenchyma, can be seen under low-power magnification (Fig 8). These nodules are peribronchiolar in >80% of cases and subpleural in 70%.[7]

Because most patients with LCH are smokers, respiratory bronchiolitis is a frequent concomitant finding.[3,14] Under high-power light microscopy, atypical histiocytes (LCs or histiocytosis X cells) are prominent (encompassing up to 50% of cells) and are surrounded by variable numbers of eosinophils, lymphocytes, plasma cells, fibroblasts, and foci of fibrosis.[3,4,6] Aggregates of these LCs comprise the key histologic feature of PLCH and may be seen within the nodular lesions, airspaces, and alveolar interstitium.[4,6,34] LCs can be identified by conventional stains (*eg*, hematoxylin-eosin) on high-power light microscopy by an experienced pathologist.[34] They are distinctive large, ovoid mononuclear phagocytes with moderate amounts of eosinophilic cytoplasm, a prominently grooved, folded nucleus, inconspicuous nucleoli, and finely dispersed chromatin (Fig 9).[3,6]

Electron microscopy, which is not necessary for clinical purposes, demonstrates distinctive 42-nm pentilaminar intracytoplasmic inclusions (termed *X bodies* or *Birbeck granules*) within LCs.[1,4,5] LCs also express the CD1a antigen (the common thymocyte antigen)[3] and stain for S100 protein.[34] LCs are distributed in normal lung but rarely constitute >4% of cells.[3,34] In PLCH, the cellular lesions are composed of LCs, admixed with other inflammatory cells. Large numbers of macrophages may be prominent in the alveolar spaces and interstitium, simulating desquamative interstitial pneumonia (DIP).[3,5–7] Eosinophils are prominent in some cases, mimicking chronic eosinophilic pneumonia.[5–7] However, in some patients, eosinophils are sparse or absent.[3] Early lesions form in terminal and respiratory bronchioles and invade and destroy the bronchial wall in the process.[1] Cavitation may represent the lumen of the preexisting bronchiole

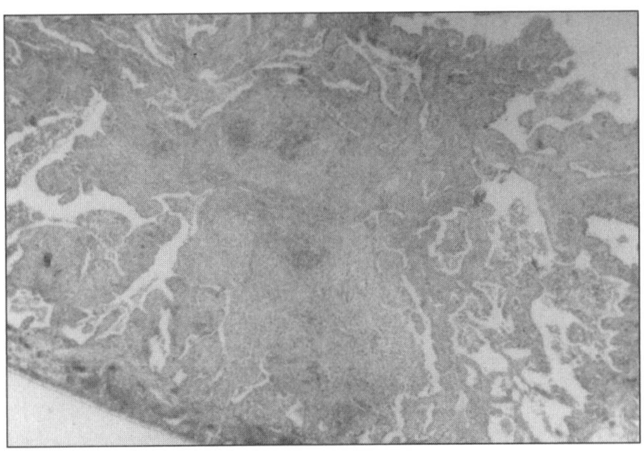

Figure 8. Photomicrograph of a subpleural granulomatous nodule in a patient with pulmonary LCH. The darker staining areas within the nodule correspond to inflammatory cellular infiltrates. The process extends into the alveolar interstitium. The pleural surface is at the lower left corner (hematoxylin-eosin, low-power magnification).

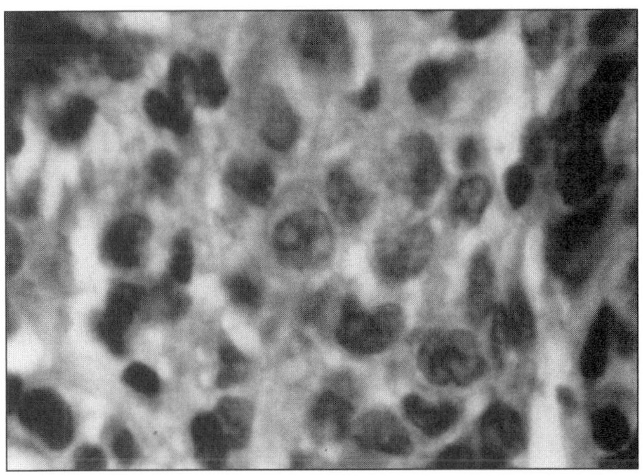

Figure 9. Photomicrograph of pulmonary LCH. Scattered atypical histiocytes (LCs) are present within a cellular nodule. LCs are moderately large cells with pale eosinophilic cytoplasm and an indented, clefted nuclei (hematoxylin-eosin, oil immersion). From Lynch JP III, Raghu G. Major disease syndromes of unknown etiology. In: Baum G, Crapo J, Karlinsky J, et al, eds. Textbook of pulmonary diseases. 7th ed. Philadelphia, PA: Lippincott Williams & Wilkins, 2004; 629–655.

destroyed by the granulomatous process.[1] As the process evolves, bronchioles and alveolar walls are destroyed and replaced by fibrotic connective tissue. Dilated and distorted bronchioles and alveolar parenchymal cysts result. Dense fibrosis (consisting of mature collagen) and intraluminal fibrosis (consisting of young, organizing connective tissue within lumens of bronchioles and alveoli) may be seen.[4,7] Intraluminal buds of connective tissue resemble COP.[7] Thus, the histopathologic features of PLCH overlap with those of other chronic ILDs. Identification of large numbers of LCs is the key to the diagnosis. However, late- or end-stage PLCH may be relatively acellular, with <5% LCs and extensive alveolar and honeycomb cysts.[1,34] In this context, distinguishing PLCH from other end-stage chronic fibrotic lung disorders is difficult, if not impossible. The retention of a nodular or stellate configuration is a clue to the diagnosis.[4,6] Because the pattern and distribution of lesions is a key to the diagnosis of PLCH, surgical (open or thoracoscopic) lung biopsies often are required to substantiate the diagnosis.[3] Transbronchial lung biopsies or BAL fluid are diagnostic in 10 to 40% of patients,[3,7] but significant potential for sampling error exists.[1,35] When bronchoscopic specimens are assessed, ancillary techniques such as S100 or CD1a stains are important to substantiate the diagnosis (discussed in the section "Immunologic Techniques " to follow).

Immunologic Techniques

Immunohistochemical stains may be invaluable in establishing the diagnosis of PLCH when light microscopic features are not definitive. Positive staining for S100 protein, CD1a antigen, and human leukocyte antigen DR are used to identify the characteristic LCs.[3,7] S100 protein can be assayed in paraffin-embedded biopsy specimens; some monoclonal antibodies recognizing the CD1a antigen require fresh or frozen tissue, but anti-CD1a antibody O10 recognizes the antigen in fixed and paraffin-embedded tissues.[1] These immunohistochemical methods are less expensive and less time-consuming than electron microscopy, and their use avoids the sampling problems associated with electron microscopy.

Large aggregates of S100-positive histiocytes in stellate nodules or granulomatous lesions are virtually pathognomonic of PLCH.[3] Small numbers of S100-positive cells may be seen in normal lung tissue or BAL fluid but rarely exceed 4% of cells.[36] Staining is most intense in active PLCH lesions and diminishes in the fibrotic regions.[36] Similarly, LCs express CD1a antigen (recognized by the monoclonal antibody OKT6), but lymphocytes and monocytes do not. Rare CD1a-positive histiocytes may be found in BAL fluid from normal smokers or patients with chronic ILDs (mean, 0.20%).[36] A finding of >4% of cells expressing CD1a in BAL fluid is relatively specific for PLCH,[1,36] but sensitivity is low (*ie*, <25%).[1] In one study, positive immunohistochemical stains to a murine monoclonal antibody (Mab O10) were demonstrated in 33 of 34 paraffin-embedded biopsies from patients with LCH.[37] LCs also express CD4 antigens and both CD1a and CD1c markers, a family of antigen-presenting molecules.[38] In addition, LCs in PLCH express surface markers associated with activation, such as B7 molecules, that are not present in normal pulmonary LCs.[1]

Pathogenesis

The pathogenesis of PLCH likely reflects an exaggerated immune response to cigarette smoke that is initiated or regulated by LCs.[30,34] LCs are specialized dendritic cells that express the CD1a receptor[39] and function to regulate pulmonary responses to exogenous (inhaled) and endogenous (self) antigens.[40] The striking bronchocentric nature of the inflammatory process suggests a reaction to inhaled antigens or irritants.[6,7] Accumulation of LCs is the earliest lesion to occur in PLCH.[1] LCs replicate in the alveolar structures and play a role in maintaining the alveolitis in PLCH.[6,7] In addition to large numbers of LCs within the cellular lesions, immune complexes and other inflammatory cells (*eg*, lymphocytes, plasma cells, eosinophils, mononuclear phagocytes, and foam cells) may be present. Interactions between these cells, in addition to the release of cytokines, may drive the immune and fibrotic response molecules.[1] LCs serve as accessory cells, activating T lymphocytes and recruiting other immune effector cells to the lung.[1,34] Tobacco smoke is strongly linked to PLCH. More than 90% of patients are smokers,[3-7,13,20] and constituents of cigarette smoke are known to serve as

T-cell mitogens, stimulate macrophage cytokine production,[41] and induce epithelial cell production of cytokines (*eg*, granulocyte-macrophage stimulating factor and transforming growth factor-β)[1,3,42] that recruit LCs and up-regulate lymphostimulatory activity of LCs.[1,34]

The number of pulmonary LCs is increased in asymptomatic smokers.[43] Cigarette smoking is associated with hyperplasia of pulmonary neuroendocrine cells and increased levels of bombesin-like peptides in the lower respiratory tract.[44] Large numbers of bombesin-positive neuroendocrine cells have been noted in open lung biopsy specimens in patients with PLCH.[44] These neuroendocrine cells may contribute to the recruitment and activation of mononuclear phagocytes and LCs to the lung and stimulate growth of fibroblasts.[3] Furthermore, cigarette smoke impairs CD10/neutral endopeptidase, an enzyme that plays a role in inactivating bombesin-like peptides.[44] In one study, exposure to cigarette smoke in mice evoked interstitial granulomatous inflammation, with features consistent with PLCH in humans.[45] After cessation of exposure, the density of pulmonary LCs in mice returned to normal levels. These data support the assumption that tobacco products are the major risk factor for PLCH.[46] However, the vast majority of cigarette smokers do *not* develop PLCH despite having an increased population of LCs, suggesting that a "second-hit" is necessary for the disease to occur.[34] T lymphocytes (predominantly $CD4^+$) are abundant in LCH lesions and associate closely with LC cells,[1] suggesting local production of antigen at these sites. The source of antigen is unknown but could be derived from cigarette smoke-damaged airway epithelium.[34]

Course and Prognosis

The natural history of PLCH is variable, but most patients improve or stabilize within 6 to 12 months of the onset of symptoms.[1,2,4-7,15,16] However, data are limited to retrospective studies, with variable treatment regimens. In 1978, French investigators reported 78 cases of PLCH.[5] Among 67 cases with follow-up data, outcomes were as follows: improved (13%), stable (40%), worse (21%), and death (25%). The following factors were associated with a worse prognosis: multisystemic generalized disease; extensive honeycombing on chest radiographs; severe reductions in DLCO, extremes of age; and multiple pneumothoraces.[4,5,13,20] In 1981, Friedman et al[4] reviewed 100 cases of PLCH confirmed by surgical lung biopsy. Follow-up was available in only 60 patients (both treated and untreated). Complete resolution of symptoms was noted in 33 patients (55%), 22 (37%) had persistent symptoms, 5 worsened, and only 1 (2%) died. The authors of a European study followed 45 patients with PLCH for a median of 6 years; 12 patients (27%) died or required lung transplantation.[13] Median survival from the time of diagnosis was 13 years. Reduced FEV_1/FVC ratio was an independent predictor of mortality by multivariate analysis.

Investigators from the Mayo Clinic identified 87 patients with *isolated* PLCH diagnosed between 1946 and 1996 (83 were adults; 84 were smokers).[47] Of these 87 patients, 74 (85%) ultimately achieved "disease-free survival." Treatment regimens included prednisone (58%), chemotherapy (10%), surgical excision (7%), or no treatment (25%). Ten patients (11%) died; an additional 3 patients developed progressive pulmonary disease. A subsequent review of 102 cases of PLCH in adults from the Mayo Clinic from 1976 to 1998 cited a median survival of 12.5 years; 5- and 10-year survival rates after the diagnosis were 74% and 64%, respectively.[21] Only 15 patients (15%) died from respiratory failure. Treatment regimens included smoking cessation (100%), administration of prednisone alone (39%), prednisone plus chemotherapeutic agents (15%), and lung transplantation (1%). Variables associated with worse survival included older age, lower FEV_1, high residual volume, low FEV_1/FVC ratio, and reduced DLCO.[21] Another study from the Mayo Clinic noted that the presence of PAH on echocardiogram markedly increased mortality (hazard ratio, 28.8).[48] This point bears emphasis because PAH is common in advanced PLCH. In one study of 21 patients with PLCH referred for lung transplantation, all patients had PAH (mean pulmonary arterial pressure of 59 mm Hg).[18]

Therapy

Because of the rarity of PLCH and its highly variable natural history, the role of therapy is controversial.[1] Smoking cessation is the primary and essential component of therapy; the role of pharmacological agents has not been studied in randomized trials.[34] For multisystemic LCH in children, the Histiocyte Society recommends treatment with vinblastine and corticosteroids (CS).[49] A variety of chemotherapeutic regimens have been used to treat disseminated LCH in children, including vinca alkaloids (*eg*, vincristine or vinblastine), etoposide, cladribine (2-chlorodeoxyadenosine), cyclophosphamide, methotrexate, cyclosporine A, and antithymocyte globulin.[47,49-53] In one study of disseminated LCH, cyclosporine A was administered alone (10 patients) or in combination with vinblastine, etoposide, prednisolone, and/or antithymocyte globulin (16 patients).[54] A single patient had a complete response, 3 had partial responses, and 22 (85%) did not respond.

In several case reports or small series of bone, skin, or disseminated LCH, anecdotal responses were achieved with 2-chlorodeoxyadenosine (2-CdA), a purine nucleoside that is toxic to lymphocytes and monocytes.[51,55-58] Further, favorable responses were noted in 3 cases of PLCH treated with 2-CdA.[56,58,59] In anecdotal cases, interleukin (IL)-2[60] and etanercept[61] were associated with favorable responses in children with disseminated LCH, but data are sparse. Moreover, PLCH in adults likely has a different pathogenesis than childhood LCH, and optimal therapy for PLCH is controversial.[30] No controlled or prospective studies have been performed. However, given the strong link between cigarette smoking and PLCH, patients must be urged in the strongest possible terms to discontinue smoking.[3] In most patients, the disease will stabilize or even improve after cessation of smoking.[3,62] Anecdotal responses have been noted in PLCH treated with CS and immunosuppressive and cytotoxic agents,[5,7,9,13,16,20] but the data may be confounded by the impact of smoking cessation or the potential for spontaneous remission.

One uncontrolled study cited radiographic improvement in 12 of 14 patients treated with prednisone for progressive PLCH; the other two patients were stable.[20] In another study, CS therapy was associated with worse survival,[13] but this finding may reflect a selection bias. In the cohort of PLCH reported from the Mayo Clinic, 54 of 102 patients (53%) were treated with prednisone (alone or combined with immunosuppressive agents).[21] Although data were not provided, the authors stated "no specific therapeutic interventions have been shown to improve survival." A multicenter therapeutic trial is needed to clarify the impact (if any) of therapy but has not been done. Radiation therapy may be effective for solitary lesions of bone but has no role in pulmonary LCH. The role of immunosuppressive or cytotoxic agents in isolated PLCH in adults has not been established.

The International Histiocyte Society initiated a registry of LCH in adults.[63] That registry identified 274 adults with LCH from 13 countries; 44 (16%) had isolated pulmonary involvement, and 188 (69%) had multisystemic disease.[63] Treatment regimens varied. The most commonly used therapies included vinblastine (with or without CS) in 30% and etoposide in 10%. Only 13 patients (30%) with isolated PLCH were treated. Five-year survival rates were 89% among patients with isolated PLCH and 92% among patients with multisystemic involvement. The impact of therapy of PLCH could not be ascertained.

Given the paucity of data and the potential for PLCH to remit spontaneously or after cessation of smoking,[1] this author reserve therapy for patients with severe, progressive, or debilitating disease. In this context, an initial trial of CS (0.5 to 1 mg/kg/d, with gradual taper) for 2 to 4 months is reasonable. Prolonged therapy should be continued *only* in patients manifesting *unequivocal* and *objective* improvement. Immunosuppressive or cytotoxic agents may be considered for patients with progressive PLCH recalcitrant to CS therapy and cessation of smoking. Pneumothoraces occur in 15% of patients with PLCH, and rate of recurrence exceeds 50% when managed conservatively by observation or chest tube without pleurodesis.[17] Early surgical pleurodesis is justified in managing pneumothoraces in PLCH patients. The incidence of PAH is relatively common in patients with PLCH[48] and may reflect a primary vasculopathy (including veno-occlusive disease).[19] Given the high incidence of PAH in PLCH, this author recommends transthoracic echocardiography in newly diagnosed cases to estimate right ventricular systolic pressures. The use of vasodilators for treating pulmonary hypertension in patients with PLCH has not been extensively studied.[18] However, two patients with PLCH treated with IV epoprostenol developed acute pulmonary edema.[18]

Lung transplantation has been successfully accomplished in PLCH patients with severe respiratory failure refractory to medical therapy.[64,65] Data from the International Society for Heart and Lung Transplantation (ISHLT) Registry from January 1995 to June 2004 identified only 39 patients with PLCH among 13,007 lung transplant recipients (0.3%).[66] French investigators reported 39 patients with PLCH who underwent LT at 7 centers in France;[65] rates of 1-, 2-, and 5-year survival were 77%, 64%, and 54%, respectively. The disease recurred in 21% but did not influence survival. Recurrent PLCH appears to be more common among those who resumed cigarette smoking[64,67,68] or patients with extrapulmonary involvement.[65] Patients must be vigorously counseled not to resume smoking after LT. Criteria for listing patients with PLCH for LT are lacking. This author believes that LT should be considered when the following factors are present: (1) severe respiratory failure despite smoking cessation (*eg*, FVC $<55\%$ predicted; $FEV_1 < 40\%$ predicted; DLCO $<40\%$ predicted); (2) need for supplemental oxygen; and (3) poor and declining quality of life; severe PAH.[69]

LAM

LAM is a rare disorder affecting exclusively women that is characterized by hamartomatous proliferation of atypical smooth muscle along lymphatics in the lung, thorax, abdomen, and pelvis.[70-73] Mean age of onset is between 30 and 45 years of age; $>90\%$ of cases have been in premenopausal women.[70,71,74-79] Clinical features include progressive airflow obstruction, pneumothorax, hemoptysis, or chylothorax.[74] LAM is exceptionally rare, with an estimated prevalence of 1 to 3 per million in the United States,[80] United Kingdom,[75] France,[71] and Singapore.[80] The cardinal features of LAM were described in 1974 and 1975 in two series comprising 32 patients[81] and 28 patients, respectively.[79] In 1990, Taylor et al[78] described 32 patients with LAM who were followed at Stanford and the Mayo Clinic. In 1995, Kitaichi and colleagues described 46 patients with LAM from Japan, Korea, and Taiwan.[77] Subsequent series from the United Kingdom,[82] France,[71] Korea,[83] and the United States[72,76] further elucidated the clinical spectrum and natural history of this disorder. In the United States, a national registry studied 230 patients enrolled into a national registry established by the National Heart, Lung, and Blood Institute (NHLBI).[72] In a separate registry (the LAM Foundation), 1,300 patients had been registered in the United States as of July 7, 2007.[74] In addition to sporadic LAM (which affects women), LAM can complicate tuberous sclerosis complex (TSC), a genetic disorder discussed later.[74] LAM occurs *virtually exclusively* in women.[74] Only four cases of biopsy-confirmed LAM have been reported in men; three had definite or probable TSC,[84-86] whereas one did not.[87]

Clinical Features

The most common symptom of LAM is dyspnea, which usually begins in the third or fourth decade of life and progresses inexorably over years.[71,72,75-78] Pneumothorax occurs in 50 to 80% of patients.[71,75-78] The rate of recurrence is $>70\%$, the highest among all chronic lung diseases.[74] Recurrent pneumothoraces in women of childbearing age may be a clue to the diagnosis. Chylous effusions, resulting from rupture of involved lymphatics of the pleura, mediastinal lymph nodes, or thoracic ducts, have been noted in 7 to 39% of women with LAM.[71,72,75-78] Chyloptysis, with expectoration of white, sticky sputum, may also occur.[72,75,81] Hemoptysis or focal alveolar hemorrhage, which is caused by obstruction of venules, occurs in 28 to 40% of patients with LAM.[71,72,75-78] The course of LAM is usually indolent but inexorable; most patients ultimately die of respiratory failure (typically >10 years after diagnosis). However, the prognosis of LAM is heterogeneous, and the impact of therapy is controversial (discussed later).

Differential Diagnosis

Because of the rarity of LAM and the nonspecificity of clinical features, the diagnosis is often delayed for 3 to 5 years after the onset of symptoms.[74,88] Symptoms may be erroneously ascribed to chronic bronchitis, asthma, emphysema, PLCH, or chronic ILD.[89] Pulmonary lesions identical to LAM may occur in patients with TSC, an autosomal-dominant familial disorder associated with mental retardation and cutaneous manifestations.[72,74,89,90] By contrast, LAM is not familial and is not associated with either cutaneous or neurologic manifestations.[75,89]

Chest Radiographic Changes

Plain chest radiographs in LAM are nonspecific but may demonstrate pneumothoraces, cystic or reticulonodular shadows, pleural effusions, or hyperinflation.[71,75-78] Pneumothorax has been noted in 39 to 53% of patients at the time of presentation and occurs in approximately 80% of patients during the course of the disease (Fig 10).[71,75-78] Reticulonodular infiltrates are evident in 47% to >85% of patients.[71,76-78] The reticulation actually represents summation of numerous cystic walls.[91] Cysts or bullae are detected in 41 to 58% of patients.[71,76-78] Hyperinflation develops as the degree of airways obstruction worsens, and may be seen in up to two thirds of patients late in the course of the disease. Pleural effusions (often chylous due to lymphatic obstruction) occur in 7 to 39% of patients.[71,72,76-78,92] Mediastinal and hilar lymphadenopathy are not features of LAM.[75,77] Chest radiographs may be normal early in the course of disease.[71,75,76]

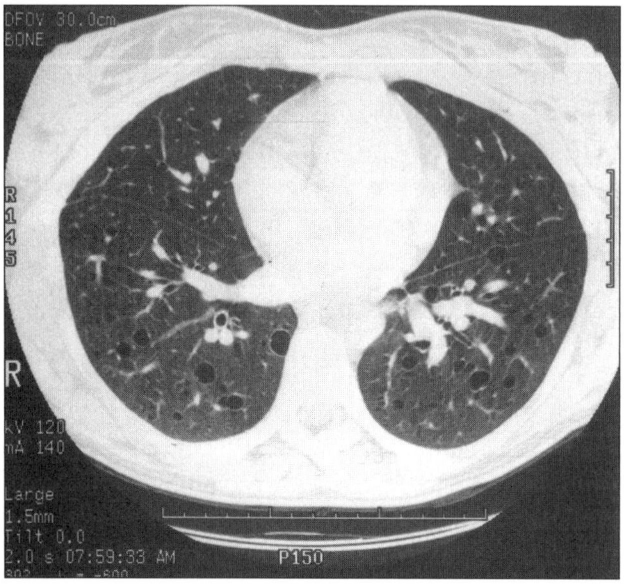

Figure 10. LAM. HRCT scan from a 33-year-old woman with a history of recurrent pneumothoraces shows numerous well-defined cysts scattered throughout the lung parenchyma.

HRCT Scans

Thin-section HRCT scans in LAM reveal numerous thin-walled cysts, ranging in size from a few millimeters to 6 cm throughout both lungs; the intervening lung parenchyma is normal (Figs 11–14).[29,71,75-78] Cysts usually are round but may assume polygonal or bizarre shapes as multiple cysts coalesce (Fig 12). In LAM, the cysts are distributed diffusely without predilection for specific

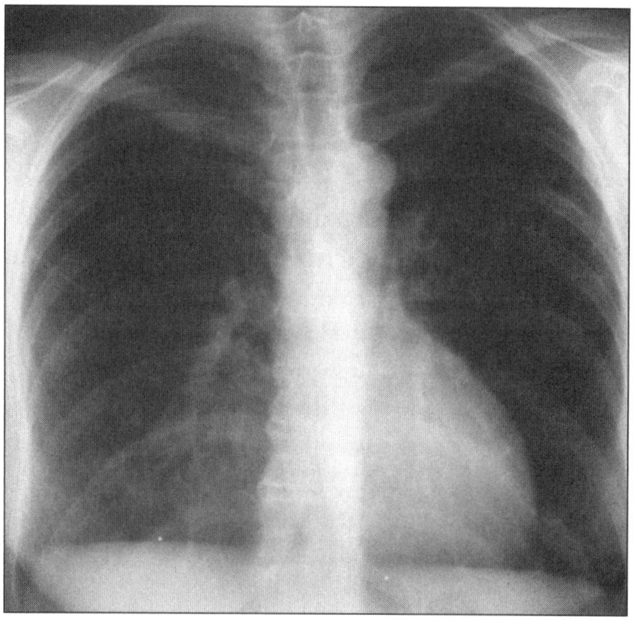

Figure 11. LAM. Posteroanterior chest radiograph demonstrating modest hyperinflation and some cystic and emphysematous changes in a 42-year-old woman with LAM. Surgical clips are present in the left lung from a previous thoracotomy for the treatment of recurrent pneumothorax.

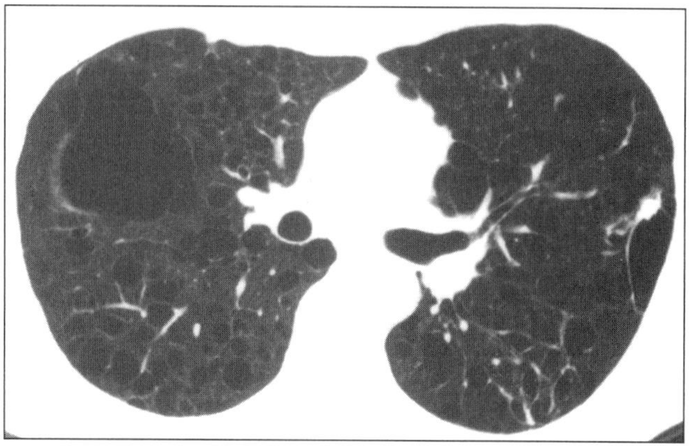

Figure 12. LAM. CT scan from the same patient demonstrating multiple thin-walled cysts of varying sizes in the lower lobes, with several large confluent cysts. Note that cysts are scattered relatively evenly throughout the lung, with neither peripheral nor central predominance. A nodular component is lacking.

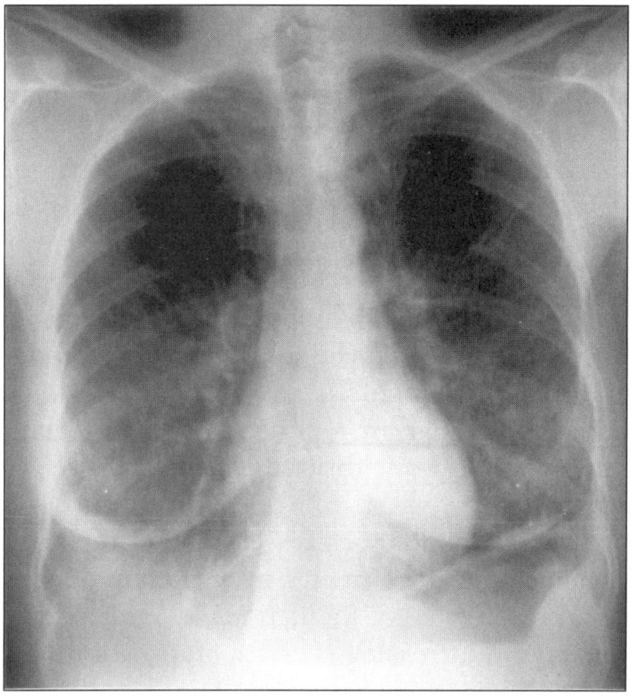

Figure 13. LAM. Posteroanterior chest radiograph from a 41-year-old woman with a history of recurrent pneumothoraces demonstrating marked hyperinflation and emphysematous changes. A reticular pattern is noted in the lower lobes, which likely reflects the walls of cysts.

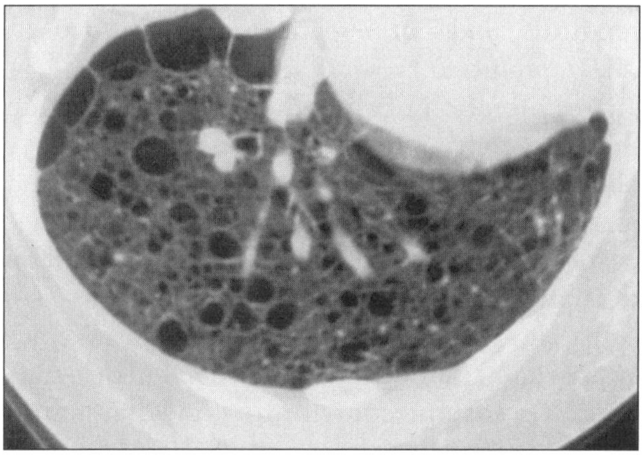

Figure 14. LAM. CT scan from the patient in Fig 13 demonstrating multiple thin-walled cystic radiolucencies throughout lung parenchyma consistent with LAM. Note that both the central and peripheral regions of the lungs are involved.

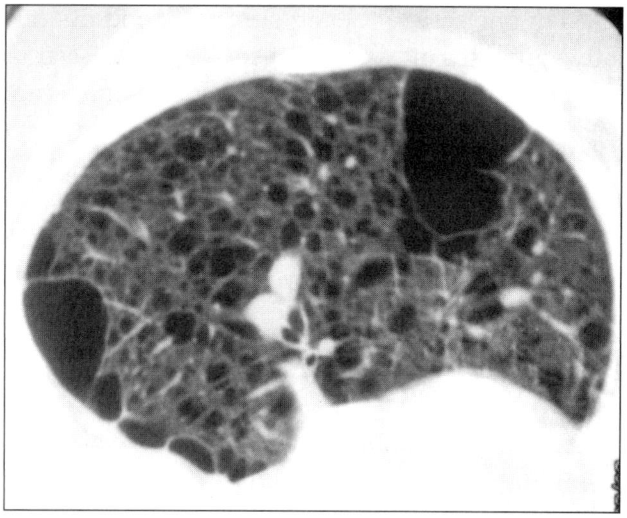

Figure 15. LAM. HRCT scan in a 44-year-old woman with LAM demonstrates multiple, thin-walled cystic radiolucencies bilaterally. Note the two large lesions, representing confluent cysts. From Lynch JP III, Raghu G. Major disease syndromes of unknown etiology. In: Baum G, Crapo J, Karlinsky J, et al, eds. Textbook of pulmonary diseases. 7th ed. Philadelphia, PA: Lippincott Williams & Wilkins, 2004; 629–655.

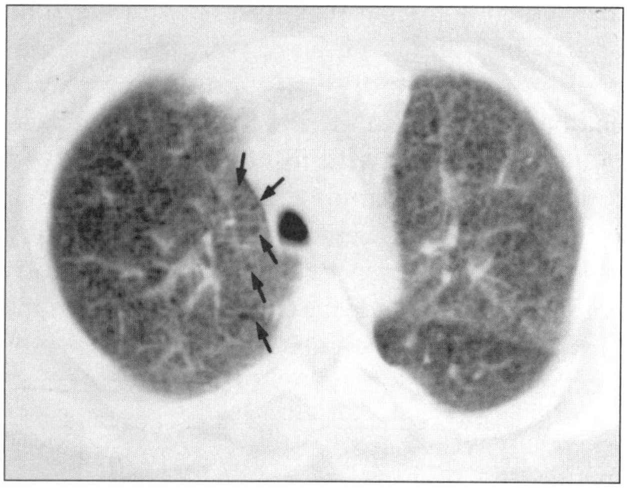

Figure 16. LAM. CT scan (upper lobes) from a 36-year-old woman demonstrating small (1 to 3 mm) round cysts throughout both lung fields, which is consistent with early changes in LAM. A diffuse background haze (ground-glass opacification) is present, which is consistent with alveolar hemorrhage. She had a 12-month history of intermittent hemoptysis. Transbronchial lung biopsy specimens demonstrated hemosiderin-laden macrophages (which is consistent with previous hemorrhage) and clusters of smooth-muscle cells (positive for HMB45), which is consistent with LAM.

regions or lobes.[91] Cavitation is not a feature of pulmonary LAM. Nodules, interstitial fibrosis, or irregular lung-pleural interfaces—features commonly observed in other chronic ILDs—are absent or a minor feature in LAM.[29] GGOs were not cited in early reports of HRCT in LAM[78,91] but were noted in 12% (8 of 66)[71] and 59% (22 of 37)[77] of patients in two more recent series. GGOs may reflect foci of alveolar hemorrhage, pulmonary hemosiderosis, or diffuse proliferation of smooth-muscle cells (Figs 15 and 16).[71,75,76] Mediastinal or intrathoracic lymphadenopathy is unusual.[29,77,93] However, retrocrural adenopathy is common, found in 26% of patients with

LAM in one series.[76] Semiquantitative and quantitative analyses of extent of disease by thin-section CT scan correlate well with physiologic parameters (*eg*, FEV_1, DLCO, and gas exchange at rest and exercise)[91,94] and exercise performance.[95] Abdominal CT may reveal (1) cysts or angiomyolipomas (AMLs) in the kidney, spleen, or pelvic organs or (2) retrocrural or para-aortic lymphadenopathy.[75,76,89,96,97]

Differential Diagnosis of HRCT

Cystic radiolucencies may be observed in pulmonary LCH, emphysema, and any chronic end-stage lung disease. However, salient differences distinguish these entities from LAM. Cysts in PLCH are preferentially distributed in the upper and mid-lung zones, and a nodular component is usually evident.[15,27] Cavitation may be observed in PLCH but is rare in LAM. Honeycomb cysts, a prominent feature of idiopathic or collagen vascular disease–associated pulmonary fibrosis, are distributed in the peripheral (subpleural) regions of the lungs and are nearly invariably accompanied by linear bands, distortion of lung parenchyma, or GGOs. In those disorders, the process is heterogeneous, with focal areas of involved lung interspersed among large areas of normal lung parenchyma. Severe, end-stage LAM may give rise to large cysts that may resemble bullous emphysema; however, the emphysematous lesions lack discernible walls and have an upper lobe predominance. The cysts in LAM are more regular and have well-formed walls.[76,78,91] Other rare causes of cystic lung disease include lymphocytic interstitial pneumonia,[98] Sjögren syndrome,[99] hypersensitivity pneumonitis,[100] amyloidosis,[99] light chain deposition disease,[101] and Birt-Hogg Dube' syndrome.[102]

Ventilation-Perfusion Lung Scans

An unusual "speckling" pattern on ventilation lung scanning was cited in 28 of 39 of patients with LAM (72%) in one study.[103] On CT scans, all 39 had pulmonary cysts. Univariate analysis showed that the extent of disease on chest radiographs and CT scans, cyst size, ventilation-perfusion abnormalities, and the degree of speckling were inversely correlated with FEV_1, DLCO, and ratio of FEV_1/FVC but not with FVC or TLC.[103]

Pulmonary Function Tests

Early in the course of LAM, spirometry may be normal.[71,72,74,77] The DLCO is reduced in >65% of patients.[71,72,76-78,104] An obstructive ventilatory defect, often with air trapping, has been cited in 29 to 78% of patients; lung volumes are normal or increased.[71,76-78,105] Restrictive defects in LAM may reflect the presence of chylous pleural effusions or effects of previous pneumothoraces or pleurodesis.[94,104] Impairments in exercise performance and gas exchange are typical[76] and correlate with the extent of cystic disease on quantitative CT scanning.[95,106]

Cardiopulmonary exercise testing typically demonstrates impairments in maximum oxygen uptake ($\dot{V}O_2$max).[107] Reductions in $\dot{V}O_2$max correlate with increasing severity of disease by CT and histologic criteria.[107] By multivariate analysis, FEV_1 and DLCO correlate with $\dot{V}O_2$max.[107] Reduced DLCO is the best predictor of exercise-induced hypoxemia.[107] In one study, exercise-induced hypoxemia occurred in 10 of 24 patients (41%) with DLCO between 60% and 70% predicted, 7 of 29 patients (21%) with DLCO between 70% and 80% predicted, and 7 of 69 patients (10%) with DLCO >90% predicted.[107]

Proliferation of smooth-muscle cells within the pulmonary interstitium may cause airways obstruction, dilation of proximal airspaces, and destruction of pulmonary capillaries. Airspace cystic lesions appear to be more important than muscular proliferation in small airways as a cause of airflow obstruction.[95] Loss of alveolar support and parenchymal interdependence may be an important contributory mechanism of airflow obstruction. In one study of 143 patients with LAM, a predominantly solid (as opposed to cystic) histologic pattern of LAM lesions in lung biopsy specimens was associated with a more rapid decrease in FEV_1.[104] Further, a positive response to bronchodilators was associated with more severe airflow obstruction and a greater rate of decline in expiratory flow.[104] Interestingly, airway inflammation did not correlate with severity of airflow obstruction or response to bronchodilators.[104]

Reductions in the FEV_1/FVC ratio and increased TLC are associated with a worse prognosis and poor survival.[77,105] By contrast, FVC, FEV_1, arterial blood gases, and alveolar-arterial gradient do not predict survival.[77,105] The rate of progression of airflow obstruction is highly variable, ranging from a few years to more than two decades.[75,78,104] A review of 47 patients with LAM in the United Kingdom cited a mean decrease in FEV_1 of 118 mL/year, but there was marked variability between patients.[82] In a retrospective review of 31 cases of LAM, French investigators cited a mean decrease in FEV_1 of 106 mL/year.[71] The largest study (comprising 275 patients with LAM in the United States followed for 5 years) cited annual decreases in FEV_1 ranging from 52 to 119 mL.[108] Overall annual rates of decrease were 1.7% predicted for FEV_1 and 2.4% predicted for DLCO. The most significant predictors of functional decrease were initial lung function and age. The rate of decrease in FEV_1 was lower in older patients. Conversely, patients with greater initial FEV_1 and DLCO (less severe disease) had more rapid decreases in DLCO.[108] In another study of LAM patients with *mild* disease, the presence of pneumothorax was associated with a lower FEV_1 and more rapid decrease in FEV_1 than those without pneumothorax.[109] These correlations were not observed in patients with more profuse cystic changes.

Although airflow obstruction is the most important factor responsible for exercise limitation, pulmonary vascular involvement plays a contributory role.[95] PAH at rest in LAM is uncommon (<10% of cases)[110] but may be elicited by exercise.[111] Taveira-DaSilva et al[111] performed echocardiography at rest and during exercise in 95 patients with LAM. By echocardiographic criteria, PAH was present in 8 patients at rest but was elicited by exercise (systolic pulmonary artery pressure >40 mm Hg) in 56 (59%). Exercise arterial oxygen saturation was the best predictor of exercise-induced PAH.[111]

Pathology

Grossly, the lungs in LAM may first appear emphysematous. However, as the disease progresses, the entire lung is replaced by cysts. Histologically, LAM is characterized by proliferation of atypical interstitial smooth muscle and thin-walled cysts within lung, renal parenchyma, uterus, or affected organs.[75,77,79,81,89] Unlike other forms of ILD, there is very little fibrosis in LAM. The smooth muscle cells are heterogeneous and may exhibit features of large spindle cells, smaller cells with little cytoplasm, or epithelioid cells.[75,89] These smooth muscle cells are often arranged in nodules or in linear fascicles.[75] The LAM cells grow in a haphazard arrangement, unlike the orderly patterns of organization of normal smooth muscle cells.[112]

In pulmonary LAM, open lung biopsies demonstrate both cystic lesions and muscular lesions (*ie*, proliferation of immature smooth muscle cells) (Fig 17).[75,77] Nodular proliferations of immature smooth muscle surround airways, blood vessels, and lymphatics and extend into bronchioles and alveolar interstitium. Destruction of alveolar parenchyma forms cysts, which are surrounded by immature smooth muscle. The walls of the cysts are typically <2 mm thick.[91] Pneumothoraces result from rupture of subpleural cysts.[71,75,77] Proliferating smooth muscle may obstruct pulmonary venules (causing focal edema and pulmonary hemorrhage) or lymphatics (leading to chylothorax).[71,75,78,79] Hemosiderin-laden macrophages within alveolar spaces or interstitium may be a clue to previous episodes of hemorrhage.[71,75,77] The extent of cystic or smooth muscle lesions on open lung biopsy has prognostic significance. Predominantly cystic LAM lesions suggest a worse prognosis and survival, whereas grades of smooth muscle proliferation or hemosiderosis do not correlate with survival.[77,105] LAM histology scores, based on the extent of replacement of

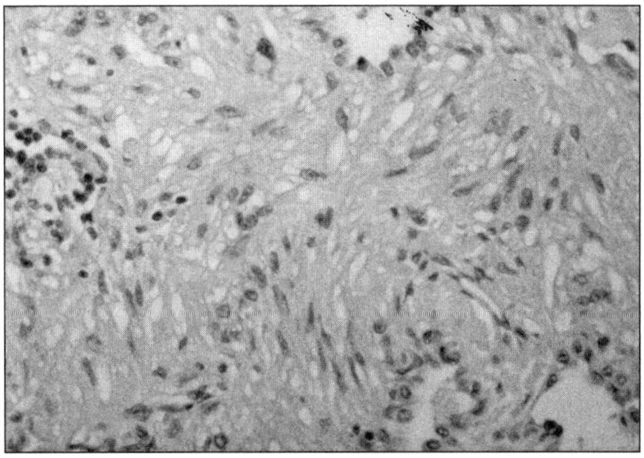

Figure 17. Photomicrograph of LAM. Open-lung biopsy specimen demonstrating the proliferation of atypical smooth-muscle cells within the alveolar interstitium, which is consistent with LAM (hematoxylin-eosin, high-power magnification).

lung tissue by cystic lesions and infiltration of LAM cells, are a predictor of death and time to transplantation.[93]

Immunohistochemical Stains and Ancillary Diagnostic Techniques

Smooth muscle cells in pulmonary LAM are similar histologically and by immunohistochemical analysis to AMLs, which are benign mesenchymal tumors consisting of blood vessels, abnormal smooth muscle, and fat.[71,75,113] Immunohistochemical stains are positive for muscle-specific actin, desmin, and human melanoma black-45 (HMB-45).[75,114] HMB-45 produces a granular pattern of staining within the cytoplasm, often with a perinuclear accentuation.[114] HMB-45 immunoreactivity in smooth muscle is highly specific for LAM, AMLs, and clear cell tumor of the lung but is never found in normal smooth muscle.[75,114] The specificity of HMB-45 may allow a diagnosis of LAM by transbronchial lung biopsy, provided the immunohistochemical marker is positive.[71,76] The immunohistochemical reactivity of LAM cells is localized more frequently in the large epithelioid cells.[93] In addition, LAM cells contain increased amounts of matrix metalloproteinases (MMPs), especially MMP-2 but also MMP-1 and MMP-9.[115] These MMPs likely play a critical role in the development of pulmonary cystic lesions in LAM.[115] Receptors for progesterone and estrogen have been noted in the nuclei of proliferating smooth-muscle cells in some patients with LAM,[71,78] but these findings are not uniform.[116] Electron microscopy of smooth cells in LAM demonstrates indented round to ovoid nuclei with prominent nucleoli, prominent microfilament bundles with dense bodies, a well-developed rough endoplasmic reticulum, and numerous clusters of intracytoplasmic, electron-dense, membrane-bound, crystalloid granules.[117] Similar cells are found in renal or hepatic AMLs.[117]

BAL Fluid

In two studies, hemosiderin-laden macrophages were found in BAL fluid in 60 to 81% of LAM patients; BAL differential counts were normal.[71,76]

Diagnosis of LAM

Historically, the diagnosis of LAM required open lung biopsy.[78,79,81] It was often diagnosed inadvertently at the time of thoracotomy for recurrent pneumothoraces.[78] The presence of innumerable small cysts throughout the lung surface without nodularity or interstitial fibrosis is virtually pathognomonic for LAM.[78] Transbronchial lung biopsy may be adequate to substantiate the diagnosis but requires a skillful pathologist to perform.[71,77,78] Unless the pathologist is familiar with the salient histologic features, the abnormal smooth muscle cells are often misinterpreted as fibrocytes. In equivocal cases, positive immunohistochemical stains (*eg*, HMB-45) may substantiate the diagnosis of LAM, provided that clinical and radiographic features (especially HRCT) are consistent.[71,75,76] The diagnosis of LAM can be established without lung biopsy provided HRCT features are characteristic, clinical criteria are consistent, and any of the following features are present: typical renal AMLs, chronic chylous ascites with abdominal lymphadenopathy, or characteristic histopathologic findings on lymph node biopsy.[71,74-76] Blood tests have no diagnostic value in LAM. However, serum vascular endothelial growth factor-D (VEGF-D) shows promise as a screen for pulmonary cyst development in women with TSC.[118]

Extrapulmonary Involvement

AMLs or cysts may involve abdominal or retroperitoneal lymph nodes, spleen, kidney, periadrenal blood vessels, liver, uterus, and ovaries.[71,75,76,97,112,113,119] Although the source of LAM cells (atypical proliferating smooth muscle cells) is not known, there is direct evidence for blood-borne and lymphatic dissemination of LAM.[74,119-121] Induction of lymphangiogenesis may be important. Lymphatic endothelial markers are expressed abundantly in LAM, including podoplanin, VEGF receptor-3, and VEGF-C.[121] VEGF-D is increased more than threefold in the serum of patients with LAM[122] and may prove to be a useful biomarker for LAM. Possible sources of LAM cells include AMLs, lymphatic or bone marrow cells, uterine or ovarian cells, or cells of neural crest origin.[74]

Renal or abdominal AMLs (HMB-45 positive) have been noted in 15 to 54% of patients with pulmonary LAM and often antedate the diagnosis of pulmonary LAM.[71,76,97,113] In one study, uterine leiomyomas were cited in 41% of patients with LAM.[71] AMLs often are incidental findings on CT, but the growth of these smooth muscle tumors may cause local pain, bleeding, chylous ascites, or compression of contiguous structures.[75,76,113] A study of 12 AMLs from women with LAM demonstrated positive estrogen receptor immunoreactivity in 10 (83%); all expressed progesterone receptors (PRs).[123] A previous study noted positive PRs in 55% of AMLs associated with TSC but in only 7% *without* LAM or TSC.[124]

AMLs are hyperechogenic on ultrasonography and reveal fat attenuation on CT.[75,76] CT scanning is the best screening test to assess the presence, size, and extent of renal or intra-abdominal cystic or angiomyolipomatous lesions in patients with pulmonary LAM.[97,113] In one prospective study, 80 patients with LAM underwent chest and abdominopelvic CT and abdominopelvic ultrasonography.[97] Intra-abdominal lesions were detected in 61 patients (76%), including renal AMLs in 43 (54%), enlarged abdominal lymph nodes in 31 (39%), lymphangiomyoma in 13 (16%), ascites in 8 (10%), dilatation of the thoracic duct in 7 (9%), and hepatic AMLs in 3 (4%).[97]

A significant correlation ($p = 0.02$) was found between enlarged abdominal lymph nodes and the severity of lung disease.[97] Ultrasonography and abdominal CT scans may have complementary roles in the diagnosis and follow-up of abdominal and pelvic manifestations of LAM.[97] Appropriate management of renal AMLs or cysts depends on size, growth rate, and the presence or absence of symptoms. AMLs often are incidental findings noted on CT but may cause pain, local bleeding, compression of renal parenchyma, and impaired renal function.[75,76,113] The risk of local complications is increased for lesions >4 cm in size.[75,113] Asymptomatic patients with lesions <4 cm in greatest dimension can be followed with yearly ultrasonography or CT; lesions >4 cm in size *or* causing symptoms should be followed no less often than at 6-month intervals.[113] Expanding or symptomatic lesions >4 cm in size should be treated with surgery or embolization.[113] Partial or total nephrectomy may be required to manage complications (*eg*, hemorrhage and refractory pain).[76,113] An increased risk of renal cell carcinoma has been noted in patients with TSC and AML.[110] The prevalence of meningiomas, which possess PRs, appears to be increased in patients with LAM and TSC.[125] In one prospective study, MRI or CT scans of the brain were performed in 250 women with LAM; lesions consistent with meningiomas on MRI were found in 8 (5 had TSC).[125]

TSC

Both LAM and TSC are caused by mutations in the tuberous sclerosis genes, *TSC1* and *TSC2*, that control cell growth, survival, and motility through the Akt/mammalian target of rapamycin signaling pathway.[74] Sporadic LAM (S-LAM) and TSC-associated LAM (TSC-LAM) share many common clinical and radiographic features. However, pulmonary manifestations are typically milder in patients with TSC-LAM.[89] Further, compared with S-LAM, patients with TSC-LAM have a lower incidence of abdominal lymphangioleiomyomas (9% vs 12%), thoracic duct dilation (0% vs 4%), pleural effusion (6% vs 12%), and ascites (6% vs 10%).[126] Additionally, patients with TSC-LAM have a greater frequency of hepatic (33% vs 2%) and renal (93% vs 32%) AMLs, previous nephrectomy (25% vs 7%), and noncalcified pulmonary nodules (12% vs 1%).[126]

TSC, an autosomal-dominant disorder with high penetrance and variable expressivity, shares some features with LAM (*eg*, extrapulmonary AMLs; hamartomatous proliferation of smooth muscle; pulmonary LAM).[74,127] TSC affects 1 in 5,800 individuals[128] and is far more common than sporadic LAM.[74] TSC affects the migration and differentiation of neural crest cells and affects multiple tissues, including skin, CNS, lymphatics, bone, and lung.[113,127] Up to 60% of cases of TSC are sporadic, with no family history.[80] Both male and female patients can be affected with TSC. Clinical features commonly observed with TSC include mental retardation, seizures, digital fibromas, sebaceous adenomas, depigmented skin lesions, sclerotic bone lesions, and cranial calcifications.[71,129] These features are not present in sporadic LAM.[75,128] The phenotypic expression of tuberous sclerosis is variable, but 75% of patients die by the age of

20 years.[113] Early prevalence studies cited pulmonary lesions indistinguishable radiographically and histopathologically from LAM in 1 to 4% of patients with TSC.[71,75,90,127] However, subsequent studies suggest that the prevalence of LAM among women with TSC is 26 to 39%.[93,128,130]

In one prospective study, screening HRCT scans were performed in 48 patients with TSC who had no pulmonary symptoms, no previous history of LAM, and normal PFTs.[93] Pulmonary cysts consistent with LAM were detected in 13 of 38 (34%) female patients but in none of 10 male patients with TSC. Similarly, in a retrospective study of 78 women with TSC, 20 (26%) had evidence of LAM (by CT in 13; by surgical lung biopsy or autopsy in 7).[130] AMLs are found in 80% of patients with TSC.[71,75,91,127] AMLs in both LAM and TSC express the antimelanoma monoclonal antibody HMB-45, suggesting a common origin from a progenitor smooth muscle cell.[71,75,113,128] Chromosomal abnormalities (13q14 and 14q24) are noted in TSC, LAM, and uterine leiomyomas.[74,128] Further, the marker for LAM cells (HMB45) is located on chromosome 12q13-15, a region frequently rearranged in uterine leiomyomas.[80] Both leiomyomas and LAM involve proliferation of smooth muscle in women of childbearing age.[74,128]

In both TSC and LAM, mutations in one of two genes (*TSC1* or *TSC2*) are present (mutations in *TSC2* are more common in both disorders).[74,128] Tumor suppressor genes (*TSC1* and *TSC2*) encode *TSC1* and *TSC2* proteins, also known as hamartin and tuberin, respectively.[74,128] In TSC, a germline mutation (*ie*, first hit) is present in all cells in the body. Neoplasms and dysplasias occur when somatic "second-hit" mutations result in loss of heterozygosity for the normal allele.[74,128] This results in loss of function of either *TSC1* or *TSC2* proteins.[128] Because TSC genes suppress tumor growth, this additional mutation allows cellular proliferation and the formation of hamartomas.[128] *TSC1* mutations in general are associated with milder manifestations of disease severity compared with *TSC2* mutations.[131] Germline mutations are present in all cells of the body in TSC or TSC-LAM, whereas in sporadic LAM, both the first-hit and second-hit mutations are confined to lesions in the lung, kidney, and lymph nodes.[74] Loss of heterozygosity for *TSC2* (but not *TSC1*) was found in renal AMLs from 7 of 14 patients with LAM without clinical features of TSC.[132] A similar lesion was found in AMLs in patients without LAM or TSC.[75] Because a germ-line mutation is not found in LAM, sequential somatic mutations of the *TSC2* gene likely occur in LAM. The relationships between LAM, TSC, and other smooth muscle proliferative disorders (*eg*, AMLs, leiomyomas) are likely complex, and additional studies are required to elucidate the genetics and pathogenetic mechanisms involved in these disorders.[74,128]

Pathogenesis

Significant advances in the understanding of the pathogenesis of the smooth-muscle proliferation in LAM have been made within the past decade.[74,128,133,134] Because LAM only affects women (with rare exceptions), estrogens likely play a key role in the pathogenesis.[70,74] Steroid receptors for estrogen were detected in LAM but not normal lungs,[134] suggesting that steroids may also play a role in LAM pathology. LAM occurs nearly invariably in premenopausal women, and exogenous or endogenous estrogens accelerate the course of the disease.[70,74] One postulate is that estrogen signals through Akt and releases the tuberin-deficient or hamartin-deficient cell from feedback inhibition, resulting in abnormal proliferation.[74]

LAM cells have high mitotic and low apoptotic activities that are important in their proliferative behavior.[80,135] LAM cells consist of two subpopulations: myofibroblast-like spindle-shaped cells and epithelioid-like polygonal cells.[70,119] Spindle-shaped cells express smooth muscle-specific proteins smooth muscle α-actin, desmin, and vimentin and display high rates of proliferation.[70] By contrast, the epithelioid-like cells exhibit lower rates of proliferation.[70] Both cell types express melanoma-associated proteins HMB-45 and CD63.[128] Until recently, LAM was considered benign. However, LAM cells may be found in multiple sites (*eg*, renal AMLs, lung, chylous effusions, lymph nodes, blood, urine, etc), suggesting metastatic behavior.[119,128,135] Recent evidence suggests that LAM is a cancer resulting from biallelic mutations at a single genetic locus, resulting in unregulated growth, lymphatic or vascular spread, and tissue destruction.[74,136]

Course and Prognosis of LAM

The course of LAM is indolent, but most patients ultimately die of respiratory failure. However, the pace of the disease is extremely variable. Early retrospective reviews[79,81] cited 5- and 10-year survival rates of only 60% and 20%, respectively. Subsequent studies noted improved survival, which likely reflects earlier diagnosis (particularly with the advent of CT scans). In 1990, Taylor et al[78] reported that 25 of 32 patients with LAM (78%) were alive a mean of 8.5 years after onset of the disease. Data from Asia cited survival rates of >70% at 5 years after the onset of LAM but only 38% (10 of 26 patients) at 8.5 years.[77] A study of 69 LAM patients from France cited survival rates (by Kaplan-Meier analysis) of 91% at 5 years, 79% at 10 years, and 71% after 15 years.[71] In a recent study of 57 LAM patients from the United Kingdom, 10-year survival from the onset of symptoms was 91%.[137] Similarly, a recent report of 227 LAM patients cited 10-year survival rate of 92%.[109]

Treatment

Because of the rarity of LAM, optimal therapy has not been determined.[72,74,108,138] No randomized or controlled studies have been performed. Corticosteroids, immunosuppressive agents, cytotoxic drugs, and radiation therapy have no role in LAM. Because LAM is exclusively a disease of women and appears to be exacerbated by estrogens, physicians should advise against pregnancy or the use of exogenous estrogens.[71,75,82,138] Historically, diverse estrogen-ablative therapies have been tried (*eg*, oophorectomy, administration of antiestrogen regimens [*eg*, progesterone, tamoxifen, androgens, lynestrenol]; luteinizing hormone–releasing hormone antagonists [*eg*, goserelin]; gonadotropin-releasing hormone agonists [*eg*, leuprolide acetate]; and somatostatin).[71,75–78,82,83] However, these therapies are of unproven benefit. Data are discouraging but are limited by retrospective analyses and small numbers of patients.

In a retrospective review from Stanford and the Mayo Clinic, oophorectomy *alone* was ineffective in all 16 patients.[78] None of 9 patients treated with tamoxifen improved; 2 of 19 treated with IM medroxyprogesterone acetate (MPA) *alone* stabilized or improved.[78] In 1995, Kitaichi et al[77] retrospectively evaluated 40 treatment courses in patients with LAM. Only 2 patients improved; 9 stabilized and 29 deteriorated. Oophorectomy or progesterone *alone* was never effective. The combination of oophorectomy and progesterone was associated with deterioration in 9, stabilization in 1, and improvement in 1. One patient improved with combined treatment with progesterone, tamoxifen, and oophorectomy. Gonadotropin-releasing hormone agonists were ineffective in all 6 patients. Tamoxifen (alone or in combination with other agents), was given to 13; only 1 improved. A review from Korea identified 21 cases of LAM seen from 1984 to 1997.[83] Follow-up for ≥12 months was available in only 10 patients, all of whom were treated with MPA and/or tamoxifen. No patient underwent oophorectomy. The disease progressed in 8 of 10; no patient improved.[83]

Tamoxifen has partial estrogen-agonist activity, which raises concerns about its potential to exacerbate the proliferative process.[75] Chu and colleagues[76] reported 35 women with LAM evaluated at the National Institutes of Health from 1995 to 1997. Fifteen patients (43%) underwent bilateral oophorectomy before their entry into the study; 28 (80%) had received medical antiestrogen therapy and 7 (20%) were untreated. Only one patient with chylothorax improved with MPA; the value of therapy in the remaining patients was not discussed.

The administration of a synthetic analog of luteinizing hormone–releasing hormone was associated with improvement in one patient with LAM described by Rossi and coworkers[139] but was ineffective in two other patients reported by Radermecker et al.[140] Triptorelin, a gonadotropin-releasing hormone analog, was ineffective in a prospective study of 11 premenopausal women with LAM.[141] Anecdotal case reports cited responses to interferon α_2b[142] and somatostatin,[143] but the value of these modalities is unproven. French investigators identified 69 women with LAM from 1973 to 1996.[71]

Diverse hormonal therapies were administered in 57 patients (84%). Treatments included progesterone (n = 46), tamoxifen (n = 22), gonadotropin-releasing hormone agonists (n = 14), somatostatin (n = 6), and oophorectomy (n = 5).[71] Among 34 patients with serial PFTs, FEV_1 improved by ≥ 15% in only 4 patients; 19 patients stabilized and 11 deteriorated. Treatment regimens used among the patients who improved included tamoxifen and progesterone in 2, progesterone in 1, and oophorectomy in 1. A retrospective analysis of 43 patients with LAM in the United Kingdom suggested that progesterone may slow the rate of decrease of pulmonary function tests (FEV_1, TLC),[82] but differences did not achieve statistical significance.

A subsequent retrospective study by these investigators analyzed factors influencing disease progression in a cohort of 57 LAM patients, 36 of whom had been treated with progesterone.[137] There was more rapid progression of dyspnea among those who became pregnant after the onset of symptoms (hazards ratio [HR] of 2.7), patients treated with progesterone (HR, 2.2) and cigarette smokers (HR, 2.0). These associations were of borderline statistical significance. These data do *not* support a beneficial effect of progesterone on lung function.

A larger study from the United States followed 275 patients with LAM for approximately 4 years.[108] Overall, 139 patients (50%) were treated with progesterone (67 PO, 72 IM). No benefit in rates of decrease in FEV_1 or DLCO were noted among patients receiving progesterone compared with untreated patients. Absolute annual decreases in FEV_1 were 59 mL among patients *not* treated with progesterone vs 119 mL/year and 76 mL/year decreases among patients treated with PO or IM progesterone, respectively. Absolute annual decreases in DLCO were 0.57 mL/min/mm Hg among patients *not* treated with progesterone vs 0.95 and 0.70 mL/min/mm Hg among patients treated with PO or IM progesterone, respectively.[108]

Italian investigators followed 36 women with LAM for a mean of 9.8 years; all received some type of estrogen ablative therapy.[144] Five- and 10-year survival rates were excellent (97% and 90%, respectively), but the impact of therapy could not be assessed. Data from these various clinical series.[71,77,78,82,83,108,137] suggest that current therapies are of limited or no value. Unfortunately, there are no clear guidelines for optimal therapy. Estrogen receptors and PRs are found in lung LAM lesions in some patients,[71,74] but the presence or absence of hormonal receptors does not correlate with response to hormonal therapy.[76,78] I do not believe that antihormonal therapies have a role to treat LAM. Sirolimus, a macrolide with immunosuppressive properties, inhibits the activity of the mammalian target of rapamycin, suppresses smooth muscle proliferation, and suppresses DNA synthesis of LAM cells *in vitro*.[128,145] Further, sirolimus induced remission of angiolipomas in two patients with TSC.[145,146] In an open-label trial, 25 patients with AMLs were treated with sirolimus for 12 months; 5 had TSC only and 18 women had LAM (sporadic or associated with TSC).[147] After 12 months of therapy, the mean volume of AML lesions decreased by nearly 50%. Further, among 11 female patients with LAM, mean FEV_1 increased above baseline by 118 mL and FVC increased by 390 mL at 12 months.[147] These beneficial effects tended to reverse after the drug was withdrawn.

In one woman with sporadic LAM, sirolimus led to complete disappearance of abdominal and pelvic masses and right chylous effusion and improved lung function.[148] Additional case reports cited improvement with sirolimus post-LT chylothorax,[149,150] retroperitoneal AML,[151] and pulmonary LAM.[150,152] These data are encouraging, but given the potential for serious adverse effects with long-term use of sirolimus, additional studies are required to ascertain the role for this agent in LAM. A 3-year randomized, placebo-controlled clinical trial evaluating sirolimus in pulmonary LAM is in progress (Multicenter International LAM Efficacy of Sirolimus Trial).[74] Recent studies found that simvastatin inhibits migration of human LAM cell cultures and inhibits LAM cell proliferation; furthermore, combined treatment with simvastatin and sirolimus abrogated cell proliferation to a greater degree than either agent alone.[128] Future studies exploring the role of statins as therapy for LAM would be of interest. Another clinical trial in progress at the NHLBI is evaluating octreotide,[74] which has shown promise for treating chylous complications in other diseases.[153]

Bronchodilators and supplemental oxygen have adjunctive roles in selected patients with pulmonary LAM.[71,75,76] Sildenafil or vasodilators have a *theoretical* role among patients with PAH complicating LAM,[111] but data are lacking.

Management of Chylous Effusions and Pneumothoraces in LAM

Pneumothoraces complicate LAM in 50 to 80% of patients; chylothoraces, in 10 to 39%.[71,72,75,76,88] Both complications may occur repetitively in individual patients, mandating an aggressive surgical approach to therapy. Thoracostomy tubes may be adequate for pneumothorax or chylothorax in some patients, but recurrences are common.[71,74,76,92] Video-assisted thoracoscopic surgery with pleurodesis is warranted for recurrent pneumothoraces or chylothoraces complicating LAM.[92] For recurrent pneumothoraces, partial pleurectomy is preferred; chemical pleurodesis should be avoided.[71] Management of chylous pleural effusions or ascites in LAM patients is difficult. Dietary fat restriction, peritoneal-jugular shunts, and sclerosing agents have been tried but are usually ineffectual.[71,75,76,92] Given the rarity of LAM, optimal management of chylous effusions is controversial. The approach should be individualized, taking into account the severity or persistence of chylothorax, comorbidities, and local expertise.[92] For refractory chylothorax, this author favors video-assisted thoracoscopic surgery with talc pleurodesis and thoracic duct ligation. In one study, placement of a pleurovenous shunt led to successful resolution of chylous pleural effusions in one LAM patient with persistent chylothoraces refractory to pleurodesis and thoracic duct ligation.[154]

LT for LAM

Single or double LT has been successful in patients with LAM and end-stage pulmonary insufficiency.[155-158] Data from the ISHLT Registry from January 1995 to June 2006 identified 175 patients with LAM among 17,616 LT recipients worldwide (1%).[159] Survival rates after LT for LAM are generally similar to other indications.[155-158] A review of 61 LAM patients who had LT in Europe from 1997 to 2007 cited 1- and 3-year survival rates of 79% and 73%, respectively.[157] Survival rates among 44 LAM patients who had LT in France between 1988 and 2006 were similar (1- and 3-year survival rates of 80% and 74%, respectively.[158] Experience in the United States (79 patients between from 1987 to 2002) was similar: 1- and 3-year survival rates of 85% and 76%, respectively.[155]

When to list LAM patients for LT is difficult because the prognosis is varies widely among patients. Guidelines for LT in LAM include the following: disease progression despite medical therapy, $FEV_1/FVC < 50\%$, $TLC > 130\%$, $FEV_1 < 30\%$, and severe cystic disease on HRCT.[80] LAM-associated complications of LT include massive operative hemorrhage caused by extensive pleural adhesions, pneumothorax in the native lung (for single lung transplant recipients), and postoperative chylothorax.[88,157,158] Previous pleurectomy or talc pleurodesis can create difficulties with tissue plane dissection and bleeding during removal of the native lung(s).[88] In one study of 80 LAM patients who had LT, pleural-related postoperative bleeding occurred in 13 of 45 patients with previous pleurodesis compared with 1 of 35 without prior pleurodesis.[88] Management strategies for chylothorax include drainage, diet containing medium-chain triglycerides, progesterone, thoracic duct ligation, pleurodesis, and pleurectomy.[74,82] The recurrence of LAM in the donor lung allograft has been noted in 3 to 8% of LT recipients.[74,157,158] Molecular techniques confirmed that foci of LAM in lung allografts were derived from the recipient,[160,161] indicating that LAM cells can migrate or metastasize despite histologically benign features.[119]

COP

COP is a rare immune disorder characterized by granulation tissue that obstructs small bronchioles and extends into the distal alveolar ducts and alveoli.[162-165] The term BOOP is synonymous,[166] but the use of this term should be discouraged.[164,167] Clinical features of COP include focal alveolar infiltrates, cough, fever, dyspnea, and a subacute course, mimicking community-acquired pneumonia.[163,164] Obliterative bronchiolitis (OB), which is characterized by obstruction of bronchioles and small airways but lacks the organizing pneumonia (OP) component, is a distinct disorder with differing clinical and radiographic features and prognosis.[164,167] OP (with or without OB) may complicate collagen vascular disease,[168,169] Sjögren syndrome,[170] inflammatory bowel disease,[171] Wegener granulomatosis,[172] lower respiratory tract infections (*eg*, legionellae, viruses, and Mycoplasma sp),[165,173] toxic fume inhalation; radiation therapy,[174] chemotherapy,[175,176] malignancy,[177,178] lung cancer,[179] or bone marrow,[180] stem cell,[181,182] or lung or heart-lung[183] transplants. It can also occur as a reaction to pharmacologic or exogenous agents.[167,184-186] Only *idiopathic* (cryptogenic) organizing pneumonia, a disorder in which no specific etiology can be established, will be discussed here.

Epidemiology

The incidence of COP is difficult to ascertain, as historically a variety of terms were used interchangeably to refer to this disorder (*eg*, OP, COP, BOOP, bronchiolitis obliterans, and resolving pneumonia). Nonetheless, COP (or idiopathic BOOP) is rare, and most referral centers see no more than two to five cases per year. In 1983, Davison and colleagues[187] described eight patients with "cryptogenic organizing pneumonia." In 1985, Epler and colleagues[166] described 67 patients with BOOP (including 50 with the idiopathic form) gleaned from >2,500 open lung biopsies performed from 1950 to 1980. A retrospective review of pathologic files at the University of Alabama identified 24 cases from 1972 to 1984; five had connective tissue disease.[188] French investigators at a leading referral center identified 16 patients with idiopathic BOOP/COP in 6 years.[189] A survey in Japan detected 29 cases of BOOP/COP from 200 hospitals from 1986 to 1988; 5 patients had connective tissue disease.[190] In a Spanish community hospital, 33 cases of COP were observed in 19 years.[179]

A survey at a leading referral hospital in Vancouver, British Columbia, from 1985 to 1992 detected 25 cases of COP.[162] This represented a prevalence of 1.2 per 10,000 admissions. Their review of 63 published papers identified 296 patients with COP (24 were single case reports). Of the published cases, 218 were idiopathic and 29 had connective tissue disease. Gudmundsson et al[191] retrospectively evaluated all biopsy-proven cases of OP diagnosed in Iceland between 1984 and 2003.[191] The mean annual incidence of OP per 100,000 population was 1.10 for COP and 0.87 for secondary OP. Most patients with idiopathic COP present in the fourth through sixth decades of life, but all ages may be affected.[162-164,166] There is no predominance by sex.[191] COP is more common in nonsmokers (2:1 ratio).[163]

Clinical Features

Predominant symptoms are cough (typically nonproductive) and dyspnea.[162,163,166] Extrapulmonary involvement does not occur, but fever, weight loss, and malaise may be prominent.[162-164,166] The course is subacute, with symptoms developing >2 weeks to 6 months.[162,163,166] An antecedent upper or lower respiratory tract infection precedes the onset of symptoms in at least one third of patients.[162,166] The constellation of these features simulates an infectious etiology. The diagnosis is often not suspected until repetitive courses of antibiotics fail. Physical examination reveals mid-inspiratory squeaks or rhonchi in 40% of patients; wheezing does not occur.[162,166] Rales may be present, but frank consolidation changes on chest auscultation are lacking.[163,164] Clubbing is not a feature of COP.[163] No consistent laboratory aberrations are present. The erythrocyte sedimentation rate is usually increased; peripheral blood leukocytosis is noted in onethird.[162,163,166]

Chest Radiographs

Focal lobar or segmental alveolar infiltrates, often with air bronchograms, are the cardinal features, observed in 60 to 80% of patients with COP (Fig 18, 19).[162,163,164,166,187] These infiltrates are often in the periphery of the lung (resembling chronic eosinophilic pneumonia)[164,192] but lack the striking upper-lobe predilection characteristic of that disorder. The infiltrates may wax and wane, even before initiation of therapy. A more diffuse pattern, associated with reticulonodular infiltrates, occurs in 20 to 30% of patients.[162,164,166] In this context, focal opacities are lacking, and the pattern resembles other chronic ILDs. Chest radiographs are normal or reveal only hyperinflation in 4 to 10% of patients.[162,163,166] Focal airspace disease with consolidation is associated with an improved prognosis and greater rate of responsiveness to

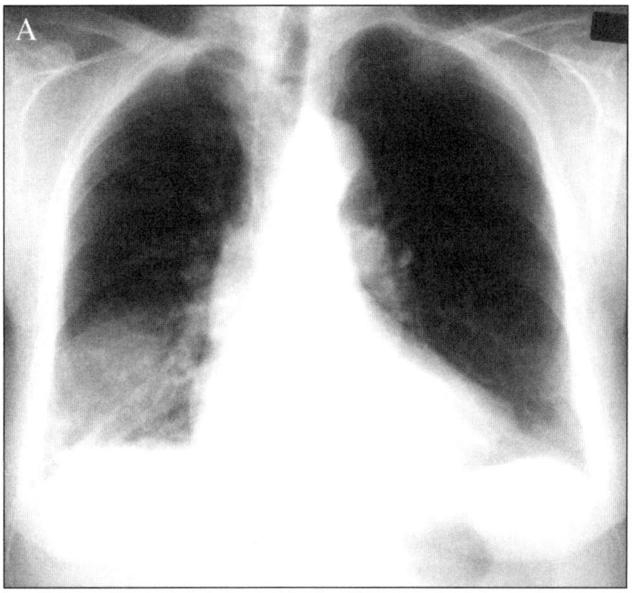

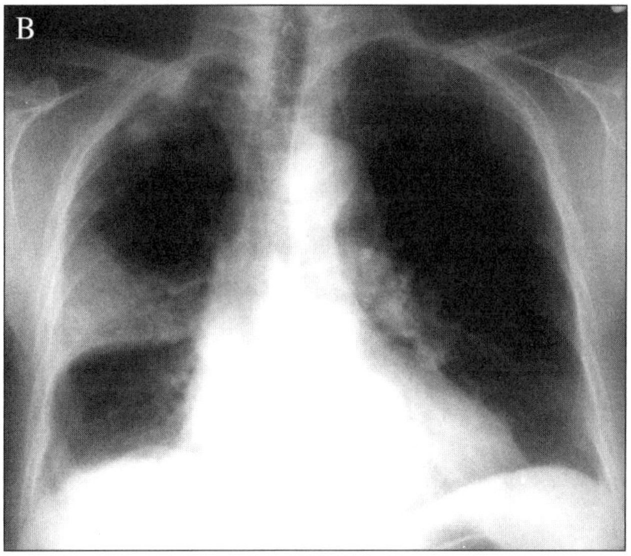

Figure 18. BOOP. *Top, A*: posteroanterior chest radiograph from a 75-year-old woman with a 6-month history of recurrent "pneumonias" demonstrating focal right lower lobe consolidation. A patchy left lower lobe infiltrate is also present. *Bottom, B*: posteroanterior chest radiograph from the same patient as in *top, A,* demonstrates right upper lobe and left lower lobe alveolar infiltrates; a patchy right lower lobe infiltrate is also present. A transbronchial lung biopsy specimen demonstrated the classic features of BOOP. Following the initiation of therapy with prednisone, 40 mg/d, complete radiographic and symptomatic resolution was evident within 3 weeks.

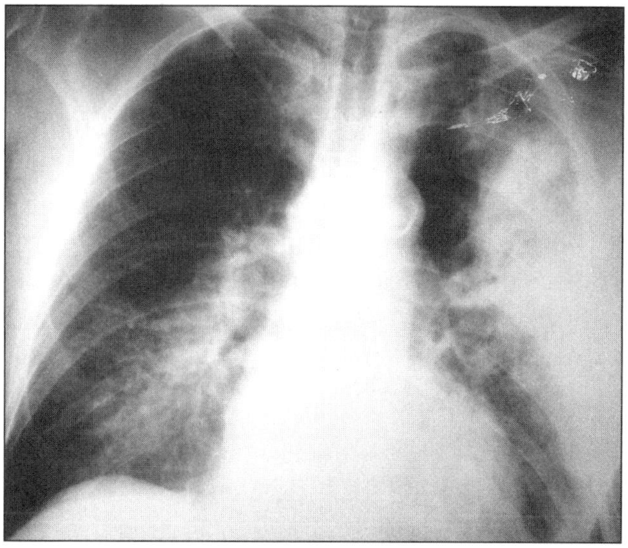

Figure 19. BOOP. Posteroanterior chest radiograph demonstrating extensive patchy alveolar infiltrates in the left lung and a patchy infiltrate in the right lower lobe in a 58-year-old man. The open-lung biopsy specimen was consistent with BOOP. After 4 weeks of therapy with prednisone, 60 mg/d, he was asymptomatic, and the infiltrates seen on chest radiographs had almost completely resolved. From Neagos GR, Lynch JP III. Making sense out of bronchiolitis obliterans. J Respir Dis 1991; 12:789-814.

corticosteroids compared with other radiographic patterns.[163] Pleural effusions, cavitation, and intrathoracic lymphadenopathy are not features of COP. However, multiple nodular mass lesions,[193] miliary lesions,[194] or cavitary nodules[195,196] have been noted in anecdotal cases.

HRCT scans depict the salient features of COP more clearly than conventional chest radiographs[163,197] but are not essential for diagnosis or management. Typically, multiple segmental or lobar dense alveolar opacities with air bronchograms are seen in the peripheral regions of the lungs.[163,192] In some cases, a feeding vessel or bronchus leading into the area of consolidation or nodular opacity may be seen. Reticulonodular infiltrates are noted in one quarter of patients. Other findings include GGOs and peribronchiolar nodules extending into the lung parenchyma in a centrifugal pattern from the involved airways.[163,192,194] Honeycombing is rare.

One study of 38 patients with COP noted the following features on CT: consolidation (87%), GGOs (58%), bronchial dilation (58%), nonseptal linear or reticular opacities (45%), nodules or mass lesions (32%), and peribronchial distribution of consolidation (29%).[192] Mediastinal lymphadenopathy may be present but is usually minor (lymph nodes <15 mm in size). The presence of consolidation on CT predicts a favorable prognosis, with complete or partial resolution with CS therapy; by contrast, reticular patterns suggest an incomplete response or progression to fibrosis.[198] Occasionally, COP presents as a solitary focal mass lesion, mimicking neoplasm.[163,199,200] In this setting, the diagnosis is usually established after surgical excision.[199,200] Medical therapy is usually not required for isolated OP noted incidentally at surgery.[200] Increased uptake of fluorodeoxyglucose on PET scan is characteristic in patients with OP;[199,201] however, this finding has no clinical value.

PFTs

PFTs in COP demonstrate reductions in lung volumes (*eg*, vital capacity and TLC) and DLCO and a widened alveolar-arterial oxygen gradient.[162-164,166] Despite the involvement of small airways, an obstructive component is rare in nonsmokers.[163,166] The lack of an obstructive defect in COP has been ascribed to the patchy nature of involvement. Some regions are completely obstructed (resulting in loss of entire units and proportionate reduction in lung volumes), whereas other units are spared. Bronchodilators generally are ineffective. These deficits usually reverse promptly with corticosteroid therapy.[162-164,166]

Histology

The cardinal histologic feature of COP is an exuberant inflammatory and fibrotic process involving terminal and respiratory bronchioles.[163,165] Tufts of granulation tissue and aggregates of neutrophils, edema, debris, fibrin, connective tissue, myofibroblasts, and fibroblasts plug the terminal bronchioles (Fig 20, 21). Inflammatory cells are present within bronchiolar lumens and extend into the peribronchiolar regions, alveolar ducts, and alveolar spaces. Mononuclear cells predominate, but scattered neutrophils and eosinophils are seen. Multinucleated giant cells are present in up to 20% of cases. Foamy alveolar macrophages within the alveolar spaces may simulate DIP.[202] The disease is patchy, but the peribronchiolar distribution (which can be identified on lower-power magnification) is a clue to the diagnosis.

Extension of the process to contiguous alveolar ducts and spaces results in the "organizing pneumonia" component (Fig 22).[163,165] Despite the presence of extensive granulation tissue and edema, the alveolar architecture is preserved and fibrosis is absent. The lesions in COP appear to be of uniform age, suggesting a stereotypic response to prior injury. By contrast, constrictive bronchiolitis, also termed OB, lacks the organizing pneumonia component of COP and is associated with a distinctly worse prognosis.[164] In OB, the small airways and bronchioles are obliterated by transmural fibrosis and inflammation, but a prominent inflammatory component is lacking.[164] The airway lumens are narrowed by a concentric deposition of collagen and fibrous connective tissue. The histologic lesions of OB may be seen as a

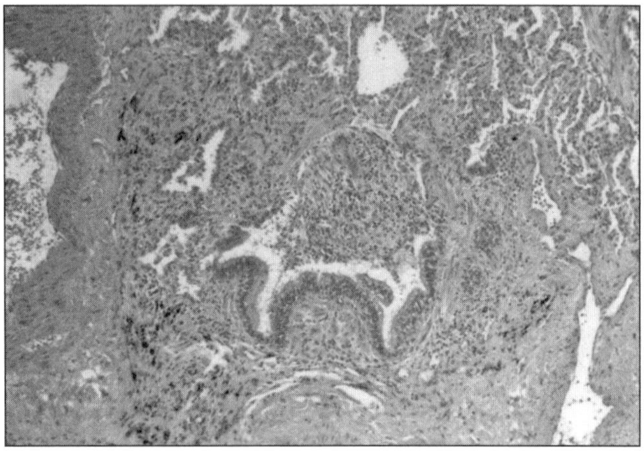

Figure 20. Photomicrograph of BOOP. Open-lung biopsy specimen demonstrating a plug of organizing granulation tissue within a respiratory bronchiole. A peribronchiolar mononuclear inflammatory cell infiltrate is also evident (hematoxylin-eosin, high-power magnification). From Neagos GR, Lynch JP III. Making sense out of bronchiolitis obliterans. J Respir Dis 1991; 12:789-814.

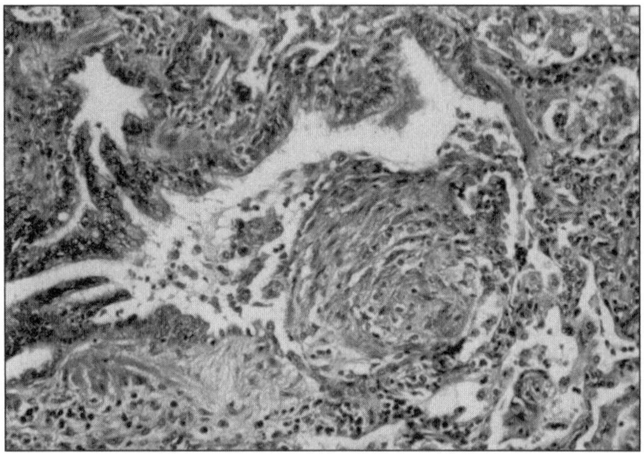

Figure 21. Photomicrograph of BOOP. Open-lung biopsy specimen demonstrating a plug of granulation tissue within the bronchioles. A peribronchiolar inflammatory cellular infiltrate is present extending into the alveolar interstitium (hematoxylin-eosin, high-power magnification).

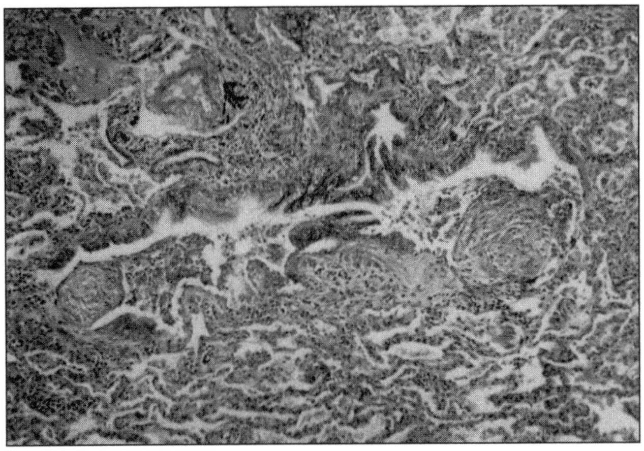

Figure 22. Photomicrograph of BOOP. Open-lung biopsy specimen demonstrating a plug of granulation tissue within the bronchioles. A peribronchiolar inflammatory cellular infiltrate is present extending into the alveolar interstitium (hematoxylin-eosin, low-power magnification). From Clinical pulmonary medicine. Boston, MA: Little Brown, 1992; 193-263.[197]

complication of rheumatoid arthritis, toxic fume inhalation, bone marrow or lung transplantation, and diverse exposures.[165,167,184,185] In contrast to COP, OB is associated with a poor prognosis and low rate of responsiveness to corticosteroids or cytotoxic agents. The course is characterized by progressive airflow obstruction, eventually resulting in respiratory failure and death. This entity is beyond the scope of this chapter.

The histologic features of COP overlap with those of several other entities, including DIP, chronic eosinophilic pneumonia, hypersensitivity pneumonitis,[163] cystic fibrosis,[203] infectious etiologies,[163] and more recently described entities such as airway centered interstitial fibrosis,[204] idiopathic bronchiolocentric interstitial pneumonia,[205] and bronchiolitis interstitial pneumonitis.[206] The differentiating features of these entities is beyond the scope of this chapter and is addressed elsewhere.[204-206] Given the patchy nature of COP, fiberoptic bronchoscopy with transbronchial biopsy is usually not adequate to establish the diagnosis with certainty. In such cases, video assisted thoracoscopic surgical lung biopsy is required. However, the diagnosis can sometimes be confirmed with transbronchial biopsy if clinical features are consistent and infectious etiologies are reliably excluded.[163,164,207] Gross macroscopic findings at the time of bronchoscopy and analysis of BAL fluid are helpful in excluding infectious etiologies. The absence of bronchitis or purulent secretions within airways and negative smears and cultures of BAL fluid makes infection less likely. BAL in COP often reveals increases in lymphocytes (20 to 40%), polymorphonuclear leukocytes (5 to 15%), or eosinophils (5%), sometimes with plasma cells or mast cells.[162-164] The CD4/CD8 ratio is decreased.[163,164] These aberrations are nonspecific, and do not distinguish COP from other infectious or immune-mediated disorders. Percutaneous CT-guided needle biopsy may establish the diagnosis in some patients with COP,[208] but caution should be applied owing to small sample size.

Pathogenesis

The pathogenesis of COP has not been elucidated but likely represents an exaggerated host response to a variety of inflammatory or injurious stimuli.[163,164] The uniformity of the histologic lesion and the peribronchiolar distribution suggest that inhaled stimuli (*eg*, possibly inhaled antigens or noxious agents) may initiate lung injury. This is followed by activation and recruitment of inflammatory cells and an attempt to repair. The frequent association of antecedent viral or respiratory tract infection in COP suggests that inhaled viral or bacterial antigens may elicit an intense local immune response.

BAL fluid in patients with COP often demonstrates lymphocytic alveolitis with expansion of $CD8^+$ cells and increased levels of Th1-related cytokines including γ-interferon, IL-12, and IL-18.[209] Newly formed intraluminal fibromyxoid tissue in COP demonstrates increased capillarization compared with fibroblastic foci of usual interstitial pneumonia (UIP).[210] Angiogenesis may be mediated by growth factors, VEGF, and basic fibroblast growth factors.[210] Regulation of angiogenesis may influence reversibility of the fibrotic lesions.

Imbalance between matrix MMPs and tissue inhibitors of metalloproteinases (TIMPs) may play a role in the airway remodeling observed in COP.[211] Concentrations of MMP-9 and TIMP-1 were increased in BAL fluid from patients with COP and UIP compared with control patients, but the highest concentrations were observed in patients with COP. Lymphocytes are important cellular sources of MMP-9. It is possible that MMP-2 preferentially degrades collagens and that TIMPs play a role in remodeling after parenchymal damage.[211] Suga et al[212] also found increased expression of MMP-9 in UIP, whereas COP cases showed predominant MMP-2 expression in BAL fluids and tissues. MMP-2 activity in COP correlated with increases in BAL lymphocytes.[212] Japanese investigators noted increased serum levels of KL-6 (a mucin-like glycoprotein) in 17 of 30 patients with COP).[213] KL-6 may be produced by damaged or regenerating type 2 epithelial cells and may be elevated in diverse idiopathic interstitial pneumonias (including UIP and nonspecific interstitial pneumonitis).[214]

The pivotal factors that initiate, direct, and regulate the inflammatory and reparative process in COP have yet to be elucidated. However, therapies that ablate the inflammatory response are usually highly efficacious in COP.

Therapy

Corticosteroids are the cornerstone of therapy for COP.[165,179,215] The optimal dosage and duration of CS therapy for COP have not been studied in randomized trials. In early studies, initial treatment with high dose prednisone (1 mg/kg/d) was advocated,[166] but lower doses (*eg*, 0.5 to 0.75 mg/kg/d) are often adequate in patients with mild-to-moderate disease.[165,179,215] Responses to CS are often dramatic (symptomatic improvement within a few days).[165] Radiographic clearing is usually evident within 1 to 4 weeks after institution of CS therapy.[162,165,166] Complete remissions occur in > 80% of patients.[165,179,214,215] In the remaining patients, minor impairments persist, but serious sequela are uncommon.

Pulmonary fibrosis occurs in < 20% of patients and death in < 5%.[162,164,166,179,215] The dose and rate of taper of CS should be individualized according to clinical symptoms, chest radiographs, and PFTs. Among responders, the dose of prednisone can be tapered to < 20 mg within 2 to 3 months.[215] Relapses may occur as the steroid is tapered or discontinued.[163,179,215] In one retrospective study, one or more relapses (mean, 2.4) occurred in 58% of 48 patients with COP.[215] Among patients experiencing multiple (≥3) relapses, the mean delay between first symptoms and treatment onset was significantly longer compared with patients who never relapsed (22 vs 11 weeks, respectively; $p = 0.02$).[215] Most relapses occurred within 1 year of the initial episode of COP; only 2 patients experienced relapses > 15 months after the initial episode.[215] Another study noted responses to steroids in 32 of 33 (97%) patients; relapses occurred in 18 (56%).[179] In both series, treatment of relapses was highly efficacious. Relapses did not affect survival or result in long-term functional morbidity.[179,215] In a recent study, relapse rates were greater in COP patients with increased serum KL-6 levels (37.5%) compared with normal KL-6 levels.[213]

Although the optimal duration of therapy has not been studied, a *minimum* of 6 to 12 months of treatment is advised.[165] This author prefers to continue *low-dose* CS (10 to 15 mg prednisone every other day) for a minimum of 12 months unless adverse effects require earlier discontinuation. Patients exhibiting a propensity to relapse each time CSs are tapered require chronic low-dose CS therapy.[164] Factors associated with a worse prognosis include a predominantly interstitial pattern on chest radiographs or HRCT[163] and lack of lymphocytosis on BAL fluid.[216] In one study, relapses were more frequent in patients with more severe hypoxemia at initial presentation.[217] In addition, relapses occurred in five of eight patients with associated disease compared with only 2 of 8 with idiopathic COP.[217]

Immunosuppressive or cytotoxic agents (*eg*, azathioprine, cyclophosphamide, cyclosporine A) are reserved for patients who do not respond or who experience adverse effects from CSs.[163,218-220] Data evaluating these agents are limited to anecdotal cases and small series. Macrolide antibiotics (particularly azithromycin) have been used to treat constrictive bronchiolitis (OB) complicating lung[183,221] or bone marrow transplantation,[180] with favorable responses noted in small series. The efficacy of macrolides reflects immunomodulatory properties[222,223] rather than antimicrobial activity. Although data are limited for COP, Stover et al[174] cited favorable responses to azithromycin in six patients with OP (three attributable to radiation therapy, three cryptogenic).[174] Others noted favorable responses with macrolide for COP,[224,225] but data are limited to a few cases. Given the favorable side effect profile of macrolide antibiotics, oral macrolides are logical therapeutic agents for patients with OP (irrespective of etiology) who are refractory to or experiencing adverse effects from CS.

Rapidly Progressive COP

A subset of patients with COP exhibit a fulminant course, with bilateral alveolar infiltrates, crackles, and severe hypoxemic respiratory failure developing within a few days or weeks.[226,227] This syndrome is rare; only 10 such patients were identified in a retrospective analysis at three medical centers from 1979 to 1992.[226] In that sentinel report, nine patients required mechanical ventilatory support. Despite CS therapy in all cases, seven patients died of progressive respiratory failure. Five patients received additional therapy with cyclophosphamide or azathioprine. Possible risk factors included underlying connective tissue disease (n = 3) and exposure to drugs or environmental agents (n = 4). Nine were current or former smokers. Histologic features of COP were present in all cases. In addition, necropsies in six patients revealed prominent alveolar septal inflammation, diffuse alveolar damage, interstitial fibrosis, and honeycombing. Korean investigators reported six patents with rapidly progressive, ultimately fatal, OP from a cohort of 45 patients with OP.[228] Because of the high mortality rate associated with rapidly progressive COP, this author recommends IV pulse methylprednisolone (1,000 mg daily for 3 days), following by high-dose prednisone (1 mg/kg/d or equivalent, with a gradual taper). The duration of therapy may be relatively brief once a clinical response has been achieved. For CS-recalcitrant patients, cyclophosphamide or azathioprine should be added.

References

1. Tazi A, Soler P, Hance AJ. Adult pulmonary Langerhans' cell histiocytosis. Thorax 2000; 55:405–416
2. Tazi A. Adult pulmonary Langerhans' cell histiocytosis. Eur Respir J 2006; 27:1272–1285
3. Vassallo R, Ryu JH, Colby TV, et al. Pulmonary Langerhans'-cell histiocytosis. N Engl J Med 2000; 342:1969–1978
4. Friedman PJ, Liebow AA, Sokoloff J. Eosinophilic granuloma of lung: clinical aspects of primary histiocytosis in the adult. Medicine (Baltimore) 1981; 60:385–396
5. Basset F, Corrin B, Spencer H, et al. Pulmonary histiocytosis X. Am Rev Respir Dis 1978; 118:811–820
6. Colby TV, Lombard C. Histiocytosis X in the lung. Hum Pathol 1983; 14:847–856
7. Travis WD, Borok Z, Roum JH, et al. Pulmonary Langerhans cell granulomatosis (histiocytosis X). A clinicopathologic study of 48 cases. Am J Surg Pathol 1993; 17:971–986
8. Soler P, Bergeron A, Kambouchner M, et al. Is high-resolution computed tomography a reliable tool to predict the histopathological activity of pulmonary Langerhans cell histiocytosis? Am J Respir Crit Care Med 2000; 162:264–270
9. Ladisch S, Gadner H. Treatment of Langerhans cell histiocytosis—evolution and current approaches. Br J Cancer Suppl 1994; 23:S41–S46
10. Willman CL, Busque L, Griffith BB, et al. Langerhans'-cell histiocytosis (histiocytosis X)–a clonal proliferative disease. N Engl J Med 1994; 331:154–160
11. Yousem SA, Colby TV, Chen YY, et al. Pulmonary Langerhans' cell histiocytosis: molecular analysis of clonality. Am J Surg Pathol 2001; 25:630–636
12. Brabencova E, Tazi A, Lorenzato M, et al. Langerhans cells in Langerhans cell granulomatosis are not actively proliferating cells. Am J Pathol 1998; 152:1143–1149
13. Delobbe A, Durieu J, Duhamel A, et al. Determinants of survival in pulmonary Langerhans' cell granulomatosis (histiocytosis X). Groupe d'Etude en Pathologie Interstitielle de la Societe de Pathologie Thoracique du Nord. Eur Respir J 1996; 9:2002–2006
14. Vassallo R, Jensen EA, Colby TV, et al. The overlap between respiratory bronchiolitis and desquamative interstitial pneumonia in pulmonary Langerhans cell histiocytosis: high-resolution CT, histologic, and functional correlations. Chest 2003; 124:1199–1205
15. Moore AD, Godwin JD, Muller NL, et al. Pulmonary histiocytosis X: comparison of radiographic and CT findings. Radiology 1989; 172:249–254
16. Selman M, Carillo G, Gaxiola M, et al. Pulmonary histiocytosis X (Eosinophilic granuloma): clinical behavior, pathogenesis, and therapeutic strategies of an unusual interstitial lung disease. Clin Pulm Med 1996; 3:191–198
17. Mendez JL, Nadrous HF, Vassallo R, et al. Pneumothorax in pulmonary Langerhans cell histiocytosis. Chest 2004; 125:1028–1032

18. Fartoukh M, Humbert M, Capron F, et al. Severe pulmonary hypertension in histiocytosis X. Am J Respir Crit Care Med 2000; 161:216–223
19. Hamada K, Teramoto S, Narita N, et al. Pulmonary veno-occlusive disease in pulmonary Langerhans' cell granulomatosis. Eur Respir J 2000; 15:421–423
20. Schonfeld N, Frank W, Wenig S, et al. Clinical and radiologic features, lung function and therapeutic results in pulmonary histiocytosis X. Respiration 1993; 60:38–44
21. Vassallo R, Ryu JH, Schroeder DR, et al. Clinical outcomes of pulmonary Langerhans'-cell histiocytosis in adults. N Engl J Med 2002; 346:484–490
22. Sadoun D, Vaylet F, Valeyre D, et al. Bronchogenic carcinoma in patients with pulmonary histiocytosis X. Chest 1992; 101:1610–1613
23. Egeler RM, Neglia JP, Puccetti DM, et al. Association of Langerhans cell histiocytosis with malignant neoplasms. Cancer 1993; 71:865–873
24. Tomashefski JF, Khiyami A, Kleinerman J. Neoplasms associated with pulmonary eosinophilic granuloma. Arch Pathol Lab Med 1991; 115:499–506
25. Neumann MP, Frizzera G. The coexistence of Langerhans' cell granulomatosis and malignant lymphoma may take different forms: report of seven cases with a review of the literature. Hum Pathol 1986; 17:1060–1065
26. Brambilla E, Fontaine E, Pison CM, et al. Pulmonary histiocytosis X with mediastinal lymph node involvement. Am Rev Respir Dis 1990; 142:1216–1218
27. Brauner MW, Grenier P, Tijani K, et al. Pulmonary Langerhans cell histiocytosis: evolution of lesions on CT scans. Radiology 1997; 204:497–502
28. Hidalgo A, Franquet T, Gimenez A, et al. Smoking-related interstitial lung diseases: radiologic-pathologic correlation. Eur Radiol 2006; 16:2463–2470
29. Koyama M, Johkoh T, Honda O, et al. Chronic cystic lung disease: diagnostic accuracy of high-resolution CT in 92 patients. AJR Am J Roentgenol 2003; 180:827–835
30. Sundar KM, Gosselin MV, Chung HL, et al. Pulmonary Langerhans cell histiocytosis: emerging concepts in pathobiology, radiology, and clinical evolution of disease. Chest 2003; 123:1673–1683
31. Crausman RS, Jennings CA, Tuder RM, et al. Pulmonary histiocytosis X: pulmonary function and exercise pathophysiology. Am J Respir Crit Care Med 1996; 153:426–435
32. Canuet M, Kessler R, Jeung MY, et al. Correlation between high-resolution computed tomography findings and lung function in pulmonary Langerhans cell histiocytosis. Respiration 2007; 74:640–646
33. Wang CW, Colby TV. Histiocytic lesions and proliferations in the lung. Semin Diagn Pathol 2007; 24:162–182
34. Vassallo R, Patel R, Aubry MC. Langerhans cell histiocytosis. In: Lynch JP III, ed. Interstitial pulmonary and bronchiolar disorders (Vol. 227). New York: InformaUSA; 2008; 733–745
35. Leslie KO, Gruden JF, Parish JM, et al. Transbronchial biopsy interpretation in the patient with diffuse parenchymal lung disease. Arch Pathol Lab Med 2007; 131:407–423
36. Chollet S, Soler P, Dournovo P, et al. Diagnosis of pulmonary histiocytosis X by immunodetection of Langerhans cells in bronchoalveolar lavage fluid. Am J Pathol 1984; 115:225–232
37. Emile JF, Wechsler J, Brousse N, et al. Langerhans' cell histiocytosis: definitive diagnosis with the use of monoclonal antibody O10 on routinely paraffin-embedded samples. Am J Surg Pathol 1995; 19:636–641
38. Tazi A, Bonay M, Grandsaigne M, et al. Surface phenotype of Langerhans cells and lymphocytes in granulomatous lesions from patients with pulmonary histiocytosis X. Am Rev Respir Dis 1993; 147:1531–1536
39. Jaksits S, Kriehuber E, Charbonnier AS, et al. CD34+ cell-derived CD14+ precursor cells develop into Langerhans cells in a TGF-beta 1-dependent manner. J Immunol 1999; 163:4869–4877
40. Banchereau J, Steinman RM. Dendritic cells and the control of immunity. Nature 1998; 392:245–252
41. Youkeles LH, Grizzanti JN, Liao Z, et al. Decreased tobacco-glycoprotein-induced lymphocyte proliferation in vitro in pulmonary eosinophilic granuloma. Am J Respir Crit Care Med 1995; 151:145–150
42. Churg A, Tai H, Coulthard T, et al. Cigarette smoke drives small airway remodeling by induction of growth factors in the airway wall. Am J Respir Crit Care Med 2006; 174:1327–1334
43. Casolaro MA, Bernaudin JF, Saltini C, et al. Accumulation of Langerhans' cells on the epithelial surface of the lower respiratory tract in normal subjects in association with cigarette smoking. Am Rev Respir Dis 1988; 137:406–411
44. Aguayo SM, King TE Jr., Waldron JA Jr., et al. Increased pulmonary neuroendocrine cells with bombesin-like immunoreactivity in adult patients

with eosinophilic granuloma. J Clin Invest 1990; 86:838–844
45. Zeid NA, Muller HK. Tobacco smoke induced lung granulomas and tumors: association with pulmonary Langerhans cells. Pathology 1995; 27:247–254
46. Wells AU, Nicholson AG, Hansell DM. Challenges in pulmonary fibrosis. 4: smoking-induced diffuse interstitial lung diseases. Thorax 2007; 62:904–910
47. Howarth DM, Gilchrist GS, Mullan BP, et al. Langerhans cell histiocytosis: diagnosis, natural history, management, and outcome. Cancer 1999; 85:2278–2290
48. Chaowalit N, Pellikka PA, Decker PA, et al. Echocardiographic and clinical characteristics of pulmonary hypertension complicating pulmonary Langerhans cell histiocytosis. Mayo Clin Proc 2004; 79:1269–1275
49. Gadner H, Grois N, Arico M, et al. A randomized trial of treatment for multisystem Langerhans' cell histiocytosis. J Pediatr 2001; 138:728–734
50. Giona F, Caruso R, Testi AM, et al. Langerhans' cell histiocytosis in adults: a clinical and therapeutic analysis of 11 patients from a single institution. Cancer 1997; 80:1786–1791
51. Saven A, Burian C. Cladribine activity in adult Langerhans-cell histiocytosis. Blood 1999; 93:4125–4130
52. Zeller B, Storm-Mathisen I, Smevik B, et al. Multisystem Langerhans-cell histiocytosis with life-threatening pulmonary involvement—good response to cyclosporine A. Med Pediatr Oncol 2000; 35:438–442
53. Braier J, Chantada G, Rosso D, et al. Langerhans cell histiocytosis: retrospective evaluation of 123 patients at a single institution. Pediatr Hematol Oncol 1999; 16:377–385
54. Minkov M, Grois N, Broadbent V, et al. Cyclosporine A therapy for multisystem Langerhans cell histiocytosis. Med Pediatr Oncol 1999; 33:482–485
55. Choi SW, Bangaru BS, Wu CD, et al. Gastrointestinal involvement in disseminated Langerhans cell histiocytosis (LCH) with durable complete response to 2-chlorodeoxyadenosine and high-dose cytarabine. J Pediatr Hematol Oncol 2003; 25:503–506
56. Goh NS, McDonald CE, MacGregor DP, et al. Successful treatment of Langerhans cell histiocytosis with 2-chlorodeoxyadenosine. Respirology 2003; 8:91–94
57. Saven A, Foon KA, Piro LD. 2-Chlorodeoxyadenosine-induced complete remissions in Langerhans-cell histiocytosis. Ann Intern Med 1994; 121:430–432
58. Pardanani A, Phyliky RL, Li CY, et al. 2-Chlorodeoxyadenosine therapy for disseminated Langerhans cell histiocytosis. Mayo Clin Proc 2003; 78:301–306
59. Aerni MR, Christine Aubry M, et al. Complete remission of nodular pulmonary Langerhans cell histiocytosis lesions induced by 2-chlorodeoxyadenosine in a non-smoker. Respir Med 2008; 102:316–319
60. Hirose M, Saito S, Yoshimoto T, et al. Interleukin-2 therapy of Langerhans cell histiocytosis. Acta Paediatr 1995; 84:1204–1206
61. Henter JI, Karlen J, Calming U, et al. Successful treatment of Langerhans'-cell histiocytosis with etanercept. N Engl J Med 2001; 345:1577–1578
62. Mogulkoc N, Veral A, Bishop PW, et al. Pulmonary Langerhans' cell histiocytosis: radiologic resolution following smoking cessation. Chest 1999; 115:1452–1455
63. Arico M, Girschikofsky M, Genereau T, et al. Langerhans cell histiocytosis in adults: report from the International Registry of the Histiocyte Society. Eur J Cancer 2003; 39:2341–2348
64. Etienne B, Bertocchi M, Gamondes JP, et al. Relapsing pulmonary Langerhans cell histiocytosis after lung transplantation. Am J Respir Crit Care Med 1998; 157:288–291
65. Dauriat G, Mal H, Thabut G, et al. Lung transplantation for pulmonary Langerhans' cell histiocytosis: a multicenter analysis. Transplantation 2006; 81:746–750
66. Hertz MI, Boucek MM, Deng MC, et al. Scientific Registry of the International Society for Heart and Lung Transplantation: introduction to the 2005 annual reports. J Heart Lung Transplant 2005; 24:939–944
67. Habbib SB, Congelton J, Carr D, et al. Recurrence of Langerhan's cell histiocytosis following bilateral lung transplantation. Thorax 1998; 53:323–325
68. Gabbay E, Dark JH, Ashcroft T, et al. Recurrence of Langerhans' cell granulomatosis following lung transplantation. Thorax 1998; 53:326–327
69. Lynch JP 3rd, Saggar R, Weigt SS, et al. Overview of lung transplantation and criteria for selection of candidates. Semin Respir Crit Care Med 2006; 27:441–469
70. Taveira-DaSilva AM, Steagall WK, Moss J. Lymphangioleiomyomatosis Cancer Control 2006; 13:276–285
71. Urban T, Lazor R, Lacronique J, et al. Pulmonary lymphangioleiomyomatosis: a study of 69 patients.

Groupe d'Etudes et de Recherche sur les Maladies "Orphelines" Pulmonaires (GERM"O"P). Medicine (Baltimore) 1999; 78:321–337

72. Ryu JH, Moss J, Beck GJ, et al. The NHLBI Lymphangioleiomyomatosis Registry: characteristics of 230 patients at enrollment. Am J Respir Crit Care Med 2006; 173:105–111
73. Johnson SR. Lymphangioleiomyomatosis. Eur Respir J 2006; 27:1056–1065
74. McCormack FX. Lymphangioleiomyomatosis: a clinical update. Chest 2008; 133:507–516
75. Johnson S. Rare diseases. 1: lymphangioleiomyomatosis: clinical features, management and basic mechanisms. Thorax 1999; 54:254–264
76. Chu SC, Horiba K, Usuki J, et al. Comprehensive evaluation of 35 patients with lymphangioleiomyomatosis. Chest 1999; 115:1041–1052
77. Kitaichi M, Nishimura K, Itoh H, et al. Pulmonary lymphangioleiomyomatosis: a report of 46 patients including a clinicopathologic study of prognostic factors. Am J Respir Crit Care Med 1995; 151:527–533
78. Taylor JR, Ryu J, Colby TV, et al. Lymphangioleiomyomatosis: clinical course in 32 patients. N Engl J Med 1990; 323:1254–1260
79. Corrin B, Liebow AA, Friedman PJ. Pulmonary lymphangiomyomatosis: a review. Am J Pathol 1975; 79:348–382
80. National Heart, Lung, and Blood Institute. Workshop Summary. Report of workshop on lymphangioleiomyomatosis. Am J Respir Crit Care Med 1999; 159:679–683
81. Silverstein EF, Ellis K, Wolff M, et al. Pulmonary lymphangiomyomatosis. AJR Am J Roentgenol Radium Ther Nucl Med 1974; 120:832–850
82. Johnson SR, Tattersfield AE. Decline in lung function in lymphangioleiomyomatosis: relation to menopause and progesterone treatment. Am J Respir Crit Care Med 1999; 160:628–633
83. Oh YM, Mo EK, Jang SH, et al. Pulmonary lymphangioleiomyomatosis in Korea. Thorax 1999; 54:618–621
84. Kim NR, Chung MP, Park CK, et al. Pulmonary lymphangioleiomyomatosis and multiple hepatic angiomyolipomas in a man. Pathol Int 2003; 53:231–235
85. Miyake M, Tateishi U, Maeda T, et al. Pulmonary lymphangioleiomyomatosis in a male patient with tuberous sclerosis complex. Radiat Med 2005; 23:525–527
86. Aubry MC, Myers JL, Ryu JH, et al. Pulmonary lymphangioleiomyomatosis in a man. Am J Respir Crit Care Med 2000; 162:749–752
87. Schiavina M, Di Scioscio V, Contini P, et al. Pulmonary lymphangioleiomyomatosis in a karyotypically normal man without tuberous sclerosis complex. Am J Respir Crit Care Med 2007; 176:96–98
88. Almoosa KF, Ryu JH, Mendez J, et al. Management of pneumothorax in lymphangioleiomyomatosis: effects on recurrence and lung transplantation complications. Chest 2006; 129:1274–1281
89. McCormack FX. Lymphangioleiomyomatosis. In: Lynch JP III, ed. Interstitial pulmonary and bronchiolar disorders (Vol. 227). New York: InformaUSA, 2008; 747–768
90. Castro M, Shepherd CW, Gomez MR, et al. Pulmonary tuberous sclerosis. Chest 1995; 107:189–195
91. Aberle DR, Hansell DM, Brown K, et al. Lymphangiomyomatosis: CT, chest radiographic, and functional correlations. Radiology 1990; 176:381–387
92. Ryu JH, Doerr CH, Fisher SD, et al. Chylothorax in lymphangioleiomyomatosis. Chest 2003; 123:623–627
93. Matsui K, Beasley MB, Nelson WK, et al. Prognostic significance of pulmonary lymphangioleiomyomatosis histologic score. Am J Surg Pathol 2001; 25:479–484
94. Avila NA, Kelly JA, Dwyer AJ, et al. Lymphangioleiomyomatosis: correlation of qualitative and quantitative thin-section CT with pulmonary function tests and assessment of dependence on pleurodesis. Radiology 2002; 223:189–197
95. Crausman RS, Lynch DA, Mortenson RL, et al. Quantitative CT predicts the severity of physiologic dysfunction in patients with lymphangioleiomyomatosis. Chest 1996; 109:131–137
96. Woodring JH, Howard RS 2nd, Johnson MV. Massive low-attenuation mediastinal, retroperitoneal, and pelvic lymphadenopathy on CT from lymphangioleiomyomatosis: case report. Clin Imaging 1994; 18:7–11
97. Avila NA, Kelly JA, Chu SC, et al. Lymphangioleiomyomatosis: abdominopelvic CT and US findings. Radiology 2000; 216:147–153
98. Johkoh T, Muller NL, Pickford HA, et al. Lymphocytic interstitial pneumonia: thin-section CT findings in 22 patients. Radiology 1999; 212:567–572
99. Jeong YJ, Lee KS, Chung MP, et al. Amyloidosis and lymphoproliferative disease in Sjögren syndrome: thin-section computed tomography findings and histopathologic comparisons. J Comput Assist Tomogr 2004; 28:776–781

100. Silva CI, Churg A, Muller NL. Hypersensitivity pneumonitis: spectrum of high-resolution CT and pathologic findings. AJR Am J Roentgenol 2007; 188:334–344
101. Colombat M, Stern M, Groussard O, et al. Pulmonary cystic disorder related to light chain deposition disease. Am J Respir Crit Care Med 2006; 173:777–780
102. Ayo DS, Aughenbaugh GL, Yi ES, et al. Cystic lung disease in Birt-Hogg-Dube syndrome. Chest 2007; 132:679–684
103. Avila NA, Chen CC, Chu SC, et al. Pulmonary lymphangioleiomyomatosis: correlation of ventilation-perfusion scintigraphy, chest radiography, and CT with pulmonary function tests. Radiology 2000; 214:441–446
104. Taveira-DaSilva AM, Hedin C, Stylianou MP, et al. Reversible airflow obstruction, proliferation of abnormal smooth muscle cells, and impairment of gas exchange as predictors of outcome in lymphangioleiomyomatosis. Am J Respir Crit Care Med 2001; 164:1072–1076
105. Crausman RS, Jennings CA, Mortenson RL, et al. Lymphangioleiomyomatosis: the pathophysiology of diminished exercise capacity. Am J Respir Crit Care Med 1996; 153:1368–1376
106. Muller NL, Chiles C, Kullnig P. Pulmonary lymphangiomyomatosis: correlation of CT with radiographic and functional findings. Radiology 1990; 175:335–9
107. Taveira-DaSilva AM, Stylianou MP, Hedin CJ, et al. Maximal oxygen uptake and severity of disease in lymphangioleiomyomatosis. Am J Respir Crit Care Med 2003; 168:1427–31
108. Taveira-Dasilva AM, Stylianou MP, Hedin CJ, et al. Decline in lung function in patients with lymphangioleiomyomatosis treated with or without progesterone. Chest 2004; 126:1867–18874
109. Steagall WK, Glasgow CG, Hathaway OM, et al. Genetic and morphologic determinants of pneumothorax in lymphangioleiomyomatosis. Am J Physiol Lung Cell Mol Physiol 2007; 293:L800–L808
110. Boehler A. Lung transplantation for cystic lung diseases: lymphangioleiomyomatosis, histiocytosis X, and sarcoidosis. Semin Respir Crit Care Med 2001; 22:509–516
111. Taveira-DaSilva AM, Hathaway OM, Sachdev V, et al. Pulmonary artery pressure in lymphangioleiomyomatosis: an echocardiographic study. Chest 2007; 132:1573–1578
112. Matsui K, Tatsuguchi A, Valencia J, et al. Extrapulmonary lymphangioleiomyomatosis (LAM): clinicopathologic features in 22 cases. Hum Pathol 2000; 31:1242–1248
113. Bernstein SM, Newell JD Jr., Adamczyk D, et al. How common are renal angiomyolipomas in patients with pulmonary lymphangiomyomatosis? Am J Respir Crit Care Med 1995; 152:2138–2143
114. Chan JK, Tsang WY, Pau MY, et al. Lymphangiomyomatosis and angiomyolipoma: closely related entities characterized by hamartomatous proliferation of HMB-45-positive smooth muscle. Histopathology 1993; 22:445–455
115. Matsui K, Takeda K, Yu ZX, et al. Role for activation of matrix metalloproteinases in the pathogenesis of pulmonary lymphangioleiomyomatosis. Arch Pathol Lab Med 2000; 124:267–275
116. Matsui K, Takeda K, Yu ZX, et al. Downregulation of estrogen and progesterone receptors in the abnormal smooth muscle cells in pulmonary lymphangioleiomyomatosis following therapy: an immunohistochemical study. Am J Respir Crit Care Med 2000; 161:1002–1009
117. Kalassian KG, Doyle R, Kao P, et al. Lymphangioleiomyomatosis: new insights. Am J Respir Crit Care Med 1997; 155:1183–1186
118. Young LR, Inoue Y, McCormack FX. Diagnostic potential of serum VEGF-D for lymphangioleiomyomatosis. N Engl J Med 2008; 358:199–200
119. Glasgow CG, Taveira-Dasilva AM, Darling TN, et al. Lymphatic involvement in lymphangioleiomyomatosis. Ann N Y Acad Sci 2008; 1131:206–214
120. Kumasaka T, Seyama K, Mitani K, et al. Lymphangiogenesis-mediated shedding of LAM cell clusters as a mechanism for dissemination in lymphangioleiomyomatosis. Am J Surg Pathol 2005; 29:1356–1366
121. Kumasaka T, Seyama K, Mitani K, et al. Lymphangiogenesis in lymphangioleiomyomatosis: its implication in the progression of lymphangioleiomyomatosis. Am J Surg Pathol 2004; 28:1007–1016
122. Seyama K, Kumasaka T, Souma S, et al. Vascular endothelial growth factor-D is increased in serum of patients with lymphangioleiomyomatosis. Lymphat Res Biol 2006; 4:143–152
123. Logginidou H, Ao X, Russo I, Henske EP. Frequent estrogen and progesterone receptor immunoreactivity in renal angiomyolipomas from women with pulmonary lymphangioleiomyomatosis. Chest 2000; 117:25–30

124. Henske EP, Ao X, Short MP, et al. Frequent progesterone receptor immunoreactivity in tuberous sclerosis-associated renal angiomyolipomas. Mod Pathol 1998; 11:665–668
125. Moss J, DeCastro R, Patronas NJ, et al A. Meningiomas in lymphangioleiomyomatosis. JAMA 2001; 286:1879–1881
126. Avila NA, Dwyer AJ, Rabel A, et al. Sporadic lymphangioleiomyomatosis and tuberous sclerosis complex with lymphangioleiomyomatosis: comparison of CT features. Radiology 2007; 242:277–285
127. Torres VE, Bjornsson J, King BF, et al. Extrapulmonary lymphangioleiomyomatosis and lymphangiomatous cysts in tuberous sclerosis complex. Mayo Clin Proc 1995; 70:641–618
128. Goncharova EA, Krymskaya VP. Pulmonary lymphangioleiomyomatosis (LAM): progress and current challenges. J Cell Biochem 2008; 103:369–382
129. Roach ES, Smith M, Huttenlocher P, et al. Diagnostic criteria: tuberous sclerosis complex: report of the Diagnostic Criteria Committee of the National Tuberous Sclerosis Association. J Child Neurol 1992; 7:221–224
130. Costello LC, Hartman TE, Ryu JH. High frequency of pulmonary lymphangioleiomyomatosis in women with tuberous sclerosis complex. Mayo Clin Proc 2000; 75:591–594
131. Sancak O, Nellist M, Goedbloed M, et al. Mutational analysis of the *TSC1* and *TSC2* genes in a diagnostic setting: genotype–phenotype correlations and comparison of diagnostic DNA techniques in Tuberous Sclerosis Complex. Eur J Hum Genet 2005; 13:731–741
132. Smolarek TA, Wessner LL, McCormack FX, et al. Evidence that lymphangiomyomatosis is caused by *TSC2* mutations: chromosome 16p13 loss of heterozygosity in angiomyolipomas and lymph nodes from women with lymphangiomyomatosis. Am J Hum Genet 1998; 62:810–815
133. Krymskaya VP. Smooth muscle-like cells in pulmonary lymphangioleiomyomatosis. Proc Am Thorac Soc 2008; 5:119–126
134. Juvet SC, Hwang D, Downey GP. Rare lung diseases I–Lymphangioleiomyomatosis. Can Respir J 2006; 13:375–380
135. Crooks DM, Pacheco-Rodriguez G, DeCastro RM, et al. Molecular and genetic analysis of disseminated neoplastic cells in lymphangioleiomyomatosis. Proc Natl Acad Sci U S A 2004; 101:17462–27467
136. Henske EP. Metastasis of benign tumor cells in tuberous sclerosis complex. Genes Chromosomes Cancer 2003; 38:376–381
137. Johnson SR, Whale CI, Hubbard RB, et al. Survival and disease progression in UK patients with lymphangioleiomyomatosis. Thorax 2004; 59:800–803
138. Johnson SR, Tattersfield AE. Clinical experience of lymphangioleiomyomatosis in the UK. Thorax 2000; 55:1052–1057
139. Rossi GA, Balbi B, Oddera S, et al. Response to treatment with an analog of the luteinizing-hormone- releasing hormone in a patient with pulmonary lymphangioleiomyomatosis. Am Rev Respir Dis 1991; 143:174–176
140. Radermecker M, Broux R, Corhay JL, et al. Failure of buserelin-induced medical castration to control pulmonary lymphangiomyomatosis in two patients. Chest 1992; 101:1724–1726
141. Harari S, Cassandro R, Chiodini J, et al. Effect of a gonadotrophin-releasing hormone analogue on lung function in lymphangioleiomyomatosis. Chest 2008; 133:448–454
142. Klein M, Krieger O, Ruckser R, et al. Treatment of lymphangioleiomyomatosis by ovariectomy, interferon alpha 2b and tamoxifen–a case report. Arch Gynecol Obstet 1992; 252:99–102
143. DeBove P, Murris-Espin M, Buscail L, et al. Somatostatin receptors in pulmonary lymphangioleiomyomatosis: therapeutic relevance. Eur Respir J 1997; 10(suppl 25):297S.
144. Schiavina M, Contini P, Fabiani A, et al. Efficacy of hormonal manipulation in lymphangioleiomyomatosis: a 20-year-experience in 36 patients. Sarcoidosis Vasc Diffuse Lung Dis 2007; 24:39–50
145. Krymskaya VP. Tumour suppressors hamartin and tuberin: intracellular signalling. Cell Signal 2003; 15:729–739
146. Wienecke R, Fackler I, Linsenmaier U, et al. Antitumoral activity of rapamycin in renal angiomyolipoma associated with tuberous sclerosis complex. Am J Kidney Dis 2006; 48:e27–e9
147. Bissler JJ, McCormack FX, Young LR, et al. Sirolimus for angiomyolipoma in tuberous sclerosis complex or lymphangioleiomyomatosis. N Engl J Med 2008; 358:140–151
148. Taille C, Debray MP, Crestani B. Sirolimus treatment for pulmonary lymphangioleiomyomatosis. Ann Intern Med 2007; 146:687–688

149. Ohara T, Oto T, Miyoshi K, et al. Sirolimus ameliorated post lung transplant chylothorax in lymphangioleiomyomatosis. Ann Thorac Surg 2008; 86:e7–e8
150. Sugimoto R, Nakao A, Yamane M, et al. Sirolimus amelioration of clinical symptoms of recurrent lymphangioleiomyomatosis after living-donor lobar lung transplantation. J Heart Lung Transplant 2008; 27:921–924
151. Morton JM, McLean C, Booth SS, et al. Regression of pulmonary lymphangioleiomyomatosis (PLAM)-associated retroperitoneal angiomyolipoma post-lung transplantation with rapamycin treatment. J Heart Lung Transplant 2008; 27:462–465
152. Chen F, Omasa M, Kondo N, et al. Sirolimus treatment for recurrent lymphangioleiomyomatosis after lung transplantation. Ann Thorac Surg 2009; 87:e6–e7
153. Kalomenidis I. Octreotide and chylothorax. Curr Opin Pulm Med 2006; 12:264–267
154. Fremont RD, Milstone AP, Light RW, et al. Chylothoraces after lung transplantation for lymphangioleiomyomatosis: review of the literature and utilization of a pleurovenous shunt. J Heart Lung Transplant 2007; 26:953–955
155. Kpodonu J, Massad MG, Chaer RA, et al. The US experience with lung transplantation for pulmonary lymphangioleiomyomatosis. J Heart Lung Transplant 2005; 24:1247–1253
156. Maurer JR, Ryu J, Beck G, et al. Lung transplantation in the management of patients with lymphangioleiomyomatosis: baseline data from the NHLBI LAM Registry. J Heart Lung Transplant 2007; 26:1293–1299
157. Benden C, Rea F, Behr J, et al. Lung transplantation for lymphangioleiomyomatosis: the European experience. J Heart Lung Transplant 2009; 28:1–7
158. Reynaud-Gaubert M, Mornex JF, Mal H, et al. Lung transplantation for lymphangioleiomyomatosis: the French experience. Transplantation 2008; 86:515–520
159. Trulock EP, Christie JD, Edwards LB, et al. Registry of the International Society for Heart and Lung Transplantation: twenty-fourth official adult lung and heart-lung transplantation report-2007. J Heart Lung Transplant 2007; 26:782–795
160. Bittmann I, Rolf B, Amann G, Lohrs U. Recurrence of lymphangioleiomyomatosis after single lung transplantation: new insights into pathogenesis. Hum Pathol 2003; 34:95–98
161. Karbowniczek M, Astrinidis A, Balsara BR, et al. Recurrent lymphangiomyomatosis after transplantation: genetic analyses reveal a metastatic mechanism. Am J Respir Crit Care Med 2003; 167:976–982
162. Alasaly K, Muller N, Ostrow DN, et al. Cryptogenic organizing pneumonia: a report of 25 cases and a review of the literature. Medicine (Baltimore) 1995; 74:201–211
163. Cordier JF. Organising pneumonia. Thorax 2000; 55:318–328
164. Ryu JH, Myers JL, Swensen SJ. Bronchiolar disorders. Am J Respir Crit Care Med 2003; 168:1277–1292
165. Cordier JF. Cryptogenic organising pneumonia. Eur Respir J 2006; 28:422–446
166. Epler GR, Colby TV, McLoud TC, et al. Bronchiolitis obliterans organizing pneumonia. N Engl J Med 1985; 312:152–158
167. Ryu JH. Classification and approach to bronchiolar diseases. Curr Opin Pulm Med 2006; 12:145–151
168. White E, Tazelaar H, Lynch JPI. Bronchiolar complications of connective tissue diseases. Semin Respir Crit Care Med 2003; 24:543–564
169. Cavallasca JA, Caubet M, Helling CA, et al. Cryptogenic organizing pneumonia (COP), as presentation of rheumatoid arthritis. Rheumatol Int 2008; 29:99–101
170. Ioannou S, Toya SP, Tomos P, et al. Cryptogenic organizing pneumonia associated with primary Sjögren's syndrome. Rheumatol Int 2008; 28:1053–1055
171. Baron FA, Hermanne JP, Dowlati A, et al. Bronchiolitis obliterans organizing pneumonia and ulcerative colitis after allogeneic bone marrow transplantation. Bone Marrow Transplant 1998; 21: 951–954
172. Uner AH, Rozum-Slota B, Katzenstein AL. Bronchiolitis obliterans-organizing pneumonia (BOOP)-like variant of Wegener's granulomatosis: a clinicopathologic study of 16 cases. Am J Surg Pathol 1996; 20:794–801
173. Wachowski O, Demirakca S, Muller KM, et al. Mycoplasma pneumoniae associated organising pneumonia in a 10 year old boy. Arch Dis Child 2003; 88:270–272
174. Stover DE, Mangino D. Macrolides: a treatment alternative for bronchiolitis obliterans organizing pneumonia? Chest 2005; 128:3611–3617
175. Radzikowska E, Szczepulska E, Chabowski M, et al. Organising pneumonia caused by transtuzumab

(Herceptin) therapy for breast cancer. Eur Respir J 2003; 21:552–555

176. Garrido M, O'Brien A, Gonzalez S, et al. Cryptogenic organizing pneumonitis during oxiliplatin chemotherapy for colorectal cancer: case report. Chest 2007; 132:1997–1999

177. Mokhtari M, Bach PB, Tietjen PA, et al Bronchiolitis obliterans organizing pneumonia in cancer: a case series. Respir Med 2002; 96:280–286

178. Martinez-Gallo M, Puy C, Ruiz-Hernandez R, et al. Severe and recurrent episodes of bronchiolitis obliterans organising pneumonia associated with indolent CD4+ CD8+ T-cell leukaemia. Eur Respir J 2008; 31:1368–1372

179. Barroso E, Hernandez L, Gil J, et al. Idiopathic organizing pneumonia: a relapsing disease. 19 years of experience in a hospital setting. Respiration 2007; 74:624–631

180. Khalid M, Al Saghir A, Saleemi S, et al. Azithromycin in bronchiolitis obliterans complicating bone marrow transplantation: a preliminary study. Eur Respir J 2005; 25:490–493

181. Freudenberger TD, Madtes DK, Curtis JR, et al. Association between acute and chronic graft-versus-host disease and bronchiolitis obliterans organizing pneumonia in recipients of hematopoietic stem cell transplants. Blood 2003; 102:3822–3828

182. Ditschkowski M, Elmaagacli AH, Trenschel R, et al. T-cell depletion prevents from bronchiolitis obliterans and bronchiolitis obliterans with organizing pneumonia after allogeneic hematopoietic stem cell transplantation with related donors. Haematologica 2007; 92:558–561

183. Belperio JA, Weigt SS, Fishbein MC, et al. Chronic lung allograft rejection: mechanisms and therapy. Proc Am Thorac Soc 2009; 6:108–121

184. Kreiss K, Gomaa A, Kullman G, et al. Clinical bronchiolitis obliterans in workers at a microwave-popcorn plant. N Engl J Med 2002; 347:330–338

185. Mann JM, Sha KK, Kline G, et al. World Trade Center dyspnea: bronchiolitis obliterans with functional improvement: a case report. Am J Ind Med 2005; 48:225–229

186. Scott AI, Sharples LD, Stewart S. Bronchiolitis obliterans syndrome: risk factors and therapeutic strategies. Drugs 2005; 65:761–771

187. Davison AG, Heard BE, McAllister WA, et al. Cryptogenic organizing pneumonitis. Q J Med 1983; 52:382–394

188. Katzenstein AL, Myers JL, Prophet WD, et al. Bronchiolitis obliterans and usual interstitial pneumonia: a comparative clinicopathologic study. Am J Surg Pathol 1986; 10:373–381

189. Cordier JF, Loire R, Brune J. Idiopathic bronchiolitis obliterans organizing pneumonia: definition of characteristic clinical profiles in a series of 16 patients. Chest 1989; 96:999–1004

190. Yamamoto M, Ina Y, Kitaichi M, et al. Clinical features of BOOP in Japan. Chest 1992; 102(1 Suppl):21S–25S.

191. Gudmundsson G, Sveinsson O, Isaksson HJ, et al. Epidemiology of organising pneumonia in Iceland. Thorax 2006; 61:805–808

192. Arakawa H, Kurihara Y, Niimi H, et al. Bronchiolitis obliterans with organizing pneumonia versus chronic eosinophilic pneumonia: high-resolution CT findings in 81 patients. AJR Am J Roentgenol 2001; 176:1053–1058

193. Akira M, Yamamoto S, Sakatani M. Bronchiolitis obliterans organizing pneumonia manifesting as multiple large nodules or masses. AJR Am J Roentgenol 1998; 170:291–295

194. Fruchter O, Solomonov A, Guralnik L, et al. An unusual radiographic manifestation of bronchiolitis obliterans organizing pneumonia. J Thorac Imaging 2007; 22:263–264

195. Haro M, Vizcaya M, Texido A, et al. Idiopathic bronchiolitis obliterans organizing pneumonia with multiple cavitary lung nodules. Eur Respir J 1995; 8:1975–1977

196. Froudarakis M, Bouros D, Loire R, et al. BOOP presenting with haemoptysis and multiple cavitary nodules. Eur Respir J 1995; 8:1972–1974

197. Pipavath SJ, Lynch DA, Cool C, et al. Radiologic and pathologic features of bronchiolitis. AJR Am J Roentgenol 2005; 185(2):354–63

198. Lee JS, Lynch DA, Sharma S, et al. Organizing pneumonia: prognostic implication of high-resolution computed tomography features. J Comput Assist Tomogr 2003; 27:260–265

199. Maldonado F, Daniels CE, Hoffman EA, et al. Focal organizing pneumonia on surgical lung biopsy: causes, clinicoradiologic features, and outcomes. Chest 2007; 132:1579–1583

200. Melloni G, Cremona G, Bandiera A, et al. Localized organizing pneumonia: report of 21 cases. Ann Thorac Surg 2007; 83:1946–1951

201. Tateishi U, Hasegawa T, Seki K, et al. Disease activity and 18F-FDG uptake in organising pneumonia:

semi-quantitative evaluation using computed tomography and positron emission tomography. Eur J Nucl Med Mol Imaging 2006; 33:906–912
202. Ryu JH, Myers JL, Capizzi SA, et al. Desquamative interstitial pneumonia and respiratory bronchiolitis-associated interstitial lung disease. Chest 2005; 127:178–184
203. Hausler M, Meilicke R, Biesterfeld S, et al. Bronchiolitis obliterans organizing pneumonia: a distinct pulmonary complication in cystic fibrosis. Respiration 2000; 67:316–319
204. Churg A, Myers J, Suarez T, et al. Airway-centered interstitial fibrosis: a distinct form of aggressive diffuse lung disease. Am J Surg Pathol 2004; 28: 62–68
205. Yousem SA, Dacic S. Idiopathic bronchiolocentric interstitial pneumonia. Mod Pathol 2002; 15:1148–1153
206. Mark EJ, Ruangchira-urai R. Bronchiolitis interstitial pneumonitis: a pathologic study of 31 lung biopsies with features intermediate between bronchiolitis obliterans organizing pneumonia and usual interstitial pneumonitis, with clinical correlation. Ann Diagn Pathol 2008; 12:171–180
207. Crestani B, Valeyre D, Roden S, et al. Bronchiolitis obliterans organizing pneumonia syndrome primed by radiation therapy to the breast: the Groupe d'Etudes et de Recherche sur les Maladies Orphelines Pulmonaires (GERM"O"P). Am J Respir Crit Care Med 1998; 158:1929–1935
208. Poulou LS, Tsangaridou I, Filippoussis P, et al. Feasibility of CT-guided percutaneous needle biopsy in early diagnosis of BOOP. Cardiovasc Intervent Radiol 2008; 31:1003–1007
209. Forlani S, Ratta L, Bulgheroni A, et al. Cytokine profile of broncho-alveolar lavage in BOOP and UIP. Sarcoidosis Vasc Diffuse Lung Dis 2002; 19:47–53
210. Lappi-Blanco E, Soini Y, Kinnula V, et al. VEGF and bFGF are highly expressed in intraluminal fibromyxoid lesions in bronchiolitis obliterans organizing pneumonia. J Pathol 2002; 196:220–227
211. Choi KH, Lee HB, Jeong MY, et al. The role of matrix metalloproteinase-9 and tissue inhibitor of metalloproteinase-1 in cryptogenic organizing pneumonia. Chest 2002; 121:1478–1485
212. Suga M, Iyonaga K, Okamoto T, et al. Characteristic elevation of matrix metalloproteinase activity in idiopathic interstitial pneumonias. Am J Respir Crit Care Med 2000; 162:1949–1956
213. Okada F, Ando Y, Honda K, et al. Comparison of pulmonary CT findings and serum KL-6 levels in patients with cryptogenic organizing pneumonia. Br J Radiol 2009; 82:212–218
214. Ishii H, Mukae H, Kadota J, et al. High serum concentrations of surfactant protein A in usual interstitial pneumonia compared with non-specific interstitial pneumonia. Thorax 2003; 58:52–57
215. Lazor R, Vandevenne A, Pelletier A, et al. Cryptogenic organizing pneumonia: characteristics of relapses in a series of 48 patients. The Groupe d'Etudes et de Recherche sur les Maladles "Orphelines" Pulmonaires (GERM"O"P). Am J Respir Crit Care Med 2000; 162:571–577
216. Costabel U, Guzman J, Teschler H. Bronchiolitis obliterans with organizing pneumonia: outcome. Thorax 1995; 50(suppl 1):559–564
217. Watanabe K, Senju S, Wen FQ, et al. Factors related to the relapse of bronchiolitis obliterans organizing pneumonia. Chest 1998; 114:1599–1606
218. Schlesinger C, Koss MN. The organizing pneumonias: an update and review. Curr Opin Pulm Med 2005; 11:422–430
219. Kobayashi I, Yamada M, Takahashi Y, et al. Interstitial lung disease associated with juvenile dermatomyositis: clinical features and efficacy of cyclosporin A. Rheumatology (Oxford) 2003; 42:371–374
220. Laszlo A, Espolio Y, Auckenthaler A, et al. Azathioprine and low-dose corticosteroids for the treatment of cryptogenic organizing pneumonia in an older patient. J Am Geriatr Soc 2003; 51:433–434
221. Verleden GM, Dupont LJ. Azithromycin therapy for patients with bronchiolitis obliterans syndrome after lung transplantation. Transplantation 2004; 77:1465–1467
222. Rubin BK, Henke MO. Immunomodulatory activity and effectiveness of macrolides in chronic airway disease. Chest 2004; 125(2 Suppl):70S–78S.
223. Labro MT, Abdelghaffar H. Immunomodulation by macrolide antibiotics. J Chemother 2001; 13:3–8
224. Kastelik JA, Greenstone M, McGivern DV, et al. Cryptogenic organising pneumonia. Eur Respir J 2006; 28:1291
225. Ichikawa Y, Ninomiya H, Katsuki M, et al. Low-dose/long-term erythromycin for treatment of bronchiolitis obliterans organizing pneumonia (BOOP). Kurume Med J 1993; 40:65–67
226. Cohen AJ, King TE Jr., Downey GP. Rapidly progressive bronchiolitis obliterans with organizing pneumonia. Am J Respir Crit Care Med 1994; 149:1670–1675

227. Perez de Llano LA, Soilan JL, Garcia Pais MJ, et al. Idiopathic bronchiolitis obliterans with organizing pneumonia presenting with adult respiratory distress syndrome. Respir Med 1998; 92:884–886

228. Chang J, Han J, Kim DW, et al. Bronchiolitis obliterans organizing pneumonia: clinicopathologic review of a series of 45 Korean patients including rapidly progressive form. J Korean Med Sci 2002; 17:179–186

Tuberculosis and Other Mycobacterial Diseases

David Ashkin, MD

Objectives:

- Become familiar with the epidemiology of tuberculosis
- Review the pathogenesis and clinical presentation of tuberculosis
- Address issues concerning the prevention of tuberculosis, including the diagnosis and treatment of tuberculosis infection
- Review issues concerning the diagnosis and treatment of tuberculosis disease
- Outline pertinent topics concerning mycobacteria other than tuberculosis (*eg*, *Mycobacterium avium* complex and *Mycobacterium kansasii*)

Key words: multidrug-resistant tuberculosis; nontuberculous mycobacteria; tuberculosis

Tuberculosis

Epidemiology

At the turn of the 20th century, tuberculosis (TB) was one of the leading causes of death in the United States. After the discovery of effective chemotherapy, the rate of TB significantly decreased at an average rate of 8% per year between 1953 and 1983. From 1985 to 1992, however, TB unexpectedly increased by approximately 20%. Factors associated with the resurgence included the HIV epidemic, increased immigration of foreign-born persons from areas of high TB incidence, an increased number of medically underserved persons (*eg*, homeless persons and drug abusers), and probably most importantly, the deterioration of the public health infrastructure for the control of TB. Associated with this increased incidence was an increase in the number of cases of drug-resistant TB.

With improvements in TB control, the overall number of cases in the United States has decreased during the last 16 years, but due to the increasing number of TB cases worldwide and the large number of international individuals arriving in the United States every year, TB remains a significant national public health problem. In 2008, there were a total of 12,898 cases of TB in the nation, with a rate of 4.2 per 100,000 persons, which is the lowest rate and total number of TB cases ever documented since national reporting began in the United States. The highest numbers of cases have been reported in California, Florida, New York, and Texas, which collectively account for 49.2% of TB cases nationally. It is estimated that approximately 15 million people are infected with TB in the United States, making for a large potential reservoir of disease in the population. The infection rate among foreign-born individuals in the United States is approximately seven times greater than that for the US-born population. Although the number of cases in the United States has been decreasing, the proportion of cases in the foreign-born population has increased from 27% in 1992 to 59% in 2008. In addition, 82% of the reported multidrug-resistant cases in the United States occurred in foreign-born individuals.

Worldwide, the rate of TB has not decreased as it has in the United States. According to the most recent statistics from the World Health Organization, the number of new cases of TB in 2007 was approximately 9.27 million worldwide, with a total prevalence of 13.7 million cases of TB disease. Ninety-five percent of TB cases occur in developing countries (especially in Africa and Asia) where HIV infection is common, and resources are scarce or unavailable to ensure proper TB treatment. It is estimated that 1.8 million people died of the disease, with a fatality rate as high as 50% in some countries with high rates of HIV coinfection. In addition, approximately one third of people in the world, or 1.86 billion people, have *Mycobacterium tuberculosis* (MTB) infection. To make matters worse, the incidence of drug-resistant TB worldwide is increasing, with new strains harboring more extensive forms of resistance (*eg*, extensively resistant TB [XDR-TB]) being more commonly recognized. During the 1990s, an estimated 30 million people died as a result of TB, making a strong argument for its being the most important pathogen in the world today.

Causative Agent of TB

TB is caused by a group of closely related mycobacteria (MTB, Mycobacterium bovis, M bovis bacillus Calmette-Guérin (BCG), Mycobacterium africanum, Mycobacterium caprae, Mycobacterium microti, Mycobacterium pinnipedii, and Mycobacterium canetti), which form the MTB complex. The MTB organism is responsible for the vast majority of cases of TB in the United States.

Transmission of MTB

The risk factors for acquiring TB infection, a prerequisite for the development of disease, are related to having contact with a source case. In the United States, important risk factors for infection are as follows: close contact with a person with TB; immigration from an endemic area (*eg*, Africa, Asia, or Latin America); exposure to untreated TB cases in congregate living facilities (*eg*, homeless shelters, correctional facilities, nursing homes, or other health-care facilities); age; and residence in high-incidence locations (*eg*, inner cities and travel to foreign endemic areas).

TB is usually spread human to human through the air by droplet nuclei, which are particles 1 to 5 μm in diameter containing MTB complex organisms. MTB enters the air when patients with active pulmonary TB cough, speak, sneeze, or sing, although coughing remains the most effective method of aerosolization. Droplet nuclei may also be produced by aerosol treatments, sputum induction, aerosolization during bronchoscopy, manipulation of lesions, or processing of tissue or secretions in the hospital or laboratory. These droplet nuclei are so small that air currents normally present in an indoor environment can keep them airborne for long periods. Individuals who are in prolonged, close contact with patients with active TB, especially in environments with poor ventilation, are most likely to inhale the organism and acquire infection (especially in congregate settings such as jails, prisons, shelters, or hospitals); however, only approximately one third of these exposed individuals acquire infection. In countries in which TB is endemic, the chances of being exposed to a person with active TB is more likely; thus, the chances for transmission are increased.

When a person inhales a droplet nucleus, which may contain 1 to 400 organisms, it usually is trapped in the upper respiratory tract and cleared. Organisms deposited on intact mucosa or skin do not invade the tissue. The smallest droplets, those measuring <5 μm, make it to the alveoli.

The chances of the transmission of MTB are influenced by the following four factors: (1) the number of organisms entering the air; (2) the concentration of organisms in the air, determined by the size of the space and the adequacy of ventilation; (3) the length of time an exposed person breathes the contaminated air; and (4) possibly the immune status of the exposed individual. Some believe that persons with HIV and others with impaired cell-mediated immunity may be more likely to acquire MTB infection after exposure than persons with normal immunity; however, disease is more likely to develop in those persons with impaired cell-mediated immunity if they have infection (discussed in the section "Pathogenesis," below).

Pathogenesis

After inhalation, the droplet nucleus is carried down the bronchial tree to a respiratory bronchiole or alveolus, where it is phagocytized by resident alveolar macrophages. The nuclei are able to survive at this primary site of infection; bacilli multiply initially within the macrophage and within 2 weeks are transported through the lymphatics to establish secondary sites. The development of an immune response, heralded by the development of delayed-type hypersensitivity during the next 4 weeks, leads to granuloma formation with a subsequent decrease in bacillary numbers. This stage of disease is called *latent TB infection* (LTBI) and is most commonly detected by a reaction to the tuberculin skin test (TST). Patients with LTBI are asymptomatic, but the condition has the potential to progress to active disease later. For most individuals with normal immune function, the proliferation of MTB is arrested once cell-mediated immunity develops, although small numbers of viable bacilli may remain within the granuloma. A primary complex can sometimes be seen on chest radiograph, but most pulmonary TB infections are clinically and radiographically inapparent. Most commonly, a positive TST result is the only indication that infection has taken place. Individuals with LTBI but not active disease are not infectious and thus cannot transmit the organism.

After TB infection, active disease develops in 3 to 5% of "immunocompetent" individuals within 2 years (defined as *progressive primary TB*, which is seen more commonly in patients with a large inoculation or immunosuppression), whereas active TB disease develops in an additional 3 to 5% of infected persons during the remainder of their lifetime. Most infected individuals are able to mount an effective immune response that encapsulates these organisms, usually for the rest of the host's life, thus preventing the progression from infection to disease. Years after the initial infection and in a small proportion of patients (approximately 5%), the immune system may not be able to contain these latent organisms, so reactivation of TB disease develops. Most cases of TB were thought to be caused by reactivation from remote infection (about 90% of cases), but studies in which the authors used DNA fingerprinting indicate that recent transmission (especially among HIV-positive individuals) probably accounts for as much as 40% of cases of TB.

Some individuals appear to be more susceptible than others to progression to TB disease. This is particularly apparent among individuals with certain medical conditions associated with varying degrees of immunosuppression (*ie*, HIV, diabetes mellitus, certain cancers, chemotherapy or immunosuppressive therapy, including tumor necrosis factor [TNF]-α blockers); silicosis; gastrectomy; old age; malnutrition; IV drug use; and renal insufficiency) and in children < 4 years old. Most of these individuals have conditions that are thought to impair cellular immunity. In fact, patients with HIV infection, with their severe defect in cellular immunity, are significantly more likely to have TB progress from infection to disease (relative risk increased 80-fold to 170-fold compared with patients without HIV infection. Unlike immunocompetent individuals, who have a 5 to 10% chance of TB progressing from infection to disease during their lifetimes, individuals patients with HIV and TB coinfection have a rate that may be as great as 8% per year. The risk of TB among anergic with HIV infection may be increased.

The partnership between HIV and TB has augmented the deadly potential of each disease. By destroying the CD4 cells of the host's immune system, HIV allows dormant TB to activate and rapidly cause disease. In response to the reactivation of TB, CD4 cells become stimulated and begin to replicate. This activation further renders the CD4 cells that are vulnerable to invasion by the HIV and allows the virus to further replicate within these cells, leading to a vicious cycle of increasing viral load and causing a further deterioration of the host's immune system. Studies have shown that the 1-year mortality rate for treated, HIV-related TB ranges from 20 to 35% and demonstrates little variation between cohorts from industrialized and developing countries.

In a person with intact cell-mediated immunity who has previously been treated for MTB, some protection against reoccurrence usually is present if MTB exposure recurs. In an otherwise-healthy, previously treated person, any organisms that are deposited in the alveoli after reexposure are likely to be killed by the cell-mediated immune response. Exceptions may occur, but in immunocompetent individuals, clinical and laboratory evidence indicates that disease produced by the inhalation of a second infecting strain is uncommon. However, reinfection has been documented both in persons without recognized immune compromise and in those with advanced HIV infection.

Classification of TB

Table 1 outlines a classification system that is used mainly as an operational framework for public health programs, which may be helpful for practicing clinicians in categorizing their patients. This classification is based on the broad host-parasite relationships as described by exposure history, infection, and disease. Table 2 reviews the US Citizenship and Immigration Services TB classification for

Table 1. *Classification of TB*

Classification	Description
0	No TB exposure, not infected
1	TB exposure, no evidence of infection
2	TB infection, no disease
3	TB, clinically active
4	TB, not clinically active
5	TB suspect (diagnosis pending)

Table 2. *US Immigrant/Refugee TB Classification**

Class	Chest Radiograph	AFB Smear	Restrictions
A: TB, infectious	Active TB	Positive	No entry to United States until treated and smears are negative
B1: TB, clinically active, not infectious	Active TB	Negative	Report to local health department for further medical evaluation within 30 d of arrival in United States
B2: TB, not clinically active	Inactive TB	Not required unless symptomatic	Same as above
No class (normal)	Normal	Not required	None

*Adapted from CDC Immigration Requirements: Technical Instructions for Tuberculosis Screening and Tuberculosis Treatment 2007. (http://www.cdc.gov/ncidod/dq/panel_2007.htm)

immigrants and refugees developed by the Centers for Disease Control and Prevention (CDC). The purpose of this classification is to identify new arrivals that are at high risk for TB and evaluate them to try to decrease the risk of active TB. It may be important for practicing physicians to be familiar with these categories because they may be asked to assist in the evaluation of such individuals.

Diagnosis and Treatment of LTBI

The TST is the most common method for identifying MTB infection in persons who do not have TB disease. Although the available TST antigens are substantially < 100% sensitive and specific for the detection of infection with MTB, no better diagnostic methods have been proven to be more effective. Blood tests approved by the US Food and Drug Administration (QuantiFERON-Gold; Cellestis Limited; Carnegie, VIC, Australia; and T-Spot. TB; Oxford Immunotec; Abingdon, UK) based on the quantification of interferon-γ released from sensitized lymphocytes in whole blood incubated overnight with antigens that are specific for MTB and control antigens hold the promise for the more specific diagnosis of LTBI.

These tests have been reported to be more specific than the TST and may be able to differentiate those individuals who may have traditionally had false-positive reactions on a TST as the result of previous exposure to nontuberculous mycobacterium (NTM) and/or BCG from those persons who truly have MTB. In fact, guidelines from the CDC now recommend that the use of such interferon-γ release assays for MTB (IGRA) may be used in all circumstances in which the TST is currently used, including contact investigations, the evaluation of recent immigrants, and sequential testing surveillance programs for infection control (*eg*, those for health-care workers). In addition, the requirement of one visit to draw the specimen (as opposed to two visits needed for conducting the TST and then subsequently to read the reaction) and a more reproducible result are also proposed advantages of the IGRA. However, the need for better definition of its performance in certain populations (*eg*, young children and immunosuppressed persons) and the need to transfer the specimen to a laboratory within 8 to 12 h are significant current drawbacks of the IGRA.

The TST is based on the fact that infection with MTB produces a delayed-type hypersensitivity reaction to certain antigens that are derived in extracts of a culture filtrate called *tuberculin*; the preparation used for testing is called *tuberculin purified protein derivative* (PPD). The diagnosis of TB infection relies on determining the size of the delayed-type hypersensitivity reaction to an intradermal injection of 0.1 mL of 5 tuberculin units of PPD (*ie*, the Mantoux method). Tests should be read 48 to 72 h after injection when the induration is at its maximum, although induration may last for up to 7 days (Erythema should not be read.) The diameter of the induration (measured transversely to the long axis of the arm) should be measured by the use of a ball-point pen. Results should be recorded as millimeters of induration. Multiple puncture tests (*eg*, the tine test) are not recommended because of their lower reliability.

Because of the lower specificity of the TST in populations with a low risk of TB infection (especially in areas with an increased prevalence of NTMs), specific cut points have been developed to improve the specificity according to the individual's risk of true TB infection and the risk of the active disease acquisition if infected.

An induration measurement of 5 mm is considered to be indicative of TB infection in patients with a high probability of infection or a high risk of disease when infection is present (*eg*, recent close contacts with TB patients, individuals with radiographic evidence of old TB, individuals with HIV infection, patients with organ transplants, patients to whom TNF-α blockers have been prescribed, and other immunosuppressed patients administered the equivalent of ≥ 15 mg of prednisone each day for > 1 month). Many reports suggesting an increased risk of progression of TB infection to active TB disease have been described in patients administered TNF blockers for conditions such as rheumatoid arthritis or inflammatory bowel disease. As such, it is generally recommended that patients who are prescribed these agents first be tested for LTBI and treated if found to have a reaction induration of > 5 mm.

Indurations measuring 10 mm are considered to be a positive result for individuals with a moderate-to-high probability of TB infection (*eg*, recent arrivals [< 5 years] from endemic areas, residents and employees of high-risk congregate settings, or mycobacterial laboratory personnel) or medical conditions that increase the likelihood of disease progression (Table 3). Patients who do not fit into these categories should be judged to have a positive reaction with indurations of 15 mm. In general, these individuals should not undergo testing for LTBI unless otherwise indicated. Persons with HIV infection may have a compromised ability to react to TSTs because of cutaneous anergy associated with progressive HIV immunosuppression. However, the usefulness of anergy testing to determine any lack of delayed-type hypersensitivity response in persons with HIV infection has not been shown to be correlated and is not recommended.

Table 3. *Medical Conditions (Other Than HIV) That Increase Risk of Progression of TB Infection*

Injection drug use
Silicosis
Diabetes mellitus
Chronic renal failure
Lymphomas, leukemias
Cancers of the head, neck and lung
Malnutrition (weight loss < 10% below ideal body weight)
Gastrectomy or jejunoileal bypass
Children younger than 4 yr who are exposed to persons at high risk for TB
Patients who receive immunosuppressive agents (including prednisone < 15 mg/d for < 1 mo and TNF blocking agents)

Confusion often arises when trying to apply the TST guidelines for LTBI in patients who have a history of vaccination with BCG. It has been shown that when a positive reaction occurs secondary to BCG vaccination, this reaction remains for at most 7 to 10 years after inoculation. Because most countries that use BCG vaccinate infants, by the time most practitioners see adults who have been vaccinated, the reaction should have waned. In those patients who have been administered a BCG vaccination, the CDC recommends ignoring the history of BCG vaccination and applying the same principles and guidelines concerning LTBI that would be used for individuals who have never been vaccinated.

Persons with negative TST reactions who are to undergo repeat annual or semiannual skin testing (*eg*, health-care workers or residents of long-term care facilities) should receive an initial two-step test. This test will help distinguish whether the development of a subsequent positive TST reaction was caused by an unrecognized booster reaction as opposed to a reaction caused by a true conversion from a recent TB exposure and subsequent infection. An example would be a person who had an initial false-negative reaction attributable to a past TB infection for which the person's immune system did not immediately react to the tuberculin. Those patients with an initial two-step test negative reaction who are found on subsequent TSTs to have an increase in the size of the reaction induration of ≥ 10 mm should be considered to have TST conversion indicative of recent infection with MTB. Two-step testing is not necessary when IGRA is used.

The identification of persons with LTBI has previously been accomplished by screening individuals or groups at variable risk for TB (*ie*, widespread programs of TST). In many situations, this screening was performed with limited consideration of the risk of TB in the population being tested. The emphasis is now on testing only those individuals who are at high risk and would benefit from treatment. To focus on groups with the highest risk of TB, the term *targeted tuberculin testing* is now being used. The dictum now is as follows: "the decision to tuberculin test is the decision to treat (and complete)." TSTs, for the most part, should not be performed in individuals for whom treatment is not contemplated. A risk of TB that is substantially greater than that in the general US population is found in persons with recent MTB infection and in those with clinical conditions associated with an increased risk of LTBI progression to active TB (Table 3). Targeted tuberculin testing should be offered only to those groups at risk and should be discouraged in those individuals at low risk. Persons infected with TB who are considered to be at high risk for the development of active TB should be offered treatment for LTBI irrespective of age.

The use of the terms *preventive therapy* and *chemoprophylaxis* has been confusing at times. To describe the intended intervention more accurately, the current guidelines recommend substituting the term *treatment of LTBI.* It is hoped that the change in nomenclature will promote a greater understanding of the concept, resulting in more widespread implementation of this important TB control strategy.

The current guideline recommends isoniazid therapy for 9 months (either 5 mg/kg/d to a maximum of 300 g, or 15 g/kg biweekly to a maximum of 900 g) for all individuals, instead of therapy for 6 months for adults and 12 months for those infected with HIV as was previously recommended. This change is based on studies that revealed 9 months of therapy to be superior to 6 months (but as effective as 12 months of therapy) in preventing the development of active disease in those persons with TB. If 9 months of isoniazid therapy cannot be accomplished, 6 months of isoniazid therapy is a less-efficacious alternative. Nine months of isoniazid therapy is recommended for children.

In response to concerns about decreased rates of completed preventive therapy, studies have shown that rifampin (10 mg/kg to a maximum of 600 mg) for 4 months or rifampin (or rifabutin) with pyrazinamide daily for 2 months in HIV-positive individuals to be effective alternatives to isoniazid. (Biweekly administration of rifampin/pyrazinamide by directly observed preventive therapy is an option if other regimens cannot be used.) However, reports of increased hepatotoxicity in patients treated with rifampin/pyrazinamide have prompted recommendations that urge a cautious and extremely limited role for this regimen, and it should only be prescribed in situations in which other recommended regimens can absolutely not be used and with close clinical and laboratory monitoring.

Before beginning therapy in patients with LTBI, active disease should be ruled out. Baseline laboratory testing is not routinely indicated for all patients at the start of or during INH therapy. It is recommended that all patients being treated for LTBI with isoniazid should receive an initial clinical evaluation and, at the least, monthly follow-up evaluations. Persons with HIV infection, pregnant women, and those in the immediate postpartum period (within 3 months of delivery), persons with a history of chronic liver disease, persons who consume alcohol regularly, and persons who are at risk for liver disease (*eg*, individuals administered other medications that affect liver function) should undergo baseline laboratory testing. Those persons with abnormal baseline liver study findings may require continued monitoring. All patients should be educated about the symptoms of hepatitis and be instructed to immediately notify the health-care provider if symptoms occur, at which time therapy should be stopped immediately and specimens for transaminase studies should be drawn. If the results are increased fivefold above the upper limit of normal or threefold above the upper limit of normal with symptoms present, treatment for LTBI should be withheld.

Clinical Manifestations, Diagnosis, and Treatment of Active TB Disease

Active TB remains primarily a disease of the pulmonary system; however, in individuals with HIV infection up to 60% of patients with TB will have extrapulmonary involvement either alone (approximately 30%) or in addition to pulmonary disease (about 33%), as opposed to 15% in individuals who are not without HIV infection. TB can occur in almost any organ, but the most common sites of extrapulmonary involvement include the pleura, lymph nodes (particularly cervical and hilar), CNS (as meningitis or tuberculoma), genitourinary system, blood, and bone marrow.

The key element in the diagnosis of TB is to have a high degree of suspicion, especially in those groups of persons who are at high risk. Early recognition of the disease is essential to stop further transmission; however, no single clinical, radiographic, or laboratory tool is sensitive or specific enough to be diagnostic, and astute clinical assessment is required. A careful history to elicit the most common symptoms of pulmonary TB (*ie*, fever, productive cough, weight loss, wasting, night sweats, shortness of breath, and occasionally hemoptysis) should be obtained. The systemic nature of many of these symptoms is caused by the cytokine release associated with the inflammatory response by the host to the organism. These symptoms are usually present for a prolonged period, characteristically weeks to months. A history of possible TB exposure risk (*eg*, previous exposure, history of homelessness, or prolonged stay in a correctional or other congregate setting, history of drug abuse, migration from an endemic area, prior PPD test) should also be elicited. Physical examination generally is not helpful in establishing the diagnosis.

Patients with prolonged symptoms, especially those who are at high risk for TB, should have a chest radiograph immediately (Table 4). Pulmonary TB in immunocompetent hosts nearly always causes abnormalities on the chest radiograph, although an endobronchial lesion may not be associated with a radiographic finding. In patients with primary TB occurring as a result of recent infection, the process is generally seen as a middle-lung or lower-lung zone infiltrate, often associated with ipsilateral hilar adenopathy. In patients with primary pulmonary pleuritis, a unilateral pleural effusion may be present. The TST result initially may be negative in these patients. Pleural fluid test findings are usually predominated by lymphocytes, are negative for acid-fast bacilli (AFB), and are positive on culture in only 50 to 60% of cases. The addition of pleural biopsy for histologic studies and culture increases the yield to approximately 80%.

Table 4. *General Indications for a Chest Radiograph To Detect TB**

- Unexplained cough (for >3 wk)
- Unexplained cough with fever (>3 d)
- Unexplained pleuritic chest pain, hemoptysis, and/or dyspnea
- Unexplained fever, night sweats, and weight loss

*From Pitchenik AE, Brooks R. The most common clinical mistakes in prevention, diagnosis and therapy of tuberculosis. In: Tuberculosis in Florida: the clinician's desktop reference. Gainesville, FL: Florida TB Control Coalition, 1999.

Pulmonary TB that develops as a result of the endogenous reactivation of LTBI in immunocompetent hosts usually causes abnormalities in the upper lobes of one or both lungs. Cavitation is common in this form of TB. The most frequent sites are the apical and posterior segments of the lung, with the right lung affected slightly more often than the left. Healing of the tuberculous lesions usually results in a scar, with the loss of lung parenchymal volume and, often, calcification. In the immunocompetent adult with TB, intrathoracic adenopathy is uncommon but may occur, especially with primary infection. As TB progresses, infected material may be spread via the airways into other parts of the lungs, causing a patchy bronchopneumonia. The erosion of a parenchymal focus of TB into a blood or lymph vessel may lead to dissemination of the organism and a miliary pattern (evenly distributed small nodules) on the chest radiograph.

Nodules and fibrotic scars are seen most commonly in old, healed TB and may contain slowly multiplying tubercle bacilli with the potential for future progression to active TB. The risk of progression is significant, and persons who have nodular or fibrotic lesions consistent with findings of previous disease found on a chest radiograph and who have a positive TST reaction should be considered high-priority candidates for the treatment of LTBI, regardless of age.

In patients with HIV infection, the nature of the radiographic findings depends to a certain extent on the degree of immunosuppression. TB that occurs in patients with HIV infection and with preserved or restored immune function tends to have the typical radiographic findings that were described in the proceeding two paragraphs. In more advanced HIV disease with associated immunosuppression, the radiographic findings become more atypical; cavitation is uncommon, and lower-lung zone or diffuse infiltrates and intrathoracic adenopathy are frequent. Clear lung fields may be present in up to 35% of patients with active TB and AIDS. Patients with symptoms or chest radiograph findings that are suspicious for TB disease should be immediately isolated if they are admitted to a health-care facility or congregate setting.

The foundation of a rapid, accurate microbiological diagnosis of TB is proper specimen collection and rapid transport to the laboratory. At least three sputum specimens should be obtained for AFB smear and culture; recent recommendations include at least one specimen to be sent for nucleic acid amplification to attempt to establish the diagnosis microbiologically. A quality sputum specimen should contain a volume of 5 to 10 mL. If the patient is unable to produce an adequate specimen, sputum induction and/or bronchoscopy should be considered (with proper infection control precautions used).

Sputum smears, the time-honored test for the diagnosis of TB, only yield a positive result for TB in approximately 50% of active cases. The advantage of the smear is that it is both rapid and cheap. The reason for its low sensitivity is the need for 10,000 to 100,000 organisms in 1 mL of specimen. In addition, the smear is not specific because other mycobacteria also may have a similar appearance. Patients with smear-positive sputa are more likely to transmit infection to contacts compared with those with smear-negative studies, although this latter group has clearly been shown to transmit infection.

Culture findings are positive in approximately 80% of cases, but unfortunately organisms take a prolonged time to grow, up to 8 weeks for solid media and 1 to 3 weeks for liquid media. At least 500 organisms per milliliter need to be present in the specimen to obtain a positive culture result. Susceptibility testing (which should be performed on all initial isolates) may take another 1 to 3 weeks, although tests that use molecular technology are now becoming available that could shorten the turn around time for susceptibility studies to 1 to 2 days.

Fifteen to twenty percent of diagnosed cases cannot be confirmed microbiologically and are considered to be culture-negative or clinical TB. In these patients, the diagnosis of TB is based on the presence of symptoms, positive TST results, a radiographic appearance compatible with TB, and an improvement in clinical status after treatment with antituberculous therapy, despite negative microbiological studies and no other etiology accounting for the illness. This is found more often in children and individuals from whom quality specimens are difficult to obtain. Bronchoscopic studies that use BAL and transbronchial biopsy, which are performed with appropriate infection control precautions, may help to establish the diagnosis and rule out other etiologies when the diagnosis is in question. When TB is strongly suspected, the initiation of presumptive antituberculous therapy is appropriate while awaiting microbiological confirmation.

Nucleic acid amplification techniques hold the promise of being able to detect a few strands of nucleic acid in a sample, amplify it, and identify the presence of TB within a matter of hours. The test is $>90\%$ sensitive and 99% specific when used in smear-positive cases. Unfortunately, in smear-negative cases, the sensitivity may only be 60 to 80%. The test has been approved by the US Food and Drug Administration for use on respiratory specimens (not approved for nonrespiratory specimens) from untreated cases. The most recent recommendations from the CDC recommend obtaining at least one (and many authorities recommend the use of multiple) specimens to improve the test sensitivity on patients suspected of having active TB disease; however, the clinician must be aware that a negative test result does not rule out the possibility of TB and that a positive test result might not guarantee a diagnosis of TB.

Since the advent and utilization of effective chemotherapy against TB in the 1950s, 95% of all individuals with pansusceptible TB who complete therapy are now cured. In those individuals with multidrug-resistant strains (resistant to at least isoniazid and rifampin) and XDR-TB (resistance to isoniazid, rifampin, a quinolone, and either capreomycin, kanamycin or amikacin), traditional chemotherapy may be ineffective in $>40\%$ of patients.

The American Thoracic Society (ATS) and the CDC recommended that four-drug therapy with isoniazid, rifampin, pyrazinamide, and either ethambutol or streptomycin be started initially in patients from areas in which isoniazid resistance exceeds 4% until susceptibility test results are available. In areas with $<4\%$ isoniazid resistance, the fourth drug may be omitted from the initial regimen. Once the results reveal susceptibility to isoniazid, rifampin, and pyrazinamide, therapy with ethambutol or streptomycin should be discontinued. After 2 months of therapy, pyrazinamide is stopped, and isoniazid and rifampin are continued for an additional 4 months for a total of 6 months of treatment (completion is also defined by the number of doses administered; Table 5).

It is important to obtain sputum cultures at the time of the completion of 2 months of therapy (called *the initial phase of treatment*) to identify patients who are at increased risk of relapse. If culture findings are not negative after 2 months of therapy and cavities are present on chest radiographs, then treatment should be extended for at least 4 months after negative results are achieved. This regimen can be administered effectively either daily or intermittently by the use of directly observed therapy (DOT; Table 5). It may also be

Table 5. *TB Treatment Options for Adults and Children With Culture-Positive Pulmonary TB Caused by Drug-Susceptible Organisms**

Initial Phase			Continuation Phase				Rating† (Evidence)‡	
Regimen	Drugs	Interval and Doses§ (Minimal Duration)	Regimen	Drugs	Interval and Doses§ ǁ (Minimal Duration)	Range of Total Doses (Minimal Duration)	HIV−	HIV+
1	INH RIF PZA EMB	7 d/wk for 56 doses (8 wk) or 5 d/wk for 40 doses (8 wk)¶	1a	INH/RIF	7 d/wk for 126 doses (18 wk) or 5 d/wk for 90 doses (18 wk)¶	182–130 (26 wk)	A (I)	A (II)
			1b	INH/RIF	Twice weekly for 36 doses (18 wk)	92–76 (26 wk)	A (I)	A (II)#
			1c**	INH/RPT	Once weekly for 18 doses (18 wk)	74–58 (26 wk)	B (I)	E (I)
2	INH RIF PZA EMB	7 d/wk for 14 doses (2 wk), then twice weekly for 12 doses (6 wk) or 5 d/wk for 10 doses (2 wk),¶ then twice weekly for 12 doses (6 wk)	2a	INH/RIF	Twice weekly for 36 doses (18 wk)	62–58 (26 wk)	A (II)	B (II)§
			2b**	INH/RPT	Once weekly for 18 doses (18 wk)	44–40 (26 wk)	B (I)	E (I)
3	INH RIF PZA EMB	Three times per week for 24 doses (8 wk)	3a	INH/RIF	Three times weekly for 54 doses (18 wk)	78 (26 wk)	B (I)	B (II)
4	INH RIF EMB	7 d/wk for 56 doses (8 wk) or 5 d/wk for 40 doses (8 wk)#	4a	INH/RIF	7 d/wk for 217 doses (31 wk) or 5 d/wk for 155 doses (31 wk)#	273–195 (39 wk)	C (I)	C (II)
			4b	INH/RIF	Twice weekly for 62 doses (31 wk)	118–102 (39 wk)	C (I)	C (II)

*Reprinted with permission from the Centers for Disease Control and Prevention from MMWR Morb Mortal Wkly Rep 2003: 52;1-77. EMB = ethambutol; RIF = rifampin; RPT = rifapentine; − = negative; + = positive.
†Ratings: A = preferred; B = acceptable alternative; C = offer when A and B cannot be given; E = should never be given.
‡Evidence: I = randomized clinical trial; II = data from clinical trials that were not randomized or were conducted in other populations; III = expert opinion.
§When DOT is used, drugs may be administered 5 days per week and the necessary number of doses adjusted accordingly. Although there are no studies that have compared five daily doses with seven daily doses, extensive experience indicates this would be an effective practice.
ǁPatients with cavitation seen on an initial chest radiograph and positive culture findings at the completion of 2 mo of therapy should receive therapy with a 7-month continuation phase (31-week; either 217 doses [daily] or 62 doses [twice weekly]).
¶Five-day-a-week administration is always given by DOT. Rating for 5 days per week regimens is AIII.
#Not recommended for HIV-infected patients with CD4+ cell counts of <100 cells/μL.
**Options 1c and 2b should be used only in HIV-negative patients who have negative sputum smears at the time of completion of 2 mo of therapy and who do not have cavitation on initial chest radiograph (see text). For patients started on this regimen and found to have a positive culture from the 2-month specimen, treatment should be extended an extra 3 mo.

used in individuals infected with HIV as well as patients with extrapulmonary disease. However, for individuals with HIV infection with a CD4 count of <100 cells/µL, daily or intermittent therapy three times a week is recommended instead of biweekly therapy as the result of reports of the development of relapse with rifampin-monoresistant disease. In addition, children with miliary TB, bone/joint TB, or tuberculous meningitis should receive a minimum of 9 to 12 months of therapy.

If pyrazinamide cannot be administered for the first 2 months, a reasonable alternative is INH and rifampin administered for 9 months. A 4-month regimen of isoniazid and rifampin is acceptable therapy for adults who have active TB and negative results of smears and cultures (*ie*, culture-negative or clinical TB).

It is essential to treat pregnant women who have active TB. Isoniazid and rifampin have been shown to be safe for use in pregnant women and should be administered. Pyrazinamide, although recommended by many authorities, has not been thoroughly studied in pregnant women and should be used at the discretion of the treating clinician. Streptomycin has been shown to be harmful to the developing fetus and should not be used.

Corticosteroids have been shown to be of benefit in preventing cardiac constriction from TB pericarditis and in decreasing neurologic sequelae resulting from TB meningitis. They may have a role in preventing bronchial stenosis in cases of diffuse endobronchial TB. The need to treat with multiple drugs for a prolonged period leads to the major obstacle facing the control of TB, *ie*, adherence to therapy. If patients do not take their medications as prescribed for the entire period, treatment failure and resistance have been shown to develop. Once medications are begun, adherence needs to be ensured.

The decrease of TB in the United States has been attributed in large part to the implementation and utilization of DOT, which has been shown to significantly improve the completion rates of TB therapy, as well as to impede the development of resistant strains. The responsibility for successful treatment has clearly been assigned by current guidelines to the public health program or private provider, not to the patient. Furthermore, it is strongly recommended that the initial treatment strategy use patient-centered case management with an adherence plan that emphasizes DOT.

Through DOT, representatives of health-care facilities (usually from the public health system) go into the community to observe and ensure that patients take their medications. Numerous studies have demonstrated that there is no reliable way to predict which patient will be adherent to therapy; therefore, all patients with active TB disease should be considered for DOT. Those who are not started on DOT should be given combination pills (*ie*, pills containing isoniazid, rifampin, and pyrazinamide together) to avoid monotherapy and the subsequent development of resistance.

Patients must be monitored for the effectiveness of treatment and toxicity. Soon after beginning therapy, patients should have an improvement in symptoms (*eg*, cough, fevers, night sweats, and weight gain). Those who do not have a symptomatic improvement or whose culture results fail to convert to negative within 2 months of treatment initiation should be evaluated for treatment failure. More than 80% of patients receiving appropriate therapy are culture negative after 2 months of treatment.

The potential reasons for treatment failure include the following: (1) resistance to prescribed medications or the use of an inadequate combination of drugs, resulting in increased drug resistance; (2) inadequate medication levels caused by malabsorption, food or drug interactions, or concurrent medical conditions; and (3) noncompliance with prescribed treatment regimens. Of these, the latter is by far the most common cause of treatment failure. It is important to seek the advice of a TB expert when patients have resistant disease, complicating concurrent medical conditions, or a lack of expected response to therapy.

Adverse reactions are not uncommon in the treatment of TB. Isoniazid, which is best known for its hepatotoxicity, also causes peripheral neuropathy, for which vitamin B_6 (pyridoxine) is prescribed as prophylaxis. Rifampin may cause hepatotoxicity in addition to muscle and joint stiffness and pain. Baseline liver function tests should be performed for all patients beginning treatment, and monthly monitoring is recommended for anyone with baseline abnormalities or concomitant liver disease. Clinical monitoring through regular inquiry of the patient as to the development systems of toxicity is recommended for all other patients. If transaminase levels become elevated and symptoms of hepatitis occur, therapy with all medications should be discontinued. Once signs and symptoms resolve or improve, medications should be reintroduced sequentially, and the patient should be monitored for the recurrence of hepatitis. Pyrazinamide can also cause hepatotoxicity as well as high uric acid levels, resulting in gout-like symptoms. Ethambutol is associated with optic neuritis, especially in doses of >20 mg/kg/d and in patients with renal insufficiency. The monthly assessment of visual acuity and color discrimination is recommended to identify patients who may have this toxicity.

Drug resistance has been increasingly recognized in the United States as well as worldwide. The most common reasons for the development of drug resistance are patient nonadherence to therapy and/or physician mistakes (*eg*, adding a single drug to an ineffective regimen). Multidrug-resistant TB is defined as strains that are resistant to at least isoniazid and rifampin. XDR-TB is defined as resistance to at least isoniazid, rifampin, a quinolone, and either capreomycin, kanamycin, or amikacin. Outbreaks of such strains have been well documented, resulting in significant rates of morbidity and mortality, especially among populations with HIV infection. The control and prevention of such outbreaks have required the expenditure of significant efforts and resources by hospital and TB control programs.

The treatment of multidrug-resistant TB is frequently unsuccessful, requiring the use of more toxic, expensive drugs, in addition to possible surgery; thus, emphasis is on the prevention. In patients with confirmed multidrug-resistant disease, therapy with at least two drugs to which the isolate is susceptible is recommended for at least 12 months after documented conversion of the cultures to negative results. Most experts recommend 18 to 24 months of total therapy. Patients with isoniazid-resistant TB can be treated with rifampin, pyrazinamide, and ethambutol for 6 to 9 months. Patients with rifampin-resistant TB should be treated with isoniazid, pyrazinamide, and ethambutol for at least 12 months after culture results convert to negative. Consultation with a TB expert is recommended for the management of drug-resistant TB.

Patients with HIV have a response to therapy similar to that of individuals without HIV infection; however, the treatment of HIV has altered TB therapy. Protease inhibitors (PIs), nonnucleoside reverse transcriptase inhibitors, and chemokine (CC motif) 5 receptor antagonists, three of the most potent agents available to control HIV, interfere with rifampin, which is the most important drug available in TB treatment. Rifampin is a potent inducer of the hepatic p450 system. For example, this induction enhances the metabolism of many of the PIs, causing reduced serum levels and leading to ineffective viral suppression, as well as the development of resistance. Conversely, many of the PIs may interfere with the metabolism of the rifamycins, causing high serum levels and potential toxicity.

On the basis of more current experience, rifabutin, which is a rifamycin derivative with less effect on the hepatic p450 system but equivalent efficacy against TB, may be used safely and effectively with the PIs. Consultation with a resource familiar with the potential pharmacokinetic interactions of these medications should be consulted to determine the best combinations and dosages for the particular patient (recent recommendations can be found at http://www.cdc.gov/tb/TB_HIV_Drugs/default.htm).

With the use of antiretroviral therapy and the subsequent improvement in the host's immune response, patients with TB disease may actually exhibit a "paradoxical" worsening of their clinical condition, which is thought to be attributable to an inflammatory response from the immune reactivation (called the *immune reconstitution inflammatory syndrome*). These patients may experience the development of new ascites, lymphadenopathy, fever, pleural effusions, or cerebral lesions. These may be life-threatening conditions, depending on the site and size of the lesion. Clinicians treating TB patients who have HIV must be aware of this phenomenon and rule out other etiologies that may be responsible for development of the lesions and/or clinical worsening. If no other etiology can be found, continued treatment for HIV and TB usually results in an improvement without further intervention. In selected cases, the use of immunomodulators (*eg*, steroids) may be indicated to slow the progression of this response.

Infection Control

Given the increased number of immunosuppressed individuals in health-care facilities, infection control efforts to stem nosocomial outbreaks of TB among patients and staff are essential. All patients who are suspected of having active TB should be immediately isolated and remain so until they are no longer infectious or until TB has been ruled out.

Airborne infection isolation rooms should have negative air pressure to prevent infected air from entering hallways and should use at least six air exchanges per hour. Health-care workers who are caring for these individuals should wear N95 masks to avoid inhaling infectious particles while working in the enclosed room. The observance of these guidelines is especially important in rooms in whim cough-inducing procedures are performed. Patients in health-care facilities can be removed from isolation once they have received medications for 10 to 14 days, they are responding clinically, and their AFB smear results are negative. Patients may be discharged from the hospital before they are removed from respiratory isolation if the following conditions are met: (1) they are returning to their previous residence (in noncongregate settings), and the health department has assessed that no vulnerable individuals (*ie*, immunocompromised persons and children <2 years of age) are present and (2) others who have been exposed have been evaluated for LTBI therapy.

Vaccination

BCG, which is an attenuated strain of *M bovis*, was first used as a vaccine in humans in the early 1920s. It has since become the most widely used vaccine preparation in the world, despite questions regarding its 0 to 80% efficacy in preventing pulmonary TB in adults. Although the data are less than ideal, numerous studies have consistently shown the effectiveness of the BCG vaccine in reducing the incidence of TB in infants and young children, particularly against potentially fatal disseminated TB. For this reason, BCG remains an important part of vaccination programs in most of the world because of its effectiveness in reducing pediatric mortality rates for disseminated TB. Its inferior efficacy in preventing TB, compared with INH treatment for LTBI, and the interference with TST has limited its use in the United States.

Diagnosis and Treatment of Pulmonary Disease Caused by NTMs

Epidemiology, Transmission, and Pathogenesis

Although not as important worldwide as TB, diseases caused by other mycobacteria appear to be more common than TB in the United States. The recognition of these organisms as pathogens is relatively recent. These organisms, characterized as the NTM, share a number of features. Unlike MTB, these NTMs are normal inhabitants of the environment (usually soil and water). Also, unlike TB, pulmonary disease and other infections caused by the NTMs are not contagious, and patients with these diseases are generally not isolated. Many clinicians believe that these organisms are opportunistic rather than virulent pathogens because some local or systemic immune impairment is required for them to cause disease.

Much remains to be understood about the pathogenesis of NTM infection and disease. It is assumed that most persons have exposure to these organisms through the environment. The aerosolization of environmental NTMs may play a role in respiratory disease, whereas ingestion may be the source of infection for children with NTM lymphadenitis and for most patients with AIDS, whose disseminated *M avium* or *Mycobacterium genavense* begins as a GI colonization. Bacteremic spread of the organism in patients with AIDS then involves multiple organ systems, including bone marrow, lymph nodes, liver, and spleen. Direct inoculation with NTM organisms from water or other material is the likely source of infection in patients with soft-tissue infections. It is not known whether NTM disease develops soon after infection or, like TB, after a period of latency.

Clinical Manifestations

Early reports concerning patients with pulmonary disease caused by NTMs involved older white men with a history of underlying lung disease. The diseases appeared to regional, with most patients from the rural southeastern United States having disease caused by *M avium*, whereas most from the central states had disease caused by *M kansasii*. NTM disease is not reportable in the United States, and an accurate incidence of the disease is limited. Severely immunosuppressed (CD4 counts of < 100 cells/µL) individuals with HIV infection are particularly susceptible to disseminated disease caused by *M avium*. Before the widespread use of highly active antiretroviral therapy, disseminated *M avium* disease developed in individuals with HIV infection who had CD4 counts of < 100 cells/µL at a rate of 20% annually. Localized pulmonary disease caused by *M avium* occurs in < 5% of cases in hosts with HIV infection. With the effective use of highly active antiretroviral therapy, however, the incidence of *M avium* disease seems to be decreasing.

Chronic pulmonary disease is the most common localized manifestation of NTMs; it usually appears in older individuals, but not all patients have a history of underlying lung disease. *M avium* complex (MAC, consisting of *M avium* and the less-common but difficult-to-distinguish *Mycobacterium intracellulare*) and *M kansasii* are the most frequent NTM pathogens causing lung disease in the United States. Other less-common NTM pathogens include *Mycobacterium abscessus*, *Mycobacterium fortuitum*, *Mycobacterium chelonae*, *Mycobacterium szulgai*, *Mycobacterium simiae*, *Mycobacterium xenopi*, *Mycobacterium malmoense*, *Mycobacterium celatum*, and *Mycobacterium asiaticum*.

Pulmonary disease caused by MAC generally is classified into the following three syndromes:

1. Upper-lobe disease that mimics reactivated TB clinically and radiographically. This syndrome is the best-known one. Patients are generally older men and have a history of COPD.
2. MAC that develops as a complication of previous bronchiectasis. This condition is usually seen in patients with a history of TB or *M kansasii* infection who present with a recurrence of symptoms and a new infiltrate in an area of old disease. These patients also tend to be older, but there is no gender predilection and no relationship to smoking-related disease. This syndrome also may occur in patients with bronchiectasis as the result of previous virus-related or bacteria-related damage or cystic fibrosis.
3. MAC with no underlying disease. These patients are predominantly women, are nonsmokers, and have interstitial rather than cavitary radiographic changes, which usually are confined to the lingula and right middle lobes (referred to as *Lady Windermere syndrome*). Some investigators have noted a progression to respiratory failure in some individuals. The finding of MAC in these patients was thought to be colonization, but recent studies that have used high-resolution CT scanning have suggested that the development of bronchiectasis in these patients is attributable to pathologic disease caused by MAC.

Signs and symptoms of NTM pulmonary disease are variable and nonspecific. They include chronic cough, sputum production, and fatigue. Less commonly, malaise, dyspnea, fever hemoptysis, and weight loss can occur, usually with advanced NTM disease. Evaluation is often complicated by the symptoms caused by coexisting lung diseases, including COPD associated with smoking, bronchiectasis, previous mycobacterial diseases, cystic fibrosis, and pneumoconiosis.

There are some differences in the radiographic features of NTM lung disease compared with those produced by MTB. NTMs tend to cause thin-walled cavities with less surrounding parenchymal infiltrate, have less bronchogenic but more contiguous spread of disease, and produce more marked involvement of the pleura over the involved areas of the lungs. Occasionally, they may produce dense pneumonic disease or a solitary pulmonary nodule without cavitation. Basal pleural disease is not often found, and pleural effusions are rare. High-resolution CT scan studies have shown that up to 90% of patients with mid- and lower-lung field noncavitary disease with MAC have associated multifocal bronchiectasis, with many patients having clusters of small (< 5 mm) nodules in associated areas of the lung (*ie*, the "tree-in-bud" pattern).

Diagnosis

In the absence of specific diagnostic features in the history, physical examination, and chest radiograph findings, culture isolation of the NTM is essential; however, because these organisms are commonly found in nature, the contamination of culture material or transient infection does occur. Thus, a single positive sputum culture finding, especially with a small numbers of organisms, is not always sufficient to diagnose NTM disease. The previous notion that individuals had true colonization with NTMs (*eg*, no tissue invasion) is now thought to probably be rare. Given the changing understanding of the disease caused by NTMs, the ATS published an official statement concerning the diagnostic criteria of NTM lung disease in HIV-seropositive and HIV-seronegative hosts. These criteria fit best with MAC, *M abscessus*, and *M kansasii* because too little is known about other NTMs to be certain how applicable these criteria would be.

The following criteria should be used to establish a diagnosis of pulmonary disease caused by NTMs. The criteria apply to symptomatic patients with infiltrate, nodular, or cavitary disease, or high-resolution CT scans that show multifocal bronchiectasis or multiple small nodules. Other etiologies for the clinical and radiologic findings should be excluded. At least three respiratory samples from each patient should be evaluated. Those having one of the following should be considered to have disease caused by NTMs:

1. Positive culture results from at least two separate expectorated sputum samples (if the results from the initial sputum samples are nondiagnostic, consider repeat sputum AFB smears and cultures); or
2. Positive culture results from at least one bronchial wash or BAL; or
3. Transbronchial or other lung biopsy specimens with mycobacterial histopathologic features (*eg*, granulomatous inflammation or AFB) and positive culture findings for NTMs or biopsy specimens showing mycobacterial histopathologic features (*eg*, granulomatous inflammation or AFB) and one or more sputum or bronchial washings that are culture positive for NTMs; or
4. Patients who are suspected of having NTM lung disease but who do not meet the diagnostic criteria should be followed up until the diagnosis is firmly established or excluded.

Expert consultation should be obtained when NTMs are recovered that are either infrequently encountered or usually represent environmental contamination. Routine susceptibility testing of all NTMs is discouraged, but such testing is warranted to obtain baseline data for unresponsive disease or when relapses occur.

Treatment

Note that making the diagnosis of NTM lung disease does not, *per se*, necessitate the institution of therapy, which is a decision based on the potential risks and benefits of therapy for individual patients.

M kansasii: Treatment for pulmonary disease caused by this organism was disappointing before the advent of rifampin therapy. With the introduction of rifamycins, the rate of treatment failures has decreased. The recommended treatment for adults consists of a regimen of daily isoniazid (300 mg); rifampin (600 mg); and ethambutol (25 mg/kg for 2 months, then 15 mg/kg for 18 months), with a minimum of 12 months of treatment after culture results are negative. Clarithromycin or rifabutin should be substituted for rifampin in HIV-positive patients who receive PIs.

M avium: The medical treatment of pulmonary disease caused by MAC in HIV-negative patients historically has been frustrating and disappointing. However, significant advances in the drugs available (*eg*, newer macrolides) have been made, and there is now greater expectation that pulmonary MAC disease can be effectively treated (defined as high rates of sputum conversion with long-term negative results on culture) with medications alone. Treatment consists of a regimen of daily clarithromycin (500 mg bid) or azithromycin (250 mg), rifampin (600 mg) or rifabutin (300 mg), and ethambutol (25 mg/kg for 2 months, then 15 mg/kg) in adults without HIV infection. Therapy with streptomycin two to three times weekly should be considered for the first 8 weeks as tolerated. Patients should be treated until culture findings are negative for 1 year.

Disseminated MAC Disease in Patients With HIV Infection: Therapy in adults should include clarithromycin, 500 mg bid, or azithromycin, 250 to 500 mg, plus ethambutol, 15 mg/kg/d. Consideration should be given to the addition of a third drug (preferably rifabutin at a dose of

300 mg/d). Therapy should be continued for life until more data become available. Prophylaxis should be administered to adults with AIDS with CD4 counts of <50 cells/ μL, especially in the presence of a history of previous opportunistic infections, consisting of rifabutin, 300 mg/d, clarithromycin, 500 mg bid, azithromycin, 1,200 mg once weekly and azithromycin, 1,200 mg once weekly, plus rifabutin, 300 mg/d.

Annotated Bibliography

American Thoracic Society, Centers for Disease Control and Prevention. Targeted tuberculin testing and treatment of latent tuberculosis infection. Am J Respir Crit Care Med 2000; 161:S221–S247

American Thoracic Society, Centers for Disease Control and Prevention. Diagnostic standards and classification of tuberculosis in adults and children. Am J Respir Crit Care Med 2000; 161:1376–1395

American Thoracic Society, Centers for Disease Control and Prevention, Infectious Diseases Society of America. Treatment of TB. Am J Respir Crit Care Med 2003; 167:603–662

American Thoracic Society, Centers for Disease Control and Prevention and the Infectious Disease Society of America. Controlling tuberculosis in the United States. MMWR Recomm Rep 2005; 54:1–81

The four official statements from the CDC and ATS that set the standards for diagnosis and treatment of TB disease and infection. They also make recommendations for public health department programs for control of the illness. Each is comprehensive and review the "science" behind the recommendations.

American Thoracic Society, Infectious Diseases Society of America. Diagnosis, treatment and prevention of nontuberculous mycobacterial diseases. Am J Respir Crit Care Med 2007; 175:367–416

An official statement from the ATS/Infectious Diseases Society of America. A very good and thorough review on NTM diagnosis and treatment.

Behr MA, Warren SA, Salamon H, et al. Transmission of *Mycobacterium tuberculosis* from patients smear negative for acid-fast bacilli. Lancet 1999; 353:444–449

A study using DNA fingerprinting that revealed that as many as 17% of TB cases may be the result of transmission from smear-negative, culture-positive patients.

Burman WJ. Issues in the management of HIV-related tuberculosis. Clin Chest Med 2005; 26:283–294

Good review of the treatment of individuals infected with HIV with TB, including necessary regimen adjustments when using HIV and TB medications concomitantly.

Centers for Disease Control and Prevention, National Institutes of Health, and the HIV Medicine Association of the Infectious Diseases Society of America. Guidelines for prevention and treatment of opportunistic infections in HIV-infected adults and adolescents. MMWR Recomm Rep 2009; 58:1–207

Most current recommendations from the CDC for the prevention and treatment of TB MAC among individuals infected with HIV.

Centers for Disease Control and Prevention. Updated guidelines on managing drug interactions in the treatment of HIV-related tuberculosis. Available at: http://www.cdc.gov/tb/TB_HIV_Drugs/default.htm.Accessed May 4, 2009

Recent recommendations concerning the concomitant administration of HIV antiretroviral agents and rifamycins.

Centers for Disease Control and Prevention. Guidelines for using the QuantiFERON-TB Gold test for detecting *Mycobacterium tuberculosis* infection, United States. MMWR Recomm Rep 2005; 54:49–55

Recent recommendations concerning the use of this test for the diagnosis of LTBI.

Colditz GA, Brewer TF, Berkey CS, et al. Efficacy of BCG vaccine in the prevention of tuberculosis: metaanalysis of the published literature. JAMA 1994; 271:698–702

A meta-analysis showing that BCG therapy is about 50% effective at preventing TB.

Mahmoudi A, Iseman MD. Pitfalls in the care of patients with tuberculosis: common errors and their acquisitions of drug resistance. JAMA 1992; 270:65–68

This classic article revealed that physicians caring for TB patients made on average 3.93 errors that subsequently contributed to the acquisition of drug resistance. The most common errors were as follows: (1) adding a single drug to a failing regimen, (2) failure to identify preexisting or acquired drug resistance, (3) initiation of an inadequate primary regimen, (4) failure to address nonadherence to therapy, and (5) inappropriate isoniazid prophylaxis. The average cost of treatment per patient was $180,000.

Narita M, Ashkin D, Hollender ES, et al. Paradoxical worsening of tuberculosis following antiretroviral therapy in patients with AIDS. Am J Respir Crit Care Med 1998; 158:157–161

Case series description of "paradoxical response" or "immune reactivation with inflammatory response" in patients with TP and HIV coinfection who received antiretroviral therapy.

Prince DS, Peterson DD, Steinger RM, et al. Infection with *Mycobacterium avium* complex in patients without predisposing conditions. N Engl J Med 1989; 321:863–868
Description of a group of patients who did not meet the previously recognized demographics for pulmonary disease caused by MAC.

Wallace RJ. Nontuberculous mycobacterial infections in the HIV-negative host. In: Rom WN, Garay S, eds. Tuberculosis. Boston, MA: Little, Brown and Company; 2004, 651–662
Well-written chapter by one of the nation's leading experts reviewing NTM in HIV-negative hosts.

Idiopathic Pulmonary Fibrosis, Nonspecific Interstitial Pneumonia/Fibrosis, and Sarcoidosis

Joseph P. Lynch III, MD, FCCP

Objectives:

- Describe the salient epidemiologic, clinical, physiologic, and radiographic features of idiopathic pulmonary fibrosis, nonspecific interstitial pneumonia/fibrosis, and sarcoidosis
- Discuss the salient features seen on high-resolution CT scans and their impact on prognosis
- Review the characteristic histopathologic features of each of these disorders and the role of transbronchial or surgical (open or thoracoscopic) lung biopsies
- Discuss the clinical role (if any) of ancillary studies such as radionuclide scanning or BAL to stage or follow up these disorders
- Review therapeutic strategies

Key words: cryptogenic fibrosing alveolitis; idiopathic pulmonary fibrosis; nonspecific interstitial pneumonia; sarcoidosis; usual interstitial pneumonia

Idiopathic Pulmonary Fibrosis

Idiopathic pulmonary fibrosis (IPF), also known as *cryptogenic fibrosing alveolitis*, is a specific form of chronic interstitial lung pneumonia associated with the histologic pattern of usual interstitial pneumonia (UIP).[1–5] Although UIP is a distinct histologic lesion,[6] this histologic pattern is not specific for IPF and can also be found in other diseases (*eg*, connective tissue diseases [CTDs]), asbestosis, and diverse occupational, environmental, or drug exposures.[2–4,7] A diagnosis of IPF can be established only when these and other alternative etiologies have been excluded.[3,4]

The cardinal features of IPF include progressive cough, dyspnea, bilateral interstitial infiltrates on chest radiographs, a restrictive ventilatory defect on pulmonary function tests (PFTs), and progressive fibrosis and destruction of the lung parenchyma.[2,3,8] The features are nonspecific and may be observed with myriad other interstitial lung diseases (ILDs).[3,4,8] The term *IPF* should be restricted to patients with the appropriate clinical features and the histologic pattern of UIP.[3,4,8] Other histologic patterns (*eg*, desquamative interstitial pneumonia [DIP][9,10]; respiratory bronchiolitis interstitial lung disease [ILD] [RBILD][10]; nonspecific interstitial pneumonia [NSIP][11–14]; acute interstitial pneumonia [AIP][15,16]; lymphoid interstitial pneumonia [LIP][17,18]; cryptogenic organizing pneumonia [COP][19]; and chronic hypersensitivity pneumonia[20,21]) are distinct entities with differing clinical expression and prognoses.[3,4] A definitive diagnosis of UIP requires surgical lung biopsy (SLB),[6] but the diagnosis of UIP can be affirmed with confidence by thin-section high-resolution CT (HRCT) scans in some patients.[22–25] IPF is one of the most frustrating disorders to manage because treatment is largely ineffective.[2,26–28]

Epidemiology

IPF is rare, but precise data regarding incidence and prevalence are lacking.[29–31] Most population-based epidemiologic surveys[29,32–35] were based on clinical diagnosis, death certificates, or diagnostic coding and lacked histologic confirmation; such studies included a mixture of ILDs, including disorders other than UIP. Studies from Europe[31–33,35] and Japan[34] cited prevalence rates of IPF ranging from 3 to 8 cases per 100,000 population. In the United States, prevalence rates range from 13 to 42 cases per 100,000.[29,30] The incidence of IPF appears to be increasing. The incidence of IPF increased progressively in the United Kingdom between 1991 and 2003.[31] Similarly, in the United States, deaths attributed to pulmonary fibrosis (PF) increased significantly from 1992 to 2003 (>28% increase).[36]

The incidence of IPF is much greater in men and in the elderly (peak onset after the sixth decade of life).[25,28–31,34,36,37] In the United States, the rate of mortality from IPF is increasing more rapidly in women than men,[36] possibly reflecting the impact of cigarette smoking. In one study in the United States, the prevalence of IPF in adults between

35 to 44 years of age was 2.7 per 100,000.[29] By contrast, the prevalence exceeded 175 per 100,000 in adults >75 years old.[29] Rates of mortality from IPF are markedly increased in the elderly. In the United States, projected deaths (per million) in 2008 were as follows: 18 (ages 45 to 54 years); 71 (ages 55 to 64 years); 306 (age 65 to 74 years); 827 (age 75 to 84 years); and 1,380 (age >85 years).[36] The incidence of idiopathic UIP is a rare occurrence in children.[3,38,39] Despite its rarity, IPF accounts for >16,000 deaths annually in the United States[36]; this mortality rate is greater than a number of malignancies, including bladder cancer, multiple myeloma, and acute myelogenous leukemia.[36]

Risk Factors for IPF

The cause of idiopathic UIP is unknown, but environmental and occupational exposures likely play etiologic roles.[40–42] IPF is more common in current or former smokers.[25,26,42–44] The degree of exposure (quantified as pack-years of smoking) is directly correlated with the occurrence of IPF.[43,45] Importantly, ever-smoking remains a risk factor for the development of IPF, even after smoking cessation.[43] In familial IPF, smoking was discovered to be the strongest associated risk factor and had an odds ratio of 3.6.[46] Risk factors for IPF cited in some studies included the following: exposure to metal and wood dusts,[34,40,44–47] organic solvents,[34] and residence in agricultural or polluted urban areas.[34,37,44] However, a study from the British Isles[33] found no evidence for an increased risk of IPF among individuals exposed to wood or metal dusts. In that study, an increased rate of mortality caused by IPF was noted in electricians, electrical engineers, firemen, and cleaners, occupations associated with exposure to potentially toxic fumes or chemicals.[33]

A meta-analysis[42] of six case-control studies found the following six exposures associated with IPF: ever-smoking, agriculture farming, livestock, wood dust, metal dust, and stone/sand. ILD is an occupational disease in coal miners; sandblasters; and workers exposed to asbestos, tungsten carbide, beryllium, and other metals,[41] suggesting that at least some cases of idiopathic UIP represent pneumoconioses. The considerable variability that exists in the development of PF among workers exposed to similar concentrations of fibrogenic/organic dusts implies that genetic factors are likely important in modulating the lung injury.[42]

Chronic aspiration secondary to gastroesophageal reflux (GER) is a possible cause (or contributory factor) in the pathogenesis of IPF.[48–50] PF is a common complication of systemic sclerosis (scleroderma), a disorder with an extremely high prevalence of esophageal dysmotility.[51] Aspiration of stomach contents (acid or not), leads to lung injury and fibrosis.[41,52] Esophageal reflux has been noted in more than two thirds of patients with IPF awaiting lung transplant (LT).[48–50,53] Importantly, 30 to 50% of IPF patients with GER have no symptoms of reflux.[48,49,53] Further, the severity of IPF does not correlate with the severity of GER.[48,49] Among LT recipients (with or without IPF), GER can cause allograft injury[52,54] and appears to be a risk factor for bronchiolitis obliterans syndrome.[54,55]

In light of these findings, aggressive treatment of GER is recommended to reduce the chance for repetitive lung injury, which may elicit fibrosis. In a small series of patients with early IPF,[48] aggressive treatment of GER was associated with stabilization or improvement of lung function. Further, retrospective studies[56,57] of LT recipients found that early fundoplication (within 3 months of LT) was associated with greater freedom from bronchiolitis obliterans syndrome and improved lung function[58] in patients with GER. Additional studies are required to assess the role of GER or aspiration in the pathogenesis or progression of IPF and therapeutic strategies to prevent or reduce GER.

Several lines of evidence suggest that genetic factors are important in the pathogenesis of IPF. Clusters of IPs/fibrosis in families (familial interstitial pneumonia [FIP]) have been noted in 0.5 to 3.7% of patients with IPF.[38,46,59–62] The mode of transmission of FIP is not known but is believed to be autosomal dominant with variable/reduced penetrance.[46,59,61,62] Familial IP is indistinguishable from nonfamilial (sporadic) IPF, but patients tend to be younger with the familial variant.[60,61,63] Interestingly, multiple types of IPs have been noted in FIP (*eg*, UIP, NSIP, DIP, COP; 46,64). In one study[46] of 78 patients with histologically confirmed FIP, histologic patterns included the following: UIP (86%), NSIP (10%), COP (2.5%), and unclassified (1.3%). Forty-five percent of pedigrees exhibited more than one histologic pattern among affected family members.[46] In familial IPF, asymptomatic

ILD may progress to symptomatic IPF during a period of decades.[64]

Interestingly, gene expression profiles of lung tissues from patients with familial IP (either UIP or NSIP) exhibit striking similarities but differ from gene expression profiles in sporadic IPF.[65–67] Mutations in genes encoding proteins involved in chronic inflammation (*ie*, chemokines, complement, and Igs); smooth-muscle markers (*ie*, smooth-muscle cells and myofibroblasts); and/or matrix mobilization and resolution[65–67] may be important in the pathogenesis of IPF. Genetic polymorphisms for interleukin (IL)-1 receptor antagonist or tumor necrosis factor (TNF)-α,[68] complement receptor,[1,69] or transforming growth factor (TGF)-β[70] may influence risk of IPF or disease progression. Interestingly, polymorphism of the angiotensinogen gene was associated with IPF progression but not with disease predisposition.[71] Mutations in the gene for surfactant protein C may cause FIP (including UIP, NSIP, and DIP.[72–76]

Germ-line mutations in the genes *hTERT* and *hTR*, which encode telomerase reverse transcriptase and telomerase RNA, were implicated in dyskeratosis congenita, a rare hereditary disorder associated with PF and aplastic anemia.[77] These mutations result in telomere shortening, which limits the replicative capacity of tissues and has been implicated in age-related disease.[78] Interestingly, older age and smoking also cause telomere shortening.[77] The authors of two studies[79,80] found that short telomeres were more common in FIP and sporadic IPF compared with control patients, even when mutations in hTERT and hTR were lacking. PF may also complicate diverse genetic disorders such as Hermansky-Pudlak syndrome.[81] familial hypocalciuric hypercalcemia,[82] and neurofibromatosis.[83] IPF occurs in white and in nonwhite populations; the prevalence among different ethnic groups has not been studied.[3] However, in the United States, mortality rates caused by IPF were greater in non-Hispanic white compared with Hispanic or black populations.[36] A retrospective study[84] of IPF in New Zealand cited a lower incidence in those of Maori or Polynesian descent than in those of European descent.

Differences in susceptibility to fibrogenic agents may reflect genetic polymorphisms.[59,60] Animal models involving different inbred strains of rodents demonstrate dramatic variability in the lung inflammatory/fibrotic response to injurious agents.[85,86] The aforementioned studies suggest that IPF is a heterogeneous disorder caused by a number of environmental/occupational exposures in combination with genetic predispositions.

Clinical Features of IPF

Initial symptoms of IPF are cough (typically nonproductive) and dyspnea.[2] Over time, the cough may become paroxysmal and debilitating, and dyspnea and exercise limitation worsen. Physical examination reveals end-inspiratory rales (often with a "Velcro" quality) in >85% of patients with IPF.[2,28] Clubbing is noted in >25% of patients.[2,3,28] Extrapulmonary involvement does not occur[2] and should suggest other disorders (particularly CTD-associated pulmonary fibrosis [PF]).[87] However, certain diseases, such as ischemia cardiac disease,[88–90] deep venous thrombosis,[88] diabetes mellitus,[91,92] and GER,[49,91] are more common in patients with IPF. The onset of the disease is usually indolent, but IPF progresses inexorably over months to years.[2,3,25,27,28]

The course is highly variable, with some patients maintaining stability for years,[2,93] whereas in others the course is rapid, with fatal respiratory failure evolving over a few months.[94] Additionally, some patients have gradual progression over years, followed by acute exacerbations associated with abrupt and often fatal hypoxemia respiratory failure.[93,95] Spontaneous remissions do not occur.[2,3] Mean survival from the onset of symptoms approximates 3 to 5 years.[25,26,28,96] Fewer than 15% of patients survive 10 years from the onset of symptoms.[25–28] Older age[27,28,96] and more severe impairments in pulmonary function or HRCT scans[27,28,96,97] are associated with a worse prognosis. Some studies[27,28,45,94,98] cited greater rates of mortality in men, but others[28] did not.

The major cause of death is respiratory failure[99,100]; surveys of deaths among IPF patients in the United Kingdom and United States noted that progression of lung disease accounted for 72%[100] and 60%[36] of deaths, respectively. Other causes include pulmonary embolism,[99,101] lung cancer,[99,101,102] cardiac failure, cerebrovascular accidents (primarily in the elderly).[101] Acute respiratory failure requiring mechanical ventilation may complicate IPF, either from infection or an acute exacerbation of the underlying disease process.[95,103–106] In this context, mortality is high (>90%). For this reason, mechanical ventilation is usually ill-advised in patients with severe IPF. Unfortunately, medical therapy has not been shown to alter the course of the disease.

Lung Cancer Complicating UIP

Lung cancer occurs in 4 to 13% of patients with IPF.[102,107–109] The risk is greater in smokers,[107,109] but the heightened risk of lung cancer is not solely a result of the effects of cigarette smoking.[102,107] Surgical resection may be curative in IPF patients with non-small cell lung cancer, but postoperative morbidity and mortality is increased.[110,111]

Acute Exacerbations of UIP

A subset of patients with IPF have an accelerated course of the disease, often as a terminal event, characterized by severe hypoxemia, dyspnea, and pulmonary infiltrates on chest radiographs or CT scans,[95,104,112–114] This syndrome has been termed *acute exacerbation of IPF.*[95] Clinical and radiographic features resemble the ARDS.[95,104,112,113] The cardinal histologic feature on lung biopsy or necropsy is diffuse alveolar damage and/or organizing pneumonia superimposed on a background of UIP.[104,113] Idiopathic AIP[15,16] exhibits similar clinical and histologic features as acute exacerbation of IPF, but it lacks the requisite features of UIP. The factors responsible for this accelerated phase of IPF are unknown, but viral infections, high concentrations of oxygen, or drug reactions are plausible etiologic factors.[16] This syndrome is usually fatal. Favorable responses have been noted with high-dose IV pulse methylprednisolone, but data are limited to anecdotal cases and small series.[15,95,104,112–114]

Laboratory Tests

Laboratory test results in IPF are nonspecific. The erythrocyte sedimentation rate is increased in 60 to 94% of patients; circulating antinuclear antibodies or rheumatoid factor have been found in 10 to 26% of patients with IPF.[2,3] These serologic studies[2,3] do not correlate with the extent or activity of the disease and do not predict therapeutic responsiveness. However, for new cases of suspected IPF, we obtain serologies for CTD (*eg*, antinuclear antibody and antibodies to SSA, SSB, Scl-70 [scleroderma], Sm, RNP, Jo-1, double-stranded DNA) and hypersensitivity pneumonitis (HP) to rule out those disorders. Elevations of the glycoprotein KL-6[115,116] and lung surfactant proteins A and D[116–118] have been noted in serum and BAL fluid in patients with IPF and may have prognostic value. These assays are available in only a few research laboratories, and additional studies are required to assess their specificity and clinical role.

Chest Radiographs

Chest radiographs in IPF typically reveal bilateral interstitial (reticular) infiltrates with a predilection for the basilar and peripheral (subpleural) regions of the lung (Fig 1).[2,3] With progression of the disease, all lung fields are affected and lung volumes decrease. Similar radiographic features may be observed in asbestosis and CTD-associated PF.[119,120] Pulmonary hypertension and cor pulmonale may be seen in far-advanced cases.[121] Intrathoracic lymphadenopathy and pleural thickening are not features seen on plain chest radiographs but may be noted on CT.[122] Chest radiographs have limited prognostic value, but serial radiographs

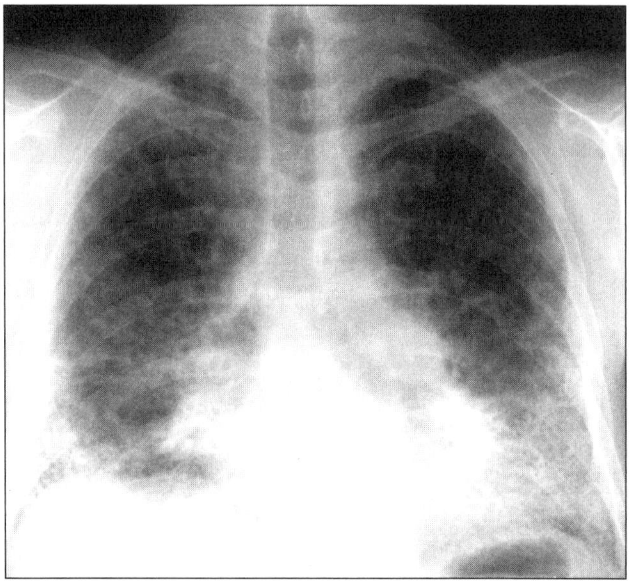

Figure 1. IPF/UIP. Posteroanterior chest radiograph from a 61-year-old man with IPF/UIP demonstrates extensive reticulonodular infiltrates with a bibasilar predominance. A mixed alveolar and interstitial pattern is evident in the lower lobes.

(including old films) may be used to gauge the pace and evolution of the disease.[2]

Thin-Section HRCT Scans

HRCT Features and Value in the Differential Diagnosis: HRCT scans, using thin (1- to 2-mm) sections without the use of contrast, are far more accurate than conventional chest radiographs in assessing the extent and nature of the disease.[123,124] HRCT has diagnostic[24,125,126] and prognostic[98,123,124,127] value and should be part of the initial evaluation of suspected ILD. The HRCT features of IPF/UIP are stereotypic and predictable and include a patchy, heterogeneous distribution with a predilection for the peripheral (subpleural) and basilar regions of the lungs; small cystic radiolucencies (*ie*, honeycomb change [HC]); coarse reticular or linear opacities (intralobular and interlobular septal lines); ragged pleural surfaces; irregular or thickened bronchial walls or pulmonary vessels; and bronchiectasis and bronchiolectasis (Figs 2-6).[23,121]

Air bronchograms (1 to 2 mm in diameter) reflect dilated peripheral airways surrounded by fibrotic lung tissue. Bronchovascular thickening, a cardinal feature of sarcoidosis, is minimal or absent in UIP.[121] Focal ground-glass opacities (GGOs)—hazy zones of increased alveolar attenuation—may be present in IPF/UIP[127] but are not a dominant feature.[23] HC is highly characteristic of IPF/UIP but may be absent in mild cases.[22,127] In severe cases, severe volume loss, anatomic distortion, and dilated pulmonary arteries are observed. Zones of

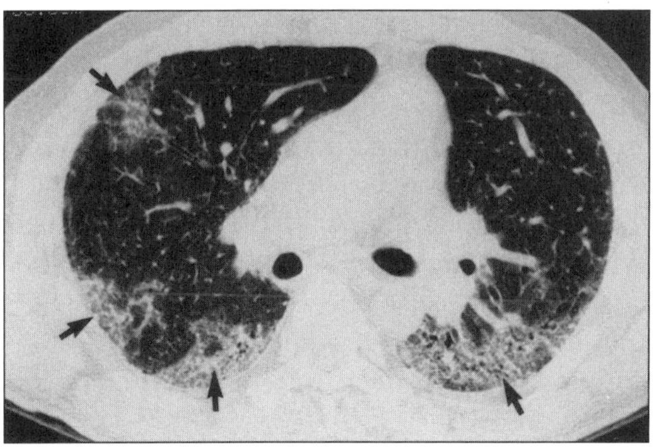

Figure 2. UIP. HRCT demonstrates foci of GGOs in the subpleural regions of the lower lobes (arrows). A few small honeycomb cysts are also present. The central portions of the lung are relatively spared.

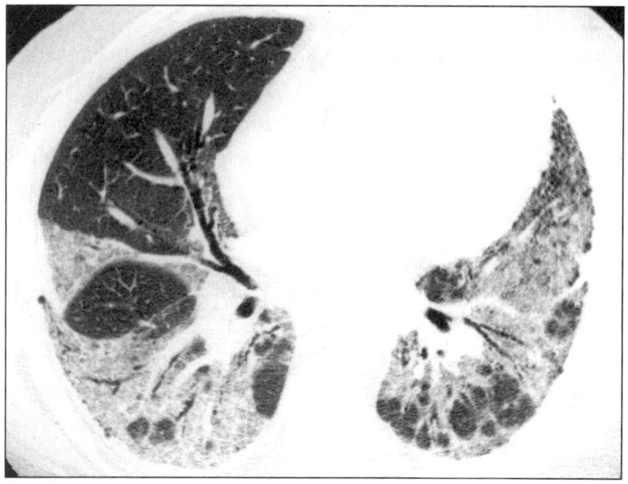

Figure 3. HRCT from a 53-year old man with UIP confirmed on open-lung biopsy specimen. Note extensive areas of GGOs with air-bronchograms in the lower lobes. Despite extensive involvement of the posterior regions of both lower lobes, the anterior portion of the left lower lobe is relatively normal, emphasizing the patchy nature of the disease.

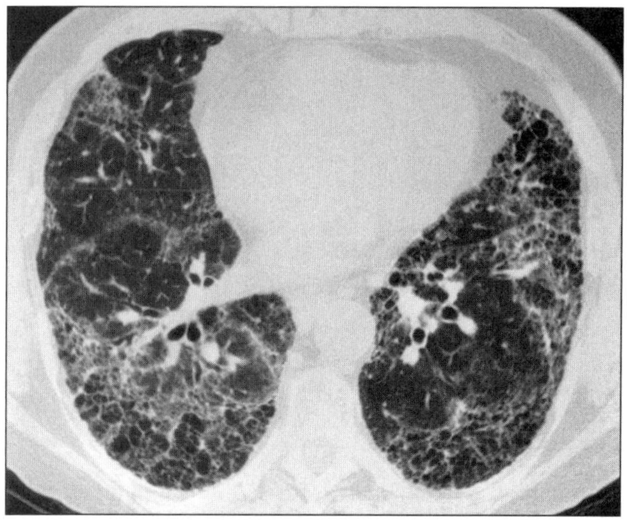

Figure 4. HRCT from a 63-year-old woman with UIP confirmed on open-lung biopsy specimen. HC is evident, particularly in the peripheral (subpleural) regions. Dilated bronchi, indicating traction bronchiectasis, are also present. There are no GGOs.

emphysema (particularly in the upper lobes) may be present concomitantly in smokers.[128–131] Mediastinal lymph node enlargement (LNE) has been noted in 53 to 93% of patients with IPF[24,132–135] but is nonspecific.[134,135] LNE in IPF usually involves only one or two nodal stations, and the nodes usually measure <15 mm.[133,135] The presence of LNE correlated with the extent of disease in some studies[133,134] but not all studies.[122,132] One study[133] noted

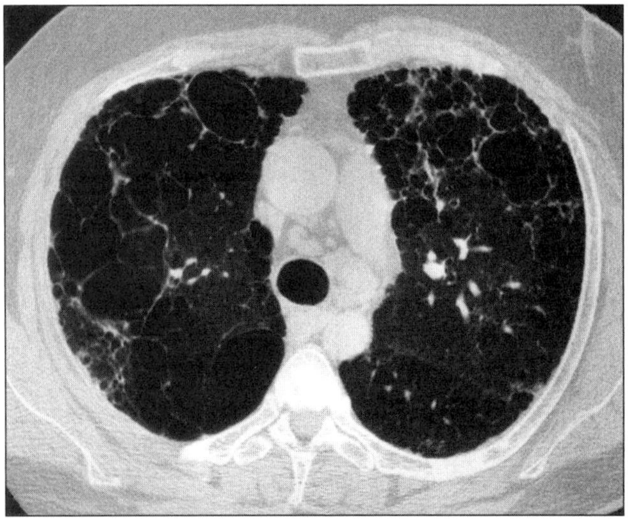

Figure 5. HRCT from a 44-year-old man with severe UIP on open-lung biopsy specimen. Note the marked cystic radiolucencies (some cysts are >3 cm in diameter) and honeycombing involving both lungs. Although most of the lung parenchyma has been destroyed, note the accentuation of the cystic disease process in the peripheral (subpleural) regions.

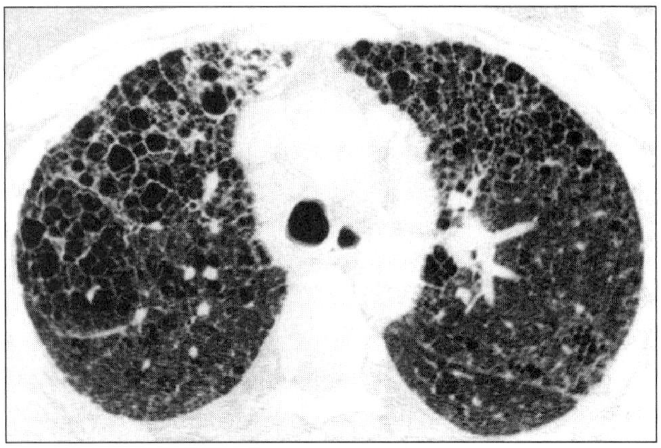

Figure 6. HRCT from a 48-year-old woman with UIP, with extensive cystic radiolucencies (honeycomb cysts) scattered throughout the lung parenchyma. Despite treatment with corticosteroids, AZA, and CP, she died of progressive respiratory failure.

that increase in LNE over time was associated with progression of fibrosis in UIP or NSIP.

Differential Diagnosis by HRCT: Focal GGOs may be observed in UIP, but the presence of predominant or extensive GGOs suggests an alternative diagnosis such as DIP,[136] HP,[4,137,138] cellular NSIP,[4,11,13,139] COP,[19] chronic eosinophilic pneumonia,[140] or pulmonary alveolar proteinosis.[141] HC is a cardinal feature of UIP[121] but is absent in AIP[15] and DIP.[4,136] Honeycombing is not a prominent feature in NSIP, but focal HC may be seen in fibrotic variants of NSIP.[22,139] Cystic radiolucencies may be observed in other disorders (*eg*, Langerhans-cell histiocytosis,[142] sarcoidosis,[143] lymphangioleiomyomatosis,[144] chronic HP,[145] LIP,[18] pneumoconiosis), but the distribution of lesions and presence of concomitant abnormalities differentiates these disorders from UIP.[146]

Can HRCT Obviate the Need for SLB in IPF?: HRCT may obviate the need for SLB, provided the CT features are classical for UIP (including presence of honeycombing.[22,24,98,125] The accuracy of a confident diagnosis of UIP by a trained observer is >95%.[22,24,98,125] However, classical features of UIP (confident diagnosis by CT) are present in only 34 to 67% of patients with histologically confirmed UIP.[2,24,125,127] Interobserver and intraobserver variability may be problematic[127]; consensus is usually reached when extensive HC and subpleural predominance are deemed to be present.[22] CT patterns overlap between UIP and fibrotic NSIP.[139] Subpleural predominance, reticulation, and HC may be found in fibrotic NSIP, and focal GGOs may be observed in UIP.[127,139] Predominant GGOs make the diagnosis of UIP unlikely.[139,147]

When CT features are typical for UIP, specificity approaches 100%.[22,24] In one study,[22] two radiologists independently assessed CT scans from a cohort of patients with either idiopathic UIP (n = 73) or NSIP (n = 23). CT scans were categorized as definite UIP, probable UIP, indeterminate, probable NSIP, or definite NSIP. CT features were typical (definite or probable) of UIP in 27 of patients (37%); with histologic UIP on SLB. Importantly, all 27 patients with a CT pattern of probable or definite UIP had histologic UIP on SLB. In contrast, only 18 of 44 patients (41%) with probable or definite NSIP on CT had histologic NSIP on SLB (59% had UIP).[22] These data suggest that CT features of UIP are associated with advanced, late-stage disease. Among patients with earlier phases of UIP, CT features may be atypical[148] or indeterminate.[22] When HRCT features are classical for UIP (including HC), SLB is not necessary. However, SLB should be performed when CT scans are nondiagnostic or atypical unless specific contraindications exist.[98]

Prognostic Value of HRCT in IPF: The prognosis of IPF can be inferred from the extent and nature (*ie*, predominant pattern) of HRCT abnormalities.[123,124,127,148,149] The extent of disease on CT correlates roughly with severity of functional impairment (*ie*, FVC and diffusing capacity of the lung for carbon monoxide [DLco])[128,150]; the pattern of CT does not.[150] When serial CT scans were performed, changes in CT were concordant with physiologic parameters (*eg*, FVC and DLco).[128,151] PFTs improved only when GGOs regressed on HRCT[128,151]; extensive fibrosis or HC on HRCT predicted the progression of disease.[123,124,151]

Early reports[149,151–154] noted that a predominant GGO pattern in patients with IPF correlated with greater rates of response to corticosteroid therapy (improvement in 33 to 44% of cases) and greater survival compared with reticular or HC patterns. However, it is likely that patients with extensive GGO who were responsive to corticosteroids had histologic patterns distinct from UIP, such as DIP,[136] NSIP,[139,155] or HP.[4,137] Combinations of patterns (*eg*, GGO, reticular, HC) may be present in individual patients.[2,121] In some patients, GGOs evolve to HC or reticular lines.[149,151,154] Reticular patterns or HC do not regress and may worsen over time.[23,128,130,149,156]

Severe HC on CT is a strong predictor of mortality (> 80% mortality within 2 years).[98,123,124] British investigators[124] evaluated prognostic variables in a cohort of 115 patients with UIP awaiting LT. By multivariate stepwise regression analysis, only DLco percentage of predicted and CT-fibrotic (CT-fib) scores independently predicted 2-year survival. Receiver operating curve analysis gave the best fit (predictive value) with a combination of DLco and CT-fib scores. The optimal points on the receiver operating curves discriminating survivors from nonsurvivors corresponded to a DLco of 39% of predicted and CT-fib scores > 2.25.[124] The curve resulting from a model combining these two parameters yielded a specificity and sensitivity of 84% and 82%, respectively, for discriminating survivors from nonsurvivors.

These data are remarkably similar to our own data.[123] We extended our experience in a cohort of 106 patients with UIP,[98] which confirmed that CT-fib score ≥ 2.0 was a significant predictor of mortality. A mean CT-fib score ≥ 2.0 in any lobe was associated with increased mortality (risk ratio, 3.35) compared with patients with a CT-fib score < 2 in all lobes. A similar finding was noted when patients were segregated by mean CT-fib ≥ 2 for all lobes (risk ratio, 2.5; $p = 0.002$). However, when the histologic diagnosis was incorporated into the model, the diagnosis of UIP was the most powerful predictor of mortality and overshadowed the predictive ability of the CT-fib score.[98]

In a multicenter prospective study[23] of 315 patients with IPF, greater CT-fib scores and lower DLco correlated with increased mortality risk (by multivariate analysis). Other investigators[148,155] noted that CT patterns typical of IPF/UIP were associated with a greater rate of mortality compared with atypical CT scans, suggesting that CT features typical of IPF reflect advanced disease. However, in a recent study,[127] the authors retrospectively reviewed 98 patients with a histologic diagnosis of UIP who underwent CT scans. Patterns of CT scans were categorized as follows: (1) definite UIP, (2) probable UIP, and (3) suggestive of alternative diagnosis. Mean survival rates were 45.7, 57.9, and 76.9 months, respectively. Median survival rates were 34.8, 43.4, and 112 months, respectively. Although these differences between groups did not achieve statistical significance, these data suggest that patients whose CT scans are interpreted as definite UIP have a worse prognosis. By multivariate analysis, the extent of traction bronchiectasis and fibrosis scores influenced prognosis. More complex HRCT scoring systems that use stereologic methods correlate well with open-lung biopsy[157] but are logistically difficult and of limited clinical utility. In summary, extensive HC or reticulation on CT and no or minimal GGO suggests a low likelihood of response to medical therapy and high mortality (98,123,124). Unless contraindications exist, these patients should be listed for LT.[158]

Several studies[128,130,155,156] assessed evolution of CT over time. Pulmonary functional parameters improved only when GGO regressed on HRCT.[128,130,156] Serial PFTs are more useful than serial CT scans to assess prognosis. In one study[155] of 60 patients with IPF, we found that increasing extent of GGO on CT (> 10% increase from baseline) at 6-month follow-up was associated with greater rates of mortality, whereas change in CT-fib score did not predict long-term survival. By multivariate analysis, decreases in FVC at 6 months and UIP diagnosis were associated with worse survival compared with patients who had stable or improved FVC or a histologic diagnosis of NSIP.[155] Changes in CT-alveolar or CT-fib scores did not contribute further information once these factors were included in the multivariate model. Given the potential for fibrosis to evolve over time, the value of CT in predicting long-term prognosis is modest.[22]

Physiology

Characteristic physiologic aberrations in IPF include reduced lung volumes (FVC and total lung capacity [TLC]) consistent with a restrictive defect; normal or increased expiratory flow rates; impaired oxygenation, and impaired gas exchange.[3,159] The DLCO is reduced, often disproportionately to other aberrations.[129,150,159] The DLCO is an indirect reflection of the pulmonary vasculature; reductions reflect destruction or loss of alveolar walls or capillaries. In nonsmokers with IPF, expiratory flow rates are preserved, and the ratio of FEV_1 to FVC is increased. When emphysema also is present, lung volumes (*ie*, FVC and TLC) are preserved, and DLCO is disproportionately reduced.[128,129,131,150]

The measurement of the DLCO is complex and varies even among individual patients. Normalizing the DLCO by the lung volume, yielding the DLCO/lung volume ratio, does not improve the predictive value of DLCO and is not necessary.[159] Reduced compliance and alterations in pressure-volume curves are characteristic of IPF,[28] but these sophisticated studies require an esophageal balloon and lack clinical value. Impaired oxygenation, which is accentuated with exercise, is a cardinal feature of IPF.[28,159,160] Early in the course of the disease, Pao_2 may be preserved at rest but invariably worsens with exercise. As the disease advances, hypoxemia at rest is a nearly universal feature. Cardiopulmonary exercise tests (CPETs) reveal hypoxemia or widened alveolar-arterial oxygen pressure difference [$P(A\text{-}a)O_2$]; reduced oxygen consumption; increased dead space; increased minute ventilation for the level of oxygen consumption; high-frequency, low-tidal volume breathing pattern; and low oxygen puls.[28,159,161,162]

Impact of Physiologic Tests on Survival

Not surprisingly, severe derangements in PFTs or oxygenation predict a worse prognosis and lower rates of survival.[2,159] Survival is worse in patients with severe impairments in vital capacity (VC) or DLCO. The 3-year rate of mortality is > 50% when VC decreases to < 60% of predicted or DLCO decreases to < 45% of predicted.[2,159] Changes in TLC are less predictive of survival.[2,159] However, the prognostic value of physiologic parameters at a single time point is limited.[93] Further, disparate results have been reported from different centers. For example, in one retrospective study[163] of 53 patients with UIP, decreased percentage of predicted DLCO was independently linked to the rate of mortality ($p = 0.01$), whereas three other studies[28,164,165] found no such relationship. In those studies, the following parameters correlated with rates of mortality: percentage of predicted FVC ($p < 0.05$) and widened $P(A\text{-}a)O_2$ ($p < 0.005$)[165]; multistage Pao_2 on CPET ($p = 0.006$)[164]; and reduced lung volumes and abnormal oxygenation during maximal exercise.[28]

British investigators[124] examined 2-year survival among a cohort of 115 IPF patients awaiting LT. The best predictors of survival (assessed at 2 years) were as follows: DLCO > 39% of predicted and less fibrosis on HRCT scan.[124] In a separate study[166] by these investigators, 116 nonsmokers with IPF were prospectively assessed to evaluate predictors of prognosis. The following variables predicted survival (by multivariate analysis): percentage of predicted TLC, percentage of predicted DLCO, age, and clearance of inhaled ^{99m}Tc-diethylenetriamine penta-acetic acid (DTPA) from the lungs.

Several investigators[28,160,167–174] have found that hypoxemia (at rest or exercise) is an independent predictor of mortality in patients with IPF or fibrotic NSIP. The 6-min walk test (6MWT) with oximetry is a noninvasive and relatively inexpensive way to ascertain prognosis and need for supplemental oxygen therapy and follow the course of IPF. We[160] performed the 6MWT in 83 patients with UIP and 22 patients with NSIP; desaturation to ≤ 88% strongly correlated with mortality. Among patients with UIP, desaturation was associated with increased risk of death (hazard ratio, 4.2; $p = 0.01$) after adjusting for age, sex, smoking, baseline DLCO, FVC, and resting oxygen saturation.[160] Further, 6-min walk distance (6MWD) correlates with percentage of predicted DLCO[124,168,170] and has prognostic value.

In one study[169] of IPF patients awaiting LT, survival time was shorter among patients with 6MWD < 350 m. A subsequent study[168] by these investigators retrospectively analyzed the utility of 6MWD as a predictor of mortality in a cohort of 454 IPF patients awaiting LT. Lower 6MWD was associated with increased mortality (assessed at 6 months) and was superior to FVC percentage of predicted as a predictor of mortality. Patients with 6MWD < 207 m had a more than fourfold-greater mortality rate than those with 6MWD ≥ 207 m, even after adjustment for demographics, FVC percentage of predicted, pulmonary hypertension, and medical comorbidities.[168] Flaherty et al[175] assessed the prognostic value of 6MWD and extent of desaturation on 6MWT in a cohort of 197 patients with IPF. By multivariate analysis, 6MWD was not a reliable predictor of mortality, but the degree of desaturation during 6MWT had greater prognostic value.

Patients with oxygen saturation ≤ 88% during their initial 6MWT had a median survival of 3.2 years compared with 6.8 years for those with baseline arterial oxygen saturation > 88% ($p = 0.006$). The prognostic value of serial changes in FVC, DLCO, 6MWD, and desaturation area (DA) varied according to the extent of desaturation on 6MWT.[175] Among patients with an oxygen saturation < 88% during 6MWT, a decrease in DLCO emerged as the only predictor of mortality; changes in FVC, DA, or walk distance were not predictive in this group. For patients with an oxygen saturation > 88% during 6MWT, decreases in FVC and increases in DA predicted subsequent mortality, whereas decreases in 6MWD and DLCO were less predictive.

These data emphasize the importance of stratifying by baseline level of desaturation when assessing prognosis. Recently, a 6-min step dose was advocated as another way of assessing exercise capacity and prognosis in patients with IPF or other ILDs.[176] Formal CPET provides additional data, including measurement of maximal oxygen uptake ($\dot{V}O_2$), an integrated measure of respiratory, cardiovascular, and neuromuscular function.[162] One recent study[161] evaluated $\dot{V}O_2$ as a predictor of survival in a cohort of 117 patients with IPF. Patients with baseline $\dot{V}O_2$ < 8.3 mL/kg/min had an increased risk of death after adjusting for age, smoking status, FVC, and DLCO. Further, $\dot{V}O_2$ was a stronger predictor than desaturation < 88% on 6MWT. However, $\dot{V}O_2$ did not predict survival when examined as a continuous variable. However, CPET with arterial cannulation is invasive, logistically difficult, difficult to perform for some patients, and lacks practical value.

Clinical-Radiographic-Physiologic Scoring Systems

Watters et al[177] developed the clinical-radiographic-physiologic (CRP) scoring system, a composite score incorporating clinical (dyspnea), radiographic (chest radiographs), and physiologic parameters to more objectively monitor the course of IPF. A modification of the CRP score (arbitrary total of 100 points) was developed; it predicted survival better than physiologic or radiographic features alone.[28] In one prospective study[28] of 238 patients with UIP, a comprehensive CRP score (obtained at the time of initial visit) was used to predict survival. Parameters included age, finger clubbing, smoking history, the extent of profusion of interstitial opacities and pulmonary hypertension on chest radiographs, percentage of predicted TLC, and Pa_{O_2} during maximal exercise. In addition, an abbreviated CRP score, excluding Pa_{O_2} during maximal exercise, was applied.

The comprehensive CRP score was superior to the abbreviated CRP score, but both scoring systems had excellent prognostic value. The modified CRP score predicted 5-year survival with remarkable accuracy.[28] Five-year survival rates at CRP scores of 20, 40, 60, and 80 points were 89%, 53%, 4%, and < 1%, respectively. The abbreviated CRP was less accurate but more adaptable to clinical practice. Although HRCT data were not included in that study, it is likely that incorporating HRCT data in place of chest radiographs would enhance the predictive value of such systems. Further, it can be argued that other parameters (*eg*, FVC or DLCO) could be substituted in place of TLC.

British investigators[165] developed a composite physiologic index (CPI) incorporating CT and physiologic parameters. The CPI score evaluated disease extent observed by CT and selected functional variables (*eg*, percentage of predicted FVC, DLCO, and FEV_1). Exercise components were not included in this index. The CPI accounts for coexisting emphysema, which may confound pulmonary functional indexes. Importantly, CPI predicted the rate of mortality better than PFTs or CT parameters in isolation. Further, the CPI was compared with the original[177] or modified[28] CRP scoring systems in 30 patients with UIP who underwent exercise testing. The CPI was a superior predictor of outcome compared with the physiologic component of the original CRP score ($p = 0.02$) and the physiologic component of the modified CRP score ($p = 0.009$). The CPI score is promising but may not be easily adapted into clinical practice settings. Additional studies using these or similar CRP scoring systems would be of interest.

What Is the Role of Sequential Physiologic Studies To Follow UIP?

Sequential physiologic studies are critical to assess the evolution of the disease. I obtain serial measurements of FVC, DLCO, and oxygen saturation (by pulse oximetry) at 3- to 4-month intervals to follow the course of the disease.[2] The FVC is logistically easy to perform, relatively inexpensive, and less variable than TLC or DLCO. Thus, FVC is an ideal parameter to follow in individual patients. Because of inherent variability, serial changes in DLCO are less reliable. Formal CPETs with arterial cannulation are inconvenient, expensive, and lack practical value.[2] Serial 6MWTs with oximetry are more convenient and cost-effective for monitoring the course of the disease[160] and assessing the need for supplemental oxygen. Although optimal parameters to assess response to therapy have not been validated, the American Thoracic Society (ATS) defined improvement as ≥10% increase in FVC or TLC, ≥15% increase in DLCO, or ≥4% increase in oxygen saturation or ≥4 mm increase in Pa_{O_2} during exercise.[3] Improvement or stability in VC or DLCO with corticosteroid therapy is associated with improved prognosis.[123,178,179] Conversely, deterioration in VC or DLCO at 3 months,[179] 1 year,[178] or later time points[180] predicts a greater rate of mortality.

In a retrospective study,[155] we assessed the value of serial PFTs in 80 patients with UIP and 29 patients with NSIP. For patients with UIP, a change in FVC was the best physiologic predictor of mortality. By multivariate analysis, ≥10% decrease in FVC at 6 months was an independent risk factor for mortality (hazard ratio, 2.47; $p = 0.006$).[155] In addition, ≥10% increase in GGO on HRCT (*ie*, CT-alveolar) at 6 months predicted a greater risk of subsequent death (relative risk, 2.88; $p = 0.001$) compared with <10% change.[155] A change in DLCO at 6 months did not add independent prognostic value. Changes in CT-fib or TLC did not predict long-term survival when adjusted for corresponding baseline values. Further, baseline alveolar-arterial gradient [$P(A\text{-}a)O_2$] was not a predictor of survival.

Collard et al[181] evaluated the prognostic value of serial clinical (dyspnea score) and physiologic parameters in 81 patients with IPF. (All had histologically confirmed UIP.) Survival correlated with dyspnea scores and pulmonary functional parameters [FVC percentage of predicted, $P(A\text{-}a)O_2$] at baseline, as well as changes in these parameters at 6- or 12-month time points. Not surprisingly, survival was worse among patients with deteriorating dyspnea scores or PFTs at 6 or 12 months.[181] British investigators[172] retrospectively reviewed the prognostic significance of histopathologic diagnoses, baseline PFTs, and serial trends in pulmonary functional indexes (*eg*, FVC, FEV_1, DLCO) at 6 and 12 months in 104 patients (UIP, $n = 63$; fibrotic NSIP, $n = 37$). Survival was better in fibrotic NSIP compared with UIP ($p = 0.001$) but not in patients with severe functional impairment. Mortality during the first 2 years was linked solely to the severity of functional impairment at presentation (*ie*, lower DLCO and FVC levels). The CPI score[165] was the strongest determinant of outcome ($p < 0.001$).[172] At 6 months, serial PFTs and histopathologic diagnosis were prognostically equivalent.[172] However, at 12 months, serial PFT trends (DLCO, FVC, FEV_1, CPI) predicted mortality better than any other covariates including histologic pattern (all $p < 0.0005$). In this context, change in DLCO provided the best prognostic information (2-year survival); histologic pattern provided no additional prognostic value. However, for late deaths (beyond 3 years), the risk of mortality was greater with UIP than with fibrotic NSIP.

Pulmonary Arterial Hypertension Complicating IPF

Pulmonary arterial hypertension (PAH) and right ventricular (RV) dysfunction are common in patients with IPF.[182–184] The pathogenesis of PAH in IPF is complex and does not correlate with lung volumes or extent of pulmonary dysfunction.[183,185–188] Pulmonary artery remodeling and proangiogenic cytokines are likely central to developing PAH in

IPF,[183,185,189] but ablation of pulmonary vessels and vasoconstriction may play contributory roles.[183] In patients with advanced IPF, PAH was noted in 20 to 84% of patients.[131,182,187,190–193] However, one prospective study[186] of patients with all stages of IPF noted PAH (mean pulmonary artery pressure [mPAP] > 25 mm Hg by right-heart catheterization [RHC]) in only 8.1%. One recent study[184] of 44 patients with IPF awaiting LT found that mPAP increased progressively over time (rate of change 3.8 mm Hg per month in the entire cohort). Baseline lung function, oxygen requirements, or mPAP did not predict the rate of change in mPAP nor which cases progressed to New York Heart Association functional class IV.

The presence of PAH is associated with markedly worse survival.[131,186,187,190,194] In one study,[190] 88 patients with IPF had estimates of systolic pulmonary artery pressure (sPAP) by transthoracic echocardiography (TTE). Increased sPAPs were noted in 84% of patients; sPAP exceeded 50 mm Hg in 27 patients (31%). Median survival was significantly worse among patients with sPAP > 50 mm Hg (0.7 years) compared with patients with sPAP ≤ 35 mm Hg (4.8 years) or sPAP of 36 to 50 mm Hg (4.1 years). Others parameters associated with worse survival by univariate analysis included male gender; lower DLCO, use of oxygen, history of coronary artery disease, and worse New York Heart Association functional class.[190] In another cohort of 79 IPF patients, 1-year mortality rates were 28% in those with PAH (defined as mPAP > 25 mm Hg by RHC) compared with 5.5% in those without PAH.[187] Another prospective study[186] evaluated 61 patients with IPF who had RHC. Five-year survival was 83% among patients with normal pulmonary artery pressure (PAP) and preserved DLCO (≥ 40% of predicted) compared with only 16% among patients with high PAP, low DLCO, or both ($p < 0.001$).[186] Several investigators[183,187,188,191,193] found that the DLCO correlates with PAH, whereas FVC or lung volumes do not.

Screening for PAH among patients with IPF is reasonable because it has prognostic value and may influence therapy. TTE is invaluable to assess RV size and function and estimate sPAP and is superior to chest CT as a predictor of PAH.[193] Severe RV hypertrophy, reduced RV function, and abnormal bowing of the interventricular septum on TTE reflect RV dysfunction. TTE may allow the estimation of sPAP, which has prognostic value. However, TTE has only modest predictive value for PAH.[193,195] In one study[195] of 106 patients with ILD, estimates of sPAP by TTE and RHC were discordant by > 10 mm Hg in 63% of patients. Accuracy improved when sPAP was < 45 mg Hg.[195]

We[193] performed TTE and RHC in 61 IPF patients; estimation of RV systolic pressure was possible in 33 patients (54%). By using a RV systolic pressure > 40 mm by RHC as a cutoff, we found that sensitivity and specificities for PAH were 76% and 38%, respectively. Exercise-induced desaturation, reduced DLCO (< 40% predicted), or need for supplemental oxygen are surrogate markers for PAH in IPF.[190,193] The FVC/DLCO ratio and oxygen saturation may be markers for PAH.[190,193] In a cohort of IPF patients.[193] a model incorporating FVC/DLCO ratio and oxygen saturation was superior to TTE (improved specificity and negative predictive value) in assessing PAH. DLCO did not contribute to mPAP prediction above and beyond oxygen saturation, whereas FVC/DLCO ratio did. However, RHC is invasive, and its role in patients with IPF is controversial. RHC is not necessary in patients with IPF when TTE results are normal but should be considered when TTE results suggest RV dysfunction or PAH.

Reduced 6MWT distance and increased plasma brain natriuretic peptide (BNP) are surrogate markers of PAH in patients with PF.[188,194] In one study,[188] 39 patients with PF and severe restrictive lung disease (FVC < 55% predicted, including 28 with UIP) underwent RHC, measurement of BNP levels, and 6MWT. Among 28 patients with IPF, increased BNP concentrations correlated with increased PAP and pulmonary vascular resistance and correlated inversely with 6MWT distance. Importantly, PFT results did not differentiate between patients with normal and elevated PAPs. Korean investigators[194] retrospectively analyzed 131 IPF patients with both TTE and plasma BNP measurements; sPAP > 40 cm H_2O was used as the threshold for PAH. Both PAH and elevated BNP were independent predictors of mortality. One-year mortality and mean survival rates were worse among patients with PAH (61% and 10.8 months) compared with 20% and 23.7 months among patients without PAH. Further, prognosis was much worse among patients with elevated BNP levels compared with those with normal BNP levels (1-year mortality

70.5% vs 23.7%; mean survival 11.0 months vs 22.5 months, respectively). The combination of both PAH and BNP was a more robust marker of mortality than either value alone. These data[188,194] suggest that plasma BNP concentration may be a useful a noninvasive marker to screen for PAH.

The impact of treating PAH in patients with IPF has not been elucidated. Favorable responses to sildenafil (a phosphodiesterase inhibitor),[192,196] prostacyclin,[182] iloprost,[197] or endothelin-1 (ET-1) receptor antagonists[198] have been noted in IPF patients with PAH, but impact on long-term outcome has not been established. A multicenter placebo-controlled trial sponsored by the Idiopathic Pulmonary Fibrosis Clinical Research Network evaluating sildenafil for severe IPF is in progress. The use of ET-1 receptor blockers has theoretical value in IPF-associated PAH,[182,183] but data are limited. In a double-blind randomized controlled trial (DBRCT),[198] 158 patients with IPF were randomized to bosentan (an endothelin-1 receptor antagonist) or placebo. Patients with severe disease (FVC $<50\%$ of predicted or DLCO $<30\%$ of predicted or $Pa_{O_2} < 55$ mm Hg) or PAH were excluded. At 12 months, bosentan was not superior to placebo with regard to the primary end point (*ie*, 6MWD); further, physiologic parameters (FVC, DLCO, arterial oxygen saturation) did not differ between groups. However, a trend in favor of bosentan was noted in secondary end points (including time to death or disease progression [hazard ratio, 0.61, $p = 0.12$] and quality of life and dyspnea scores).[198] Another randomized controlled trial (RCT)[199] evaluating bosentan among IPF patients with severe disease or PAH is in progress (Bosentan Use in Interstitial Lung Disease [BUILD-3]). Mediators such as TGF-β, TNF-α, platelet-derived growth factor, and other profibrotic cytokines may be involved in the pathogenesis of IPF-associated PAH.[183,200] Therapies targeting specific cytokines are worthy of study,[201] but data are lacking.

Histologic Features

The histologic pattern of UIP observed in patients with IPF[3,5,6] can be found in other etiologies (*eg*, CTD, asbestosis, and diverse occupational, environmental, or drug exposures).[3,6] Historically, UIP was considered a subset of patients with IPF,[202] but current recommendations restrict the term *IPF* to patients with idiopathic UIP.[3,6] In 2002, the ATS and European Respiratory Society published a classification schema recognizing seven idiopathic interstitial pneumonias (IIPs): UIP; NSIP, organizing pneumonia, AIP, RBILD, DIP, and LIP (Table 1).[4] UIP is the most common of the IIPs, comprising 47 to 71% of cases; NSIP accounts for 13 to 48% of cases.[3,96,98,147,148,203–205] Clinical, physiologic, and radiographic features of UIP and NSIP overlap; further, fibrotic NSIP and UIP may be difficult to distinguish even by experienced pathologists.[155,172,204,206,207] The remaining IIPs are less common and exhibit clinical features that are in sharp contrast to UIP. Salient features of these other IIPs are reviewed elsewhere (*eg*, DIP,[10] RBILD,[9,208] NSIP,[11,209,210] AIP,[4,16,112] COP,[19] and LIP[17,18]). The literature is confusing, however, because these variants were often included in series of IPF, even though clinical, radiographic, and prognostic features are disparate.

UIP: The histologic diagnosis of UIP requires an SLB, preferably with wedge biopsies from two or three sites.[7,211] Care should be taken to avoid the worst areas (*ie*, areas with advanced HC).[7,211] Cardinal features of UIP that distinguish this entity from other IIPs are temporal heterogeneity, profusion of fibroblastic foci (FF), and HC.[3,5,6] UIP exhibits both geographic and temporal heterogeneity. The lesions are bilateral but patchy and exhibit a striking predilection for the basilar and peripheral (subpleural) regions of the lung. This nonuniform distribution can be appreciated at low-power magnification (Fig 7, *top*).

In addition to geographic heterogeneity, the lesions also exhibit temporal nonuniformity. Areas of active injury, inflammation, and fibroblastic

Table 1. *Classification of IIPs**

Histologic Pattern	CRP Diagnosis
UIP	IPF/cryptogenic fibrosing alveolitis
NSIP	NSIP (provisional)
OP	COP
Diffuse alveolar damage	AIP
Repiratory bronchiolitis	RB-ILD
DIP	DIP
LIP	LIP

*Adapted from Amer J Respir Crit Care Med.[4]

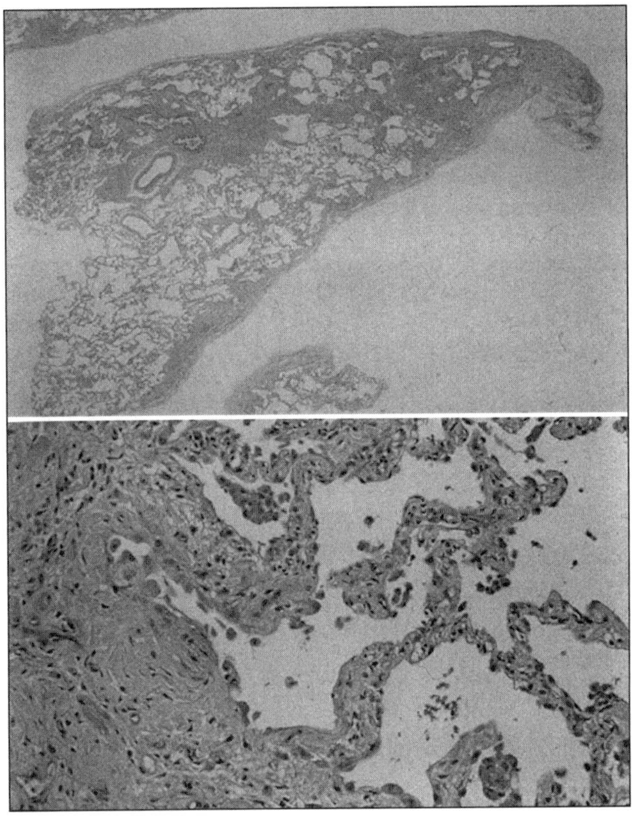

Figure 7. *Top*: Photomicrograph of UIP in open-lung biopsy specimen. Patchy subpleural fibrosis with dense scarring cause remodeling of lung architecture. Note the marked heterogeneity (hematoxylin-eosin) [reproduced with permission from Lynch et al, J Respir Dis 2000; 21;197–214]. *Bottom*: Photomicrograph of UIP in an open-lung biopsy specimen. Fibrosis shows heterogeneity with dense eosinophilic collagen and a loose FF. The adjacent lung is relatively unaffected. These findings are consistent with UIP (hematoxylin-eosin) [reproduced with permission from Lynch et al, J Respir Dis 2000; 21;197–214].

proliferation coexist with areas of dense (old) fibrosis. Even within the same lobe, alternating zones of interstitial inflammation, fibrosis, HC, and normal lung can be observed. Alveolar walls are thickened by excessive collagen, extracellular matrix, patchy mononuclear cell infiltrates (*eg*, lymphocytes, plasma cells), and fibroblasts.[3,6] Intra-alveolar macrophages may be observed but are not conspicuous. Scattered neutrophils or eosinophils may be present. These inflammatory changes are not prominent and are usually confined to areas of collagen deposition or HC.[6]

The variability of UIP is also evident when the nature of the fibrosis is examined. Zones of "old," relatively acellular collagen bundles are interspersed with aggregates of actively

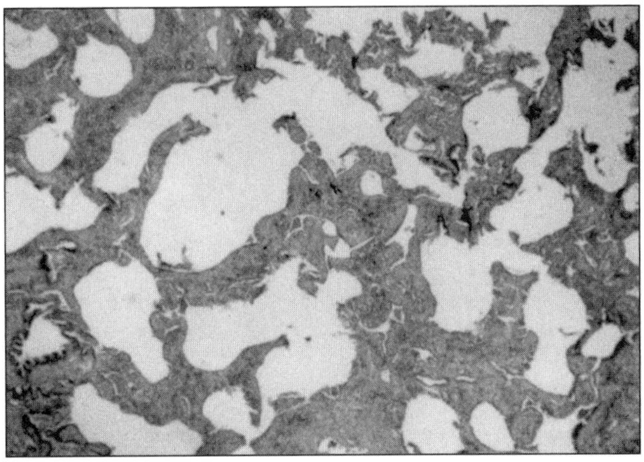

Figure 8. Photomicrograph of IPF. Open-lung biopsy specimen reveals end-stage honeycomb lung. The large cystic airspaces represent destroyed and coalescent alveolar septae. Minimal inflammatory cells are present at this late phase [reproduced with permission from Lynch JP III, Strieter RM. In: Internal medicine for the specialist. Montvale, NJ: Medical Economics, 1988; 61–84].

proliferating myofibroblasts and fibroblasts. These aggregates, termed *fibroblast foci*, develop in areas of previous lung injury and are associated with active collagen synthesis. FF are not pathognomonic but are necessary for the diagnosis of UIP (Fig 7, *bottom*).[6] Small cystic radiolucencies (termed *honeycomb cysts*) within the subpleural regions reflect irreversible scarring and architectural remodeling.[5,6] HC is an essential and often prominent feature of UIP but is not specific because it may be a sequela of severe lung injury caused by diverse causes.[4] In late phases of UIP, the lung architecture is destroyed and replaced by large cystic air spaces (remnants of previous alveoli) and dense scar. Such cases are termed *end-stage fibrosis* or *honeycomb lung* (Fig 8).[5] Secondary features include pulmonary hypertensive changes, smooth-muscle hypertrophy and hyperplasia, type II pneumocyte proliferation and hyperplasia, bronchiolectasis, and traction bronchiectasis. Subpleural fat and metaplastic bone reflect severe disease.[203] Focal emphysematous blebs may be present in smokers.

DIP: DIP is a histologic syndrome characterized by dense collections of alveolar macrophages within air spaces (Fig 9), a homogeneous pattern, preserved alveolar architecture, and minimal or absent fibrosis or honeycombing.[4,10,212] A significant interstitial component is lacking and is overshadowed by the intra-alveolar component. The striking

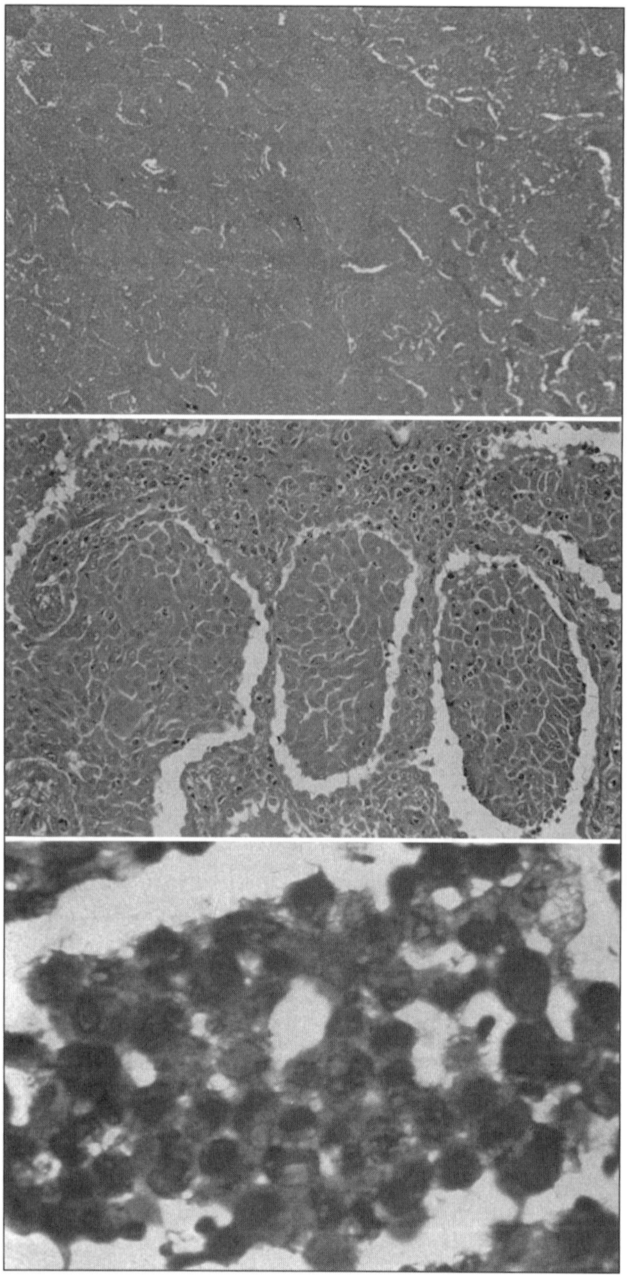

Figure 9. *Top*: Photomicrograph of DIP. Open-lung biopsy specimen demonstrates extensive and diffuse filling of the alveolar spaces with alveolar macrophages. A single lymphoid aggregate is present. The alveolar architecture is preserved [reproduced with permission from Lynch et al, J Respir Dis 2000; 21;197–214]. *Center*: Photomicrograph (high power) of DIP showing dense aggregates of alveolar macrophages filling the alveolar spaces. The alveolar walls are thickened, but the alveolar architecture is preserved. Fibrosis or honeycomb cysts are absent [reproduced with permission from Lynch et al, J Respir Dis 2000; 21;197–214]. *Bottom*: DIP. Dense aggregates of alveolar macrophages fill alveolar spaces (hematoxylin-eosin) [reproduced with permission from Lynch et al, J Respir Dis 2000; 21;197–214].

heterogeneity and peripheral distribution characteristic of UIP are lacking in DIP. The uniformity of the lung lesion in DIP suggests a reaction to an inhaled stimulus rather than persistent alveolar injury characteristic of UIP. More than 90% of patients with DIP are smokers, suggesting that constituents of tobacco play a pathogenic role.[10,212] Chest radiographs typically demonstrate reduced lung volumes and nonspecific linear or reticulonodular interstitial infiltrates; in one fourth of patients, bibasilar, hazy GGOs are present.[9]

HRCT scans demonstrate diffuse GGO, often with bibasilar or subpleural predominance; HC is absent.[10] The average age of onset of symptoms for patients with DIP is approximately 40 years.[10,212] PFTs demonstrate a restrictive defect, with reduced DLCO.[10,212] Prognosis is generally good, with long-term survival exceeding 90% at 5 years.[10,212] Although most patients are treated with corticosteroids, spontaneous improvement may occur.[10,212] Cessation of cigarette smoking is mandatory. Most patients improve or stabilize with the administration of corticosteroids,[9,10,212] but progressive, even fatal, respiratory failure can ensue. The role of cytotoxic and other immunosuppressive agents has not been studied.

RBILD

RBILD, grouped with the IIPs, is characterized by dense collections of pigmented alveolar macrophages within respiratory bronchioles but sparing the distal lung parenchyma.[9,212,213] Honeycombing and severe fibrosis are not found. The pathologic lesion *respiratory bronchiolitis* was originally described in an autopsy series of young cigarette smokers who died of nonpulmonary causes. The lesions were subsequently termed *small airways disease* or *smoker bronchiolitis*. Histologic features overlap with DIP, but DIP is more uniform and extensive than RBILD and exhibits a striking intra-alveolar component.[9,212] DIP and RBILD share common histologic features and occur almost exclusively in smokers,[9,213,214] suggesting a common pathogenesis. Patients with RBILD are generally young (age <45 years) and present with mild symptoms of cough, dyspnea, or sputum production.[9,213] Chest radiographs demonstrate small irregular opacities ("dirty lungs") or reticular or reticulonodular infiltrates but are normal in up to 28% of patients.[9,212] HRCT scans reveal numerous 2- to 3-mm irregular peribronchiolar nodules; GGOs or emphysema may also be present.[9,213] PFTs reveal reduced DLco and mild airflow obstruction; lung volumes are variable.[9]

The course of RBILD is indolent or stable, and prognosis is generally excellent. However, data are limited. Cessation of cigarette smoking is essential.[9,212] Improvement and even complete resolution often occurs after the cessation of cigarette smoking.[9,212] Corticosteroids are required in a minority of patients. Late fibrosis or fatalities are rare. However, British investigators[215] identified 10 patients with RBILD from 1980 to 1998, 7 of whom were treated with prednisolone, which was combined with azathioprine or cyclophosphamide in 6 patients. Despite cessation of smoking and aggressive therapy, the condition of three patients deteriorated. Thus, the spectrum of RBILD is broader than the original descriptions.[216,217]

AIP: AIP, originally described by Hamman and Rich in 1944, is a syndrome characterized by rapidly progressive respiratory failure (often within a few days) and histologic features of diffuse alveolar damage on lung biopsy.[15,16] Although this entity is distinct from IPF, some patients with IPF undergo an accelerated phase and histologic features consistent with AIP.[95,115,218] Clinical features of AIP include bilateral alveolar infiltrates, an acute and rapid course, hypoxemic respiratory failure requiring mechanical ventilatory support, extensive GGOs on HRCT, a high mortality rate (>50%), and potential responsiveness to high-dose corticosteroids.[15,16,115,218]

An acute viral-like prodrome often precedes the onset of AIP; fever is present in up to 50% of patients.[15,16] Histologic features include hyaline membranes, fibrinous exudate, epithelial-cell necrosis, and interstitial and intra-alveolar edema.[6,16] As the process organizes and undergoes repair, type II cells proliferate along alveolar walls, hyaline membranes, and air space exudates resorb; and FBs proliferate within the alveolar interstitium and spaces.[6] The histologic features of AIP are nonspecific and are found with myriad disorders, including ARDS, inhalation or drug-induced injury, collagen vascular diseases, or infections.[6] Mortality rates with idiopathic AIP range from 50 to 88%.[15,16] Although data are limited, sustained and complete remissions have been achieved with the administration of high-dose corticosteroids.[6,15,16,115,218] Patients surviving the initial episode may heal with no sequelae or with variable degrees of fibrosis.[15,16] Recurrent, even fatal, episodes of AIP may occur months or years after the initial episode.[15] Although data are limited, aggressive treatment with high-dose IV pulse methylprednisolone is warranted for patients with AIP.

NSIP/Fibrosis: In 1994, Katzenstein proposed the term *NSIP/fibrosis* to describe lung biopsy results from immunocompetent patients with clinical syndromes resembling IPF[219] but with histologic features distinct from UIP, DIP, RBILD, AIP, or LIP.[6] An inciting cause was not identified in most patients, but some had underlying CTD, drug reactions, or HP.[219] In the sentinel report,[219] the prognosis of NSIP was distinctly better than IPF. An international ATS/European Respiratory Society consensus statement[4] on the classification of IIPs published in 2002 recognized NSIP as a distinct histopathological pattern found in response to occupational exposures, CTD, or as an idiopathic form. NSIP likely represents a stereotypic response to diverse injuries or toxins. The relationship between NSIP and UIP remains uncertain.[5,14,220]

Histopathology of NSIP

Salient histologic features of idiopathic NSIP included varying degrees of inflammation and fibrosis that are temporally uniform, *ie*, occurring over a single time span (Fig 10).[219] The temporal uniformity in NSIP suggests a response to a single insult. Scattered foci of organizing pneumonia are noted in nearly 50% of patients; prominent accumulation of intra-alveolar macrophages mimicking DIP is observed in one third of cases.[219] The key histologic feature distinguishing NSIP from UIP is its temporal uniformity.[6,209] In NSIP, the lesions appear to be of similar age, whereas in UIP, new and old lesions are present concomitantly.[6] Varying degrees of fibrosis and inflammation are observed in NSIP and UIP, but honeycombing, a prominent feature of UIP, is rare in patients with NSIP.[5,148,203,210] UIP is characterized by heterogeneity, greater destruction of the alveolar architecture, extensive fibrosis, and minimal intra-alveolar inflammation.[5,6]

Clinical Manifestations of NSIP

Clinical manifestations of NSIP are similar to IPF, with bibasilar crackles, cough, dyspnea, interstitial infiltrates, reduced DLco, and a restrictive defect on PFT results.[13,14,210,220] Because clinical

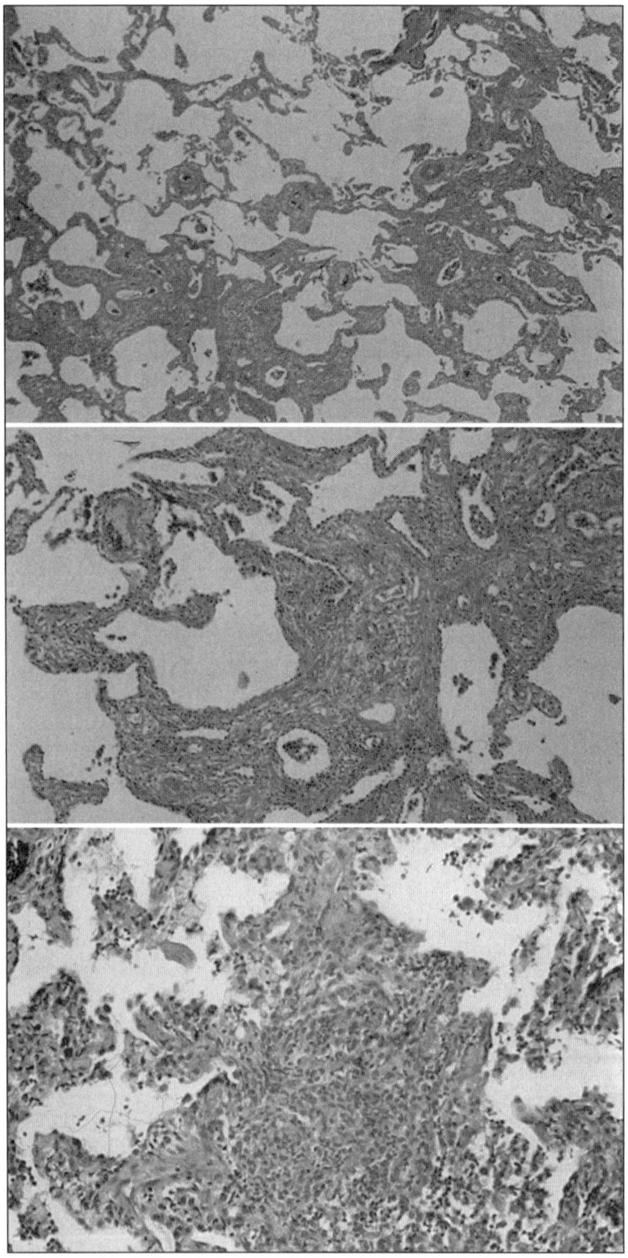

Figure 10. *Top*: Photomicrograph of NSIP. Open-lung biopsy specimen shows patchy interstitial fibrosis that lacks the subpleural distribution and temporal heterogeneity of UIP [reproduced with permission from Lynch et al, J Respir Dis 2000; 21;197–214]. *Center*: Photomicrograph of NSIP. Open-lung biopsy specimen. The alveolar septae are thickened by fibrosis and interstitial chronic inflammation (hematoxylin-eosin) [reproduced with permission from Lynch et al, J Respir Dis 2000; 21;197–214]. *Bottom*: Photomicrograph of NSIP. Open-lung biopsy specimen. Prominent interstitial inflammation without dense scarring is evident. Some pneumocytes are hyperplastic. These inflammatory features are consistent with the cellular form of NSIP [reproduced with permission from Lynch et al, J Respir Dis 2000; 21;197–214].

and radiographic features overlap with IPF, it is highly likely that examples of NSIP were included in historical series of IPF. However, NSIP and IPF differ in several important respects. The onset of NSIP may be subacute, evolving over a few weeks, whereas IPF evolves over years.[13] Fever, noted in one third of patients with NSIP, is not found in IPF. Clubbing is found in 10 to 40% of patients with NSIP but in 66 to 93% of patients with IPF.[12,147,148] Compared with patients with IPF, patients with NSIP are younger, and there is a slight female predominance in NSIP.[12,14,147,148] BAL lymphocytosis is common in NSIP[147,221] but rare with IPF.[147,222] However, significant overlap exists between NSIP and IPF.[223] HRCT features of NSIP and IPF/UIP differ.[11,147,148,222] Bilateral GGOs are characteristic in NSIP but rare in IPF/UIP.[147] HC, a cardinal feature of UIP, is absent or sparse in NSIP.[20,147,148,222] Most importantly, the prognosis of NSIP is much better than IPF/UIP.[14] Some patients with NSIP improve either spontaneously or in response to corticosteroid or immunosuppressive therapy. In striking contrast, improvement is rare in IPF (< 10%), even with aggressive therapy.[2,13,27,163,204]

In several early studies,[96,98,147,148,152,203] 5-year survival with NSIP exceeded 70%, compared with < 30% with IPF. It is highly likely that many patients in earlier publications labeled as IPF but manifesting GGO on HRCT, BAL lymphocytosis, or "steroid responsiveness" in fact represented cases of NSIP.[151,153,224,225] Subsequent studies[13,147,203] suggest that the designation *NSIP* is excessively broad. Segregation by histologic features into cellular nonspecific interstitial pneumonia (cellular NSIP) or fibrotic forms of NSIP identifies patient subsets with differing prognoses.[147,203] Patients with the cellular form have more GGOs and less honeycombing on HRCT, a greater rate of corticosteroid responsiveness, and lower rates of mortality.[147,203]

Although NSIP has a better prognosis than IPF, mortality with fibrotic NSIP is high. British investigators[204] monitored 28 patients with idiopathic NSIP up to 10 years after SLB. At a median follow-up of 42 months, 17 patients (61%) had died; median survival was only 52 months. These data suggest that earlier studies[98,147,203] citing survival rates > 90% with NSIP were overly optimistic. Similarly, a retrospective review[172] of 104 patients with IPF reclassified 61 patients as having UIP and 43 (41%) as having fibrotic NSIP. At a median follow-up of 32 months, 25 of 43 NSIP patients (48%) had died vs 48 deaths among 61 patients with UIP (79%).

Furthermore, the prognosis of fibrotic NSIP patients with severe functional impairment is poor. Among NSIP patients with DLCO <35% of predicted, 3-year survival was < 50%.[172] Korean investigators[221] cited 5-year survival rates of 56% among 48 patients with fibrotic NSIP and 34% among 131 patients with UIP. Further, early studies[147,203,226,227] cited favorable responses to corticosteroids (alone or combined with immunosuppressive agents) in 60 to 83% of patients, whereas subsequent studies[98,148,204] were less sanguine (response rates of 25 to 40%). Short-term (*ie*, 2-year) survival rates underestimate long-term mortality associated with NSIP.[172,204,221] Additional studies are required to further elucidate the clinical features, outcomes and rate of progression associated with NSIP and histologic subsets (*eg*, cellular or fibrotic forms).

SLB

The optimal staging and role of SLBs in patients with IPF are controversial. Video-assisted thoracoscopic surgery (VATS) lung biopsies are required to establish the diagnosis of UIP unequivocally,[7,228,229] but many clinicians are reluctant to subject patients to the morbidity of surgery, particularly when therapeutic options for IPF are of limited value.[124] Although VATS is relatively safe, acute exacerbation in respiratory status was noted in 2.1% of 236 patients undergoing SLB for ILD.[230] SLB was associated with rapid deterioration in respiratory status (consistent with acute exacerbations) in 3 to 4% of patients with idiopathic NSIP or CTD-associated ILD.[231]

Despite these caveats, SLB can be justified in otherwise-stable patients given the potential for serious toxicities associated with aggressive immunosuppressive therapy and the prognostic value of SLB. Clinical surveys have found that SLB is performed in less than onethird of patients with IPF.[124,232,233] Within the past decade, HRCT has increasingly been used in lieu of SLB to diagnose UIP/IPF.[27,124,148] However, SLB remains the "gold standard" for the diagnosis of UIP and assessment of prognosis.[6] The role of SLB in clinical practice is threefold: (1) to rule out other etiologies, (2) to better define the pattern of IIP (primarily UIP vs NSIP), and (3) to better define prognosis.

VATS is less invasive than open-lung biopsies and provides adequate histologic material.[7,97,164] VATS can often be performed in the outpatient setting with minimal morbidity.[234] Tissue should be obtained from at least two sites (*eg*, upper and lower lobes of the same lung); representative areas should be sampled (*ie*, avoid normal or very fibrotic areas).[97,98,164,206] Specific histologic features or subtypes of IIPs have prognostic value.[6,98,164,204] Establishing the histologic diagnosis of UIP is a strong predictor of increased mortality and poor response to therapy when compared with other IIPs.[6,27,96–98] In one prospective study,[164] long-term survival was worse in patients with greater degrees of FF, whereas the degree of alveolar cellularity or alveolar wall fibrosis did not affect survival. In a cohort of 53 patients with UIP, British investigators[163] confirmed that increasing FF correlated with rate of mortality ($p = 0.006$) and decreases in FVC and DLCO at 6 months and 12 months. Neither the extent of established fibrosis nor intra-alveolar macrophage accumulation correlated with outcome.[163] In contrast, in a cohort of 99 patients with idiopathic UIP, we[235] found that the extent of FF, established fibrosis, or intra-alveolar macrophage accumulation did not predict survival. Another study[236] of 43 patients with IPF found no relationship between profusion of FF on SLB and survival.

Variation in histologic features in individual patients limits the prognostic accuracy of even SLB.[97,205,206] Although SLB is touted as a "gold standard," a minute fraction of the lung parenchyma is sampled. Evaluation of SLB is subject to interobserver and intralobar variation, even by expert pulmonary pathologists.[97,204,206] Further, discriminating UIP from fibrotic NSIP is difficult.[203,204] More importantly, foci of UIP and NSIP may be found within the same lobe in individual patients.[97,205] A confident diagnosis of UIP or NSIP may be difficult to make, particularly by pathologists lacking expertise in pulmonary histology. Importantly, HRCT may corroborate the diagnosis of UIP, provided that radiographic features are classic.[22,125] Further, the extent and pattern of changes on HRCT have prognostic value.[123,124,127,146,150]

Although the decision to perform VATS lung biopsy should be individualized, we favor VATS biopsy (if no contraindications exist) in patients with recent onset of ILD of unknown cause, when transbronchial lung biopsies (TBBs) are nondiagnostic. However, VATS biopsy is not warranted in patients who have a prolonged course (>2 years) and clinical, physiologic, and HRCT features that are characteristic of IPF/UIP.[3,125] Moreover, the risk of VATS lung biopsy is excessive in elderly (>70 years old) or debilitated patients, particularly when clinical and HRCT features strongly suggest UIP. In such patients, HRCT is sufficient to determine an approach to therapy. Bronchoscopy with TBBs is most useful to diagnose alternative causes of ILD (*eg*, sarcoidosis, Langerhans-cell granulomatosis [LCG], pulmonary alveolar proteinosis, lymphangitic carcinomatosis, COP). Because of the small sample size (2 to 5 mm), TBBs cannot substantiate the diagnosis of UIP, DIP, or NSIP and cannot be used to assess the extent of inflammation or fibrosis.

BAL

BAL is useful to exclude alternative etiologies that may mimic IPF (*eg*, specific infections such as *Pneumocystis carinii*, Mycobacteria, and fungi, PAP, and LCG)[237] but has no role to diagnose or stage IPF.[3,4,223,238] Increases in polymorphonuclear leukocytes, mast cells, alveolar macrophages, and myriad cytokines are noted in BAL fluid from patients with IPF; lymphocyte numbers are usually normal.[238] However, BAL cell profiles in IPF do not predict prognosis or therapeutic responsiveness.[3,238] BAL has yielded significant insights into the pathogenic mechanisms responsible for IPF, but BAL is of doubtful clinical value in assessing the extent or activity of IPF.[166,238]

Radionuclide Scans

^{67}Ga citrate scanning has been used as a surrogate marker of alveolar inflammation (alveolitis) in IPF and other inflammatory pulmonary disorders. Increased intrapulmonary uptake of ^{67}Ga was associated with a more cellular biopsy in some early studies. However, even with careful quantification,^{67}Ga scans failed to predict responsiveness to therapy.[2] ^{67}Ga scans are expensive and inconvenient because scanning is performed 48 h after injection. Despite initial enthusiasm for its application, ^{67}Ga scanning is of no practical value. The clearance of ^{99}Tc-DTPA aerosol is accelerated in IPF and is a marker of increased lung permeability.[166,239,240] British investigators[239] found that normal DTPA clearance in patients with IPF was associated with stable lung function; survival was not analyzed. In contrast, accelerated clearance of the fast component (*ie*, reduced $t_{0.5}$F) was an independent predictor of mortality in patients with idiopathic UIP.[166] In that study,[166] age and DLCO were the most important predictors of survival, followed by percentage of predicted TLC and $t_{0.5}$F.

Thus, the incremental practical value of $t_{0.5}$F appears to be small. Further, increased clearance of DTPA occurs in smokers and patients with other inflammatory lung disorders; its prognostic value is debatable.[240] Clearance of inhaled pertechnegas (an aerosol of ^{99}Tc-labeled carbon particles) is increased (compared with normal control subjects) in IPF, HP, and CTD-associated PF but not sarcoidosis,[241] consistent with increased alveolar capillary permeability. Increased metabolic activity may be noted by PET scans in patients with IPF.[156] At present, radionuclide imaging studies have no role in the management of IPF.

Pathogenesis

The pathogenesis of IPF is complex and likely involves myriad components, including repetitive lung injury (particularly to alveolar epithelial cells [AECs]), destruction of subepithelial basement membranes, inflammation, cytokines and chemokines, exaggerated deposition of collagen and extracellular matrix, recruitment and proliferation of fibroblasts, inappropriate wound-healing response, and excessive angiogenesis.[242] The fibrotic/inflammatory process in UIP has been likened to abnormal wound healing,[243,244] with a vigorous fibroblastic response to AEC injury occurring. Injury of AECs and destruction of the subepithelial basement membranes lead to local recruitment, differentiation, and proliferation of fibroblasts.[242] Excessive deposition of collagen and extracellular matrix contributes to the fibrotic process.[242,245]

A complex interplay between inflammatory and mesenchymal cell populations amplifies and perpetuates the fibrotic response.[242,245] Early theories of pathogenesis suggested that a heightened inflammatory response led to injury and fibrosis. Current theories suggest a primary role for FB dysregulation; inflammatory cells may play a contributory, albeit minor, role.[242,245] Soluble mediators (cytokines) produced by fibroblasts and AECs amplify and perpetuate the fibrotic response. TGF-β likely plays a critical role in IPF.[242,245] Other cytokines that appear to be involved in the pathogenesis include TNF-α, platelet-derived growth factor, connective tissue growth factor, IL-8, and CXC chemokines.[242,245] Other possible mediators of the fibrotic process in IPF include integrin-mediated intercellular adhesion molecules, surfactant proteins, proteases, leukotrienes, oxygen radicals, and myriad soluble mediators.[2,242,243]

The relative deficiency of γ-interferon (γ-IFN), a cytokine that inhibits collagen synthesis and fibrosis, may contribute to the fibroproliferative process.[2] The signals responsible for initiating and perpetuating this process are not known. However, the so-called FF in IPF/UIP may be the leading edge of the inflammatory/fibrotic process.[6] Further, AEC death is most prominent immediately adjacent to FF.[246] Mesenchymal cells that form FFs in IPF/UIP are activated and display a contractile phenotype, commonly referred to as *myofibroblasts*.[247] Myofibroblast differentiation and fate are controlled by soluble growth factors such as TGF-β_1 and matrix-derived signals.[245] Myofibroblasts in the lung in IPF may be derived from extrapulmonary fibrocytes and bone marrow-derived progenitor cells.[248]

Under the influence of TGF-β_1, myofibroblasts display increased production of collagen, vimentin, β-actin, and tissue inhibitors of metalloproteinases,[2] leading to a bias toward excessive matrix production and wound contraction in UIP. Additionally, a proangiogenic environment may favor fibrosis in IPF.[249] IL-8 and γ-IFN--inducible protein-10 (IP-10), members of the CXC chemokine family, affect fibrosis via angiogenic mechanisms.[245] IL-8 stimulates neovascularization, whereas IP-10 inhibits angiogenesis. In humans with IPF, IL-8 is markedly elevated in BAL fluid and serum,[250] whereas IP-10 levels in IPF lung biopsies are reduced compared with control patients.[251] Genetic factors may be important in the pathogenesis of the disease and its clinical expression.[59] Differences in gene expression may influence the severity and course of the disease.[59,94]

Selman et al[94] examined gene expression profiles in 88 patients with slowly progressing IPF (symptoms > 24 months) and 26 patients with the rapid variant (symptoms < 6 months). Two genes, adenosine 2B receptor and prominin-1/CD133, were expressed more strongly in the rapid group. It is evident that the pathophysiology of IPF is complex, with diverse cell types/mediators participating in the initiation, orchestration, perpetuation, and evolution of the inflammatory/fibrotic process. Unfortunately, as will be discussed in greater detail below, therapeutic strategies designed to ablate inflammatory responses have had little or no impact on the outcome of IPF/UIP. In light of this, novel therapies targeted against FB proliferation or other profibrotic mediators are being investigated (discussed later in this chapter).

Therapy

The management of patients with IPF is frustrating because the disease progresses inexorably and treatment has not been shown to alter the natural history of the disease.[2,27,252] Initial treatment strategies, based on the concept that inflammation was a key factor in the pathogenesis of IPF, involved the administration high-dose corticosteroids and/or immunosuppressive agents.[27,164,224,225,253,254] However, RCTs were not performed. Several early studies[224,225,253,255] cited response rates of 10 to 30% with corticosteroids, but these older studies included a mix of histologic entities (*eg*, UIP, DIP, RBILD, NSIP, HP, etc) and cannot be extrapolated to UIP.

Other studies[96,147,148,204 256] that included patients with UIP cited response rates of 0 to 17%. Importantly, a survival benefit with corticosteroid therapy has not been demonstrated.[13,26,27,57,164] Unfortunately, the administration of corticosteroids is associated with a plethora of adverse effects, particularly in elderly or debilitated patients.[179,258] Given the significant toxicities, the administration of corticosteroids in high doses should not be used to treat IPF.[179] Similarly, immunosuppressive or cytotoxic agents have not been shown to influence mortality or clinical outcomes.[1,2,27,199,259–262] Anecdotal responses to azathioprine[202,262] or cyclophosphamide[261,263] were noted in early studies, but the preponderance of data suggest that these agents are ineffective as therapy for IPF.[2,26,27,259 260] Several large retrospective studies[26,27,164,264] failed to document survival benefit with any form of therapy.

Expert Consensus Statements and Recommendations for Therapy: International consensus statements conclude that existing therapies are of unproven benefit but acknowledge that physicians may wish to treat patients with deteriorating disease.[3,232] Both statements advocated an individualized approach to therapy. For patients requiring treatment, the British Thoracic Society Committee advocated combining prednisolone (0.5 mg/kg/d, with taper) plus azathioprine (2 to 3 mg/kg/d) as initial therapy.[232] The ATS statement recommended combining prednisone (0.5 mg/kg/d for 4 weeks, with subsequent taper) with either oral azathioprine (2 to 3 mg/kg/d) or oral cyclophosphamide (2 mg/kg/d).[3] For patients unable to take corticosteroids, azathioprine or cyclophosphamide alone are used. These recommendations represented a substantial departure from earlier regimens, which advocated much greater doses of corticosteroids.[45,225,262] Therapy should be continued for 6 months unless adverse effects develop and require modification or discontinuation of therapy. Prolonging treatment beyond 6 months should be limited to patients who improve or remain stable. It should be emphasized that these recommendations[3,232] reflect expert opinion but have not been validated in clinical trials.

My Recommendations for Therapy for IPF: Given the lack of survival benefit, and potentially serious toxicities of corticosteroids or immunosuppressive therapy, I rarely recommend therapy for IPF. However, treatment may be offered to patients with severe symptoms and a declining course, provided that the pros and cons of therapy are discussed honestly. We emphasize to patients that no therapy has been proven to influence survival or clinically important outcomes. For patients exhibiting a subacute or deteriorating course and/or surrogate markers of alveolitis (GGO on CT scan), we offer oral azathioprine, 2 to 3 mg/kg/d, alone or combined with low-dose prednisone, 20 mg every other day or equivalent.

Azathioprine does not cause bladder injury or bladder carcinomas and has less oncogenic potential than cyclophosphamide.[265] Because of its suppressive effects on bone marrow, CBC and platelet counts should be obtained every 2 weeks for the first 6 weeks and then every 4 to 8 weeks thereafter. Significant anemia, leukopenia ($<3,500/\mu L$) or thrombocytopenia ($<120,000/\mu L$) warrants dose reduction. Azathioprine should be used with caution in patients receiving allopurinol, and the dose should be reduced by at least 50%.[265] After 6 months, efficacy should be examined. Unless there is unequivocal and objective improvement, we discontinue therapy after a 6-month trial. Further, treatment is discontinued among patients experiencing side effects or disease progression. Cyclophosphamide has potentially serious toxicities,[265] and we do not use cyclophosphamide for IPF. Mycophenolate mofetil and other immunosuppressive agents have been used by some clinicians, but these agents have not been evaluated in clinical trials.

In contrast to the dismal responses noted with immunosuppressive or cytotoxic therapy in IPF/UIP, favorable responses to corticosteroids (alone or combined with azathioprine) have been noted with NSIP, particularly cellular variants.[210,220] For NSIP, either cellular or fibrotic, I recommend a course of therapy with corticosteroids and azathioprine for a minimum of 6 months. Patients who are intolerant of azathioprine or in whom azathioprine fails may be switched to mycophenolate mofetil or cyclophosphamide, but published data in this regard are lacking.

Novel Therapeutic Options: TNF-α antagonists (*eg*, etanercept and infliximab) have been tried in some cases of PF (idiopathic and CTD-associated), but data are limited. In a recent prospective, multicenter trial,[266] 84 patients with IPF were randomized to etanercept (twice weekly) or placebo. At 48 weeks, there were no significant differences in primary end points (physiologic parameters) between groups, but trends favoring etanercept were observed in some secondary end points.[266] Anecdotal responses to infliximab were noted in case reports[267,268] of CTD-associated pulmonary fibrosis. However, TNF-α antagonists are expensive and have serious potential toxicities.[268,269] Additional studies are required before endorsing these agents for IPF.

Novel and Future Therapies: Major advances await the development of novel therapies that prevent fibroproliferation and enhance alveolar reepithelialization.[201,245] Agents that have been tested in pilot studies include interferons, *N*-acetylcysteine (NAC), and pirfenidone (5-methyl-1-phenyl-2-[1H]-pyridine).

γ-IFN-1b: γ-IFN-1b is an endogenous cytokine that down-regulates the expression of TGF-β and may have antifibrotic effects.[201] Initial studies[270,271] employing recombinant γ-IFN-1b were encouraging, but the INSPIRE trial, which randomized 800 patients with mild-to-moderate IPF to recombinant γ-IFN-1b or placebo in a 2:1 ratio, showed no benefit. The study was ended because of "futility" in March 2007 (InterMune, Brisbane, CA).

NAC: NAC is an antioxidant that stimulates glutathione synthesis, attenuates fibrosis in animal models,[272] and augments glutathione levels in BAL in patients with IPF.[273] A phase III multicenter, double-blind, placebo-controlled trial (European Idiopathic Pulmonary Fibrosis International Group Exploring *N*-acetylcysteine [NAC] I Annual)[274] in Europe evaluated the efficacy of oral NAC in IPF. In this study, all patients received conventional therapy with prednisone, 0.5 mg/kg/d, with taper, plus azathioprine, 2 mg/kg/d. Patients were then randomized to oral NAC, 1,800 mg/d, or placebo. At the end of 1 year, PFT results had deteriorated in both cohorts. However, the rates of decrease in FVC and DLCO were less in patients receiving NAC ($p < 0.05$).[274] However, these changes in PFTs were small (absolute difference in FVC of 4.8% and in DLCO of 5.1%) and of doubtful clinical significance. The benefit if any of NAC as therapy for IPF remains controversial. Nonetheless, NAC is inexpensive and has few side effects, making this an attractive option for IPF.[275] A multicenter RCT sponsored by the Idiopathic Pulmonary Fibrosis Clinical Research Network is planned to address the impact of NAC in IPF.

Pirfenidone: Pirfenidone (5-methyl-1-phenyl-2-[1H]-pyridine) attenuates pulmonary fibrosis in animal models, reduces synthesis of collagen I and III and TNF-α, inhibits TGF-β-stimulated collagen synthesis, decreases extracellular matrix, and blocks the mitogenic effect of profibrotic cytokines.[201,276]. In a phase II open-label trial,[277] 54 consecutive patients with IPF were treated with pirfenidone. Conventional therapy failed in 46; 8 were untreated. With pirfenidone, 1- and 2-year survival rates were 78% and 63%, respectively. After 6 months of therapy, PFT results appeared to stabilize, but results are difficult to interpret because follow-up PFTs were not performed in all patients.

In another nonrandomized trial,[278] 13 patients with PF (idiopathic, $n = 11$; associated with scleroderma, $n = 2$) were treated with oral pirfenidone for 1 year. At 2-year follow-up, nine patients had died and two patients remained stable; the disease had progressed in the remaining two patients. Further, in a cohort[279] of 11 patients with PF complicating Hermansky-Pudlak syndrome, pirfenidone was associated with a slower rate of decrease in PFTs (*ie*, FVC, FEV_1, DLCO) compared with 10 patients receiving placebo.

A phase II RCT[280] compared pirfenidone to placebo (2:1 ratio) in a cohort of 107 patients with IPF. The study was discontinued prematurely because acute exacerbations were noted in five patients receiving pirfenidone (14%) compared with no cases in the placebo group. The primary end point (change in lowest oxygen saturation on 6MWT > 6 or 9 months) was not met. There were no significant differences between groups in rate of mortality, TLC, DLCO, or resting Pao_2. The rate of decrease in FVC at 9 months was lower in the pirfenidone group ($p = 0.037$), but differences between groups were small and of doubtful clinical significance. These studies[277–280] are insufficient to assess the efficacy of pirfenidone but support the need for additional therapeutic trials. Pirfenidone has been approved for use in Japan based on a randomized trial, but published data are not available. Currently, pirfenidone is not commercially available elsewhere. Two placebo-controlled DBRCTs evaluating pirfenidone as therapy for IPF were recently completed in the United States (InterMune, Brisbane, CA) but have not yet been published.

ET-1 Receptor Antagonists: ET-1, a potent pulmonary vasoconstrictor, displays profibrotic effects and may play a role in the pathogenesis of IPF.[281] Bosentan, an ET-1 receptor antagonist, reduced collagen deposition in animal models (bleomycin-induced pulmonary fibrosis),[282] but its efficacy in humans with IPF has not yet been shown. Results of a multicenter DBRCT[198] evaluating BUILD-1 were recently published. In that study, 158 patients with IPF were randomized to bosentan or placebo. Patients with severe pulmonary dysfunction (FVC < 50% of predicted or DLCO < 35% of predicted) or concomitant PAH were excluded. At 12 months, the 6MWT worsened in both groups (no significant differences between groups). Mean changes from baseline in FVC at 12 months were −6.4% and −7.7% in the bosentan and placebo groups, respectively. Mean changes from baseline in DLCO at 12 months were −4.3% and −5.8% in the bosentan and placebo groups, respectively. A trend in favor of bosentan was noted in the secondary end point of time to death or disease progression (hazard ratio, 0.63; $p = 0.12$). A larger DBRCT (BUILD-3) assessing the impact of bosentan vs placebo in IPF is in progress. Further, a DBRCT assessing ambrisentan (another ET-1 receptor antagonist) is planned.

Phosphodiesterase-4 Inhibitors: Sildenafil, a phosphodiesterase-4 inhibitor, has been shown to be effective to treat idiopathic PAH.[283] Data regarding sildenafil for PAH complicating IPF are limited to anecdotal cases and small series. In an open-label RCT, 16 patients with PAH secondary to PF underwent right-heart catheterization to assess the acute hemodynamic effects of vasodilators.[192] Eight patients received sildenafil (50-mg oral dose), and eight received the maximal tolerated dose of IV epoprostenol. Pulmonary vascular resistance decreased equally in both groups: epoprostenol (−36.9%), sildenafil (−32.5%). Importantly, epoprostenol increased intrapulmonary ventilation/perfusion mismatching, whereas sildenafil maintained ventilation/perfusion matching and improved Pao_2. However, this study only assessed parameters 60 min after ingestion of sildenafil. Long-term effects of sildenafil in patients with ILD (with or without PAH) are not known. Anecdotal responses were noted in small series[196,284] of patients with IPF and PAH, but these data are inadequate to assess the role of sildenafil for patients with ILD. A randomized trial evaluating the impact of sildenafil in patients with IPF is in progress (ClinicalTrials.gov identifier: NCT00352482).

Anticoagulants: Inflammation and vascular injury in IPF may lead to a prothrombotic state that could exacerbate lung injury.[285] Japanese investigators[286] randomized 56 IPF patients to anticoagulants (warfarin) or placebo. Three-year survival and freedom from acute exacerbations were improved in the anticoagulated group. However, the dropout rate was high, and it is possible that selection bias may have influenced the study. Given the risk associated with anticoagulation therapy, additional studies involving greater numbers of patients are required before endorsing this form of therapy.

Novel (Future) Agents: Unfortunately, current therapies for IPF are of unproven efficacy. Novel agents with potential antifibrotic properties have theoretical value but have not yet been evaluated in IPF.[199,201,244,272] Agents that are currently being studied in IPF include imatinib mesylate, sirolimus, captopril, inhaled iloprost, and other inhibitors of fibrotic growth factors.[199,285,287]

LT: LT is the best option for patients with severe IPF.[158,252,288,289] Early listing for transplantation is urged in patients with progressive IPF because the waiting time for procuring donor organs may exceed 2 years.[158] Patients with severe functional impairment (*eg*, FVC < 60% of predicted, DLCO < 40% of predicted), oxygen dependency, and/or a deteriorating course should be referred promptly for transplantation. The decision as to when to list should be left to the transplant center, according to local waiting times. Unfortunately, many patients with severe IPF die while awaiting organs.[158]

Data from the International Society of Heart and Lung Transplantation (ISHLT) Registry[290] cited 1-, 3-, and 5-year survival rates of 68%, 52%, and 50%, respectively, among IPF patients after LT. Initial studies[291,292] from single centers noted similar mortality rates with single lung transplants (SLTs) and bilateral sequential lung transplants (BSLTs). However, a review[289] of 821 patients who received LTs for IPF (636 SLT, 185 BSLT) in the United States between 1994 and 2000 reported significantly better early (1-month) and late (3-year) survival rates with SLT compared with BSLT. When posttransplant survival was reanalyzed contingent on survival to 1 month, survival by procedure type (SLT vs BSLT) was similar.

The reason for the increased mortality with BSLT likely reflects an increase in surgical problems in the early transplant period with BSLT. Data from the ISHLT Registry[293] for recipients with IPF noted improved survival with BSLT vs SLT ($p = 0.03$); survival rates were similar up to 3 years but diverged thereafter. The most recent data from the ISHLT[294] cited lower survival rates at 3 months after LT among patients with IPF (84%) or idiopathic PAH (74%) compared with those with cystic fibrosis (90%) and COPD (91%). Among patients surviving to 1 year, IPF and COPD had the worst long-term survival, most likely reflecting older age and comorbidities.[294]

Secondary PAH is not a contraindication to LT, but its presence may influence the operative and perioperative management. Whelan et al[295] reviewed 830 patients with IPF who underwent transplantation between 1995 and 2002 in the IHSLT registry; 77% had SLT and 23% had BSLT. By multivariate analysis, mean PAP and BSLT were independent risk factors for mortality. Among SLT recipients, there was a linear relationship between PAP and 90-day mortality. However, only 8.3% of patients with SLT had mPAP >40 mm Hg. The decision as to which procedure (*ie*, SLT or BSLT) should be done depends on the expertise of the local transplant program.[158] However, given the improved survival with BSLT among patients with idiopathic PAH,[293] most centers perform BSLT for IPF patients with secondary PAH.

Adjunctive Therapy: Supplemental oxygen is critical to optimize quality of life and enhance exercise capacity in patients with IPF[296]; impact on survival has not been studied. However, continuous oxygen ameliorates pulmonary vasoconstriction and may delay the clinical development of cor pulmonale. Judicious use of diuretics may be necessary to control peripheral edema in patients with cor pulmonale. The role of vasodilators in patients with secondary PAH is controversial.[192,297]

What Is the Relationship Between NSIP and UIP?

Controversy exists as to whether NSIP is a separate disease entity or a continuum of disease related to IPF/UIP.[5,13,209,220] Histologic features of NSIP overlap, and distinguishing fibrotic NSIP from UIP is difficult.[98,204,206] More importantly, both NSIP and UIP may coexist in individual patients. Review of SLB from patients with IIPs observed both NSIP and UIP (*ie*, discordant UIP) in 13 to 26% of patients.[97,205] Further, both NSIP and UIP may be observed in PF complicating CTDs.[298–301] NSIP and UIP may represent different points in the progression of a single disease or may represent distinct (albeit overlapping) processes. It is possible that cellular NSIP represents an early phase that may progress to fibrotic NSIP and ultimately UIP. If so, the survival advantage of NSIP may simply represent lead-time bias.[155,172] Until these questions are answered, I approach NSIP as a potential reversible lesion, with both inflammatory and fibrotic components. Unless specific contraindications exist, I treat NSIP with a combination of corticosteroids, 40 mg/d for 1 month, with gradual taper, and azathioprine, 2 mg/kg/d, for a 6-month trial. Responders are continued on medical therapy, often for prolonged periods. Patients in whom therapy fails and who exhibit a deteriorating course are listed for LT. (Criteria for listing are similar to IPF.)

Sarcoidosis

Sarcoidosis is a poorly understood granulomatous disease that involves the lung and intrathoracic lymph nodes in >90% of patients.[302–306] However, virtually any organ can be affected.[307] Skin involvement, peripheral lymphadenopathy, and eye involvement each occur in 20 to 30% of patients.[304] Clinically significant involvement of spleen,[308] liver,[308] heart,[309] CNS,[310–312] or bone[313] occurs in 2 to 7% of patients.[304] The clinical expression and course are heterogeneous. One third or more of patients are asymptomatic, with incidental findings of bilateral hilar lymphadenopathy (BHL) on chest radiographs. Symptoms are protean, reflecting the site of organ involvement. The natural history is usually favorable. Spontaneous remissions occur in nearly two thirds of patients, and a waxing and waning course is common.[303,305,306] The presence of acute inflammatory manifestations (*ie*, erythema nodosum, polyarthritis, and fever), termed *Löfgren syndrome*, portends an excellent prognosis, with high rates (>85%) of spontaneous remission.[302,314–317] Factors associated with poor prognosis and more aggressive disease include black race, osseous involvement, lupus pernio (disfiguring nasolabial cutaneous lesions), chronic hypercalcemia, and chronic pulmonary sarcoidosis.[303–306,314] Ethnic, geographic, and genetic factors influence prognosis.[317–319]

Löfgren syndrome is three to six times more common in women.[317,320] Black race is associated with a greater rate of chronic progressive disease, worse long-term prognosis, extrapulmonary involvement, and greater risk of relapses.[314,316,321–323] In 10 to 15% of patients with sarcoidosis, the course is chronic and progressive, resulting in permanent damage and fibrosis of affected organs; 1 to 6% of patients die of sarcoidosis.[303–306,314] Lower mortality rates (0 to 0.5%) have been cited in nonreferral settings, when the diagnosis was made as part of routine radiographic screening.[324,325] An epidemiologic study[31] in the United Kingdom identified 1,019 cases of sarcoidosis between 1991 and 2003. Mortality rates at 3 years and 5 years for patients with sarcoidosis were 5% and 7%, respectively, compared with 2% and 4% among age- and gender-matched controls without sarcoidosis. Causes of death were not reported.

Epidemiology

Sarcoidosis is worldwide in distribution, but its prevalence varies according to racial and geographic factors. Sarcoidosis is four to eight times more common in black than in white patients.[326–328] In North America and Europe, prevalence rates of 10 to 20 cases per 100,000 persons have been cited.[327,329] In Scandinavia and certain parts of the British Isles, prevalence rates exceed 80 cases per 100,000.[329,330] The incidence is much lower (<2 per 100,000) in southern Europe.[329,331] Sarcoidosis has infrequently been reported in Central or South America or Africa, but whether this represents underrecognition or reduced prevalence of the disease is not known. More than two thirds of patients present between the ages of 20 and 40 years.[332] There is a slight female predominance.[306,327] Sporadic cases within families are well recognized.[332,333] Familial sarcoidosis (defined as having first- or second-degree relatives with sarcoidosis) occurs in 17% of African-American patients with sarcoidosis, compared with 6% among white patients.[327]

Data from the multicenter ACCESS study[326] noted that the familial relative risk of sarcoidosis was greatest among siblings, followed by grandparents, and then parents. A specific genetic defect has not been identified, but genes of the major histocompatibility complex locus on chromosome 6p are believed to be involved.[334] The inheritance pattern is likely complex, with heterogeneous alleles, polymorphisms, and linkages.[335,336] The cause of sarcoidosis remains elusive, but genetic, environmental, and infectious causes have been suggested.[305] Specific genetic polymorphisms may influence prognosis. Human leukocyte antigen DQB1*0201 is a marker for a good prognosis in Dutch and British patients with sarcoidosis.[337] Polymorphisms of the C-C chemokine receptor gene (CCR2 haplotype 2) are associated with Löfgren syndrome and a good prognosis in Dutch patients.[338]

Histopathology

The histologic hallmark of sarcoidosis is the noncaseating (nonnecrotizing) granuloma composed of epithelioid cells and multinucleated giant cells, surrounded by a cuff of lymphocytes and plasma cells (Fig 11).[306,339] Fibrosis is present in varying degrees (Fig 12). Disruption and destruction of parenchyma may be prominent. Because mycobacterial and fungal granulomas can cause nonnecrotizing granulomas, special stains for acid-fast bacilli and fungi should be performed to exclude these infectious etiologies. In the respiratory tract, sarcoid granulomas are often situated in the submucosa of bronchioles and along bronchovascular bundles (Fig 13).[306,339] Coalescent granulomata may give rise to confluent mass lesions, nodules, or consolidation of lung parenchyma.[303] Exuberant granulomatous inflammation may infiltrate and destroy affected organs, leading to significant and irreparable loss of function. In the lung, progression to end-stage fibrosis (honeycomb lung) can occur.

Fiberoptic bronchoscopy with TBB is the preferred diagnostic procedure to diagnose pulmonary sarcoidosis. Diagnostic yields are 60 to 95%.[303] To avoid sampling error, I obtain several biopsy

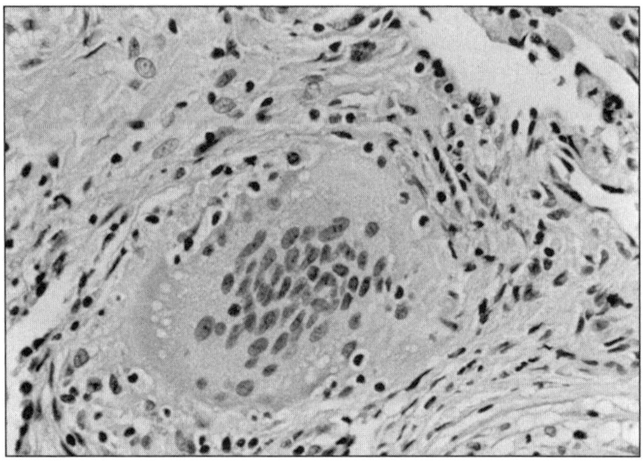

Figure 11. Sarcoidosis. Photomicrograph of TBB specimen. Multinucleated giant-cell in the center of a granuloma, surrounded by lymphocytes and mononuclear cells in the periphery (hematoxylin-eosin) [reproduced with permission from Lynch JP III, Strieter RM. In: Internal medicine for the specialist. Montvale, NJ: Medical Economics, 1994; 38–62].

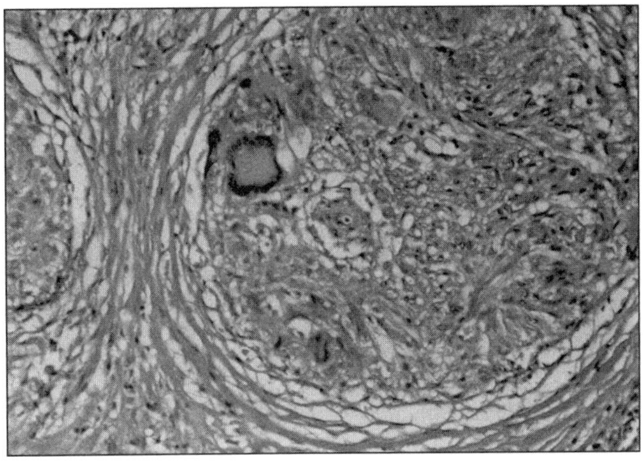

Figure 12. Sarcoidosis. Photomicrograph of TBB specimen, showing "burned out" granuloma demonstrating nonnecrotizing granuloma containing multinucleated giant cells and epithelioid cells in the center. In the periphery, no significant inflammatory cells are present, but concentric rings of collagen encircle the granuloma (hematoxylin-eosin) [reproduced with permission from Lynch JP III, Strieter RM. In: Internal medicine for the specialist. Montvale, NJ: Medical Economics, 1994; 38–62].

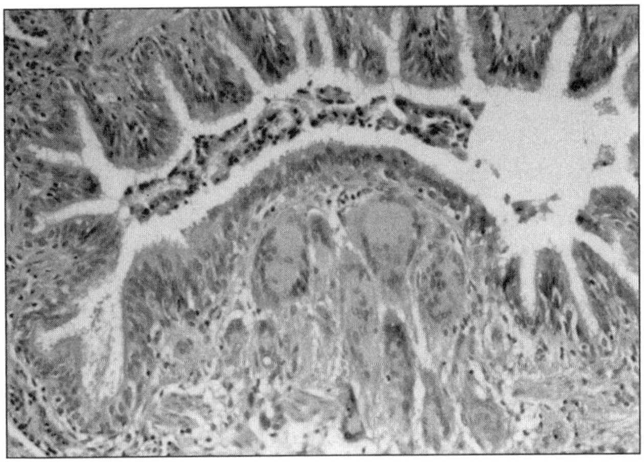

Figure 13. Sarcoidosis. Photomicrograph of endobronchial lung biopsy specimen showing prominent multinucleated giant cells within the submucosa underlying the bronchioles (hematoxylin-eosin) [reproduced with permission from Lynch JP III, Strieter RM. In: Immunologically mediated pulmonary disease. Philadelphia, PA: Lippincott-Williams and Wilkins, 1991; 189–216].

specimens from both the upper and lower lobes at the time of initial diagnostic bronchoscopy. When TBBs are nondiagnostic, mediastinoscopic lymph node biopsies may substantiate the diagnosis, provided that enlarged mediastinal lymph nodes are present. However, mediastinoscopy as a routine, initial diagnostic procedure for hilar lymphadenopathy is not cost-effective and has a potential for patient morbidity.[340]

Percutaneous needle aspiration may be an alterative to surgical biopsies. In one study[341] of 19 patients with suspected sarcoidosis, endosonography-guided fine-needle aspiration (FNA) of enlarged mediastinal lymph nodes demonstrated nonnecrotizing granulomas in 100%; 1 patient had tuberculosis (sensitivity and specificity rates of 100% and 94%, respectively). Experience with this technique is limited. In another series,[342] transbronchial FNA (TBFNA) with a 26-gauge needle revealed cytological features consistent with sarcoidosis in 88 of 116 patients (76%) with mediastinal or hilar adenopathy. Sensitivity of TBFNA cytology in this context was 79%; specificity was 92%. Complications of TBFNA include the following: pneumothoraces (10 to 60%) or hemoptysis (5 to 10%).[343] Tambouret et al[344] performed 32 percutaneous FNA biopsies from a variety of sites (*eg*, lymph nodes, salivary glands, lung, liver) in 28 patients with sarcoidosis; all aspirates showed granulomatous inflammation. Simultaneous or subsequent excisional biopsies confirmed the diagnosis in 17 patients.[344] Thus, FNA biopsy can be an alternative to surgical biopsies in selected patients. The optimal approach to diagnosing mediastinal lymph nodes (*ie*, TBFNA or CT-guided FNA) depends on the expertise and preference of the local institution. SLB (*ie*, VATS or open) is rarely necessary to diagnose sarcoidosis. Biopsy of extrapulmonary sites may be appropriate when specific lesions or abnormalities are identified (*eg*, lymphadenopathy, skin lesions, abnormal liver enzymes).[304,307]

Laboratory Features

Laboratory features are nonspecific. Hypercalcemia occurs in 1 to 4% of patients, and hypercalciuria in 15 to 40%.[304–306,345] These derangements in calcium metabolism reflect enhanced production of 1,2-dihydroxycalciferol by mononuclear phagocytes from sarcoid granulomas.[304] Polyclonal hypergammaglobulinemia occurs in 30 to 80% of patients with chronic disease.[304–306,314,345] Serum angiotensin-converting enzyme (ACE) levels are elevated in 30 to 80% of patients with sarcoidosis.[303,306,345] False-positive results are uncommon (<10%), but increased serum ACE can occur in active histoplasmosis and other granulomatous processes. The use of serum ACE as a surrogate marker of disease activity is discussed later.

Chest Radiographs

Abnormalities are present on chest radiographs in >90% of patients with sarcoidosis.[303] BHL, often associated with enlargement of right paratracheal lymph nodes, is the classic radiographic feature, observed in more than two thirds of patients (Fig 14).[143,303] Pulmonary parenchymal infiltrates are present in 25 to 50% of patients.[303] Pulmonary parenchymal infiltrates are typically bilateral and patchy, with a predilection for the mid- and upper lung zones (Fig 15). Multiple focal nodular or alveolar opacities in the upper lobes may mimic tuberculosis and fungal pneumonia. Other disorders that preferentially involve the upper lobes include LCG, cystic fibrosis, silicosis, and chronic eosinophilic pneumonia. Cavitation is rare.[346] Pleural effusions occur in <2% of patients.[303] Pleural thickening on plain chest radiographs is rare and usually reflects longstanding chronic disease. Diffuse reticulonodular or miliary infiltrates may be indistinguishable from other chronic ILDs (*eg*, IPF, pneumoconiosis, pulmonary alveolar proteinosis, lymphangitic carcinomatosis; Fig 16). Progression of the lung lesion results in distortion and destruction of the lung architecture, with upward retraction of the hila, broad coarse septal bands, bullae,

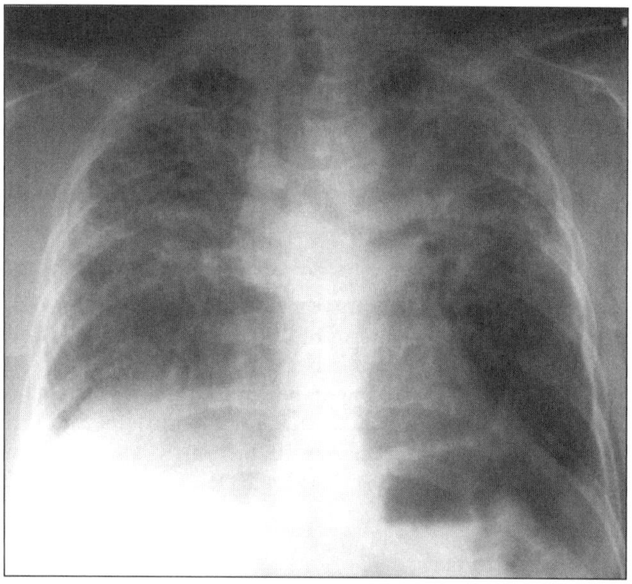

Figure 15. Stage II sarcoidosis. Chest radiograph demonstrating extensive cystic radiolucencies (honeycombing) and fibrosis preferentially affecting upper lobes of both lungs. Linear fibrotic strands and volume loss are noted throughout. In addition, BHL is present.

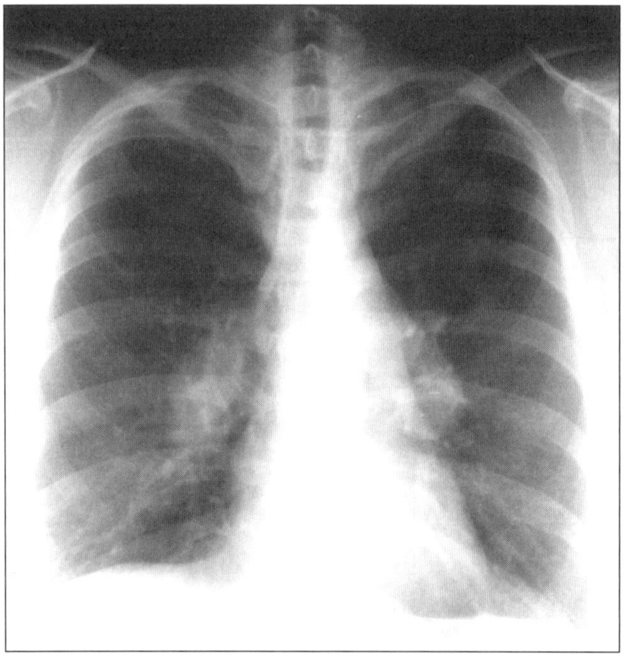

Figure 14. Sarcoidosis (stage I). Chest radiograph demonstrating extensive bilateral hilar and right paratracheal lymphadenopathy.

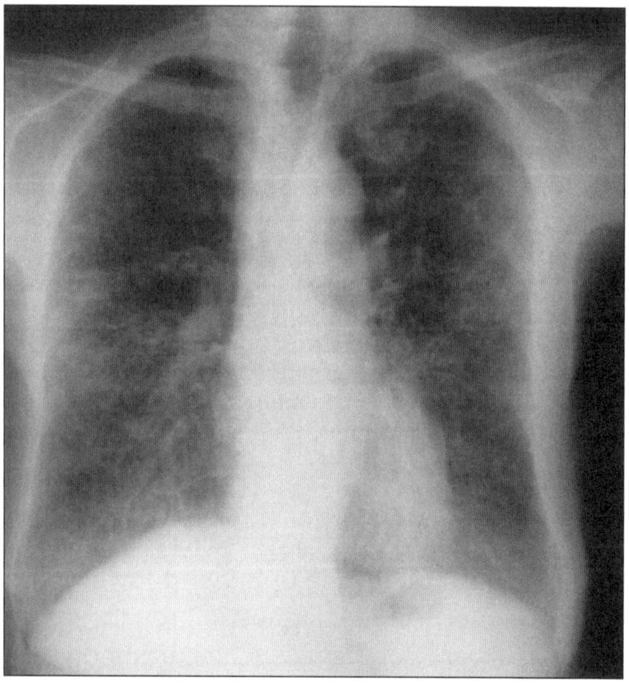

Figure 16. Stage III sarcoidosis. Chest radiograph demonstrates patchy reticulonodular densities throughout both lung fields. Lung volumes are well preserved. There is no definite lymphadenopathy.

and end-stage honeycomb lung (Fig 17, *top*). With far advanced disease, mycetomas, bullous emphysema, and pulmonary hypertension may be observed (Fig 17, *bottom*). Calcification of hilar or mediastinal nodes may be seen in long-standing sarcoidosis.

Radiographic Classification System

The radiographic staging system developed more >4 decades ago continues to be useful prognostically. This schema applies the following criteria on plain chest radiographs: stage 0, normal; stage I, BHL without parenchymal infiltrates; stage II, BHL plus parenchymal infiltrates; and stage III, parenchymal infiltrates without intrathoracic lymphadenopathy.[303] Some investigators advocate defining patients with extensive destruction, fibrosis, and volume loss as stage IV. This radiographic staging system may be useful as a prognostic guide, although significant variability exists. Spontaneous remissions occur in 60 to 90% of patients with stage I disease, 40 to 70% with stage II, and 10 to 20% with stage III.[302,303,347] Serious sequela are rare with stage I sarcoidosis but may be appreciable in other stages. Virtually all fatalities caused by pulmonary sarcoidosis occur in patients with radiographic stage II, III, or IV disease.[303] The course of the disease is usually dictated within the first 18 to 24 months of onset.[303] Spontaneous remissions occur in up to 40% within the first 6 months[347,348]; >80% of spontaneous remissions occur within the first 2 years.[349] Persistence of radiographic infiltrates beyond 2 years suggests that spontaneous remissions are unlikely to occur, and strongly warrants consideration of corticosteroid therapy.[349] In some patients, the course is chronic, with multiple exacerbations or disease progression over the course of years.[303,322,323]

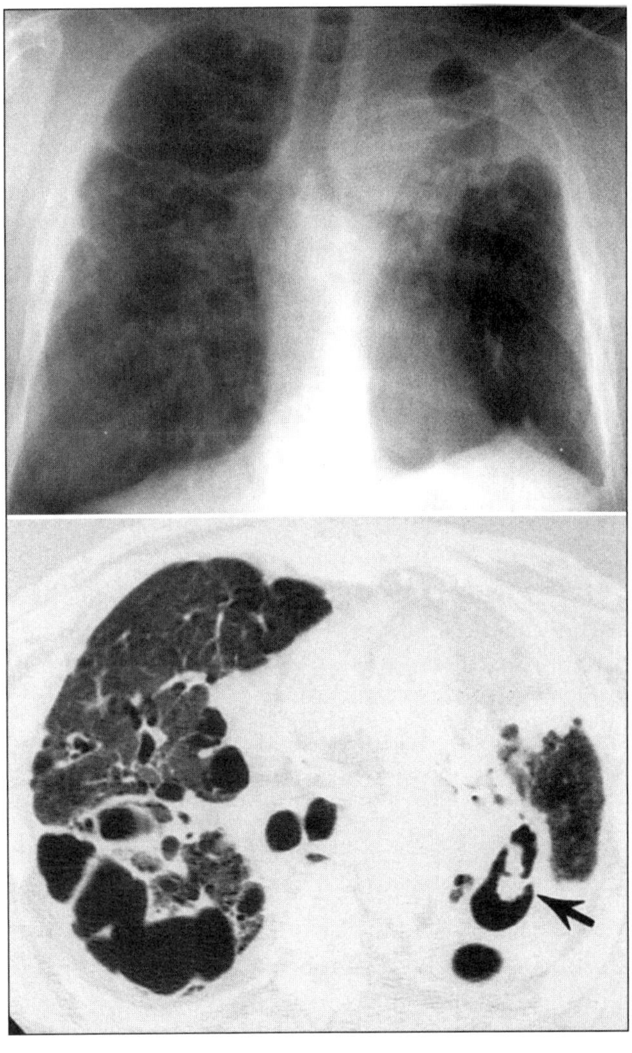

Figure 17. *Top*: Stage IV sarcoidosis. Posteroanterior chest radiograph demonstrates extensive cystic, bullous, and fibrotic changes; upward retraction of the hilum; and extensive pleural thickening in the left apex. Note surgical clips on the left lung from a previous left upper lobe lobectomy for a mycetoma. *Bottom*: HRCT demonstrating a mycetoma (arrow) in the superior segment of the left lower lobe in the same patient as in Fig 17, *top*, 8 months after resection a left upper lobe mycetoma. Note the bullae and cystic changes in the remaining lung parenchyma.

Chest CT

Chest CT is far more sensitive than conventional chest radiography in delineating parenchymal details or detecting the extent of intrathoracic lymphadenopathy.[143,350] Hilar or mediastinal lymph adenopathy is present in 47 to 94% of patients with sarcoidosis.[351] The most commonly involved nodal stations (in order of decreasing frequency) are as follows: right lower paratracheal, right hilar, subcarinal, and aortopulmonary window.[351] Routine CT scanning is not required to diagnose or stage sarcoidosis and is not cost-effective.[350] However, CT may be helpful in patients with atypical manifestations or with normal chest radiographs but with clinical suspicion of disease.[143,350] The use of 1- to 2-mm slice HRCT scans is superior to conventional CT in depicting parenchymal lesions and discriminating alveolitis from fibrosis.[143,352] Characteristic HRCT features of sarcoidosis include the following: nodular opacities and micronodules (<3 mm in diameter) along bronchovascular bundles, central bronchovascular thickening and nodularity, confluent nodular opacities with air bronchograms, GGOs, crowding and central retraction of bronchi and vessels near the hilae, and pleural or subpleural nodules.[143]

Nodules are present in > 80% of patients with sarcoidosis and represent aggregates of granulomas.[143,351,353] Irregularity or thickening of bronchovascular bundles, occasionally with a beaded appearance, is a cardinal sign of pulmonary sarcoidosis.[351] GGOs were noted in 16 to 83% of patients with sarcoidosis[351,353]; granulomatous and fibrotic lesions may give rise to this CT feature.[351] Progression of the sarcoid lung lesion may form conglomerate masses, architectural distortion, and cystic destruction (Fig 18). Cavitation was noted on CT in 2.7% of patients with sarcoidosis, typically in patients with advanced disease.[346] In a retrospective study[346] of 23 patients with cavitary sarcoidosis, 52 were in radiographic stage IV); 48% had severe extrapulmonary involvement. Active lesions (*eg*, consolidation or GGO) were present concomitantly in 19 patients (83%).[346] Wall thickening during follow-up suggests an infectious complication (particularly aspergillomas).[346] Other nonspecific features include irregular interfaces; thickened alveolar septae or pleural surfaces; traction bronchiectasis; and distortion or displacement of vessels, bronchi, or interlobar tissues.

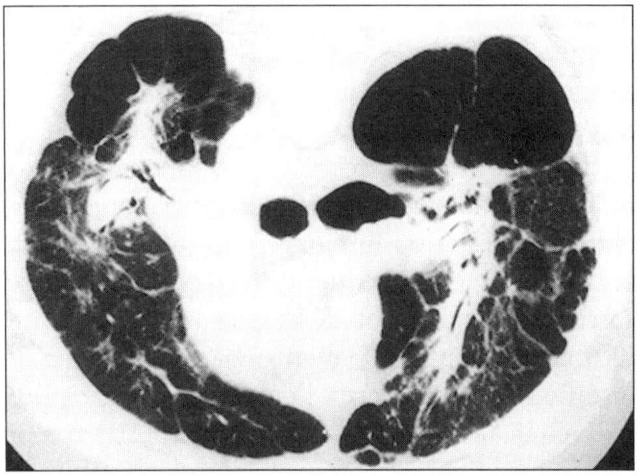

Figure 18. HRCT scan from a 48-year-old man with severe, chronic pulmonary sarcoidosis. Cuts at the level of the main carina show areas of bronchial thickening and consolidation centrally, in an axial distribution. Large cystic, bullous changes are evident in the posterior lung fields. The lung architecture is distorted.

In sarcoidosis, the preferential distribution of parenchymal lesions along bronchovascular bundles and lymphatics with an upper-lobe predominance[143] contrasts sharply with IPF/UIP, which has a predilection for the basilar and subpleural (peripheral) regions of the lungs.[253] Emphysema may be observed in advanced stage sarcoidosis (typically stage IV) but is more extensive in smokers.[354] CT features of airflow obstruction may include a mosaic pattern of attenuation; bronchial wall or peribronchiolar thickening; bronchial distortion, compression, or stenosis; and bronchiectasis.[355] Fibrosis and conglomerate masses may be present concomitantly, particularly in patients with bronchial distortion.[355] Specific CT features have prognostic significance. Focal nodular, alveolar, or GGOs suggest an active inflammatory component. In contrast, distortion of lung parenchyma, volume loss, linear bands, bronchiectasis, cystic radiolucencies, and bullae are characteristic of end-stage fibrosis.[143]

Because of its expense, I do not advocate routine HRCT in the diagnosis or staging of sarcoidosis. However, HRCT has a role in selected patients in assessing prognosis and determining the likelihood of response to therapy. Patients with extensive fibrosis, honeycombing, and lung distortion are not likely to respond to therapy with corticosteroids or immunosuppressive agents. By contrast, patients with large focal alveolar opacities and a ground-glass pattern are better candidates for therapy. CT patterns may evolve over time. Serial CT in 40 patients with pulmonary sarcoidosis showed several distinctive evolutionary patterns.[356] Macroscopic nodules often disappeared or decreased in size at follow-up. Consolidation and GGO resolved in some patients but evolved into honeycombing in other patients (associated with a decrease in FVC). A conglomeration pattern shrank and evolved into bronchial distortion and a decline in FEV_1/FVC ratio. Given the imprecise correlations between CT and physiologic parameters, direct measurement of PFTs is critical to assess the extent and degree of pulmonary functional impairment.

PFTs

Restrictive ventilatory defects are observed in 30 to 60% of patients with pulmonary sarcoidosis.[303] Airway obstruction, with reduced FEV_1 and expiratory flow rates, occurs in 9 to 40% of patients.[355,357] A prospective study[358] noted airflow limitation (defined as <70% FEV_1/FVC ratio) in 20 of 228 (8.8%) consecutive Japanese patients with sarcoidosis. Airflow limitation was more common in men, smokers, and those patients classified as radiographic stage IV. Airflow obstruction may reflect submucosal or endobronchial inflammation, parenchymal distortion, bronchostenosis, or exaggerated bronchial reactivity.[303,355,359,360] Increased airway hyperreactivity in response to methacholine is common in patients with sarcoidosis.[359,361] The DLCO is the most sensitive of the PFT parameters,[359] but the degree of impairment is less severe in sarcoidosis than in IPF.[302] Hypoxemia is unusual but may be present in patients with advanced disease. CPET findings are abnormal in up to 50% of patients with sarcoidosis, even when static PFT results are normal.[362] In one study, significant associations were noted between chest radiographic stage and TLC, DLCO, $P(A\text{-}a)O_2$, and change in Po_2 with exercise.[363] However, CPETs are logistically cumbersome and have limited practical value.

PFTs at a single time point cannot discriminate active from inactive disease and do not correlate with histology. However, serial PFTs are important to follow the course of the disease and assess response to therapy. VC improves more frequently than DLCO, TLC, or arterial oxygenation.[302] Changes in VC and DLCO are concordant in >90 of patients.[302,316] A prospective study[316] in the United States of 193 sarcoid patients cited excellent concordance between changes in FVC and FEV_1. Given the variability of DLCO and the expense of obtaining lung volumes, spirometry and flow-volume loops are the most useful and cost-effective parameters to follow the course of pulmonary sarcoidosis. FVC is the most sensitive indicator of disease progression (or resolution). Spirometry should be repeated at 6-month intervals for the first 2 years, even in patients with minimal or no pulmonary symptoms. Patients with pulmonary symptoms or derangements in pulmonary function require more frequent studies. Deteriorating pulmonary function or persistence of severe derangements warrants a trial of corticosteroid therapy, regardless of whether radiographic abnormalities are present.

Ancillary Studies

Serum ACE levels, radionuclide scans, and BAL cell profiles have been used to more accurately determine the extent and activity of the disease, but their role remains controversial. Serum ACE levels, ^{67}Ga scans, and BAL may reflect different stages or components of the disease process. Further, serum ACE levels and ^{67}Ga scans may reflect the macrophage component, which may not necessarily correlate with BAL lymphocytosis or lymphokine release.

ACE: ACE, an enzyme normally produced by endothelial cells, is produced in exaggerated amounts by sarcoid granuloma macrophages.[303] Serum ACE levels may reflect total body granuloma burden but are not sensitive to active localized disease. Changes in serum ACE often parallel the course of the disease and may be used to guide treatment decisions, provided clinical information is taken into account. Isolated elevations of serum ACE in the absence of clinical symptoms do not require therapy. Importantly, serum ACE levels may be normal in patients with active disease.[302] I obtain a baseline serum ACE level in patients with sarcoidosis and obtain serial levels in selected patients when clinical criteria are inadequate to judge disease activity.

^{67}Ga Citrate Scans: ^{67}Ga citrate scans were used as a surrogate marker of disease activity in sarcoidosis and other inflammatory pulmonary disorders. ^{67}Ga is taken up avidly by activated alveolar macrophages, and intrapulmonary uptake of ^{67}Ga may be a marker of active alveolar inflammation (alveolitis). Characteristic patterns of uptake have been noted in sarcoidosis (*eg*, increased uptake in lacrimal, salivary, and parotid glands and hilar and mediastinal lymph nodes).[364,365] However, ^{67}Ga scans are expensive, inconvenient, difficult to quantitate, and lack prognostic value.[364,365] I see no role for ^{67}Ga scanning in either the initial staging or longitudinal follow-up of patients with sarcoidosis. However, ^{67}Ga scanning may have a limited role in patients with normal chest radiographs and suspected sarcoidosis to detect clinically silent extrathoracic sites of ^{67}Ga uptake and provide sites for biopsies.[365,366] PET scans may demonstrate increased metabolic activity in patients with pulmonary[365] or extrapulmonary sarcoidosis (*eg*, bone,[367] cardiac,[368] or

neural sites[369]). However, the clinical value of PET is uncertain.[351]

BAL: BAL has provided significant insights into the pathogenesis of sarcoidosis.[370] BAL in sarcoidosis demonstrates increased numbers of activated lymphocytes (typically $CD4^+$ T cells), alveolar macrophages, and myriad proinflammatory cytokines and mediators.[370,371] BAL lymphocytosis is present in $>85\%$ of patients with pulmonary sarcoidosis; granulocytes are normal or low.[237,302,370] BAL reveals increased numbers of activated T lymphocytes (predominantly $CD4^+$) and activated macrophages, with reduced T suppressor cells ($CD8^+$), in patients with active pulmonary sarcoidosis.[370–372] In late phases of sarcoidosis, neutrophils and/or mast cells may be increased.[373] BAL cell profiles are not specific for sarcoidosis but narrow the differential diagnosis.[237,370] Importantly, BAL cell profiles fail to predict prognosis or responsiveness to corticosteroid therapy.[302,370] High levels of T lymphocytes or lymphokines may reflect active alveolitis but do not imply that deterioration will inevitably occur.[302] Because of the waxing and waning nature of sarcoidosis, BAL has limited prognostic value. Marked increases in $CD4^+$ lymphocytes, consistent with an intensive alveolitis, are characteristic of Löfgren syndrome, yet spontaneous remissions occur in $>85\%$ of patients in this setting.[302,315] Serial bronchoscopy is invasive, expensive, and impractical for sequential evaluation of sarcoidosis.

Pathogenesis

The inciting signals responsible for the exuberant granulomatous response and its subsequent progression to fibrosis (or resolution) have not been identified. Interactions between activated mononuclear phagocytes (*eg*, monocytes and macrophages) and activated T-helper/inducer lymphocytes are responsible for the induction and evolution of the granulomatous process.[371,372] At sites of active disease, striking increases in helper/inducer ($CD4^+$) lymphocytes and increased $CD4^+/CD8^+$ ratios and increased release of diverse lymphokines (consistent with a T-helper type 1 [Th1] response), monokines, and biochemical markers have been noted.[371,372] Early in the course, Th1 cytokines (*eg*, γ-IFN and IL-2) predominate at sites of disease activity; this compartmentalization of the immune response (with a Th1 cytokine bias) may abate as the disease remits.[371,372] Lung T cells from patients with active pulmonary sarcoidosis release several cytokines that contribute to the induction of the immune response and facilitate T-cell replication and mononuclear phagocyte activation.[371,372] Alveolar macrophages from patients with pulmonary sarcoidosis are activated, enhance antigen presentation, express receptors for IL-2, and release growth factors that promote fibroblast recruitment and proliferation.[371] Macrophages play a dual role in orchestrating the sarcoid lung lesion by producing monokines that may either amplify or down-regulate the inflammatory process.

Therapy

Corticosteriods are the mainstay of therapy and may produce dramatic remissions in patients with severe or progressive sarcoidosis.[302,374] Favorable responses to corticosteroid therapy are achieved in 60 to 90% of patients with symptomatic sarcoidosis, but relapses occur in 16 to 74% of patients after the cessation of therapy.[302,303,348,374,375] Long-term efficacy is less clear. Because of the potential for spontaneous resolution and the toxicities associated with corticosteroid therapy, indications for treatment are controversial. Several prospective studies performed in the 1970s failed to show a favorable effect on long-term prognosis. Although several studies suggested short-term improvement with corticosteroid therapy, relapses often occurred after the cessation of therapy. The lack of efficacy may reflect the study designs because patients with stage I disease, minimal or no symptoms, and normal lung function were often enrolled into treatment trials. In most of these studies, high rates of improvement or stabilization were noted in both treated and untreated patients.

The long-term impact of corticosteroid therapy is difficult to assess because of the high rate of spontaneous remissions as well as inclusion of patients with irreversible disease. These data cannot be extrapolated to patients with severe or progressive pulmonary disease who are the best candidates for therapy. A multicenter, randomized trial of stage II or III sarcoidosis sponsored by the British Thoracic Society found that corticosteroid therapy in patients with persistent radiographic infiltrates after an initial 6-month observation period was associated with improved lung function, chest radiographs, and symptoms compared with untreated controls.[347]

Among 149 patients with stage II or III pulmonary sarcoidosis eligible for the study, 33 patients required immediate corticosteroid therapy for control of symptoms and were excluded. In addition, 58 patients whose chest radiographs improved spontaneously within 6 months of entry served as an untreated observation group. The remaining 58 untreated patients with persistent radiographic infiltrates after 6 months were randomly assigned to be administered routine corticosteroids for 18 months (n = 27) or selective therapy only (to control symptoms or deteriorating pulmonary symptoms; n = 31). No placebo group was included. The dose of corticosteroids in the treated group was modest (*ie*, prednisolone, 30 mg/d for 1 month, tapered to 10 mg by 4 months; maintenance therapy with 10 mg/d was continued for 9 months). Incremental doses were permitted as necessary to maximize radiographic improvement.

The results affirmed the benefit of regular treatment with corticosteroid therapy in patients with radiographic stage II or III disease who failed to spontaneously remit during the 6-month period of observation. These data support the use of corticosteroid therapy for patients with stage II or III disease whose condition does not improve spontaneously within a reasonable period. The optimal observation period before deciding on therapy has not been determined. A period of not more than 6 to 18 months is appropriate because spontaneous remission beyond this point is unlikely. More immediate institution of therapy is warranted for patients with severe or deteriorating symptoms or pulmonary dysfunction.

Corticosteroids have potential toxicity, and routine therapy for patients with mild or no symptoms is inappropriate. Indications for therapy should be circumscribed and focused. Despite the lack of consensus regarding efficacy of therapy, there is little doubt that corticosteroids dramatically suppress or reverse the disease in some cases. Corticosteroids are warranted for myocardial,[309] CNS,[312] or ophthalmologic (*eg*, uveitis) complications of sarcoidosis.[304,307] Corticosteroids are also indicated for chronic hypercalcemia (to avert late complications of nephrocalcinosis and nephrolithiasis) and for severe or progressive pulmonary or extrapulmonary dysfunction.

The dose and duration of therapy need to be individualized. Chronic disease of mild-to-moderate severity can be treated with modest dosages (*eg*, 40 mg every other day for 3 to 4 months, with subsequent taper). Greater doses (*eg*, prednisone 1 mg/kg/d for 4 weeks, with a gradual taper) are appropriate for myocardial or CNS manifestations. The duration of therapy and the rate of taper need to be individualized according to clinical response and presence or absence of adverse effects. A 3-month trial of corticosteroids is usually adequate to judge efficacy. If no objective response has been shown within this time, corticosteroids can be tapered and discontinued. In contrast, among responders, corticosteroids should be continued, albeit in a tapering regimen, for 12 to 18 months. Relapses may occur as the steroid dosage is reduced or discontinued. In such cases, escalation of the dose may be efficacious. Long-term corticosteroids are indicated only for patients who have shown unequivocal response to therapy yet relapse with attempts to stop therapy.

Inhaled Corticosteroids: Inhaled corticosteroids were associated with anecdotal responses in patients with mild pulmonary sarcoidosis, but firm data supporting their efficacy are lacking. In one double-blind, placebo-controlled trial in Finland,[376] 189 patients with pulmonary sarcoidosis (stage I, II, or III) were randomly assigned to receive either oral prednisone for 3 months followed by inhaled budesonide or placebo. Among patients with stage II disease, chest radiographic findings did not differ between groups. Differences in PFTs (FVC, DLCO) between groups were minimal. A trend toward improvement in DLCO was noted in corticosteroid-treated patients with stage II disease. These differences were small and did not achieve statistical significance. Changes in FVC over time were similar between groups.

Long-term follow-up from the Finnish study,[377] which randomized patients with stage I and II newly diagnosed (<3 months) sarcoidosis to immediate treatment with placebo or prednisolone for 3 months followed by inhaled budesonide for 15 months found no differences in treated or placebo groups in chest radiographs at 1 year. However, at 5 years, patients in the placebo cohort had lower mean FVC and DLCO and worse chest radiograph findings compared with treated patients. Differences between groups were small, and the significance of these observations is not clear.

In another double-blind trial, British investigators[378] randomly assigned 44 adults with stage II or III pulmonary sarcoidosis to inhaled fluticasone (1,000 μg bid) or placebo for 6 months. Approximately 75% were administered oral corticosteroids at the start of the study. No significant differences in PFTs, mean dose of oral corticosteroid, or chest radiograph findings were detected at any time point. These studies[376–378] suggest that inhaled corticosteroids have minimal value as the primary therapy for pulmonary sarcoidosis. However, given their low toxicity, a trial of an inhaled corticosteroid is reasonable in patients with significant endobronchial inflammation, cough, or persistent pulmonary symptoms.

Immunosuppressive or Cytotoxic Agents: Immunosuppressive or cytotoxic agents (*eg*, methotrexate, azathioprine, cyclosporine, chlorambucil, cyclophosphamide, and leflunomide) have been used, with anecdotal successes, in patients in whom treatment is failing or who are experiencing side effects from corticosteroids. However, randomized trials evaluating these agents are lacking, and the best agent has not been determined.

Immunosuppressive Agents: Both azathioprine and methotrexate may be useful for sarcoidosis refractory to corticosteroids or as steroid-sparing agents in patients requiring high-dose corticosteroids for control of the disease.

Azathioprine: azathioprine (2 to 3 mg/kg/d), alone or combined with corticosteroids, has been associated with anecdotal successes in sarcoidosis, even in patients in whom corticosteroid therapy is failing. However, randomized trials have not been performed. Further, studies directly comparing azathioprine with alternative agents for sarcoidosis are lacking. In two early studies,[379,380] 10 of 20 patients in whom corticosteroid therapy is failing responded to azathioprine. In another retrospective study,[381] 8 of 14 patients with neurosarcoidosis responded to azathioprine. Diab et al[382] treated seven patients with a combination of prednisone and azathioprine; all patients improved. In contrast, investigators from South Africa found azathioprine to be of marginal benefit in a retrospective study[383] of 10 patients with pulmonary sarcoidosis. All had shown only partial (n = 6) or no (n = 4) response to corticosteroids. The addition of azathioprine (100 to 150 mg/d) plus low-dose corticosteroids was associated with significant and sustained improvement in lung function in only two patients; two additional patients had transient improvement and a steroid-sparing effect. Two patients in whom azathioprine therapy failed subsequently responded to cyclosporine A (CsA) and high-dose corticosteroids. No patient who did not respond to high-dose corticosteroids responded to azathioprine. German investigators[384] treated 11 patients with chronic sarcoidosis with azathioprine plus prednisolone. All had symptomatic improvement; chest radiographs improved in nine patients, and PFT results improved in seven patients. Late relapses (8 to 22 months) occurred in three patients. Although these data are limited, I believe azathioprine may be useful as a steroid-sparing agent or in selected patients with severe or progressive sarcoidosis refractory to corticosteroids. Extensive clinical experience with azathioprine in organ transplant recipients and other immune disorders suggests that serious late sequela associated with chronic azathioprine use are uncommon.[265]

Methotrexate: Methotrexate, a folic acid antagonist with both immunosuppressive and anti-inflammatory effects, has been efficacious for both pulmonary and extrapulmonary sarcoidosis.[385,386] Methotrexate can be administered parenterally (intramuscularly) or orally as a pulse once weekly. Dosages ranging from 10 to 25 mg/wk have been used. In uncontrolled studies[387,88] by investigators from the University of Cincinnati who evaluated > 230 patients, favorable responses to methotrexate were cited in 52 to 66% of patients. Relapses were frequent with cessation of therapy but usually responded to reinstitution of methotrexate.

Although these studies are not definitive, methotrexate has a role as a steroid-sparing agent in sarcoidosis. Because of potential toxicities, methotrexate should be restricted to patients requiring unacceptably high doses of corticosteroids (> 20 mg/d prednisolone or equivalent) or experiencing serious side effects from corticosteroids. In this context, a 4- to 6-month trial of methotrexate is reasonable. I initiate therapy with 7.5 mg once weekly and escalate the dose by 2.5-mg increments weekly (to a maximal dose of 20 mg) until a clinical response or toxicity has occurred.

Serious adverse effects are rare (< 1% of patients), but side effects requiring cessation of therapy occur in 3 to 15% of cases.[265]

Adverse effects of methotrexate are dose dependent and may be minimized by the addition of folic acid (1 mg/d). Adverse effects associated with methotrexate include GI effects (*eg*, nausea, vomiting, and diarrhea), stomatitis (*eg*, mucosal or oral ulcers), and rash. Less common complications, each occurring in 1 to 4% of patients, include megaloblastic anemia, leukopenia, or thrombocytopenia; opportunistic infections; and interstitial pneumonitis.[265,389]

In contrast to the alkylating agents, methotrexate is not carcinogenic. Methotrexate is teratogenic and cannot be used in patients at risk of conception. The most worrisome side effect is hepatic cirrhosis, which may occur in up to 2% of patients with long-term use (> 2 years).[265] The risk of permanent liver disease with long-term use of methotrexate (> 2 years) has not been defined in patients with sarcoidosis. A series[390] of 68 patients with chronic sarcoidosis treated with long-term (> 2 years) methotrexate therapy cited histologic features consistent with MTX toxicity in 14 patients (21%). Importantly, serial liver function tests were not useful in determining which patients would have methotrexate toxicities.

Contraindications to methotrexate include ethanol abuse, concomitant liver disease, history of hepatitis, patients unable to adhere to dosing schedules, renal failure, active infection, anemia, and leukopenia. Serial transaminase levels, CBC counts, and platelet counts should be monitored every 4 to 8 weeks in patients receiving methotrexate. Persistent or progressive rises in hepatic enzymes, thrombocytopenia, or leukopenia warrant discontinuation of therapy or reduction of the dose. Given its potential for late, irreversible hepatotoxicity, methotrexate should be continued beyond 6 months only in patients demonstrating unequivocal objective improvement. Enthusiasm for its use needs to be tempered by the high rates of relapse noted on cessation of therapy. I prefer azathioprine for patients with chronic, progressive sarcoidosis requiring long-term treatment (> 1 year).

Leflunomide: Leflunomide has been used to treat sarcoidosis, but data are sparse. One nonrandomized trial[391] cited responses in 25 of 32 sarcoid patients (78%) treated with leflunomide (alone or combined with methotrexate). Leflunomide appears to be less toxic than methotrexate and may be an alternative to methotrexate, but data are sparse.

Mycophenolate Mofetil: Responses to mycophenolate mofetil were noted in anecdotal cases of extrapulmonary sarcoidosis,[392,393,394] but data are lacking in pulmonary sarcoidosis.

CsA: CsA, a fungal decapeptide that exhibits relatively selective inhibitory effects on T-cell activation, proliferation, and lymphokine release, would be expected to be an ideal agent for treating sarcoidosis. However, despite anecdotal responses in some corticosteroid-resistant patients,[383] CsA has been disappointing as therapy for pulmonary sarcoidosis. In a study[395] from the National Institutes of Health, eight patients with symptomatic pulmonary sarcoidosis received oral CsA, 10 mg/kg/d, for 6 months. Despite inhibitory effects on T-cell proliferation and cytokine release *in vitro*, pulmonary function or BAL results did not change.

In one study,[396] six patients with corticosteroid-refractory CNS sarcoidosis were treated with CsA plus corticosteroids for 6 months. No patient achieved complete remission, but a steroid-sparing effect was suggested. A subsequent study[381] by these investigators cited favorable responses in 11 of 14 patients with neurosarcoidosis treated with CsA. A randomized controlled trial by Wyser and coworkers[397] showed no benefit with oral CsA, 5 to 7 mg/kg/d, combined with prednisone as compared with prednisone alone in a cohort of 37 patients with pulmonary sarcoidosis. Adverse effects (particularly renal insufficiency and infections) and relapses were greater in the patients receiving combined therapy.[397] CsA is very expensive and is associated with numerous toxicities (*eg*, hypertension, renal insufficiency, hirsutism, neuropathies, disorders in lipids, heightened susceptibilities to infections, and lymphoproliferative disorders).[265] In light of the myriad complications associated with its use and the lack of demonstrated efficacy, cyclosporine has at best a marginal role as salvage therapy for patients with severe, progressive sarcoidosis refractory to corticosteroids. Topical cyclosporine eye drops may be effective for sarcoid conjunctivitis.[398]

Alkylating Agents

Published data regarding alkylating agents (*eg*, cyclophosphamide, chlorambucil) for the treatment of sarcoidosis are limited to sporadic case reports and small retrospective series, Chlorambucil, an alkylating agent of the nitrogen mustard class, was associated with favorable responses in nonrandomized studies (primarily in patients experiencing adverse effects from corticosteroids).[399–401] However, chlorambucil is oncogenic and has numerous toxicities.[265] Given the availability of alternative therapeutic agents, chlorambucil has no role in the treatment of sarcoidosis.

Cyclophosphamide: Cyclophosphamide (oral or pulse) has rarely been used to treat sarcoidosis. Anecdotal responses have been noted, but data are limited to a few case reports and small series.[312,374,402,403] Lower and colleagues[312] cited favorable responses in 8 of 10 patients treated with IV pulse cyclophosphamide for neurosarcoidosis, 8 of whom had concomitant lung involvement. Previous therapy included corticosteroids in all 10 and methotrexate in 8. Thus, cyclophosphamide has a role for severe sarcoidosis refractory to corticosteroids or other immunosuppressive agents. However, in light of its oncogenic potential, particularly in relatively young patients, I reserve cyclophosphamide for severe sarcoidosis refractory to corticosteroids and azathioprine or methotrexate.

Other Antiinflammatory and Immunomodulatory Agents

Nonsteroidal antiinflammatory agents (*eg*, indomethacin and phenylbutazone) have been used to treat the acute articular manifestations of sarcoidosis, but have no role in treating more severe cases of pulmonary or extrapulmonary sarcoidosis.

Antimalarial Drugs: Antimalarial drugs (*eg*, chloroquine and hydroxychloroquine) have immunomodulating properties and are efficacious in treating rheumatoid arthritis, systemic lupus erythematosus, and diverse immune-mediated diseases. Antimalarials concentrate in cells of the reticuloendothelial system and melanin-containing tissues (*eg*, skin, spleen, leukocytes, kidney) and are preferentially concentrated in epithelioid, mononuclear, and giant cells comprising sarcoid granulomata. Anecdotal responses have been noted with the antimalarials for cutaneous,[404] osseous,[374] and neurologic[405] sarcoidosis and sarcoid-induced hypercalcemia.[406,407]

The role of antimalarials in treating pulmonary sarcoidosis is less well established. However, a randomized trial[408] of 23 patients with symptomatic pulmonary sarcoidosis (radiographic stage II or III) suggested benefit with chloroquine. Sixteen of the 23 patients had previously been treated with high-dose corticosteroids, without sustained improvement. All 23 patients were treated with high-dose chloroquine (750 mg/d) for 6 months. Five patients withdrew from the study before the 6-month acute phase (three as the result of intolerable side effects). After 6 months, the dose of chloroquine was tapered by 250 mg every 2 months. Eighteen patients were then randomly assigned to a maintenance group (chloroquine, 250 mg/d; n = 10) or observation group (no chloroquine; n = 8).

After the initial 6-month treatment with high-dose chloroquine, symptoms, PFT results, serum ACE levels, and Ga^{67} scan findings improved. After randomization, the rate of decline in PFTs was slower, and there were fewer relapses in patients receiving maintenance chloroquine vs no chloroquine therapy. Studies comparing chloroquine with chloroquine therapy have not been performed. The major toxicity of antimalarials is ocular (particularly chloroquine); dizziness and nausea may also occur.[408] Unfortunately, prolonged administration of chloroquine can lead to irreversible retinopathy and blindness. Given the potential serious ocular toxicity associated with chloroquine, hydroxychloroquine, which is less toxic, is preferred. The dose of hydroxychloroquine is 200 mg once or twice daily for a 6-month trial. Long-term maintenance therapy (100 to 400 mg/d) is reserved for patients manifesting unequivocal responses. Slit-lamp examinations should be done by an ophthalmologist every 9 months to rule out ocular toxicity. The combination of hydroxychloroquine with corticosteroids or immunosuppressive agents may enhance immunomodulatory effects compared with any of these agents alone.

Alternative Therapies: Anecdotal responses have been cited with thalidomide (a sedative with teratogenic properties),[409,410] melatonin,[411] and pentoxifylline[412] in patients with sarcoidosis, but the value of these agents is unproven. Pentoxifylline and dexamethasone suppressed release of TNF-α from sarcoid alveolar macrophages *in vitro*, but *in vivo* data were lacking.[413]

TNF-α: TNF-α inhibitors (particularly infliximab) have been used, with anecdotal success, to treat refractory sarcoidosis (particularly lupus pernio and extrapulmonary cases).[414–427] Data in pulmonary sarcoidosis are limited.[422,428,429] In a recent multicenter trial,[422] 138 patients with chronic pulmonary sarcoidosis were randomized to placebo or infliximab, 3 mg/kg, or infliximab, 5 mg/kg, at weeks 0, 2, 6, 12, 18, and 24. At 24 weeks, the primary end point change in FVC percentage of predicted was slightly greater among infliximab-treated patients (2.5% above baseline) compared with placebo-treated patients (no change). This difference, although statistically significant, is of doubtful clinical significance. Treatment with TNF inhibitors is very expensive and has been associated with a heightened risk of tuberculosis,[430] other opportunistic infections, and other adverse effects, [431–434] including lymphoma development.[435] Currently, additional studies are required to establish the role of TNF-α inhibitors (*eg*, infliximab, etanercept, or adalimumab) as therapy for sarcoidosis.

Pulmonary Hypertension

Pulmonary hypertension is a rare complication of sarcoidosis but may occur in patients with advanced radiographic stages.[195,436–439] Although data are limited, favorable responses to short- and long-term vasodilators have been cited (*eg*, inhaled nitric oxide, IV epoprostenol, and oral calcium-channel blockers).[437] Supplemental oxygen should be administered for patients with hypoxemia.

LT

SLT or BLT has been successfully accomplished in patients with severe pulmonary sarcoidosis refractory to aggressive medical therapy.[158,438,440–442] From January 1995 to June 2006, 438 adults worldwide had received LT for sarcoidosis.[293] Long-term survival rates after LT for sarcoidosis are generally similar to other indications.[441] Recurrence of sarcoid granulomas within the lung allografts is common but rarely causes clinical symptoms.[443] Deciding when to list patients for LT is difficult because predicting life expectancy in individual patients is difficult.[438,444] However, waiting time for organs can be prolonged, and 27 to 53% of patients with end-stage pulmonary sarcoidosis die while awaiting transplantation.[438,440,445] Typically, patients with sarcoidosis referred for LT have severe impairment in PFTs (mean percentage of predicted FVC $<$ 44%; mean percentage of predicted FEV_1 $<$ 38%).[440,445]

In one study[438] of patients with sarcoidosis awaiting LT, the following factors were associated with increased mortality on the waiting list: Pao_2 $\leq$ 60 mm Hg, mean PAP $\geq$ 35 mm Hg, cardiac index $\leq$ 2 L/min/m^2, and right atrial pressure $\geq$ 15 mm Hg. A retrospective review[445] of 405 sarcoid patients listed for LT in the United States noted three variables that were independently associated with increased mortality: black race, amount of supplemental oxygen needed, and mPAP. Pulmonary arterial hypertension is an ominous sign in sarcoidosis, and warrants referral for LT. Invasive aspergillosis may complicate LT among sarcoid patients with preexisting mycetomas.[158]

References

1. Lynch J III, Fishbein MC, Saggar R, et al. Idiopathic pulmonary fibrosis. Exp Rev Respir Med 2007; 1:377–390
2. Lynch JP 3rd, Saggar R, Weigt SS, et al. Usual interstitial pneumonia. Semin Respir Crit Care Med 2006; 27:634–651
3. American Thoracic Society. Idiopathic pulmonary fibrosis: diagnosis and treatment. International consensus statement. American Thoracic Society (ATS), and the European Respiratory Society (ERS). Am J Respir Crit Care Med 2000; 161:646–664
4. American Thoracic Society/European Respiratory Society International Multidisciplinary Consensus Classification of the Idiopathic Interstitial Pneumonias. This joint statement of the American Thoracic Society (ATS), and the European Respiratory Society (ERS) was adopted by the ATS board of directors, June 2001 and by the ERS Executive Committee, June 2001. Am J Respir Crit Care Med 2002; 165:277–304
5. Katzenstein AL, Mukhopadhyay S, Myers JL. Diagnosis of usual interstitial pneumonia and distinction from other fibrosing interstitial lung diseases. Hum Pathol 2008; 39:1275–1294

6. Katzenstein AL, Myers JL. Idiopathic pulmonary fibrosis: clinical relevance of pathologic classification. Am J Respir Crit Care Med 1998; 157:1301–1315
7. Lai CK, Wallace WD, Fishbein MC. Histopathology of pulmonary fibrotic disorders. Semin Respir Crit Care Med 2006; 27:613–622
8. King TE Jr. Clinical advances in the diagnosis and therapy of the interstitial lung diseases. Am J Respir Crit Care Med 2005; 172:268–279
9. Ryu JH, Colby TV, Hartman TE, et al. Smoking-related interstitial lung diseases: a concise review. Eur Respir J 2001; 17:122–132
10. Ryu JH, Myers JL, Capizzi SA, et al. Desquamative interstitial pneumonia and respiratory bronchiolitis-associated interstitial lung disease. Chest 2005; 127:178–184
11. Hartman TE, Swensen SJ, Hansell DM, et al. Nonspecific interstitial pneumonia: variable appearance at high-resolution chest CT. Radiology 2000; 217:701–705
12. Flaherty KR, Martinez FJ, Travis W, et al. Nonspecific interstitial pneumonia (NSIP). Semin Respir Crit Care Med 2001; 22:423–434
13. Martinez FJ. Idiopathic interstitial pneumonias: usual interstitial pneumonia versus nonspecific interstitial pneumonia. Proc Am Thorac Soc 2006; 3:81–95
14. Travis WD, Hunninghake G, King TE Jr., et al. Idiopathic nonspecific interstitial pneumonia: report of an American Thoracic Society project. Am J Respir Crit Care Med 2008; 177:1338–1347
15. Vourlekis JS, Brown KK, Cool CD, et al. Acute interstitial pneumonitis: case series and review of the literature. Medicine (Baltimore) 2000; 79: 369–378
16. Bouros D, Nicholson AC, Polychronopoulos V, et al. Acute interstitial pneumonia. Eur Respir J 2000; 15:412–418
17. Koss MN, Shigemitsu H. Lymphocytic interstitial pneumonia (LIP) and other pulmonary lymphoproliferative disorders. In: Lynch JP III, ed. Interstitial pulmonary and bronchiolar disorders (Vol 227). New York: InformaUSA, 2008; 403–428
18. Nicholson AG. Lymphocytic interstitial pneumonia and other lymphoproliferative disorders in the lung. Semin Respir Crit Care Med 2001; 22: 409–422
19. Cordier JF. Cryptogenic organising pneumonia. Eur Respir J 2006; 28:422–446
20. Silva CI, Muller NL, Lynch DA, et al. Chronic hypersensitivity pneumonitis: differentiation from idiopathic pulmonary fibrosis and nonspecific interstitial pneumonia by using thin-section CT. Radiology 2008; 246:288–297
21. Selman M, Mejia M, Pardo A. Hypersensitivity Pneumonitis. In: Lynch JP III, ed. Interstitial pulmonary and bronchiolar disorders (Vol 227). New York: InformaUSA, 2008; 267–288
22. Flaherty KR, Thwaite EL, Kazerooni EA, et al. Radiological versus histological diagnosis in UIP and NSIP: survival implications. Thorax 2003; 58:143–148
23. Lynch DA, Godwin JD, Safrin S, et al. High-resolution computed tomography in idiopathic pulmonary fibrosis: diagnosis and prognosis. Am J Respir Crit Care Med 2005; 172:488–493
24. Hunninghake GW, Lynch DA, Galvin JR, et al. Radiologic findings are strongly associated with a pathologic diagnosis of usual interstitial pneumonia. Chest 2003; 124:1215–1223
25. Antoniou KM, Hansell DM, Rubens MB, et al. Idiopathic pulmonary fibrosis: outcome in relation to smoking status. Am J Respir Crit Care Med 2008; 177:190–194
26. Hubbard R, Johnston I, Britton J. Survival in patients with cryptogenic fibrosing alveolitis: a population-based cohort study. Chest 1998; 113:396–400
27. Douglas WW, Ryu JH, Schroeder DR. Idiopathic pulmonary fibrosis: impact of oxygen and colchicine, prednisone, or no therapy on survival. Am J Respir Crit Care Med 2000; 161:1172–1178
28. King TE Jr, Tooze JA, Schwarz MI, et al. Predicting survival in idiopathic pulmonary fibrosis: scoring system and survival model. Am J Respir Crit Care Med 2001; 164:1171–1181
29. Coultas DB, Zumwalt RE, Black WC, et al. The epidemiology of interstitial lung diseases. Am J Respir Crit Care Med 1994; 150:967–972
30. Raghu G, Weycker D, Edelsberg J, et al. Incidence and prevalence of idiopathic pulmonary fibrosis. Am J Respir Crit Care Med 2006; 174:810–816
31. Gribbin J, Hubbard RB, Le Jeune I, et al. Incidence and mortality of idiopathic pulmonary fibrosis and sarcoidosis in the UK. Thorax 2006; 61:980–985
32. Hubbard R, Johnston I, Coultas DB, et al. Mortality rates from cryptogenic fibrosing alveolitis in seven countries. Thorax 1996; 51:711–716

33. Harris JM, Cullinan P, McDonald JC. Occupational distribution and geographic clustering of deaths certified to be cryptogenic fibrosing alveolitis in England and Wales. Chest 2001; 119:428–433
34. Iwai K, Mori T, Yamada N, et al. Idiopathic pulmonary fibrosis: epidemiologic approaches to occupational exposure. Am J Respir Crit Care Med 1994; 150:670–675
35. Scott J, Johnston I, Britton J. What causes cryptogenic fibrosing alveolitis? A case-control study of environmental exposure to dust. BMJ 1990; 301:1015–1017
36. Olson AL, Swigris JJ, Lezotte DC, et al. Mortality from pulmonary fibrosis increased in the United States from 1992 to 2003. Am J Respir Crit Care Med 2007; 176:277–284
37. Mannino DM, Etzel RA, Parrish RG. Pulmonary fibrosis deaths in the United States, 1979–1991: an analysis of multiple-cause mortality data. Am J Respir Crit Care Med 1996; 153:1548–1552
38. Thomas AQ, Lane K, Phillips J 3rd, et al. Heterozygosity for a surfactant protein C gene mutation associated with usual interstitial pneumonitis and cellular nonspecific interstitial pneumonitis in one kindred. Am J Respir Crit Care Med 2002; 165:1322–1328
39. Fan LL, Kozinetz CA. Factors influencing survival in children with chronic interstitial lung disease. Am J Respir Crit Care Med 1997; 156: 939–942
40. Baumgartner KB, Samet JM, Coultas DB, et al. Occupational and environmental risk factors for idiopathic pulmonary fibrosis: a multicenter case-control study: collaborating centers. Am J Epidemiol 2000; 152:307–315
41. Garantziotis S, Schwartz DA. Host-environment interactions in pulmonary fibrosis. Semin Respir Crit Care Med 2006; 27:574–580
42. Taskar VS, Coultas DB. Is idiopathic pulmonary fibrosis an environmental disease? Proc Am Thorac Soc 2006; 3:293–298
43. Baumgartner KB, Samet JM, Stidley CA, et al. Cigarette smoking: a risk factor for idiopathic pulmonary fibrosis. Am J Respir Crit Care Med 1997; 155:242–248
44. Hubbard R, Lewis S, Richards K, et al. Occupational exposure to metal or wood dust and aetiology of cryptogenic fibrosing alveolitis. Lancet 1996; 347:284–289
45. Schwartz DA, Van Fossen DS, Davis CS, et al. Determinants of progression in idiopathic pulmonary fibrosis. Am J Respir Crit Care Med 1994; 149:444–449
46. Steele MP, Speer MC, Loyd JE, et al. Clinical and pathologic features of familial interstitial pneumonia. Am J Respir Crit Care Med 2005; 172: 1146–1152
47. Miyake Y, Sasaki S, Yokoyama T, et al. Occupational and environmental factors and idiopathic pulmonary fibrosis in Japan. Ann Occup Hyg 2005; 49:259–265
48. Sweet MP, Patti MG, Leard LE, et al. Gastroesophageal reflux in patients with idiopathic pulmonary fibrosis referred for lung transplantation. J Thorac Cardiovasc Surg 2007; 133:1078–1084
49. Raghu G, Freudenberger TD, Yang S, et al. High prevalence of abnormal acid gastro-oesophageal reflux in idiopathic pulmonary fibrosis. Eur Respir J 2006; 27:136–142
50. Patti MG, Tedesco P, Golden J, et al. Idiopathic pulmonary fibrosis: how often is it really idiopathic? J Gastrointest Surg 2005; 9:1053–1056, discussion 6–8
51. Highland KB, Garin MC, Brown KK. The spectrum of scleroderma lung disease. Semin Respir Crit Care Med 2007; 28:418–429
52. D'Ovidio F, Mura M, Tsang M, et al. Bile acid aspiration and the development of bronchiolitis obliterans after lung transplantation. J Thorac Cardiovasc Surg 2005; 129:1144–1152
53. D'Ovidio F, Singer LG, Hadjiliadis D, et al. Prevalence of gastroesophageal reflux in end-stage lung disease candidates for lung transplant. Ann Thorac Surg 2005; 80:1254–1260
54. Blondeau K, Mertens V, Vanaudenaerde BA, et al. Gastro-oesophageal reflux and gastric aspiration in lung transplant patients with or without chronic rejection. Eur Respir J 2008; 31:707–713
55. Belperio JA, Weigt SS, Fishbein MC, et al. Chronic lung allograft rejection: mechanisms and therapy. Proc Am Thorac Soc 2009; 6:108–121
56. Cantu E 3rd, Appel JZ 3rd, Hartwig MG, et al. J. Maxwell Chamberlain Memorial Paper: early fundoplication prevents chronic allograft dysfunction in patients with gastroesophageal reflux disease. Ann Thorac Surg 2004; 78:1142–1151; discussion 1151
57. Hartwig MG, Appel JZ, Davis RD. Antireflux surgery in the setting of lung transplantation:

strategies for treating gastroesophageal reflux disease in a high-risk population. Thorac Surg Clin 2005; 15:417–427

58. Davis RD Jr., Lau CL, Eubanks S, et al. Improved lung allograft function after fundoplication in patients with gastroesophageal reflux disease undergoing lung transplantation. J Thorac Cardiovasc Surg 2003; 125:533–542
59. du Bois RM. Genetic factors in pulmonary fibrotic disorders. Semin Respir Crit Care Med 2006; 27:581–588
60. Grutters JC, du Bois RM. Genetics of fibrosing lung diseases. Eur Respir J 2005; 25:915–927
61. Marshall RP, Puddicombe A, Cookson WO, et al. Adult familial cryptogenic fibrosing alveolitis in the United Kingdom. Thorax 2000; 55:143–146
62. Lawson WE, Loyd JE. The genetic approach in pulmonary fibrosis: can it provide clues to this complex disease? Proc Am Thorac Soc 2006; 3:345–349
63. Garcia CK, Raghu G. Inherited interstitial lung disease. Clin Chest Med 2004; 25:421–433
64. Rosas IO, Ren P, Avila NA, et al. Early interstitial lung disease in familial pulmonary fibrosis. Am J Respir Crit Care Med 2007; 176:698–705
65. Yang IV, Burch LH, Steele MP, et al. Gene expression profiling of familial and sporadic interstitial pneumonia. Am J Respir Crit Care Med 2007; 175:45–54
66. Kaminski N. Microarray analysis of idiopathic pulmonary fibrosis. Am J Respir Cell Mol Biol 2003; 29(3 Suppl):S32–S36
67. Selman M, Pardo A, Barrera L, et al. Gene expression profiles distinguish idiopathic pulmonary fibrosis from hypersensitivity pneumonitis. Am J Respir Crit Care Med 2006; 173:188–198
68. Whyte M, Hubbard R, Meliconi R, et al. Increased risk of fibrosing alveolitis associated with interleukin-1 receptor antagonist and tumor necrosis factor-alpha gene polymorphisms. Am J Respir Crit Care Med 2000; 162:755–758
69. Zorzetto M, Ferrarotti I, Trisolini R, et al. Complement receptor 1 gene polymorphisms are associated with idiopathic pulmonary fibrosis. Am J Respir Crit Care Med 2003; 168:330–334
70. Xaubet A, Marin-Arguedas A, Lario S, et al. Transforming growth factor-beta1 gene polymorphisms are associated with disease progression in idiopathic pulmonary fibrosis. Am J Respir Crit Care Med 2003; 168:431–435
71. Molina-Molina M, Xaubet A, Li X, et al. Angiotensinogen gene G-6A polymorphism influences idiopathic pulmonary fibrosis disease progression. Eur Respir J 2008; 32:1004–1008
72. Nogee LM, Dunbar AE 3rd, Wert SE, et al. A mutation in the surfactant protein C gene associated with familial interstitial lung disease. N Engl J Med 2001; 344:573–579
73. Cameron HS, Somaschini M, Carrera P, et al. A common mutation in the surfactant protein C gene associated with lung disease. J Pediatr 2005; 146:370–375
74. Hamvas A, Nogee LM, White FV, et al. Progressive lung disease and surfactant dysfunction with a deletion in surfactant protein C gene. Am J Respir Cell Mol Biol 2004; 30:771–776
75. Whitsett JA. Genetic basis of familial interstitial lung disease: misfolding or function of surfactant protein C? Am J Respir Crit Care Med 2002; 165:1201–1202
76. Whitsett JA, Weaver TE. Hydrophobic surfactant proteins in lung function and disease. N Engl J Med 2002; 347:2141–2148
77. Armanios MY, Chen JJ, Cogan JD, et al. Telomerase mutations in families with idiopathic pulmonary fibrosis. N Engl J Med 2007; 356:1317–1326
78. Hao LY, Armanios M, Strong MA, et al. Short telomeres, even in the presence of telomerase, limit tissue renewal capacity. Cell 2005; 123:1121–1131
79. Alder JK, Chen JJ, Lancaster L, et al. Short telomeres are a risk factor for idiopathic pulmonary fibrosis. Proc Natl Acad Sci USA 2008; 105:13051–13056
80. Cronkhite JT, Xing C, Raghu G, et al. Telomere shortening in familial and sporadic pulmonary fibrosis. Am J Respir Crit Care Med 2008; 178:729–737
81. Brantly M, Avila NA, Shotelersuk V, et al. Pulmonary function and high-resolution CT findings in patients with an inherited form of pulmonary fibrosis, Hermansky-Pudlak syndrome, due to mutations in HPS-1. Chest 2000; 117:129–136
82. Auwerx J, Boogaerts M, Ceuppens JL, et al. Defective host defence mechanisms in a family with hypocalciuric hypercalcaemia and coexisting interstitial lung disease. Clin Exp Immunol 1985; 62:57–64
83. Riccardi VM. Von Recklinghausen neurofibromatosis. N Engl J Med 1981; 305:1617–1627

84. Young LM, Hopkins R, Wilsher ML. Lower occurrence of idiopathic pulmonary fibrosis in Maori and Pacific Islanders. Respirology 2006; 11:467–470
85. Churg A. The uptake of mineral particles by pulmonary epithelial cells. Am J Respir Crit Care Med 1996; 154:1124–1140
86. Ortiz LA, Lasky J, Hamilton RF Jr., et al. Expression of TNF and the necessity of TNF receptors in bleomycin-induced lung injury in mice. Exp Lung Res 1998; 24:721–743
87. Nunes H, Uzunhan Y, Valeyre D, et al. Connective tissue disease-associated interstitial lung disease. In: Lynch JP III, ed. Interstitial pulmonary and bronchiolar disorders (Vol 227). New York: Informa-USA, 2008; 429–486
88. Hubbard RB, Smith C, Le Jeune I, et al. The association between idiopathic pulmonary fibrosis and vascular disease: a population-based study. Am J Respir Crit Care Med 2008; 178:1257–1261
89. Kizer JR, Zisman DA, Blumenthal NP, et al. Association between pulmonary fibrosis and coronary artery disease. Arch Intern Med 2004; 164:551–556
90. Ponnuswamy A, Manikandan R, Sabetpour A, et al. Association between ischaemic heart disease and interstitial lung disease: a case-control study. Respir Med 2009; 103:503–507
91. Gribbin J, Hubbard R, Smith C. Role of diabetes mellitus and gastro-oesophageal reflux in the aetiology of idiopathic pulmonary fibrosis. Respir Med 2009; 103:927-931
92. Enomoto T, Usuki J, Azuma A, et al. Diabetes mellitus may increase risk for idiopathic pulmonary fibrosis. Chest 2003; 123:2007–2011
93. Martinez FJ, Safrin S, Weycker D, et al. The clinical course of patients with idiopathic pulmonary fibrosis. Ann Intern Med 2005; 142:963–967
94. Selman M, Carrillo G, Estrada A, et al. Accelerated variant of idiopathic pulmonary fibrosis: clinical behavior and gene expression pattern. PLoS ONE 2007; 2:e482
95. Collard HR, Moore BB, Flaherty KR, et al. Acute exacerbations of idiopathic pulmonary fibrosis. Am J Respir Crit Care Med 2007; 176: 636–643
96. Bjoraker JA, Ryu JH, Edwin MK, et al. Prognostic significance of histopathologic subsets in idiopathic pulmonary fibrosis. Am J Respir Crit Care Med 1998; 157:199–203
97. Flaherty KR, Travis WD, Colby TV, et al. Histopathologic variability in usual and nonspecific interstitial pneumonias. Am J Respir Crit Care Med 2001; 164:1722–1727
98. Flaherty KR, Toews GB, Travis WD, et al. Clinical significance of histological classification of idiopathic interstitial pneumonia. Eur Respir J 2002; 19:275–283
99. Daniels CE, Yi ES, Ryu JH. Autopsy findings in 42 consecutive patients with idiopathic pulmonary fibrosis. Eur Respir J 2008; 32:170–174
100. Rudd RM, Prescott RJ, Chalmers JC, et al. British Thoracic Society Study on cryptogenic fibrosing alveolitis: response to treatment and survival. Thorax 2007; 62:62–66
101. Panos RJ, Mortenson RL, Niccoli SA, et al. Clinical deterioration in patients with idiopathic pulmonary fibrosis: causes and assessment. Am J Med 1990; 88:396–404
102. Le Jeune I, Gribbin J, West J, et al. The incidence of cancer in patients with idiopathic pulmonary fibrosis and sarcoidosis in the UK. Respir Med 2007; 101:2534–2540
103. Stern JB, Mal H, Groussard O, et al. Prognosis of patients with advanced idiopathic pulmonary fibrosis requiring mechanical ventilation for acute respiratory failure. Chest 2001; 120:213–219
104. Parambil JG, Myers JL, Ryu JH. Histopathologic features and outcome of patients with acute exacerbation of idiopathic pulmonary fibrosis undergoing surgical lung biopsy. Chest 2005; 128:3310–3315
105. Saydain G, Islam A, Afessa B, et al. Outcome of patients with idiopathic pulmonary fibrosis admitted to the intensive care unit. Am J Respir Crit Care Med 2002; 166:839–842
106. Mallick S. Outcome of patients with idiopathic pulmonary fibrosis (IPF) ventilated in intensive care unit. Respir Med 2008; 102:1355–1359
107. Hubbard R, Venn A, Lewis S, et al. Lung cancer and cryptogenic fibrosing alveolitis: a population-based cohort study. Am J Respir Crit Care Med 2000; 161:5–8
108. Daniels CE, Jett JR. Does interstitial lung disease predispose to lung cancer? Curr Opin Pulm Med 2005; 11:431–437
109. Aubry MC, Myers JL, Douglas WW, et al. Primary pulmonary carcinoma in patients with idiopathic pulmonary fibrosis. Mayo Clin Proc 2002; 77:763–770

110. Kawasaki H, Nagai K, Yoshida J, et al. Postoperative morbidity, mortality, and survival in lung cancer associated with idiopathic pulmonary fibrosis. J Surg Oncol 2002; 81:33–37
111. Kumar P, Goldstraw P, Yamada K, et al. Pulmonary fibrosis and lung cancer: risk and benefit analysis of pulmonary resection. J Thorac Cardiovasc Surg 2003; 125:1321–1327
112. Swigris JJ, Brown KK. Acute interstitial pneumonia and acute exacerbations of idiopathic pulmonary fibrosis. Semin Respir Crit Care Med 2006; 27:659–667
113. Kim DS, Park JH, Park BK, et al. Acute exacerbation of idiopathic pulmonary fibrosis: frequency and clinical features. Eur Respir J 2006; 27: 143–50
114. Suh GY, Kang EH, Chung MP, et al. Early intervention can improve clinical outcome of acute interstitial pneumonia. Chest 2006; 129:753–761
115. Yokoyama A, Kohno N, Hamada H, et al. Circulating KL-6 predicts the outcome of rapidly progressive idiopathic pulmonary fibrosis. Am J Respir Crit Care Med 1998; 158:1680–1684
116. Ohnishi H, Yokoyama A, Kondo K, et al. Comparative study of KL-6, surfactant protein-A, surfactant protein-D, and monocyte chemoattractant protein-1 as serum markers for interstitial lung diseases. Am J Respir Crit Care Med 2002; 165:378–381
117. Takahashi H, Shiratori M, Kanai A, et al. Monitoring markers of disease activity for interstitial lung diseases with serum surfactant proteins A and D. Respirology 2006; 11 Suppl:S51–S54
118. Takahashi H, Fujishima T, Koba H, et al. Serum surfactant proteins A and D as prognostic factors in idiopathic pulmonary fibrosis and their relationship to disease extent. Am J Respir Crit Care Med 2000; 162:1109–1114
119. Kocheril SV, Appleton BE, Somers EC, et al. Comparison of disease progression and mortality of connective tissue disease-related interstitial lung disease and idiopathic interstitial pneumonia. Arthritis Rheum 2005; 53:549–557
120. Lynch JP III, Orens J, Kazerooni EA. Collagen vascular diseases. In: Sperber M, ed. Diffuse lung diseases: a comprehensive clinical-radiological overview. London: Springer-Verlag, 1999; 325–355
121. Elliot TL, Lynch DA, Newell JD Jr., et al. High-resolution computed tomography features of nonspecific interstitial pneumonia and usual interstitial pneumonia. J Comput Assist Tomogr 2005; 29:339–345
122. Franquet T, Gimenez A, Alegret X, Rodriguez-Arias JM. Mediastinal lymphadenopathy in cryptogenic fibrosing alveolitis: the effect of steroid therapy on the prevalence of nodal enlargement. Clin Radiol 1998; 53:435–438
123. Gay SE, Kazerooni EA, Toews GB, et al. Idiopathic pulmonary fibrosis: predicting response to therapy and survival. Am J Respir Crit Care Med 1998; 157:1063–1072
124. Mogulkoc N, Brutsche MH, Bishop PW, et al. Pulmonary function in idiopathic pulmonary fibrosis and referral for lung transplantation. Am J Respir Crit Care Med 2001; 164:103–108
125. Hunninghake GW, Zimmerman MB, Schwartz DA, et al. Utility of a lung biopsy for the diagnosis of idiopathic pulmonary fibrosis. Am J Respir Crit Care Med 2001; 164:193–196
126. Aziz ZA, Wells AU, Hansell DM, et al. HRCT diagnosis of diffuse parenchymal lung disease: inter-observer variation. Thorax 2004; 59:506–511
127. Sumikawa H, Johkoh T, Colby TV, et al. Computed tomography findings in pathological usual interstitial pneumonia: relationship to survival. Am J Respir Crit Care Med 2008; 177:433–439
128. Xaubet A, Agusti C, Luburich P, et al. Pulmonary function tests and CT scan in the management of idiopathic pulmonary fibrosis. Am J Respir Crit Care Med 1998; 158:431–436
129. Doherty MJ, Pearson MG, O'Grady EA, et al. Cryptogenic fibrosing alveolitis with preserved lung volumes. Thorax 1997; 52:998–1002
130. Wells AU, King AD, Rubens MB, et al. Lone cryptogenic fibrosing alveolitis: a functional-morphologic correlation based on extent of disease on thin-section computed tomography. Am J Respir Crit Care Med 1997; 155:1367–1375
131. Cottin V, Nunes H, Brillet PY, et al. Combined pulmonary fibrosis and emphysema: a distinct underrecognised entity. Eur Respir J 2005; 26:586–593
132. Souza CA, Muller NL, Lee KS, et al. Idiopathic interstitial pneumonias: prevalence of mediastinal lymph node enlargement in 206 patients. AJR Am J Roentgenol 2006; 186:995–999
133. Attili AK, Kazerooni EA, Gross BH, et al. Thoracic lymph node enlargement in usual interstitial pneumonitis and nonspecific-interstitial

pneumonitis: prevalence, correlation with disease activity and temporal evolution. J Thorac Imaging 2006; 21:288–292
134. Jung JI, Kim HH, Jung YJ, et al. Mediastinal lymphadenopathy in pulmonary fibrosis: correlation with disease severity. J Comput Assist Tomogr 2000; 24:706–710
135. Niimi H, Kang EY, Kwong JS, et al. CT of chronic infiltrative lung disease: prevalence of mediastinal lymphadenopathy. J Comput Assist Tomogr 1996; 20:305–308
136. Hartman TE, Primack SL, Swensen SJ, et al. Desquamative interstitial pneumonia: thin-section CT findings in 22 patients. Radiology 1993; 187:787–790
137. Hartman TE. The HRCT features of extrinsic allergic alveolitis. Semin Respir Crit Care Med 2003; 24:419–426
138. Lacasse Y, Selman M, Costabel U, et al. Clinical diagnosis of hypersensitivity pneumonitis. Am J Respir Crit Care Med 2003; 168:952–958
139. MacDonald SL, Rubens MB, Hansell DM, et al. Nonspecific interstitial pneumonia and usual interstitial pneumonia: comparative appearances at and diagnostic accuracy of thin-section CT. Radiology 2001; 221:600–605
140. Marchand E, Cordier JF. Idiopathic chronic eosinophilic pneumonia. Semin Respir Crit Care Med 2006; 27:134–141
141. Trapnell BC, Whitsett JA, Nakata K. Pulmonary alveolar proteinosis. N Engl J Med 2003; 349:2527–2539
142. Tazi A. Adult pulmonary Langerhans' cell histiocytosis. Eur Respir J 2006; 27:1272–1285
143. Lynch III JP. Computed tomographic scanning in sarcoidosis. Semin Respir Crit Care Med 2003; 24:393–418
144. Johnson SR. Lymphangioleiomyomatosis. Eur Respir J 2006; 27:1056–1065
145. Sahin H, Brown KK, Curran-Everett D, et al. Chronic hypersensitivity pneumonitis: CT features comparison with pathologic evidence of fibrosis and survival. Radiology 2007; 244:591–598
146. Zisman DA, Kazerooni E, Flaherty K, et al. Idiopathic pulmonary fibrosis: role of high-resolution thin-section computed tomographic scanning. In: Lynch JP III, ed. Idiopathic pulmonary fibrosis. New York, NY: Marcel Dekker Press, 2004; 237–252
147. Nagai S, Kitaichi M, Itoh H, et al. Idiopathic nonspecific interstitial pneumonia/fibrosis: comparison with idiopathic pulmonary fibrosis and BOOP. Eur Respir J 1998; 12:1010–1019
148. Daniil ZD, Gilchrist FC, Nicholson AG, et al. A histologic pattern of nonspecific interstitial pneumonia is associated with a better prognosis than usual interstitial pneumonia in patients with cryptogenic fibrosing alveolitis. Am J Respir Crit Care Med 1999; 160:899–905
149. Akira M, Sakatani M, Ueda E. Idiopathic pulmonary fibrosis: progression of honeycombing at thin-section CT. Radiology 1993; 189:687–691
150. Wells AU, Hansell DM, Rubens MB, et al. Functional impairment in lone cryptogenic fibrosing alveolitis and fibrosing alveolitis associated with systemic sclerosis: a comparison. Am J Respir Crit Care Med 1997; 155:1657–1664
151. Wells AU, Rubens MB, du Bois RM, et al. Serial CT in fibrosing alveolitis: prognostic significance of the initial pattern. AJR Am J Roentgenol 1993; 161:1159–1165
152. Wells AU, Cullinan P, Hansell DM, et al. Fibrosing alveolitis associated with systemic sclerosis has a better prognosis than lone cryptogenic fibrosing alveolitis. Am J Respir Crit Care Med 1994; 149:1583–1590
153. Wells AU, Hansell DM, Rubens MB, et al. The predictive value of appearances on thin-section computed tomography in fibrosing alveolitis. Am Rev Respir Dis 1993; 148:1076–1082
154. Hartman TE, Primack SL, Kang EY, et al. Disease progression in usual interstitial pneumonia compared with desquamative interstitial pneumonia: assessment with serial CT. Chest 1996; 110:378–382
155. Flaherty KR, Mumford JA, Murray S, et al. Prognostic implications of physiologic and radiographic changes in idiopathic interstitial pneumonia. Am J Respir Crit Care Med 2003; 168:543–548
156. Misumi S, Lynch DA. Idiopathic pulmonary fibrosis/usual interstitial pneumonia: imaging diagnosis, spectrum of abnormalities, and temporal progression. Proc Am Thorac Soc 2006; 3:307–314
157. Coxson HO, Hogg JC, Mayo JR, et al. Quantification of idiopathic pulmonary fibrosis using computed tomography and histology. Am J Respir Crit Care Med 1997; 155:1649–1656

158. Lynch JP 3rd, Saggar R, Weigt SS, et al. Overview of lung transplantation and criteria for selection of candidates. Semin Respir Crit Care Med 2006; 27:441–469
159. Martinez FJ, Flaherty K. Pulmonary function testing in idiopathic interstitial pneumonias. Proc Am Thorac Soc 2006; 3:315–321
160. Lama VN, Flaherty KR, Toews GB, et al. Prognostic value of desaturation during a 6-minute walk test in idiopathic interstitial pneumonia. Am J Respir Crit Care Med 2003; 168:1084–1090
161. Fell CD, Liu LX, Motika C, et al. The prognostic value of cardiopulmonary exercise testing in idiopathic pulmonary fibrosis. Am J Respir Crit Care Med 2009; 179:402–407
162. Lama VN, Martinez FJ. Resting and exercise physiology in interstitial lung diseases [review]. Clin Chest Med 2004; 25:435–453, v
163. Nicholson AG, Fulford LG, Colby TV, et al. The relationship between individual histologic features and disease progression in idiopathic pulmonary fibrosis. Am J Respir Crit Care Med 2002; 166:173–177
164. King TE Jr., Schwarz MI, Brown K, et al. Idiopathic pulmonary fibrosis: relationship between histopathologic features and mortality. Am J Respir Crit Care Med 2001; 164:1025–1032
165. Wells AU, Desai SR, Rubens MB, et al. Idiopathic pulmonary fibrosis: a composite physiologic index derived from disease extent observed by computed tomography. Am J Respir Crit Care Med 2003; 167:962–969
166. Mogulkoc N, Brutsche MH, Bishop PW, et al. Pulmonary (99m)Tc-DTPA aerosol clearance and survival in usual interstitial pneumonia (UIP). Thorax 2001; 56:916–923
167. Timmer SJ, Karamzadeh AM, Yung GL, et al. Predicting survival of lung transplantation candidates with idiopathic interstitial pneumonia: does Pao_2 predict survival? Chest 2002; 122:779–784
168. Lederer DJ, Arcasoy SM, Wilt JS, et al. Six-minute-walk distance predicts waiting list survival in idiopathic pulmonary fibrosis. Am J Respir Crit Care Med 2006; 174:659–664
169. Kawut SM, O'Shea MK, Bartels MN, et al. Exercise testing determines survival in patients with diffuse parenchymal lung disease evaluated for lung transplantation. Respir Med 2005; 99:1431–1439
170. Eaton T, Young P, Milne D, et al. Six-minute walk, maximal exercise tests: reproducibility in fibrotic interstitial pneumonia. Am J Respir Crit Care Med 2005; 171:1150–1157
171. Miki K, Maekura R, Hiraga T, et al. Impairments and prognostic factors for survival in patients with idiopathic pulmonary fibrosis. Respir Med 2003; 97:482–490
172. Latsi PI, du Bois RM, Nicholson AG, et al. Fibrotic idiopathic interstitial pneumonia: the prognostic value of longitudinal functional trends. Am J Respir Crit Care Med 2003; 168:531–537
173. Hallstrand TS, Boitano LJ, Johnson WC, et al. The timed walk test as a measure of severity and survival in idiopathic pulmonary fibrosis. Eur Respir J 2005; 25:96–103
174. Caminati A, Bianchi A, Cassandro R, et al. Walking distance on 6-MWT is a prognostic factor in idiopathic pulmonary fibrosis. Respir Med 2009; 103:117–123
175. Flaherty KR, Andrei AC, Murray S, et al. Idiopathic pulmonary fibrosis: prognostic value of changes in physiology and six-minute-walk test. Am J Respir Crit Care Med 2006; 174:803–809
176. Dal Corso S, Duarte SR, Neder JA, et al. A step test to assess exercise-related oxygen desaturation in interstitial lung disease. Eur Respir J 2007; 29:330–336
177. Watters LC, King TE, Schwarz MI, et al. A clinical, radiographic, and physiologic scoring system for the longitudinal assessment of patients with idiopathic pulmonary fibrosis. Am Rev Respir Dis 1986; 133:97–103
178. Hanson D, Winterbauer RH, Kirtland SH, et al. Changes in pulmonary function test results after 1 year of therapy as predictors of survival in patients with idiopathic pulmonary fibrosis. Chest 1995; 108:305–310
179. Flaherty KR, Toews GB, Lynch JP 3rd, et al. Steroids in idiopathic pulmonary fibrosis: a prospective assessment of adverse reactions, response to therapy, and survival. Am J Med 2001; 110:278–282
180. Schwartz DA, Helmers RA, Galvin JR, et al. Determinants of survival in idiopathic pulmonary fibrosis. Am J Respir Crit Care Med 1994; 149:450–454
181. Collard HR, King TE Jr., Bartelson BB, et al. Changes in clinical and physiologic variables predict survival in idiopathic pulmonary fibrosis. Am J Respir Crit Care Med 2003; 168:538–542

182. Nathan SD, Noble PW, Tuder RM. Idiopathic pulmonary fibrosis and pulmonary hypertension: connecting the dots. Am J Respir Crit Care Med 2007; 175:875–880
183. Patel NM, Lederer DJ, Borczuk AC, et al. Pulmonary hypertension in idiopathic pulmonary fibrosis. Chest 2007; 132:998–1006
184. Nathan SD, Shlobin OA, Ahmad S, et al. Serial development of pulmonary hypertension in patients with idiopathic pulmonary fibrosis. Respiration 2008; 76:288–294
185. Colombat M, Mal H, Groussard O, et al. Pulmonary vascular lesions in end-stage idiopathic pulmonary fibrosis: histopathologic study on lung explant specimens and correlations with pulmonary hemodynamics. Hum Pathol 2007; 38:60–65
186. Hamada K, Nagai S, Tanaka S, et al. Significance of pulmonary arterial pressure and diffusion capacity of the lung as prognosticator in patients with idiopathic pulmonary fibrosis. Chest 2007; 131:650–656
187. Lettieri CJ, Nathan SD, Barnett SD, et al. Prevalence and outcomes of pulmonary arterial hypertension in advanced idiopathic pulmonary fibrosis. Chest 2006; 129:746–752
188. Leuchte HH, Neurohr C, Baumgartner R, et al. Brain natriuretic peptide and exercise capacity in lung fibrosis and pulmonary hypertension. Am J Respir Crit Care Med 2004; 170:360–365
189. Voelkel NF, Douglas IS, Nicolls M. Angiogenesis in chronic lung disease. Chest 2007; 131:874–879
190. Nadrous HF, Pellikka PA, Krowka MJ, et al. Pulmonary hypertension in patients with idiopathic pulmonary fibrosis. Chest 2005; 128:2393–2399
191. Nathan SD, Shlobin OA, Ahmad S, et al. Pulmonary hypertension and pulmonary function testing in idiopathic pulmonary fibrosis. Chest 2007; 131:657–663
192. Ghofrani HA, Wiedemann R, Rose F, et al. Sildenafil for treatment of lung fibrosis and pulmonary hypertension: a randomised controlled trial. Lancet 2002; 360:895–900
193. Zisman DA, Ross DJ, Belperio JA, et al. Prediction of pulmonary hypertension in idiopathic pulmonary fibrosis. Respir Med 2007; 101:2153–2159
194. Song JW, Song JK, Kim DS. Echocardiography and brain natriuretic peptide as prognostic indicators in idiopathic pulmonary fibrosis. Respir Med 2009; 103:180–186
195. Arcasoy SM, Christie JD, Ferrari VA, et al. Echocardiographic assessment of pulmonary hypertension in patients with advanced lung disease. Am J Respir Crit Care Med 2003; 167:735–740
196. Collard HR, Anstrom KJ, Schwarz MI, et al. Sildenafil improves walk distance in idiopathic pulmonary fibrosis. Chest 2007; 131:897–899
197. Dandel M, Lehmkuhl HB, Mulahasanovic S, et al. Survival of patients with idiopathic pulmonary arterial hypertension after listing for transplantation: impact of iloprost and bosentan treatment. J Heart Lung Transplant 2007; 26:898–906
198. King Jr TE, Behr J, Brown KK, et al. A randomized placebo-controlled trial of bosentan in patients with idiopathic pulmonary fibrosis. Am J Respir Crit Care Med 2008; 177:75–81
199. Daniels CE, Ryu JH. Treatment of idiopathic pulmonary fibrosis. Semin Respir Crit Care Med 2006; 27:668–676
200. Agostini C, Gurrieri C. Chemokine/cytokine cocktail in idiopathic pulmonary fibrosis. Proc Am Thorac Soc 2006; 3:357–363
201. Thannickal V, Flaherty K, Hyzy R, et al. Emerging drugs for idiopathic pulmonary fibrosis. Expert Opin Emerging Drugs 2005; 10:707–727
202. Winterbauer RH, Hammar SP, Hallman KO, et al. Diffuse interstitial pneumonitis: clinicopathologic correlations in 20 patients treated with prednisone/azathioprine. Am J Med 1978; 65:661–672
203. Travis WD, Matsui K, Moss J, Ferrans VJ. Idiopathic nonspecific interstitial pneumonia: prognostic significance of cellular and fibrosing patterns: survival comparison with usual interstitial pneumonia and desquamative interstitial pneumonia. Am J Surg Pathol 2000; 24:19–33
204. Nicholson AG, Colby TV, du Bois RM, et al. The prognostic significance of the histologic pattern of interstitial pneumonia in patients presenting with the clinical entity of cryptogenic fibrosing alveolitis. Am J Respir Crit Care Med 2000; 162:2213–2217
205. Monaghan H, Wells AU, Colby TV, et al. Prognostic implications of histologic patterns in multiple surgical lung biopsies from patients with idiopathic interstitial pneumonias. Chest 2004; 125:522–526
206. Thomeer M, Demedts M, Behr J, et al. Multidisciplinary interobserver agreement in the diagnosis of idiopathic pulmonary fibrosis. Eur Respir J 2008; 31:585–591

207. Nicholson AG, Addis BJ, Bharucha H, et al. Interobserver variation between pathologists in diffuse parenchymal lung disease. Thorax 2004; 59:500–505
208. Portnoy J, Veraldi KL, Schwarz MI, et al. Respiratory bronchiolitis-interstitial lung disease: long-term outcome. Chest 2007; 131:664–671
209. Nicholson AG, Wells AU. Nonspecific interstitial pneumonia: nobody said it's perfect. Am J Respir Crit Care Med 2001; 164:1553–1554
210. Flaherty KR, Martinez FJ. Nonspecific interstitial pneumonia. Semin Respir Crit Care Med 2006; 27:652–658
211. Visscher DW, Myers JL. Histologic spectrum of idiopathic interstitial pneumonias. Proc Am Thorac Soc 2006; 3:322–329
212. Caminati A, Harari S. Smoking-related interstitial pneumonias and pulmonary Langerhans cell histiocytosis. Proc Am Thorac Soc 2006; 3:299–306
213. Vassallo R, Jensen EA, Colby TV, et al. The overlap between respiratory bronchiolitis and desquamative interstitial pneumonia in pulmonary Langerhans cell histiocytosis: high-resolution CT, histologic, and functional correlations. Chest 2003; 124:1199–1205
214. Fraig M, Shreesha U, Savici D, et al. Respiratory bronchiolitis: a clinicopathologic study in current smokers, ex-smokers, and never-smokers. Am J Surg Pathol 2002; 26:647–653
215. Moon J, du Bois RM, Colby TV, et al. Clinical significance of respiratory bronchiolitis on open lung biopsy and its relationship to smoking related interstitial lung disease. Thorax 1999; 54:1009–1114
216. Myers JL, Veal CF Jr., Shin MS, et al. Respiratory bronchiolitis causing interstitial lung disease: a clinicopathologic study of six cases. Am Rev Respir Dis 1987; 135:880–884
217. Yousem SA, Colby TV, Gaensler EA. Respiratory bronchiolitis-associated interstitial lung disease and its relationship to desquamative interstitial pneumonia. Mayo Clin Proc 1989; 64:1373–1380
218. Akira M, Hamada H, Sakatani M, et al. CT findings during phase of accelerated deterioration in patients with idiopathic pulmonary fibrosis. AJR Am J Roentgenol 1997; 168:79–83
219. Katzenstein AL, Fiorelli RF. Nonspecific interstitial pneumonia/fibrosis: histologic features and clinical significance. Am J Surg Pathol 1994; 18:136–147
220. Flaherty K. Nonspecific Interstitial Pneumonitis (NSIP). In: Lynch JP III, ed. Interstitial pulmonary and bronchiolar disorders (Vol 227). New York: InformaUSA; 2008, 365–378
221. Jegal Y, Kim DS, Shim TS, et al. Physiology is a stronger predictor of survival than pathology in fibrotic interstitial pneumonia. Am J Respir Crit Care Med 2005; 171:639–644
222. Kim TS, Lee KS, Chung MP, et al. Nonspecific interstitial pneumonia with fibrosis: high-resolution CT and pathologic findings. AJR Am J Roentgenol 1998; 171:1645–1650
223. Veeraraghavan S, Latsi PI, Wells AU, et al. BAL findings in idiopathic nonspecific interstitial pneumonia and usual interstitial pneumonia. Eur Respir J 2003; 22:239–244
224. Turner-Warwick M, Haslam PL. The value of serial bronchoalveolar lavages in assessing the clinical progress of patients with cryptogenic fibrosing alveolitis. Am Rev Respir Dis 1987; 135:26–34
225. Watters LC, Schwarz MI, Cherniack RM, et al. Idiopathic pulmonary fibrosis: pretreatment bronchoalveolar lavage cellular constituents and their relationships with lung histopathology and clinical response to therapy. Am Rev Respir Dis 1987; 135:696–704
226. Cottin V, Donsbeck AV, Revel D, et al. Nonspecific interstitial pneumonia: individualization of a clinicopathologic entity in a series of 12 patients. Am J Respir Crit Care Med 1998; 158:1286–1293
227. Park JS, Lee KS, Kim JS, et al. Nonspecific interstitial pneumonia with fibrosis: radiographic and CT findings in seven patients. Radiology 1995; 195:645–648
228. Tiitto L, Heiskanen U, Bloigu R, et al. Thoracoscopic lung biopsy is a safe procedure in diagnosing usual interstitial pneumonia. Chest 2005; 128:2375–2380
229. Lettieri CJ, Veerappan GR, Helman DL, et al. Outcomes and safety of surgical lung biopsy for interstitial lung disease. Chest 2005; 127:1600–1605
230. Kondoh Y, Taniguchi H, Kitaichi M, et al. Acute exacerbation of interstitial pneumonia following surgical lung biopsy. Respir Med 2006; 100:1753–1759
231. Park IN, Kim DS, Shim TS, et al. Acute exacerbation of interstitial pneumonia other than idiopathic pulmonary fibrosis. Chest 2007; 132:214–220

232. The diagnosis, assessment and treatment of diffuse parenchymal lung disease in adults. Introduction. Thorax 1999; 54(Suppl 1):S1–S14
233. Johnston ID, Gomm SA, Kalra S, et al. The management of cryptogenic fibrosing alveolitis in three regions of the United Kingdom. Eur Respir J 1993; 6:891–893
234. Chang AC, Yee J, Orringer MB, et al. Diagnostic thoracoscopic lung biopsy: an outpatient experience. Ann Thorac Surg 2002; 74:1942–1946, discussion 6–7
235. Flaherty KR, Colby TV, Travis WD, et al. Fibroblastic foci in usual interstitial pneumonia: idiopathic versus collagen vascular disease. Am J Respir Crit Care Med 2003; 167:1410–1415
236. Hanak V, Ryu JH, de Carvalho E, et al. Profusion of fibroblast foci in patients with idiopathic pulmonary fibrosis does not predict outcome. Respir Med 2008; 102:852–856
237. Welker L, Jorres RA, Costabel U, et al. Predictive value of BAL cell differentials in the diagnosis of interstitial lung diseases. Eur Respir J 2004; 24:1000–1006
238. Nagai S, Handa T, Ito Y, et al. Bronchoalveolar lavage in idiopathic interstitial lung diseases. Semin Respir Crit Care Med 2007; 28:496–503
239. Wells AU, Hansell DM, Harrison NK, et al. Clearance of inhaled 99mTc-DTPA predicts the clinical course of fibrosing alveolitis. Eur Respir J 1993; 6:797–802
240. Singh S, Wells AU, du Bois R. Other imaging techniques for idiopathic interstitial pneumonias. In: Lynch JP III, ed. Idiopathic pulmonary fibrosis. New York, NY: Marcel Dekker, 2004; 237–252
241. Thomeer MJ, Dehaes B, Mortelmans L, et al. Pertechnegas lung clearance in different forms of interstitial lung disease. Eur Respir J 2002; 19: 31–36
242. Lynch JP III, Madihara R, Fishbein MC, et al. Idiopathic pulmonary fibrosis. In: Lynch JP III, ed. Interstitial pulmonary and bronchiolar disorders. Vol. 227. New York: InformaUSA, 2008; 333–364
243. Selman M, King TE, Pardo A. Idiopathic pulmonary fibrosis: prevailing and evolving hypotheses about its pathogenesis and implications for therapy. Ann Intern Med 2001; 134:136–151
244. Maher TM, Wells AU, Laurent GJ. Idiopathic pulmonary fibrosis: multiple causes and multiple mechanisms? Eur Respir J 2007; 30:835–839
245. Selman M, Thannickal VJ, Pardo A, et al. Idiopathic pulmonary fibrosis: pathogenesis and therapeutic approaches. Drugs 2004; 64:405–430
246. Uhal BD, Joshi I, Hughes WF, et al. Alveolar epithelial cell death adjacent to underlying myofibroblasts in advanced fibrotic human lung. Am J Physiol 1998; 275:L1192–L1199
247. Kuhn C, McDonald JA. The roles of the myofibroblast in idiopathic pulmonary fibrosis: ultrastructural and immunohistochemical features of sites of active extracellular matrix synthesis. Am J Pathol 1991; 138:1257–1265
248. Lama VN, Phan SH. The extrapulmonary origin of fibroblasts: stem/progenitor cells and beyond. Proc Am Thorac Soc 2006; 3:373–376
249. Keane MP, Belperio JA, Burdick MD, et al. ENA-78 is an important angiogenic factor in idiopathic pulmonary fibrosis. Am J Respir Crit Care Med 2001; 164:2239–2242
250. Keane MP, Arenberg DA, Lynch JP 3rd, et al. The CXC chemokines, IL-8 and IP-10, regulate angiogenic activity in idiopathic pulmonary fibrosis. J Immunol 1997; 159:1437–1443
251. Keane MP, Belperio JA, Arenberg DA, et al. IFN-gamma-inducible protein-10 attenuates bleomycin-induced pulmonary fibrosis via inhibition of angiogenesis. J Immunol 1999; 163:5686–5692
252. Williams TJ, Wilson JW. Challenges in pulmonary fibrosis: 7–Novel therapies and lung transplantation. Thorax 2008; 63:277–284
253. Lynch JP III, Wurfel M, Flaherty K, et al. Usual interstitial pneumonia. Semin Respir Crit Care Med 2001; 22:357–387
254. Nagai S, Kitaichi M, Hamada K, et al. Hospital-based historical cohort study of 234 histologically proven Japanese patients with IPF. Sarcoidosis Vasc Diffuse Lung Dis 1999; 16:209–214
255. Tukiainen P, Taskineu E, Holsti P, et al. Prognosis of cryptogenic fibrosing alveolitis. Thorax 1983; 38:349–355
256. Douglas WW, Ryu JH, Swensen SJ, et al. Colchicine versus prednisone in the treatment of idio pathic pulmonary fibrosis: a randomized prospective study. Members of the Lung Study Group. Am J Respir Crit Care Med 1998; 158:220–225
257. Mapel DW, Samet JM, Coultas DB. Corticosteroids and the treatment of idiopathic pulmonary fibrosis: past, present, and future. Chest 1996; 110:1058–1067

258. Lynch JP 3rd, White E, Flaherty K. Corticosteroids in idiopathic pulmonary fibrosis. Curr Opin Pulm Med 2001; 7:298–308
259. Collard HR, Ryu JH, Douglas WW, et al. Combined corticosteroid and cyclophosphamide therapy does not alter survival in idiopathic pulmonary fibrosis. Chest 2004; 125:2169–2174
260. Zisman DA, Lynch JP 3rd, Toews GB, et al. Cyclophosphamide in the treatment of idiopathic pulmonary fibrosis: a prospective study in patients who failed to respond to corticosteroids. Chest 2000; 117:1619–1626
261. Johnson MA, Kwan S, Snell NJ, et al. Randomised controlled trial comparing prednisolone alone with cyclophosphamide and low dose prednisolone in combination in cryptogenic fibrosing alveolitis. Thorax 1989; 44:280–288
262. Raghu G, Depaso WJ, Cain K, et al. Azathioprine combined with prednisone in the treatment of idiopathic pulmonary fibrosis: a prospective double-blind, randomized, placebo- controlled clinical trial. Am Rev Respir Dis 1991; 144:291–296
263. Kolb M, Kirschner J, Riedel W, et al. Cyclophosphamide pulse therapy in idiopathic pulmonary fibrosis. Eur Respir J 1998; 12:1409–1414
264. Selman M, Carrillo G, Salas J, et al. Colchicine, D-penicillamine, and prednisone in the treatment of idiopathic pulmonary fibrosis: a controlled clinical trial. Chest 1998; 114:507–512
265. Lynch JP 3rd, McCune WJ. Immunosuppressive and cytotoxic pharmacotherapy for pulmonary disorders. Am J Respir Crit Care Med 1997; 155:395–420
266. Raghu G, Brown KK, Costabel U, et al. Treatment of idiopathic pulmonary fibrosis with etanercept: an exploratory, placebo-controlled trial. Am J Respir Crit Care Med 2008; 178:948–955
267. Bargagli E, Galeazzi M, Rottoli P. Infliximab treatment in a patient with rheumatoid arthritis and pulmonary fibrosis. Eur Respir J 2004; 24:708
268. Antoniou KM, Mamoulaki M, Malagari K, et al. Infliximab therapy in pulmonary fibrosis associated with collagen vascular disease. Clin Exp Rheumatol 2007; 25:23–28
269. Ostor AJ, Crisp AJ, Somerville MF, et al. Fatal exacerbation of rheumatoid arthritis associated fibrosing alveolitis in patients given infliximab. BMJ 2004; 329:1266
270. Ziesche R, Hofbauer E, Wittmann K, et al. A preliminary study of long-term treatment with interferon gamma-1b and low-dose prednisolone in patients with idiopathic pulmonary fibrosis. N Engl J Med 1999; 341:1264–1269
271. Raghu G, Brown KK, Bradford WZ, et al. A placebo-controlled trial of interferon gamma-1b in patients with idiopathic pulmonary fibrosis. N Engl J Med 2004; 350:125–133
272. Thannickal VJ, Flaherty KR, Martinez FJ, et al. Idiopathic pulmonary fibrosis: emerging concepts on pharmacotherapy. Expert Opin Pharmacother 2004; 5:1671–1686
273. Behr J, Maier K, Degenkolb B, et al. Antioxidative and clinical effects of high-dose N-acetylcysteine in fibrosing alveolitis: adjunctive therapy to maintenance immunosuppression. Am J Respir Crit Care Med 1997; 156:1897–1901
274. Demedts M, Behr J, Buhl R, et al. High-dose acetylcysteine in idiopathic pulmonary fibrosis. N Engl J Med 2005; 353:2229–2242
275. Hunninghake GW. Antioxidant therapy for idiopathic pulmonary fibrosis. N Engl J Med 2005; 353:2285–2287
276. Oku H, Shimizu T, Kawabata T, et al. Antifibrotic action of pirfenidone and prednisolone: different effects on pulmonary cytokines and growth factors in bleomycin-induced murine pulmonary fibrosis. Eur J Pharmacol 2008; 590: 400–408
277. Raghu G, Johnson WC, Lockhart D, et al. Treatment of idiopathic pulmonary fibrosis with a new antifibrotic agent, pirfenidone: results of a prospective, open-label Phase II study. Am J Respir Crit Care Med 1999; 159:1061–1069
278. Nagai S, Hamada K, Shigematsu M, et al. Open-label compassionate use one year-treatment with pirfenidone to patients with chronic pulmonary fibrosis. Intern Med 2002; 41:1118–1123
279. Gahl WA, Brantly M, Troendle J, et al. Effect of pirfenidone on the pulmonary fibrosis of Hermansky-Pudlak syndrome. Mol Genet Metab 2002; 76:234–242
280. Azuma A, Nukiwa T, Tsuboi E, et al. Double-blind, placebo-controlled trial of pirfenidone in patients with idiopathic pulmonary fibrosis. Am J Respir Crit Care Med 2005; 171:1040–1047
281. Gross TJ, Hunninghake GW. Idiopathic pulmonary fibrosis. N Engl J Med 2001; 345:517–525
282. Park SH, Saleh D, Giaid A, et al. Increased endothelin-1 in bleomycin-induced pulmonary fibrosis and the effect of an endothelin receptor

antagonist. Am J Respir Crit Care Med 1997; 156:600–608
283. Galie N, Ghofrani HA, Torbicki A, et al. Sildenafil citrate therapy for pulmonary arterial hypertension. N Engl J Med 2005; 353:2148–2157
284. Madden BP, Sheth A, Wilde M, et al. Does sildenafil produce a sustained benefit in patients with pulmonary hypertension associated with parenchymal lung and cardiac disease? Vasc Pharmacol 2007; 47:184–188
285. Walter N, Collard HR, King TE Jr. Current perspectives on the treatment of idiopathic pulmonary fibrosis. Proc Am Thorac Soc 2006; 3:330–338
286. Kubo H, Nakayama K, Yanai M, et al. Anticoagulant therapy for idiopathic pulmonary fibrosis. Chest 2005; 128:1475–1482
287. Noth I, Martinez FJ. Recent advances in idiopathic pulmonary fibrosis. Chest 2007; 132:637–650
288. Nathan SD, Saggar R, Lynch JP III. Lung transplantation for interstitial lung disorders. In: Lynch JP III, Ross D, eds. Lung and heart-lung transplantation (Vol 227). New York: Taylor and Francis, 2006; 165–204
289. Meyer DM, Edwards LB, Torres F, et al. Impact of recipient age and procedure type on survival after lung transplantation for pulmonary fibrosis. Ann Thorac Surg 2005; 79:950–957, discussion 7–8
290. Trulock EP, Edwards LB, Taylor DO, et al. The registry of the International Society for Heat and Lung Transplantation: twenty-first official adult heart transplant report---2004. J Heart Lung Transplant 2004; 23:804–815
291. Meyers BF, Lynch JP, Trulock EP, et al. Single versus bilateral lung transplantation for idiopathic pulmonary fibrosis: a ten-year institutional experience. J Thorac Cardiovasc Surg 2000; 120:99–107
292. Charman SC, Sharples LD, McNeil KD, et al. Assessment of survival benefit after lung transplantation by patient diagnosis. J Heart Lung Transplant 2002; 21:226–232
293. Trulock EP, Christie JD, Edwards LB, et al. Registry of the International Society for Heart and Lung Transplantation: twenty-fourth official adult lung and heart-lung transplantation report-2007. J Heart Lung Transplant 2007; 26:782–795
294. Christie JD, Edwards LB, Aurora P, et al. Registry of the International Society for Heart and Lung Transplantation: twenty-fifth official adult lung and heart/lung transplantation report–2008. zJ Heart Lung Transplant 2008; 27:957–969
295. Whelan TP, Dunitz JM, Kelly RF, et al. Effect of preoperative pulmonary artery pressure on early survival after lung transplantation for idiopathic pulmonary fibrosis. J Heart Lung Transplant 2005; 24:1269–1274
296. Harris-Eze AO, Sridhar G, Clemens RE, et al. Oxygen improves maximal exercise performance in interstitial lung disease. Am J Respir Crit Care Med 1994; 150:1616–1622
297. Olschewski H, Ghofrani HA, Walmrath D, et al. Inhaled prostacyclin and iloprost in severe pulmonary hypertension secondary to lung fibrosis. Am J Respir Crit Care Med 1999; 160:600–607
298. Douglas WW, Tazelaar HD, Hartman TE, et al. Polymyositis-dermatomyositis-associated interstitial lung disease. Am J Respir Crit Care Med 2001; 164:1182–1185
299. Bouros D, Wells AU, Nicholson AG, et al. Histopathologic subsets of fibrosing alveolitis in patients with systemic sclerosis and their relationship to outcome. Am J Respir Crit Care Med 2002; 165:1581–1586
300. Nakamura Y, Chida K, Suda T, et al. Nonspecific interstitial pneumonia in collagen vascular diseases: comparison of the clinical characteristics and prognostic significance with usual interstitial pneumonia. Sarcoidosis Vasc Diffuse Lung Dis 2003; 20:235–241
301. Tansey D, Wells AU, Colby TV, et al. Variations in histological patterns of interstitial pneumonia between connective tissue disorders and their relationship to prognosis. Histopathology 2004; 44:585–596
302. Lynch JP 3rd, Ma YL, Koss MN, et al. Pulmonary sarcoidosis. Semin Respir Crit Care Med 2007; 28:53–74
303. Lynch III JP, Kazerooni EA, Gay SE. Pulmonary sarcoidosis. Clin Chest Med 1997; 18:755–785
304. Lynch III J, Baughman R, Sharma O. Extrapulmonary sarcoidosis. Semin Respir Infect 1998; 13:229–254
305. Newman LS, Rose CS, Maier LA. Sarcoidosis. N Engl J Med 1997; 336:1224–1234
306. Statement on sarcoidosis. Joint Statement of the American Thoracic Society (ATS), the European Respiratory Society (ERS), and the World Association of Sarcoidosis and Other Granulomatous Disorders (WASOG) adopted by the ATS Board of Directors and by the ERS Executive Committee,

February 1999 [review]. Am J Respir Crit Care Med 1999; 160:736–755

307. Judson MA. Extrapulmonary sarcoidosis. Semin Respir Crit Care Med 2007; 28:83–101
308. Judson MA. Hepatic, splenic, and gastrointestinal involvement with sarcoidosis. Semin Respir Crit Care Med 2002; 23:529–541
309. Deng J, Baughman R, Lynch III JP. Cardiac involvement in sarcoidosis. Semin Respir Crit Care Med 2002; 23:513–528
310. Kidd D, Beynon HL. The neurological complications of systemic sarcoidosis. Sarcoidosis Vasc Diffuse Lung Dis 2003; 20:85–94
311. Allen RK, Sellars RE, Sandstrom PA. A prospective study of 32 patients with neurosarcoidosis. Sarcoidosis Vasc Diffuse Lung Dis 2003; 20:118–125
312. Lower EE, Broderick JP, Brott TG, et al. Diagnosis and management of neurological sarcoidosis. Arch Intern Med 1997; 157:1864–1868
313. Zisman DA, Shorr A, Lynch JP III. Sarcoidosis involving the musculoskeletal system. Semin Resp Crit Care Med 2002; 23:555–570
314. Neville E, Walker A, James DG. Prognostic factors predicting the outcome of sarcoidosis: an analysis of 818 patients. Q J Med 1983; 208:525–533
315. Mana J, Gomez-Vaquero C, Montero A, et al. Lofgren's syndrome revisited: a study of 186 patients. Am J Med 1999; 107:240–245
316. Judson MA, Baughman RP, Thompson BW, et al. Two year prognosis of sarcoidosis: the ACCESS experience. Sarcoidosis Vasc Diffuse Lung Dis 2003; 20:204–211
317. Grunewald J, Eklund A. Sex-specific manifestations of Lofgren's syndrome. Am J Respir Crit Care Med 2007; 175:40–44
318. Pietinalho A, Ohmichi M, Lofroos AB, et al. The prognosis of pulmonary sarcoidosis in Finland and Hokkaido, Japan: a comparative five-year study of biopsy-proven cases. Sarcoidosis Vasc Diffuse Lung Dis 2000; 17:158–166
319. Chappell AG, Cheung WY, Hutchings HA. Sarcoidosis: a long-term follow up study. Sarcoidosis Vasc Diffuse Lung Dis 2000; 17:167–173
320. Baughman RP, Teirstein AS, Judson MA, et al. Clinical characteristics of patients in a case control study of sarcoidosis. Am J Respir Crit Care Med 2001; 164:1885–1889
321. Johns CJ, Schonfeld SA, Scott PP, et al. Longitudinal study of chronic sarcoidosis with low-dose maintenance corticosteroid therapy: outcome and complications. Ann N Y Acad Sci 1986; 465:702–712
322. Johns CJ, Michele TM. The clinical management of sarcoidosis: a 50-year experience at the Johns Hopkins Hospital. Medicine (Baltimore) 1999; 78:65–111
323. Gottlieb JE, Israel HL, Steiner RM, et al. Outcome in sarcoidosis: the relationship of relapse to corticosteroid therapy. Chest 1997; 111:623–631
324. Reich JM. Mortality of intrathoracic sarcoidosis in referral vs population-based settings: influence of stage, ethnicity, and corticosteroid therapy. Chest 2002; 121:32–39
325. Huhti E, Poukkula A, Lilja M. Prognosis for sarcoidosis in a defined geographical area. Br J Dis Chest 1987; 81:381–390
326. Rybicki BA, Iannuzzi MC, Frederick MM, et al. Familial aggregation of sarcoidosis: a case-control etiologic study of sarcoidosis (ACCESS). Am J Respir Crit Care Med 2001; 164:2085–2091
327. Rybicki BA, Major M, Popovich J Jr., et al. Racial differences in sarcoidosis incidence: a 5-year study in a health maintenance organization. Am J Epidemiol 1997; 145:234–241
328. Rybicki BA, Iannuzzi MC. Epidemiology of sarcoidosis: recent advances and future prospects. Semin Respir Crit Care Med 2007; 28: 22–35
329. Hosoda Y, Yamaguchi M, Hiraga Y. Global epidemiology of sarcoidosis: what story do prevalence and incidence tell us? Clin Chest Med 1997; 18:681–694
330. Hillerdal G, Nou E, Osterman K, et al. Sarcoidosis: epidemiology and prognosis: a 15-year European study. Am Rev Respir Dis 1984; 130:29–32
331. Mana J, Badrinas F, Morera J, et al. Sarcoidosis in Spain. Sarcoidosis 1992; 9:118–122
332. Rybicki BA, Maliarik MJ, Major M, et al. Epidemiology, demographics, and genetics of sarcoidosis. Semin Respir Infect 1998; 13:166–173
333. McGrath DS, Daniil Z, Foley P, et al. Epidemiology of familial sarcoidosis in the UK. Thorax 2000; 55:751–754
334. Schurmann M, Lympany PA, Reichel P, et al. Familial sarcoidosis is linked to the major histocompatibility complex region. Am J Respir Crit Care Med 2000; 162:861–864
335. Schurmann M, Reichel P, Muller-Myhsok B, et al. Results from a genome-wide search for predisposing genes in sarcoidosis. Am J Respir Crit Care Med 2001; 164:840–846

336. Petrek M, Drabek J, Kolek V, et al. CC chemokine receptor gene polymorphisms in Czech patients with pulmonary sarcoidosis. Am J Respir Crit Care Med 2000; 162:1000–1003
337. Sato H, Grutters JC, Pantelidis P, et al. HLA-DQB1*0201: a marker for good prognosis in British and Dutch patients with sarcoidosis. Am J Respir Cell Mol Biol 2002; 27:406–412
338. Spagnolo P, Renzoni EA, Wells AU, et al. C-C chemokine receptor 2 and sarcoidosis: association with Lofgren's syndrome. Am J Respir Crit Care Med 2003; 168:1162–1166
339. Rosen Y. Pathology of sarcoidosis. Semin Respir Crit Care Med 2007; 28:36–52
340. Reich JM, Brouns MC, O'Connor EA, et al. Mediastinoscopy in patients with presumptive stage I sarcoidosis: a risk/benefit, cost/benefit analysis. Chest 1998; 113:147–153
341. Fritscher-Ravens A, Sriram PV, Topalidis T, et al. Diagnosing sarcoidosis using endosonography-guided fine-needle aspiration. Chest 2000; 118:928–935
342. Smojver-Jezek S, Peros-Golubicic T, Tekavec-Trkanjec J, et al. Transbronchial fine needle aspiration cytology in the diagnosis of mediastinal/hilar sarcoidosis. Cytopathology 2007; 18:3–7
343. Zwischenberger JB, Savage C, Alpard SK, et al. Mediastinal transthoracic needle and core lymph node biopsy: should it replace mediastinoscopy? Chest 2002; 121:1165–1170
344. Tambouret R, Geisinger KR, Powers CN, et al. The clinical application and cost analysis of fine-needle aspiration biopsy in the diagnosis of mass lesions in sarcoidosis. Chest 2000; 117: 1004–1011
345. Lynch JP III. Pulmonary sarcoidosis: current concepts & controversies. Compr Ther 1997; 23:197–210
346. Hours S, Nunes H, Kambouchner M, et al. Pulmonary cavitary sarcoidosis: clinico-radiologic characteristics and natural history of a rare form of sarcoidosis. Medicine (Baltimore) 2008; 87:142–151
347. Gibson GJ, Prescott RJ, Muers MF, et al. British Thoracic Society Sarcoidosis study: effects of long term corticosteroid treatment. Thorax 1996; 51:238–247
348. Hunninghake GW, Gilbert S, Pueringer R, et al. Outcome of the treatment for sarcoidosis. Am J Respir Crit Care Med 1994; 149:893–898
349. Romer FK. Presentation of sarcoidosis and outcome of pulmonary changes. Dan Med Bull 1982; 29:27–32
350. Mana J, Teirstein AS, Mendelson DS, et al. Excessive thoracic computed tomographic scanning in sarcoidosis. Thorax 1995; 50:1264–1266
351. Nunes H, Brillet PY, Valeyre D, et al. Imaging in sarcoidosis. Semin Respir Crit Care Med 2007; 28:102–120
352. Drent M, De Vries J, Lenters M, et al. Sarcoidosis: assessment of disease severity using HRCT. Eur Radiol 2003; 13:2462–2471
353. Nishimura K, Itoh H, Kitaichi M, et al. CT and pathological correlation of pulmonary sarcoidosis. Semin Ultrasound CT MR 1995; 16:361–370
354. Terasaki H, Fujimoto K, Muller NL, et al. Pulmonary sarcoidosis: comparison of findings of inspiratory and expiratory high-resolution CT and pulmonary function tests between smokers and nonsmokers. AJR Am J Roentgenol 2005; 185:333–338
355. Naccache JM, Lavole A, Nunes H, et al. High-resolution computed tomographic imaging of airways in sarcoidosis patients with airflow obstruction. J Comput Assist Tomogr 2008; 32:905–912
356. Akira M, Kozuka T, Inoue Y, et al. Long-term follow-up CT scan evaluation in patients with pulmonary sarcoidosis. Chest 2005; 127:185–191
357. Lavergne F, Clerici C, Sadoun D, et al. Airway obstruction in bronchial sarcoidosis: outcome with treatment. Chest 1999; 116:1194–1199
358. Handa T, Nagai S, Fushimi Y, et al. Clinical and radiographic indices associated with airflow limitation in patients with sarcoidosis. Chest 2006; 130:1851–1856
359. Subramanian I, Flaherty K, Martinez F. Pulmonary function testing in sarcoidosis. In: Baughman RP, ed. Sarcoidosis (vol 210). New York, NY: Taylor and Francis Group, 2006; 415–433
360. Shorr AF, Torrington KG, Hnatiuk OW. Endobronchial involvement and airway hyperreactivity in patients with sarcoidosis. Chest 2001; 120:881–886
361. Mihailovic-Vucinic V, Zugic V, Videnovic-Ivanov J. New observations on pulmonary function changes in sarcoidosis. Curr Opin Pulm Med 2003; 9:436–441
362. Miller A, Brown LK, Sloane MF, et al. Cardiorespiratory responses to incremental exercise in sarcoidosis patients with normal spirometry. Chest 1995; 107:323–329
363. Medinger AE, Khouri S, Rohatgi PK. Sarcoidosis: the value of exercise testing. Chest 2001; 120: 93–101

364. Mediwake R, Wells A, Desai D. Radiological imaging in sarcoidosis. In: Baughman RP, ed. Sarcoidosis (Vol 210). New York: Taylor and Francis Group, 2006; 365–398
365. Mana J, Vankroonenburgh M. Nuclear imaging techniques in sarcoidosis. Eur Respir Monograph 2005; 10:284–300
366. Tanabe Y, Ohuchi Y, Ogawa T. Muscular and myocardial involvement in sarcoidosis: the usefulness of Ga-67 imaging. Clin Nucl Med 2002; 27:749–752
367. Aberg C, Ponzo F, Raphael B, et al. FDG positron emission tomography of bone involvement in sarcoidosis. AJR Am J Roentgenol 2004; 182:975–977
368. Takeda N, Yokoyama I, Hiroi Y, et al. Positron emission tomography predicted recovery of complete A-V nodal dysfunction in a patient with cardiac sarcoidosis. Circulation 2002; 105: 1144–1145
369. Dubey N, Miletich RS, Wasay M, et al. Role of fluorodeoxyglucose positron emission tomography in the diagnosis of neurosarcoidosis. J Neurol Sci 2002; 205:77–81
370. Costabel U, Guzman J, Albera C, et al. Bronchoalveolar lavage in sarcoidosis. In: Baughman RP, ed. Sarcoidosis (Vol 210). New York: Taylor and Francis Group, 2006; 399–414
371. Zissel G, Prasse A, Muller-Quernheim J. Sarcoidosis: immunopathogenetic concepts. Semin Respir Crit Care Med 2007; 28:3–14
372. Semenzato G, Bortoli M, Brunetti E, et al. Immunology and pathophysiology. In: In: Baughman RP, ed. Sarcoidosis (Vol 210). New York: Taylor and Francis Group, 2006; 49–63
373. Ziegenhagen MW, Rothe ME, Schlaak M, et al. Bronchoalveolar and serological parameters reflecting the severity of sarcoidosis. Eur Respir J 2003; 21:407–413
374. Baughman RP, Sharma OP, Lynch JP III. Sarcoidosis. is therapy effective? Semin Respir Infect 1998; 13:255–273
375. Sharma OP. Pulmonary sarcoidosis and corticosteroids. Am Rev Respir Dis 1993; 147:1598–1600
376. Pietinalho A, Tukiainen P, Haahtela T, et al. Oral prednisolone followed by inhaled budesonide in newly diagnosed pulmonary sarcoidosis: a double-blind, placebo-controlled multicenter study: Finnish Pulmonary Sarcoidosis Study Group. Chest 1999; 116:424–431
377. Pietinalho A, Tukiainen P, Haahtela T, et al. Early treatment of stage II sarcoidosis improves 5-year pulmonary function. Chest 2002; 121:24–31
378. du Bois RM, Greenhalgh PM, Southcott AM, et al. Randomized trial of inhaled fluticasone propionate in chronic stable pulmonary sarcoidosis: a pilot study. Eur Respir J 1999; 13:1345–1350
379. Pacheco Y, Marechal C, Marechal F, et al. Azathioprine treatment of chronic pulmonary sarcoidosis. Sarcoidosis 1985; 2:107–113
380. Sharma O, Hughs DTD, James DG, et al. Immunosuppressive therapy with azathioprine in sarcoidosis. In: Levnisky L, Macholoa F, eds. Fifth International Conference on Sarcoidosis and Other Granulomatous Disorders, Prague, Czech Republic, 1971; 635–637
381. Agbogu BN, Stern BJ, Sewell C, et al. Therapeutic considerations in patients with refractory neurosarcoidosis. Arch Neurol 1995; 52:875–879
382. Diab SM, Karnik AM, Ouda BA, et al. Sarcoidosis in Arabs: the clinical profile of 20 patients and review of the literature. Sarcoidosis 1991; 8:56–62
383. Lewis SJ, Ainslie GM, Bateman ED. Efficacy of azathioprine as second-line treatment in pulmonary sarcoidosis. Sarcoidosis Vasc Diffuse Lung Dis 1999; 16:87–92
384. Muller-Quernheim J, Kienast K, Held M, et al. Treatment of chronic sarcoidosis with an azathioprine/prednisolone regimen. Eur Respir J 1999; 14:1117–1122
385. Baughman RP, Winget DB, Lower EE. Methotrexate is steroid sparing in acute sarcoidosis: results of a double blind, randomized trial. Sarcoidosis Vasc Diffuse Lung Dis 2000; 17:60–66
386. Baughman RP, Lower EE. A clinical approach to the use of methotrexate for sarcoidosis. Thorax 1999; 54:742–746
387. Lower EE, Baughman RP. Prolonged use of methotrexate for sarcoidosis. Arch Intern Med 1995; 155:846–851
388. Baughman RP, Lower EE. Steroid-sparing alternative treatments for sarcoidosis. Clin Chest Med 1997; 18:853–864
389. Zisman DA, McCune WJ, Tino G, et al. Drug-induced pneumonitis: the role of methotrexate. Sarcoidosis Vasc Diffuse Lung Dis 2001; 18:243–252
390. Baughman RP, Koehler A, Bejarano PA, et al. Role of liver function tests in detecting methotrexate-induced liver damage in sarcoidosis. Arch Intern Med 2003; 163:615–620

391. Baughman RP, Lower EE. Leflunomide for chronic sarcoidosis. Sarcoidosis Vasc Diffuse Lung Dis 2004; 21:43–48
392. Moudgil A, Przygodzki RM, Kher KK. Successful steroid-sparing treatment of renal limited sarcoidosis with mycophenolate mofetil. Pediatr Nephrol 2006; 21:281–285
393. Choudhary A, Harding SP, Bucknall RC, et al. Mycophenolate mofetil as an immunosuppressive agent in refractory inflammatory eye disease. J Ocul Pharmacol Ther 2006; 22:168–175
394. Stern BJ, Corbett J. Neuro-ophthalmologic manifestations of sarcoidosis. Curr Treat Options Neurol 2007; 9:63–71
395. Martinet Y, Pinkston P, Saltini C, et al. Evaluation of the in vitro and in vivo effects of cyclosporine on the lung T-lymphocyte alveolitis of active pulmonary sarcoidosis. Am Rev Respir Dis 1988; 138:1242–1248
396. Stern BJ, Schonfeld SA, Sewell C, et al. The treatment of neurosarcoidosis with cyclosporine. Arch Neurol 1992; 49:1065–1072
397. Wyser CP, van Schalkwyk EM, Alheit B, et al. Treatment of progressive pulmonary sarcoidosis with cyclosporin A: a randomized controlled trial. Am J Respir Crit Care Med 1997; 156:1371–1376
398. Akpek EK, Ilhan-Sarac O, Green WR. Topical cyclosporin in the treatment of chronic sarcoidosis of the conjunctiva. Arch Ophthalmol 2003; 121:1333–1335
399. Kataria YP. Chlorambucil in sarcoidosis. Chest 1980; 78:36–43
400. Israel HL, McComb BL. Chlorambucil treatment of sarcoidosis. Sarcoidosis 1991; 8:35–41
401. Israel HL, Fouts DW, Beggs RA. A controlled trial of prednisone treatment of sarcoidosis. Am Rev Respir Dis 1973; 107:609–614
402. Demeter SL. Myocardial sarcoidosis unresponsive to steroids: treatment with cyclophosphamide. Chest 1988; 94:202–203
403. Doty JD, Mazur JE, Judson MA. Treatment of corticosteroid-resistant neurosarcoidosis with a short-course cyclophosphamide regimen. Chest 2003; 124:2023–2026
404. Zic JA, Horowitz DH, Arzubiaga C, et al. Treatment of cutaneous sarcoidosis with chloroquine: review of the literature. Arch Dermatol 1991; 127:1034–1040
405. Sharma OP. Neurosarcoidosis: a personal perspective based on the study of 37 patients. Chest 1997; 112:220–228
406. Adams JS. Hypercalcemia and hypercalciuria. Semin Respir Med 1992; 13:402–410
407. Adams JS, Diz MM, Sharma OP. Effective reduction in the serum 1,25-dihydroxyvitamin D and calcium concentration in sarcoidosis-associated hypercalcemia with short-course chloroquine therapy. Ann Intern Med 1989; 111:437–438
408. Baltzan M, Mehta S, Kirkham TH, et al. Randomized trial of prolonged chloroquine therapy in advanced pulmonary sarcoidosis. Am J Respir Crit Care Med 1999; 160:192–197
409. Baughman RP, Judson MA, Teirstein AS, et al. Thalidomide for chronic sarcoidosis. Chest 2002; 122:227–232
410. Carlesimo M, Giustini S, Rossi A, et al. Treatment of cutaneous and pulmonary sarcoidosis with thalidomide. J Am Acad Dermatol 1995; 32:866–869
411. Cagnoni ML, Lombardi A, Cerinic MC, et al. Melatonin for treatment of chronic refractory sarcoidosis. Lancet 1995; 346:1229–1230
412. Zabel P, Entzian P, Dalhoff K, et al. Pentoxifylline in treatment of sarcoidosis. Am J Respir Crit Care Med 1997; 155:1665–1669
413. Tong Z, Dai H, Chen B, et al. Inhibition of cytokine release from alveolar macrophages in pulmonary sarcoidosis by pentoxifylline: comparison with dexamethasone. Chest 2003; 124:1526–1532
414. Meyerle JH, Shorr A. The use of infliximab in cutaneous sarcoidosis. J Drugs Dermatol 2003; 2:413–414
415. Mallbris L, Ljungberg A, Hedblad MA, et al. Progressive cutaneous sarcoidosis responding to anti-tumor necrosis factor-alpha therapy. J Am Acad Dermatol 2003; 48:290–293
416. Katz JM, Bruno MK, Winterkorn JM, et al. The pathogenesis and treatment of optic disc swelling in neurosarcoidosis: a unique therapeutic response to infliximab. Arch Neurol 2003; 60:426–430
417. Roberts SD, Wilkes DS, Burgett RA, et al. Refractory sarcoidosis responding to infliximab. Chest 2003; 124:2028–2031
418. Pettersen JA, Zochodne DW, Bell RB, et al. Refractory neurosarcoidosis responding to infliximab. Neurology 2002; 59:1660–1661
419. Yee AM, Pochapin MB. Treatment of complicated sarcoidosis with infliximab anti-tumor necrosis

factor-alpha therapy. Ann Intern Med 2001; 135:27–31
420. Baughman RP, Lower EE. Infliximab for refractory sarcoidosis. Sarcoidosis Vasc Diffuse Lung Dis 2001; 18:70–74
421. Baughman RP, Iannuzzi M. Tumour necrosis factor in sarcoidosis and its potential for targeted therapy. BioDrugs 2003; 17:425–431
422. Baughman RP, Drent M, Kavuru M, et al. Infliximab therapy in patients with chronic sarcoidosis and pulmonary involvement. Am J Respir Crit Care Med 2006; 174:795–802
423. Baughman RP, Lower EE. Novel therapies for sarcoidosis. Semin Respir Crit Care Med 2007; 28:128–133
424. Pritchard C, Nadarajah K. Tumour necrosis factor alpha inhibitor treatment for sarcoidosis refractory to conventional treatments: a report of five patients. Ann Rheum Dis 2004; 63:318–320
425. Utz JP, Limper AH, Kalra S, et al. Etanercept for the treatment of stage II and III progressive pulmonary sarcoidosis. Chest 2003; 124:177–185
426. Haley H, Cantrell W, Smith K. Infliximab therapy for sarcoidosis (lupus pernio). Br J Dermatol 2004; 150:146–149
427. Khanna D, Liebling MR, Louie JS. Etanercept ameliorates sarcoidosis arthritis and skin disease. J Rheumatol 2003; 30:1864–1867
428. Doty JD, Mazur JE, Judson MA. Treatment of sarcoidosis with infliximab. Chest 2005; 127:1064–1071
429. Saleh S, Ghodsian S, Yakimova V, et al. Effectiveness of infliximab in treating selected patients with sarcoidosis. Respir Med 2006; 100:2053–2059
430. Keane J, Gershon S, Wise RP, et al. Tuberculosis associated with infliximab, a tumor necrosis factor alpha-neutralizing agent. N Engl J Med 2001; 345:1098–1104
431. Ioannou Y, Isenberg DA. Current evidence for the induction of autoimmune rheumatic manifestations by cytokine therapy. Arthritis Rheum 2000; 43:1431–1442
432. Chung ES, Packer M, Lo KH, et al. Randomized, double-blind, placebo-controlled, pilot trial of infliximab, a chimeric monoclonal antibody to tumor necrosis factor-alpha, in patients with moderate-to-severe heart failure: results of the anti-TNF Therapy Against Congestive Heart Failure (ATTACH) trial. Circulation 2003; 107:3133–3140
433. Mann DL, McMurray JJ, Packer M, et al. Targeted anticytokine therapy in patients with chronic heart failure: results of the Randomized Etanercept Worldwide Evaluation (RENEWAL). Circulation 2004; 109:1594–602
434. Kavanaugh A, St Clair EW, McCune WJ, Braakman T, Lipsky P. Chimeric anti-tumor necrosis factor-alpha monoclonal antibody treatment of patients with rheumatoid arthritis receiving methotrexate therapy. J Rheumatol 2000; 27:841–850
435. Brown SL, Greene MH, Gershon SK, et al. Tumor necrosis factor antagonist therapy and lymphoma development: twenty-six cases reported to the Food and Drug Administration. Arthritis Rheum 2002; 46:3151–3158
436. Shorr AF, Helman DL, Davies DB, et al. Pulmonary hypertension in advanced sarcoidosis: epidemiology and clinical characteristics. Eur Respir J 2005; 25:783–788
437. Preston IR, Klinger JR, Landzberg MJ, et al. Vasoresponsiveness of sarcoidosis-associated pulmonary hypertension. Chest 2001; 120:866–872
438. Arcasoy SM, Christie JD, Pochettino A, et al. Characteristics and outcomes of patients with sarcoidosis listed for lung transplantation. Chest 2001; 120:873–880
439. Nunes H, Humbert M, Capron F, et al. Pulmonary hypertension associated with sarcoidosis: mechanisms, haemodynamics and prognosis. Thorax 2006; 61:68–74
440. Shorr AF, Davies DB, Nathan SD. Outcomes for patients with sarcoidosis awaiting lung transplantation. Chest 2002; 122:233–238
441. Nathan S, Saggar R, Lynch J. Lung transplantation for interstitial lung disorders. In: Lynch JP III, Ross DJ, eds. Lung and heart-lung transplantation (Vol 217). New York: Taylor and Francis, 2006; 165–204
442. Shah L. Lung transplantation in sarcoidosis. Semin Respir Crit Care Med 2007; 28:134–140
443. Martinez FJ, Orens JB, Deeb M, et al. Recurrence of sarcoidosis following bilateral allogeneic lung transplantation. Chest 1994; 106:1597–1599
444. Shorr AF, Helman DL, Davies DB, et al. Sarcoidosis, race, and short-term outcomes following lung transplantation. Chest 2004; 125:990–996
445. Shorr AF, Davies DB, Nathan SD. Predicting mortality in patients with sarcoidosis awaiting lung transplantation. Chest 2003; 124:922–928

Pulmonary Vasculitis and Alveolar Hemorrhage Syndromes

Ulrich Specks, MD

Objectives:

- Review the spectrum of pulmonary vasculitides and their clinical manifestations
- Describe the clinical spectrum of antineutrophil cytoplasmic antibody (ANCA)-associated vasculitis and review treatment principles
- Review the clinical presentation and management of Churg-Strauss syndrome (CSS)
- Discuss the differential diagnosis of diffuse alveolar hemorrhage (DAH)
- Review specific diseases that can cause DAH

Key words: alveolar hemorrhage; antibasement membrane disease; antineutrophil cytoplasmic antibodies; Behçet disease; Churg-Strauss syndrome; Goodpasture syndrome; Henoch-Schönlein purpura; idiopathic pulmonary hemosiderosis; microscopic polyangiitis; Takayasu arteritis; temporal arteritis; vasculitis; Wegener granulomatosis

Pulmonary Vasculitis

Pulmonary vasculitis is usually a manifestation of a systemic disorder leading to inflammation of vessels of different sizes by a variety of immunologic mechanisms. Vasculitis can be separated into primary and secondary vasculitis. The primary systemic vasculitides are a heterogeneous group of syndromes of unknown etiology that share a clinical response to immunosuppressive therapy. Their wide spectrum of frequently overlapping clinical manifestations is defined by the size and location of the affected vessels as well as by the nature of the inflammatory infiltrate. Secondary vasculitis may occur in the context of a well-defined underlying disorder or have a specific etiology, such as collagen vascular disease, infection, therapeutic, or illicit drug use.

Most classification schemes and definitions of the vasculitides are based on the size of the most prominently affected vessels. Definitions, nomenclature, and classification schemes are currently under review and may change. Physicians should be familiar with two sets of criteria and definitions. First, the 1990 criteria[1,2] of the American College of Rheumatology for the classification of vasculitis were developed to allow the separation of patients with one form of vasculitis from those with another and not to serve as diagnostic criteria. Second, the nomenclature and definitions put forth by the Chapel Hill consensus conference[3] in 1992 acknowledge the presence of ANCA and separate classic polyarteritis nodosa from microscopic polyangiitis and ANCA-associated vasculitis. It is important to recognize that not all respiratory symptoms occurring in patients with vasculitis are caused by the inflammation of pulmonary vessels.

Urticarial Vasculitis

Urticarial vasculitis (UV) is a systemic disorder characterized by urticaria associated with arthralgias in 60% of patients, arthritis in 28% of patients, abdominal pain in 25% of patients, and glomerulonephritis in 5% of patients. Angioedema, fever, uveitis, episcleritis, and seizures may also occur.[4,5] Hypocomplementemia is present in 38% of patients, and this hypocomplementemic form of UV has been associated with pulmonary complications not directly caused by vasculitis. Obstructive pulmonary disease, which occurs in up to two thirds of these patients, is thought to result from a combination of smoking and an unknown immunologic process. Emphysematous changes in the basal regions may occur in some patients.[6] UV with or without hypocomplementemia can also occur in patients with systemic lupus erythematosus (SLE).

Giant Cell Arteritis

Giant-cell arteritis (GCA), also called *temporal arteritis*, *cranial arteritis*, and *granulomatous arteritis*, is a generalized inflammatory disorder involving large- and medium-sized arteries.[1] It is the most common form of vasculitis in the Northern hemisphere, and it appears to affect predominantly elderly patients. The typical features of the disease include new-onset headache, a palpably tender or nodular temporal artery with decreased pulsation, and an increased erythrocyte sedimentation rate (ESR). Granulomatosus inflammation of the vessel wall is found in 60% of temporal artery biopsy specimens. GCA and polymyalgia rheumatica are thought to be part of a disease spectrum. The clinical illness appears gradually with the development of nonspecific systemic symptoms such as low-grade fever, malaise, and weight loss. Headache, which is variable but often severe, is the most common symptom in GCA. Amaurosis fugax is observed in 20% of patients and visual loss in 10%. It is now recognized that the aorta may also be affected by the disease.[7]

Respiratory symptoms have been reported in up to 25% of patients,[8] but they rarely require management by a pulmonologist. Cough, hoarseness, and throat pain usually resolve promptly with glucocorticoid therapy. However, respiratory symptoms may be the initial presentation of GCA. Therefore, this possibility should be considered in any elderly patient with new onset of cough, hoarseness, or throat pain without other identifiable cause, and it is reasonable to measure the ESR in such patients.[9] Isolated cases with pleural effusion or multinodular pulmonary lesions have also been reported in GCA. Such cases are difficult to interpret. Particularly in the later situation, Wegener granulomatosis (WG) should be considered in the differential diagnosis because it may also present with temporal arteritis.[10] Therapy of GCA continues to rely heavily on the use of glucocorticoids without a proven alternative.[11] The glucocorticoid-sparing role of methotrexate for GCA remains controversial.[12]

Takayasu Arteritis

Takayasu arteritis (TA) is a large-vessel vasculitis affecting predominantly the aorta and its major branches in young patients.[13] TA has also been called *pulseless disease, aortic arch syndrome,* or *reversed coarctation.* The disease affects mostly young adult women. It is not limited to patients of Asian decent. Early disease manifestations include constitutional symptoms, low-grade fever, and arthralgias. Variable pulses of the extremities and claudication of affected vascular territories are typical. Renovascular hypertension, pulmonary hypertension, and ischemia of affected organs may be the more disabling complications of this chronically relapsing disease.

Pulmonary complications are the result of a unique arteriopathy predominantly of the large- and medium-size pulmonary vessels. Progressive defects in the outer media of the arteries and ingrowth of granulation tissue-like capillaries associated with thickened intima and subendothelial smooth-muscle proliferation lead to pulmonary artery stenoses and occlusion as well as pulmonary hypertension in up to one half of all patients. The inflammatory infiltrate of the vessel wall is predominantly lymphoplasmacytic with variable amounts of giant cells. The involvement of pulmonary arteries is common but often asymptomatic. It is detectable by conventional angiography, perfusion scan, or magnetic resonance angiography. Chest roentgenograms are often normal, but CT scans may show areas of low attenuation as a result of regional hypoperfusion, subpleural reticulolinear changes, and pleural thickening. Fistula formation between pulmonary artery branches and bronchial arteries, as well as nonspecific inflammatory interstitial lung disease, have also been reported.

Therapy for TA consists primarily of immunosuppression with glucocorticoids. Other immunosuppressive agents, including methotrexate, are used in conjunction with glucocorticoids for remission induction and as glucocorticoid-sparing agents for remission maintenance. Unfortunately, many patients relapse when the glucocorticoid dose is reduced to <15 mg/d. The use of anti-tumor necrosis factor-α agents has been reported as beneficial in patients refractory to standard therapy.[14] Vascular bypass procedures may be beneficial in severe disease, but beneficial results are only temporary.[15]

Classic Polyarteritis Nodosa

Since its formal separation from microscopic polyangiitis, this form of vasculitis, which affects predominantly medium-sized vessels, is diagnosed rarely.[16] Polyarteritis nodosa (PAN) does not affect capillaries. Therefore, it does not cause glomerulonephritis or alveolar hemorrhage (AH). However, classic PAN can on rare occasions affect the bronchial or bronchiolar arteries. Most cases of classic PAN diagnosed are associated with viral infections, specifically hepatitis B and C. Consequently, antiviral therapy plays a prominent role in the management of such cases in addition to immunosuppression. Classic PAN is far less likely to reoccur than microscopic polyangiitis and therefore can generally be treated with a shorter course of immunosuppression.[17]

ANCA-Associated Vasculitis

The primary systemic small vessel vasculitides are WG, microscopic polyangiitis (MPA), and the CSS. In contrast to the other forms of systemic vasculitis with predilections for larger vessels, most patients with active WG and MPA and more than half of patients with active CSS have ANCA. Of all systemic vasculitides, the ANCA-associated vasculitides are most likely to cause respiratory manifestations. WG and MPA will be discussed together here because the same diagnostic and therapeutic principles apply; CSS will be discussed separately.

The Chapel Hill Consensus Nomenclature has defined WG as "granulomatous inflammation involving the respiratory tract, and necrotizing vasculitis affecting small to medium-sized vessels (*ie,* capillaries, venules, arterioles, and arteries)."[3] Histopathologic documentation of granulomatous involvement of the respiratory tract is not explicitly required. Roentgenographic evidence or clinical examination findings highly predictive of granulomatous pathology are sufficient. Consequently, the diagnosis of WG depends on a correlation of clinical, pathologic, and serologic features.

MPA is defined as a "necrotizing vasculitis with few or no immune deposits, affecting small vessels (*ie,* capillaries, venules, or arterioles). Necrotizing arteritis involving small and medium-sized arteries may be present. Necrotizing glomerulonephritis is very common; pulmonary capillaritis resulting in AH occurs frequently."[3] The vasculitis of MPA is indistinguishable from that of WG, and there may be substantial clinical overlap. The literature needs to be interpreted with this in mind. In fact, the therapeutic approach to patients with WG and MPA is governed by the same principles, and most ongoing clinical studies and therapeutic trials combine both diseases.

For treatment stratification, a patient's disease activity is categorized as limited disease or severe disease. Severe disease is either life threatening or threatening an organ with irreversible loss of function. Consequently, patients with any of the following disease manifestations should be labeled as having severe disease: AH, glomerulonephritis, eye involvement (except mere episcleritis), and nervous system involvement, including sensorineural hearing loss. Limited disease includes essentially all patients who have nonsevere disease.

The term *limited disease* used in the United States comprises what European investigators have referred to as *early systemic disease* as well as *localized disease*. Although this separation is not based on well-defined biological distinctions, most disease manifestations leading to the categorization as severe disease are caused by capillaritis. In contrast, most symptoms leading to the classification as limited disease are the result of necrotizing granulomatous inflammation. Patients with limited WG have a longer disease duration, a greater likelihood of experiencing an exacerbation of previous disease after a period of remission, and a greater prevalence of destructive upper respiratory tract disorders (*eg,* saddle-nose deformity).[18] Tracheobronchial involvement also distinguishes WG from MPA; it may represent unique treatment challenges (discussed later in this section).

Histopathologic features that define WG and separate it from MPA include discrete or confluent necrotizing granulomatous inflammation with vasculitis. Fibrinoid necrosis, microabscesses, focal vasculitis, thrombosis, and fibrous obliteration of the vascular lumen may be observed. Giant cells are a hallmark of the necrotizing granulomatous inflammation of WG. Other histopathologic findings, including bronchiolitis obliterans organizing pneumonia, bronchocentric inflammation, and a marked number of eosinophil infiltrates, are atypical features that have also been described in WG.

The etiology of ANCA-associated vasculitis remains unknown. Occupational exposures have been suggested as possible etiologic factors, including inhalation of silica-containing compounds, grain dust, and heavy metals.[19–22] Infection has been linked to the onset of the disease as well as to relapses.[23] A multifactorial genetic predisposition may also contribute to the development of ANCA-associated vasculitis.[24] Genetic polymorphisms in the PR3 molecule as well as its expression on neutrophils may influence the induction and course of WG. Along the same line, heterozygotes for the P_1* Z variant of the α_1-antitrypsin gene are reported to have a sixfold-greater risk for developing the disease than the general population. Last not least, ANCAs seem to play a pathogenic role for the development of vasculitis.[25]

The characteristic disease manifestation of WG affecting the respiratory tract is caused by necrotizing granulomatous inflammation. Ear, nose, and throat symptoms are initially noted by >85% of patients. These may include rhinorrhea, purulent or bloody nasal discharge, nasal mucosal drying and crust formation, epistaxis, and otitis media. Deep facial pain from paranasal sinus involvement, nasal septal perforation, and ulceration of the vomer are important signs. *Staphylococcus aureus* is frequently detected in the nose and sinuses and has been linked to relapses of the disease.[26] Other signs include aphthous lesions of the nasal and oral mucosa and inflammation and destruction of the nasal cartilage leading to a saddle-nose deformity. Ulcerated lesions of the larynx and trachea are present in 30% of untreated cases and may produce hemoptysis.

The median age of patients is 45 years, the male/female ratio is about equal, and >90% of patients are white. The clinical presentation varies from subacute nonspecific respiratory illness to rapidly progressive AH syndrome. Pulmonary symptoms are usually associated with unilateral or bilateral abnormalities on the chest radiograph, including infiltrates, nodules, or mass lesions that may or may not cavitate. The nodules range from a few millimeters to several centimeters in size. Solitary nodules may also occur. Unusual manifestations include lymphadenopathy, lobar consolidation, and large pleural effusions. Tracheobronchial lesions are common, and they may be asymptomatic or mistaken for asthma.[27,28] Pulmonary function tests and inspiratory and expiratory flow-volume loops may aid in follow-up.

Patients with ANCA-associated vasculitis have variable degrees of elevated of ESR or C-reactive protein. If WG or MPA are suspected, it is crucial to obtain a urine analysis and microscopy and measure serum creatinine because early renal involvement may be clinically silent yet progress rapidly.

In WG and MPA, ANCAs that cause a cytoplasmic immunofluorescence pattern (C-ANCA) on ethanol-fixed neutrophils are caused by antibodies reacting with proteinase 3 (PR3; PR3-ANCA). In contrast, a variety of antibodies can cause a perinuclear immunofluorescence pattern (P-ANCA) on ethanol-fixed neutrophils. Only those that also react with myeloperoxidase are of interest in the context of ANCA-associated vasculitis. Maximal diagnostic accuracy of ANCA testing requires corroboration of a positive target antigen specific test result (PR3-ANCA or myeloperoxidase-ANCA) by immunofluorescence, and *vice versa*.[29] Only the PR3-ANCA with C-ANCA combination and the myeloperoxidase-ANCA with P-ANCA combination are sensitive and specific for ANCA-associated vasculitis.[30–32]

The clinical utility, *ie*, positive and negative predictive values of ANCA testing for WG and MPA, are critically dependent on the pretest probability of the disease in the patient tested as well as on the analytical accuracy of the test method.[33] If applied in patients with clinical features indicating a high pretest probability of WG or MPA, ANCA testing has a very high positive predictive value. However, occasional false-positive ANCA test results have been reported in a variety of infections. Particularly, subacute bacterial endocarditis may represent a diagnostic dilemma because it may mimic small-vessel vasculitis clinically and has been reported with C-ANCA/PR3-ANCA.[34] Other infections reported with ANCA either do not have the right pairing of immunofluorescence test results with its corresponding antigen specificity or their clinical features are distinct from WG or MPA.[23] In patients undergoing evaluation for necrotizing glomerulonephritis with or without AH, ANCA may occur in conjunction with anti-glomerular basement membrane antibodies (anti-GBMs).[35] These ANCAs are usually of the myeloperoxidase-ANCA variety. The presence of anti-GBM seems to determine the prognosis in such double-positive patients.[35]

Most patients with severe WG or MPA have a positive ANCA test (sensitivity >95%), but up to 30% of patients with limited WG may not have detectable ANCA.[36] Although there is an association between ANCA titers and disease activity, changes in ANCA levels do not reliably predict the disease activity in individual patients. Therefore, serial titers of ANCA should not be used to plan long-term therapy.[37]

Standard therapy for WG and MPA currently follows the same basic principles. Methotrexate, 25 mg, once a week in combination with oral prednisone is now the standard of care for patients with limited WG.[38] However, there is only one prospective randomized trial[39] in which the authors compared methotrexate with cyclophosphamide for remission induction in such patients. The trial conducted by the European Vasculitis Study Group (EUVAS) showed that methotrexate is indeed noninferior to cyclophosphamide for remission induction, but the side effects were less. The trial[39] also documented that early discontinuation of immunosuppression in patients with ANCA-associated vasculitis is fraught with a high rate of relapse. The largest reported group of patients with limited WG was treated with methotrexate for remission induction in the context of the Wegener's Granulomatosis Etanercept Trial (WGET).[40] More than 90% of patients achieved remission with this regimen, and >70% achieved a sustained remission (lasting >6 months). These rates are equivalent to those achieved with cyclophosphamide in severe disease (discussed to follow).

Cyclophosphamide at a dose of 2 mg/kg/d in combination with prednisone remains the standard of care for patients with severe WG or MPA. In contrast to the original regimen introduced by Fauci,[40a] the consensus now is to limit the duration of cyclophosphamide therapy to the first 3 to 6 months. Once remission has been induced and the prednisone taper is well under way, cyclophosphamide should be switched to either azathioprine, which is preferred in patients with renal involvement and any degree of renal insufficiency, or methotrexate. The first option is supported by the results of a randomized trial conducted by the EUVAS that showed azathioprine is as good as cyclophosphamide for remission maintenance to 18 months.[41] A randomized controlled trial[42] has shown that methotrexate and azathioprine are equivalent for remission maintenance.

Mycophenolate mofetil (MMF) represents another alternative to methotrexate and azathioprine for remission maintenance.[43] However, this agent is significantly more expensive, and the available published reports indicate that a substantial number of patients also relapse while receiving this agent.[43] In the absence of randomized trials comparing the different remission maintenance agents, it remains unclear to what extent the reported results with MMF are tainted by patient selection. The use of MMF for remission maintenance can only be supported for patients in whom methotrexate and azathioprine has failed or who have contraindications for both agents. The WGET trial, [40] in which methotrexate was used for remission maintenance, confirmed that long-term remission remains an elusive goal for many patients; remission was maintained in less than half of the patients.

Whenever cyclophosphamide is used for remission induction, consideration should be given to the patient's fertility. Young men should be offered sperm banking before therapy is initiated. If time allows, ovarian protection should be offered to young women in addition to minimizing the cumulative exposure as much as possible.[44]

Recent data from the EUVAS group[44a] indicate that the IV application of cyclophosphamide is as effective as oral application and maybe safer. Earlier studies[44b] had indicated that safety was improved because of a lower cumulative dose with IV cyclophosphamide but that a greater relapse rate was observed after discontinuation. In the author's experience-based opinion, IV cyclophosphamide should be avoided in the ICU setting. However, its use is preferred over oral cyclophosphamide in patients with questionable compliance, in young women with fertility issues, and in patients who have GI problems with oral cyclophosphamide application.

In patients with MPA who have myeloperoxidase-ANCA and mild renal disease (creatinine <3 to 5 mg/d) and no other life- or organ-threatening disease manifestations, MMF may represent an alternative to cyclophosphamide provided that careful observation is guaranteed.[45] This statement is based on results from a randomized controlled trial in 35 patients from China in which the authors compared oral MMF (1.5 to 2 g/d) with IV cyclophosphamide (0.75 to 1.0 g/m^2 once monthly).[45] In addition, all patients received IV methylprednisolone bolus therapy, 0.5 g/d for 3 days, followed by oral prednisone, 0.6 to 0.8 mg/kg for 4 weeks tapered by 5 mg/wk to 10 mg/d. This study showed that the efficacy of these regimens was equivalent, but MMF was better tolerated than cyclophosphamide.[45]

For some patients with WG and MPA, the combination of glucocorticoids and cyclophosphamide may not be sufficient to induce a remission quickly. Plasma exchange (PLEX) should be considered early in patients who present with rapidly progressive glomerulonephritis and renal failure as well as in patients who present with DAH. PLEX is currently supported by two studies.[46,47] The EUVAS investigators conducted the Methylprednisolone Versus Plasma Exchange Trial in patients who presented with a serum creatinine level of ≥5.5 mg/dL.[46] In addition to standard therapy for severe disease (oral prednisone and cyclophosphamide), patients were randomized to either receive three pulses of IV methyl-prednisolone or 2 weeks of PLEX (7 × 60 mL/kg). PLEX was clearly superior to methylprednisolone with respect to renal recovery.[46] A single-center cohort study[47] of 20 patients presenting with AH described 100% survival of the patients when PLEX was added to standard immunosuppressive therapy. If AH is uncontrolled despite aggressive immunosuppressive therapy and PLEX, the use of recombinant activated factor VII may be considered.[48,49]

The term *refractory disease* is commonly used to describe patients who have persistent disease activity on the maximal tolerated dose of cyclophosphamide or who have contraindications for the use of cyclophosphamide. A variety of agents have been proposed for use in addition or instead of the failing regimen in such patients. Small case series and uncontrolled trials have suggested some efficacy of infliximab in such patients.[50,51] However, infliximab therapy was associated with a high frequency of infections with bad outcomes.[50,51] The authors of WGET[40] showed that etanercept had no effect for remission induction or maintenance when used in addition to standard therapy. Moreover, significantly more malignancies were observed in the etanercept arm among patients who had received cyclophosphamide.[52] As a consequence, the use of etanercept in patients who have received or are receiving cyclophosphamide is contraindicated. Given all the available data, there is no convincing rationale for the use of anti-tumor necrosis factor therapy in patients with WG.

A novel promising treatment approach has recently emerged. B lymphocytes are thought to be instrumental in the pathogenesis of autoimmune disease including ANCA-associated vasculitis. B lymphocytes can be depleted with the chimeric monoclonal antibody targeting CD20, rituximab, that is selectively expressed on the surface of B lymphocytes. A retrospective analysis of the compassionate use of rituximab and a small prospective pilot trial have shown that this agent was successful in inducing remission and allowing discontinuation of glucocorticoids in patients with refractory disease.[53,54] Other single case reports and small series with short-term follow-up support these observations.[54a] This experience has led to an ongoing large randomized placebo-controlled trial that compares rituximab to cyclophosphamide for remission induction in patients with severe ANCA-associated vasculitis (www.clinicaltrials.gov). There are several reports on the use of other agents in patients with refractory disease. Antithymoglobulin has some efficacy but significant side effects.[54b] Dispergualine is an agent available in Japan and Europe but not in the United States.[54c]

The management of large airway involvement in WG may represent unique challenges. Subglottic stenosis may require dilation procedures paired with local injection of long-acting glucocorticoids with or without mitomycin C.[55] Stenosis of the large airways may require bronchoscopic interventions, including dilation by rigid bronchoscope, Nd:YAG treatment, and the placement of silicone airway stents.[27,28]

Complications are responsible for the significant rate of morbidity and mortality seen in patients with WG and MPA. Both the disease and the treatment lead to organ damage. In the National Institutes of Health report on 158 patients, permanent complications developed in 86% of patients from WG itself, including end-stage renal disease, chronic pulmonary dysfunction, diminished hearing, destructive sinus disease, saddle-nose deformities, proptosis, and blindness. Among the treated patients, 42% experienced permanent treatment-related problems, including chemical (drug-induced) cystitis, osteoporotic fracture, bladder cancer, myelodysplasia, and avascular necrosis.[56] Reflecting more recent standard practice, in 180 patients in WGET,[57] damage that occurred despite (or because of) therapy included visual impairment, hearing loss, nasal blockade, pulmonary fibrosis, hypertension, renal insufficiency, peripheral neuropathy, gonadal failure, and diabetes mellitus. Only 11% of the enrolled patients did not exhibit a single point on the vascular damage index (which was developed from 61 various items) after 1 year of study enrollment.[57] The WGET also concluded that patients with limited WG are at a greater risk of WG-related damage than are those with severe disease.[57]

In the same cohort of 180 patients with WG, the incidence rate of venous thromboembolism was found to be high when compared with available rates in the general population, patients with lupus, and patients with rheumatoid arthritis.[58] This increased risk of thromboembolic disease has also been documented for the other ANCA-associated vasculitides.[59]

A high frequency of echocardiographic abnormalities attributable to WG and associated increased mortality was observed in a study[60] of 85 patients with confirmed WG. In 26 of these 73 patients with echocardiographic abnormalities (36%), the lesions appeared directly related to WG and consisted of regional wall motion abnormalities in 17 patients (65%), left ventricular systolic dysfunction with decreased ejection fraction in 13 patients (50%), and pericardial effusion in 5 patients (19%). Other findings included valvulitis, left ventricular aneurysm, and a large intracardiac mass.[60]

Churg-Strauss Syndrome

The Chapel Hill Consensus definition for CSS is "eosinophil-rich and granulomatous inflammation involving the respiratory, and necrotizing vasculitis affecting small to medium-sized vessels, and associated with asthma and eosinophilia."[3] CSS is included among the ANCA-associated vasculitides, but only 40 to 70% of patients with active CSS have detectable ANCA.[61–63] CSS is primarily distinguished from WG and MPA by a high prevalence of asthma and peripheral blood and tissue eosinophilia. Three distinct disease phases of the disease have been described.[64] The first is a prodromal allergic phase with asthma. This phase may last for a number of years. Second is an eosinophilic phase with prominent peripheral and tissue eosinophilia. This phase may also last a number of years, and the manifestations may remit and recur during this time period. The differential diagnosis for patients in this phase of the disease includes parasitic infection and chronic eosinophilic pneumonia. The third vasculitic phase consists of systemic vasculitis and may be life threatening. The three phases are not seen in all patients, do not necessarily occur in this order, and may even concur. However, asthma usually predates vasculitic symptoms by a mean of 7 years (range 0 to 61 years).[61] Formes frustes of CSS have also been described with eosinophilic vasculitis and/or eosinophilic granulomas in isolated organs without evidence of systemic disease.[65]

Pulmonary parenchymal involvement occurs in 38% of patients. Transient alveolar-type infiltrates are most common. These have a predominantly peripheral distribution and are indistinguishable from infiltrates found in chronic eosinophilic pneumonia. Occasionally, nodular lesions may be seen in CSS. In contrast to WG and MPA, AH is exceedingly rare.[61] Renal involvement in CSS is less prominent than in WG on MPA and does not generally lead to renal failure. In contrast, peripheral nerve involvement, typically in the form of mononeuritis multiplex, is more frequent. Skin, heart, CNS, and abdominal viscera may also be involved.

The classic histopathologic picture consists of necrotizing vasculitis, eosinophilic tissue infiltration, and extravascular granulomas. However, not all features are found in every case, and they are not pathognomonic of the condition. Particularly the finding of a Churg-Strauss granuloma on skin biopsy should not be confused with the diagnosis of CSS. This type of necrotizing extravascular granuloma may be seen in CSS as well as in other systemic autoimmune diseases, including WG and rheumatoid arthritis.

If ANCAs are present, they are usually P-ANCA reacting with myeloperoxidase.[61] The ANCA status appears to correlate with disease activity.[61] Recent studies suggest a more vasculitic disease phenotype in the presence of ANCA, but not all studies have found this, and there remains substantial overlap of organ manifestations between patients with CSS who are ANCA positive and those who are ANCA negative.[61–63]

In recent years, significant attention has been devoted to CSS detected in patients by the use of leukotriene receptor antagonists. Available case studies and limited population-based incidence estimates suggest that these agents may lead to unmasking of vasculitic symptoms in asthmatic patients by allowing dose reductions or discontinuation of oral glucocorticoid therapy. There is no evidence suggesting that these agents cause CSS.

The prognosis of CSS is better than that of WG or MPA because the overall rate of mortality is lower and not significantly different from the normal population.[61] Most deaths are secondary to cardiac involvement.

Systemic glucocorticoids remain the mainstay of therapy for CSS. There are no clinical trials that provide clear guidance. It seems most appropriate to treat CSS according to the principles applied to the management of ANCA associated vasculitis. Accordingly, cyclophosphamide should be added to glucocorticoids for remission induction in all patients with disease manifestations that threaten the patient's life or the function of a vital organ, *ie*, particularly those with central- or peripheral-nerve involvement, glomerulonephritis, heart involvement, or AH. Methotrexate, azathioprine, or MMF have been used as glucocorticoid-sparing agents in less-severe disease and for remission maintenance. Refractory disease and disease dominated by difficult-to-control eosinophilic inflammation have been reported to respond to interferon- therapy.[66] However, continued long-term interferon- therapy may be necessary, and this treatment carries the risk of substantial toxicity. Rituximab has also been used successfully in CSS.[67,68]

Idiopathic Pauci-Immune Pulmonary Capillaritis

This is a diagnosis of exclusion in patients presenting with diffuse AH as a result of capillaritis in the absence of symptoms or serologic evidence of any detectable underlying systemic disorder.[69] Direct immunofluorescence studies of the lung tissue reveal no immune deposits. This isolated pauci-immune pulmonary capillaritis is histopathologically indistinguishable from that of ANCA-associated vasculitis. These patients are best treated with an immunosuppressive regimen according to the guidelines for severe WG or microscopic polyangiitis.

Behçet Disease

Behçet disease (BD) is a rare chronically relapsing systemic inflammatory disorder characterized by aphthous oral ulcers and at least two or more of the following: aphthous genital ulcers, uveitis, cutaneous nodules or pustules, or meningoencephalitis. Reported prevalence of the disease is 1:16,000 in Japan and 1:20,0000 in the United States. There is a strong association with the major histocompatibility complex antigen HLA-B51.[70] The mean age of patients at the onset of BD is 35 years; most studies have reported a predominance of men with the disease over women. Respiratory manifestations are common in BD and include cough, hemoptysis, chest pain, and dyspnea.[71] Hemoptysis is often massive and fatal. The vasculitis of BD is immune complex mediated and may affect vessels of all sizes. Secondary thrombosis with major venous occlusion can occur. Thrombosis may not be preventable in BD by anticoagulation, but aspirin 80 mg/d, has been advocated. Destruction of the elastic lamina of pulmonary arteries causing aneurysm formation, secondary erosion of bronchi, and arterial-bronchial fistulae may result in massive hemoptysis. CT or MR angiography are used to detect pulmonary artery aneurysms. Recurrent pneumonia as well as bronchial obstruction as a consequence of mucosal inflammation have also been described.

Therapy of the underlying disease consists of immunosuppression.[72] Prednisone alone may not be sufficient to control the vasculitis. The addition of other drugs, such as colchicine, chlorambucil, methotrexate, cyclosporin, or azathioprine, is recommended. The use of biological agents, in particular anti-tumor necrosis factors agents, has also been reported. The addition of azathioprine or cyclophosphamide to glucocorticoids may result in the resolution of pulmonary aneurysms. Once pulmonary arteritis has been identified, anticoagulation should be avoided. The prognosis of pulmonary involvement is poor. Approximately one third of patients die within 2 years of pulmonary involvement, most from fatal pulmonary hemorrhage. Embolization therapy may be used as treatment and prevention of hemorrhage from pulmonary artery aneurysms.

Henoch-Schönlein Purpura

Henoch-Schönlein purpura (HSP), also known as *anaphylactoid purpura* or *allergic purpura*, is a syndrome that is characterized by acute purpura, arthritis, colicky abdominal pain, and nephritis. Pathologic findings include acute arteriolitis and venulitis in the superficial dermis and the bowel.

Proliferative and necrotizing glomerulonephritis is usually mild. A similar type of renal lesion is seen in patients with infective subacute bacterial endocarditis, WG, SLE, PAN, and Goodpasture syndrome.

Immunofluorescence microscopy shows large deposits of IgA in the skin and kidney. Although HSP is more common in children (mean age of patients, 17 years), adults may also be affected. Palpable purpura, which are usually distributed over the buttocks and lower extremities, and fever are generally the first signs. The purpura may precede, accompany, or follow arthralgias and abdominal colic. The triad of purpura, arthritis, and abdominal pain is present in approximately 80% of patients. Joint involvement is typically monoarticular and transient, involves the large joints, and causes pain that is out of proportion to the objective evidence of synovitis. Peritonitis and melena are common. Pulmonary manifestations of HSP are rare. Only 26 cases have been reported to date, and capillaritis has been documented histopathologically only in a minority of them.[73] IgA deposits along the pulmonary capillary walls, analogous to those found in vessels of the skin and glomeruli of affected kidneys, are pathognomonic for HSP.

Secondary Vasculitis

Many of the rheumatologic diseases exhibit a secondary vasculitic process in the organs involved. Infectious processes, particularly secondary to infection with Aspergillus and Mucor sp, invade vascular structures and produce secondary vasculitis. Certain drugs and chemicals can induce vasculitis. Other uncommon secondary vasculitic entities include benign lymphocytic angiitis and granulomatosis, bronchocentric granulomatosis, and necrotizing sarcoid angiitis.

AH Syndromes

Diffuse hemorrhage into the alveolar spaces is sometimes called alveolar hemorrhage syndrome. The clinical course of AH is unpredictable and may progress rapidly to respiratory failure; it is always potentially life threatening. Consequently, its consideration needs to be an integral part of the differential diagnostic evaluation of patients with alveolar infiltrates on chest roentgenogram. The symptoms of AH are nonspecific. Patients usually seek care because of dyspnea and cough, possibly associated with fever. Diffuse alveolar infiltrates on chest roentgenogram are the first diagnostic hallmark. Depending on the severity of the disease process at the time of evaluation, anemia and hypoxemia may be prominent. Hemoptysis is a common presenting symptom of AH, but it may be absent in up to onethird of patients with AH.[74]

AH can result from a variety of underlying or associated conditions that cause a disruption of the alveolar-capillary basement membrane integrity. Mechanisms leading to AH include immunological inflammatory conditions causing immune-complex deposition or capillaritis (*eg*, Goodpasture syndrome, SLE, ANCA-associated vasculitis); direct chemical/toxic injury (*eg*, from toxic or chemical inhalation, abciximab use, all-*trans*-retinoic acid, trimellitic anhydride, or smoking crack cocaine); physical trauma (*eg*, pulmonary contusion); and increased vascular pressure within the capillaries (*eg*, mitral stenosis or severe left ventricular failure). AH is best confirmed by BAL. Progressively more bloody return indicates alveolar origin of the blood.[75] The presence of $>20\%$ hemosiderin-laden macrophages among the total number of alveolar macrophages recovered by BAL is reported to indicate AH, even in the absence of ongoing active bleeding.[76] Pulmonary AH is significantly associated with the following: thrombocytopenia ($<50{,}000$ cells/μL), other abnormal coagulation variables, renal failure (creatinine concentration, ≥ 2.5 mg/dL), and a history of heavy smoking. The diagnostic approach to the patient presenting with AH is aimed at the rapid identification of the underlying cause and at prompt implementation of appropriate therapy.

Exposure to inhalational toxins such as trimellitic anhydride or pyromellitic dianhydrate, drug abuse (including crack cocaine abuse), and smoking should be identified. The medical history will also uncover preexisting comorbidities that can cause AH, including mitral stenosis, coagulation disorders, recent bone marrow or hematopoietic stem-cell transplantation, preexisting autoimmune disorders, and therapeutic drugs. Similarly, the initial physical examination should include a careful search for signs of comorbidities and possible systemic autoimmune disorders.

Initial blood and urine testing should screen for other organ involvement, particularly kidney involvement (CBC, chemistry group, urine analysis and microscopy), and determine the current coagulation status (activated partial thromboplastin time, international normalized ratio). Baseline markers of inflammation (ESR and C-reactive protein) are helpful to monitor subsequent responses to therapy. At the same time, specific serologic testing for potential underlying systemic disease processes should be initiated. This includes testing for ANCA, anti-GBM antibodies, anti-nuclear antibodies, anti--double-stranded DNA antibodies, rheumatoid factor, and anti-phospholipid antibodies, as well as determination of complement and creatinine kinase levels. The decision to obtain a biopsy specimen needs to be considered carefully, with one weighing the risks of the biopsy procedure, the likelihood of obtaining a diagnostic piece of tissue, the likelihood of the biopsy findings to alter the therapeutic approach, and the risks associated with the chosen therapy.

The AH syndromes can be broadly separated into those in which AH is caused by or associated with pulmonary capillaritis and those that lack pulmonary capillaritis (bland histology). Pulmonary capillaritis refers to the specific histopathologic finding of alveolar wall infiltration with inflammatory cells centered on capillary walls and small veins.[77] The inflammatory cells are predominantly neutrophils, but eosinophils or monocytes may also be encountered. Capillaritis usually causes fibrinoid necrosis of alveolar and vessel walls and may culminate in the destruction of the underlying lung architecture.[77] The interstitial infiltration by neutrophils seen in the context of capillaritis needs to be distinguished from the predominant intra-alveolar neutrophilic infiltration commonly associated with active infections. Another hallmark of capillaritis is the presence of pyknotic cells and nuclear fragments from neutrophils undergoing apoptosis. This feature, referred to as *leukocytoclasis*, allows the distinction of true capillaritis from neutrophil margination related to surgical trauma, which can simulate capillaritis.[78] Most of the syndromes associated with pulmonary capillaritis leading to AH have been discussed in the "Pulmonary Vasculitis" section of this chapter. The subsequent paragraphs will describe a few unique syndromes or conditions that may also be associated with AH.

Anti-Basement Membrane Antibody Disease (Goodpasture Syndrome)

Anti-basement membrane antibody disease (ABMA), also known as anti-GBM disease or Goodpasture syndrome, is a rare autoimmune disease characterized by the presence of autoantibodies directed against the NC1-domain of the $\alpha 3$ chain of basement membrane collagen type IV. This epitope is only accessible for autoantibodies in the basement membranes of kidneys and lungs.[79] Diffuse AH occurs in about one half of patients with ABMA. It is thought to require an additional inhalational injury, particularly smoking, for the development of the pulmonary manifestation of this disease.[80,81] Isolated AH in the absence of renal disease is rare in ABMA. Circulating autoantibodies to basement membrane are detectable in the serum, but the diagnosis of ABMA hinges on the histopathologic documentation of linear IgG deposits along the basement membranes in lung or kidney. ABMA is arguably not a vasculitis. Bland pulmonary hemorrhage is the most frequently described histopathologic pattern in diffuse AH associated with ABMA. However, capillaritis as a secondary histopathologic feature has been encountered in some patients.[82] Early implementation of immunosuppressive therapy in conjunction with PLEX is the key to a favorable outcome in patients with ABMA.[83] The pulmonary outcome of ABMA is generally favorable, whereas chronic renal failure is common.[81]

Vasculitides

The various primary vasculitis syndromes that may cause AH have been discussed in detail previously. It is worth reiterating here is that the most common cause of pulmonary renal syndrome defined as AH with glomerulonephritis is ANCA-associated vasculitis, either WG or MPA. In contrast, AH is rare in the context of CSS.

SLE and Other Collagen Vascular Disorders

The disease manifestations of SLE are highly variable. Pulmonary capillaritis leading to diffuse AH is rare in SLE but is usually a severe complication of the disease. Direct immunofluorescence microscopy reveals prominent immune complex deposits in the affected tissue of patients with

SLE, including the lungs. Hence, the development of pulmonary capillaritis in SLE is thought to be immune complex mediated. The onset of diffuse AH in patients with SLE is usually abrupt, and it is seldom the first sign of the disease. In the overwhelming majority of patients, the rapid development of pulmonary infiltrates is associated with fever. Hemoptysis may be absent in up to one half of the patients. Consequently, the differentiation of diffuse AH from infection may be difficult in SLE and may require a diagnostic BAL. Mechanical ventilation, infection, and cyclophosphamide therapy were identified by univariate analysis as negative prognostic factors in one cohort.[74] The reported mortality of diffuse AH in SLE ranges from 0 to 90%.[84–87] Treatment consists of glucocorticoids and cyclophosphamide. The use of PLEX has been suggested, but its benefit remains unproven.

In all other types of collagen vascular or connective tissue disorders, respiratory complications are very common. However, pulmonary capillaritis presenting as diffuse AH is rare. Isolated cases have been reported with polymyositis, rheumatoid arthritis, and mixed connective tissue disease.[88,89] Consequently, serologic testing performed as part of an evaluation of diffuse AH should include studies aimed at the identification of these potential underlying disease entities.

Antiphospholipid Syndrome

Antiphospholipid syndrome (APS) is defined by arterial and venous thromboses or recurrent miscarriages occurring in patients with anti-phospholipid antibodies (anticardiolipin antibodies, lupus anticoagulant, or both). If APS occurs in the context of another autoimmune disease, malignancy, or drug exposure, it is labeled *secondary APS*. In the absence of other coexisting disorders, it is considered primary.[90] Hypercoagulability can cause pulmonary embolism and infarction, pulmonary microthrombosis, and pulmonary arterial thrombosis with secondary pulmonary hypertension as consequence.[91–93] However, primary pulmonary hypertension as well as ARDS have also been reported as complications of APS.

Diffuse AH is rare in APS. The clinical presentation is nonspecific and consists of cough, dyspnea, fever, and bilateral pulmonary infiltrates. Diffuse AH can also occur in the context of ARDS, and hemoptysis is absent in more than half of the reported patients with APS and AH. Therefore, an early BAL may help in the differential diagnosis. Tissue necrosis from microthrombosis as well as pulmonary capillaritis have been implicated as cause of AH in APS. Like in SLE, the capillaritis of APS is immune-complex mediated. Most patients respond to glucocorticoids.[91] Yet, the coexistence of thrombosis and capillaritis with AH represents a therapeutic dilemma because anticoagulation may need to be interrupted to control the hemorrhage. Early PLEX in addition to immunosuppressive therapy should be considered in patients with APS and AH.

Mitral Valve Disease

Diffuse AH is a well-known feature of mitral stenosis, even though the possibility is rarely considered in clinical practice.[94] Severe mitral insufficiency can also produce AH. Hemoptysis can be the presenting feature. It is caused either by the rupture of dilated and varicose bronchial veins early in the course of mitral stenosis or as a result of the stress failure of pulmonary capillaries. In surgically untreated patients, recurrent episodes of AH may lead to chronic hemosiderosis of the lungs, fibrosis, and punctuate calcification/ossification of the lung parenchyma.

Idiopathic Pulmonary Hemosiderosis

Idiopathic pulmonary hemosiderosis (IPH) is a rare disorder of unknown cause. It is a diagnosis of exclusion. Many cases reported before the discovery of ANCA probably represented ANCA-associated vasculitis. Most cases diagnosed as IPH today are probably associated with gluten-sensitive sprue (celiac disease). The combination of AH and celiac disease has also been called *Lane-Hamilton syndrome*.[95] In contrast to diffuse AH of other etiologies, the AH of IPH may be subtle and not necessarily associated with hemoptysis. Iron deficiency anemia is a hallmark of IPH. It is thought to be caused by recurrent lung hemorrhage or malabsorption of iron in the GI tract or both. IPH can occur in children or young adults. Patients suspected of IPH should be tested for anti-gliadin antibodies, particularly because GI symptoms may be absent or very subtle. Most patients with IPH attributable to celiac disease respond to a gluten-free diet and do not need immunosuppressive therapy.[95] Repeated AH in IPH has been reported to progress to lung fibrosis; early appropriate therapy may prevent this outcome.[96]

Toxic AH

AH can result from toxic fume inhalation or from blood-borne toxins. Fumes or dust of trimellitic anhydride (a component of certain plastics, paints, and epoxy resins) cause acute rhinitis and asthmatic symptoms if exposure is minor; with greater exposure, AH occurs.[97, 98] The trimellitic anhydride-hemoptysis anemia syndrome occurs after high-dose exposure to fumes.[99, 100] Isocyanates have caused lung hemorrhage. Illicit drug use, particularly crack cocaine inhalation, has also been linked to AH.[101]

Many medications have been associated with the development of AH,[102] including drugs with antiplatelet or anticoagulant effects such as abciximab; immunosuppressive and chemotherapeutic agents such as D-penicillamine, sirolimus,[103] and all-*trans*-retinoic acid[104]; antithyroid drugs such as propyl-thiouracil; or continuous IV infusion of epoprostenol for primary pulmonary hypertension.[100]

AH After Bone Marrow Transplantation

DAH occurs in both allogeneic and autologous hematopoietic stem-cell transplantation recipients (bone marrow transplantation [BMT]), usually during the first 30 days, with most episodes occurring around day 12 after BMT.[105–107] Recipients of autologous BMT are at greater risk than recipients of allogeneic BMT. AH and diffuse alveolar damage are the two major complications after BMT. The overall incidence of diffuse alveolar damage is 5 to 7%. An autopsy series[108] has found diffuse AH in 24% of recipients after BMT. Risk factors for the development of AH include intensive conditioning chemotherapy and older age (> 40 years).

Post-BMT AH is a form of noninfectious pneumonitis characterized by sudden onset of dyspnea, nonproductive cough, fever, and hypoxemia. Hemoptysis is rare, and its absence may lead to incorrect diagnosis. Many cases are identified only at autopsy.[109] The clinical presentation is nonspecific. Chest imaging shows diffuse but patchy alveolar densities with central predominance. Lung biopsy is rarely indicated. BAL is important to detect AH and to exclude infections. Diffuse AH is a potentially fatal respiratory complication with a reported mortality in excess of 50%.[105,110] Standard therapy consists of high-dose parenteral corticosteroids.

Miscellaneous Causes of AH

Pulmonary lymphangioleiomyomatosis is an uncommon cause of AH syndrome. A significant number of patients with pulmonary veno-occlusive disease, the development of AH may occur.[111,112] and pulmonary capillary hemangiomatosis has also been described as a possible cause of AH.[113] Tumor emboli have also been associated with AH.[114]

References

1. Hunder GG, Arend WP, Bloch DA, et al. The American College of Rheumatology 1990 criteria for the classification of vasculitis: introduction. Arthritis Rheum 1990; 33:1065–1067
2. Hunder GG. The use and misuse of classification and diagnostic criteria for complex diseases. Ann Intern Med 1998; 129:417–418
3. Jennette JC, Falk RJ, Andrassy K, et al. Nomenclature of systemic vasculitides: the proposal of an international consensus conference. Arthritis Rheum 1994; 37:187–192
4. Schwartz HR, McDuffie FC, Black LF, et al. Hypocomplementemic urticarial vasculitis: association with chronic obstructive pulmonary disease. Mayo Clin Proc 1982; 57:231–238
5. Wisnieski JJ, Baer AN, Christensen J, et al. Hypocomplementemic urticarial vasculitis syndrome: clinical and serologic findings in 18 patients. Medicine (Baltimore) 1995; 74:24–41
6. Ghamra Z, Stoller JK. Basilar hyperlucency in a patient with emphysema due to hypocomplementemic urticarial vasculitis syndrome. Respir Care 2003; 48:697–699
7. Bongartz T, Matteson EL. Large-vessel involvement in giant-cell arteritis. Curr Opin Rheumatol 2006; 18:10–17
8. Machado EB, Michet CJ, Ballard DJ, et al. Trends in incidence and clinical presentation of temporal arteritis in Olmsted County, Minnesota, 1950–1985. Arthritis Rheum 1988; 31:745–749

9. Larson TS, Hall S, Hepper NGG, et al. Respiratory tract symptoms as a clue to giant cell arteritis. Ann Intern Med 1984; 101:594–597
10. Nishino H, DeRemee RA, Rubino FA, et al. Wegener's granulomatosis associated with vasculitis of the temporal artery: report of five cases. Mayo Clin Proc 1993; 68:115–121
11. Mazlumzadeh M, Hunder GG, Easley KA, et al. Treatment of giant cell arteritis using induction therapy with high-dose glucocorticoids: a double-blind, placebo-controlled, randomized prospective clinical trial. Arthritis Rheum 2006; 54:3310–3318
12. Mahr AD, Jover JA, Spiera RF, et al. Adjunctive methotrexate for treatment of giant cell arteritis: an individual patient data meta-analysis. Arthritis Rheum 2007; 56:2789–2797
13. Seo P, Stone JH. Large-vessel vasculitis. Arthritis Rheum 2004; 51:128–139
14. Hoffman GS, Merkel PA, Brasington RD, et al. Anti-tumor necrosis factor therapy in patients with difficult to treat Takayasu arteritis. Arthritis Rheum 2004; 50:2296–2304
15. Maksimowicz-McKinnon K, Clark TM, Hoffman GS. Limitations of therapy and a guarded prognosis in an American cohort of Takayasu arteritis patients. Arthritis Rheum 2007; 56:1000–1009
16. Watts RA, Jolliffe VA, Carruthers DM, et al. Effect of classification on the incidence of polyarteritis nodosa and microscopic polyangiitis. Arthritis Rheum 1996; 39:1208–1212
17. Guillevin L, Lhote F. Distinguishing polyarteritis nodosa from microscopic polyangiitis and implications for treatment. Curr Opin Rheumatol 1995; 7:20–24
18. Stone JH. Limited versus severe Wegener's granulomatosis: baseline data on patients in the Wegener's granulomatosis etanercept trial. Arthritis Rheum 2003; 48:2299–2309
19. Duna GF, Cotch MF, Galperin C, et al. Wegener's granulomatosis: role of environmental exposures. Clin Exp Rheumatol 1998; 16:669–674
20. Lane SE, Watts RA, Bentham G, et al. Are environmental factors important in primary systemic vasculitis? A case-control study. Arthritis Rheum 2003; 48:814–823
21. Albert D, Clarkin C, Komoroski J, et al. Wegener's granulomatosis: possible role of environmental agents in its pathogenesis. Arthritis Rheum 2004; 51:656–664
22. Hogan SL, Cooper GS, Savitz DA, et al. Association of silica exposure with anti-neutrophil cytoplasmic autoantibody small-vessel vasculitis: a population-based, case-control study. Clin J Am Soc Nephrol 2007; 2:290–299
23. Capizzi SA, Specks U. Does infection play a role in the pathogenesis of pulmonary vasculitis? Semin Respir Infect 2003; 18:17–22
24. Kallenberg CG, Rarok A, Stegeman CA. Genetics of ANCA-associated vasculitides. Cleve Clin J Med 2002; 69:SII61–SII63
25. Jennette JC, Falk RJ. New insight into the pathogenesis of vasculitis associated with antineutrophil cytoplasmic autoantibodies. Curr Opin Rheumatol 2008; 20:55–60
26. Stegeman CA, Cohen Tervaert JW, Sluiter WJ, et al. Association of chronic nasal carriage of *Staphylococcus aureus* and higher relapse rates in Wegener granulomatosis. Ann Intern Med 1994; 120:12–17
27. Daum DE, Specks U, Colby TV, et al. Tracheobronchial involvement in Wegener's granulomatosis. Am J Respir Crit Care Med 1995; 151:522–526
28. Polychronopoulos VS, Prakash UB, Golbin JM, et al. Airway involvement in Wegener's granulomatosis. Rheum Dis Clin North Am 2007; 33:755–775
29. Savige J, Gillis D, Benson E, et al. International consensus statement on testing and reporting of antineutrophil cytoplasmic antibodies (ANCA). Am J Clin Pathol 1999; 111:507–513
30. Merkel PA, Polisson RP, Chang Y, et al. Prevalence of antineutrophil cytoplasmic antibodies in a large inception cohort of patients with connective tissue disease. Ann Intern Med 1997; 126:866–873
31. Russell KA, Wiegert E, Schroeder DR, et al. Detection of anti-neutrophil cytoplasmic antibodies under actual clinical testing conditions. Clin Immunol 2002; 103:196–203
32. Vassilopoulos D, Niles JL, Villa-Forte A, et al. Prevalence of antineutrophil cytoplasmic antibodies in patients with various pulmonary diseases or multiorgan dysfunction. Arthritis Rheum 2003; 49:151–155
33. Mandl LA, Solomon DH, Smith EL, et al. Using antineutrophil cytoplasmic antibody testing to diagnose vasculitis: can test-ordering guidelines improve diagnostic accuracy? Arch Intern Med 2002; 162:1509–1514
34. Choi HK, Lamprecht P, Niles JL, et al. Subacute bacterial endocarditis with positive cytoplasmic antineutrophil cytoplasmic antibodies and anti-proteinase 3 antibodies. Arthritis Rheum 2000; 43:226–231

35. Rutgers A, Slot M, van Paassen P, et al. Coexistence of anti-glomerular basement membrane antibodies and myeloperoxidase-ANCAs in crescentic glomerulonephritis. Am J Kidney Dis 2005; 46:253–262
36. Finkielman JD, Lee AS, Hummel AM, et al. ANCA are detectable in nearly all patients with active severe Wegener's granulomatosis. Am J Med 2007; 120:643 e649–e614
37. Finkielman JD, Merkel PA, Schroeder D, et al. Antiproteinase 3 antineutrophil cytoplasmic antibodies and disease activity in Wegener granulomatosis. Ann Intern Med 2007; 147:611–619
38. Specks U. Methotrexate for Wegener's granulomatosis: what is the evidence? Arthritis Rheum 2005; 52:2237–2242
39. De Groot K, Rasmussen N, Bacon PA, et al. Randomized trial of cyclophosphamide versus methotrexate for induction of remission in early systemic antineutrophil cytoplasmic antibody-associated vasculitis. Arthritis Rheum 2005; 52:2461–2469
40. The WGET Research Group. Etanercept plus standard therapy for Wegener's granulomatosis. N Engl J Med 2005; 352:351–361
40a. Fauci AS, Haynes BF, Katz P, et al. Wegener's granulomatosis: prospective clinical and therapeutic experience with 85 patients for 21 years. Ann Intern Med 1983; 98:76–85
41. Jayne D, Rasmussen N, Andrassy K, et al. A randomized trial of maintenance therapy for vasculitis associated with antineutrophil cytoplasmic autoantibodies. N Engl J Med 2003; 349:36–44
42. Pagnoux C, Mahr A, Hamidou MA, et al. Azathioprine or methotrexate maintenance for ANCA-associated vasculitis. N Engl J Med 2008; 359:2790–2803
43. Koukoulaki M, Jayne DR. Mycophenolate mofetil in anti-neutrophil cytoplasm antibodies-associated systemic vasculitis. Nephron Clin Pract 2006; 102: c100–c107
44. Somers EC, Marder W, Christman GM, et al. Use of a gonadotropin-releasing hormone analog for protection against premature ovarian failure during cyclophosphamide therapy in women with severe lupus. Arthritis Rheum 2005; 52:2761–2767
44a. de Groot K, Harper L, Jayne DR, et al. Pulse versus daily oral cyclophosphamide for induction of remission in antineutrophil cytoplasmic antibody-associated vasculitis: a randomized trial. Ann Intern Med 2009; 150:670–680
44b. de Groot K, Adu D, Savage CO. The value of pulse cyclophosphamide in ANCA-associated vasculitis: meta-analysis and critical review. Nephrol Dial Transplant 2001; 16:2018–2027
45. Hu W, Liu C, Xie H, et al. Mycophenolate mofetil versus cyclophosphamide for inducing remission of ANCA vasculitis with moderate renal involvement. Nephrol Dial Transplant 2008; 23:1307–1312
46. Jayne DR, Gaskin G, Rasmussen N, et al. Randomized trial of plasma exchange or high-dosage methylprednisolone as adjunctive therapy for severe renal vasculitis. J Am Soc Nephrol 2007; 18:2180–2188
47. Klemmer PJ, Chalermskulrat W, Reif MS, et al. Plasmapheresis therapy for diffuse alveolar hemorrhage in patients with small-vessel vasculitis. Am J Kidney Dis 2003; 42:1149–1153
48. Betensley AD, Yankaskas JR. Factor VIIa for alveolar hemorrhage in microscopic polyangiitis. Am J Respir Crit Care Med 2002; 166:1291–1292
49. Henke D, Falk RJ, Gabriel DA. Successful treatment of diffuse alveolar hemorrhage with activated factor VII. Ann Intern Med 2004; 140:493–494
50. Lamprecht P, Voswinkel J, Lilienthal T, et al. Effectiveness of TNF-alpha blockade with infliximab in refractory Wegener's granulomatosis. Rheumatology (Oxford) 2002; 41:1303–1307
51. Booth A, Harper L, Hammad T, et al. Prospective study of TNFalpha blockade with infliximab in anti-neutrophil cytoplasmic antibody-associated systemic vasculitis. J Am Soc Nephrol 2004; 15:717–721
52. Stone JH, Holbrook JT, Marriott MA, et al. Solid malignancies among patients in the Wegener's Granulomatosis Etanercept Trial. Arthritis Rheum 2006; 54:1608–1618
53. Keogh KA, Wylam ME, Stone JH, et al. Induction of remission by B lymphocyte depletion in eleven patients with refractory antineutrophil cytoplasmic antibody-associated vasculitis. Arthritis Rheum 2005; 52:262–268
54. Keogh KA, Ytterberg SR, Fervenza FC, et al. Rituximab for refractory Wegener's granulomatosis: report of a prospective, open-label pilot trial. Am J Respir Crit Care Med 2006; 173:180–187
54a. Golbin JM, Specks U. Targeting B lymphocytes as therapy for ANCA-associated vasculitis. Rheum Dis Clin North Am 2007; 33:741–754
54b. Schmitt WH, Hagen EC, Neumann I, et al. Treatment of refractory Wegener's granulomatosis with

antithymocyte globulin (ATG): an open study in 15 patients. Kidney Int 2004; 65:1440–1448
54c. Flossmann O, Baslund B, Bruchfeld A, et al. Deoxyspergualin in relapsing and refractory Wegener's granulomatosis. Ann Rheum Dis 2009; 68:1125–1130
55. Lebovics RS, Hoffman GS, Leavitt RY, et al. The management of subglottic stenosis in patients with Wegener's granulomatosis. Laryngoscope 1992; 102:1341–1345
56. Hoffman GS, Kerr GS, Leavitt RY, et al. Wegener granulomatosis: an analysis of 158 patients. Ann Intern Med 1992; 116:488–498
57. Seo P, Min YI, Holbrook JT, et al. Damage caused by Wegener's granulomatosis and its treatment: prospective data from the Wegener's Granulomatosis Etanercept Trial (WGET). Arthritis Rheum 2005; 52:2168–2178
58. Merkel PA, Lo GH, Holbrook JT, et al. High incidence of venous thrombotic events among patients with Wegener granulomatosis: the Wegener's Clinical Occurrence of Thrombosis (WeCLOT) study. Ann Intern Med 2005; 142: 620–626
59. Allenbach Y, Seror R, Pagnoux C, et al. High frequency of venous thromboembolic events in Churg-Strauss syndrome, Wegener's granulomatosis and microscopic polyangiitis but not polyarteritis nodosa: a systematic retrospective study on 1130 patients. Ann Rheum Dis 2009; 68:564–567
60. Oliveira GH, Seward JB, Tsang TS, et al. Echocardiographic findings in patients with Wegener granulomatosis. Mayo Clin Proc 2005; 80:1435–1440
61. Keogh KA, Specks U. Churg-Strauss syndrome: clinical presentation, antineutrophil cytoplasmic antibodies, and leukotriene receptor antagonists. Am J Med 2003; 115:284–290
62. Sinico RA, Di Toma L, Maggiore U, et al. Prevalence and clinical significance of antineutrophil cytoplasmic antibodies in Churg-Strauss syndrome. Arthritis Rheum 2005; 52:2926–2935
63. Sable-Fourtassou R, Cohen P, Mahr A, et al. Antineutrophil cytoplasmic antibodies and the Churg-Strauss syndrome. Ann Intern Med 2005; 143:632–638
64. Lanham JG, Elkon KB, Pusey CD, et al. Systemic vasculitis with asthma and eosinophilia: a clinical approach to the Churg-Strauss syndrome. Medicine 1984; 63:65–81
65. Churg A, Brallas M, Cronin SR, et al. Formes frustes of Churg-Strauss syndrome. Chest 1995; 108:320–323
66. Tatsis E, Schnabel A, Gross WL. Interferon-a treatment of four patients with the Churg-Strauss syndrome. Ann Intern Med 1998; 129:370–374
67. Koukoulaki M, Smith KG, Jayne DR. Rituximab in Churg-Strauss syndrome. Ann Rheum Dis 2006; 65:557–559
68. Pepper RJ, Fabre MA, Pavesio C, et al. Rituximab is effective in the treatment of refractory Churg-Strauss syndrome and is associated with diminished T-cell interleukin-5 production. Rheumatology (Oxford) 2008; 47:1104–1105
69. Jennings CA, King TE Jr., Tuder R, et al. Diffuse alveolar hemorrhage with underlying isolated, pauciimmune pulmonary capillaritis. Am J Respir Crit Care Med 1997; 155:1101–1109
70. Verity DH, Marr JE, Ohno S, et al. Behçet's disease, the Silk Road and HLA-B51: historical and geographical perspectives. Tissue Antigens 1999; 54:213–220
71. Uzun O, Akpolat T, Erkan L. Pulmonary vasculitis in Behçet disease: a cumulative analysis. Chest 2005; 127:2243–2253
72. Kurokawa MS, Yoshikawa H, Suzuki N. Behcet's disease. Semin Respir Crit Care Med 2004; 25:557–568
73. Nadrous HF, Yu AC, Specks U, et al. Pulmonary involvement in Henoch-Schönlein purpura. Mayo Clin Proc 2004; 79:1151–1157
74. Zamora MR, Warner ML, Tuder R, et al. Diffuse alveolar hemorrhage and systemic lupus erythematosus: clinical presentation, histology, survival, and outcome. Medicine (Baltimore) 1997; 76:192–202
75. Robbins RA, Linder J, Stahl MG, et al. Diffuse alveolar hemorrhage in autologous bone marrow transplant recipients. Am J Med 1989; 87:511–518
76. De Lassence A, Fleury-Feith J, Escudier E, et al. Alveolar hemorrhage: diagnostic criteria and results in 194 immunocompromised hosts. Am J Respir Crit Care Med 1995; 151:157–163
77. Colby TV, Fukuoka J, Ewaskow SP, et al. Pathologic approach to pulmonary hemorrhage. Ann Diagn Pathol 2001; 5:309–319
78. Kadokura M, Colby TV, Myers JL, et al. Pathologic comparison of video-assisted thoracic surgical lung biopsy with traditional open lung biopsy. J Thorac Cardiovasc Surg 1995; 109:494–498

79. Salama AD, Pusey CD. Immunology of anti-glomerular basement membrane disease. Curr Opin Nephrol Hypertens 2002; 11:279–286
80. Donaghy M, Rees AJ. Cigarette smoking and lung haemorrhage in glomerulonephritis caused by autoantibodies to glomerular basement membrane. Lancet 1983; 2:1390–1393
81. Lazor R, Bigay-Game L, Cottin V, et al. Alveolar hemorrhage in anti-basement membrane antibody disease: a series of 28 cases. Medicine (Baltimore) 2007; 86:181–193
82. Lombard CM, Colby TV, Elliott CG. Surgical pathology of the lung in anti-basement membrane antibody-associated Goodpasture's syndrome. Hum Pathol 1989; 20:445–451
83. Levy JB, Turner AN, Rees AJ, et al. Long-term outcome of anti-glomerular basement membrane antibody disease treated with plasma exchange and immunosuppression. Ann Intern Med 2001; 134:1033–1042
84. Schwab EP, Schumacher HR, Freundlich B, et al. Pulmonary alveolar hemorrhage in systemic lupus erythematosus. Semin Arthritis Rheum 1993; 23:8–15
85. Koh WH, Thumboo J, Boey ML. Pulmonary haemorrhage in Oriental patients with systemic lupus erythematosus. Lupus 1997; 6:713–716
86. Santos-Ocampo AS, Mandell BF, Fessler BJ. Alveolar hemorrhage in systemic lupus erythematosus: presentation and management. Chest 2000; 118:1083–1090
87. Chang MY, Fang JT, Chen YC, et al. Diffuse alveolar hemorrhage in systemic lupus erythematosus: a single center retrospective study in Taiwan. Ren Fail 2002; 24:791–802
88. Schwarz MI, Sutarik JM, Nick JA, et al. Pulmonary capillaritis and diffuse alveolar hemorrhage: a primary manifestation of polymyositis. Am J Respir Crit Care Med 1995; 151:2037–2040
89. Schwarz MI, Zamora MR, Hodges TN, et al. Isolated pulmonary capillaritis and diffuse alveolar hemorrhage in rheumatoid arthritis and mixed connective tissue disease. Chest 1998; 113:1609–1615
90. Wilson WA, Gharavi AE, Koike T, et al. International consensus statement on preliminary classification criteria for definite antiphospholipid syndrome: report of an international workshop. Arthritis Rheum 1999; 42:1309–1311
91. Gertner E. Diffuse alveolar hemorrhage in the antiphospolipid syndrome: spectrum of disease and treatment. J Rheumatol 1999; 26:805–807
92. Asherson RA, Cervera R, Piette JC, et al. Catastrophic antiphospholipid syndrome; clinical and laboratory features of 50 patients. Medicine (Baltimore) 1998; 77:195–207
93. Espinosa G, Cervera R, Font J, et al. The lung in the antiphospholipid syndrome. Ann Rheum Dis 2002; 61:195–198
94. Woolley K, Stark P. Pulmonary parenchymal manifestations of mitral valve disease. Radiographics 1999; 19:965–972
95. Agarwal R, Aggarwal AN, Gupta D. Lane-Hamilton syndrome: simultaneous occurrence of coeliac disease and idiopathic pulmonary haemosiderosis. Intern Med J 2007; 37:65–67
96. Buschman DL, Ballard R. Progressive massive fibrosis associated with idiopathic pulmonary hemosiderosis. Chest 1993; 104:293–295
97. Grammer LC, Shaughnessy MA, Zeiss CR, et al. Review of trimellitic anhydride (TMA) induced respiratory response. Allergy Asthma Proc 1997; 18:235–237
98. Grammer LC, Ditto AM, Tripathi A, et al. Prevalence and onset of rhinitis and conjunctivitis in subjects with occupational asthma caused by trimellitic anhydride (TMA). J Occup Environ Med 2002; 44:1179–1181
99. Herbert FA, Orford R. Pulmonary hemorrhage and edema due to inhalation of resins containing trimellitic anhydride. Chest 1979; 76:546–551
100. Ogawa A, Matsubara H, Fujio H, et al. Risk of alveolar hemorrhage in patients with primary pulmonary hypertension-anticoagulation and epoprostenol therapy. Circ J 2005; 69:216–220
101. Garcia-Rostan y Perez GM, Garcia Bragado F, Puras Gil AM. Pulmonary hemorrhage and antiglomerular basement membrane antibody-mediated glomerulonephritis after exposure to smoked cocaine (crack): a case report and review of the literature. Pathol Int 1997; 47:692–697
102. Schwarz MI, Fontenot AP. Drug-induced diffuse alveolar hemorrhage syndromes and vasculitis. Clin Chest Med 2004; 25:133–140
103. Vlahakis NE, Rickman OB, Morgenthaler T. Sirolimus-associated diffuse alveolar hemorrhage. Mayo Clin Proc 2004; 79:541–545
104. Nicolls MR, Terada LS, Ruder RM, et al. Diffuse alveolar hemorrhage with underlying pulmonary capillaritis in the retinoic acid syndrome. Am J Respir Crit Care Med 1998; 158:1302–1305

105. Afessa B, Tefferi A, Litzow MR, et al. Diffuse alveolar hemorrhage in hematopoietic stem cell transplant recipients. Am J Respir Crit Care Med 2002; 166:641–645
106. Yen KT, Lee AS, Krowka MJ, et al. Pulmonary complications in bone marrow transplantation: a practical approach to diagnosis and treatment. Clin Chest Med 2004; 25:189–201
107. Afessa B, Peters SG. Major complications following hematopoietic stem cell transplantation. Semin Respir Crit Care Med 2006; 27:297–309
108. Roychowdhury M, Pambuccian SE, Aslan DL, et al. Pulmonary complications after bone marrow transplantation: an autopsy study from a large transplantation center. Arch Pathol Lab Med 2005; 129:366–371
109. Sharma S, Nadrous HF, Peters SG, et al. Pulmonary complications in adult blood and marrow transplant recipients: autopsy findings. Chest 2005; 128:1385–1392
110. Lewis ID, DeFor T, Weisdorf DJ. Increasing incidence of diffuse alveolar hemorrhage following allogeneic bone marrow transplantation: cryptic etiology and uncertain therapy. Bone Marrow Transplant 2000; 26:539–543
111. Cohn RC, Wong R, Spohn WA, et al. Death due to diffuse alveolar hemorrhage in a child with pulmonary veno-occlusive disease. Chest 1991; 100:1456–1458
112. Rabiller A, Jais X, Hamid A, et al. Occult alveolar haemorrhage in pulmonary veno-occlusive disease. Eur Respir J 2006; 27:108–113
113. Tron V, Magee F, Wright JL, et al. Pulmonary capillary hemangiomatosis. Hum Pathol 1986; 17:1144–1150
114. Almagro P, Julia J, Sanjaume M, et al. Pulmonary capillary hemangiomatosis associated with primary pulmonary hypertension: report of 2 new cases and review of 35 cases from the literature. Medicine (Baltimore) 2002; 81:417–424

Notes

Women's Issues in Pulmonary Medicine

Stephanie M. Levine, MD, FCCP

Objectives:

- Review the normal respiratory and cardiovascular physiology of pregnancy
- Review the management of asthma in pregnancy
- Review the management of venous thromboembolism in pregnancy
- Review the management of tuberculosis and other respiratory infections in pregnancy
- Review the causes and management of acute respiratory failure in pregnancy
- Discuss the statistics regarding smoking and the epidemiology of lung cancer in women
- Review disorders unique to women, *eg*, catamenial diseases and lymphangioleiomyomatosis

Key words: acute respiratory failure; asthma; lung cancer; pregnancy; venous thromboembolism; women

This chapter will focus on pulmonary diseases unique to women, including issues surrounding pregnancy, as well as diseases that may have different epidemiology and/or prognosis in women. Common pulmonary problems with different treatment plans in the pregnant or lactating woman and causes and management of acute respiratory failure in the pregnant patient will be reviewed. Other diseases that occur exclusively or are more prevalent in women, such as lymphangioleiomyomatosis (LAM), are discussed, but they are primarily covered elsewhere in this course.

Physiology of Pregnancy

During pregnancy, the body undergoes anatomic and physiologic changes affecting both the respiratory and cardiovascular systems. It is important that the pulmonologist be familiar with these normal physiologic changes (Tables 1, 2).

Respiratory

The upper respiratory tract undergoes changes during pregnancy, including hyperemia of the airway mucosa, increased secretion production,

Table 1. *Normal Respiratory Physiologic Changes in Pregnancy*

Variables	Changes
Pulmonary function	
Expiratory reserve volume	Decreased
Residual volume	Decreased
Functional residual capacity	Decreased
Total lung capacity	Mildly decreased
Inspiratory capacity	Increased
Vital capacity	No change
Tidal volume	Increased
Respiratory rate	No change, mild increase
Minute ventilation	Increased
Peak flow	No change
FEV_1	No change
Lung compliance	No change
Total respiratory compliance	Decreased
Diffusion capacity	Increase followed by decrease
Gas exchange	
$Paco_2$	Decreased to 28 to 32 mm Hg
Pao_2	Increase followed by decrease
pH	Increased to 7.40 to 7.45
Serum bicarbonate	Decreased to 18 to 21 mEq/L
Alveolar-arterial gradient	Mildly increased
Oxygen consumption	Increased
Carbon dioxide production	Increased

Table 2. *Normal Cardiovascular Physiologic Changes in Pregnancy*

Variables	Change
Cardiac output	Increased
Heart rate	Increased
Stroke volume	Increased
Systemic vascular resistance	Decreased
Pulmonary vascular resistance	Decreased
BP	Decreased
Blood volume	Increased
RBC volume	Increased, but less than blood volume
Hematocrit	Dilutional decrease
Serum protein levels	Decreased

and mucosal edema, particularly accentuated in the third trimester. Patients can have upper respiratory tract symptoms secondary to the aforementioned, including epistaxis, nasal stuffiness, hoarseness, and voice changes. Nasal polyposis and allergic rhinitis can begin or become exacerbated during pregnancy. These changes are primarily caused by the production of estrogen. The health-care provider should be aware of these changes when performing procedures such as endotracheal intubation and/or nasopharyngeal tube placement.

The thoracic cage also undergoes anatomic changes during pregnancy. The diaphragm becomes elevated up to an average of 4 cm above normal at full-term pregnancy. However, diaphragmatic dysfunction caused by pregnancy is unusual because, concurrent with these changes, there is a widening of the lower rib cage and alteration of the abdominal muscles; thus, diaphragmatic excursion is actually maintained or increased.

Pulmonary Function Tests: The major change in pulmonary function testing in pregnancy is a progressive decrease in the expiratory reserve volume by 8 to 40% and a decrease in residual volume by 7 to 22%, both changes attributable to the enlarging uterus and diaphragmatic elevation. Because of these changes, functional residual capacity is, in turn, decreased by 10 to 25% by the third trimester of pregnancy. Total lung capacity may decrease slightly, inspiratory capacity increases, and vital capacity does not change significantly during pregnancy. The decrease in residual volume with a relatively maintained total lung capacity results in a low ratio of residual volume to total lung capacity. Closure of the small airways during normal tidal breathing caused by the reduction in functional residual capacity can result in changes in ventilation/perfusion matching and gas exchange discussed below.

Tidal volume increases significantly during pregnancy by 150 mL to a final value of 450 to 600 mL, or a 30 to 50% increase in the average patient. This increase is most likely to the result of a direct progesterone-mediated increase in central respiratory drive and enhancement of the hypercapnic ventilatory drive. There is little or no change in respiratory rate during pregnancy, and tachypnea is an unusual finding. Because of the increase in tidal volume, there is a significant increase in resting minute ventilation from 6 L in the nonpregnant state to 9 L at full term (or 20 to 50% above baseline).

There are no significant changes in peak flow rates, FEV_1, airway resistance, or maximum voluntary ventilation during pregnancy. Although lung compliance does not change significantly during pregnancy, there is a reduction in total respiratory compliance caused by a reduction in chest wall compliance because of an elevated diaphragm caused by uterine enlargement by the third trimester. Diffusion capacity of the lung for carbon monoxide may increase slightly in the first trimester, followed by a slight decrease later in pregnancy, likely the result of alterations in pulmonary vascular volume.

Gas Exchange: Gas exchange in pregnancy is characterized by a mild compensated respiratory alkalosis secondary to an increase in minute ventilation out of proportion to maternal needs. Thus, normal $Paco_2$ values are lower, 28 to 32 mm Hg, and serum bicarbonate is compensatorily decreased to 18 to 21 mEq/L. Normal pH is slightly alkalemic at 7.40 to 7.45. Pao_2 is slightly elevated, 100 to 105 mm Hg, with a slight decrease at term to 100 mm Hg. There is normally an increase of 5 to 10 mm Hg in in alveolar-arterial gradient above baseline, especially in the supine position. Oxygen consumption increases by 20 to 30% during pregnancy, with a concomitant increase in carbon dioxide production by 30 to 35%. These changes are attributable to increased maternal and fetal metabolic requirements and increases in work of breathing and cardiac output. During delivery, oxygen consumption can increase to 40 to 100% above baseline.

Sleep-Disordered Breathing: Because of the above-normal physiologic changes during pregnancy, in particular the estrogen-related changes in upper airway patency, the incidence of snoring increases during pregnancy. Most studies also suggest that there is an increased incidence and severity of sleep-disordered breathing during pregnancy, which increases as pregnancy progresses. Obstructive sleep apnea during pregnancy may develop in patients predisposed to sleep-disordered breathing, and patients with preexisting obstructive sleep apnea may have worsening severity of disease. Untreated, this worsening may lead to complications of maternal hypertension and fetal growth retardation. Continuous positive airway pressure has been used for treatment, same as in the nonpregnant individual.

Cardiovascular

The cardiovascular system probably undergoes the most significant changes during pregnancy, including an increase in cardiac output, beginning in the first trimester and peaking at about the 25th to 32nd week at 30 to 50% above normal. This increased is attributable to both a change in heart rate as well as stroke volume and a decrease in systemic vascular resistance, partially as the result of shunting of blood to the low-resistance placental bed and perhaps increased levels of vasodilator mediators. Pulmonary vascular resistance also decreases. Both systolic and particularly diastolic pressures are reduced. Postural hypotension may be apparent, particularly in the third trimester when the uterus can compress the inferior vena cava (IVC), impeding venous return to the heart. During delivery, cardiac output may be further augmented by an additional 10 to 15% as the result of catecholamine release.

Total blood and plasma volume increases up to 35 to 50% of normal, peaking in the mid-third trimester with a lesser increase in RBC volume (approximately 20 to 40%). The result is hemodilution with a relative decrease in hemoglobin, hematocrit (approximately a 12% decrease), and relative RBC volume, *ie*, the anemia of pregnancy. There is also a dilutional decrease in serum protein levels, resulting in a decrease of 5 mm Hg in plasma oncotic pressures, predisposing patients to edema formation, including pulmonary edema. There is an approximate total body fluid expansion of 6 to 8 L of water divided among the fetus, amniotic fluid, and intracellular and extracellular spaces, and an increase in plasma volume of 1 to 1.5 L. These changes in fluid status are likely the result of increased mineralocorticoid production and/or hormonally mediated vasodilation.

Dyspnea During Pregnancy

Up to twothirds of pregnant women report dyspnea during pregnancy. Although the etiology of this normal physiologic dyspnea is not clearly defined, it is most commonly reported in the first and second trimesters, with improvement toward the end of the third trimester. These findings support the fact that dyspnea is not purely related to mechanical enlargement of the uterus. Marked progesterone elevations early in pregnancy, resulting in direct brainstem stimulation and hyperventilation and an alteration in the sensitivity to carbon dioxide, likely contribute to the sensation of dyspnea. The normal anemia of pregnancy may also contribute to the sensation of dyspnea. One must also be aware of concomitant heart disease manifested in pregnant women. Mitral stenosis and other stenotic lesions may become apparent during pregnancy, particularly in the third trimester when blood volume is at its maximum, and right-to-left shunts tend to worsen.

Treatment of Specific Pulmonary Diseases in the Pregnant Patient

Asthma, pulmonary embolism (PE), and infections such as tuberculosis (TB) are can be present the pregnant patient. It is important that the pulmonologist be aware of the management of these conditions in pregnancy, including the acceptable pharmacologic treatments.

US Food and Drug Administration Drug Classification

Acceptable pharmaceutical agents in pregnancy have been classified by the US Food and Drug Administration. A category A drug means that well-controlled drug studies in pregnant women have failed to demonstrate any risk to the fetus, and the possibility of fetal harm appears remote. A category B drug indicates that animal drug studies have shown that there was no demonstrated fetal risk, but controlled drug studies have not been performed in pregnant women, or animal reproduction studies have shown an adverse effect that was not confirmed in studies conduced in pregnant women. A category C agent is a drug for which studies in animals have revealed adverse effects on the fetus, including teratogenicity, and there are no controlled studies in women; or that studies in women and animals are not available. These drugs can be used if the potential benefit of the drug outweighs the potential risk to the fetus. A category D agent is a drug for which studies have shown positive evidence of human fetal risks, but in certain situations, these drugs may be of benefit if the risk is outweighed by potential gain. Category X agents are those drugs in which animals or humans have demonstrated fetal abnormalities and/or there is evidence of fetal risks based on human experience and clearly the risk outweighs the benefit of the drug (*eg*, thalidomide).

Asthma

Of the approximate 10 to 12 million asthmatic patients in the United States, a significant number are of childbearing age. Asthma affects up to 7% of pregnant women.[1] Poorly controlled asthma can result in and small but increased risks of preterm labor and birth, preeclampsia, congenital anomalies, intrauterine growth retardation, and low birth weight, as well as increased maternal morbidity, such as placenta previa. These effects are likely attributable to hypoxemia, resulting in decreased placental blood flow. General medical teaching states that asthma gets worse in one third of patients during pregnancy, onethird of patients improve and have fewer frequent asthma exacerbations, and approximately one third have no change in the frequency or severity of asthma. The best predictor of asthma severity in pregnancy is the severity of asthma in the nonpregnant state and the course of asthma in previous pregnancies. Asthma tends to be less severe in the first and latter third trimesters and worse in the middle of pregnancy (*ie*, gestational weeks 17 to 36). Asthma may also worsen during delivery and in the postpartum period. Gastroesophageal reflux, sinusitis, and allergic rhinitis leading to worsening asthma should be carefully evaluated in the pregnant asthmatic.

The treatment of chronic asthma in pregnancy is similar to that of the nongravid asthmatic. In 1993, the National Asthma Education Program sponsored by the National Heart, Lung, and Blood Institute developed guidelines for the treatment of the pregnant asthmatic patient, subsequently revised in 2004.[2] In 2008, the Global Initiative for Asthma was updated and outlines treatment on a spectrum of control from controlled to partly controlled to uncontrolled asthma.[3] In general, patients whose asthma is well controlled on an appropriate medical regimen before pregnancy can remain on this regimen if it continues to be well controlled during pregnancy.

Short-acting selective β_2-agonists are indicated for intermittent (well-controlled) asthma (albuterol has been the drug most widely studied in pregnancy and is the preferred agent). These agents are category C. Low-dose inhaled corticosteroids are the preferred agent for initiating treatment for mild persistent asthma (partly controlled) in the pregnant patient. Alternative treatments include leukotriene receptor antagonists (not zileuton) or low-dose theophylline.

Budesonide (category B) and beclomethasone (category C) are the best-studied inhaled corticosteroids, and budesonide is the preferred agent. Patients with moderate persistent asthma (partly controlled) should be treated with low-dose inhaled budesonide or beclomethasone with a long-acting β_2-agonist (such as salmeterol). Medium-dose inhaled corticosteroids are another alternative for the treatment of moderate persistent asthma (partly controlled), and a long-acting β_2-agonist can be added if needed. Patients already maintained on other inhaled corticosteroids can be continued on those agents. Other than budesonide, all other inhaled corticosteroids are category C agents. Patients maintained on salmeterol for control of moderate persistent asthma prior to pregnancy can remain on this agent. Salmeterol has not been well studied in pregnancy and is listed as category C. Oral theophylline or a leukotriene receptor antagonist can be added if the asthma remains poorly controlled.

Severe persistent asthma (poorly controlled) should be managed with high-dose inhaled corticosteroids and a long-acting β_2-agonist. Systemic corticosteroids (category C) can also be used for control of severe and acute exacerbations of asthma. Earlier studies raised the concern of increased risk of prematurity and low-birth-weight infants with the use of systemic corticosteroids, but this may have been related to the severity of asthma in these patients rather than the medications used. Other studies have shown a 0.3% incidence of congenital malformations, an increased incidence of cleft palate, and increased risk of preeclampsia with the use of systemic corticosteroids. Patients who are receiving systemic corticosteroids require careful evaluation for gestational diabetes. In the steroid-dependent asthmatic, stress-dose corticosteroids should be administered during labor and delivery.

Theophylline (category C) has been used safely in pregnancy, although clearance in the third trimester may be reduced, and there is decreased protein binding of the drug. There are few data examining the use of leukotriene receptor antagonists during pregnancy, but montelukast and zafirlukast can be used in patients demonstrating a previous response to these agents. Both are listed as category B agents. Zileuton (category C) has been associated with teratogenicity in animals and should be avoided. Terbutaline and other parenteral β-agonists administered near term can cause tocolytic pulmonary edema and are often avoided, although terbutaline is a category B agent. Prostaglandin $F_2\alpha$ used for uterine atony should be avoided in asthmatics because it can cause bronchoconstriction. Omalizumab, an IgE inhibitor, is rated pregnancy category B, and can be considered for improved control of poorly controlled asthma.

The management of acute asthma and status asthmaticus is the same as in the nonpregnant asthmatic. For acute asthma, anticholinergic agents are also permissible (category B). On the basis of the normal compensated respiratory alkalosis of pregnancy, when evaluating the pregnant asthmatic in the midst of an acute episode, a $Paco_2$ of 35 mm Hg could indicate fatigue and impending ventilatory failure. Intubation should be considered with a $Paco_2$ of approximately 42 mm Hg consistently because this relative acidosis places the fetus at risk. Heliox has been used for the treatment of status asthmaticus. Epinephrine is not recommended for use during pregnancy because of concern for uteroplacental vasoconstriction.

Venous Thromboembolism in Pregnancy

PE is a leading cause of nonobstetric maternal mortality. Some studies have suggested that PE can account for 20 to 50% of maternal deaths. The spectrum of venous thromboembolism (VTE) can affect 0.05 to 0.1% of pregnancies. Although earlier studies suggested an increased incidence of deep-venous thrombosis (DVT) in the third trimester and postpartum period, subsequent studies have supported an equal distribution of DVT throughout pregnancy and suggest that DVT may be as common or more common antepartum as postpartum.

Pregnant women are at increased risk of VTE during pregnancy (some reports suggest as much as five times greater) because of a combination of all three componentsthe Virchow triad. There is increased venous stasis, hypercoagulability, and endothelial disruption of pelvic and uteroplacental vessels during delivery. The hypercoagulability in pregnancy is caused by alterations in levels of clotting factors (increases in fibrinogen, factors I, II, VII, VIII, IX, X, and XII); possibly decreased fibrinolytic activity; decreases in protein S levels; and a progressive increase throughout pregnancy in activated protein-C resistance. The increase in venous stasis is mechanical as the result of reduced venous flow in the lower-extremity and pelvic vessels from the compression of the IVC by the gravid uterus, and there is an interesting predominance of left lower-extremity DVT (approximately 90%), likely attributable to greater compression of the left iliac vein by the right iliac artery. There is also a predominance of iliofemoral DVT that is more likely to embolize. Other risk factors for VTE in pregnancy include prolonged bed rest; cesarean delivery (a twofold risk increase as compared with vaginal delivery); preeclampsia; advanced maternal age; obesity; multiparity; and previous VTE and thrombophilia. Despite the increased risks of VTE, an episode of thrombosis during pregnancy should still prompt a thrombophilic evaluation.

The most commonly used and best diagnostic test for determining DVT in pregnancy is Doppler ultrasound, although test results may be impaired and false-positive results can occur. Additionally, problems such as difficulty in detecting iliac, pelvic, and calf thromboses exist. The sensitivity and specificity of this study may be improved when performed in the left lateral decubitus position. Venography (<50 millirad fetal exposure) is rarely used for the diagnosis of DVT. The utility of the d-dimer assay in pregnancy is limited because elevations may occur normally in pregnancy, but it is likely of some utility in the case of low clinical suspicion and in earlier stages of pregnancy.

The diagnosis of suspected PE in pregnancy is similar to that in the nonpregnant individual. Ventilation/perfusion scanning can be used (6- to 30-millirad fetal exposure); however, a smaller dose of radioisotope is recommended, and when possible, the perfusion scan should be performed without the ventilation scan to further minimize radiation exposure. There are limited data evaluating the role of CT angiography for the diagnosis of PE in the pregnant patient, but it appears safe, and it is often performed if Doppler study results are negative. Pulmonary angiography should be used when indicated as the "gold standard" test for the diagnosis of PE (<50 millirad fetal exposure for a brachial approach, and 220 to 375 millirad for a femoral approach).

There are several important caveats to treating VTE during pregnancy, and this topic is included in the eighth American College of Chest Physicians evidenced-based clinical practice guidelines on anticoagulation.[4] Heparin is the anticoagulant agent of choice for both treatment and prophylaxis during pregnancy because it does not cross the placenta, and low-molecular-weight heparin (LMWH; category B) or unfractionated heparin (UFH; category C) can be safely used (level of evidence Grade 1A). LMWH is the preferred agent with (Grade 2C). For treatment of VTE, LMWH at weight-adjusted doses or UFH IV for 5 days, followed by adjusted-dose UFH subcutaneously to maintain the activated partial thromboplastin time (APTT) in the therapeutic range or adjusted LMWH is recommended (Grade 1A).

Some authors suggest that anti-Xa levels should be used to monitor LMWH therapy and in some cases of full-dose heparin anticoagulation, rather than APTT because of alterations in fibrinogen and Factor VIII that can make APTT results less reliable. High doses of UFH may be required. Anticoagulation should be continued throughout pregnancy (grade 1B) and 6 weeks postpartum to complete a total of 6 months of anticoagulation (grade 2C). Warfarin can be safely used in the postpartum period. In some unique situations, such as prophylaxis for mechanical heart valves, warfarin can be used after the 13th week of pregnancy until the mid-third trimester without complications. There is a paucity of data on the use of the pentasaccharide agents in pregnancy.

One should be aware of the significant complications with prolonged heparin use, including heparin-induced thrombocytopenia. Osteoporosis can also be a complication in patients receiving long-term therapy with heparin. LMWH may be associated with a lower incidence of osteoporosis and heparin-induced thrombocytopenia. Heparinoids can be used in cases of heparin-induced thrombocytopenia.

Warfarin (category X) crosses the placental barrier, particularly between 6 to 10 gestational weeks, and is associated with poor fetal epiphyseal cartilage formation, chondrodysplasia, and fetal nasal hypoplasia. CNS abnormalities have also been described, including malformations, optic atrophy, and microhemorrhages with warfarin use at any time during pregnancy. The use of warfarin is permissible during lactation. After an episode of VTE, anticoagulation should be continued with warfarin for 4 to 6 weeks after delivery or to complete 3 months of anticoagulation.

Thrombolytic agents are relatively contraindicated during pregnancy, especially near term and within 2 weeks postpartum because of the risk of hemorrhage. However, published case reports of successful use exist. IVC filter placement can be performed, although suprarenal placement is recommended because the left ovarian vein empties into the left renal vein.

The management of labor and delivery in the fully anticoagulated patient can be difficult. Epidural anesthesia should be used with caution in fully anticoagulated patients because epidural hematomas may result. Most patients receiving LMWH or UFH should have anticoagulation stopped 24 h before elective induction (grade 1C). Patients at high risk for recurrent VTE should be switched to UFH at least 24 h before expected induced delivery to safely discontinue anticoagulation 6 to 8 h before the expected delivery.

The indications for prophylaxis for VTE in pregnancy are the same as those in the nonpregnant individual, with some of the following specific recommendations.[4] Patients with a history of a single previous VTE related to a clear transient risk factor, but not with additional risk factors other than pregnancy currently, should undergo close surveillance during pregnancy and prophylactic anticoagulation in the 4- to 6-week postpartum period (grade 1C). Patients with a history of idiopathic VTE should receive prophylaxis with LMWH or UFH or close surveillance during pregnancy and anticoagulation in the 4- to 6-week postpartum period (grade 1C). Patients with any type of thrombophilia are at increased risk for VTE in pregnancy, but patients with antithrombin deficiency are particularly at risk for VTE and should receive antepartum prophylaxis and postpartum prophylactic anticoagulation (grade 2C).

Most authors, and the guidelines, suggest that patients with a history of VTE during a previous pregnancy should undergo surveillance or receive prophylaxis for VTE in subsequent pregnancies in addition to postpartum anticoagulation prophylaxis (grade 2C) because the recurrence rate can be as high as 12%. Patients with a history of two or more episodes of VTE should receive anticoagulation during pregnancy and be converted to long-term anticoagulation postpartum (grade 2C). Patients requiring long-term warfarin anticoagulation before pregnancy should be converted to UFH or LMWH when pregnancy is planned, or as early in pregnancy as possible if not planned. The article by Bates et al[4] contains specific recommendations for unique situations, such as patients with mechanical heart valves.

LMWH heparin or UFH are the agents of choice for prophylaxis, used at prophylactic doses of prophylactic UFH (5,000 U subcutaneously q12h), or intermediate-dose UFH (subcutaneously q12h after anti-Xa levels), or prophylactic LMWH (subcutaneously q24h following peak anti-Xa levels). LMWH is the preferred prophylactic agent (grade 2C).

TB in Pregnancy

With increases in the rates of TB in the United States, largely resulting from increases in HIV infection and increases in foreign-born immigrants, there has been an increase in TB cases in childbearing adults and children. The actual incidence of TB in pregnancy is not completely clear but can be in the range of 1% in poverty-stricken inner-city areas with poor access to prenatal health care. The prognosis of TB in pregnant women has been debated. At one time, it was thought that TB had an increased incidence of dissemination in the pregnant woman. Most data support that there is no difference in the susceptibility to infection, course of disease, obstetrical outcome, prognosis, and incidence of TB in nonpregnant or pregnant women unless immunosuppression coexists.

Treatment of active TB in pregnancy is similar to that of treatment in the nonpregnant individual with a few caveats.[5] Drugs approved in pregnant patients include isoniazid (INH), rifampin, and ethambutol. These drugs all cross the placenta but have not been shown to have teratogenic effects. In general, pyrazinamide, streptomycin, and ethionamide should be avoided in pregnancy. There are situations in which treatment with these other drugs may outweigh the potential risks of using these agents. The teratogenicity of streptomycin is primarily fetal ototoxicity as the result of nerve damage, congenital auditory malformations, and/or congenital deafness. Pyrazinamide has been avoided traditionally in the United States because it has not been well studied in pregnancy, but it is used routinely by the World Health Organization and the International Union Against Tuberculosis and Lung Disease.

Thus, standard treatment for active TB should include INH, rifampin, and ethambutol for 9 months because the regimen does not contain pyrazinamide. These same drugs can be continued during lactation without compromise to the infant. It the patient has infection with a potentially drug-resistant organism, then the addition of pyrazinamide should be considered pending results of susceptibility testing. Patients with INH-resistant TB can be treated rifampin and ethambutol. Therapeutic abortion may have to be considered in patients with multidrug-resistant TB. It is a standard recommendation that pyridoxine always be administered with INH during pregnancy to decrease the incidence of INH neurotoxicity (optic and peripheral neuropathy).

Chemoprophylaxis for latent TB infection (LTBI) is somewhat more controversial.[6] Because it appears that pregnancy does not increase the risk for active TB in patients with LTBI, many health-care workers would delay prophylactic treatment until after delivery in an HIV-negative patient with clear chest radiograph findings who is not a recent converter, and who is not in another high-risk group. However, most authorities recommend 9 months of INH prophylaxis if the patient is in a high-risk LTBI group. Routine purified protein derivative (PPD) testing during pregnancy has fallen out of favor at most medical centers and is not used unless in an endemic TB area or unless the patient is in a high-risk group, such as those with HIV infection.

Children <5 years of age with LTBI are at high risk of progression to disease and/or more severe and/or disseminated disease; they require 9 months of INH prophylaxis. If a child is exposed to a mother with active TB, he or she should be separated from the mother (only until the mother is deemed not contagious), undergo PPD skin testing and a chest radiograph, and be placed on

INH therapy for 8 to 12 weeks even if the skin test result is negative. At that time, the PPD should be repeated. If the PPD result remains negative, INH can be discontinued; if results are positive, 9 months of INH prophylaxis should be administered.

Pneumonia in Pregnancy

In general, the incidence of bacterial pneumonia in the pregnant woman is similar to that in the nonpregnant woman. Pneumonia may complicate 1.2 to 2.7 per 1,000 deliveries and may be more frequent in inner cities. Preterm labor, preterm delivery, and respiratory failure can result. The Maternal mortality rate can be as great as 4%.

Several small epidemiologic studies examining the bacterial organisms responsible for community-acquired pneumonia in the pregnant patient show the spectrum to be similar to that in the nonpregnant woman, and similar empiric therapies can be used. The cephalosporins and penicillins can be safely used in pregnancy (all are category B). Quinolones are category C agents. The macrolides are category B and C agents. The tetracyclines are category D agents and should be avoided. The sulfonamide drugs are category C agents and are usually reserved for infections such as *Pneumocystis pneumonia*.

A few specific organisms responsible for pneumonia in pregnancy deserve mention. In pregnancy, cell-mediated immunity may be altered, and thus, infections with fungal and viral organisms can be more severe and life threatening. The risk of dissemination with coccidioidomycosis, as well as mortality, is likely increased during pregnancy (20% vs 0.2% in the nonpregnant individual), although this has not been borne out consistently in all studies.[7] It is generally thought that dissemination is more likely if the infection is acquired in the third trimester. Treatment includes amphotericin or a liposomal derivative. Both agents are category B agents. The majority of the azoles are classified as category C.

Of the viral agents, *Varicella zoster* is the most feared during pregnancy. Although this illness is usually self-limited and benign in children, in the nonexposed adult pregnant patient, the mortality rate associated with *Varicella pneumonia* may approach 35%. Infection is most severe in the third trimester. Patients present with fever and rash and, and pneumonia can develop rapidly. A typical chest radiograph shows miliary and nodular infiltrates, usually resolving within 14 days. The end radiographic result of such pneumonia is often calcified, but physiologically insignificant, nodules. Acyclovir (category B) can be safely used during pregnancy and should be begun with the first sign of Varicella infection.

Influenza virus can also be more severe during pregnancy, although some data suggest that the rate of mortality associated with influenza during pregnancy may be similar to that in the nonpregnant woman. The antiinfluenza drugs are category C agents. Influenza vaccine is made from inactivated virus. Women at high risk should be immunized for influenza during pregnancy regardless of the stage of pregnancy. All other pregnant women should be vaccinated after the first trimester.

Acute Respiratory Failure in Pregnancy

Hemodynamics

As pregnancy progresses, cardiac output can become positionally dependent because of the gravid uterus potentially obstructing the IVC and reducing venous return. This is particularly true in the third trimester and is most notable in the supine position. Severe hypotension can result. This effect is reduced in the full or partial left lateral decubitus position, allowing the uterus to be displaced from the IVC. This can be an important factor in the resuscitation of the hypotensive pregnant patient. Because of low colloid oncotic pressure, invasive monitoring with pulmonary artery pressures may have to be interpreted with caution, and pulmonary edema can result at a lower pulmonary artery occlusion pressure.

Sepsis

In addition to non—obstetric-related causes of sepsis in the pregnant patient, sepsis can result from endometritis, pelvic thrombophlebitis, and septic abortion and from procedures such as amniocentesis and/or infection of cesarean or episiotomy incisions. It is important to recall that baseline hemodynamic parameters in a nonseptic pregnant individual, *ie*, high cardiac output and low systemic vascular resistance, can be confused with the hemodynamics of sepsis.

Mechanical Ventilation

The principles of mechanical ventilation in the pregnant patient are similar to those in the non-pregnant woman. Intubation may be more difficult because of edema of the upper airway, a reduced airway caliber, and an increased risk for aspiration and bleeding; therefore, smaller endotracheal tubes may be required. Tidal volumes may have to be reduced as the result of reduced chest wall compliance from the gravid uterus, and greater peak pressures may be required to overcome chest wall stiffness. Gas exchange goals should be to maintain $Paco_2$ in the pregnant eucapnic range of 28 to 32 mm Hg with a $Pao_2 > 90$ mm Hg to prevent fetal hypoxemia. A further reduction in $Paco_2$ can lead to reduced uterine blood flow and fetal hypoxemia. The fetus is very sensitive to hypoxemia, and attempts to compensate for maternal hypoxia by divergence of maternal blood flow to essential tissues, a leftward shift in the oxyhemoglobin dissociation curve, and high avidity of fetal hemoglobin for oxygen. Noninvasive mechanical ventilation has not been well studied in pregnancy, but its utility may be limited by the increased risk of aspiration and narrow airway caliber in this population.

Amniotic Fluid Embolism

Amniotic fluid embolism (AFE) is a rare but catastrophic complication of pregnancy. The incidence of AFE ranges between 1 in 8,000 and 1 in 80,000 pregnancies, with an associated 80 to 90% mortality rate responsible for 10 to 20% of maternal deaths in the peripartum period. Risk factors for AFE include advanced maternal age, multiparity, premature rupture of membranes, and meconium staining of amniotic fluid. The use of uterine stimulants and tumultuous labor may also be risk factors. The risk of AFE extends 48 h into the immediate postpartum period and has also been reported to develop during abortions and placental abruption. The pathophysiology of AFE is not completely known, but postulated mechanisms include true mechanical obstruction of the pulmonary vasculature with fetal squamous cells and other debris, alveolar capillary leak caused by a release of mediators during delivery, pulmonary edema caused by left ventricular failure, and an anaphylactic reaction to exposure of the mother to fetal antigens.

AFE presents catastrophically with the acute onset of tachypnea, dyspnea, tachycardia, cyanosis, hypotension, hypoxemia likely caused by ventilation/perfusion abnormalities, and hemodynamic collapse. Seizures can occur. Disseminated intravascular coagulation can develop in 40 to 80% of patients, and hemorrhage can be the initial presentation. In the majority (70%) of those patients who survive the initial event, ARDS will develop. AFE is often followed by some transient left ventricular dysfunction, as supported by studies using pulmonary artery catheters.

The diagnoses of AFE is one of exclusion but can be supported in the appropriate clinical setting with the presence of fetal squamous cells and lanugo hairs in the maternal circulation, although these can also be present under normal conditions and are not pathognomonic for this diagnosis. Treatment is supportive with intubation, mechanical ventilation, vasopressors, sedation, neuromuscular blockade, and pulmonary artery catheter placement. Factor replacement may be required for hemorrhage.

Venous Air Embolism

Venous air embolism can occur during normal delivery, with placenta previa, and during abortion. It has also been reported during oral genital sex and during gynecologic procedures using air insufflation. One percent of maternal deaths are thought to be from venous air embolism. The usual sites of air entry are at the subplacental venous sinuses, during the antepartum or peripartum period, followed by entry into the venous circulation. In the right ventricle, air can obstruct the pulmonary blood flow, resulting in cardiopulmonary collapse. In general, it is thought that 100 mL of air can lead to mortality. Recruitment and activation of neutrophils, protein aggregation at the turbulent air blood interface and obstruction of pulmonary arterial vessels by microemboli also contribute to the pathophysiology of venous air embolism.

Patients with venous air embolism present with profound hypotension, as well as nonspecific signs of coughing, dizziness, tachypnea, dyspnea, tachycardia, and diaphoresis. Respiratory arrest soon follows, and the rate of mortality can increase to 90%. The classic but rarely heard cardiac mill-wheel murmur audible over the precordium is supportive of the diagnosis of venous air embolism. ARDS may develop. Other findings include mental status changes, coma, seizures, stroke, myocardial infarction, and thrombocytopenia. Bubbles may be visualized in the retinal arterioles, and subdermal air may be present. Air in the heart or great vessels is occasionally seen on the chest radiograph.

Treatment includes recognition of the syndrome, followed by placing the patient in the left lateral decubitus position so that the air bubble is removed from the entrance to the right ventricular outflow tract. Cases of aspiration of air from the right heart using a pulmonary artery or central venous catheter have been reported. Patients should receive ventilation with 100% oxygen to facilitate removal of nitrogen, which comprises a significant (up to 80%) of gas content in the embolus. The use of hyperbaric oxygen therapy should be considered. There are anecdotal reports of using heparin to treat microemboli and corticosteroids to decrease pulmonary edema in this syndrome.

Tocolytic Pulmonary Edema

Until recently, β-adrenergic agents were widely used in obstetrics for inhibition of preterm labor, often administered in combination with corticosteroids to promote fetal lung development. The most common agents used were β_2-selective agents such as terbutaline, ritodrine, and isoxsuprine; and tocolytic pulmonary edema developed in as many as 4 to 5% of patients receiving these agents. Currently, many obstetricians use magnesium for treatment of preterm labor, which has resulted in a decrease in this entity.

Usually, symptoms of tocolytic pulmonary edema develop within 24 h but occur more commonly 48 h after initiation of therapy. They can also develop within 24 h after discontinuation of the drug. Those patients who receive prolonged tocolytic therapy with concomitant infusions of crystalloid volume, those with multiple gestations, and those with preeclampsia are more at risk for tocolytic pulmonary edema. The mechanisms of tocolytic pulmonary edema include possible fluid overload, direct cardiac toxicity, alterations, and reductions in colloid oncotic pressure and/or increased pulmonary capillary permeability.

Patients with tocolytic pulmonary edema typically present with dyspnea, tachycardia, tachypnea, chest pain, crackles, and the presence of pulmonary edema on chest radiograph. This syndrome reverses quickly, usually 12 to 24 h after recognition and discontinuation of the offending agent. The prognosis is excellent. Transient use of oxygen and diuretics may be needed.

Aspiration

Aspiration historically has been a significant problem in obstetrics and is estimated to account for 2% of maternal mortality in the United States. The classic description was made by Mendelson (in 1946), who described large volumes of gastric contents entering the tracheobronchial tree in women undergoing labor and delivery. Because of this large volume of aspiration of low pH-containing gastric contents, ARDS and chemical pneumonitis subsequently developed. Immediate asphyxia was also described.

The obstetric patient is at risk for aspiration for many reasons, including progesterone-induced relaxation of lower esophageal sphincter tone, an increase in intragastric pressure caused by mechanical compression by the gravid uterus, as well as by frequent examinations, a decrease in gastric emptying during parturition, and being in the supine position. In some cases, alterations in mental status caused by sedation and a reduction in vocal chord closure possibly related to analgesia used during labor may also contribute to an increased risk of aspiration.

There is a correlation between the volume of gastric contents aspirated, the acidity of the aspirate, the presence of particulate matter, the bacterial load, and the host resistance on the progression and severity of clinical symptoms. It is thought that the low pH (<2.5) of the aspirate is the major inciting pathogenic process for disease because of a chemical pneumonitis, although large volumes, particularly those containing food particles, can be clinically significant even with greater pH levels. ARDS can result. A small subgroup of patients will have immediate respiratory arrest and death after aspiration as the result of uncorrectable hypoxemia. In those cases in which small volumes of gastric contents are aspirated, symptoms may be delayed until 6 to 24 h after the event. Bacterial pneumonia can develop 24 to 72 h after the aspiration.

Treatment is supportive. As in the nonpregnant patient, there is no role for prophylactic antibiotics or corticosteroids when treating this aspiration syndrome. Resolution usually occurs over the next 4 to 5 days unless secondary superinfection develops. Bronchoscopy may be indicated when witnessed aspiration with large food particles has occurred. The chances of aspiration can be reduced by the use of regional anesthesia, restricting oral intake at the time of delivery and cricoid pressure if endotracheal intubation is required.

ARDS

ARDS is defined similarly in the pregnant as in the nonpregnant individual. In addition to the causes of ARDS discussed elsewhere in this course, there is a long list of ARDS etiologies unique to or associated with pregnancy. These include placental abruption, air embolism, amniotic fluid embolism, aspiration, eclampsia, septic abortion, and the dead fetus syndrome.

Pulmonary Edema

Pulmonary edema can accompany preeclampsia/eclampsia in approximately 3% of cases. Pulmonary edema may develop more frequently in the immediate postpartum period. Risk factors include advanced age and multigravity. Mechanisms for preeclampsia-related pulmonary edema include increased left ventricular afterload, myocardial dysfunction, the alterations in colloid oncotic pressure discussed earlier, as well as fluid overload. There may also be a component of increased pulmonary capillary permeability. Management is approached in the standard manner with oxygen, diuresis, control of hypertension, and mechanical ventilation, if required. Invasive hemodynamic monitoring may be required.

Peripartum Cardiomyopathy

Pregnancy-related cardiomyopathy can develop in 1 in 1,300 to 1 in 4,000 deliveries, and usually presents in the third trimester or up to 6 months postpartum. Risk factors include advanced age, multiple gestations, preeclampsia, and African-American race. Patients typically present with dyspnea, orthopnea, peripheral edema, pulmonary edema, tachycardia, and a cardiac gallop. The chest radiograph shows cardiomegaly and pulmonary edema, and echocardiography demonstrates global hypokinesis. Prognosis is variable, and approximately 30% of these patients recover, 30% may have residual cardiac damage, and 30% may require heart transplantation. The cause of death is often thromboembolism from left ventricular thrombus. The recurrence of cardiomyopathy with subsequent pregnancies is common.

Primary Pulmonary Hypertension

Patients with pulmonary hypertension, either secondary or primary, are at increased risk for maternal (35 to 50%) and fetal mortality during pregnancy. The risk appears to be greatest in the immediate peripartum period, when a large amount of blood volume is "autotransfused" from the uteroplacental bed back to the maternal circulation. Acute right-heart failure can result. Patients with primary pulmonary hypertension should be counseled against becoming pregnant and encouraged to seek termination of pregnancy and permanent forms of birth control. Those patients wishing to continue with their pregnancy should be managed with medications such as inhaled nitric oxide and/or IV or inhaled prostacyclin during the peripartum period. Placement of a pulmonary artery catheter should be strongly considered during delivery. Long-term management could include epoprostenol (prostacyclin, a category B agent) or sildenafil (category B), but the oral endothelin receptor blocker agents such as bosentan are contraindicated as the result of teratogenicity (category X).

Tobacco and Lung Disease in Women

Tobacco

At the end of the 19th century and beginning of the 20th century, cigarette smoking and tobacco use were limited primarily to male subjects and were thought to be socially unacceptable for women.

However, in the early 20th century, with the advent of the suffrage movement, numerous ad campaigns promoted the use of tobacco by women, including well-known advertisements with the famous slogan "You've come a long way, baby." Tobacco smoking began to be associated with the educated and/or liberated American woman, a concept further promoted by the advertising of the tobacco industry. The use of tobacco products by women increased dramatically after World War II and peaked in 1965, when the prevalence of smoking among women approached 35%. Currently, 18.1% of women and 23.9% of men smoke.

The initial 1964 landmark US Public Health Surgeon General's Report on Smoking and Health primarily addressed smoking and respiratory health in men. However, in 1980, the Surgeon General's Report on the Health Consequences for Smoking for Women was released. This report concluded that women demonstrate the same dose—response relationships with cigarette smoking as do men, and that the risk of lung cancer increases with the increasing number of cigarettes smoked per day, earlier ages of cigarette smoking, longer duration of smoking, greater tar and nicotine content of cigarettes, and inhalation of cigarette smoke.

The study predicted that rates of mortality in women from lung cancer may be comparable with that experienced by men, that there would be a rapid increase in lung cancer rates in women similar to that seen in men 25 years previously, and that lung cancer death rates in women would surpass those of breast cancer by the early 1980s. The study also found that the incidence of other respiratory conditions such as influenza was 20% greater in ever-smoking women than in nonsmoking women, that there was an increase in death rates attributable to COPD in smoking women compared with nonsmoking women, and that this death rate correlated with the number of cigarettes smoked. Finally, the study concluded that women smokers had worse pulmonary function than ex-smokers or never-smokers and that the severity of decrease in pulmonary function was dose related to the number of cigarettes smoked.

The follow-up 2001 Surgeon General Report on Women and Smoking[8] found the following: (1) in 1998, 22% of women smoked cigarettes; (2) lung cancer is the leading cause of cancer deaths in women, and 90% of these deaths are related to smoking; and (3) in 2000, 25% of cancer deaths in women were caused by cancer of the lung. The study also stated that the risk of lung cancer increases with quantity, duration, and intensity of smoking.

Lung Cancer

Lung cancer has become the leading cause of cancer deaths in both men and women in the United States, surpassing death rates in women as the result of breast cancer in 1987. More than 80 to 90% of lung cancers in women are related to tobacco use and, thus, are preventable. In 2007, 26% of cancer deaths in women were caused by cancer of the lung. Although breast cancer affects a large number of women per year, lung cancer has a significantly worse prognosis, with greater mortality rates. In 2007, > 71,000 women died of cancer of the lung and bronchus as compared with 40,480 deaths caused by breast cancer. In 2007, > 114,600 women were diagnosed with lung cancer. Lung cancer incidence rates in women began to level off from the mid-1990s to early 2000 and are now decreasing; however, death rates in women from lung cancer continue to increase and are just now reaching the plateau seen in men in the 1980s. It is expected that the death rates from lung cancer in men and women will approach unity in the next 5 to 10 years.

Of the different cell types, adenocarcinoma is the most common cell type of lung cancer in both smoking and nonsmoking women, regardless of age and is the most common cell type in young people and in nonsmokers of both sexes. A possible increase in the susceptibility of tobacco carcinogens in women has been a highly debated topic. Some studies have indicated that there is an increase in the relative risk for lung cancer developing in smoking women than in men; other studies have not been able to support this. Yet other studies have shown that there is an increased odds ratio of tobacco-related lung cancer in women only for some certain types of lung cancer. For example, it appears that smoking women have a greater odds ratio for small cell carcinoma developing than do men. There are many postulated reasons as to why women may have an increased susceptibility to tobacco carcinogens, including the fact that there may be an increased frequency of mutations in the P53 and other tumor suppressor genes in women than in men; in addition, a greater promutagenicity

DNA level (CP450), greater levels of DNA adducts, and decreased capacity for DNA repair have been observed in women.

In addition, hormones (estrogens) and hormonal replacement may play a role in the variable susceptibility to tobacco carcinogens, particularly with adenocarcinoma. In never-smokers, age adjusted incidence rate is greater for women 14.4 to 20.8/100,000 person years as compared with men 4.8 to 13.7/100,000. Other risk factors for lung cancer in women include a family history of lung cancer; occupational exposures to compounds such as asbestos, cadmium, beryllium, silicosis, radon; and previous lung disease as are found in men. In general, women with lung cancer have a better prognosis and equal or better survival with treatment than do men, regardless of cell type and stage.

COPD

Cigarette smoking is the major cause of COPD in women, and the risk increases with the amount and duration smoked. Ninety percent of COPD mortality among women in the United States is attributable to smoking. Mortality rates attributable to COPD among men now appear to be have reached a plateau, whereas COPD mortality rates among women continue to increase. A total of 1.5 to 3.6 times more women are hospitalized with COPD than are men. The current prevalence of COPD in women is greater than or equal to that in men, and this may be underestimated because several studies have suggested that COPD is less frequently diagnosed in women.

This finding parallels the trends previously discussed in lung cancer. Because the slope of this curve is steeper than that seen in men, it is possible that women are more vulnerable to tobacco-induced COPD. Studies in these regards have been conflicting, but most indicate that women with exposure to tobacco smoke have more severe COPD and more lung function impairment with fewer pack-years of tobacco use than do men. It does seem clear that COPD develops in women at an earlier age than it does men. Some of the postulated mechanisms for this increased prevalence include small air airway size, which alters the distribution of toxins contained in tobacco, hormonal mechanisms, and variations in cytochrome P450 levels.

In children who have prenatal exposure to environmental tobacco smoke from a smoking mother, studies have shown that fetal lung development is affected. These children have more airway obstruction, increased airway hyperresponsiveness, and alterations in lung maturation and lung growth. There is a small decrement in birth weight and increased risk of intrauterine growth retardation and other obstetric complications. Those children exposed to environmental tobacco smoke in the postnatal period have an increased incidence of cough, wheezes, respiratory illnesses, and infection. Pulmonary function is decreased slightly, and there is an increase in airway responsiveness. These children tend to have an increase in childhood asthma, earlier development of asthma, and more severe asthma. Other studies have shown that atopy tends to develop in children exposed to environmental tobacco smoke, which can result in worsening asthma. There have also been correlations found between environmental tobacco smoke and obstructive apnea in children and sudden infant death syndrome in infants.

Catamenial Pneumothorax and Hemoptysis

Catamenial complications by definition develop during menstruation. Catamenial pneumothorax occurs very rarely and is usually recurrent. Patients are usually in their late 20s to >30 years of age when they initially present. Symptoms develop within 24 to 48 h of the onset of menstrual flow. The pneumothoraces are often on the right side and are often associated with pelvic endometriosis. The mechanisms of air entry into the pleural space may be to the result of a defect at the site of pleural or diaphragmatic endometriosis or may be by air gaining access to the peritoneal cavity during menstruation and then subsequently entering the pleural cavity through a diaphragmatic defect. The diagnosis is fairly straightforward when a pneumothorax develops during the first 48 h of menstrual flow. Treatment includes ovulation-suppressing drugs. Patients wishing to conceive or who do not want ovulation suppressed should undergo thoracotomy with repair of diaphragmatic defects, if present, followed by pleurodesis. Catamenial hemothorax has also been described.

Catamenial hemoptysis is thought to occur as the result of endometriosis in the lung parenchyma. It is usually a cause of scant hemoptysis but can, in some cases, be severe. Treatment includes hormonal suppression and/or resection of lung parenchyma involved with endometriosis.

Hormone-Replacement Therapy and the Risk of Venous Thromboembolic Disease

The cardiovascular disease risks of hormone-replacement therapy (HRT) in women have been addressed by several large studies.[9,10] In the Women's Health Initiative Study, the risk of VTE (both DVT and PE) was significantly increased in those women receiving HRT. There were 34 VTE events per 10,000 person-years in the HRT group vs 16 VTE events/10,000 person-years in the non-HRT group. The hazard ratio was 2.11 (confidence interval, 1.58 to 2.82). In the Heart and Estrogen/Progestin Replacement Study, there was a twofold increase in VTE risk in the women receiving HRT. One of the possible explanations for these findings may be an increase in activated protein C resistance with the use of HRT. The results at longer follow-up, at 3 years after discontinuation of HRT, suggest that cardiovascular risks return to a level comparable with those patients who did not receive HRT, but an increased incidence of malignancy is being found in those women who had received HRT.[11]

LAM

LAM is covered extensively in other portions of this syllabus but will be reviewed briefly here. LAM is a rare disease (prevalence 1 to 2/million) affecting premenopausal women with a mean age of 35 years. The disorder is characterized by proliferation of atypical smooth muscle in the bronchovasculature, lymphatics, and interstitium of the lung, as well as the abdomen and pelvis. Typically, these smooth-muscle cells stain positive with the monoclonal antibody HMB-45 (a melanoma-related tumor marker).

Clinically, patients present with symptoms of dyspnea, cough, chest pain, and hemoptysis. The physical examination may reveal decreased breath sounds, crackles, and sometimes ascites and/or abdominal masses. Spontaneous pneumothoraces and/or chylothoraces may also be presenting findings. Radiographically, LAM is characterized by cyst formation and chronic interstitial infiltrates. Hyperinflation develops as the disease progresses. Pleural effusions and pneumothoraces may also be present. High-resolution CT can reveal diffuse, homogenous cystic disease with cysts ranging from a few millimeters to ≥1 cm in size (6-cm cysts have been reported); characteristically, nodularity, as seen in eosinophilic granuloma, is absent. Pulmonary function testing most commonly shows mixed obstructive and restrictive physiology with an elevated total lung capacity and residual volume and a reduced diffusion capacity, but up to one third of patients can have normal pulmonary function.

Complications of LAM include recurrent pneumothoraces in > 50% of patients, chylous effusions in approximately onethird of patients, chylous ascites, and renal angiomyolipomas in up to 50% of patients. These latter tumors can develop in the kidneys or in other solid organs (uterus, ovaries, liver, spleen) and are composed of blood vessels, smooth muscle, and fat.

The diagnosis of LAM can be suspected by the clinical presentation and characteristic radiographic appearance and confirmed by lung biopsy with HMB-45 staining, either transbronchial, thoracoscopic, or surgical. The major entities in the differential diagnosis are other causes of cystic lung disease with preserved lung volume, particularly eosinophilic granuloma and cystic sarcoidosis.

The prognosis with LAM is variable, but median survival is often reported to be 8 to 10 years. The cause of death is usually respiratory failure. Treatment for LAM has included hormonal manipulation with the use of antiestrogen agents (such as tamoxifen), progesterone agents, luteinizing hormone-releasing hormone analogs, and/or oophorectomy with variable results. Patients should avoid estrogens and pregnancy. Lung transplantation has been performed for LAM, although disease recurrence has been documented.

Recently, sirolimus, acting via suppression of mammalian target of rapamycin signaling, has been studied with a primary end point of decreasing angiomyolipoma volume at 12 months.[12] In this small study, there was a 50% reduction in angiomyolipoma size in patients receiving therapy with sirolimus, but the tumor size increased after discontinuation of treatment. An interesting secondary finding in the study was an improvement in spirometry of 5 to 10% in FEV_1 and FVC, which was only partially sustained after discontinuation of sirolimus.

References

1. Schatz M. The efficacy and safety of asthma medications during pregnancy. Semin Perinatol 2001; 25:145–152
2. National Asthma Education and Prevention Program. Report of the Working Group on Asthma and Pregnancy: management of asthma during pregnancy; update 2004. Bethesda, MD; National Institutes of Health, 2005; 1–57; NIH publication 05–3279
3. GINA Report: Global Strategy for Asthma Management and Prevention. Available at: http://www.ginasthma.com/Guidelineitem.asp??l1=2&l2=1&intId=60. Accessed February 16, 2009
4. Bates SM, Greer I, Pabinger I, et al. Venous thromboembolism, thrombophilia, antithrombotic therapy, and pregnancy: American College of Chest Physicians Evidence-based clinical practice guidelines (8th edition). Chest 2008; 133:844S–886S
5. American Thoracic Society/Centers for Disease Control and Prevention/Infectious Diseases Society of America. Treatment of tuberculosis. Am J Respir Crit Care Med 2003; 167:603–662
6. ATS Official Statement. Targeted tuberculin testing and treatment of latent tuberculosis infection. Am J Respir Crit Care Med 2000; 161:S221–S247
7. Ramsey PS, Ramin KD. Pneumonia in pregnancy. Obstet Gynecol Clin North Am 2001; 28:553–569
8. Surgeon General's report: women and smoking; a report of the Surgeon General, 2001. Available at: www.cdc.gov/tobacco/sgr. Accessed February 16, 2009
9. Rossouw JE, Anderson GL, Prentice RL, et al. Risks and benefits of estrogen plus progestin in healthy postmenopausal women: principal results from the Women's Health Initiative randomized controlled trial. JAMA 2002; 288:321–333
10. Hulley S, Furberg C, Barrett-Connor E, et al. Noncardiovascular disease outcomes during 6.8 years of hormone therapy: heart and Estrogen/Progestin Replacement Study follow-up (HERS II). JAMA 2002; 288:58–66
11. Heiss G, Wallace R, Anderson GL, et al. Health risks and benefits 3 years after stopping randomized treatment with estrogen and progestin. JAMA 2008; 299:1036–1045
12. Bissler JJ, McCormack FX, Young LR, et al. Sirolimus for angiomyolipoma in tuberous sclerosis complex or lymphangioleiomyomatosis. N Engl J Med 2008; 358:140–51

Annotated Bibliography

Andres RL, Miles A. Venous thromboembolism and pregnancy. Obstet Gynecol Clin North Am 2001; 28:613–630

This is a review of this subject.

American Thoracic Society/Centers for Disease Control and Prevention/Infectious Diseases Society of America. Treatment of tuberculosis. Am J Respir Crit Care Med 2003; 167:603–662

This statement includes a section on the treatment of TB in pregnancy.

ATS official statement. Targeted tuberculin testing and treatment of latent tuberculosis infection. Am J Respir Crit Care Med 2000; 161:S221–S247

This statement includes a section on the treatment of LTBI in pregnancy.

Bain C, Feskanich D, Speizer FE, et al. Lung cancer rates in men and women with comparable histories of smoking. J Natl Cancer Inst 2004; 96:826–834

An article suggesting that there is no sex difference in rates of lung cancer with comparable smoking histories.

Bates SM, Greer I, Pabinger I, et al. Venous thromboembolism, thrombophilia, antithrombotic therapy, and pregnancy: American College of Chest Physicians Evidence-based clinical practice guidelines (8th edition). Chest 2008; 133:844S–886S

This is the most recent evidence-graded consensus conference regarding antithrombotic agents in pregnancy.

Bissler JJ, McCormack FX, Young LR, et al. Sirolimus for angiomyolipoma in tuberous sclerosis complex or lymphangioleiomyomatosis. N Engl J Med 2008; 358: 140–151

This article describes the results of the trial using sirolimus.

Chapman KR. Chronic obstructive pulmonary disease: are women more susceptible than men? Clin Chest Med 2004; 25:331–341

An article presenting evidence to support the question.

Chapman KR, Tashkin DP, Pye DJ. Gender bias in the diagnosis of COPD. Chest 2001; 119:1691–1695

A discussion of sex differences in the diagnosis of COPD.

Collop NA, Adkins D, Phillips BA. Gender differences in sleep and sleep-disordered breathing. Clin Chest Med 2004; 25:257–268

This article includes a section on sleep-disordered breathing in pregnancy.
Deblieux PM, Summer WR. Acute respiratory failure in pregnancy. Clin Obstet Gynecol 1996; 39:143–152
This is a review of causes of respiratory failure in pregnancy.
Elkus R, Popovich JL. Respiratory physiology in pregnancy. Clin Chest Med 1992; 13:555–565
This is an overview of the normal physiologic adaptation of the respiratory system to pregnancy.
Fu JB, Kau TY, Severson RK, et al. Lung cancer in women: analysis of the national surveillance, epidemiology, and end results database. Chest 2005; 127:768–777
More information is provided on this subject.
Gazdar AF, Thun MJ. Lung cancer, smoke exposure, and sex. J Clinical Oncol 2007; 25:469–471
An interesting editorial discussing the issues of tobacco exposure, lung cancer, and sex.
GINA Report: Global Strategy for Asthma Management and Prevention. Available at: http://www.ginasthma.com/Guidelineitem.asp??l1=2&l2=1&intId=60. Accessed February 16, 2009
The most recent guidelines for asthma classification and treatment.
Greer IA. Thrombosis in pregnancy: maternal and fetal issues. Lancet 1999; 353:1258–1265
This is a thorough review in this area, with a detailed discussion of the thrombophilias.
Greer IA. Prevention and management of venous thromboembolism in pregnancy. Clin Chest Med 2003; 24:123–137
This is a review article on this subject.
Heiss G, Wallace R, Anderson GL, et al. Health risks and benefits 3 years after stopping randomized treatment with estrogen and progestin. JAMA 2008; 299:1036–1045
This article describes the health risks and benefits found at 3-year follow-up of women who had formerly received HRT.
Hulley S, Furberg C, Barrett-Connor E, et al. Noncardiovascular disease outcomes during 6.8 years of hormone therapy: Heart and Estrogen/Progestin Replacement Study follow-up (HERS II). JAMA 2002; 288:58–66
Results of the Heart and Estrogen/Progestin Replacement Study are provided, including risks of VTE with HRT.
Jemal A, Siegel R, Ward E, et al. Cancer statistics, 2008. CA Cancer J Clin 2008; 58:71–96
An update on 2008 cancer statistics including incidence and mortality.
Lapinsky SE, Kruczynski K, Slutsky AS. Critical care in the pregnant patient. Am J Respir Crit Care Med 1995; 152:427–455
This is an excellent comprehensive review of this subject.
McCormack FX. Lymphangioleiomyomatosis: a clinical update. Chest 2008; 133:507–516
This is a good review article on this topic.
Moore J, Baldisseri MR. Amniotic fluid embolism. Crit Care Med 2005; 33:279s–285s
This is a good review of this topic.
Murphy VE, Gibson PG, Smith R, Clifton VL. Asthma during pregnancy: mechanisms and treatment implications. Eur Respir J 2005; 25:731–750
National Asthma Education and Prevention Program. Report of the Working Group on Asthma and Pregnancy: management of asthma during pregnancy; update 2004. Bethesda, MD: National Institutes of Health, 2005; 1–57
This is an updated report on this subject from the National Institutes of Health.
Nelson-Piercy C. Asthma in pregnancy. Thorax 2001; 56:325–328
This is a review of this topic.
Patel JD, Bach PB, Kris MG. Lung cancer in US women: a contemporary epidemic. JAMA 2004; 291:1763–1768
This is a review article on this subject.
Pereira A, Krieger BP. Pulmonary complications of pregnancy. Clin Chest Med 2004; 25:299–310
This is a review of this general topic.
Position statement: the use of newer asthma and allergy medications during pregnancy. Ann Allergy Asthma Immunol 2000; 84:475–480
This is another review on this topic.
Ramsey PS, Ramin KD. Pneumonia in pregnancy. Obset Gynecol Clin North Am 2001; 28:553–569
This is a good review in this area.
Rossouw JE, Anderson GL, Prentice RL, et al. Risks and benefits of estrogen plus progestin in healthy postmenopausal women: principal results from the Women's Health Initiative randomized controlled trial. JAMA 2002; 288:321–333
Results of the Women's Health Initiative are presented, including risks of VTE with HRT.
Schatz M. The efficacy and safety of asthma medications during pregnancy. Semin Perinatol 2001; 25:145–152
This article describes published consensus recommendations regarding the pharmacologic management of asthma during pregnancy.
Schatz MM, Zeiger RS, Harden K, et al. The safety of asthma and allergy medications during pregnancy. J Allergy Clin Immunol 1997; 100:301–306
This is a review of the use and safety of asthma medications used during pregnancy.
Surgeon General's report: women and smoking; a report of the Surgeon General, 2001. Available at: www.cdc.gov/tobacco/sgr. Accessed February 16, 2009

Tan KS, Thomson NC. Asthma in pregnancy. Am J Med 2000; 109:727–733

This is a good review of this subject.

Tanoue LT. Cigarette smoking and women's respiratory health. Clin Chest Med 2000; 21:47–65

This article reviews epidemiology of smoking and smoking-related diseases in women.

Thomas L, Doyle LA, Edelman MJ. Lung cancer in women: emerging differences in epidemiology, biology, and therapy. Chest 2005; 128:370–381

An update on the epidemiology, biology, and therapy of lung cancer in women.

Unterborn J. Pulmonary function testing in obesity, pregnancy, and extremes of body habits. Clin Chest Med 2001; 22:759–768

This chapter includes a subsection on pulmonary function testing in pregnancy.

Wendel PJ. Asthma in pregnancy. Obstet Gynecol Clin North Am 2001; 28:537–551

This article discusses the pathophysiology of asthma and the effects of asthma on pregnancy and vice versa, and reviews the National Asthma Education Program guidelines for the treatment of asthma in pregnancy.

Notes

Occupational Asthma

William S. Beckett, MD, FCCP

Objectives:

- Provide a clinical definition of occupational asthma
- Show the relationship of occupational asthma to the larger realm of adult asthma
- Outline mechanisms by which asthma develops from exposures in the work setting
- Discuss the evaluation of a patient with possible occupational asthma
- Review the management of a patient with confirmed occupational asthma

Key words: asthma; irritant asthma; occupational asthma; occupational lung disease; reactive airways dysfunction syndrome; work-related asthma

This chapter expands on the introduction to occupational asthma by Dr. Sidney Braman in the chapter "Asthma" earlier in this publication. It addresses the American Board of Internal Medicine Pulmonary Disease Certification "Occupational and Environmental Disease" content category topics of "Occupational Asthma," "Byssinosis," "Reactive Airways Dysfunction Syndrome," and "Work/Disability Evaluation."

Clinical Definition of Occupational Asthma

From Dr. Braman's chapter on "Asthma," we read that: "Allergens and occupational factors are considered the most important causes of asthma.... Asthma that is precipitated by a particular occupational environment and not by stimuli outside the workplace is called occupational asthma. Two types of asthma have been described: asthma that follows a latent period of exposure to either a high- or low-molecular-weight sensitizing antigen, and asthma that follows a latent period of exposure to workplace irritants. One form of irritant asthma is called *reactive airways dysfunction syndrome*, a condition that usually results from the sudden inhalation of a large dose of a highly irritating substance."[1–3]

In addition, individuals with a history of asthma may experience a recurrence of asthma after years of being asymptomatic when they are challenged with an irritant or allergen in the workplace. This has been termed *work-aggravated asthma* and, from the point of view of medical management, is similar to other forms of occupational asthma.

Because the workplace environment contributes to the severity of asthma in these patients, the chest physician's challenge is to determine whether a change in the workplace environment will improve or cure the patient's occupational asthma or whether, conversely, in the patient with nonoccupational asthma, it will have no effect. This determination usually requires a clear statement in the medical record as to whether the patient's asthma is or is not occupational. A diagnosis of occupational asthma often presents problems to the patient and employer, requiring a major change in employment. If nonoccupational, it is safe to allow the patient to continue in the same job, focusing on better medical management.

Frequency of Cases

Reliable data show that the proportion of new cases of occupational asthma in North American adults is approximately 9 to 15%, or 1 in 6 to 1 in 10 new-onset cases of asthma.[4] Any patient who is employed and who presents with new-onset asthma should thus be questioned about occupational exposures.

Natural History of Occupational Asthma

Numerous useful reviews, both brief and comprehensive, are available.[5–11] Typically, asthma will begin weeks to years after working with a new substance that can cause asthma. Symptoms may be minor or intermittent at first and gradually increase as the patient's sensitization increases, sometimes to the point where the patient has nightly wheezing and orthopnea.

Table 1. *Most Frequently Reported Specific Causes or Contributors to Work-Related Asthma in the United States**

Di-isocyanates
Stainless steel welding plume
Formaldehyde
Paint
Pesticides
Natural rubber latex
Chlorine
Glutaraldehyde
Diesel exhaust
Epoxy resins
Acrylates
Wood dust

*From Jajosky et al. MMWR Morb Mortal Wkly Rep 1999; 48(suppl): No SS-3.

In some cases, patients will have had childhood asthma that remitted in adolescence, but for others, this onset of asthma will be the first. The cardinal feature is the onset of asthma while working with inhalational exposure to a substance that can cause asthma, although there is emerging evidence that repeated skin contact with some substances can result in respiratory sensitization. Although there is some literature to suggest that the early diagnosis of occupational asthma leads to less severity and improved chances for complete remission, the published literature in this area is uncertain.

Causes of Occupational Asthma

More than 400 substances have been identified as causes of occupational asthma.[12,13] Examples of a few of the most commonly reported causes in the United States are shown in Table 1.

Other Risk Factors for Occupational Asthma

Specific gene polymorphisms are associated with an increased risk for the development of asthma for a few causes of occupational asthma, but testing for these is not clinically useful. A history of atopy or cigarette smoking is a risk factor for sensitization to high-molecular-weight substances (*eg*, biologically derived antigens, such as proteins from laboratory animals or wheat flour) but not for sensitization to others (*eg*, low-molecular-weight chemicals like isocyanates).

Pathophysiology, Histopathology, and Physiologic Mechanisms

In these respects, occupational asthma does not differ, or differs only in minor ways, from other types of asthma.[14,15] Please refer to the "Asthma" chapter in this publication by Dr. Braman for a comprehensive discussion.

Clinical Features of Occupational Asthma

Useful Diagnostic Measures

History: The combination of the following four elements of the patient's medical history has a 64% positive predictive value in the diagnosis of occupational asthma[16]: current diagnosis of asthma; and onset of asthma after entering the workplace; association between symptoms of asthma and work; and workplace exposure to an agent known to give rise to occupational asthma. Allergic rhinitis to the offending substance often precedes the onset of lower respiratory tract symptoms.

Physical Examination: Wheeze is usually present minutes to hours after a significant exposure and is absent between exacerbations.

Pulmonary Function Testing: Comprehensive, evidence-based reviews of diagnostic approaches to occupational asthma[17,18] recommend the following tests in addition to a medical history and physical examination:

Methacholine challenge: improves the diagnostic accuracy of an asthma diagnosis (84% sensitivity, 48% specificity).

- Immunology testing: tests for serum-specific IgE (*ie*, blood radioallergosorbent tests or skin- prick tests) are available through reference laboratories (*eg*, Mayo Clinic Laboratory; Rochester, MN) for a large number of common high-molecular-weight substances. Some allergists also have skin-prick testing reagents for some of the large -molecular-weight substances. However, there is no specific IgE for many of the less common low-molecular-weight substances. A positive test result for a specific IgE to the suspected antigen increases the diagnostic certainty of occupational asthma. When preexisting or subclinical asthma is exacerbated by work, a similar approach is taken.[19]

- Measurement of peak expiratory flow rate with the use peak flowmeters: the recording of portable peak expiratory flow rates (best of three blows) four times per day during days at work and days away from work may also help to distinguish occupational from nonoccupational asthma because reversible airflow obstruction is necessary to the diagnosis of asthma, and an occupationally related pattern may be evident. Clinical interpretation by visual comparison of the patient's exposure history has been found to be as accurate as computer-based interpretation.

Treatment of Occupational Asthma

As with all asthma, the treatment goal is to remove the patient from exposure to triggers and to minimize symptoms by controlling asthma with medications that have the least adverse effects for the patient. Once diagnosed, the main difference between treating occupational and nonoccupational asthma is removing the patient from exposure. This treatment begins with notifying the patient and, with the patient's permission, the employer, and trying to identify a specific exposure that can be successfully avoided. It is usually much to the patient's advantage to continue working for the same employer, but in circumstances in which the offending agent has been removed, the reduction of air levels has been achieved or, in some cases, respiratory protection has been added. The assistance of an occupational medicine specialist or an industrial hygienist may be necessary at this point.

Reduction or elimination of exposure alone may be enough to bring resolution of asthma. However, in >50% of recognized cases, patients require ongoing therapy with medications. The guidelines for treatment follow the standard approaches, as outlined in the chapter "Asthma" by Dr. Braman in this syllabus.

Byssinosis

Byssinosis is a form of occupational asthma that is caused by the inhalation of dust released when processing the cotton plant (including the leaves and Gram-negative bacterial endotoxin associated with the cotton fibers but not the cotton fibers themselves). Symptoms are intermittent and tend to improve with continued exposure through the work week, then return after a weekend away from exposure. Unlike other types of occupational asthma, severe cases may be associated with episodic fever on exposure.

Work/Disability Evaluation

In the case of occupational asthma, a most difficult initial decision may be in determining whether it is safe to allow the patient to return to work, or whether he or she can return with specific work restrictions. Once a diagnosis of occupational asthma is made, it is often important for the treating physician to determine whether disability is present and, if so, to what extent.

For any pulmonary patient who presents with a request for disability evaluation, the physician must first decide whether the lung disease is nonoccupational (in which case federal Social Security Administration disability criteria apply if the patient is totally disabled), or whether it is occupational (*ie*, caused by the job) in which state-specific worker compensation disability rules may apply.

American Medical Association Guides

Many states require the physician to apply the criteria of the *Guides to the Evaluation of Permanent Impairment*[20] in rating the degree of disability for all occupational conditions including lung disease. Although for most conditions the guides focus on permanent pulmonary function loss, for asthma more emphasis is placed on the frequency and severity of exacerbations despite maximal medical therapy.

Social Security Disability

For the patient who is unable to work at all because of lung disease, whether occupational or nonoccupational, Social Security Administration disability criteria may apply. These criteria are available on the Internet.[21] In brief, total disability from asthma is considered when

> Attacks (as defined in section 3.00C), in spite of prescribed treatment and requiring physician intervention, occur at least once every

2 months or at least six times a year. Each inpatient hospitalization for longer than 24 h for control of asthma counts as two attacks, and an evaluation period of at least 12 consecutive months must be used to determine the frequency of attacks.

Fatal Occupational Asthma

Although infrequently reported, fatal cases of occupational asthma[22] have occurred in patients for whom the association with the workplace was not made in a timely fashion or who returned to be reexposed at work against medical advice.

Annotated References

Reactive Airways Dysfunction Syndrome

1. Alberts WM, do Pico GA. Reactive airways dysfunction syndrome. Chest 1996; 109:1618–1626
   Comprehensive review that discusses reactive airways dysfunction syndrome as a distinct subset of IIA.
2. Bardana EJ. Reactive airways dysfunction syndrome (RADS): guidelines for diagnosis and treatment and insight into likely prognosis. Ann Allergy Asthma Immunol 1999; 83:583–586
   Excellent short review with a balanced discussion of the controversial areas of this disorder.

Irritant Asthma

3. Tarlo SM. Workplace respiratory irritants and asthma. Occup Med 2000; 15:471–484
   Tarlo uses a more inclusive definition of IIA.

Frequency of Cases of Occupational Asthma

4. Balmes J, Becklake M, Blanc P, et al. American Thoracic Society statement: occupational contribution to the burden of airway diseases. Am J Respir Crit Care Med 2003; 167:787–797
   Brief reviews of occupational asthma are presented.
5. Chan-Yeung M, Malo J-L. Occupational asthma. N Engl J Med 1995; 333:107–112
6. Tarlo SM, Liss GM. Occupational asthma: an approach to diagnosis and management. Can Med Assoc J 2003; 168:867–871

   These short-but-complete reviews are recommended for those whose review time is limited. Each review takes a little different tack but covers essentially the same material.

Comprehensive Reviews: Occupational Asthma

7. Tarlo SM, Boulet LP, Cartier A, et al. Canadian Thoracic Society: guidelines for occupational asthma. Can Respir J 1998; 5:289–300
   Perhaps the clearest, most clinically useful review addressing diagnosis.
8. Mapp CE, Boschetto P, Maestrelli, et al. State of the art: occupational asthma. Am J Respir Crit Care Med 2005;172:280–305
   A "state-of-the-art" article that is full of facts. This updates the classic Chan-Yeung and Lam state-of-the-art article from 1986.
9. Chan-Yeung M, Malo JL, Tarlo SM. Proceedings of the first Jack Pepys occupational asthma symposium. Am J Respir Crit Care Med 2003; 167:450–471
   A 2003 review of the subject is presented from luminaries in the field.
10. Nicholson PJ, Cullinan P, Taylor AJ, et al. Evidence based guidelines for the prevention, identification, and management of occupational asthma. Occup Environ Med 2005; 62:290–299
11. Rachiotis G, Savani R, Brant A, et al. Outcome of occupational asthma after cessation of exposure: a systematic review. Thorax 2007; 62:147–152
    Sources of information on causes are listed.
    To know whether the materials your patient works with are known to cause asthma, ask the patient to bring you materials safety data sheets from work or request these yourself from the employer under the Occupational Safety and Health Administration "Right to Know" law. The employer must provide them within 15 business days.
12. SIRI MSDS index. Available at: http://siri.org/msds/index.php. Accessed April 22, 2009
    If you know only the brand names or product names of the substances, you can quickly get the chemical names from the material safety data sheets online at SIRI.org.
13. Sommaire. Tables of agents and substances that can cause asthma. Available at: http://www.remcomp.fr/asmanet/asmapro/agents.htm#start. Accessed April 22, 2009
    Once you know the chemical names, you can check them against the >400 known causes of occupational asthma

on-line at "ASMAPRO," which includes links to PubMed and references to the medical literature.

Mechanisms of Occupational Asthma

14. Mapp CE, Boschetto P, Miottoi D, et al. Mechanisms of occupational asthma. Ann Allergy Asthma Immunol 1999; 83:645–664
15. Sastre J, Vandenplas O, Park HS. Pathogenesis of occupational asthma. Eur Respir J 2003; 22:364–373
Both articles discuss the known facts and the proposed theories of the pathogenetic mechanisms at work in occupational asthma.

Diagnosis, Evaluation, Management

16. Malo J-L, Ghezzo H, L'Arqueveque J, et al. Is the clinical history a satisfactory means of diagnosing occupational asthma? Am Rev Respir Dis 1991; 143:528–532
17. Tarlo S, Balmes J, Balkisoon R, et al. Management of occupational asthma: an ACCP evidence-based clinical guideline. Chest 2008; 134(3 suppl):1S–41S
The most detailed (very long) evidence-based approach to date. It uses an expert panel review of the current literature. It is recommended that methacholine challenge tests and specific IgE assays or skin-prick tests (when available) be used to improve diagnostic accuracy.
18. Nicholson PJ, Cullinan P, Taylor AJ, et al. Evidenced based guidelines for the prevention, identification and management of occupational asthma. Occup Environ Med 2005; 62:290–299
Similar guidelines from the United Kingdom that place more emphasis on the use of serial portable peak flow measurements four times daily both at work and away from work in the confirmation of suspected diagnosis. It emphasizes asking patients about the occurrence of allergic rhinitis preceding asthma.
19. Friedman-Jimenez G, Petsonk L, Szeinuk J, et al. Work-related asthma. Am J Ind Med 2000; 37:121–141
A detailed review that can be downloaded free from http://www3.interscience.wiley.com/cgi-bin/fulltext/67501287/PDFSTART

Work/Disability Evaluation

20. American Medical Association. The respiratory system. In: Robert Rondinelli, ed. Guides to the evaluation of permanent impairment. 6th ed. Chicago, IL: AMA Press, 2007
This rating system is the one most widely required by individual state worker compensation systems. You will need to check with your state to determine whether these or other medical guidelines apply.
21. Disability Evaluation Under Social Security. Baltimore, MD: Social Security Administration, June 2006; Publication No. 64–039. Available at: http://www.ssa.gov/disability/professionals/bluebook/3.00-Respiratory-Adult.htm#3.03%20Asthma. Accessed March 29, 2009

Fatal Occupational Asthma

22. Ortega HG, Kreiss K, Schill DP, et al. Fatal asthma from powdering shark cartilage and review of fatal occupational asthma literature. Am J Ind Med 2002; 42:50–54

Notes

Diseases Related to High Altitude and Diving and Near-Drowning: Basics of Hyperbaric Medicine

Igor Aksenov, MD, PhD; and Michael Strauss, MD

Objectives:

- Understand the physiology and pathophysiology of diving and high-altitude pulmonary-related problems
- Describe the main diseases related to high altitude, their diagnosis, management, and prevention
- Discuss the different types of diving, contraindications to diving, and the evaluation and management of common medical problems of diving
- Explain the pathophysiology of drowning and near-drowning
- Appreciate the mechanisms of hyperbaric oxygen therapy and its indications and contraindications

Key words: altitude; barotrauma; decompression; diving; drowning; high-altitude diseases; hyperbaric oxygen; medical problems of diving

Diseases Related to High Altitude

High-Altitude Physiology

Ascent in altitude results in a decrease in barometric pressure and corresponding decreases in Po_2. The barometric pressure at sea level is 760 mm Hg, whereas on the summit of Mount Everest (altitude 8,848 m or 29,029 feet) it is approximately 250 mm Hg. This correlates with a 67% decrease in Po_2 from approximately 159 mm Hg at sea level to 53 mm Hg at the top of Mount Everest.

Acclimatization is a process of adjustment to high altitude and low inspired oxygen that allows minimizing effects of hypoxia. The initial response to hypoxia is increased alveolar ventilation, which is called the *hypoxic ventilatory response*. The hypoxic ventilatory response causes a reduction in the alveolar Pco_2 and an increase in the alveolar Po_2 with subsequent increase in arterial oxygen content. Increased alveolar ventilation also causes respiratory alkalosis, which leads to increased renal bicarbonate elimination and metabolic acidosis. However, the renal compensation is only partial and therefore respiratory alkalosis persists. The adjustments of the cardiovascular system to high altitude include increases in cardiac output and pulmonary artery pressure, improved ventilation/perfusion matching, as well as selective vasodilatation and vasodilatation that improves oxygen delivery to the brain and heart. In the brain, hypoxia induces cerebral vasoconstriction, which is attenuated by hypocapnia-induced cerebral vasoconstriction. The final result is small increase in cerebral blood flow in proportion to tissue hypoxia. Hypoxia also induces secretion of renal-generated erythropoietin, which stimulates RBC production in bone marrow. However, it takes 10 to 14 days to increase the mass of the RBCs from this effect. Changes at the tissue and cell level include improvement in oxidative metabolism in mitochondria and hypoxia-induced factor-1α signaling of vascular endothelial growth factor. Vascular endothelial growth factor, in turn, stimulates angiogenesis.

High-Altitude Illness

The term *high-altitude illness* encompasses three conditions that occur as a result of acute exposure to hypobaric hypoxia during rapid ascent in altitude. These conditions include acute mountain sickness (AMS), high-altitude cerebral edema (HACE), and high-altitude pulmonary edema (HAPE). Long-term exposure to high altitude may result in the development of chronic mountain sickness (CMS).

AMS: AMS represents the most common form of altitude illness. It usually occurs 6 to 48 h after rapid ascents to attitudes >8,000 feet (2,440 m). The exact mechanism of AMS is unknown, but it appears to result from hypoxia-induced cerebral vasodilation. Some studies suggest that vasogenic brain edema and increased blood-brain barrier permeability contribute to the pathogenesis of AMS.

Typical symptoms of AMS include headache, dizziness, fatigue, malaise, anorexia, nausea, vomiting, and difficulty sleeping. Findings from the physical examination may include tachycardia, mild crackles in the chest with auscultation, and peripheral edema. These findings are nonspecific and are not necessary to make a diagnosis of AMS. The diagnosis of AMS is established from the clinical symptoms in the setting of ascent to altitude. AMS can be exacerbated by strenuous physical activity, alcohol consumption, and use of sedative medications.

A slow ascent that makes it possible to acclimatize gradually to altitude is the best way to prevent AMS. The general rule is that at altitudes >3,000 m (9,840 feet), the climber should spend the night at an altitude <300 m (984 feet) greater than the previous night. Adequate hydration and rest are important as well. Medications that can be used for the prevention of AMS include acetazolamide and dexamethasone. Acetazolamide (125 mg po bid starting a day before ascent) promotes acclimatization by stimulating bicarbonate diuresis and respiration. Acetazolamide is contraindicated in patients with known sulfa allergy. Dexamethasone, unlike acetazolamide, does not have effects on acclimatization. Mechanisms to explain how this drug benefits AMS are unknown. It may be related to reduction of cerebral blood volume or decreased capillary permeability. Dexamethasone has a rapid onset of action. However, it is important to remember that cessation of this drug may result in a recurrence of symptoms. Other drugs that may help prevent AMS include theophylline and temazepam.

Appropriate treatment of AMS is important because it can progress to HACE. First and most important, climbers with AMS symptoms should stop their ascent, rest and, if possible, descend >300 m (>984 feet). Other measures include oxygen supplementation and adequate fluid intake. Acetazolamide and dexamethasone both are effective in treatment of AMS. In general, acetazolamide should be considered as a first-line agent, and dexamethasone should be administered to climbers with sulfa allergy. Acetazolamide and dexamethasone can also be used as a combination if one has rapid progression of symptoms.

HACE: HACE is a potentially fatal neurologic condition. It is a more severe form of AMS. HACE usually occurs within hours or days after arrival at altitude. It has been reported to occur at altitudes as low as 2,750 m (9,022 feet). It is manifested by neurologic symptoms and signs such as headache, loss of coordination, ataxia, confusion, hallucinations, stupor, and coma. Physical examination findings may demonstrate papilledema, truncal ataxia, and cranial nerve palsies. Death usually occurs from brain herniation. Symptoms of HACE are nonspecific, and other diagnoses such as meningitis, encephalitis, intoxications, electrolyte imbalances, and glucose disturbances should be considered in the differential diagnosis.

The best prevention of HACE is slow ascent. Acetazolamide prophylaxis is recommended for individuals with a previous HACE history. HACE is a medical emergency and requires immediate interventions. Descent to a lower altitude should be initiated without delay. The patient should be administered oxygen and dexamethasone (8 mg IV, IM, or po). If descent is not possible, hyperbaric oxygen therapy (HBOT) in a portable chamber can be a life-saving treatment if this equipment is available on the mountain.

HAPE: HAPE is a form of noncardiogenic, hydrostatic pulmonary edema. It is potentially fatal and accounts for more deaths than any other high-altitude illness. HAPE occurs 2 to 3 days after rapid ascent to altitudes >2,590 m (8,500 feet). Some individuals are more predisposed to HAPE than others. The most important pathophysiologic mechanism of HAPE is hypoxic pulmonary vasoconstriction. This causes acute pulmonary hypertension, pulmonary capillary stress fractures and, eventually, the development of pulmonary edema. The release of cytokines and inflammatory mediators may play a role in the pathogenesis of HAPE, but it appears to be a secondary reaction to the hydrostatic injury. Other proposed mechanisms for HAPE include decreased nitric oxide synthesis and increased sympathetic tone in the pulmonary vasculature.

Symptoms of HAPE may occur gradually after AMS, but they can also present rapidly without any other signs. Clinical findings include nonproductive cough, fatigue, and dyspnea. Cough may become productive with pink, frothy sputum. Affected individuals may have mental status changes, lethargy, and coma secondary to hypoxemia. Physical examination findings include tachycardia and crackles on auscultation of the chest. Chest radiograph may show enlarged pulmonary arteries and patchy or homogenous infiltrates that commonly involve the right middle lobe and both lower lobes of the lungs.

As with AMS and HACE, the best method to prevent HAPE is a slow ascent that provides adequate time for acclimatization. Medications that can be used for prophylaxis include nifedipine, dexamethasone, phosphodiesterase inhibitors, and salmeterol. A placebo-controlled study of nifedipine in alpinists with previous manifestations of HAPE showed a significant decrease in development of HAPE when compared with the use of placebo. Phosphodiesterase inhibitors promote pulmonary vasodilation and reduce pulmonary artery pressure. One study showed that sildenafil improved exercise performance at altitude. However, only tadalafil was shown to reduce the incidence of HAPE. Prophylactic inhalation of high doses of the β-agonist salmeterol was associated with a decreased incidence of HAPE.

Treatment of HAPE includes immediate descent, high-flow oxygen, rest, and the administration of medications such as nifedipine, sildenafil, tadalafil, and dexamethasone. Nifedipine should be used carefully because it can lower systemic BP and reduce cerebral perfusion pressure. The use of HBOT while at altitude, if available, can be a life-saving intervention.

CMS (Monge Disease): CMS or *Monge disease* is observed in inhabitants who reside at high altitudes. This disorder was originally described in Andean mountain residents. It is caused by erythropoietin-induced increased production of RBCs in response to hypoxia. Findings in CMS include headache, dizziness, lethargy, insomnia, memory problems, cyanosis, fluid retention, and parasthesias. Pulmonary hypertension and congestive heart failure may develop. CBC typically demonstrates increased levels of hemoglobins and hematocrits. Definite treatment of CMS is a return to a lower altitude. Symptoms can be reduced by oxygen administration, phlebotomy, and acetazolamide.

Altitude and Air Travel in Hypoxemic Patients

Commercial airplanes usually fly at altitudes of 3,000 m (10,000 feet) to 12,200 m (40,000 feet). The Federal Aviation Administration requires that cabin pressures be maintained at pressures equivalent to altitudes less than 2,438 m (8,000 feet), although this maximum may be breached in emergencies. At 2,438 m, the Po_2 is equivalent to breathing 15.1% oxygen at sea level. Because of this, patients with underlying lung disease may become hypoxic, and patients who are already receiving oxygen may require increased oxygen supplementation. According to guidelines published by the British Thoracic Society, patients with the following conditions/risk factors should be assessed prior to permitting commercial air travel:

- Severe COPD or asthma;
- Severe restrictive lung disease (including chest wall and respiratory muscle disease), especially with hypoxemia and/or hypercapnia;
- Cystic fibrosis;
- History of air travel intolerance with respiratory symptoms (dyspnea, chest pain, confusion or syncope);
- Comorbidity with other conditions worsened by hypoxemia (cerebrovascular disease, coronary artery disease, heart failure);
- Pulmonary tuberculosis;
- Within 6 weeks of hospital discharge for acute respiratory illness;
- Recent pneumothorax;
- Risk of or previous venous thromboembolism; and
- Preexisting requirement for oxygen or ventilator support.

The preflight assessment should include the following: (1) history and physical examination; (2) spirometry, and (3) oxygen saturation by pulse oximetry (Spo_2) measurement. Blood gas tensions are preferred in patients with known or suspected hypercapnia. In-flight oxygen is not recommended if the patient's room-air Spo_2 is $>95\%$. In those patients who have a resting sea level Spo_2 of 92 to 95% with additional risk factors, hypoxic challenge testing is recommended. If the sea level Spo_2 is $<92\%$, then in-flight oxygen is recommended. Patients who receive supplemental oxygen at sea level should increase the flow while at cruising altitude. Additional risk factors for flying in commercial aircraft include hypercapnia, $FEV_1 < 50\%$ of predicted, lung cancer, and the need for ventilator support.

Currently, there are several methods to predict in-flight PaO_2, including the following:

1. Predicting hypoxemia from equations: These equations are helpful as a screening test. The equations have been derived almost exclusively from patients with COPD, and they do not predict response to exercise.
2. Measurement of PaO_2 or SpO_2 under hypobaric conditions: This method is the most precise one, but it requires depressurization in a hypobaric chamber, which is not usually an option in most clinical settings and pulmonary function laboratories.
3. The high-altitude stimulation test reproduces in-flight hypoxia by changing the fraction of inspired oxygen (FIO_2). In general, an altitude of 1,520 m (5,000 feet) is equivalent to FIO_2 of 17%; 2,438 m (8,000 feet) to FIO_2 of 15%; and 3,048 m (10,000 feet) to FIO_2 of 14%. This is a simple and accurate test that can be performed in most pulmonary function laboratories. If the predicted in-flight PaO_2 decreased < 50 mm Hg, then supplemental oxygen is recommended.

Federal Aviation Administration rules do not allow passengers to carry their own oxygen tanks or liquid oxygen on commercial flights. However, patients can bring portable battery-powered oxygen concentrators. Patients should have a letter from a physician with an explanation of their medical condition(s) and their oxygen requirements for commercial air travel.

Diving Medicine

Types of Diving

Sports diving includes a spectrum of diving types ranging from breath-hold snorkeling to use of closed-circuit self-contained underwater breathing apparatus (SCUBA) gear (Table 1). Deep technical diving, surface supply diving, and saturation diving are not considered recreational types of diving and are not included in Table 1. The distinction between the sports diver and the commercial diver is no longer as clear as it was in the past when commercial divers used equipment that was unavailable to the sports diver. Today, in our opinion, the main distinction between the commercial and the sports diver is the former gets paid for his or her diving activity, whereas the sports diver does not.

Medical Clearance and Contraindications for Diving

Diving requires good physical and mental health. Medical standards are different for breath-hold, recreational SCUBA diving, and commercial divers.

Breath-Hold/Snorkel Diving: Generally, there are no medical requirements to participate in this type of diving. Fitness is the key to safe breath-hold diving. If there are any fitness issues, the diver should be screened with the use of standards similar to those for a sedentary person who decides to start a conditioning/aerobic exercise program.

Recreational SCUBA Diving: In the United States, according to the Professional Association of Dive Instructors, no mandatory medical examination is required. However, Professional Association of Dive Instructors as well as other diving certification organizations require candidates who take their SCUBA diving training programs complete a medical history questionnaire. If any of the history questions are checked as being present, then an evaluation and clearance by a physician is usually required before the diving candidate is allowed to continue recreational SCUBA diving training. For those >40 years of age, especially if fitness for diving is a concern, a prediving training physical examination is recommended preferably with a stress ECG study.

The physical examination of a potential SCUBA diver should be directed toward identification of ear, nose, and throat problems that could interfere with pressure equilibration during descents and ascents, as well as cardiovascular and pulmonary diseases that would contribute to heart problems caused by the physical demands of diving and pulmonary overpressure syndromes with depth changes, respectively. Obesity significantly increases the risks of decompression sickness (DCS) because nitrogen is lipid soluble. Mental health issues must not be overlooked because the ability to follow instructions, avoid panic, and remain

Table 1. *Types of Sports Diving*

Type	Breathing Equipment	Advantages	Disadvantages	Comments
Breath-holding	Snorkel	Freedom	Depth limited by breath-hold time	Probably the largest number of participants
SCUBA	Regulator and tank; open circuit*	Extends bottom time	Inefficient use of air supply†	The majority of recreational SCUBA diving
Enriched-air nitrox	Regulator and tank; open circuit	Reduced chances of decompression sickness	Increased chances of oxygen toxicity	Less fatigue
Rebreather	Closed circuit‡	Prolongs underwater times	Many hours of training; increased hazards	Equipment costs about $5,000–$10,000

*Open circuit: After inhaling compressed gas from the SCUBA tanks via the regulator, the diver exhales each breath into the water

†Efficiency: This is a very inefficient use of the gas supply because 79% of the contents of the tank is the inert gas nitrogen. Each inhalation contains 21% oxygen, whereas there is 16% oxygen in the exhaled gas. Consequently, only 5% of the air in the SCUBA tank is used for the body's respiration and ventilation needs, whereas 95% is exhaled into the water.

‡Closed circuit: The gas supply recycles through breathing bags while carbon dioxide is absorbed in the rebreather circuit. Oxygen is added (usually via sensor controls) at a rate sufficiently to meet the diver's oxygen requirements.

clearheaded are essential for safe diving. Individuals who abuse alcohol or who are using street drugs should not be permitted to dive. Prescription medications or conditions for which they are prescribed may be relative or absolute constraindications. For example, if the patient with anxiety receives sedative medications, then he or she should not dive because (1) anxiety during diving may cause rapid ascent and result in serious problems (see next section) and (2) effects of sedative medications may be increased under pressure. Conditions such as diabetes and asthma are relative contraindications to diving, and clearance to recreational SCUBA dive with these conditions is contingent on the patient's insight to their problems and how well they manage these conditions.

Commercial Diving: This type of diving has specific standards. In the United States, these standards are provided by the Association of Diving Contractor Standards (1994), the United States Navy, the Occupational Safety and Health Administration, the National Oceanographic and Atmospheric Administration, and the American Academy of Underwater Sciences (for scientific divers). Divers working under the auspices of these organizations are required to pass regular medical examinations. The exact standards are based on the tasks that diver has to perform. In addition to the information required for the recreational SCUBA diver, attention has to be given to the health of the patient's back as well as the presence of deformities or other musculoskeletal problems that limit mobility and strength. For those divers who perform long and/or deep dives or have had recurrent episodes of DCS imaging studies for dysbaric osteonecrosis should be performed periodically. These latter divers also seem so be prone to plaque-like lesions in their brains and spinal cords that resemble those seen in multiple sclerosis. Consequently, careful neurologic screening of the commercial diver is essential, and if there is any question of neurologic impairments, screening with magnetic resonance should be done.

Pulmonary contraindications for all types of diving include symptomatic asthma requiring long-term use of medications, COPD, pulmonary infections, history of spontaneous pneumothorax, pulmonary cysts and scars, and pulmonary fibrosis. These conditions significantly increase the risk of extraalveolar air (pulmonary overpressure) syndromes. Epilepsy is also an absolute contraindication for all types of compressed gas diving because of the risk of seizures from alterations in the partial pressure of the breathing gases.

Diving-Related Medical Problems

Ear and Sinus Barotrauma: Barotraumas are the most frequent problems of divers. Ear squeeze is the common terminology used to describe this problem. The middle ear spaces and sinus cavities are embedded in the skull bones. The tympanic membrane separates the middle ear space from the external ear canal. The Eustachian tube provides a passage to the middle ear space from the back of the nasopharynx, whereas the ostia of the sinuses provide connections to the sinus cavities and make it possible to equilibrate pressures in these structures. Problems arise when these channels become occluded, and the diver is unable to equilibrate pressure in the middle-ear spaces and sinus cavities as the ambient pressures change with descents and ascents. The Boyle law quantifies these pressure-volume effects, stating that as pressures of a confined gas increase, the volumes decrease and vice versa.

The ear and sinus cavities are lined with well-vascularized respiratory epithelium. As a pressure differential develops, the vessels dilate and the ear drum distends inward (stage 1 of ear barotrauma). This generates pain. The next stage (stage 2) in the progression is leakage of fluid from the vessels into the middle ear space. This leaking causes muted hearing. In stage 3, rupture of blood vessels with bleeding into the middle-ear space occurs. Sputum may become blood tinged. Perforation of the ear drum is the final step (stage 4) in the progression. Because water may then fill the ear canal, pain may resolve because the middle-ear space becomes a fluid-filled cavity and the pressure differential is obliterated. However, cold water entering the middle-ear space can cause vertigo, lead to disorientation, and generate uncontrollable panic. During ascent, reverse ear squeezes may occur as the result of expansion of the air in closed space. Dizziness and vertigo may be associated with this especially if unilateral. This condition is termed *alternobaric vertigo*.

The diver himself or herself should be responsible for first-line interventions for ear and sinus squeezes. At the first sign of ear pain, descent should be halted. Ascending a few feet may help to "clear" the ears. If equilibration is not achieved, the diver should return to the surface. Over-the-counter vasoconstrictor medications (for example, pseudoephedrine) both orally and via nasal installation can reduce congestion and may allow the diver to continue the dive. In most cases, the aforementioned measures are sufficient to facilitate equilibration of pressure in the middle-ear spaces and sinus cavities and to continue diving activities.

If symptoms persist or the ear drum perforates, the diver should be evaluated by a physician. Fluid may need to be drained from the middle-ear space (tympanotomy). If a perforation occurs, the diver must not re-enter the water until the ear drum has healed (*ie*, approximately 2 to 3 weeks) because of the risk of inducing infection into the middle-ear space. If the drum is perforated, antibiotics are prescribed in conjunction with decongestants. If middle-ear equilibration problems recur, antihistamines for those with allergies may be helpful. Any persistent vertigo, dizziness, nausea, or hearing loss symptoms are serious and warrant immediate medical attention. They may be caused by round or oval window ruptures or injury to the inner-ear structures from DCS.

Extraalveolar Air (Pulmonary Overpressure) Syndromes: Problems arising from extraalveolar air are of three types: subcutaneous/mediastinal emphysema, pneumothorax, and arterial gas embolism (AGE). These occur infrequently. AGE is one of the most serious of all diving problems because immediate recompression may be required to prevent irreparable brain damage. AGE is not related to the depth or the duration of the dive. It has been reported after breathing a compressed gas from depths as shallow as eight feet and then breath-holding while coming to the surface. Extraalveolar air syndromes are caused by air retention in the lungs either as the result of breath-holding or from pathological conditions such as asthma or emphysematous blebs. As ambient pressure decreases with ascent, gas in the lung expands, as explained by the Boyle law.

Subcutaneous/mediastinal emphysema occurs when alveoli rupture and air dissects into the tissues of the mediastinum, upper trunk, and/or neck. If the air dissects into the pleural space, a pneumothorax may result. Finally, if air expansion in the lungs occurs explosively as the result of an uncontrolled ascent, concomitant rupture of alveoli and adjacent blood vessels allow air to pass directly into the bloodstream. The air bubbles become emboli, are carried to the brain, and occlude its circulation. Consequently, the symptoms of AGE can be the same as any of those seen with a cerebral vascular accident.

Cessation of diving activities until the signs and symptoms of subcutaneous/mediastinal emphysema resolve is usually all that is required to manage these problems. Rarely, these conditions interfere with breathing. If so, oxygen inhalation should be instituted. For pneumothorax and AGE, breathing of pure oxygen should be initiated immediately. The symptoms of AGE remit completely in approximately 50% of patients while breathing pure oxygen. After they are extricated from the water, possibly with pneumothorax and AGE, and are awaiting transportation to a medical center, patients may require first-line treatment for shock, seizures, and cardiac arrest. Re-expansion of the lung with placement of a chest tube is required for a pneumothorax that has caused > 20% collapse of the lung. Hyperbaric oxygen recompression therapy is the definitive treatment for AGE.

Two measures prevent extraalveolar air syndromes. First, medical screenings before starting diving should be performed to detect asthma and other chronic lung conditions that may trap air during ascent. Second, dive training to teach buoyancy control and avoiding panic are essential to prevent unscheduled, uncontrolled ascents. The majority of AGE events occur in inexperienced divers.

DCS: DCS, which is sometimes referred to as the *bends* or *caisson disease*, is caused by bubble formation in tissues. The Dalton law (*ie*, the total pressure in a gas system is the sum of the partial pressures of the contained gases) explains how changes of pressure with descent and ascent alter the partial pressures of the gases in the breathing medium. For example, with a dive to a depth of 33 feet (10 m; equivalent to 2 absolute atmospheres [atm abs]) the partial pressures of the oxygen and nitrogen in the breathing medium double. Ordinarily, this has little effect on oxygenation of tissues, but if the pressure is increased 10-fold, the increased Po_2 could lead to a seizure as the result of oxygen toxicity. An increase in the partial pressure of nitrogen has different effects. This inert gas is forced into all body tissues in direct proportion to its partial pressure in the breathing medium Henry law. The rate of on-gassing (process of gas entering the tissue due to the increased pressure) depends on depth (pressure gradient), duration, gas mixture, and perfusion (blood flow). If the pressure of nitrogen is so great that it exceeds the ability of the tissue to off-gas (process of gas leaving the tissue due to the decreased pressure) it in an orderly fashion, bubbles form in the tissue, and DCS results. As the diver ascends, the bubbles expand (the Boyle law).

Presentations of DCS are variable and not always predictable. DCS has a wide variety of presentations, from skin itches to joint pains, and from paralysis to unconsciousness. Sometimes, the symptoms of DCS are so similar to those of AGE that it is difficult to make the exact diagnosis. In such situations, the term *decompression illness* is used to encompass both possibilities. The symptoms of DCS arise from the location in which the bubbles form. If bubbles form in the extremely fast (with respect to on-gassing and off-gassing of nitrogen) lung tissues where it is exchanged with the ambient air, respiratory distress termed *the chokes* occurs. If bubbles form in the blood stream during transport of the nitrogen released from the tissues to the lungs and block circulation, bends shock or symptoms caused by the occlusion of the blood supply to critical organs such as the heart, brain, and spinal cord occur. These presentations are similar to those of AGE; hence, the utilization of the term *decompression illness*. If bubbles form in peripheral and/or noncritical tissues, itching, rash, joint pain, paresthesias, and/or fatigue occur.

As in AGE, the breathing of pure oxygen should be instituted as soon as the diagnosis of DCS is suspected. If the patient is alert, fluid administration and ingestion of a single dose of an antiplatelet agent such as aspirin are recommended. Oxygen breathing helps to "wash out" the nitrogen, whereas fluids and aspirin help to maintain the circulation of blood. The diver should be kept at rest. In remote areas, returning to the water and breathing pure oxygen at a depth of 33 feet and then gradually ascending, although controversial, is recommended by some authorities in diving medicine.

Hyperbaric oxygen recompression is the definitive treatment for DCS. If there are residual symptoms after the initial hyperbaric oxygen recompression treatment, repetitive treatments should be administered until the symptoms resolve completely or plateau over a 3- to 7-day period.

DCS is prevented by the use of safe diving practices. Factors such as fitness, adequate hydration, and following dive computer (or dive tables) profiles are fundamental to safe diving. Other specific measures include the following: (1) limiting ascent rates to 1 foot every 2 s; (2) taking a 3-min rest stop at 15 feet; (3) avoiding repetitive dives at the end of the day, when fatigued and/or chilled; (4) taking a 1-day break after 3 or 4 days of repetitive, consecutive dives each day; (5) not flying for at least 24 h after the last SCUBA dive; (6) avoiding alcoholic beverages during the dive activities; and (7) and using common sense to avoid interfering with the orderly off-loading of nitrogen; for example, not wearing constrictive bands, falling asleep with joints in hyperflexed positions, or exercising excessively.

Other Indirect Effects of Pressure: Nitrogen Narcosis, Oxygen Toxicity, Carbon Dioxide Toxicity, Carbon Monoxide Poisoning, and High-Pressure Nervous System Syndrome: These problems occur infrequently, are invariable associated with the bottom phase of the dive, and are usually associated with the use of special equipment such as closed-circuit (rebreather) SCUBA or special gas (pure oxygen, nitrox [enriched air nitrox] or helium-oxygen mixtures). A summary of these conditions is presented in Table 2.

Near-Drowning and Drowning: Any time consciousness is lost in the water, the victim is at risk of drowning. Aspiration often is associated with drowning because the breathing reflexes are usually the last to remain after a hypoxic injury to the brain. If the victim is rescued and resuscitated, then the incident is labeled a *near-drowning*. Whereas aspiration and the resulting lung injury can be managed effectively with appropriate interventions, the consequences of hypoxic brain injury are usually irreversible and can range from imperceptible to a persistent vegetative state.

The brain is the most critical organ in the body with respect to injury from oxygen deprivation. After 4 min of anoxia, brain injury is likely to occur. Although breath-holding for several minutes is

Table 2. *Additional Problems Associated With Indirect Effects of Pressure*

Condition	Etiology	Symptoms	Management	Prevention
Nitrogen narcosis, *ie*, "rapture of the deep"	Narcotic effects from breathing this gas under pressure. Each 50 feet of descent is roughly equivalent to the effects from drinking one martini.	Confusion, irrational actions, stupor, syncope. Victim may panic and ascend in an uncontrolled fashion. Complications include AGE, DCS, and/or drowning.	Ascent; the dive buddy needs to control the victim's ascent to avoid complications. Symptom resolve immediately with ascent.	Adhere to safe depth limits (< 130 feet). Use helium for deep dives.
Oxygen toxicity, *ie*, "oxygen hit"	Breathing oxygen under increased pressure. Seizure threshold is a function of depth, duration, activity, and the environment, *eg*, cold water, poor visibility, currents.	Anxiety, tunnel vision, tinnitus, muscle twitching, and seizures.	Ascent, breathe gas with lower oxygen content, *eg*, air instead of pure oxygen or nitrox mixtures.	Adhere to strict depth limits when diving with pure oxygen (33 feet for 30 min) and table limits with nitrox mixtures.
Carbon dioxide toxicity	Increased carbon dioxide from problems with carbon dioxide absorber or work in unventilated spaces (tunnel and caisson workers).	Headache, increased respiratory rate, feelings of suffocation, syncope. Burns in mouth from soda lime.	Ventilate by breathing fresh air. Terminate dive if rebreather (with carbon dioxide absorber) equipment is used.	Strict adherence to safety and set-up protocols when using rebreather equipment. Ensure adequate ventilation when working in closed spaces.
Carbon monoxide poisoning	Contamination of air supply with exhaust fumes from internal combustion engines	Headache, confusion, collapse, syncope, coma, and death	Surface; breathe pure oxygen; hyperbaric oxygen;	Ensure gas supply is free of contamination.
High-pressure nervous system syndrome	Diving deeper than 650 feet with helium-oxygen mixtures	Tremors, in-coordination, syncope	Ascent	Add small amounts of nitrogen to the breathing gas.

possible, the interruption of the perfusion of the brain for more than a moment or so, for example, in a third-degree heart block, leads to immediate loss of consciousness. Conversely, loss of consciousness associated with water immersion has "protective effects" in terms of preservation of brain function. This is ascribed to the oxygen-conserving effects of the diving reflex and hypothermia from immersion in cold water. Remarkable recoveries have been reported from near-drowning, even after the victim has been immersed for >30 min.

Consequently, the adage "never say drowned" is very appropriate for two reasons: first, remarkable recoveries that have been observed; and second, the primary cause of the patient's presentation should be identified. Once the primary cause is identified, appropriate management becomes logical. For example, if the diver loses consciousness while at the bottom phase of the dive, then hyperbaric oxygen recompression therapy is essential to offload the inert gas present in the tissues and prevent complications of decompression illness (*ie*, DCS and/or AGE). In addition, concurrent optimal management of the pulmonary and brain injuries from near-drowning must be administered.

Basics of HBOT

Mechanisms of Hyperbaric Oxygen

The Undersea and Hyperbaric Medical Society gives the following definition of HBOT: The patient breathes 100% oxygen intermittently while the pressure of the treatment chamber is increased to >1 atm abs. Treatment pressures range from 1.4 to 3 atm abs. Treatments may be performed in a single-person chamber (monoplace) or multiplace chamber (*ie*, may hold two or more people). Breathing 100% oxygen at 1 atm abs or exposing isolated parts of the body to 100% oxygen does not constitute HBOT.

Hyperbaric oxygen has two primary mechanisms that account for the therapeutic and the undesirable side effects of this treatment modality: (1) the mechanical effect caused by pressurization (bubble size reduction a la the Boyle law), and (2) hyperoxygenation. A hyperbaric oxygen exposure at 2 atm abs increases plasma and tissue oxygen tensions 10-fold, the blood oxygen content by 125%, and the diffusion of oxygen through tissue fluids by a threefold factor. The main side effect from the mechanical effect is barotrauma as discussed under the section "Diving Medicine." A hyperbaric oxygen toxicity seizure is a very rarely occurring side effect from hyperoxygenation.

Secondary mechanisms occur as a result of tissue hyperoxygenation but are clear and distinct from hyperoxygenation itself. The secondary effects include, but are not limited, to the following: (1) vasoconstriction to reduce posttraumatic edema; (2) enhancement of host factor functions such as fibroblast activity, angiogenesis, leukocyte oxidative killing, and bone remodeling for wound healing that was unable to occur in the hypoxic environment; (3) microbiological effects such as bacteriostasis, cessation of toxin production, toxin inactivation, and augmentation of certain antibiotics; (4) mitigation of the reperfusion injury by perturbing the neutrophil-capillary endothelium adhesion mechanism; and (5) gas washout for management of DCS and carbon monoxide poisoning.

Indications for HBOT

The following 13 indications are approved uses of hyperbaric oxygen therapy as defined by the Hyperbaric Oxygen Therapy Committee of the Undersea and Hyperbaric Medical Society:

- Air or gas embolism;
- Carbon monoxide poisoning, carbon monoxide poisoning complicated by cyanide poisoning;
- Clostridial myositis and myonecrosis (gas gangrene);
- Crush injury, compartment syndrome, and other acute traumatic ischemia;
- DCS;
- Enhancement of healing in selected problem wounds;
- Exceptional blood loss (anemia);
- Intracranial abscess;
- Necrotizing soft-tissue infections;
- Osteomyelitis (refractory);
- Delayed radiation injury (soft-tissue and bony necrosis);
- Skin grafts and flaps (compromised); and
- Thermal burns.

Contraindications for HBOT

Absolute contraindications for HBOT include the following:

1. Untreated pneumothorax: Air in the pleural space can increase in size as pressure decreases during ascent.
2. The concomitant administration of doxorubicin or cis-platinum: HBOT can increase the cytotoxic effect of these medications.
3. Disulfiram: This medication blocks the production of superoxide dismutase, a protective antioxidant against oxygen toxicity.
4. Bleomycin: This drug increase pulmonary toxicity in patient undergoing HBOT.
5. Mafenide acetate: A carbonic anhydrate inhibitor that is used in burn wounds. It causes metabolic acidosis as the result of carbon dioxide buildup, causing peripheral vasodilation.
6. Premature infants: Oxygen in premature infants can cause retrolental fibroplasia, leading to blindness.

Suggested Reading

High-Altitude--Related Disorders

Barry PW, Pollard AJ. Altitude illness. BMJ 2003; 326: 915–919

Bärtsch P, Maggiorini M, Ritter M, et al. Prevention of high-altitude pulmonary edema by nifedipine. N Engl J Med 1991; 325:1284–1289

Gallagher SA, Hackett PH. High-altitude illness. Emerg Med Clin North Am 2004; 22:329–355

Ghofrani HA, Reichenberger F, Kohstall MG, et al. Sildenafil increased exercise capacity during hypoxia at low altitudes and at Mount Everest base camp: a randomized, double-blind, placebo-controlled crossover trial. Ann Intern Med 2004; 141:169–177

Grocott MP, Martin DS, Levett DZ, et al. Arterial blood gases and oxygen content in climbers on Mount Everest. N Engl J Med 2009; 360:140–149

Hackett PH, Roach RC. High-altitude illness. N Engl J Med 2001; 345:107–114

Sartori C, Allemann Y, Duplain H, et al. Salmeterol for the prevention of high-altitude pulmonary edema. N Engl J Med 2002; 346:1631–1636

Schoene RB. Illnesses at high altitude. Chest 2008; 134:402–416

Air Travel in Hypoxemic Patients

Aerospace Medical Association, Air Transport Medicine Committee. Medical guidelines for air travel, second edition. Aviat Space Environ Med 2003; 74:A1–A19

British Thoracic Society Standards of Care Committee. Managing passengers with respiratory disease planning air travel: British Thoracic Society recommendations. Thorax 2002; 57:289–304

Dine CJ, Kreider ME. Hypoxia altitude simulation test. Chest 2008; 133:1002–1005

Mohr LC. Hypoxia during air travel in adults with pulmonary disease. Am J Med Sci 2008; 335:71–79

Mortazavi MJ, Eisenberg MJ, Langleben D, et al. Altitude-related hypoxia: risk assessment and management for passengers on commercial aircraft. Aviat Space Environ Med 2003; 74:922–927

Diving-Related Disorders

Brubakk AO, Neuman TS, eds. Bennett and Elliott's physiology and medicine of diving. Edinburgh: Saunders, 2003

Melamed Y, Shupak A, Bitterman H. Medical problems associated with underwater diving. N Engl J Med 1992; 326:30–35

Strauss MB, Aksenov IV. Diving medicine: questions physicians often ask. Consultant Live. Part I: 2004; 44:961–963; and Part II: 44:1167–1171. Available at: http://www.consultantlive.com/display/article/10162/34671. Accessed April 23, 2009

Strauss MB, Aksenov IV. Diving science: essential physiology and medicine for divers. Champaign, IL: Human Kinetics, 2004

Strauss MB, Aksenov IV. Medical problems of diving and the primary care physician: Part I. Primary Care Reports 2002; 8:164–171

Strauss MB, Aksenov IV. Medical problems of diving and the primary care physician: Part II. Primary Care Reports 2002; 8:172–188

Strauss MB, Aksenov IV. Medical problems of diving and the primary care physician: Part III. Primary Care Reports 2002; 8:185–191

HBOT

Kindwall EP, Whelan H, eds. Hyperbaric Medicine Practice, 3rd ed. Flagstaff, AZ: Best Publishing Company, 2008

The Undersea and Hyperbaric Medical Society (UHMS). Hyperbaric Oxygen Therapy Committee. Guidelines: indications for hyperbaric oxygen. Kensington, MD: UHMS, 2000. Available at: http://www.uhms.org/ResourceLibrary/Indications/tabid/270/Default.aspx. Accessed March 19, 2009

Notes

Notes